with contributions by

WILLIAM E. BENSON
S. ARTHUR BORUCHOFF
GARY N. FOULKS
ARTHUR S. GROVE, JR.
CHARLES R. LEONE, JR.
FRANCIS A. L'ESPERANCE, JR.
J. ARCH MCNAMARA
DENIS M. O'DAY
ROBERT D. REINECKE
J. JAMES ROWSEY
JERRY A. SHIELDS
GEORGE L. SPAETH
WILLIAM S. TASMAN
GEORGE W. WEINSTEIN
RICHARD P. WILSON

Illustrations by Mark Weakley

Second Edition

OPHTHALMIC SURGERY:
Principles & Practice

Edited by

GEORGE L. SPAETH, M.D.

Director of Glaucoma Service and Research Laboratory,
Wills Eye Hospital;
Professor of Ophthalmology,
Thomas Jefferson Medical College,
Philadelphia, Pennsylvania

1990

W. B. SAUNDERS COMPANY

Harcourt Brace Jovanovich, Inc.

Philadelphia, London, Toronto, Montreal, Sydney, Tokyo

W. B. SAUNDERS COMPANY
Harcourt Brace Jovanovich, Inc.

The Curtis Center
Independence Square West
Philadelphia, PA 19106

Library of Congress Cataloging-in-Publication Data

Ophthalmic surgery: principles & practice / edited by George L.
Spaeth: with contributions by William E. Benson . . . [et al.];
illustrations by Mark Weakley–2nd ed.
  p.   cm.

Includes bibliographies and index.

ISBN 0–7216–2467–7

1. Eye—Surgery.   I. Spaeth, George L., 1932–
II. Benson, William Edmunds.
   [DNLM: 1. Eye—surgery.   WW 168 0615]

RE80.0655 1990   617.7'1–dc20

DNLM/DLC   89–6117

Listed here is the latest translated edition of this book together with
the language of the translation and the publisher
Italian—*First edition*—Verduci Editore, Rome, Italy

Acquisition Editor: Richard Zorab
Manuscript Editor: Barbara Hodgson
Production Manager: Frank Polizzano
Illustration Coordinator: Joan Sinclair
Indexer: Dian Witt

OPHTHALMIC SURGERY: Principles and Practice   ISBN 0–7216–2467–7

Last digit is the print number: 9   8   7   6   5   4   3   2   1

This book is dedicated to my family.

CONTRIBUTORS

WILLIAM E. BENSON, M.D.
Professor of Ophthalmology, Jefferson Medical College of Thomas Jefferson University. Attending Surgeon, Wills Eye Hospital, Thomas Jefferson University Hospital, and Chestnut Hill Hospital, Philadelphia, Pennsylvania.
Retinal Detachment; Vitrectomy

S. ARTHUR BORUCHOFF, M.D.
Associate Clinical Professor of Ophthalmology, Harvard Medical School. Surgeon in Ophthalmology, Massachusetts Eye and Ear Infirmary, Boston, Massachusetts.
Corneal Surgery

GARY N. FOULKS, M.D.
Professor of Ophthalmology, Duke University School of Medicine. Attending Surgeon, Duke University Eye Center, Durham, North Carolina.
Corneal Surgery

ARTHUR S. GROVE, Jr., M.D.
Assistant Professor of Ophthalmology, Harvard University Medical School. Associate Surgeon in Ophthalmology and Consultant in Orbital and Plastic Surgery, Massachusetts Eye and Ear Infirmary, Boston, Massachusetts.
Surgery of the Orbit

CHARLES RUSSELL LEONE, Jr., M.D.
Clinical Professor of Ophthalmology, University of Texas Health Science Center at San Antonio. Attending Ophthalmologist, St. Luke's Lutheran Hospital, Methodist Hospital, and Humana Hospital, San Antonio, Texas.
Plastic Surgery

FRANCIS A. L'ESPERANCE, Jr., M.D.
Professor of Clinical Ophthalmology, Columbia University College of Physicians and Surgeons. Attending Ophthalmologist, Edward S. Harkness Eye Institute, Columbia-Presbyterian Medical Center, New York, New York.
Ophthalmic Lasers: Current Status

J. ARCH McNAMARA, M.D., F.R.C.S.C.
Instructor in Ophthalmology, Jefferson Medical College of Thomas Jefferson University. Assistant Surgeon, Retina Service, Wills Eye Hospital; Attending Surgeon, Chestnut Hill Hospital, Philadelphia, Pennsylvania; Associate Staff Surgeon, Our Lady of Lourdes Hospital, Camden, New Jersey.
Vitrectomy

DENIS M. O'DAY, M.D., F.A.C.S.

Professor of Ophthalmology, Vanderbilt University School of Medicine. Director of the Corneal and External Disease Service, Vanderbilt University Hospital, Nashville, Tennessee.
Intraocular Infections

ROBERT D. REINECKE, M.D.

Professor of Ophthalmology, Jefferson Medical College of Thomas Jefferson University. Senior Surgeon, Wills Eye Hospital, Philadelphia, Pennsylvania.
Extraocular Muscles

J. JAMES ROWSEY, M.D.

Clinical Professor of Ophthalmology, University of Oklahoma McGee Eye Institute. Attending Surgeon, Presbyterian Hospital, Oklahoma City, Oklahoma.
Radial Keratotomy: Principles and Practice

JERRY A. SHIELDS, M.D., F.A.C.S.

Professor of Ophthalmology, Jefferson Medical College of Thomas Jefferson University. Director, Ocular Oncology Service, Wills Eye Hospital, Philadelphia, Pennsylvania.
Therapeutic Approaches to Intraocular Tumors

GEORGE L. SPAETH, M.D.

Professor of Ophthalmology, Jefferson Medical College of Thomas Jefferson University. Director, William and Anna Goldberg Glaucoma Service, and Attending Surgeon, Wills Eye Hospital; Attending Surgeon, Chestnut Hill Hospital, Philadelphia, Pennsylvania.
Introduction; Phases of the Surgical Procedure; Fundamental Surgical Procedures; Instrumentation, Sutures, and Standard Ophthalmic Procedures; Glaucoma Surgery; Ophthalmic Conditions Requiring Prompt Care

WILLIAM TASMAN, M.D.

Professor and Chairman, Department of Ophthalmology, Jefferson Medical College of Thomas Jefferson University. Codirector, Retina Service, and Ophthalmologist-in-Chief, Wills Eye Hospital; Consultant in Ophthalmology, Children's Hospital of Philadelphia, Attending Surgeon, Chestnut Hill Hospital, Philadelphia, Pennsylvania.
Retinal Photocoagulation

GEORGE W. WEINSTEIN, M.D.

Professor and Jane McDermott Shott Chairman, Department of Ophthalmology, West Virginia University School of Medicine. Chief of Ophthalmology Service, West Virginia University Hospital, Morgantown, West Virginia.
Cataract Surgery

RICHARD P. WILSON, M.D.

Associate Professor, Jefferson Medical College of Thomas Jefferson University. Attending Surgeon, Wills Eye Hospital, Philadelphia, Pennsylvania.
Anesthesia

ACKNOWLEDGMENTS

This text reflects the influence and help of many people: my parents, whose lives have been models for me; my teachers, such as Otto Krayer, Irving H. Leopold, Ludwig von Sallmann, James Shipman, and especially to my father, Edmund B. Spaeth, and my brother Philip G. Spaeth, who understood that knowledge develops value only when it is shared, and who enthusiastically shared their knowledge and experience; too many of them have received too little recognition. It is my hope that these good teachers and others like them are content with the awareness that they have made the world a better place.

PREFACE
To The First Edition

The ophthalmic surgeon really can improve the quality of life. He or she has the ability to restore a productive and enjoyable life by removing a cataract, transplanting a cornea, removing bloody vitreous, or reconstructing an injured person's face; sight can be preserved by repairing a ruptured globe or relieving excessive intraocular pressure; function and appearance can be improved by correcting a deviated eye; and life may be maintained by treating malignant tumors.

It is not surprising that ophthalmic surgeons find a deep satisfaction in their work.

The competent surgeon is both knowledgeable and experienced. No novice can be a great surgeon; but experience alone is not adequate. Knowledge is the foundation on which surgical competence is built. The purpose of this text is to bring together in one book those things the ophthalmic surgeon needs to know to practice his or her craft well.

Competent surgeons may not always agree regarding either principles or practice. In order to provide information that is broadly based, the contributors to this text have been selected because they are knowledgeable, experienced, articulate, catholic, and come from different backgrounds. Personal preferences, unintentional omissions, and even idiosyncrasies are not completely avoidable. To provide balance, and to assure that the information given is pertinent, each chapter has been reviewed by another author. In addition, some chapters have been further reviewed by other experts of great skill and experience. I'm grateful to these reviewers for their invaluable contributions. They have added to the final appearance of the work. They should not, however, be held accountable for the final rendering, which is entirely the editor's responsibility. Those to whom particular thanks go include Philip Knapp, M.D. (Extraocular Muscles); P. Robb McDonald, M.D. (Cataract Surgery); Peter Watson, M.D. (Glaucoma Surgery); and Max Fine, M.D. (Corneal Surgery).

Mark Weakley is the principal illustrator for this text. Virtually all of the unsigned drawings were made by him, and he has my thanks for being so deeply concerned with depicting precisely each author's intent. Deborah Randall provided other illustrations; her professional skill and invariable completion of work prior to the time it was expected made it a particular pleasure to work with her.

This text reflects the influence and help of many people: my father, whose surgical text and whose life both are models for me; Otto Krayer, whose personal brilliance and intellectual breadth inspired me at medical school (How will I ever forget his question kindly but seriously posed to me at our first meeting—"What is the purpose of a physician?"); Irving H. Leopold, who keeps asking the right questions; Ludwig von Sallmann, simultaneously a fine clinician, teacher, and investigator; and James Shipman, who understood that the value of knowledge develops only when it is shared. Heartfelt thanks go to Kate McVay and Mary Ann

Sammartino, who, despite many other responsibilities, kept this text going through numerous visions and revisions; to the contributing authors for the thought, effort, and expense of preparing their valuable chapters; to Lisette Bralow and Erika Shapiro of the W. B. Saunders Company, who have been grand to work with; and to all teachers who have enthusiastically shared their knowledge and experience, many of whom have received little reward other than the awareness that they have made the world a better place.

GEORGE L. SPAETH, M.D.
Philadelphia

PREFACE
To The Second Edition

The purpose of this text is to bring together in one manageable, affordable book the knowledge that ophthalmic surgeons need to practice their craft well.

The favorable response to the first edition of this text and the dramatic changes in ophthalmic surgery since 1982 indicated the need for a new edition. Every chapter has been revised; some have been completely rewritten. New chapters have been added on keratorefractive and laser surgery. The chapter on cataract surgery provides detailed description of lens implantation and extracapsular techniques. The use of laser surgery is covered completely.

We hope and believe this second edition will find a useful place in offices, clinics, operating rooms, medical schools, and hospitals around the world.

GEORGE L. SPAETH, M.D.
Philadelphia

CONTENTS

10

11

12

13

14

VITRECTOMY 400

J. Arch McNamara and William E. Benson

15

SURGERY OF THE ORBIT 421

Arthur S. Grove, Jr.

16

PLASTIC SURGERY 528

Charles R. Leone, Jr.

17

EXTRAOCULAR MUSCLES 638

Robert D. Reinecke

18

THERAPEUTIC APPROACHES TO INTRAOCULAR TUMORS

Jerry A. Shields

19

OPHTHALMIC CONDITIONS REQUIRING PROMPT CARE

George L. Spaeth

I

PRINCIPLES OF OPHTHALMIC SURGERY

1

INTRODUCTION

by George L. Spaeth

The techniques of ophthalmic surgery have proliferated so rapidly that a single surgeon cannot possibly be fully competent in all aspects. Nevertheless, most surgical eye diseases can be properly managed with relatively few procedures. The average ophthalmic surgeon need not be competent in every aspect of surgery in order to give good care. For example, a surgeon who is fully proficient in peripheral iridectomy, trabeculectomy, cataract extraction through a clear corneal incision, and cyclophotocoagulation can provide most glaucoma patients fine care.

In this text we have emphasized *selectivity*. For example, peripheral iridectomy with thermal sclerostomy is the only standard full-thickness filtration procedure described. The choice is not meant to imply that other, similar procedures are of lesser worth. It is, rather, a statement that peripheral iridectomy with thermal sclerostomy is probably *as satisfactory* as any other operative procedure in its class, and that experience with other operations of a similar nature is unnecessary for the average surgeon.

Inclusion of a procedure in the text should not be taken as tacit comment that all surgeons ought to be performing this procedure. All surgeons vary in the range and comprehensiveness of their competency: some are better craftsmen, some are better technicians, and some have better judgment.

A selection of classic, comprehensive, and specialized texts is included (see references).

THE ARTISAN, THE TECHNICIAN, AND THE COMPLETE SURGEON

That both art and science are essential parts of medical practice is a well-established concept. It is also clear that the development of technology is a characteristic feature of the past hundred years. This period stressed the scientific method as a fundamental aspect of medical care. During the latter half of the 19th century the image of the surgeon changed from prognosticator to effective medical scientist. Before that time the surgeon was revered and rewarded primarily because of his ability to support his patient during difficult times; this required mastery of the art, or craft, of medicine. Many individuals benefited as well from the mechanical skills of surgeons, but all too often the limitations of the technology of the time predetermined that the result would be of limited help. Thus the great surgeon of the past was fundamentally a great artisan or craftsman.

Craftmanship requires knowledge of the tools and materials used in performing one's craft. In the craft of surgery these include surgical instruments, anesthesia, knowledge of the treatment of injury and disease, and the indications for and techniques used in many types of operative procedures. The surgeon must also understand the patient—his nature, needs, and wishes—and the unique qualities of each patient and each interaction.

The artisan is personally involved with his or

her work, which therefore carries with it a subjective component. The artisan or craftsman recognizes that each work created is unique. The technologist, on the other hand, attempts to remove himself as much as possible from his work. Technology implies objectivity, standardization, and uniformity of results. The results of the technologist are relatively easy to measure, and hence performance is relatively easy to evaluate. On the other hand, the quality of the artist's or craftsman's product is difficult to measure. Is, for example, Cellini's rococco salt cellar a "better job" than Cro-Magnon man's flint arrowhead or Calder's starkly simple mobiles? Furthermore, the *process* of creating is as important to the craftsman as the product itself. The artisan surgeon learned by apprenticeship. He taught by example. His major activity was demonstrating care. His product was not so much "cure" as it was "care."

Great surgeons today are still great artisans, but the technological revolution has dramatically changed the surgeon's role. It provided the means for him to be more effective. No longer did the surgeon study the arts, but rather physics, chemistry, and statistics. Truly astounding improvements in the surgical product resulted from this technology revolution. Unfortunately the art of medicine has been neglected. Even the science (e.g., the methodology of the scientifically designed clinical trial) is still not adequately used. As a result, the surgeon does not have as much scientifically valid information to answer his basic questions as could be hoped for: Which suture is best for cataract extraction? When should a hyphema be drained? These are among the hundreds of still unanswered questions. They are unanswered because the surgeon has not brought to his craft the lessons of the technological and scientific revolution. Clinical impression, apprenticeship, and example continue to be the primary sources of information for the surgeon. Thus, in response to the question "Why do you do X?" the surgeon's answer is almost invariably either "Because X is the way I was trained" or "Because X seems to work for me."

Even though fundamental questions still are unanswered, the ability of the surgeon to be effective has increased dramatically. The benefit to the patient of intraocular lens implantation can be literally "miraculous."

But technology by itself is inadequate and incomplete. What is needed, especially in the coming years, is the conjunction of the art of the craftsman with the science of the technician. Fortunately the two methodologies are not mu-

tually exclusive; in fact, they are complementary. *First and foremost, the humanity and grace of the surgeon as master craftsman must not be lost.* Both attributes are necessary.

The learned surgeon realizes all too well that even now the ability to cure completely is only seldom within his grasp, and recognizes that the patient is often more disabled by the emotional reaction to the disease than by the disease itself. He understands the uniqueness of each patient and each patient's response to disease. He recognizes the critical importance of the relationship between patient and surgeon. The responsibility of the surgeon is still to support the patient during difficult times, to comfort, and to care. Superimposed on this responsibility is an obligation for him to assess his craftsmanship in a scientifically valid way, to know the *science* of surgery as well as the craft. We must add the skills of the technician to those of the craftsman. We must learn more about both our tools and our material, that is, our patients, and how they interact. The medical student needs to learn about human nature and the human condition, while at the same time becoming a superb technician. Both attributes are necessary.

Students who consider medicine as a career should be encouraged to spend their time learning who they are, why they are, and how they relate to the spiritual and material world in and around them, and especially to other people. Technical skills grow best when grafted on a whole, healthy, vital tree; considered by themselves, technical skills become lifeless tools, appropriated primarily for the profit of those who possess them. Such is the antithesis of caring.

A surgeon should not be timid. He must act decisively and authoritatively—this is an integral part of the craft. He must consider and balance the available information, making sure that he uses appropriate means to obtain as much information as necessary to make a prudent decision, and then he must act. If the surgeon is unsure whether the visual field has really deteriorated in a glaucomatous patient who appears to be under marginal control, the field should be repeated; if the surgeon is unsure regarding the quality of the visual field examination, the test should be repeated by someone who is able to assure a valid examination. We are accountable for what we do not do as well as for what we do. All too frequently physicians and surgeons hide unjustifiably under the cloak of "First, do no harm." The truly caring surgeon must be willing to risk harm to achieve an anticipated improvement. To let, for example, a glaucoma patient's vision slip away because the surgeon is afraid of the risks of surgery is as damaging to the patient as it is to perform a procedure that is unnecessary.

To sum up, we hope that this text will help all surgeons bring to their craft adequate knowledge of surgical technique. The provision of that information is a primary purpose of this volume. We have attempted to make the material as accurate and objective as possible. We also hope that every surgeon will recognize his or her obligation to develop new knowledge, and to use, whenever feasible, the methodology of the valid clinical trial. Were we all to do so we could become far more effective craftsmen than we currently are. It is further hoped that there will be sufficient agreement with the content of this text that it can serve as a set of guidelines to be used appropriately by surgeons to judge the quality of their own performance and the performance of others. We are not only obligated to perform well ourselves, but, as members of a privileged profession, we must also assure that we do everything within our power to protect patients from those who are unknowledgeable or unscrupulous, or both. When we fail to act corporately in such a manner we fail society just as seriously as we fail our patient individually when we act incompetently or in a manner that is not in the patient's best interest.

INPATIENT VERSUS OUTPATIENT SURGERY

Whether surgery is best performed in an outpatient or inpatient setting is based on what is deemed best for the patient. "Best" includes cost, convenience, competence, and the assurance that complications can be correctly handled. *Value* is the critical consideration. It is not in the best interest of the patient to provide care that is unnecessarily costly or unnecessarily risky. *The decision regarding the need to hospitalize, like the need to refer, must be made by the patient in concert with the physician.* The true cost of surgery cannot be measured merely by the expense of the procedure. Surgery that is performed "better" in the broadest sense of the word results in a better outcome, avoiding subsequent procedures, hospitalizations, loss of function, and loss of wages. A procedure that temporarily seems cheaper may, in the long run, be vastly more expensive, both for the patient and for society.

Decisions regarding the appropriate setting for care *must* be made on a case-by-case basis. They cannot be appropriately made by a clerk or even by another physician who is not fully acquainted with the details of the case. The patient's surgeon, as an advocate for the patient, must act in a way that is intended to be in the best interest of the patient. In today's experimental medical health care system this responsibility of the surgeon will inevitably bring him or her into direct conflict with regulations set up by hospitals, third party payers, and state and federal agencies.

ALTERNATIVE SYSTEMS OF CARE

Systems intended to streamline and lower the cost of surgery are being developed. For example, preoperative and postoperative care is delegated by some surgeons to associates, employees, or even nonmedical practitioners. Whether such systems are proper is determined by two major considerations: first, the quality of the care and, second, the relation to what the patient wants. Not all patients want the same type of care; some prefer the most complex and most expensive, and others would choose simpler, less expensive care. The surgeon must not misrepresent the services offered. The patient must understand fully just what the surgeon will and will not do. A clearly articulated contract must be established. If the patient gets what he or she wants, the physician-patient relationship may be proper.

In actuality the matter is far more complex. The fears and anxieties, the apparent ignorance in comparison with the physician, all of these put the patient in a vulnerable position, one that can all too easily be exploited by the physician or health care providers. An ancient tradition has evolved in which groups of healers put self-imposed regulations on the behavior of the members in their group. Present-day professional codes of ethics reflect these behavioral guides, all of which have one aspect in common: protection of the patient. However, a problem implicit in this system is that it largely relies on what the healer considers best for the patient; this may diverge from the patient's own beliefs.

We are currently witnessing the working out of the tensions involved in changing health care systems. The goal is to incorporate the patient's wishes and at the same time maintain the physician's high standards of performance and integrity. To date this goal has seen successes on both sides. But it is against this shifting backdrop that decisions need to be judged, as to whether or not they are appropriate. As long as the ultimate standard is a sincere effort to put the interest of the patient first, the behavior is probably appropriate.

REFERRAL

Many factors enter the decision of where and by whom a particular surgical procedure is best performed. A most important consideration is that the patient have confidence in his or her surgeon. Admittedly, some patients will not have confidence in anybody, but such situations are rare.

Whenever feasible, surgery should be performed at a facility close to the patient's home. The surgical experience itself can be upsetting, and the support that comes from familiar surroundings is nourishing, especially for the very young and the very old. When surgery is performed at a distance from the patient's home, postsurgical complications can make the situation difficult, the patient asking himself whether it is worth continuing the difficult and tiring trips to the operating surgeon, or concluding that it is wiser—or at any rate overwhelmingly more convenient—to return to the local physician. Surgery also tends to be more expensive when performed at a distance.

On the other hand, some factors favor referral, *even* in cases in which the patient has confidence in the local surgeon. If the patient or the local surgeon believes that another surgeon is more competent in performing the procedure required, the consideration of a referral should definitely arise. It has been demonstrated that substantially fewer postoperative complications occur in referral centers than in peripheral institutions. Furthermore, and a factor not to be underestimated, although most patients are aware that complete success is not an invariable part of surgical treatment and are, therefore, prepared to accept results less desirable than hoped for, the entire foundation for such acceptance on the part of the patient is unwavering faith that the quality of care received was satisfactory. Many people are unable to cope with a poor result unless they profoundly believe that they have had "the best care." Surgeons who find themselves caring for a patient who is frankly, or even peripherally, skeptical about the competence of their surgeon

are courting catastrophe for themselves and for their patients when they decide to proceed themselves with the surgery. No surgeon is obligated to perform surgery when referral services are reasonably available.

When the facilities or the personnel for competent surgery are not available, it is often better to avoid surgery. A patient with useful vision but uncontrolled glaucoma will not be helped by a botched filtering procedure; nor will the person with 20/200 vision caused by keratoconus or vitreous hemorrhage be benefited by a poorly performed corneal graft or vitrectomy.

THE CLINICAL TRIAL

The basic principles of the valid clinical trial are as follows:

1. To limit variables
2. To eliminate bias
3 To make specific and sensitive measurements
4. To study comparable groups by valid statistical methods

First, let us consider, for example, the surgeon who is trying to decide whether to use silk or nylon for cataract extraction. Available information does not answer his question. He must design a study that will measure *only* the effect of the suture material itself; that is, he must first limit the variables. Thus he cannot use silk in one manner and nylon in another; for example, he cannot use seven interrupted silk sutures and two running nylon sutures, for were he to do so, he would be studying the technique of placing suture material and not the type of suture material itself. He cannot use steroids postoperatively in the eyes of patients sutured with silk and not in those in whom nylon was used. With the one exception of the type of suture material used, *every aspect* of the surgical technique must ideally be the same in the two groups studied.

Second, he must eliminate bias. Bias can be of several types. It may occur in the design, the operation, or the interpretation phases of the study. The surgeon who wants to prove that nylon is preferable to silk would consciously or unconsciously evaluate patients differently, being more critical regarding the use of silk. When a reaction was between "mild" and "moderate," the case with the nylon suture would be considered "mild," whereas the silk suture would be graded as "moderate." This type of bias is generally understood, and masking techniques can help to eliminate it. Nevertheless, masked surgical studies are seldom done.

Bias can invalidate a study in many other ways. For example, if the surgeon decided to use silk for his first hundred cases and nylon for the second hundred cases, the results would be unfairly biased in favor of the nylon because the surgeon would be likely to improve his surgical technique during the period of time of the study. On the other hand, if the surgeon had never used nylon but was very familiar with silk, it would not be fair to compare the surgical result in patients in whom nylon was used by the surgeon for the first time with those in whom he had used the suture with which he was far more comfortable. Or consider the surgeon who decides to use silk on his Monday cases and nylon on his Friday cases, believing that to be a convenient way of "randomizing" the study. But it is quite possible that knowingly or unknowingly he has traditionally scheduled more difficult cases on Monday, so that complications will not occur over the weekend. Therefore, the patients are not truly randomized, and the groups are not validly comparable.

To eliminate bias one must use a system that assures true randomness of selection and objectivity of evaluation.

Third, the surgeon must make measurements that are sensitive and specific enough to reflect accurately what is actually happening. For example, the surgeon may decide that the criterion of the "success" of his cataract extraction is postoperative visual acuity. Assume that the results show the mean visual acuity postoperatively in the patients in whom silk was used (Group S) and in those in whom nylon was used (Group N) to be the same. The surgeon, therefore, concludes that there is no difference between the groups, and thus that the silk and nylon sutures are equally "good." However, measurement of visual acuity may, in fact, be too crude a standard by which to determine subtle differences in the two results. For example, the mean astigmatic correction in Group N could be larger than that in Group S, perhaps even twice as large, with statistical significance of P less than .001. If this were the case, it would be clear that a real difference did exist in the surgical result obtained when using silk sutures versus that obtained when using nylon. Thus, for this experiment, determining the degree of acuity was not an adequately sensitive measurement for finding the real difference that occurred.

Fourth, for the results of a clinical trial to be valid the surgeon must study comparable groups. The surgeon cannot validly conclude, because no endophthalmitis developed in his 7000 cases using silk sutures, and Dr. X reported 3 cases of endophthalmitis in his 13,000 cases using nylon, that silk is a better suture. It is highly unlikely that two groups unequal in size that have as their only common denominator the need for cataract extraction will be sufficiently similar that they can be validly compared. Although this seems so obvious that it is almost embarrassing to mention, it is surprising how many articles appear in ophthalmic journals each month in which one author states that his procedure is "better" because his results were superior to those of Dr. X. Even assuming that both surgeons limited the variables, eliminated bias, and measured accurately enough to detect actual differences, comparisons between the two groups are little more than "interesting" unless the two populations studied are truly comparable. Furthermore, comparison must be made using valid statistical methods. Only by using such techniques can the investigator accurately assess the likelihood that the observed finding was a consequence of the variable tested and not a chance occurrence.

Of equal importance is the lack of significance of a negative result. Assume, for the sake of argument, that silk suture causes severe hypersensitivity reactions in 2 per cent of cases, whereas nylon causes no hypersensitivity reactions. At the end of a study comparing silk and nylon sutures the surgeon identifies in Group S two cases that have had troublesome allergic reactions, but no cases in Group N. When he analyses the data by standard statistical methods, he finds that Group S and Group N are not statistically different; therefore, he concludes that the tendency of the two sutures to cause allergic reactions is the same. But in fact his study did not prove *that*; his study showed only that he did not have enough cases to observe differences of a small, but perhaps real magnitude. The statement "This study did not reveal any difference between Group N and Group S" *must not* be interpreted as saying that Group N and Group S are the same. One cannot generalize negative findings any more than one can say that because all dogs are animals, all animals are dogs.

An important point regarding the interpretation of statistical results is that one must keep in mind the difference between *mathematical* significance and *clinical* significance. For example, Group S may have had a final astigmatic correction of 0.87 plus or minus 0.1 diopters, while Group N showed 1.00 plus or minus 0.1 diopters of postoperative astigmatism. The difference is highly significant statistically, but clinically it makes virtually no difference whether a patient has a cylinder of 0.87 or one of 1.00 diopters. Therefore, to conclude that silk is a better suture than nylon because it was shown statistically that it produced less astigmatism *is mathematically correct, but clinically incorrect.*

It is important to provide *absolute numbers* when presenting data. Percentages are not adequate. A paper stating that "67 per cent of patients treated with operation Q improved" may sound convincing until the reader learns that only three cases were treated.

The reader must also beware of imprecise statements. For example, the period of follow-up will influence the nature and validity of the results. A statement such as "cases were reexamined up to 18 months after surgery" is of little value. Perhaps only one case was examined 18 months postoperatively, all the others having been reevaluated 1 month after surgery. This could be entirely possible within the framework of the sentence given, so the reader must be careful not to assume that the reevaluation of all cases was made 18 months after surgery.

This discussion of clinical trials is brief, but it should indicate to the reader that the vast bulk of published and oral communication regarding surgical results represents only "clinical impression." The impression may be valid, but it may equally well be fallacious. We surgeons are so eager to have results that we forget that the method of study determines the validity. If we would restrict ourselves to correctly studying one thing at a time, the fund of useful information would increase far more rapidly than it is currently. Taking the nylon sutures versus silk sutures question as an example, if we wanted to determine which was better for cataract extraction, we would first master the techniques of using both silk and nylon sutures. Next, we would use one or the other suture in the same way in strictly comparable groups, varying nothing else and introducing cases randomly. Finally, using measurements that were sufficiently specific and sensitive to indicate the changes that had occurred, we would analyze the data by statistically valid techniques. Even after we had carried out such an elegant clinical trial, however, we would still not be justified in generalizing our conclusions too broadly. All that we could state with authority would be

that either silk or nylon *appeared* to be better when used in a particular way in a particular population by a particular surgeon. However, because the conclusion would probably be valid as a result of our having fulfilled the four basic requirements of the clinical trial, it would serve as a block on which further studies could be built. Such investigations can be done by any surgeon who designs and manages his study well.

TRAINING REQUIRED TO BECOME A PRACTICING OPHTHALMIC SURGEON

The ophthalmic surgeon is first a member of an amazing and magnificent universe, second a person, third a physician, and fourth an ophthalmic surgeon. It is all too easy, as our time becomes preoccupied by the daily excitement and real rewards of practicing ophthalmology, to pervert this order and distort our perspectives. Our first responsibility is to be conscious of the universal interconnectedness of everything, or to a universal God, and the second, to our species and the fundamental unit of that species, the family in the most comprehensive sense—our loved ones and all those who need us. Third, as physicians we have a special obligation toward those who need help with their emotional and physical health. Fourth, we are ophthalmic surgeons. Proper training thus begins in the home and progresses to a comprehensive education that assures the development of social skills and stresses the humanities and their interrelations with the sciences, and finally to the specifics of health and disease.

Ophthalmic patients are afflicted with a full range of conditions that require medical, surgical, and emotional care. Although ophthalmic surgery demands special training and skills, without which surgeons cannot practice their craft properly, the ophthalmic surgeon must first possess the general knowledge regarding health and disease that is needed by all physicians. This is usually acquired by satisfactory completion of an accredited medical school program, with an additional year of general medical and surgical experience before starting a full-time residency in ophthalmology.

Specific training in ophthalmic surgery begins with the residency period. Ideally, the resident's surgical experience should span the entire 3 years of this training, during which considerable time is spent in the role of assistant to senior instructors. Later the trainee should perform as the primary surgeon in a wide variety of ophthalmic operative procedures. One satisfactory mode of progression is that shown in Table 1–1.

No matter how carefully planned and supervised the program, complications will inevitably occur; the intelligent ophthalmic surgeon should learn from these unfortunate events. In fact, the surgeon who has not had broad exposure to the complications of surgery will not be adequately prepared to cope with them when they occur. It should be remembered that the skillful teacher can lead the neophyte surgeon through difficult experiences; the confidence that grows out of the knowledge of the correct way to handle such situations is an essential component of the fully developed surgeon. Furthermore, learning surgeons must develop first-hand familiarity with the humbling truth that the surgical result may be less beneficial than hoped for by the patient or the surgeon, or both. Training programs that avoid cases of great complexity or cases in which a poor result could seriously hamper the patient's life style cannot claim to be doing more than a superficial job of introducing the physician to the field of surgery.

The resident's first really difficult procedure should, if at all possible, be performed in a setting in which the necessary supervision and support are present. Considerable experience with such surgery is preferable before the surgeon is allowed to be "on his own." Both the surgeon who completes a residency training program and the patient who expects to benefit from his encounter with the surgeon are justified in believing that the ophthalmologist who finishes an accredited ophthalmic residency

TABLE 1–1. Optimal Mode of Training Ophthalmic Surgeons

1. Practical experience in a supervised clinic (helping to diagnose and select patients for surgery)
2. Observation of surgery
3. Practice with eye bank and animal eyes
4. Further observation as first assistant to surgeons teaching full range of preoperative, operative, and postoperative care
5. Highly supervised surgical experience incorporating diagnosis, examination techniques, indications for surgery, details of surgical techniques, and continuing postoperative care
6. Broad surgical experience with gradually increasing autonomy
7. Experience teaching surgical procedures, including preoperative and postoperative care

TABLE 1–2. Aspects of the Accomplished Craftsman

Understands the *purposes* of the craft.
Knows the *technical* aspects of the craft.
Is familiar with the *materials* used.
Recognizes the *limitations* of the craft.

program should be able satisfactorily to manage the great majority of surgical problems with which he will be confronted.

Many or most of the details, and even some of the principles, learned by the student will change with time. The ophthalmic surgeon must maintain a highly flexible approach to the learning situation. Modifications and improvements develop at such a remarkable rate that every surgeon must realize that a technique widely used today will probably be outdated in the near future. A large number and variety of postgraduate courses are now available; these should be used by the mature surgeon. Constant self-criticism (not self-doubt) and reevaluation of principles and practice are required for continuing growth.

A profound understanding of himself or herself and his or her world is the final element that leads to the development of the surgeon as a great craftsman and a great contributor to the world (Table 1–2).

REFERENCES

Historical Reviews

1. Bartisch, G.: Ophthalmodouleia: das ist Augendienst. Dresden, Stöckel, 1583.
2. Weiner, M., Alvis, B. Y.: Surgery of the Eye. Philadelphia, W. B. Saunders Co., 1931.
3. Spaeth, E. B.: Principles and Practice of Ophthalmic Surgery. Philadelphia, Lea & Febiger, 1939.

Recommended Readings in General and Specific Areas

4. Arruga, H.: Ocular Surgery. Translated from the third Spanish edition by Hogan, M. J., Chaparro, L. E. New York, McGraw-Hill, 1952. Third English edition translated from fourth Spanish edition by Hogan, M. J., Chaparro, L. E. Barcelona, Salvat Editores; New York, McGraw-Hill, 1962.
5. Berens, C., King, J. H.: An Atlas of Ophthalmic Surgery. Philadelphia, J. B. Lippincott Co., 1961.
6. Stallard, H. H.: Eye Surgery. Bristol, John Wright & Sons, Ltd., 1946. (Fifth edition, published 1973.)
7. Miller, S. J.: Eyes. 3rd ed. Operative Surgery Series. London, Butterworths, 1976.
8. Troutman, R. C.: Microsurgery of the Anterior Segment of the Eye. St. Louis, C. V. Mosby Co., 1974.
9. Amoils, S. P.: Cryosurgery in Ophthalmology. Chicago, Year Book Medical Publishers, 1975.
10. L'Esperance, F. A.: Ocular Photocoagulation: A Stereoscopic Atlas. St. Louis, C. V. Mosby Co., 1975.

11. Mitsui, Y.: Ganka shujutsu no tehodoki (Techniques in Ophthalmological Surgery). Tokyo, Kanehara Shuppan, 1975.
12. Machemer, R.: Vetrectomy: A Pars Plana Approach. Current Ophthalmology Monographs Set. New York, Grune & Stratton, 1975.
13. Proceedings of Fourth Ophthalmic Microsurgery Study Group, Lund, Sweden, July 4–7, 1972; Surgery of the Iris and the Ciliary Body. Palm, E., Mackensen, G., eds. *In* Advances in Ophthalmology, Vol. 30. Basel, S. Karger, 1975.
14. Peyman, G. A., Sanders, D. R.: Advances in Uveal Surgery, Vitreous Surgery, and the Treatment of Endophthalmitis. New York, Appleton-Century-Crofts, 1975.
15. Beard, C.: Ptosis. 2nd ed. St. Louis, C. V. Mosby Co., 1976.
16. Fox, S. A.: Ophthalmic Plastic Surgery. 5th ed. New York, Grune & Stratton, 1976.
17. Guibor, P. (ed.): Oculoplastic Surgery and Trauma. New York, Stratton Intercontinental, 1976.
18. Jones, L. T., Wobig, J. L.: Surgery of the Eyelids and Lacrimal System. Birmingham, Aesculapius Publishing Co., 1976.
19. Reeh, M. J., et al.: Practical Ophthalmic Plastic and Reconstructive Surgery. Philadelphia, Lea & Febiger, 1976.
20. Soll, D. B., Asbell, R. L. (eds.): Management of Complications in Ophthalmic Plastic Surgery. Birmingham, Aesculapius Publishing Co., 1976.
21. Fifth Symposium of the Ophthalmic Microsurgery Study Group. London, June 1974: Microsurgery of Cataract Vitreous and Astigmatism. Kersley, J., Pierse, D., (eds.). *In* Advances in Ophthalmology, Vol. 33. Basel, S. Karger, 1976.
22. Tessier, P., et al. (eds.): Symposium on Plastic Surgery in the Orbital Region, Vol. 12. St. Louis, C. V. Mosby Co., 1976.
23. Zweng, H. C. (ed.): Recent Advances in Photocoagulation. Boston, Little, Brown & Co., 1976.
24. Fasanella, R. M. (ed.): Eye Surgery: Innovations and Trends, Pitfalls, Complications. Springfield, Ill., Charles C Thomas, 1977.
25. Helveston, E. M.: Atlas of Strabismus Surgery. St. Louis, C. V. Mosby Co., 1977.
26. Krasnov, M. M.: Mikrochirurgie der Glaukome. Leipzig, Thieme, 1977.
27. Rougier, J., et al.: Chirurgie Plastique Orbitopalpebrale. Paris, Masson, 1977.
28. Troutman, R. C.: Microsurgery of the Anterior Segment of the Eye: The Cornea, Vol. 2. St. Louis, C. V. Mosby Co., 1977.
29. Weinstein, G. W., Drews, R. C.: The Surgery of Intraocular Lenses. Thorofare, N.J., C. B. Slack, 1977.
30. Emery, J. M. (ed.): Current Concepts in Cataract Surgery: Selected Proceedings of the Fifth Biennial Cataract Surgical Congress. St. Louis, C. V. Mosby Co., 1978.
31. Katzin, H., Klein, R.: New Aspects of Vitreous Surgery. New York, Intercontinental Publications, 1978.
32. Klein, R., Katzin, H.: Microsurgery of the Vitreous: Comparisons of Instrumentation, Techniques and Philosophies. Baltimore, Williams & Wilkins, 1978.
33. Lim, A. M. (eds.): Fison's Retinal Detachment Surgery. Basel, S. Karger, 1978.
34. Macomber, W. B. (ed.): Symposium on Orbital and Eyelid Surgery. Philadelphia, W. B. Saunders Co., 1978.
35. Meltzer, M. A.: Plastic Surgery of the Eye. *In* Intercontinental Handbook Series. Schachat, W. S. (ed.). New York, Intercontinental Publications, 1978.
36. Tenzel, R. R. (ed.): Ocular Plastic Surgery. Boston, Little, Brown & Co., 1978.
37. Girard, L. J.: Ultrasonic Fragmentation for Intraocular Surgery. St. Louis, C. V. Mosby Co., 1979.
38. Iliff, C. E., Iliff, W. J., Iliff, N. T.: Oculoplastic Surgery. Philadelphia, W. B. Saunders Co., 1979.
39. Lim, A., Constable, I. J.: Colour Atlas of Ophthalmic Surgery. Boston, Houghton Mifflin Professional Pubs., 1979.
40. Machemer, R., Asbert, T. M.: Vitrectomy. 2nd ed. Current Ophthalmology Monographs. New York, Grune & Stratton, 1979.
41. Meltzer, M. A.: Ophthalmic Plastic Surgery for the General Ophthalmologist. Baltimore, Williams & Wilkins, 1979.
42. Montandon, D., Maillard, G.-F.: Plastiques et Réconstructions Orbito-Palpébrales. Geneva, Editions Médicine et Hygiène, 1979.
43. Tessier, P. A.: Plastic Surgery of the Eye and Orbit. (Translated by S. A. Wolfe.) Paris, Masson, 1979.
44. Jaffe, N. S.: Cataract Surgery and Its Complications. 4th ed. St. Louis, C. V. Mosby Co., 1984.
45. Luntz, M. H., et al.: Glaucoma Surgery. Baltimore, Williams & Wilkins, 1984.
46. Hersh, P. S.: Ophthalmic Surgical Procedures. Boston, Little, Brown & Co., 1988.
47. Engelstein, J. M. (ed.): Cataract Surgery: Current Options and Problems. Orlando, Fla., Grune & Stratton, 1984.
48. Heilmann, K., Paton, D.: Atlas of Ophthalmic Surgery. Stuttgart, Georg Thiem Verlag, 1985.
49. Menezo, J. L.: Microcirugia de la Catarata. Barcelona, Ediciones Scriba, 1983.
50. Rice, T. A., et al. (eds.): Ophthalmic Surgery. 4th ed. St. Louis, C. V. Mosby Co., 1984.
51. Waltman, S. R. (ed.): Surgery of the Eye. New York, Churchill Livingstone, 1988.
52. Barraquer, J., Rutllan, J.: Microsurgery of the Cornea. Barcelona, Ediciones Scriba, S.A., 1984.
53. Bigar, F. (ed.): Microsurgery update 1982-1984. *In* Developments in Ophthalmology, Vol. 11. Basel, S. Karger, 1985.

2

PHASES OF THE SURGICAL PROCEDURE

by George L. Spaeth

THE SURGICAL EVENT

The surgical event encompasses far more than just the time spent in the operating room.[1] *The surgical event starts with the decision to do surgery and does not end until the changes initiated by the surgery are stable.* The operating surgeon is reponsible for the entire surgical event. He or she may delegate care during that period, but must continue to supervise all care. Thus the technician, a junior physician, or an optometrist may refract a patient 2 months after cataract surgery, and may even order the appropriate correction. The responsibility for the correction, however, continues to be the operating surgeon's, and therefore, he or she is accountable. If transfer of care to a different practitioner is anticipated, the details must be arranged and agreed on by the patient before the performance of the surgical procedure.

DIAGNOSIS

The first step in the proper performance of surgery is correct diagnosis. Correct diagnosis demands adequate evaluation of the patient. Unless this evaluation provides the surgeon with the information needed to make an appropriate decision, optimal results will not be achieved.

Because facilities vary widely from place to place, there may be circumstances in which it may not be feasible to obtain the most sensitive diagnostic examinations possible for a particular patient. When this is the case, the surgeon must remember the shortcomings of the examination and must not credit the data with false validity. Consider, for example, the patient on appropriate medical therapy who has an intraocular pressure of 40 mm Hg, and moderately advanced glaucomatous cupping of the optic nerve head; equipment for a visual field examination is not available, but confrontation fields fail to document field loss. Under such circumstances the surgeon would be ill-advised to rely on the confrontation field as reliable evidence of normal function. Although clearly other factors also must be considered in the patient just described, surgery would appear to be the most reasonable option, despite the *apparently* normal visual fields.

In the overwhelming majority of cases it is, however, possible to gather enough valid information to arrive at a reasonably sure diagnosis. All appropriate efforts should be made; it is my impression that the most common cause of an unsatisfactory surgical result is inadequate evaluation of the patient and the patient's expectations.

PREPARATION OF THE PATIENT

The surgeon must adequately prepare the patient, and in some instances the patient's family, for any proposed surgery. The idea of surgery on the eyes is, for most people, frightening. Blindness is generally disabling to the spirit as well as to the body. It is the ophthalmologist's duty, therefore, to explain tactfully to the patient the nature of his problem and to mention the available options for managing it. Such a discussion should include the possibility of treatment by nonsurgical means, the nature of surgical options with attention toward reasonable prognosis, the effect the surgery would probably have on the patient's life style, the probability of partial or total disability, and the anticipated costs.

The surgeon should remember that a surgical procedure can be considered a violation of the patient's "privacy" in the strictest sense of the word. The patient should make the ultimate decision as to whether or not surgery is to be performed and by whom. It is the physician's responsibility to advise the patient that he has a condition that necessitates surgery, to offer the possibility of a surgical correction, and to provide enough information to permit the patient to make an appropriate decision. The information should be presented in a clear-cut, reassuring manner, so that the patient will not automatically shy away from the idea of necessary surgery. The risks of performing surgery should be explained, but always in a format in which they are weighed against the risks of *not* performing surgery. It is a mistake to tell a patient that he has an X per cent chance of losing sight in surgery without also telling him that he has about a Y per cent chance of losing sight if the surgery is *not* performed. When such comparative risks are explained, the patient will, in most instances, make a decision in line with the surgeon's own opinion.

In some cases a patient is reluctant to make the surgical decision himself. The physician must then take on this burden. In my experience this is a rare event. It usually indicates incomplete discussion between the surgeon and the patient. When the surgeon believes that his patient is unable to decide what is in her own best interest, the surgeon usually underestimates the patient and overestimates his own rights and abilities. Patients must be encouraged to participate in deciding on which option is most appropriate. When the patient chooses not to do so, it is not only the physician's right, but his *obligation* to make what he or she judges to be the most reasonable decision.

When a patient differs in his conclusion from that of the surgeon, it is quite possible that it is because of lack of confidence in the surgeon. In such instances the surgeon is probably best advised to ask the patient if a consultation is desired. He should not wait for the patient to request such a consultation, for patients are frequently reluctant to do this.

A variety of forms can be used to help provide the patient with the necessary information regarding his diagnosis, hospitalization, and recovery. Although brochures prepared by professional firms and various agencies are available, it is a relatively simple thing for each surgeon to prepare such forms himself. The forms are then more likely to be fully pertinent. Such information, however, should never be considered a substitute for direct communication between the patient and the surgeon.

INFORMED CONSENT

Informed consent involves important medical and ethical considerations as well as the more strictly legal ones. The following discussion deals primarily with the ethical aspects of informed consent, with the meaning of the phrase, and with its importance for the patient, the physician, and the medical profession.[1]

Informed consent is, in many ways, at the heart of the American system of medical and surgical practice. It essentially means that the patient understands the risks and the benefits involved in a proposed procedure. Such understanding demands knowledge and discussion. It also requires a two-way contract between the patient and the surgeon. The patient and the physician become partners, both of whom are primarily interested in the patient's health. The enhancement of this partnership as a meaningful relationship may be the best way to ensure high-quality medical care.

In the Commonwealth of Pennsylvania informed consent is defined as

the consent of a patient to the performance of health care services by a physician or podiatrist: Provided: That prior to the consent having been given, the physician or podiatrist has informed the patient of the nature of the proposed procedure or treatment and of those risks and alternatives to treatment of diagnosis that a reasonable patient would consider material to the decision whether or not to undergo treatment or diagnosis.

Exceptions to the rule exist, and the law states that physicians will not be held liable for failing to obtain informed consent in the following circumstances:

a. In the case of an emergency that prevents consulting the patient.

b. When furnishing the information to the patient would have resulted in a seriously adverse effect on the patient or on the therapeutic process, to the material detriment of the patient's health.

c. In the case of a minor, when in the physician's judgment an attempt to secure the consent of the parent or legal guardian would result in delay of treatment that would increase the risk to the minor's life or health.

Consent for the treatment of minors should be obtained from the patient's parent or guardian, although exceptions may be made if the minor is (a) 18 years of age or older, (b) one who has graduated from high school, (c) one who has married, or (d) one who has been pregnant.*

Informed consent is not merely the obtaining of a signature on a piece of paper.[2-4] In fact, the act of having a patient sign a written consent for surgery unfortunately sometimes serves as means to avoid obtaining truly informed consent.

The form can improperly substitute for the actual consent. This is rather like the practice of going to church in order to avoid the more difficult responsibilities of being a participating member of a religious faith.

Some physicians appear to believe that the major purpose of obtaining a signed "informed consent" is to prevent malpractice suits. The extreme mental and emotional stress that often accompanies such lawsuits makes prevention of them a deservedly important goal. However, simply because a patient signs a form stating that he gives permission for a particular operation does not eliminate the possibility of litigation. The patient may state at a later date that he did not really understand the form. In fact, it has been shown that patients forget more than they recall the information given to them preoperatively.[5] An informed consent form in itself will not effectively prevent malpractice suits from being filed.

On the other hand, the process of obtaining true informed consent—that is, the meaningful interchange of information, anticipations, hopes, and fears that should precede a request for the patient to sign any form—does help to limit the likelihood that suit will be brought at a later date. It must be remembered that the form is only documentation of the discussion; the form is not the consent.

*Source: Pennsylvania Health Insurance Corporation Bulletin #2B, November 1978.

Some patients, of course, will bring suit even when the physician has been expert, thorough, and caring in obtaining informed consent; a properly executed consent form may provide protection for the surgeon or his institution at a later date.

Failure to obtain adequate informed consent is not the basis for many malpractice claims—only 2.5 per cent according to one study.[6] Most plaintiffs' lawyers plead lack of informed consent as a last-resort allegation in weak cases, and do not, as a rule, use it as a primary charge against a negligent doctor.

Paradoxically, there are risks to the patient in obtaining informed consent. The individual who stands to be helped by cataract extraction, for example, may decline surgery when he hears his surgeon say, "You may lose your eye." Information itself changes people's moods and feelings. The suggestible patient who is fully informed of the difficulties that occasionally plague people with unilateral aphakia may effectively convince himself that he cannot be rehabilitated. Were such a person less completely apprised of the possible risks, he would probably manage quite satisfactorily. Furthermore, some patients who are functioning well become incapacitated when burdened with greater knowledge of their illness. We must remember that both the manner of obtaining informed consent and the information itself can be damaging to the patient.

The effects on the physician, and consequently on the patient, of a litigative climate should also be recalled. The anxieties produced in the physician by this situation are not conducive to good medical practice.

Surgical care should *never* be based solely on medicolegal considerations. The surgeon must, in each case, exercise his reasonable judgment based on his understanding of the case. This is not to say that the surgeon should be unaware of what is considered to be "standard practice." The surgeon is in fact unlikely to be found negligent when practicing according to the accepted standard. In a case in which the surgeon chooses to deviate from this standard, he should be aware that he is making such a deviation and be able to justify it. When standard care is not chosen, the proper concern is not whether litigation will ensue, but rather why such a deviation is in the patient's best interest. The history of medicine makes it clear that *standard* levels of care are not always *optimal* levels of care. The conscientious physician must constantly be evaluating the benefits and risks of the care he is offering. It is often the case that improvement in care will result only when deviations from that standard are made. Such alterations must be reasonable and in the best interests of the patient.

One of the prerequisites to obtaining informed consent is sufficient knowledge on the part of both doctor and patient (see Table 2–1). The physician must adequately understand the medical and surgical aspects of the case under consideration. He must also have a reasonable comprehension of the patient's needs and wishes. Both the patient and the surgeon should compare the anticipated risks and benefits of not performing surgery.

Not only must the surgeon have an adequate knowledge of the medical aspects of the case, but he must also be aware of his own motivations with regard to such questions as why he chose to perform or not to perform surgery. The major intent of the surgeon should be to help the patient. However, the surgeon is subjected to the full range of influences that affect human decisions; occasionally some may be of almost overwhelming weight. Included among these are pressures from the patient or the patient's family and friends, economic considerations, hope of acquiring new knowledge, curiosity regarding a new instrument or procedure, prestige associated with performing particularly difficult surgery, and the pleasure of conquering a difficult challenge. None of these is a justifiable reason for surgery, since none passes the criteria that are the standard for ethical care, specifically, *is the action thought to be in the best interest of the patient and is the action agreeable to the patient.* On the other hand, there are considerations that may put pressure on the surgeon to avoid operating;

these include concern that surgery will damage the patient, timidity based on previous unfortunate experiences with similar surgery, worry that an unfavorable result will bring damaging litigation, and reluctance to refer the patient elsewhere for economic or psychological reasons. Thus the pressures are not solely economic. To perform surgery is stressful and fatiguing. When compensation for the performance of surgery is present, whether in the form of academic promotion, public acclaim, or economic reward, the surgeon will be driven toward electing to do surgery; when compensation is inadequate, or when the physician may be penalized for operating unsuccessfully, then the desire to perform surgery is greatly diminished. The latter case is by no means necessarily preferable to the former. To deny a patient the possibility for improvement by means of surgery is just as unfortunate as to perform surgery when it is not likely to help. The patient has the best chance of receiving proper treatment in a system in which (a) the surgeon is knowledgeable regarding both medical care and himself, (b) rewards and punishments are acceptable to both patients and physicians alike, and (c) the patient is knowledgeable enough to assess the quality of his care.[3]

Some patients do not want to be informed. Occasional patients will be articulate about this, saying something like, "Doctor, don't tell me anything; just do what you need to do." In such a situation it is usually best for the physician to try to determine why the patient does not want to know. There may be a significant underlying emotional difficulty that, in some cases, may be more important than the patient's ophthalmic problem. When the patient remains adamant about not knowing, the surgeon may understandably be reluctant to proceed with recommended treatment, recognizing that although he may have the patient's consent, it is not truly an informed consent. Nevertheless, under such circumstances the surgeon should not delay in proceeding with what, in his opinion, appears to be the appropriate therapy. He should probably put a note on the patient's chart to the effect that the patient specifically asked not to be informed of the details. In most cases such a patient's request should be honored, for the patient may well know himself better than the physician does, and may anticipate that a recitation of the risks of the surgery, even if done compassionately, might induce such fear that the patient would decide against doing what in fact would be in his own best interest. Such a patient may well prefer to trust

TABLE 2–1. Requirements for Obtaining Appropriate Informed Consent

1. Sufficient knowledge by the surgeon:
   a. Adequate understanding of the medical and surgical aspects of the case under consideration.
   b. Adequte understanding of the patient's needs and wishes.
   c. Adequate understanding of the surgeon's own motivations.
2. Willingness of the surgeon to discuss matters with the patient.
3. Willingness of the patient to discuss matters with the surgeon.
4. Ability of the surgeon to communicate information to the patient and of the patient to comprehend it.
5. Sufficient time for discussion of the patient's and surgeon's concerns, and for the information to be assimilated.

completely the physician's recommendation. Clearly such trust should never be exploited. It should be honored, and in such a case the physician should feel free to follow his own recommendations. One person's feelings about informed consent are expressed in the newspaper article in Figure 2–1.[6]

Physicians are not always cognizant of the absolutely central role they play in patient care. Physicians and surgeons have not been replaced by computers, or computed tomography scanners, or surgical microscopes. These technological masterpieces occasionally get in the way of the physician-patient relationship, and may even substitute for particular aspects of it, but they can never meaningfully replace it.

In summary, informed consent is an essential part of medical practice, for four rather different reasons. First, it is the physician's ethical responsibility to be honest with the patient.[1] Second, it is the patient's right to make decisions regarding his or her destiny, and the patient is not in a position to do this without appropriate knowledge. Third, the process of obtaining informed consent is one of the most important practical ways of assuring high standards and improving quality of medical care. Finally, the physician is legally obligated to obtain such consent.

PREOPERATIVE STUDIES

Adequate knowledge of the patient's state of health before performance of surgery is clearly essential to achieving a successful result. For example, the presence of an enlarged prostate could lead to serious urinary retention in patients who require the use of agents that induce marked diuresis. A history should be taken preoperatively that includes questions about systemic medications being taken by the patient, known or suspected allergies and drug reactions, bleeding abnormalities, and previous surgical experiences. Pertinent questions should also be asked regarding the patient's general health and family and social life. A brief, but skillful physical examination is usually appropriate. Laboratory studies should be limited to those that bear directly on the patient's state of health. The need for these will clearly vary with the patient, the anticipated surgical procedure, and the facilities available.

For cases in which general anesthesia is thought advisable, the anesthesiologist should evaluate the patient preoperatively. Even when only local anesthesia is to be used, a visit from the anesthesiologist or nurse is helpful.

PREOPERATIVE CULTURES AND ANTIBIOTICS

Preoperative cultures are not indicated for most patients who require extraocular or intraocular surgery. However, when an infection is present or suspected, appropriate cultures may be pertinent.

The use of topical antibiotics preoperatively in the management of clean surgical cases is a controversial subject. Although topical preoperative antibiotics may function to decrease the number of bacteria in the conjunctival sac, and thereby reduce the statistical likelihood of contamination, they will not sterilize the conjunctiva. Adversely, they expose the patient to the risk of developing a drug allergy, and they may aid in the growth of resistant strains of organisms.

Antibiotics administered orally, parenterally, or periocularly are used by some ophthalmologists. The efficacy of this practice has not been determined; however, the risks probably outweigh the potential advantages. There is no evidence that trimming the eyelashes decreases periocular bacterial flora.

More detailed discussion of the prevention and management of infection is presented in Chapter 6.

PREPARING AND DRAPING THE SURGICAL FIELD

Neither the skin nor the conjunctival surfaces can be truly sterilized without causing undue trauma to the tissues themselves. Proper preparation can, however, markedly reduce the bacterial count and remove irritating debris. The method of preparing the surgical field used at the Wills Eye Hospital in Philadelphia follows.

1. Two cotton fluffs are saturated with Betadine scrub soap solution diluted with sterile saline solution. Holding one fluff in each hand, both eyes are scrubbed, starting at the inner canthus. Working in a circular motion the adnexa, lashes, lids, brows, nose, and cheek are washed, extending inferiorly so that the upper lip is included and superiorly as far as the hairline, for a total of 5 minutes. Two clean

────────────── **Terminal Candor** ──────────────

The Patient Looks at His Doctor

By DONALD C. WILSON

When I first took my as-yet undiagnosed cancer to my doctor I was laying a time-bomb in his lap. Now looking back on that encounter I know I have put an agonizingly demanding task before him. As I come to the realization of the probable course of this illness I find myself wanting two people from the one physician. I want a technical professional. That is, I want the best medical help available. Second, I want a human professional, that is, one who will deal with me not as a disease but as a human.

Until recently that was an aspect of medicine that medical schools didn't spend much time on. But with cancer's reminder to medicine that it still has a long way to go, the human aspects of patient care loom large. When **curing** is beyond the physicians's reach, **caring** moves to the front burner. It would seem then, that medicine is as much an art as it is a science.

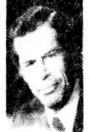

D. C. Wilson

From where I sit somewhere between the initial diagnosis and whatever the end may be, my respect for the medical profession is enhanced by what I have seen in the doctors with whom I have had to do. That experience has led me to some high expectations of the physician as a human professional. Specifically, from my doctor I have come to want five things.

1. I want my doctor to be in touch with his own or her own feelings. Before he can be aware of what I am going through, he needs to be aware of his own experience, particularly, his experience of failure. For if my case is fatal, it does mark a defeat for all that he has been trained to do. He has defined his vocation as a healer, and as Dr. S. E. Adelman writes, cancer "defeats my whole picture of the world, in which I am all-powerful, defying disease, knowing more than the layman, initiate into the secrets of disease, immune to old fears and superstitions." His tools, his education, his support system, most important, his own expectations, have equipped him for success. The dying patient confronts him with guilt and with a painful reminder of his own mortality. If the patient is "brave" the doctor may be able to suppress his emotions. But when anxiety breaks through the patient's defenses, then his demands on the physician's own involvement increase. I don't expect my doctor to welcome failure, but I do need him to face it — and to go on with me from there.

2. I want my doctor to be in touch with my feelings. When, for instance, he is explaining the diagnosis I am apt to hear only what I am prepared to hear. As the doctor is tempted to deny, so is the patient. The psyche has a way of censoring its own intake. My doctor needs to know that he may have to go over the same ground at a later time. Parents recognize how selective children can be in listening to instructions: "I didn't hear you tell me to clean the garage!" So my doctor needs to know where I am when he is telling me.

In a deeper sense I want my doctor to be aware of my feelings. If there is anyone who has a greater stake in my case than the doctor, it is I. I want my doctor to recognize my role in our relationship. To the extent that my physician enables me to mobilize all the resources of body, mind, and faith he is performing the highest arts of the healing profession. Norman Cousins in The Saturday Review (2/18/78) quotes Dr. Gerald Looney of the Medical College of the University of Southern California: "Nothing is more out of date than the notion that doctors can't learn from their patients . . . I teach my students to listen very carefully to their patients . . . That's what good medical practice is all about." I suspect that as the course of the disease progresses and the patient's ability to function independently becomes more and more restricted, it will become correspondingly essential for the patient to have a say in making decisions about those choices still open.

Next week we will look at three other areas of ministry that my contact with competent physicians has taught me to expect.

Dr. Wilson is a former pastor in Lancaster and has been ill with cancer more than three years. This series of columns appears each Wednesday and Friday. Questions or comments may be mailed to Dr. Wilson in care of the Intelligencer Journal, 8 W. King St., Lancaster, Pa. 17604.

A

FIGURE 2–1. (Courtesy of Mrs. Donald C. Wilson and the *Lancaster Intelligencer Journal.*)

---

fluffs are saturated with saline solution with the excess wrung out, and are used to wipe off the Betadine scrub, working from the inner canthus and using only one wipe of the widest stroke possible.

2. Two toothettes saturated in Betadine skin preparation solution paint the previously scrubbed area, starting at the upper lid margins and working superiorly to the forehead and the hairline. Two new toothettes are saturated in Betadine solution to paint the previously scrubbed area, including the lower lid margins and extending inferiorly over the cheek to include the upper lip.

3. With two cotton fluffs the painted area from the inner canthus to the hairline is wiped, using only one wipe of the widest possible stroke.

4. A large sterile drape is placed over the chest of the patient, so that its superior margin reaches well up onto the chin. Three sterile drapes are placed under the patient's head, and using the smallest of these, the head is wrapped in a modified turban style. A moist eye pad is placed on the lid of the opposite closed eye, in order to keep the eye closed and protected.

5. Argyrol may be instilled at the start of the preparation procedure. Although this does not sterilize the eye, it does coagulate the mucus and other debris on the conjunctiva, making it easier to remove this later using swabs and irrigation.

6. The surgeon makes certain that the external surfaces are absolutely dry and that no excess Argyrol or saline solution remains in the cul-de-sacs. The surgeon then places a barrier drape from his tray onto the surgical field and unfolds this appropriately. If the patient is under local anesthesia, the instrument stand placed over the patient's chest serves as a tent

——Terminal Candor——

Patient Looks at His Doctor—II

By DONALD C. WILSON

In our last column I stated that my contact with physicians in the course of my illness had led me to a magnificent respect for the medical profession and to some high expectations from its practitioners. Specifically, I have come to want in my doctor an awareness of his own feelings about death. Second, I want him or her to be aware of my feelings as a patient. In addition —

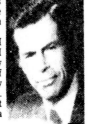

D. C. Wilson

3. I want my doctor to be honest. By this I mean I want to be told the facts and in detail. I want my diagnosis by name; I want to know what my prospects are; I want the details of the treatment, the side-effects of the therapy and the physical limitations that are foreseen. The doctor may tell me too much; he may not tell me enough. What I can't stand from him is a lie.

Candor is the basis for our relationship and it has to last the course. The patient who, following the initial diagnosis and treatment, has a recurrence, presents the doctor with an even more complex psychological problem. When this happens, writes Dr. Benjamin F. Rush Jr. of the New Jersey Medical School, "the surgeon tumbles from his high place." Well, the know-how for a cure may be out of human reach but the integrity of the patient/doctor relationship becomes all the more important. If trust has been absent before, it will be hard to generate it now. On the other hand, trust that has been built from the start may be one of the most potent resources during the terminal period.

4. I want my doctor to involve my family in the treatment. They are already involved in the illness. If I know one thing about my condition and my family knows another, our communication is diminished. When there is discouraging news I am not sure that I will be alert to cover all the bases. Here the physician must keep control. One professor of medicine, Laurens P. White of California, puts it this way explicitly: "I make it a point to try not to discuss diagnosis and prognosis with the family without the patient being present. In this way everybody knows at the same time what everybody else knows, but, more importantly, everybody knows that everybody knows, and that different stories are not being given to different people."

B

But the doctor's role as a human professional goes beyond conveying the relevant information. When the doctor lets the patient and family know that he is including the family in his care, that assurance gives encouragement to each of them in their own respective roles. A family group can be compared to a mobile hanging from the ceiling. Every move by one member prompts a corresponding movement of every other member and the whole family. Other health-care professionals can play a part in harmonizing these movements — nurse, clergy, social-worker. But for the physician as executive director of the caring ministry there is no substitute.

5. I want my doctor with me to the end. Let me tell you a secret. When I ask my doctor how long it will be to the end I am not necessarily asking for a calendar date. What I am really concerned with is whether the physician will be with me all the way. I can think of no more heartening answer than: "I don't know how long you are going to live, but I'll tell you this — that however long it takes and whatever it takes, we will go through this together."

I expect to need him as a fellow-human after he has outlived his capacity as a technician. If he sees that his usefulness to me is ended when he has no new treatment to prescribe, he is not only deserting me but he is denying the value of his own humanity.

A five-year-old boy suspected he wasn't going to get well and asked his doctor. The doctor told him he was very sick and the treatment had not been effective. He asked the boy if he was afraid. The boy asked the doctor if he was afraid. They both decided they were not. When the boy told his parents that everything would be all right, they asked him how he knew. "Because my doctor loves me," was the reply.

The Apostle Paul told us that "love is patient and kind." Impending death that prompts the doctor to wonder where he failed prompts the patient to wonder if he is worth it. The patience and kindness then forthcoming from the doctor can mark the difference between prolonging life and prolonging dying. It ought to be the right of each of us to live until we die.

Dr. Wilson is a former pastor in Lancaster and has been ill with cancer more than three years. This series of columns appears each Wednesday and Friday. Questions or comments may be mailed to Dr. Wilson in care of the Intelligencer Journal, 8 W. King St., Lancaster, Pa. 17604.

FIGURE 2–1 *Continued*

pole to keep the barrier drape elevated from the patient's face, keeping the patient far more comfortable. The surgeon then incises the barrier drape, making sure that the width of the incision extends well past the inner and outer canthi. The edges of the drape are retracted approximately 1 cm from the lid margins and pressed firmly to the skin. The edges of the drape can be placed close to the lid margins or wrapped under the lid margins. The scissors used to incise the drape are given to the circulating nurse.

Barrier drapes permit far greater isolation of the surgical field than was possible with previous draping techniques. They have the disadvantage of being virtually airtight, however, and consequently it is essential that there be a means of removing the carbon dioxide that builds up underneath the drape and providing additional oxygen throughout the operative procedure. Some drapes are flammable, and appropriate precautions must be taken. In addition, fine forceps can pick up fragments of lint from disposable paper drapes. These fragments can produce marked inflammation.

ANESTHESIA

Adequate anesthesia is important to the successful outcome of a surgical procedure. Previous practice has generally been to administer medication (e.g., a sedative, an antiemetic, and an analgesic) before the surgery, to produce a loss of anxiety and a general feeling of well-being. However, it is not at all certain that such medication is in fact necessary. Experiences with outpatient surgery suggest that many patients need little or even no premedication. The general tendency now is either to use general anesthesia or to use minimal sedation in association with local anesthesia. The surgeon who uses potent medication such as Innovar must consider that his patient is receiving the equivalent of general anesthesia and take appropriate preoperative, postoperative and intraoperative precautions. Procedures performed under local anesthesia are probably best accomplished when there is careful psychological preparation of the patient, an appropriately soothing and confidence-inspiring atmosphere during the preoperative and operative periods, excellent technique of administration of the local anesthetic agent, and administration of the minimal amount of short-acting medication. The goal is to have the patient relaxed and cooperative during surgery, and completely alert and ready for ambulation (should that be appropriate) immediately after surgery.

Principles regarding the use of anesthesia and anesthetic techniques are discussed in detail in Chapter 5.

OPERATIVE TECHNIQUES

General principles that apply to virtually all operative techniques are discussed in Chapter 3. Specific principles and techniques are covered in each of the individual chapters dealing with the subspecialties.

POSTOPERATIVE CARE

The final phase of the surgical procedure begins at the conclusion of the operation and extends through the postoperative recovery phase until the patient's healing is complete.

Bedrest and Patching

With modern suturing techniques severe restriction of activity in the early postoperative period is seldom necessary, even after intraocular surgery.[8, 9] Early ambulation should be encouraged, to prevent the host of problems that arise with prolonged bedrest, a special concern in the elderly. Most patients should be up and about the same day as surgery.

Modern wound closure also reduces the need for eye patches. Although a firm patch may make a patient more comfortable by preventing movement of the lids and excess tearing, it has the negative effect of increasing the temperature around the eye, thus providing a better environment for bacterial growth. The use of eye patches should be discontinued as soon as the patient can function comfortably without them. The use of a perforated shield or protective glasses to prevent an inadvertent bump to the eye is still recommended.

Postoperative Medication

There is no "routine" postoperative medication to fit the needs of all patients. Each and every case must be considered separately. The surgeon must be familiar with the advantages and disadvantages of various therapeutic agents. The tremendous importance of proper postoperative medication cannot be over-emphasized. A successful operative procedure can be ruined by incorrect postoperative therapy; on the other hand, a marginally successful operation can often be salvaged by proper medication. (This emphasis on postoperative care was a teaching of E. B. Spaeth.) Sedation and analgesia should be kept to a minimum. Aspirin in any form is often contraindicated because of its tendency to encourage bleeding. When sedation is required, pentobarbital is often effective and has the additional benefit of minimizing postoperative nausea and vomiting. Medications should not be used as a substitute for the psychological support and reassurance that can come from all those who participate in the patient's postoperative care, but most essentially from the surgeon himself.

Discharge and Rehabilitation

Time of discharge varies with the surgery and the patient. For cases in which outpatient follow-up is possible, early discharge is encouraged.

The surgeon's task is not complete until the patient has been fully rehabilitated. This aspect of the surgical procedure, especially for patients who undergo cataract extraction, may be the most challenging; it may persist for the remainder of the patient's life.

One of the weakest aspects of many present-day training programs is the lack of exposure of

TABLE 2–2. Causes for a Surgical Result That is Less Than Optimal

Due to the Surgeon (partially controllable by the medical profession)
  Poor surgeon-patient relationship
  Poor diagnostic skill
  Lack of technical knowledge or skill
  Insufficient medical care
  Inadequate facilities
  Lack of surgical judgment

Due to the Medical Setting (partially controllable by the medical profession and the administration of the hospital)
  Poor facilities
  Inadequate nursing care

Due to the Patient (partially controllable by public education)
  Ignorance of the disease
  Unwillingness to understand the disease
  Refusal to cooperate in a program of appropriate treatment

Due to the Nature of the Disease Itself (partially controllable by increased knowledge)

Due to External Forces
  Societal conditions that could be controlled (e.g., malnutrition)
  Conditions that appear to be uncontrollable (e.g., accidents)

the learning surgeon to the patient in the postoperative period. The neophyte simply does not have the chance to see the unfortunate and long-lasting distress often caused by so-called successful, but ill-chosen surgery. *The art of proper selection of surgery demands exposure to patients in the postoperative period.* An additional problem in this regard is that the inexperienced surgeon may fail to fully realize the great need for immediate recognition of complications, together with institution of remedial steps, and the tremendous importance of reassuring and comforting the patient.

The recognition and management of specific complications are dealt with later in this text. As we conclude this brief introduction to the general aspects of ophthalmic surgery, it is pertinent, however, to review some of the general causes for the unfortunate events that may reduce the benefits of a surgical experience. These are listed in Table 2–2.

Probably the single most important factor that affects the surgical outcome is the character of the surgeon, which largely determines the nature of the other characteristics listed. There is a deep fundamental validity in the inscription on the monument in the Sanctuary of Aesculapius:

These are the duties of a physician; first [to repeat] the Paeonian chants and to heal his mind and give assistance to himself before giving it to anyone [else], and not to look upon [his patient] or make approaches in a manner contrary to divine laws and to the oath. He would cure with moral courage and with the proper moral attitude. He would not [be spiritually] unequipped when as helper he handles lovely matrons and maidens, burn in his breast with desire [in a manner unworthy of a true] physician. . . . Having become such a one in his judgment, he would be like God saviour equally of slaves, of paupers, of rich men, of princes, and to all a brother, such help he would give. For we are all brothers. Therefore he would not hate anyone, nor would he harbor envy in his mind, nor increase his pretensions.*

REFERENCES

1. American Academy of Ophthalmology Code of Ethics, San Francisco, 1989.
2. Stanley, B., Guido, J., Stanley, M., et al.: The elderly patient and informed consent. JAMA, 252:1302, 1984.
3. Ost, D. E.: The "right" not to know. J. Med. Philos., 9:301, 1984.
4. Bockelmann, P.: Zur rechtlichen situation bei prophylaktischen Massnahmen in der Ophthalmologie. Klin. Mbl. Augenheilk., 173:129, 1978.
5. Curran, W. J.: Law-Medicine Notes: Malpractice claims: New data and new trends. N. Engl. J. Med., 300:26, 1979.
6. Wilson, P. C.: Lancaster Intelligencer Journal, 1978.
7. Antiemetics and postoperative nausea and vomiting. Med. Lett. Drugs Therap., 3:50, 1961.
8. Galin, M., Irving, B.: Immediate ambulation and discharge after cataract extraction. Trans. Am. Acad. Ophthalmol. Otolaryngol., 78:43, 1974.
9. Editorial: Ambulatory outpatient surgery: A statement of principles. Can. J. Ophthalmol. 20:165, 1985.

*Translated by James H. Oliver. Bull. History of Medicine, 7:315, 1939.

PRINCIPLES OF SURGERY
Determination of the Goal
Development of a Plan
Adaptability
Visualization of the Surgical Field
Minimization of Trauma
Restoration of Tissues
Economy
Control
Development and Improvement

3

FUNDAMENTAL SURGICAL PROCEDURES

by George L. Spaeth

PRINCIPLES OF SURGERY

To this point we have considered some of the matters that lead to the surgical decision. We have also discussed the general principles that apply to the surgical experience in its broadest sense. The patient's point of view has been stressed. In this chapter we deal more specifically with the principles of the surgical technique itself (Table 3–1).

1. Determination of the Goal. The surgeon must know the goal of the surgery. The method of performing surgery is important, but the ultimate goal is a different consideration. One may become so involved with the disease and with the surgical technique that one forgets the importance of the process itself and of the surgical result one is trying to achieve. Consider, for example, the patient whose bilateral, asymmetrically advanced cataracts have caused visual incapacitation. The dense, mature cata-

TABLE 3–1. Nine Principles of Surgery

1. Clear knowledge of purpose
2. Well-defined plan of surgery
3. Adaptability and flexibility of surgeon
4. Good visualization of surgical field
5. Minimization of trauma
6. Restoration of tissues to normal state
7. Economy
8. Control
9. Continued development and improvement

racts preclude any visualization of the ocular fundus. In this person the goal is the achievement of clinically useful vision. Extraction of the cataract in the eye with the worst vision is a conspicuous step toward reaching this objective; however, a successful cataract extraction in itself is not the objective. Failure to note the presence of a significant esotropia, or the difference of 6 diopters of refractive error between the two eyes would doom the patient to a visually unsatisfactory result, no matter how "perfect" the cataract extraction. Other specific examples help to clarify this seemingly obvious point. Consider a patient with a blepharoptosis that followed a trabeculectomy performed in conjunction with large-sector iridectomy. The ptosis is so severe that it interferes with acuity, and the patient wants to be relieved of the problem. The objective, then, is visual improvement. The patient also has marked nuclear sclerosis. The surgeon performs a ptosis procedure with an excellent cosmetic result. However, the patient, to the surgeon's surprise, is unhappy. The patient is unhappy because the acuity has improved little, if at all, and glare is more of a problem than it was before the surgery. It is important for the surgeon's and the patient's goals to be consistent. Or consider the patient with far-advanced visual field loss and an intraocular pressure of 47 mm Hg. The objective of the surgery is to lower pressure so that the vision may be preserved. The surgeon knows that if the intraocular pressure remains at 47, the small amount of visual field will rapidly be lost. The patient may understand that the primary purpose of the surgery is to preserve sight, and be surprised and disappointed when, after the operation, the surgeon is relatively pleased with an intraocular pressure of 12 and acuity that has only deteriorated two lines.

2. Development of a Plan. After a clear definition of the primary and ancillary objectives, the surgeon develops a plan designed to achieve the desired goals, keeping in mind the multiplicity of factors involved. During the planning of surgery the plan may need modification; at this point the initial purpose of the surgery again must be carefully considered. The surgeon should not make the error of substituting the plan for the primary objective. Also, it must be recognized that events during the performance of surgery may make it necessary to modify the surgeon's aim. It is essential to keep in mind that the major purpose of the plan is to achieve the objective of the patient. The surgeon's objectives must be in line with that goal.

3. Adaptability. It is not always possible to proceed exactly according to plan. When complications, foreseen or unforeseen, develop it is usually necessary to modify the plan so that the most important objective can be achieved. Whereas the fundamental goal in a patient having a cataract extraction may be the achievement of excellent visual acuity, that objective may change to preservation of a comfortable, cosmetically satisfactory eye after the development of an expulsive choroidal hemorrhage. Similarly, a fundamental goal in an elderly patient with ataxia and Alzheimer's disease may be restoration of useful vision without the need for glasses, the plan being to remove the cataract and implant a posterior chamber intraocular lens. However, major difficulties with the posterior capsule occurring at the time of the cataract extraction may make it unwise to implant an intraocular lens, and it may be more prudent to modify the plan and settle for a different goal, specifically to remove the cataract and achieve as healthy an eye as possible, with a thought that a secondary implant may be placed at a later date.

4. Visualization of the Surgical Field. Seeing clearly is not just a matter of using an instrument with adequate or even high magnification. It also requires proper lighting, correct positioning of the hands, skillful assistantship, correct positioning of the patient, and competence in the use of appropriate optical aids. Many of the improvements in modern surgical technique

TABLE 3–2. Advantages of the Modern Operating Microscope

1. Magnification capacities
    Increased power
    Variable power that is easily controlled by surgeons
2. Illumination capacities
    Coaxial
    Oblique
    Slit
    Variable intensity
    Filtered
3. Accessories easily added
    Keratometer
    Camera (still, movie, or television)
    Stereotaxis apparatus
    Specialized illumination (including laser)
    Motorized equipment
4. Field of view can be virtually identical for the assistant and the surgeon

have stemmed from the persistent demand of surgeons to see better.

The better able the surgeon is to see what he is doing, the better are the chances for a satisfactory result. To see clearly requires accurate focus, adequate extent and depth of field, good stereopsis, proper magnification, and appropriate illumination. Modern operating microscopes, by enhancing the quality of these five elements, have made possible and extended the range of surgical procedures, such as strip-

TABLE 3–3. Disadvantages of the Operating Microscope*

1. Limited view of operative field
    Small field with high magnification
    Small depth of focus with high magnification
    Where view not parfocal surgeon or assistant may obstruct each other, and surgical field may not be similar
    Where view parfocal assistant may lack stereopsis
2. Illumination problems
    Reflexes difficult to remove
    Excessive brightness and heat may damage patient's tissue
    Excessive brightness may cause retinal fatigue in surgeon
2. Immobility of instrument
    Awkward position to perform surgical maneuvers
    Inability to see certain areas
    Need for total immobility of the patient
4. Greater time expended in operating room
    Time required to set up and disassemble instrument
    Surgical operating time usually greater
5. Sterilization difficult
6. Expensive
7. Maintenance costs high
8. Not always available
9. Mechanical or electrical failures not always possible to prevent and may require prolonged time to correct

*This list applies to most presently available mounted operating microscopes. The problems are not all intrinsic, and modifications could overcome some of them.

ping of vitreoretinal membranes. The advantages of the advanced operating microscope, outlined in Table 3–2, are impressive; however, for each benefit there is a corresponding problem (Table 3–3). The operating microscope is not required for every procedure; in fact, many operations are better performed without it. Furthermore, the confident surgeon has learned how to use the advantages and minimize the disadvantages of the operating microscope.

Adequate magnification for many procedures, such as most of those performed by the ocular plastic surgeon, can be supplied by the operating loupe (Table 3–4). Most loupes provide magnification ranging from 1.5× to 4×. The loupes may be appropriate for use by the assistant, who needs to see well enough to know what the surgeon is doing, and yet wants the advantage of mobility and a virtually unobstructed field. The loupes manufactured by

Zeiss and by Keeler are satisfactory (Fig. 3–1), the former having the advantage of being of smaller size and lighter weight. Both can be fitted onto a spectacle that incorporates the surgeon's own correction.

When tissue manipulations require the ability to distinguish smaller distances (e.g., in the range of 0.3 mm), higher magnification is needed. This can be provided by a head-mounted microscope. The magnification of such instruments ranges from 3× to 10×. Although this is adequate for many procedures, and significant advantages are associated with the use of such mobile optical aids (ease of focusing, opportunity for the surgeon to position himself in a way that makes manipulations comfortable, the ability to change positions of view), there are serious problems associated with their use (Table 3–4). The surgeon must hold his head absolutely still while operating; if he does not, he will be troubled by a bothersome "against"

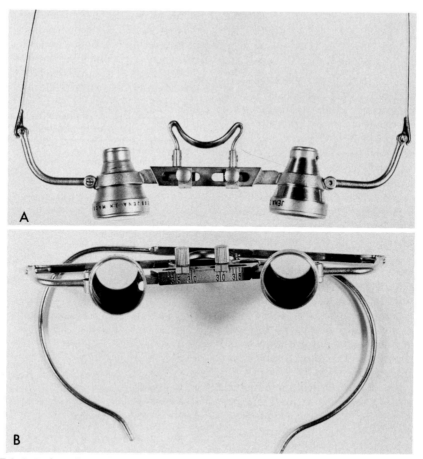

FIGURE 3–1. Traditional Zeiss loupe of 2.5× magnification. The working distance is 20 cm, the diameter of field 50 mm, and the depth of field 6 mm. This is an excellent instrument for extraocular ophthalmic surgical procedures.

TABLE 3–4. Advantages and Disadvantages of the Loupe*

ADVANTAGES	DISADVANTAGES
Complete mobility	Small field unless ocular very close to lashes
Ease of focus	Variable magnification not readily possible
Little time required for preparation	Cannot be used in very high magnifications
Excellent for assistant's use	Does not provide slit-beam illumination
Little problem adjusting illumination	Cannot accommodate special accessories (e.g., camera, keratometer)
Relatively low cost	Discomfort and inconvenience caused by necessity to tighten headband in
Readily available	order to hold loupe firmly
No sterilization problems	

*In contrast to a mounted microscope of similar magnification ($6 \times$ — $8 \times$).

movement. Moreover, the lack of accessories available with the more complex ceiling-mounted scopes can also be limiting. For example, slit illumination is difficult to obtain, and photographic documentation is less satisfactory. One of the most disturbing aspects of use of the head-mounted microscope is the discomfort that almost invariably develops after about 45 minutes' operating time; at that point the surgeon may need to remove the scope in order to relieve the ischemia caused by the tight headband. A major limitation of the loupe, however, is that it does not have variable magnification. As a result, the surgeon using such an instrument during the performance of a procedure that requires a variety of manipulations is operating with magnification that is not optimal for some of the steps involved. For example, during a cataract extraction accurate placement of the sutures is best done with a magnification of at least $8 \times$, but when the sutures are tied a lower magnification is preferable for visualization of the wider field. A head-mounted microscope cannot easily provide both. A further major disadvantage is the inability of the assistant to see exactly the same field being viewed by the surgeon.

Satisfactory head-mounted microscopes include the Beckerscope (Storz) (Fig. 3–2) and the prism loupes manufactured by Keeler and Zeiss. Both of these latter microscopes can have their magnification varied, the former from $3 \times$ to $7 \times$, and the latter from $3 \times$ to $8 \times$. Such adjustments, however, cannot be made with the ease that characterizes the mounted microscopes. The working distance of all three instruments is about 250 cm, which is satisfactory. Depth and diameter of field are not less than

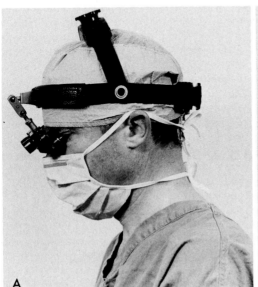 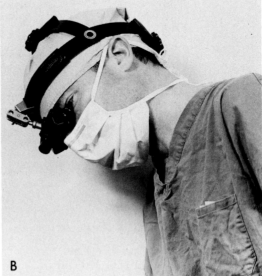

FIGURE 3–2A and B. The "Beckerscope" (Storz) provides $8 \times$ magnification with a 28 mm field. It is useful for procedures which require more magnification than is obtainable with the Zeiss loupe (Fig. 3–1), yet are facilitated by the surgeon's being able to "look around the corner." The oculars must be close to the eye (A) in order to obtain the full diameter of field.

those obtained with the mounted microscopes. A fiberoptic illuminator can be attached to the Keeler loupe.

Halfway between the full-capacity mounted microscopes and the powerful loupes just described are the portable microscopes, such as the Mentor CM-III (Codman-Shurtleff) (Fig. 3–3). This is mounted on an adjustable stand that can be attached to the ceiling, wall, table, or floor. Magnification ranges from 4.2× to 14×, and the field size is commensurate with the magnification (30.0 mm for the lowest and 17.4 mm for the highest). The working distance of 200 mm is satisfactory. The cost of the instru-

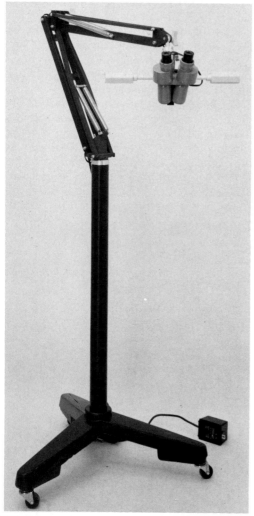

FIGURE 3–3. This microscope (Mentor CM-III) provides magnification of up to 14×. Sterilizable handles permit the surgeon to alter the orientation of the microscope during the procedure. The instrument can be easily mounted to the edge of a table or other firm support. However, stability is only fair.

ment is competitive with that of many loupes, and is a fraction of that of a complex ceiling-mounted microscope. The unit has built-in illumination of moderate intensity. Magnification is varied by changing oculars (four are available). Sterilizable handles can be attached to the microscope to aid in focusing.

The portable microscope has the disadvantage that, in most cases, the stability of the mount is not entirely satisfactory. With high magnification it is difficult to keep the field in sharp focus. Additionally, changing the position of the scope is time-consuming. When using a loupe this is obviously not a problem, and with the ceiling-mounted instrument, changing the direction of view is currently so inconvenient that the surgeon learns to adjust to working from a single position. The illumination supplied with a Mentor CM-III is adequate only for extraocular procedures. Accessories such as an assistant's scope cannot be added.

Current ophthalmic surgery simply could not be accomplished without the modern operating microscope. Great credit should be given to the surgeons who led the profession and the manufacturing houses to the awareness of the new world of surgical technique that could become possible with improved visualization. Troutman of Brooklyn, Barraquer of Barcelona, Harms of Tübingen, Mackensen of Freiburg—these surgeons deserve the thanks of all who require or perform surgery on the eye. Many others have made important contributions, including Pierse, Roper-Hall, McPherson, Draeger, Dannheim, Machmer, Paton, Kelman, and Peyman, to name but a few. Nor should the vital role of Zeiss, Keeler, and Weck manufacturing firms be forgotten. The optical companies have also responded with fine products; Nikon, Codman and Shurtleff, Topcon, and Rodenstock are among the innovative manufacturers whose products are available in many parts of the world. We now believe that optimal training of the ophthalmic surgeon demands consistent and persistent practice in using a fully developed operating microscope. Although the techniques required to use these instruments are specialized and can be achieved only with practice and supervision, the benefits are well worth the trouble. The surgeon trained with an operating microscope can quickly adjust to using a high-power loupe for those procedures that are in fact best performed without an operating microscope; however, one cannot easily go in the other direction.

The major limitation of all the instruments currently available is the drastic restriction of

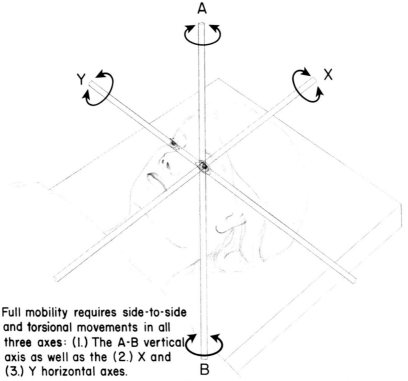

Full mobility requires side-to-side and torsional movements in all three axes: (1.) The A-B vertical axis as well as the (2.) X and (3.) Y horizontal axes.

FIGURE 3–4. The ideal operating microscope would allow the surgeon to change the direction of gaze along all three of the axes illustrated. Modern operating microscopes permit surgeon-controlled focusing along the A-B axis, and horizontal excursions parallel with the X and Y axes. Furthermore, manual rotation around the A-B axis and limited tilting related to the X and Y axes are also possible.

mobility enforced on the surgeon. Although modern instruments permit surgeon-controlled focusing in both vertical and horizontal (X-Y) directions, the important torsional movements are either impossible or so cumbersome that they are usually not altered once surgery has begun. If one observes a surgeon operating with a loupe, the extent of these torsional movements, made in all three axes around the patient's eye, is readily apparent (Fig. 3–4). The major new technique that must be mastered by the surgeon who wants to use the higher magnification and better illumination afforded by the operating microscope, then, is adjusting to this lack of mobility.

Microsurgery is usually a bit more time-consuming than loupe-assisted surgery; one reason for this is the additional time needed to prepare the microscope for the surgeon. I prefer to do this before scrubbing, as it saves time and reduces the likelihood of contamination.

When using an operating microscope the surgeon must be comfortably seated; once a position is taken, it cannot be easily changed without losing or compromising the view. Thus

there is no substitute for taking the time needed to get completely comfortable, with the operating table, the surgeon's chair, and the microscope all properly adjusted. The surgeon's stool should be easy to adjust, preferably by the surgeon himself. Armrests are useful but of little help unless they, too, can be easily positioned to ensure the most relaxed position of the hands during surgery.

The patient should be completely immobile. This may demand general anesthesia, although many individuals are able to be sufficiently still even when awake. But to try using an operating microscope with a moving patient guarantees a less than optimal result. The patient who is not under anesthesia must be kept completely comfortable; otherwise, he will not be able to withstand the procedure without undue difficulty. For example, the patient who is given mannitol 1 hour preoperatively will become restless during a prolonged procedure under local anesthesia unless he is allowed to empty his bladder immediately before the surgery. It is essential that anesthetic agents be of adequate duration.

The patient's head ideally should be placed

on a readily adjustable rest that extends out from the remainder of the operating table, permitting the surgeon to position himself more comfortably.

The microscope should be checked and adjusted as completely as possible before the start of surgery. The illumination should be in working order. The oculars should be adjusted for pupillary diameter, refractive correction, and anticipated "near-myopia"; soft rubber "blinders" should be used by most surgeons who do not wear glasses, as these will help to keep the oculars the correct distance from the eyes. Any required accessories (camera, assistant's microscope, observer tube, etc.) should be attached and aligned. The microscope should be in the center of its horizontal excursions (X-Y), and the vertical focus, in the middle of its range.

At the start of the operative procedure itself the surgeon's view should be centered on the area where it will be most required. For example, when starting an intraocular cataract extraction, the center of the field should be a few millimeters superior to the pupillary axis. The magnification should be at the lowest power (around $3\times$) for placement of the superior rectus suture and for general orientation to the surgical field. The power can then be zoomed down during the procedure to provide the optimal balance of magnification with adequate depth and diameter of field.

Throughout the procedure the surgeon must consider what type of illumination is best for each step involved, and adjust the light source accordingly. Oblique illumination has the advantage of providing bright light that is relatively free from glare, and of enhancing depth perception. If slit-beam illumination is required, it should be readied before the start of surgery. Coaxial light, although it diminishes depth perception and throws more light onto the posterior pole of the retina than does oblique illumination, is essential for procedures in which a red reflex is needed, as with phacoemulsification, or when light must be directed into the depths of the globe. The intensity of illumination should *not* automatically be put at the highest level and left there. In fact, just enough light should be used to give optimal visualization, since bright light introduces problems in itself, such as retinal fatigue of the surgeon and retinal damage for the patient; this is a particular concern in patients who already have serious loss of visual acuity, such as those with advanced glaucoma. The surgeon should be especially cautious when using bright coaxial illumination for a prolonged period in a patient

in whom the anterior segment has not been altered because the full intensity will be focused on the retina.

It is not just the high magnification of the operating microscope that makes it unique. If it were, the learning surgeon could master its technique by prior practice with a high-powered loupe or a portable instrument. It is, rather, the ability to modify the instrument during the operative procedure that is the major distinction between the operating microscope and the less complex instruments. The beginning surgeon should have access to a practice microscope that possesses a full range of regulatory controls, for it is not until the surgeon can control the zoom, the X-Y, and the fine focus with his foot as comfortably as if he were merely altering the position of his head (that is, almost unconsciously) that he can become fully proficient in microsurgery. These techniques cannot be learned with an instrument that does not have such controls (Figs. 3–5 through 3–8).

The placement of the hands under the mounted microscope is slightly different from the positioning used with a loupe. Because with the microscope the view is relatively fixed and usually comes from a superior position, the hands must be held flatter and more to the side. This position is facilitated by specially designed instruments. In addition, the hands cannot be moved more than a few millimeters. Recall that at a mere $4\times$ magnification, the diameter of the field for most instruments is only about 5 cm, and the depth of field only 2.5 mm. This field decreases rapidly with increasing magnification, so that with a moderately high magnification (e.g., $10\times$) the diameter is only 2 cm and the depth 0.6 mm (Fig. 3–6 and Table 3–5). At $20\times$ the field has lessened to 1 cm and 0.4 mm. Clearly movements of the hands when working in such a restricted field must be similarly small. In practice, the hands should move almost not at all. They should rest firmly but lightly on the patient's brow or forehead, or be supported by an armrest. Movements are largely made with the fingers.

Correct placement of the many components involved in microsurgery is vital to smooth and efficient performance. A suggested set-up is shown in Figure 3–9. This allows each member of the operating team to function well without interfering with the others. When the patient is under local anesthesia the drapes should be held elevated above the patient's face with a Mayo stand; this ensures adequate space for breathing and diminishes the patient's anxiety.

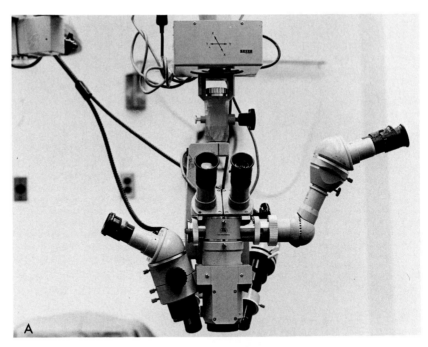

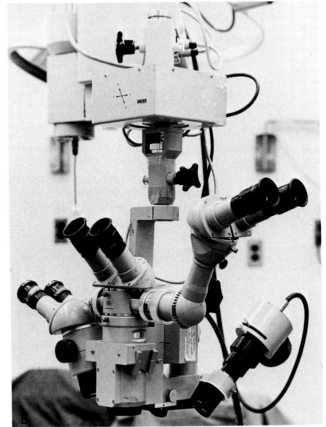

FIGURE 3–5. A wide variety of accessories can be added to many operating microscopes. Attached to the Zeiss op-Mi 6S shown here are an assistant's scope, a beam splitter, an observer's scope, a slit illuminator, and a fiberoptic coaxial illuminator. This microscope is the basic unit as used in the Wills Eye Hospital.

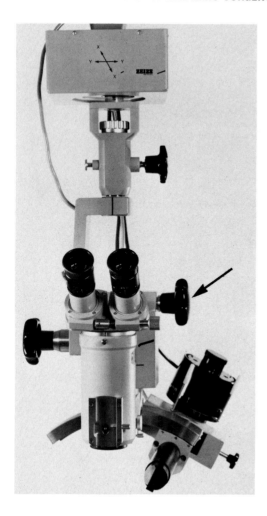

FIGURE 3–6. Direction of view can be altered while using modern operating microscopes. The microscope shown here can be rotated around the A-B vertical axis by loosening the superior blocking knob. Tilt (not true rotation) around the Y axis is accomplished by twisting the knob at the side of the microscope (arrow). Rotation around the X axis is not possible with this instrument. Side-to-side motion along the horizontal X and Y axes and vertical motion along the vertical A-B axis can be controlled by the surgeon through activation of motorized units. In the unit shown, the direction of the slit beam can be varied by motorized control.

Providing a constant supply of oxygen under the drapes ensures adequate oxygenation. However, hypercapnia, not hypoxia, is usually the cause for anxiety in the patient who is awake and covered with drapes. A suction scavenger under the drapes, to remove the expired carbon dioxide, is advisable.

5. Minimization of Trauma. Damage to the patient and to the patient's tissues occurs in many ways (Table 3–6). Ironically, operating

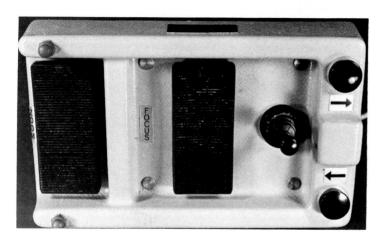

FIGURE 3–7. Foot controls for the operating microscope shown in Figure 3–9. *A*, The foot pedal controls are for the zoom, fine focus, X-Y motion, and coarse focus (from left to right, respectively).

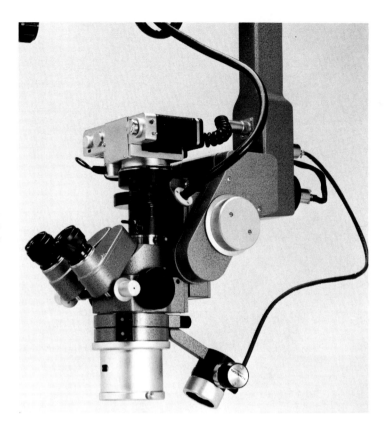

FIGURE 3–8. An operating microscope (Topcon OMS-80) adapted for still photography. The flash can be positioned so that the reflex does not obscure the image.

with excessive caution may result in a greater degree of trauma. The prolonged procedure that often characterizes the timid surgeon subjects the patient to the irritating components of irrigating solutions, to airborne infection, to increased contact with possibly contaminated instruments, to the stresses of lying immobile, to the trauma of light, and to the effects of increased amounts of anesthetic agents. On the other hand, the excessively aggressive surgeon may inflict trauma by cutting more deeply or more extensively than required, by cutting tissue, and by being unrealistic regarding his own surgical ability.

Especially in their learning stages, *surgeons should consciously slow the rate of their move-ments*. Rapid motions are less well controlled, cause more mistakes, and prolong the operating time.

6. Restoration of Tissues. The restoration of tissues to their normal state requires proper reconstruction of tissue planes. The surgeon should not be satisfied with incomplete or inaccurate repositioning of tissue. For example, sutures used in closing a corneal laceration should be placed deeply enough to achieve apposition of the entire length of the corneal edges. This principle cannot be fulfilled without excellent visualization; often special optical aids are required.

7. Economy. Economy—of motion, of materials, of procedures, and so on—applies to all aspects of the surgical process and relates to the other principles as well: no procedure should be done that is not considered necessary; motions should be as efficient as they can be; blood vessels should be cauterized with just enough heat to cause coagulation; equipment should not be unnecessarily expensive—simple instruments should be preferred to complex, costly ones that do not provide better results; operating room time should be used efficiently; and so on.

Related to this principle of economy is satis-

TABLE 3–5. Relationship Between Magnification, Diameter, and Depth of Field with a Gallilean Microscope

| MAGNIFICATION | FIELD (in mm) | |
	Diameter	Depth
2×	100	8.0
4×	50	2.5
10×	20	0.6
20×	10	0.4

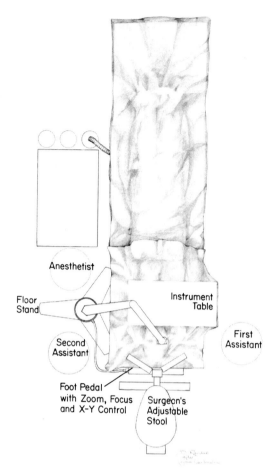

FIGURE 3–9. Suggested set-up for a floor-mounted microscope when operating on the right eye. The goal is to provide maximum freedom of action for the surgeon, the assistants, the anesthetist, and the nurses, along with maximum stability and comfort for both surgeon and patient.

faction with an adequate result. Although this concept may seem to condone mediocre surgery, it in fact does not. The surgeon should aim for a perfect result. However, he must acknowledge the virtual impossibility of achieving a truly perfect operative result, and must know when he has achieved a result close enough to perfect that further attempts are not advisable. That is, he must be able to recognize when additional effort may actually be counterproductive, serving only to jeopardize an already satisfactory situation. This is a hard aspect of surgery to teach and to learn. For example, when have enough sutures been placed? When is the anterior chamber deep enough that it does not need to be re-formed with saline solution? Determining the correct answers to such questions is essential to achieving an optimal surgical result.

TABLE 3–6. Ways in Which the Patient Can Be Traumatized During Surgery

1. Delay in initiating surgery
2. Improper preoperative care, including failure to perform all appropriate laboratory studies
3. Faulty preoperative cleansing and antisepsis
4. Effects of anesthesia
   Local toxicity
   Systemic reactions
   Immobility of the patient
   Postoperative inactivity
5. Manipulation of tissue
   Cautery
   Crushing
   Cutting
   Freezing
   Tearing
6. Exposure of tissue to irritating substances
   Air
   Blood
   Drugs
   Implanted materials
   Irrigating solutions
   Sutures
7. Exposure of tissue to infectious agents
8. Improper application of operative dressing
9. Inadequate attention to emotional needs
10. Operative maloccurrence

8. Control. The factor of control in surgery is closely linked with the principle of economy, as well as with the other principles. For example, trauma inflicted by the surgeon is minimized by the use of controlled, economical movements and the elimination of unnecessary activity. Control also refers to the entirety of the surgical event. The surgeon must be in control of the whole procedure, including the surgical team, the nursing staff, and the anesthetic assistants, in addition to having the requisite knowledge of the patient, the patient's disease, and the appropriate surgical techniques. The surgeon who finds himself in the operating room as a patient will not forget the experience and will better understand the necessity of having all operating room activities directed toward the well-being of the patient.

Finally, the surgeon must have full self-control.

9. Development and Improvement. To be a competent ophthalmic surgeon demands continuing modification of surgical skills. The surgeon who merely maintains the surgical ability achieved at the completion of residency training will, within several years, be performing substandard surgery. Although it is comfortable and tempting to continue to use a series of techniques that "work well," the competent surgeon must always be slightly changing. It is not prudent suddenly to make major alterations in surgical methodology. Rather, the surgeon should consciously and systematically alter one aspect of the procedure at a time. Such alterations should not be made without extensive preparation.

One of the most important, but least appreciated, aspects of a teaching institution is the accountability that results from the presence of residents in training. These young physicians quickly become aware of what constitutes good surgery. Surgeons in such programs have the advantage of constant scrutiny by knowledgeable colleagues. Furthermore, it is relatively easy for a surgeon in such an institution to observe colleagues and learn from them. This rarely describes accurately the situation of the ophthalmologist who performs surgery in a private surgicenter or a small community hospital and who seldom has the opportunity to perform surgery with a variety of knowledgeable ophthalmologists who are not likely to have a conflict of interest. On the other hand, ophthalmologists who work in such environments remarkably free of constraint may find it easier to be innovative.

It is thus not surprising that what seems like a disproportionate number of modern surgical advances have originated with private ophthalmologists practicing in such settings. When those advances are made at the expense of the patients, however, the cost for their development may be unnecessarily high.

REFERENCES

1. Boberg-An, J.: A new motorized chair for ophthalmic microsurgery. Am. J. Ophthalmol., 75:321, 1973.
2. Calkins, J. L., Hochheimer, B. F.: Retinal light exposure from ophthalmoscopes, slit lamps, and overhead surgical lamps. An analysis of potential hazards. Invest. Ophthalmol. Vis. Sci., 19:1009, 1980.
3. Crock, G. W., Pericic, L., Rajendran, B., et al.: A new system of microsurgery for human and experimental corneal grafting. II. Clinical and experimental applications. Br. J. Ophthalmol., 62:81, 1978.
4. Dannheim, R.: Symposium: Microsurgery of the outflow channels trabeculectomy. Trans. Am. Acad. Ophthalmol. Otolaryngol., 76:375, 1972.
5. Draeger, J.: Technical advances in ophthalmic microsurgery. An. Inst. Barraquer, 10:199, 1971–1972.
6. Fechner, P. U., Barth, R.: Effect on the retina of an air cushion in the anterior chamber and coaxial illumination. Am. J. Ophthalmol., 96:600, 1983.
7. Flynn, H. W., Jr., Brod, R. D.: Protection from operating microscope–induced retinal phytotoxicity during pars plana vitrectomy. Arch. Ophthalmol., 106:1032, 1988.
8. Hochheimer, B. F.: A possible cause of chronic cystic maculopathy. The operating microscope. Ann. Ophthalmol., 13:153, 1981.
9. Hoerenz, P.: The design of the surgical microscope—Part I. Ophthalmic Surg., 4 1(1):40, 1973.
10. Hollis, D. S.: Ophthalmology, felines and microsurgery. Ann. Ophthalmol., 5:1339, 1973.
11. Irvine, A. R., Copenhagen, D. R.: The focal nature of retinal illumination from the operating microscope. Arch. Ophthalmol., 103:549, 1985.
12. Irvine, A. R., Alvarado, J. A., Wood, I. S., et al.: Light-induced maculopathy from the operating microscope: An experimental study. Trans. Am. Ophthalmol. Soc., 82:239, 1984.
13. Khwarg, S. G., Linstone, F. A., Daniels, S. A., et al.: Incidence, risk factors, and morphology in operating microscope light retinopathy. Am. J. Ophthalmol., 103:255, 1987.
14. Jaeger, W., Kratzer, B.: Stereomikroskopbrille für operative Eingriffe am Auge. Klin. Monatsbl. Augenheilkd., 169:656, 1976.
15. Littmann, H.: Two new motorized surgical microscopes with physiologically adapted control of magnification. Klin. Monatsbl. Augenheilkd., 157:61, 1970.
16. Lücke, A., Remé, C.: Lichtschäden in der Netzhaut-Zusammenfassung experimenteller und klinischer Ergebnisse. Klin. Monatsbl. Augenheilkd., 184:77, 1984.
17. Machemer, R., Parel, J. M.: An improved microsurgical ceiling-mounted unit and automated television. Am. J. Ophthalmol., 85:205, 1978.
18. Mackensen, G.: Microsurgical manipulations in classical ocular surgery. An. Inst. Barraquer, 10:225, 1971–1972.
19. McIntyre, D. J.: Phytotoxicity: The eclipse filter. Ophthalmology, 92:364, 1985.
20. Martinez, M., Paton, D.: A new portable microscope for ophthalmic surgery. Ophthalmic Surg., 1:28, 1970.
21. Oosterhuis, J. A., Biessel, W. J.: Die Prismenlupenbrille als vergrosserndes Sehhilfsmittel für Schwachsichtige und als Operationsbrille. Klin. Monatsbl. Augenheilkd., 174:519, 1979.
22. Peyman, G. A., Urban, J.: A new operating microscope for extraocular and intraocular surgery. Am. J. Ophthalmol., 77:575, 1974.
23. Peyman, G. A., Erickson, E. S., May, D. R.: Slit illumination system and contact lens support ring for use with operating microscope. Ophthalmic Surg., 3:29, 1972.
24. Peyman, G. A., Ericson, E. S., May, D. R.: Micromanipulator arc system for intravitreal surgery. Am. J. Ophthalmol., 75:706, 1973.
25. Pierse, D. J., Steele, A. D. M.: A new headrest for ophthalmic microsurgery. Am. J. Ophthalmol., 85:253, 1978.
26. Remky, H., Ulrich, H.: Strength of illumination adequate for magnification of the microsurgical field. Klin. Monatsbl. Augenheilkd., 162:103, 1973.
27. Schwarts, L. K., Norris, J. L.: A corneal shield to prevent light-inducing maculopathy during cataract surgery. Am. J. Ophthalmol., 97:658, 1984.
28. Smith, R.: Microsurgical methods in glaucoma. Trans. Ophthalmol. Soc. U.K., 92:759, 1972.
29. Troutman, R. C.: Microsurgery for keratoplasty: Development and techniques. Int. Ophthalmol. Clin., 10:297, 1970.
30. Troutman, R. C., Kelly, S., Kaye, D., Clahane, A. C.: The use and preliminary results of the Troutman surgical keratometer in cataract and corneal surgery. Trans. Am. Acad. Ophthalmol. Otolaryngol., 83:232, 1977.

4

INSTRUMENTATION, SUTURES, AND STANDARD OPHTHALMIC PROCEDURES

by George L. Spaeth

INSTRUMENTATION

General Principles

The special techniques used when operating with a microscope require special instruments. The fixed direction of gaze prevents the surgeon from looking around obstructing objects, such as fingers or instruments. Consequently the tools of surgery must be designed so that they do not obscure the surgical field when held in comfortable positions. Additionally, protection of the tissue and the delicacy of suture material require instruments that will hold securely but atraumatically. Lastly, the instruments must enhance the surgeon's ability to perform the miniature manipulations of microsurgery. For example, a trabeculectomy flap of 0.1-mm thickness cannot be sutured with the desired degree of accuracy using a forceps with 0.3-mm teeth. On the other hand, the delicate 0.1-mm-toothed Bonn forceps is not appropriate for grasping a thick, sliding skin flap. Such a forceps would hold the tissue poorly, increase the likelihood of tearing it, and probably be ruined in the unsuccessful effort.

It is beyond the scope of this text to discuss in full detail the use of all ophthalmic instruments. The reader is referred to other texts for excellent and exhaustive coverage.[1-6] However, the fundamental principal that underlies all successful instruments can be presented quite simply. To be of optimal value, an instrument must permit the surgeon to accomplish the desired manipulation with the greatest possible ease, rapidity, repeatability, safety, and economy. For placement of a corneal suture, for example, the ideal needle holder would be one that holds the suture totally immobile with minimal pressure on the needle, has a surface that transmits, without slipping, the motion imparted by the surgeon's fingers to the needle, has its jaws positioned so that the simplest rotation motion of the needle holder with the finger causes the needle to follow exactly the desired arc through the tissue, and so on.

Surgical Trays

At the Wills Eye Hospital many surgeons use the operating rooms. The head nurse has developed surgical trays that fit the needs of most. The makeup of these trays is shown in Tables 4–1 through 4–10. The trays do not include every instrument needed by every surgeon, but they do provide the great bulk of the tools necessary for most procedures. The number of

TABLE 4–1. Basic Supplies for All Trays

Barrier drape
Weck-cell sponges
Wrapped cotton applicators
Saline solution in cup
Balanced salt solution in squeeze bottle
#21 Irrigating tip
#25 Needle
#18 Needle
2-ml Syringe
2 × 4 Sponges
Eye pad
Tetracaine dropper
Drape scissors

TABLE 4–2. Macro Cataract Tray

1	Graefe fixation forceps
1	Lister forceps
1	Fine serrated dressing forceps (straight)
1	Castroviejo forceps 0.3
1	Graefe curved iris forceps
1	Arruga capsule forceps
1	Nugent tying forceps
1	Bard-Parker handle
1	Beaver handle
1	#64 Beaver blade
1	Westcott scissors
1	Kalt needle holder
1	Castroviejo needle holder
1	Williams speculum
1	Spatula, combination 1–2 mm
1	Rizzuti retractor
1	Knapp lens loop
1	Muscle hook #1
1	Halsted hemostat
1	Olive tip irrigator

TABLE 4–3. Cataract/Glaucoma Micro Tray

1	Bonn forceps 0.12
1	Castroviejo forceps 0.3
1	Castroviejo forceps 0.12
1	Colibri forceps 0.12
1	Kelman forceps
1	Lister forceps
1	Curved McPherson tying forceps
1	Smooth forceps
1	Straight McPherson tying forceps
2	Straight Harms tying forceps
1	Bard-Parker knife handle
1	Castroviejo mini blade breaker
1	Razor blade
1	Barraquer-DeWecker scissors
1	Left Castroviejo micro scissors
1	Right Castroviejo micro scissors
1	Suture scissors
1	Troutman suture-tying scissors
1	Westcott scissors
1	Castroviejo needle holder
1	Kalt needle holder
1	Troutman-Barraquer needle holder
1	Barraquer wire speculum
1	Beaver handle with screw
1	Beaver handle without screw
1	Caliper
1	21-gauge cannula
1	27-gauge cannula
1	30-gauge cannula
1	Hartman straight mosquito clamp
1	Iris spatula
1	Lens hook
1	Lens loop
1	Muscle hook #1

TABLE 4–4. Keratoplasty Micro Tray/Special Stainless Steel Tray

1	Bonn forceps 0.12
1	Colibri forceps 0.12
1	Castroviejo forceps 0.12
1	Castroviejo forceps 0.3
1	Curved McPherson suture-tying forceps
1	Lister forceps
1	Pollack forceps
1	Smooth forceps
1	Straight McPherson suture-tying forceps
1	Blade breaker
1	Razor blade
1	Barraquer-DeWecker iris scissors
1	Left Katzin mini scissors
1	Right Katzin mini scissors
1	Suture scissors (curved)
1	Left Troutman mini scissors
1	Right Troutman mini scissors
1	Westcott scissors
1	Castroviejo needle holder
1	Kalt needle holder
1	Troutman-Barraquer needle holder
1	Barraquer spatula
1	Double-ended spatula
1	Barraquer wire speculum (adult)
1	Elliot handle for trephines
	Trephines (wrapped individually in special containers)
1	Straight Halsted hemostat
1	Martinez dissector
1	Muscle hook #1
1	21-gal cannula gauge

instruments placed on a tray should be kept to the minimum. This is more economical and also reduces the amount of wear on the instruments. Additionally, the less cluttered the tray, the easier it is to find the needed instrument.

The fine tips of microsurgical instruments need to be protected. This can be economically done by using sections from discarded intravenous tubing. The instrument tip is gently placed into the tubing, which should be cut into sections long enough to give complete protection.

Special trays for holding microsurgical instruments are helpful (Fig. 4–1). The instruments should not bump against one another on these trays or elsewhere; the tray shown in Figure 4–1 holds the instruments securely but gently in place and also assures a free supply of air to them and protects them from catching on cloth wrapping. Larger and less delicate instruments can be stored in the more standard cloth-wrapped trays (Tables 4–1 and 4–11).

TABLE 4–5. Retina-Vitreous Tray

2	Delicate Bishop-Harman forceps
1	Castroviejo forceps 0.5
1	Fixation forceps
1	Nugent forceps
1	Lister forceps
1	Smooth forceps
1	Bard-Parker knife handle
1	Beaver knife handle
1	Curved Mayo scissors
1	Curved Stevens scissors
1	Straight Stevens scissors
1	Suture scissors
1	Westcott scissors
1	Barraquer-DeWecker needle holder w/clasp
1	Castroviejo needle holder
1	Kalt needle holder
2	Curved Halsted hemostats
2	Straight Halsted hemostats
1	Arruga retractor
1	Fisher retractor
1	Lid retractor #1
1	Schepens retractor
1	2-Prong retractor
1	4-Prong retractor
2	Large Barraquer-DeWecker specula
1	Williams speculum
1	Large speculum
1	Caliper
1	Curette #2
1	21-gauge cannula
1	Gass hook
1	Lid plate
1	Muscle hook #1
2	Serrefines
2	Small towel clamps

TABLE 4–6. Basic Muscle Tray

2	Castroviejo forceps
2	Castroviejo locking forceps
1	Delicate Bishop-Harman forceps
1	Exterior delicate Bishop-Harman forceps
1	Harms forceps
1	Lister forceps
1	Left Aebli scissors
1	Right Aebli scissors
1	Suture scissors
1	Westcott scissors
1	Castroviejo needle holder
1	Kalt needle holder
1	Curved Halsted hemostat
1	Straight Halsted hemostat
2	Green hooks
2	Muscle hooks #1
2	Muscle hooks #3
2	Stevens hooks
1	Caliper
1	21-gauge cannula
1	Lid retractor #0
1	Lancaster speculum

TABLE 4–7. Lid Surgery

1	Castroviejo forceps
1	Delicate Bishop-Harman forceps
1	Fixation forceps
1	Lister forceps
1	Smooth forceps
1	Curved Mayo scissors
1	Curved Stevens scissors
1	Straight Stevens scissors
1	Suture scissors
1	Westcott scissors
1	Castroviejo needle holder
1	Kalt needle holder
2	2-Prong retractors
2	4-Prong retractors
2	6-Prong retractors
1	Lid retractor #3
1	Muscle hook #1
1	Muscle hook #3
2	Bard-Barker knife handles
1	Caliper
1	Curette #1
2	Curved Halsted hemostats
1	Double-ended spatula
1	21-gauge cannula
1	Lid plate
2	Small towel clamps

TABLE 4–8. Minor Lid Tray

1	Castroviejo forceps
1	Delicate Bishop-Harman forceps
1	Fixation forceps
1	Lister forceps
1	Smooth forceps
1	Curved Mayo scissors
1	Curved Stevens scissors
1	Straight Stevens scissors
1	Suture scissors
1	Westcott scissors
1	Castroviejo needle holder
1	Kalt needle holder
1	Lid retractor #1
2	2-Prong retractors
2	4-Prong retractors
1	Curved Halsted hemostat
1	Straight Halsted hemostat
1	Bard-Barker knife handle
1	Caliper
1	Curette
1	21-gauge cannula
1	Lid plate
1	Muscle hook #1
1	Small towel clamp

TABLE 4–9. Bone Tray

3	Straight Halsted forceps
6	Straight Hartman forceps
2	Curved Hartman forceps
1	Kelly clamp
3	Kerrison punches (0-1-2)
1	Bone biter
1	Rongeur
1	Double-action rongeur

TABLE 4–10. Dacryocystorhinostomy Tray

1 Lacrimal probe set 0000–000–7–8
1 Periosteal elevator
1 Freer knife
1 Straight lacrimal needle
1 Curved lacrimal needle
1 2-mm Chisel
1 4-mm Chisel
1 2-mm Gouges
1 4-mm Gouges
1 2-mm Osteotome
1 4-mm Osteotome
1 ENT osteotome
1 Mallet
1 Hartman punch
1 Kerrison punch #0
1 Kerrison punch #1
1 Suture scissors

TABLE 4–11. Procedure for Wrapping Trays

1. Place stainless steel Mayo tray in a green linen pillow case.
2. Arrange appropriate instruments on tray.
3. Use (2) double-thickness wrappers (two layers of material sewn together equals one wrapper) to wrap tray.
4. Make sure proper sterilization indicator is placed in thickest fold of wrapper.
5. Use sterilization tape to secure linen and to show exposure to sterilizing agent.
6. Label type of tray, expiration date, and initials on tape.

Sterilization

For surgical instruments to function well they must be properly cleaned, sterilized, and stored. This is especially true for microsurgical instruments. Cleaning is best accomplished with an ultrasonic cleaner, which should contain trays that keep the instruments separated during the cleaning procedure; fine tools should not be thrown in all together in the ultrasonic bath. After being cleaned in the ultrasonic bath the instruments should be air-dried and carefully placed in appropriate wrappers or on the appropriate tray.

Most microsurgical instruments can be sterilized satisfactorily in an autoclave. The water should be distilled, to prevent deposition of salts. Sharp instruments are better preserved by sterilization in ethylene oxide. This technique is more time-consuming, and an adequate period for elimination of the gas must be permitted after the sterilization has been completed. Plastics and other materials that may be damaged by heat or moisture are also best

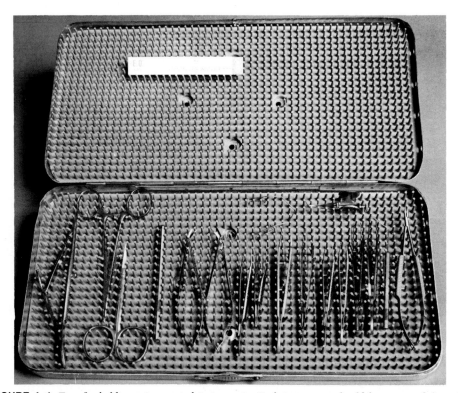

FIGURE 4–1. Tray for holding microsurgical instruments. Each instrument should be separated from the one nearest it by at least one row of flexible supports. Note that the two corneal scissors are not properly positioned, as they contact each other.

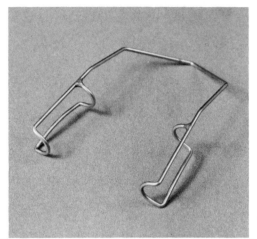

FIGURE 4–2. Barraquer colibri lid speculum. This comes in a variety of sizes. If too large a speculum is chosen, excessive tension will be placed on the lids, causing a rise in intraocular pressure.

sterilized with ethylene oxide. A variety of sterilizing solutions are available in which instruments can be soaked, but they are not as effective as autoclaving or ethylene oxide, and should not ordinarily be used for sterilization.

Instruments Used in Ophthalmic Surgery

A few commonly used instruments are described here. Additional commentary is made in the chapters describing specific surgical procedures.

Lid Speculum

The lid speculum is used to separate the lids as gently as possible without causing distress to the patient, pressure on the globe, or interference with the surgery. For most purposes the Barraquer wire colibri speculum fills the bill admirably (Fig. 4–2). This speculum comes in sizes for adults and children, but still should be adjusted for each individual by narrowing or widening the angle of the arms. If the speculum is inserted between the lids with too great an angle, the spring of the wire can exert considerable pressure against the lids and cause a substantial rise of intraocular pressure. In cases in which the Barraquer speculum does not provide needed lid separation with sufficient gentleness, or when the surgeon requires maximum control of the lids, sutures can be placed in the lid margins and the sutures retracted with appropriate force. This allows retracting the lids up from the globe as well as separating them. A small locking instrument can be used to hold the sutures in a position that will keep the lids separated, but this tends to minimize the benefit of using the lid sutures, and they are best held by an assistant. The only significant disadvantages with the suture method are the need to have a separate assistant to handle the upper and lower sutures themselves, and the trauma inflicted to the lid margins by the placement of the sutures. The lids may also be retracted by small individual hooks that fit over the lid margins; these are attached to threads that permit them to be individually and appropriately retracted, providing satisfactory exposure.

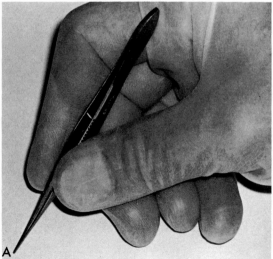
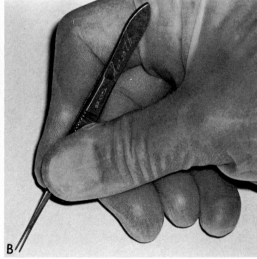

FIGURE 4–3. *A,* Utility dressing forceps with a single stop. *B,* Excessive pressure on the handle will cause the tips to splay.

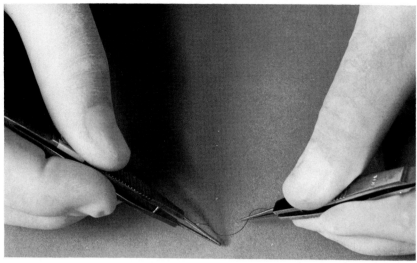

FIGURE 4–4. Incorrect method of holding forceps. The forceps in the right hand are held too high on the handle, so that the force will not be transmitted well to the tips of the Harms tying forceps. The thumb and index fingers of both hands are placed incorrectly on the instruments. Compare with Figure 4–5.

Forceps

For forceps to be useful, the tips must come firmly in contact with each other. Many of the newer instruments have double stops on the inner surfaces to help assure that the tips do not become splayed when excessive pressure is exerted on the handle (Fig. 4–3). If the fingers are placed too high on the double-stopped forceps, sufficient pressure is not exerted on the end of the forceps to allow it to function well (Fig. 4–4). If the fingers are held too close to the tips, which is an unlikely mistake, the tips will splay open in a manner similar to that shown in Figure 4–3. The correct technique, using McPherson tying forceps as an example, is shown in Figure 4–5.

When operating under a mounted microscope it is advantageous to use instruments with angled tips. This permits the surgeon to hold the instrument firmly while still keeping his fingers out of the field. Figure 4–6 shows an angled, fine-toothed 0.12-mm Barraquer colibri forceps being held in the correct position. Note that the view of the surgical field is superior to

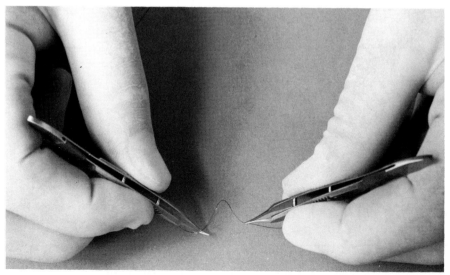

FIGURE 4–5. Correct method of holding forceps. The thumb and index finger are placed in apposition between the double stops, assuring firm, even pressure with the tips.

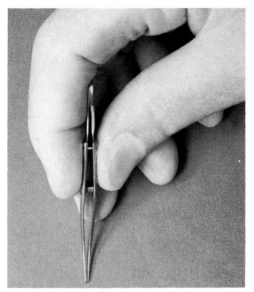

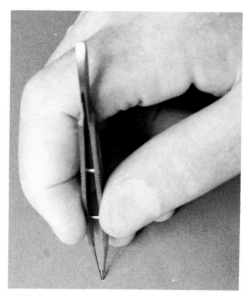

FIGURE 4–6. Angled forceps allow good visualization of the tips. (See also Figures 4–10 and 4–11.)

FIGURE 4–7. Straight instruments tend to obscure the surgical field.

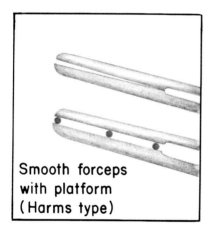

Smooth forceps
with platform
(Harms type)

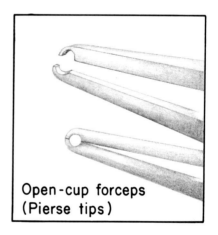

Open-cup forceps
(Pierse tips)

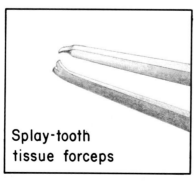

Splay-tooth
tissue forceps

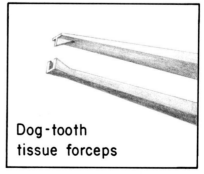

Dog-tooth
tissue forceps

FIGURE 4–8. The tips of microsurgical instruments have a variety of holding surfaces. Platforms of one of the Harms forceps (top) do not meet properly, and thus will not hold suture firmly. The Bonn and Castroviejo forceps have splay-tooth tips. Both the splay-tooth and the dog-tooth types will penetrate thin tissue such as conjunctiva.

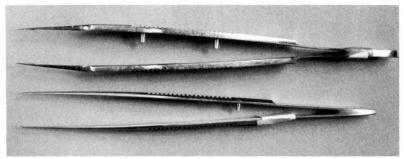

FIGURE 4–9. *Top:* Castroviejo fine-toothed (0.12 mm) tissue forceps with tying platforms. *Bottom:* Von Graefe fixation forceps. Notice difference in position of teeth.

that in Figure 4–7, in which a straight Castroviejo forceps is shown. The longer-handled Castroviejo forceps is more useful than the colibri when the surgeon needs to reach down "into a hole." For example, grasping the cornea when placing corneoscleral sutures on the nasal side of an eye in a deep socket, especially in a person with a large nose, can be difficult unless the surgeon uses an instrument with long handles, such as the Castroviejo straight forceps.

Forceps tips vary, depending on the use of the instrument. The tips can have right-angled or projecting teeth of different sizes (Fig. 4–8). For cataract, cornea, or glaucoma surgery the best size is usually 0.12 mm. A single tooth typically opposes two teeth of similar size, although other combinations have been used and have certain advantages. For example, a forceps with two teeth on each side and a space between each of them has been recommended for suturing fine tissue; this structure permits placing the suture directly between the teeth of the forceps, in line with the handles, thus preventing rocking and distortion of the tissue, which invariably occur when the suture is placed to the side of the forceps bite.[7]

The Graefe forceps has long protuberant teeth that bite well into the sclera, so that the instrument is useful for firmly fixating the intact globe (Fig. 4–9). In contrast, the teeth of the Castroviejo forceps are at right angles to the handles and are better suited for fixating cut edges, such as the cornea. When grasping an edge of thin tissue it is helpful to use the single tooth on the cut edge and the double teeth on the surface of such incisions. The Pierse-Hoskins forceps has a tip with an indentation, permitting tissue to be squeezed into the concavity and giving good holding ability safely (Fig. 4–8). It has the advantage of grasping well without causing penetration of the tissue. Thus the angled Pierse-Hoskins colibri-type forceps, shown in Figure 4–10, is especially useful in glaucoma surgery, for handling scleral flaps in trabeculectomies, and for handling the conjunctiva in any type of filtering operation.

Four of the most frequently used forceps are shown in Figure 4–11. The *Lister* is an excellent heavy instrument for placing the superior rectus suture or holding thick tissue firmly, as one does with Tenon's capsule during enucleation. The *Barraquer* and the *Castroviejo* forceps are the workhorses of most microsurgical procedures. Those shown have tying platforms that permit effective instrument tying of suture material as small as 9–0. The *Bonn* forceps is even

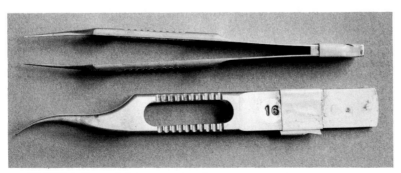

FIGURE 4–10. Angled Pierse-Hoskins forceps. Tips are shown in Figure 4–8.

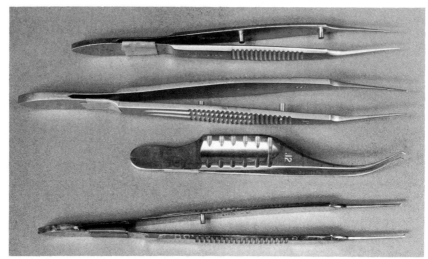

FIGURE 4–11. Four of the most frequently used forceps in ophthalmic surgery. *From top to bottom:* The Bonn, the Castroviejo, the Barraquer colibri, and the Lister.

more delicate and is especially well suited to corneal microsurgery.

When holding tissue that tends to slip, but in which one wants to be sure holes are not made by the teeth, the dressing forceps seen in Figure 4–12 are helpful. These are the forceps most frequently used on conjunctival tissue in glaucoma or retinal surgery. The tips of the handles have fine horizontal serrations that hold tissue well. The tips, however, are easily splayed if the bite of tissue is too thick or the bend in the handles too great, or if the surgeon squeezes too firmly. Such forceps should not be used to hold fine fragile suture material, such as 8–0 chromic collagen or fine nylon, as the serrations will cut the suture. When the surgeon wants to use such fine suture material, a smooth-tipped forceps is preferable; it may even be used for holding the tissue itself (Fig. 4–12).

Knife Handles and Blades

Three types of knife handles are shown in Figure 4–13: the Bard-Parker, the Beaver, and the blade breaker. The Bard-Parker blades are excellent for plastic surgery or for other macroscopic procedures; they are not fine enough for most microsurgical procedures. The Beaver blades come in a wide variety of styles and provide the surgeon with almost all the types of cutting edges required for microsurgery. The handle can be angled or rounded; the angled type is slightly preferable for flat cutting (such as that required in the development of a scleral flap), and the rounded handle for motions in which torsion may be required (as in placing a curved corneoscleral groove before a cataract extraction). The blade breaker allows the surgeon easily to fashion a knife of exquisite sharpness freshly for each case. The handle shown in Figure 4–13 permits breaking the blade and

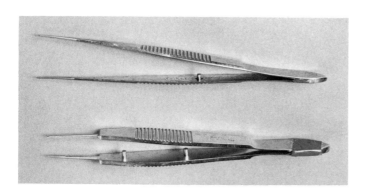

FIGURE 4–12. *Top:* Utility dressing forceps with very fine horizontal serrations at tips of handles. *Bottom:* Harms straight tying forceps.

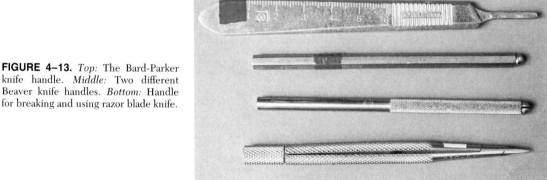

FIGURE 4–13. *Top:* The Bard-Parker knife handle. *Middle:* Two different Beaver knife handles. *Bottom:* Handle for breaking and using razor blade knife.

holding the blade for use. The instrument shown has straight jaws, but the tips may be angled at around 45 degrees to the handle in order to provide greater ease of visualization of the blade when using a mounted microscope.

As pointed out by Troutman, the ideal razor blade for use with the blade breaker is hard and brittle with a high carbon content.[1] Thus the thin, hardened stainless steel blade is preferable to the softer chromium or platinum stainless blade. The shape of the blade fragment can be varied by the manner in which the blade breaker grasps the intact razor blade (Fig. 4–14). If one wants a narrow, long fragment, the blade is grasped near the edge, whereas a shorter, wider blade can be obtained by including the razor in the full width of the blade breaker tips (Fig. 4–14A and B).

When using a blade for cutting, such as the #67 Beaver blade shown in Figure 4–15, the blade should be held absolutely parallel to the direction in which the cut is being made. This will produce the cleanest and straightest incision. The blade should not be torted; the position in Figure 4–16 is incorrect.

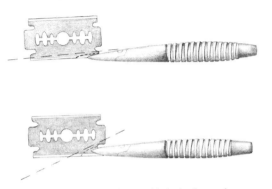

FIGURE 4–14. Shape of razor blade knife can be varied by method of breaking blade. The thinner and longer the desired fragment, the closer to the cutting surface the blade should be grasped.

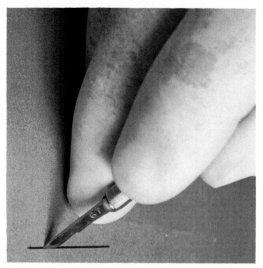

FIGURE 4–15. The #67 Beaver blade is held correctly here, with the direction of the cut and the blade exactly parallel.

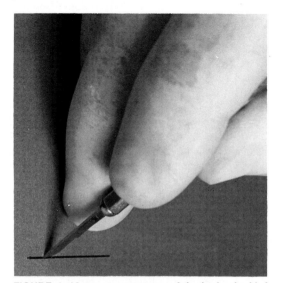

FIGURE 4–16. Incorrect position of the knife, the blade being torted away from the axis of the incision.

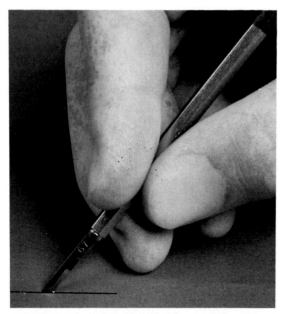

FIGURE 4–17. Blade held so that the rounded portion of the tip serves as the cutting surface.

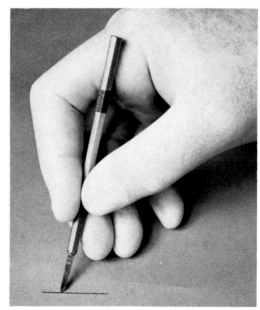

FIGURE 4–18. For precise cutting, only the tip of the blade is used. This allows a square-edged incision, i.e., the external and internal widths of it are equal.

The surgeon should also be aware of the portion of the blade with which he is cutting. The #67 Beaver blade has a sharp point at the end of the curved blade (Figs. 4–15 through 4–19). This allows the surgeon to use the blade in a variety of ways. For example, when separating tissue planes, extreme sharpness is often not necessary, and may even be detrimental. The curved portion of the blade is useful for such dissection, as when reflecting normal conjunctiva from the corneoscleral sulcus, or developing a limbus-based conjunctival flap from underlying sclera in an area of previous surgery (Fig. 4–17). In the latter case a sharp tip is likely to cut too deeply or too superficially, or to pull tissue with it; a scissor is prone to cause buttonholes.

In contrast, the tip of the #67 Beaver blade permits more precise cutting (Fig. 4–18). For example, in fashioning the edges of a scleral flap the tip of the blade is used to ensure that the incision does not extend further than needed. Tilting the angle of the handle allows the surgeon to cut most precisely (Fig. 4–19). However, the sharp tip is more likely than the rounded portion of the blade to catch tissue.

The motion of the fingers should vary, depending on the blade used and the surgeon's goal. When using a rounded blade such as the #64 Beaver, the axis of the knife pivots around the place where the handle is held (Fig. 4–20). Thus the tip of the knife handle and the tip of

the blade move in opposite directions. Such a motion causes the tip of the blade potentially to describe an arc, resulting in an incision that is deeper centrally than at the edges. This can be avoided by keeping the blade firmly against the third finger, which rests against the surface

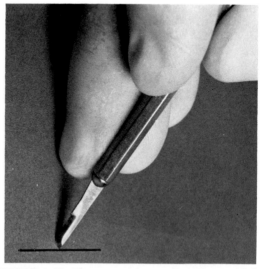

FIGURE 4–19. The most precise incision, using a blade such as the #67 Beaver, is accomplished with the blade held as shown. The direction of cutting is from right to left in the picture. The disadvantage of this method is that the tip can penetrate underlying tissues, such as the choroid under the sclera, more easily than when the knife is used as shown in Figure 4–17.

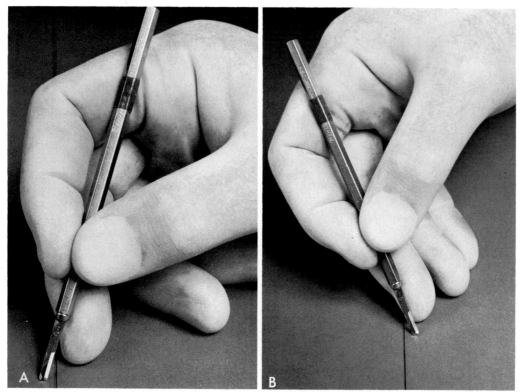

FIGURE 4–20. Note that the rounded #64 Beaver blade is pivoted around the point where it is held by the thumb and index finger (*A*), the tip of the blade moving in one direction and the handle in the other (*B*).

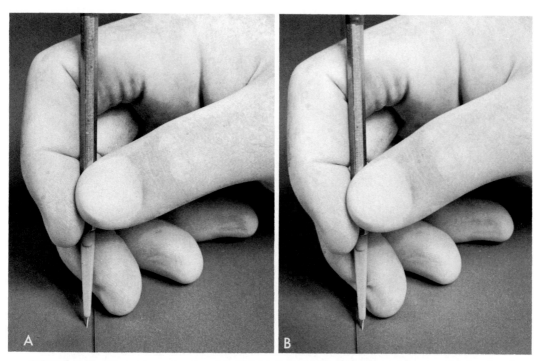

FIGURE 4–21. When using a sharply pointed blade, the handle is pulled forward between the thumb and index finger, with the immobile third finger used as a guide. The handle is not rotated. This is the manner in which a razor blade fragment would be used.

to be incised and guides the depth of the incision, keeping it constant.

A very sharp blade (such as a razor blade) should usually be used by pulling the entire knife forward, so that the handle pivots little, if at all (Fig. 4–21).

The principle of moving the blade without changing the axis of the handle also applies when performing motions such as those required to make a paracentesis opening into the cornea. The correct technique is shown in Figure 4–22. The third and fourth fingers rest firmly on the surface of the face, and the knife-needle or Wheeler knife is advanced in a horizontal plane by the thumb and index finger, with the third finger used as a guide. This permits an extremely controlled motion.

A similar motion is used when the surgeon wants to obtain a beveled cut, as with a kera-tome blade (Fig. 4–23).

When cutting tissue in a lamellar manner, as in the development of corneal or scleral flaps, the blade should be held as parallel as possible to the direction of the tissue plane to be formed. Thus, holding the blade as shown in Figure 4–24A would permit an easier development of the flap than would be possible if the blade were held in the more angled manner shown in Figure 4–24B. Angled blades such as the "hockey stick" can be helpful in this regard. The obvious fact that cutting requires motion should be remembered. Neophytes—and sometimes even more experienced surgeons—may confuse slowness with caution. The surgeon

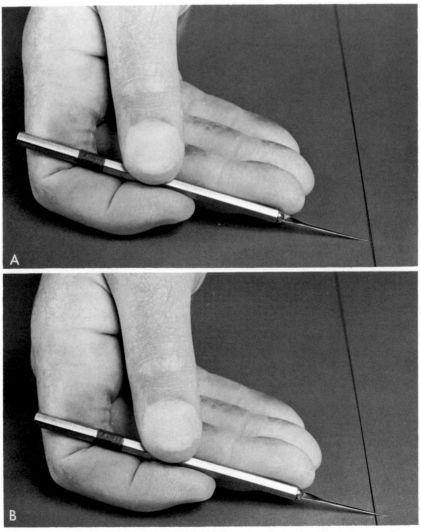

FIGURE 4–22. Certain cutting motions require the blade to be advanced without changing the axis of the handle. Here the thumb and index finger advance the knife-needle, with the third finger used as a guide.

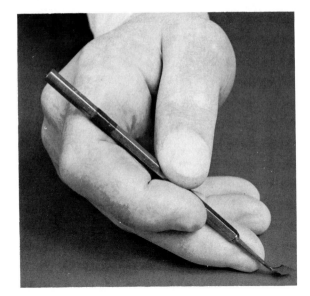

FIGURE 4–23. Angulation of the blade facilitates lamellar incisions. This type of keratome blade would be advanced without changing the axis of the handle, using a motion similar to that shown in Figure 4–22.

should decide exactly the nature of the incision to be made, including length, depth, and bevel; the hands should then be correctly placed, and finally the incision should be decisively made.

Attempts to pull a blade slowly through tissue cause compression, but not cutting, and do not help in achieving the desired goal.

New methods of cutting tissue have been

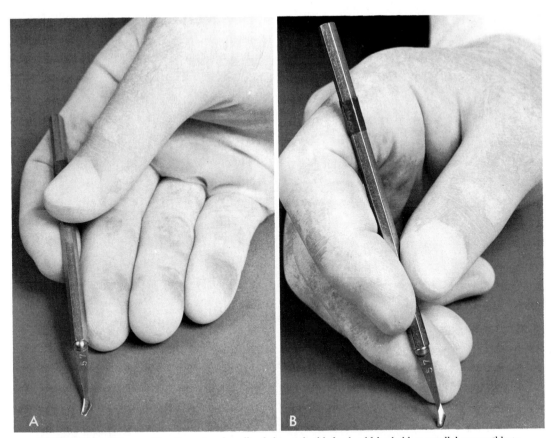

FIGURE 4–24. When cutting tissue in a lamellar fashion, the blade should be held as parallel as possible to the plane in which the tissue is being dissected, as shown in A. Assuming this plane to be parallel to the surface, the knife is correctly held in A and incorrectly held in B.

introduced in an attempt to keep trauma and deformation of tissue to an absolute minimum. These include the diamond knife and a variety of moving blades.[8] These do have advantages, although their cost is great. However, the increased sharpness is occasionally of real help.

Some knives are equipped with guards to permit making incisions of precisely measured depths. These are necessary when performing procedures such as radial keratotomy.

Scissors

Just as eye surgery requires a variety of knives, so different styles of scissors are also necessary. Figure 4–25 shows three of the more commonly used types of scissors. The *Stevens tenotomy scissors* has sturdy handles of varying lengths, and blunted tips. It is extensively used in extraocular surgery. Scissors with sharp curved tips are frequently used for cutting sutures or for incising the barrier drape at the start of the procedure. The ring-handled instruments are sturdier and provide for a firmer grip of the scissors. However, they do not permit the delicacy of operation possible with spring-handled instruments. The *Westcott spring-handled scissors* has a variety of uses. The instrument shown in Figure 4–25 has slightly blunted tips, making it especially useful for developing conjunctival flaps or cutting extraocular muscles. The surgeon should be sure that the hinged eyelet connector of the spring-handled instrument is correctly engaged before use; if it is not, the spring action will not work correctly.

The tips of scissors can be protected in a manner similar to that used to guard forceps, utilizing sections cut from discarded intravenous tubing.

The size of the scissors, including the length of the handle and the length of the tips, should be appropriate for the function required. Enucleation scissors, for example, have long, husky curved handles and tips. The Castroviejo straight keratoplasty scissors has handles that are long enough to permit a firm grip, while still permitting the instrument to be managed well under an operating microscope (Fig. 4–26). The Barraquer-DeWecker iris scissors is made with 7-mm blades that allow it to be used in tight places. Barraquer iris scissors are also available with longer blades, more closely resembling the older, larger DeWecker iris scissors. Both tips of the blades can be blunt, one can be blunt and one sharp, or both can be sharp. When using any of the DeWecker-type scissors it is important to tighten the knob at the heavy end of the handle, to be sure that the blades engage each other correctly.

The *Vannas scissors* (Fig. 4–27) is a small scissors routinely used in ophthalmic surgery. It is manufactured with blades that are straight,

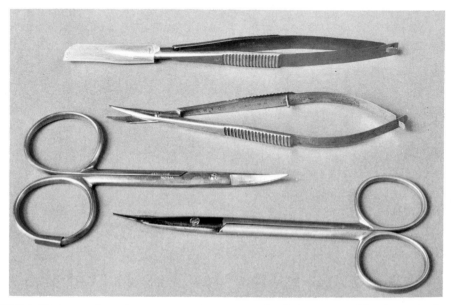

FIGURE 4–25. Frequently used scissors. *Top:* Westcott spring-handled scissors. *Middle:* Sharp-tipped suture scissors. *Bottom:* Stevens tenotomy scissors.

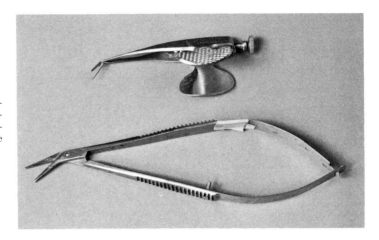

FIGURE 4–26. The Barraquer-De-Wecker iris scissors (*top*) and the Castroviejo straight keratoplasty scissors (*bottom*). The different handles facilitate use in different circumstances.

curved, or angled, and with tips that are sharp or blunt.

Extremely fine scissors for use intraocularly are essential for certain procedures (Fig. 4–28).

Scissors for cutting a curved corneoscleral incision usually have a curve that parallels the curve of the incision itself (Fig. 4–29A). These scissors have a right and a left pair, permitting cutting to the left or the right with the greatest ease. The blades need to be correctly angled from the handle to allow maximum ease of cutting. The corneal scissors shown in Figure 4–29B is being correctly held in order to cut toward the left. The inferior blade that is inserted into the anterior chamber should be slightly longer than the superior blade.

Spatulas and Irrigating Tips

Three frequently used spatulas are shown in Figure 4–30. The *Wheeler double-ended spatula* has malleable blunt tips. The *Castroviejo double-ended cyclodialysis spatula* has thin blades that are rather broad (0.5 to 1.0 mm wide). The *Troutman-Barraquer iris spatula* is rounded and blunted and is especially appropriate for disengaging synechias or sweeping an

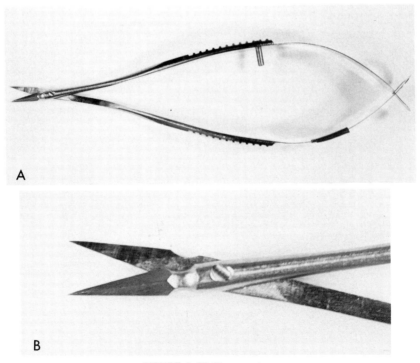

FIGURE 4–27. Vannas scissors.

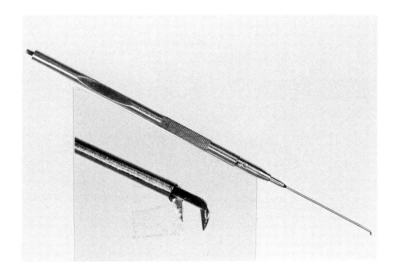

FIGURE 4–28. Extremely fine scissors are used intraocularly for a variety of purposes, such as sphincterotomies, section of intraocular lens haptics, and section of vitreous bands. Long-bladed scissors such as the Stern-Gills are especially useful for radial iridotomy and sphincterotomy.

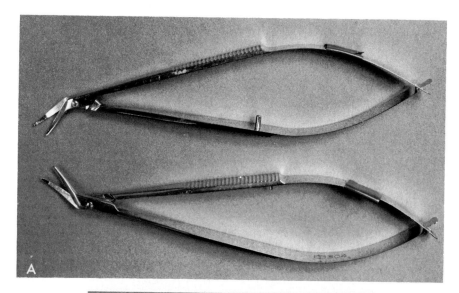

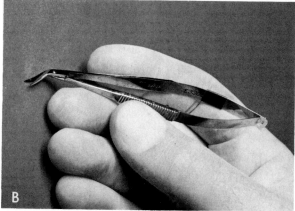

FIGURE 4–29. *A*, Left-cutting and right-cutting (top and bottom respectively) curved corneoscleral scissors. *B*, Left-handed corneoscleral scissors.

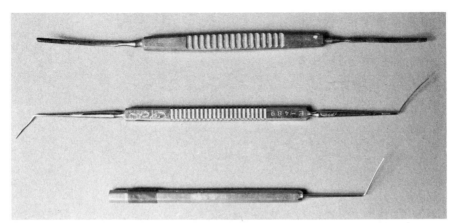

FIGURE 4–30. *Top:* Wheeler double-ended spatula. *Middle:* Castroviejo double-ended cyclodialysis spatula. The shorter (left-hand) end has been bent improperly out of the correct curvature seen with the longer blade. *Bottom:* Troutman-Barraquer iris spatula with rounded blade and blunted tip.

incision clear of vitreous. It is fine enough to be placed through a previously made knife-needle track in the cornea (Fig. 4–30).

Irrigating tips need to be correctly fashioned for the particular use intended. The *Bishop-Harman irrigator* can easily be attached to a squeeze bottle of balanced salt solution and used to keep the eye moist throughout the procedure (Fig. 4–31). Blunted at the tip, it is also useful for repositing iris. This can be done by using the tip alone, or, where advantageous, by directing a gentle stream through the irrigator and using the saline solution as the repositing force. The olive-tipped irrigator is especially useful for placing alpha-chymotrypsin under the iris (Fig. 4–31). The surgeon should have available in the operating room sterile blunt-tipped irrigating needles of small bore, preferably 27 and 30 gauge. These are most useful if angled in a manner similar to the

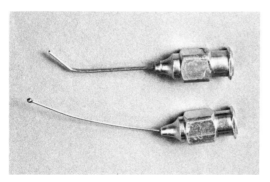

FIGURE 4–31. *Top:* Bishop-Harman irrigating tip with flat blunt surfaces; usually #21 size is used for external irrigation; a 27- or 30-gauge is best for entering through a previous paracentesis. *Bottom:* Olive-tipped irrigator.

Bishop-Harman #21 irrigating tip shown in Figure 4–31. The fine irrigating needles can be placed through paracentesis incisions in order to introduce saline solution, air, or gas.

Needle Holders

Needle holders come in a variety of forms appropriate for the uses to which they are put.[10] The *Kalt locking needle holder* grasps large needles such as those swedged onto 4–0 suture material. The jaws are wide, around 0.75 or 1.0 mm, in order to permit gripping the needle firmly. The Kalt needle holder is a good instrument for placing a 4–0 black silk suture under the superior rectus (the "bridle suture"). Needle holders designed to handle fine suture material will have their blades sprung apart if they are used with such large needles. The lock on the Kalt helps when the surgeon needs to perform a movement as gross as the placement of the bridle suture. The thumb should be placed immediately adjacent to the lock, so that the lock is easily disengaged after the needle has been placed (Fig. 4–32).

For finer suture material a nonlocking needle holder with finer jaws is essential. The presence of a lock requires the surgeon to squeeze the needle holder firmly after the suture has been placed; this motion will almost always cause an additional and undesired motion of the needle. Thus, for microsurgery, locking needle holders are not appropriate. Two useful nonlocking needle holders are shown in Figure 4–33.

The blades of the needle holder should be angled so that the needle can be passed through a proper arc merely by rotation of the fingers. This requires a rounded handle. Figure 4–34A

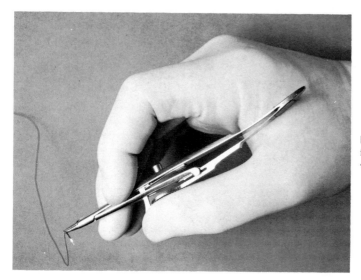

FIGURE 4–32. Kalt locking needle holder for use with large suture material, such as 4–0 size.

and *B* indicates how proper torsion of the needle holder is produced by rolling the needle holder between the index finger and the thumb. As this is done, the tip of the needle holder is automatically slightly advanced. This fine finger movement is different from that used with the Kalt needle holder, in which the fingers remain rigid and the wrist rotates. The Moria needle holder (Fig. 4–33) has a similar structure but heavier jaws than the Weck-Barraquer; this allows a bit firmer grasp, while retaining the delicacy provided by finger rotation. The Trout-man-Barraquer needle holder has jaws angled at 45 degrees. Correct placement of the suture with this instrument requires a motion different from that used with the Barraquer needle holders. Because of the angle of the jaws, rolling the Troutman needle holder with the fingers will not move the needle in a proper arc. The needle must be driven forward at the same time that the fingers are rotated (Fig. 4–34).

Tying Forceps

Tying forceps are necessary in microsurgery if sutures are to be tied securely, safely, and deftly. The Harms straight tying forceps are excellent for sutures larger than 9–0; they can even be used for 9–0 or 10–0 when reaching over the nose, or in a position where a long handle is helpful (Fig. 4–35). For suture material smaller than 8–0 the McPherson forceps are ideal (Fig. 4–35): one forceps should be straight and the other angled. The forceps must be properly held between the two stops in order to keep the tips in firm apposition (see Figs. 4–4 and 4–5).

SUTURES AND SUTURE TYING

Ophthalmic surgery would not be possible today without the magnificent suture material

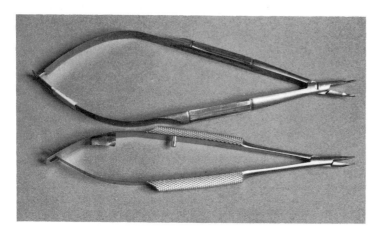

FIGURE 4–33. Weiss-Moria and Weck-Barraquer nonlocking needle holders. These are excellent microsurgical needle holders.

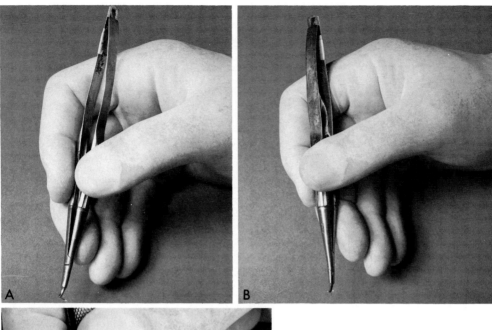

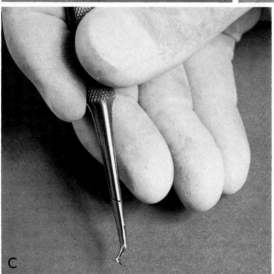

FIGURE 4–34. Use of the needle holder. *A* and *B* show the arc the needle traverses if the needle holder is merely rotated between the fingers. The more angled the jaws of the needle holder, the more complex must be the movement required to drive the needle through its proper arc (*C*).

FIGURE 4–35. The Harms straight tying forceps (top two instruments) can be used for all of the sutures used in ophthalmic surgery. The McPherson forceps (bottom two instruments) are especially useful with 8–0, 9–0, and 10–0 suture material.

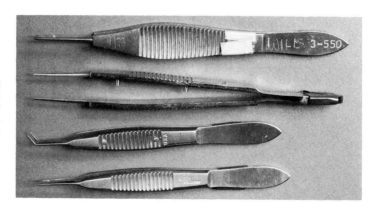

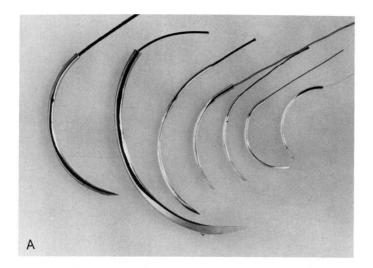

A

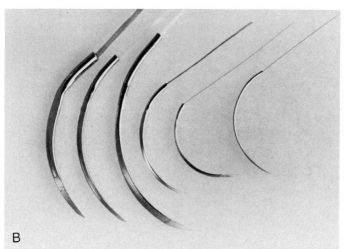

B

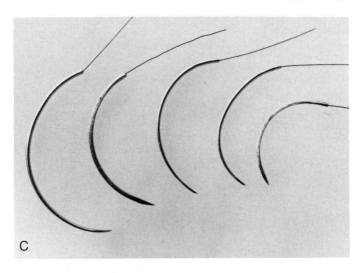

C

FIGURE 4–36. Selected commonly used needles and sutures. *A*, Various sutures. From left to right: 4-0 silk, C-1; 5-0 silk, PS-2; 6-0 silk, C-2; 6-0 polyglactin, S-14; 8-0 silk TG-100-8; 8-0 nylon TG-175-8; and 10-0 polyglactin GS-9. The C-1 is a tapered needle, 13 mm long, 3/8 curvature (135 degrees), 0.25 mm (10 mil) thick. The C-2 is the same size and shape except for a reverse cutting needle. The S-14 spatula needle is 1/4 wide (112 degrees), 8.7 mm long, and 0.33 mm thick (13 mil). The TG-100 is also a 1/4 wide needle (100 degrees), 6.6 mm long, 0.2 mm in diameter (8 mil) with a spatula needle. The TG-175 is a 1/2 wide needle (175 degrees), 7.1 mm long, and also 8 mil in diameter with a spatula needle. *B*, Absorbable sutures. From left to right: 4-0 chromic gut S-4, 5-0 gut S-14, 6-0 gut G-1, 8-0 chromic collagen TG-140-8, 10-0 polyester TG-160-6, and 11-0 CU-11. The S-4 is a spatula-tipped, 1/4 wide needle of 112 degrees curvature, a radius of 0.43 mm, and length of 9.1 mm. The S-14 is a spatula needle of similar curvature and length thinner (0.33 mm). The G-1 is a reverse cutting needle of similar thickness with more curvature (3/8 wide, 135 degrees). The TG-160 is a spatula, 1/2 wide, 160 degrees, 5.5 mm long, and 0.2 mm (8 mil) thick needle. The CU-11 needle is longer, thinner, and less curved. *C*, 10-0 Nylon sutures on spatula needles. From left to right: CU-2, TG-160-6, CU-5, CU-8, TG-160-4-3m. The needles are all 1/2 wide except for the CU-8, which has a compound curve to assist in making a small deep bite. The TG-160 has a curvature of 160 degrees, is 4.3 mm long, and is 0.12 mm (0.4 mil) with a radius of 1.5 mm. The CU-8 is more tapered, with a thinner tip and a thicker base (1.5 mm (6 mil)); it is longer (4.8 mm) and has two radii of curvature (1.3/2.5 mm).

developed during the past three decades. A fine suture such as 8–0, 9–0, or 10–0, swaged onto a sharp needle hardly larger than the suture, permits strong and accurate reapposition of tissues. The wide variety of available suture materials and needles (Fig. 4–36) gives the surgeon a flexibility that enlarges the range of feasible procedures.[11–31]

The goal is to aid the incision or wound to heal by primary union, that is, by first intention, so that the tissue is restored as completely as possible to its presurgical condition. The surgeon chooses a suture with the minimum amount of tensile strength necessary to do the job. The suture is inserted as atraumatically as possible and secured so that the least amount of tissue distortion is produced. The material chosen should last long enough to assure that the incision will heal securely and will be appropriately tolerated by the tissues.

No suture is without disadvantages.[32–43] In 1935 Rea reported watching Lapersonne in Paris place a corneoscleral suture, and described his own good results with a #1 white silk suture threaded onto a #4 needle dipped in sterilized paraffin.[44] The response of his listeners was highly disapproving. Theoretically, the surgeons criticizing Rea's use of the corneoscleral suture in cataract surgery were correct; it would be ideal were it possible for the incision to heal perfectly without the use of suture material. Unfortunately this is not a reasonable goal in ophthalmic surgery. The surgeon must evaluate each patient and choose the size and type of suture material most likely to promote healing. Plain surgical gut, for example, is an easily absorbed suture, but causes rather marked tissue reaction. At the other extreme, steel produces minimal tissue reaction but is difficult to work with. A slowly absorbing suture such as nylon has an obvious advantage when securing a tissue that heals slowly, such as cornea. On the other hand, rapidly absorbable sutures have obvious advantages in cases in which later removal would be difficult.

Other circumstances must also be considered in order to obtain the best surgical result. Wound healing often is delayed if the patient has a chronic disease such as anemia, cancer, or diabetes mellitus. The very old and the malnourished patient also heals less satisfactorily. Sutures that absorb slowly should be used in such cases.

Additionally, medications that alter wound healing affect the type of suture chosen. When drugs such as corticosteroids or 5-fluorouracil are used, which reduce the tendency of tissues to heal, appropriate sutures must be chosen.

The tensile strength of the different suture material does not differ markedly, and is not usually the factor responsible for preferring one type of material to another. On the other hand, tensile strength varies markedly with the size of the suture (Table 4–13). Thinner suture material is also more likely to pull through the tissue; this should be remembered in those rare situations in which it is necessary forcibly to oppose tissue. The thicker the suture material, the more likely it is to cause an inflammatory response, and to distort and deform the tissue.

Braiding the material used in manufacturing a suture increases the strength of the final suture. The braided suture has a greater surface friction and pulls through tissue less easily than does a monofilament or a twisted suture. Braided suture tends to unravel, which can be a problem when the suture is manipulated. But in addition, the interstices in the braid can serve as a passage through which fluid can ooze out or bacteria enter. Braided suture, because of its greater friction, tends to tie more securely.

Softness is usually a desirable characteristic in a suture. For example, the cut ends of fine silk cause virtually no irritation, in contrast to the sharp, stiff ends of nylon or Prolene, which, although less reactive, produce great discomfort for the patient and tend to erode through the overlying tissue. When integrity of the overlying tissue is desired, as with a conjunctival flap in a glaucoma procedure, such a tear through the tissue can turn a surgical success into a failure.

Synthetic sutures, especially nylon (polyamide) and Mersilene (polyester), have a high degree of resiliency, which results in a tendency for the suture to untie spontaneously. Dacron, a braided suture, and monofilament Prolene (polypropylene) are easier to tie, and hold a knot better. The synthetic absorbable sutures (polyglactin 910 and polyglycolic acid) also tend to untie spontaneously, especially the fine monofilament polyglactin 910. These sutures with high resiliency, especially when manufactured in a monofilament form, require three (or in rare instances four) throws on the first knot, and a square knot firmly placed over the first knot. Four throws are preferable. These slippery sutures are especially appropriate for use with a slip knot (see p. 60).

Nylon and polypropylene are highly elastic, and tend to stretch when being tied, especially with smaller sutures such as 9–0 or 10–0. In fact, all fine sutures stretch, including the synthetic absorbable sutures and, to a lesser extent, silk, although the elasticity of nylon is greater than that of these other materials. An elastic suture has the advantage that the suture can "give" somewhat in the immediate postoperative period, when the tissue is swollen; this elasticity reduces the likelihood that the suture will cut through the swelling tissue. However, the more elastic the suture, the more difficult it is for the surgeon to be sure that the proper degree of tension has been placed on the incision. When any fine suture is used the surgeon must be especially careful to avoid pulling the suture too tightly, but especially when using nylon. Because nylon and polypropylene remain in the tissue for many months, the result of a suture tied too tightly is persisting deformation of the incision. Obviously this can cause much unwanted astigmatism. Or, it can result in the suture pulling through the tissue, predisposing to wound dehiscence.

Because fine monofilament sutures tend to slip easily on themselves when tied, the surgeon must be careful to avoid snugging-up the initial throws too tightly. The first knot, with two or three rows, should be placed so that just the desired amount of tension and no more is present; in fact the initial knot should be slightly less tight than needed. When the second throw is placed and pulled up firmly to make a square knot, there is always some slippage, resulting in a tighter knot than was present after the first throw. The surgeon then places the third throw, also pulling that tightly in order to secure the suture from untying. With materials such as 9–0 polyglactin 910 or other materials that have a strong "memory" a fourth throw should be placed unless it is essential to have a smaller knot.

The slip knot offers the surgeon many advantages, and the technique should be mastered by all surgeons (see Fig. 4–38). Using a slip knot allows the surgeon to adjust the suture to the precise tension desired. Furthermore, because there is only one throw placed on the first knot, the final knot, even with four throws placed, tends to be smaller than with the surgeon's knot, making it easier to bury.

All sutures cause some inflammatory response.[22–24, 32, 33, 35–41, 43, 46, 47] In some instances this may not be completely undesirable. In others, such as keratoplasty, the less inflammation the better. The extent of reaction caused by a suture is not merely a factor of the suture material. It is also influenced by the amount of suture used. In this regard it should be recalled

TABLE 4–12. Correlation Between Designation of Suture Size, Actual Suture Size, and Volume of Suture

DESIGNATION OF SUTURE SIZE	SUTURE DIAMETER	SUTURE VOLUME (πr^2)
10-0	13–25μ	132–420μ²
9-0	25–38μ	420–1133μ²
8-0	38–51μ	1133–2042μ²
7-0	51–76μ	2042–4534μ²
6-0	76–102μ	4534–8176μ²

that the volume of the suture increases logarithmically with increasing diameter (Table 4–12). For example, the amount of material in an 8–0 suture is ten times greater than that in a 10–0 suture. It is understandable that there is, therefore, considerably greater reaction with larger than with smaller sutures. The tissue in which the suture is placed is also a factor. For example, polyglycolic acid sutures tend to cause less reaction and be better tolerated in corneoscleral incisions than in skin.

It is not generally appreciated that there is a great diversity in the size of sutures that have the same grade. A large 9–0 suture is more similar in size to a small 10–0 suture than a small 10–0 suture is to a large 10–0 suture. There tends to be little difference between the sutures made by an individual company. Therefore, the surgeon should be familiar with the differences between the various brands of suture as well as the various types.

Some commonly used sutures are shown in Figure 4–36.

Absorbable Sutures (Table 4–13)

The rate at which sutures lose tensile strength and the rate at which they are absorbed are two different considerations (Table 4–13).[21, 23, 46] A suture can lose tensile strength rapidly and yet remain in tissue for a prolonged period. This behavior is characteristic of gut and collagen, which may still be present a year after being placed, long after they have lost any significant holding ability. Conversely, a suture may retain adequate tensile strength long enough to permit wound healing and then rapidly absorb. This behavior is seen with the synthetic absorbable sutures. Adequate holding strength may last for up to 3 weeks, after which the suture may disappear 1 to 2 weeks later.

Both surgical gut and collagen consist of processed strands of collagen. These sutures are relatively quickly digested by the body en-

TABLE 4–13. Basic Structure of Absorbable and Slowly Absorbable Sutures

TYPE OF SUTURE	BASIC MATERIAL
Absorbable Sutures	
Surgical gut (plain or chromicized)	Submucosa of sheep intestine or serosa of beef intestine
Surgical collagen (plain or chromicized)	Flexor tendon of beef
Rattail tendon	Rattail tendon
Polyglactin 910	Copolymer of lactide and glycolide
Polyglycolic acid	Homopolymer of glycolide
Polydioxanone	Polymer of polyester $(C_4H_6O_3)_x$
Sutures That Absorb Slowly or Not at All	
Braided silk	Degummed silk
Virgin silk	Natural, sericin-coated silk filaments
Stainless steel wire	Specially formulated iron-nickel-chromium alloy
Nylon	Polymer of polyamide
Polyester fiber	Polymer of terephthalic acid and glycolethylene
Polypropylene	Polymer of propylene

zymes. Plain gut or collagen cannot be expected to have enough tensile strength to support an incision for longer than a week. Treatment with chromium salt solution conditions the collagen to resist enzymatic degradation, thus prolonging by a factor of about two the absorption time. Chromicized sutures cause less tissue reaction and are less irritating during the early stages of wound healing.[32, 33] Gut and collagen sutures are best sterilized with radioactive cobalt irradiation, as heat causes loss of tensile strength. The sutures pass well through tissue, as they are of monofilament smoothness. In the larger sizes gut is as strong as other suture material (Table 4–14). However, 8–0 collagen is quite brittle and breaks easily when manipulated.

Synthetic absorbable sutures are made from polyglactin 910, polyglycolic acid, and polydioxanone. By and large the rate of absorption of these sutures is more predictable than with surgical gut or collagen. A variety of reports show that the synthetic absorbable sutures are satisfactory for many ophthalmic uses.[12–20, 25, 26, 28, 29, 47] The finer suture material retains its strength about as long as the heavier suture, but the extremely fine 11–0 polyglactin 910 absorbs more rapidly (specifically after around 13 days) when used in corneal incisions. It is my impression from clinical experience that the synthetic absorbable sutures maintain their holding capacity when used in corneoscleral incisions when they are placed under a conjunctival flap. In such a situation they appear to have adequate tensile strength for about 3 to 4 weeks. After this they disappear rapidly. Tissue reaction tends to be less than with silk or gut, although excessive inflammation may occur.[34, 43, 48] Polyglactin 910 is available in braided (5–0 to 9–0) and monofilament (9–0 to 10–0) forms. The suture is strong even in fine sizes.

Nonabsorbable Sutures

Nonabsorbable sutures are strands of material that resist enzymatic degradation of living tissue. Many of them are not truly "nonabsorbable," and eventually deteriorate.[24, 36, 37] For example, nylon is not a permanent suture and as such is probably not ideal for uses where a truly permanent holding ability is necessary. Fine silk suture is even more rapidly degraded (see Table 4–15).

Virgin silk suture is made from several natural silk filaments drawn together and twisted to form a strand of small diameter (8–0 or 9–0). The individual silk filaments are allowed to remain embedded in the natural sericin coating that is present in silk as it is made by the silkworm. It provides a smooth suture that pulls through tissue with remarkable ease. Normally a pale cream color, its visibility may be enhanced by coloring it with methylene blue. It may also be dyed by the manufacturer.

Braided silk is manufactured by braiding

TABLE 4–14. Knot-Pull Tensile Strength of Selected Sutures (kg)*

MATERIAL SIZE	AVERAGE DIAMETER mm	STEEL	POLYPRO-PYLENE	MONO-FILAMENT NYLON	BRAIDED DACRON	VIRGIN SILK	BRAIDED SILK	GUT	POLYGLACTIN 910
10–0	0.02	—	0.03	0.03	—	—	—	—	0.04
9–0	0.03	—	0.06	0.05	—	—	—	—	0.09
8–0	0.05	0.17	0.14	0.09	—	0.07	0.08	—	0.14
6–0	0.10	0.4	0.3	0.3	0.3	—	0.3	0.28	0.4
4–0	0.20	2.0	1.3	1.0	1.2	—	0.8	0.9	1.5

*Modified from information supplied by Alcon, Inc., Ethicon, Inc., and Ullerick, K., Muxfeld, H.: Ber. Dtsch. Ophthalmol. Ges., 70:331, 1970.

TABLE 4–15. Comparison of Suture Materials

SUTURE MATERIAL	RELATIVE TENSILE STRENGTH*	RELATIVE HOLDING DURATION†	RELATIVE TISSUE REACTION‡	EASE OF HANDLING	SPECIAL KNOT REQUIRED	BEHAVIOR OF EXPOSED ENDS	AVAILABLE SIZES‖
Surgical gut or collagen							
Plain	6	1 week	4+	Good	No	Stiff	4-0–6-0
Chromic	6	<2 weeks	3+	Good	No	Stiff	4-0–8-0
Polyglactin 910							
Braided	9	2 weeks	2+	Good	Yes	Stiff	4-0–9-0
Monofilament	9	2 weeks	2+	Good	Yes	Stiff	9-0–10-0
Polyglycolic acid	9	2 weeks	2+	Good	Yes	Stiff	
Polydioxanone	9	4–6 weeks	2+	Good	Yes	Stiff	4-0–10-0
Silk							
Virgin	7	2 months	3+	Excellent	No	Softest	8-0–9-0
Braided	8	2 months	3+	Good	No	Soft	4-0–9-0
Polyamide (Nylon)	9	6 months	1+	Fair#	Yes§	Stiff & sharp	8-0–11-0
Polypropylene	10	>12 months	1+	Fair**	Yes	Stiff & sharp	4-0–6-0, 9-0–10-0
Polyester	10	>12 months	1+	Fair	Yes	Stiff	4-0–6-0

*The higher the number, the greater the relative tensile strength. Strength varies with size of material; estimates in this table apply mainly to size 8–0 sutures (see Table 4–12).

†Holding duration will vary with location and size of suture, health of patient, medications used, etc. The time given in this table is an average of the time at which about 30 per cent of tensile strength is lost.

‡1+ indicates least inflammatory response, 4+ greatest.

§The surgeon must consider whether special care is needed to assure that the knot will remain tight.

‖With needles appropriate for ophthalmic use. Sizes available will vary from time to time.

#Moderately elastic.

**Highly elastic.

dyed silk fibers that have had their natural sericin coating removed. The braiding helps to assure uniformity of diameter and slightly higher tensile strength than is present with virgin silk; however, some of the previously mentioned disadvantages of braided suture are present. The knots are easy to tie, and they hold securely. The cut ends of the suture material tend to lie flat, but are slightly more rigid than with virgin silk. Both tend to produce little discomfort unless used in exposed cornea. Softer virgin silk, however, causes less difficulty than does the braided silk. Both have excellent handling characteristics. All silk produces a moderate inflammatory response in tissue.[21, 43] Rarely a patient will show a marked intolerance. The tendency to develop a fistula around the suture is especially great with silk and may cause a serious problem.

Nylon suture is a polymer of amides manufactured synthetically. This polyamide suture may come in at least two polymeric forms having slightly different characteristics.[37] Nylon is manufactured in a braided form in the 4–0 and 5–0 sizes, but this suture is seldom used in ophthalmic surgery. Monofilament nylon has a high tensile strength and causes minimal tissue reaction.[38, 39] It is not permanent, and is degraded slowly *in vivo* so that it loses at least 15 percent of its tensile strength yearly.[36, 37] It is highly elastic, a property that presents the

surgeon with both advantages and disadvantages. Knots must be tied with special care in order not to make them too tight and yet to pull them firmly enough so that they do not spontaneously untie. Slip knots can be helpful.[45]

Polyester fibers can be braided into a multifilament strand of high tensile strength (see Tables 4–14 and 4–15). The polyester suture retains its tensile strength for more prolonged periods than does nylon. It elicits a minimal tissue reaction. Because of its braided nature it holds a bit more securely when being tied than does nylon. However, it tends to drag tissue with it as it is pulled through.

Polypropylene is an extremely inert material that may be truly "permanent" (Tables 4–14 and 4–15).[30] It is manufactured as a monofilament strand. It appears to be as well tolerated in tissue as nylon, producing little tissue response. Because the suture material is deformed as it is tied, polypropylene tends to hold a knot better than most other synthetic suture materials. The cut ends are sharp and stiff. Polypropylene is an even more elastic suture than nylon.

Tables 4–14 and 4–15 summarize the characteristics of some of the sutures frequently used in ophthalmic surgery. Steel is seldom used, but is included as a basis for reference of tensile strength. Table 4–16 lists some trade names.

TABLE 4–16. Trade Names of Some Ophthalmic Sutures*

SUTURE MATRIAL	TRADE NAME
Polyglactin 910	Vicryl (Ethicon, Inc.)
Polyglycolic acid	Dexon-N (Davis and Geck, Inc.)
Polyamide (nylon)	Ethilon (Ethicon, Inc.)
	Dermalon (Davis and Geck, Inc.)
	Supramid (Kunststoffwerk Alfred Huber)
	Perlon (Perlon Trademark Association)
Polyester (Dacron)	Mersilene (Ethicon, Inc.)
Polypropylene	Prolene (Ethicon, Inc.)
Polydioxanone	PDS (Ethicon, Inc.)

*Note: Not all suture-manufacturing companies use trademarks.

Because nylon and Prolene are resilient and wiry, special techniques must be used for tying the knot, and the cut ends of the suture must be buried in the tissue in order to avoid troublesome symptoms that could persist for months. The elasticity of Prolene and, to a lesser extent, nylon can also prove to be a problem, especially with suture materials finer than 8–0. Until the surgeon becomes fully familiar with 10–0 nylon or Prolene, for example, there is a great tendency to secure the sutures more tightly than necessary. As a result the incision becomes distorted in the area of the excessively tight suture. In fact this is a problem with all suture material size 9–0 or smaller, regardless of its type. Silk and polyglactin 910 must also be placed with special care so that they are not pulled too tightly. When using fine sutures special care must be taken to avoid the pulling of the suture through the tissue (cheese-wire effect).[49] A variety of methods have been suggested, including running or through-and-through suturing techniques.[49–52]

Tying Sutures

Surgeon's Knot

One method of tying a suture is shown in Figure 4–37. The end of the suture to which the needle is still attached is grasped with the straight forceps (Fig. 4–37-1). The suture is held obliquely, neither exactly parallel nor at right angles to the jaws of the forceps. The angled forceps are then placed in the V made by the two ends of the suture, and the long end is wrapped around the angled tip (Fig. 4–37-2). The tip is angled, so wrapping the suture is most easily accomplished. One, two, three, or four throws are placed, depending on the size and type of suture and the tension on the incision (Fig. 4–37-3). With 10–0 nylon, 9–0 nylon, or 9–0 polyglactin three are usually adequate. Three throws may also be necessary with 9–0 virgin silk, but two are enough if the tissue is in good apposition. With larger silk sutures two throws usually suffice. With smoother-surfaced material three throws may be required, even when using suture material larger than 9–0.

After the correct number of throws have been wound around the angled end of the forceps, the angled end is rotated to reach the loose end of the suture (Fig. 4–37-4). It is often helpful to delay cutting this other end until after it has been grasped; then it can be cut directly on the forceps. This loose end should be just long enough to permit easy grasping and prevent it from being accidentally pulled through the incision. With fine sutures the short end should be about 1 cm long. The angled forceps now picks up this cut short end near its very tip. If the suture is short and dry, it tends to stick up away from the surface of the globe, making it easier to grasp. When the suture is lying on the surface it is best picked up by angling the forceps so that only the tip of the instrument touches the suture, or by sliding one jaw of the forceps under the end and then closing them. Once the short end has been grasped it is pulled in exactly the opposite direction from its origin (Fig. 4–37-5). The fingers, then, move in opposite directions, pulling the first tie down firmly and squarely (Fig. 4–37-6). The instruments should not bend the suture sharply, as this may break it, especially if it is fragile, as are 8–0 chromic collagen and 9–0 silk. The suture as it is secured should make a straight line, so that the ends are being pulled exactly away from each other (Fig. 4–37-6).

After the proper tension has been placed on the incision the short end is released. The surgeon must remember that this first knot will tighten slightly as the second throw is placed. Therefore, this first knot should be slightly looser than needed at the conclusion of tying the knot. The angled forceps are again placed in the center of the V made by the two sutures (Fig. 4–37-7). The long end is wrapped once around the tip, which is then rotated to grasp the short cut end (Fig. 4–37-8 and 9). The fingers then move back to the position they were in before the first throw, again pulling away from each other in a straight line (Fig. 4–37-10). Before pulling the second tie tight, the surgeon checks the first tie to be sure it has not

Text continued on page 62

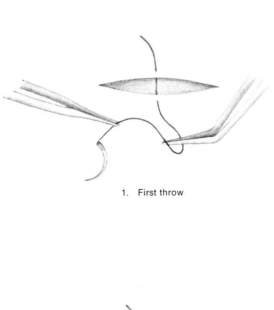

1. First throw

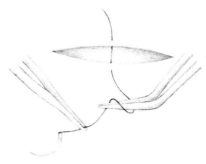

2. First throw completed

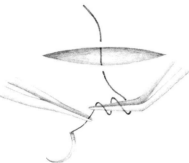

3. Second throw

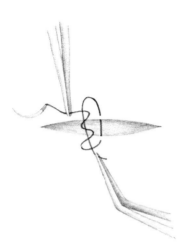

4. Jaws opened to grasp free suture

5. Ends pulled opposite positions of origins

FIGURE 4–37. Steps followed in tying surgeon's knot with one angled and one straight McPherson tying forceps.

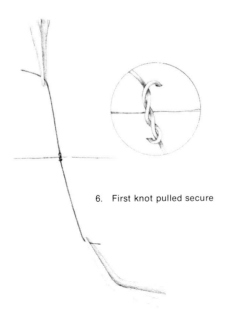

6. First knot pulled secure

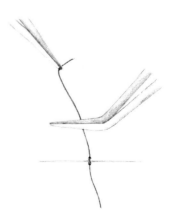

7. Start of second knot

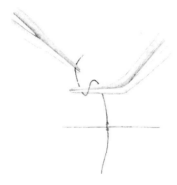

8. Single throw placed

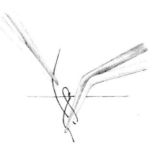

9. Angled forceps reaches over to grasp end of loose suture

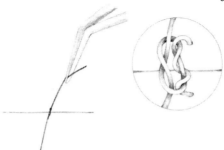

10. Second throw tightened by pulling opposite direction from prior position

FIGURE 4–37 *Continued*

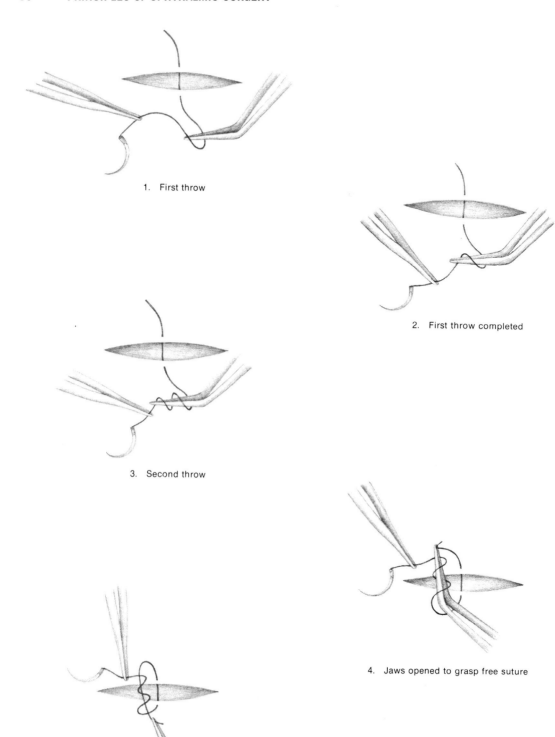

1. First throw

2. First throw completed

3. Second throw

4. Jaws opened to grasp free suture

5. Ends pulled opposite positions of origins

FIGURE 4–38. Method of tying a slip knot. Note that the second throw must exactly duplicate the first. Then a square knot is made with the third throw. A fourth square throw should be added.

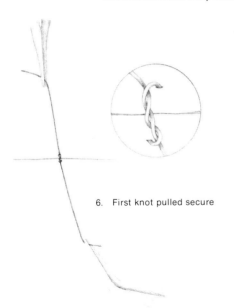

6. First knot pulled secure

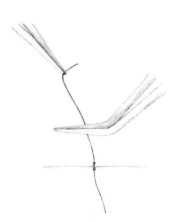

7. Start of second knot

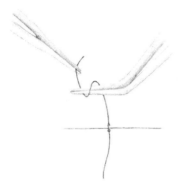

8. Single throw placed

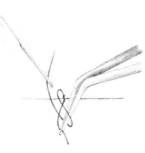

9. Angled forceps reaches over to grasp end of loose suture

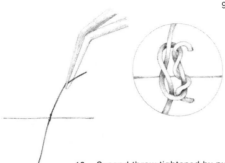

10. Second throw tightened by pulling opposite direction from prior position

FIGURE 4–38 *Continued*

slipped and is not too tight. The second tie is then gradually secured until it is entirely firm. The short end is released, and a third tie is placed, again by pulling the ends away from the place of origin. This third tie is gradually pulled tight, but as firmly as the suture will reasonably stand without being broken. Some surgeons prefer to place a fourth tie, especially with resilient monofilament sutures.

Slip Knot

The method of tying a slip knot is shown in Figure 4–38. This technique has the advantage of producing a smaller knot that is easier to bury and less likely to erode. Additionally, it allows the surgeon to place the knot with an accurate determination of the exact desired degree of tightness. Its disadvantages are that it requires four throws; it cannot be used to oppose tissue forcibly, as the knot tends to break; and it is not particularly suitable for suture materials with a high degree of friction.

The first tie of the slip knot is placed the same way as for a surgeon's knot, with the important exception that only one throw is placed. After this the left hand holding the straight tying forceps is returned to its initial position before placing the first tie. The tying forceps in the right hand releases the suture end. The second tie is then placed in the same

manner as the first tie. This may require some rather adept finger work, reaching "under" the end of the sutures being held with the left hand in order to pick up the free end, which is now on the same side of the incision as the suture being held in the left hand. After the throw of the second tie is placed, the third throw is tied the same as the second tie in a surgeon's knot. That is, this third tie must complete the square knot (Fig. 4–38). A fourth tie is then always placed to complete the slip knot. Some surgeons prefer to place a fifth single-throw square knot in addition, especially when tying sutures that have great resilience and little surface friction, such as 10–0 nylon and polypropylene.

Cutting and Burying Sutures

Regardless of what type of knot is tied, the final tie should be pulled firmly in order to assure that the knot is compressed as tightly as possible.

If the surgeon intends to bury the knot, the ends should be individually cut with a razor blade or another sharp instrument directly on the knot so that the ends are as short as possible (Fig. 4–39). The free hand ends may be cut either "up" or "down." The knife should be held so that the knot is always visible; it must

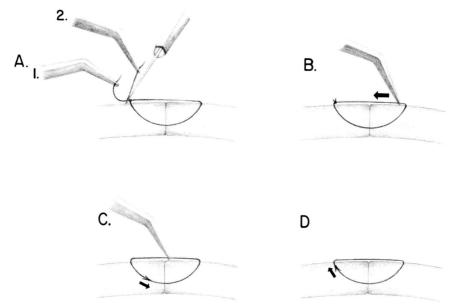

FIGURE 4–39. Method of cutting and burying fine synthetic suture material. *A,* The ends are individually cut on the knot with a sharp blade. *B,* The suture is grasped at the end opposite the knot and pulled toward the knot, which slides into the tissue (*C*). *D,* The suture is returned slightly toward its original position so that the cut ends do not serve as a barb holding the suture in place. The knife should be held so the knot is always visible; it must not obscure the view or else the end cannot be cut with certainty directly on the knot.

not obscure the view or else the end cannot be cut with certainty directly on the knot. After both ends have been cut short the suture should be carefully grasped with a smooth tying forceps and rotated so that the knot is buried in the depths of the tissue (Fig. 4–39B and C). If this is difficult, the surgeon should try pulling the suture in the opposite directions. Sometimes holding the edge of the incision with a fine-toothed forceps also helps. Once the suture knot has been buried it should be pulled back slightly toward its original position, reversing the direction of the cut ends, which facilitates removal of the suture if this should be necessary at a later date (Fig. 4–39D). If nylon or Prolene suture ends protrude and cause signs or symptoms, they can be shortened by burning them with an argon laser beam. If the sutures are too tight, especially fine, darkly colored sutures, they can easily be released in most instances by burning them with an argon laser beam.[53] This is greatly facilitated by using a Hoskins lens, which gives greater magnification and flattens the tissue, providing a much better view and allowing the heat of the laser beam to be more clearly focused on the suture. Suggested appropriate settings are 500 mW and a spot size of 50 or 100 μm for 0.1 seconds.

It is not always necessary to cut sutures directly on the knot; however, where this is not done it is usually desirable to leave the ends quite long, around 5 mm, so that they will lie flat and not erode. This is not a suitable technique if the ends will rub against the cornea.

SURGICAL NEEDLE

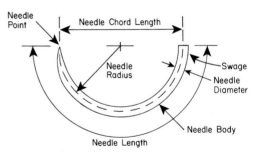

FIGURE 4–40. Basic points for consideration when choosing a surgical needle.

Needles

The basic characteristics of the needle used in ophthalmic surgery are shown in Figure 4–40. The specifications of some of the needles used in ophthalmic surgery are shown in Table 4–17[55] and Figure 4–36.

To accomplish the different goals in ophthalmic surgery the surgeon must use different needles. The size and curvature of the needle depends on the particular need. For example, when placing sutures in a clear corneal incision anterior to a filtering bleb, one chooses a short, fine needle with marked curvature, such as the GS-16 (see Table 4–17). In contrast, the larger S-14 needle with a one-quarter–circle curvature is ideal for strabismus surgery (Table 4–18). On the other hand, a long (10 to 13 mm)

TABLE 4–17. Needle Specifications*

NEEDLE	CURVATURE	CHORD LENGTH	RADIUS (mm)	WIRE DIAMETER (mm)	NEEDLE LENGTH (mm)
		Reverse-Cutting			
G-1	135°	8.80	4.76	0.33	11.50
G-2	180°	4.76	2.38	0.432	9.12
G-3	155°	9.30	4.76	0.432	13.09
G-6	110°	6.50	3.97	0.203	7.93
G-7	165°	5.52	2.78	0.203	7.93
		Spatula			
S-2	180°	4.76	2.38	0.432	9.12
S-4	112°	7.24	4.36	0.432	9.12
S-12	180°	4.76	2.38	0.330	8.73
S-14	112°	7.24	4.37	0.330	8.73
GS-8	97°	5.95	3.96	0.203	6.55
GS-9	137°	5.17	2.78	0.203	6.55
GS-10	175°	4.80	2.38	0.203	7.14
GS-14	160°	4.00	2.00	0.203	5.50
GS-15	137°	4.70	2.50	0.145	6.00
GS-16	175°	4.00	2.00	0.145	6.00
GS-17	140°	4.75	2.54	0.150	6.19
GS-18	175°	4.57	2.28	0.150	6.98
GS-19	160°	4.00	2.00	0.150	5.50

*Modified from material supplied by Ethicon, Inc.

TABLE 4–18. Selected Needles

	TYPE OF TIP	CURVATURE Wide	CURVATURE Degree	Radius	NEEDLE LENGTH (mm)	NEEDLE DIAMETER (mm)	SUTURE TYPE
Ethicon Type 55							
TG-160	Spatula	½	160	1.5	4.3	.09	Nylon, polyester, black silk, virgin silk, polyglactin, polypropylene
TG-140	Spatula	⅜	140	2.5	6.2	.12	Nylon, polyglactin, polypropylene, virgin silk, polyester
TG-4-6	Spatula	Compound		1.4/2.5	4.8	.12	Nylon
TG-100	Spatula	¼	97	4.0	6.6	.20	Nylon, chromic gut, braided silk, polyglactin
S-24	Spatula	¼	90	5.1	8.3	.33	Nylon, polyester, polyglactin
S-14	Spatula	¼	112	4.4	8.7	.33	Chromic gut, plain gut, polyester, braided silk, braided polyglactin
S-4	Spatula	¼	112	4.4	9.1	.43	Chromic gut, plain gut, polyester

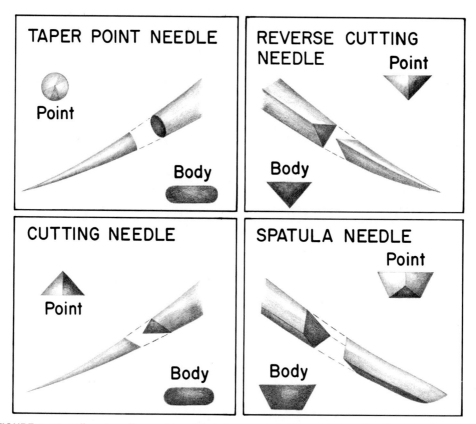

FIGURE 4–41. Different needles used in ophthalmic surgery. *A,* Taper-point needle. This is used primarily on easily penetrated tissue in which the smallest possible hole is desired. *B,* The cutting needle. The conventional cutting needle has two opposing cutting edges with a third on the inside curvature of the needle. *C,* Reverse cutting needle. Here the third cutting edge is located on the outer curvature of the needle. This is used to penetrate tough tissue such as sclera. *D,* Spatula needle. The flat surface helps to keep this needle in the proper lamellar plane. (Modified from material supplied by Ethicon, Inc.)

taper-point needle with a three-eighths–circle curvature is excellent for placing the superior rectus bridle suture.

The different shapes of some of the needles themselves are shown in Figures 4–36 and 4–41, which show the taper-point, conventional cutting, reverse cutting, and spatula needles (Fig. 4–41A through D). The spatula needle is especially useful in ophthalmic microsurgery. The sharp, flat, "side-cutting" needle is designed to travel through the cornea or sclera without penetrating more deeply or cutting out of the tissue, as would more likely be the case with a reverse cutting or conventional cutting needle (Fig. 4–41D).

STANDARD OPHTHALMIC PROCEDURES

The Bridle Suture

The placement of a suture under one of the rectus muscles can aid considerably in positioning the globe correctly. As most intraocular surgery is performed at the 12 o'clock position on the globe, this most often involves the superior rectus muscle. The same principle is applied by placing an inferior rectus suture for surgery at the 6 o'clock position, and so on.

The eye can be rotated inferiorly by being grasped at the inferior limbus with a dressing forceps and being pulled gently in an inferior direction. This makes it a bit easier to see the area of the superior rectus insertion. In most cases, however, this is not necessary. A safer technique, which avoids the possibility of tearing the conjunctiva, is to lift the upper lid with the side of the 4–0 needle, which needs to be held securely, preferably in a Kalt needle holder.

A husky-toothed forceps such as the Lister is placed under the upper lid as shown in Figure 4–42A. Note that the tips are held approximately 2 mm apart; they are not widely spread. Once the tips have been positioned 6 to 8 mm superior to the limbus, the handle of the forceps is pivoted superiorly so that the forceps is now held perpendicular to the globe. With the tips slightly spread, the forceps are pushed firmly against the globe and the tips closed, with the superior rectus muscle being grasped just posterior to the insertion of the rectus tendon onto the globe (Fig. 4–42B). The forceps are then rotated inferiorly once again, and the globe is pulled inferiorly, with the tips of the forceps

exposed (Fig. 4–42C). A 4–0 black silk suture, swaged onto a long, husky, non-cutting, tapered needle, is then placed onto the muscle, as close to the globe as possible without penetrating (Fig. 4–42D and E).

If a globe is penetrated, it is a major complication that needs to be handled immediately. Indirect ophthalmoscopy should be performed to determine the extent of the penetration. If the needle has reached intraocularly, then a localized scleral buckling procedure may be appropriate, with placement of cryo or cautery to produce the localized adhesion.

Preplacement of Sutures

It may be advantageous to place suture material before complete penetration of an incision. This is especially applicable to corneoscleral incisions. Preplacement of the suture allows the most exact alignment of the incision and assures that the suture is not too deep. Separation of the incision is also facilitated, permitting more precise completion of the incision through the deepest layers.

The incision for a preplaced suture should be made slightly deeper than the depth at which one wants to place the needle. Thus, if the surgeon wants to have the needle approximately halfway through the tissue, the incision should be made through approximately three-quarters the thickness of the tissue. Once proper depth of the incision has been reached, the suture is placed. The tip of the needle is placed against the surface of the tissue so that it will enter in a perpendicular direction (Fig. 4–43A). The needle is then rotated along its arc, the tip penetrating the incised tissue at the desired depth (Fig. 4–43B). The tip must be clearly visible in the depth of the incision (Fig. 4–43C). If it is not, the suture will be difficult to retrieve. The tip of the needle is then directed toward the external surface of the tissue before entering the opposite side of the incision; this motion assures that the suture will be able to be retracted later. The needle then proceeds through its arc to exit on the surface. The suture is drawn through the tissue, with an allowance of about 4 inches of suture material on each side of the incision.

A smooth-tipped tying forceps such as the Harms or the McPherson is introduced into the incision, so that it grasps the suture at the point at which it traverses the incision at its base (Fig. 4–43D). As the suture is retrieved from the incision, the loop that is formed is kept

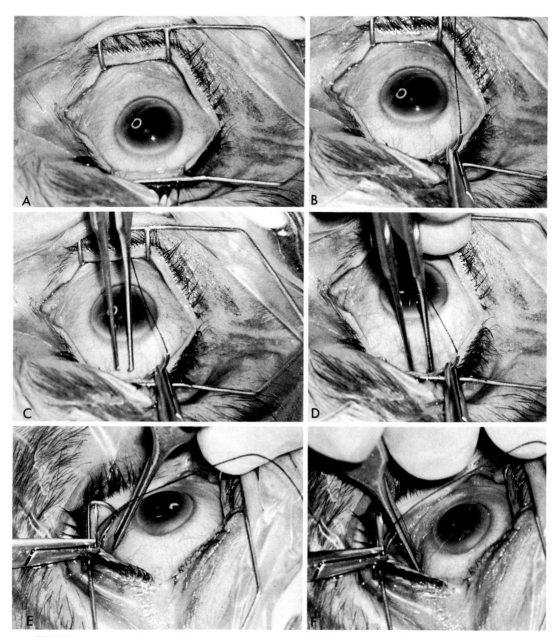

FIGURE 4–42. Technique of placing a superior rectus muscle bridle suture. *A,* The eye with a Barraquer colibri speculum in place. Note that the superior rectus muscle is well hidden by the upper lid (lower portion of photograph). *B,* The needle of a single-armed 4–0 black silk suture is used to retract the upper lid, allowing better visualization of the area in which the superior rectus suture is to be placed. *C,* The tips of a Lister forceps are held tangential to the superior portion of the globe, approximately 2 mm apart. *D,* The forceps are moved superiorly so that the tips extend past the insertion of the superior rectus muscle, that is, about 12 mm superior to the limbus. *E,* Side view showing the lid held superiorly by the needle of the 4–0 black silk suture and the Lister forceps in its initial position. *F,* The handle of the forceps is rotated superiorly while the tips are pressed firmly against the globe. Note the indentation of the globe caused by the pressure of the forceps. When the forceps have been rotated to the position shown, the tips are closed around the superior rectus muscle.

taut. A tying forceps grasps one strand of the taut, looped suture close to the incision and pulls it toward the loose suture lying on the surface of the tissue on the same side of the incision. The assistant performs a similar ma-

neuver on the other side of the taut loop. The portion of the suture pulled out of the incision is then grasped in conjunction with the suture lying on the surface of the tissue to form a traction suture (Fig. 4–43*E* and *F*). The two

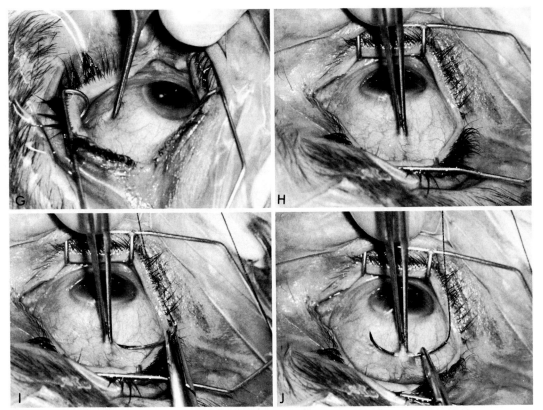

FIGURE 4–42 *Continued G,* After the muscle has been firmly grasped, the forceps are again rotated inferiorly and the globe is pulled inferiorly. *H,* Surgeon's view of the proper grasp of the superior rectus muscle. *I,* The needle of the 4–0 black silk suture is placed under the superior rectus muscle, not through its belly. *J,* Proper position of the needle deep to the forceps and between the globe and the superior rectus muscle belly.

(See Figure 11–81 for a schematic representation of the technique of inserting a superior rectus muscle bridle suture.)

traction sutures are pulled at right angles to each other to separate the incision (Fig. 4–43F). This provides excellent visualization of the depth of the incision. Furthermore, it keeps the suture out of the way as the incision is completed (Fig. 4–43G).

The preplaced suture should not be used as a substitute for fixation of the tissue elsewhere. Excessive traction will cause lamellar tissue splitting.

After the incision has been completed, the sutures can be used to provide gentle traction, to allow prolapse of underlying tissue, as would be suitable in performing a peripheral iridectomy. If such traction is not required, the tying forceps holding the edges of the loop may be released and the suture grasped at its needle end and pulled through the tissue, eliminating the loop. The incision may then easily be ex-

tended without fear of cutting the suture. When the surgeon wants to close the incision permanently, the suture is tied according to a standard method.

Paracentesis

The presence of a nonleaking opening into the anterior chamber is of great assistance in intraocular surgery. Such an opening permits re-formation of the anterior chamber with saline solution or air, deepening of the anterior chamber, irrigation of the anterior chamber, and restoration to normal or even increased levels of intraocular pressure. All of these maneuvers can occasionally be of great value, and may even transform a surgical failure into a surgical success (Table 4–19). When paracentesis is correctly performed, the risk is virtually negligible,

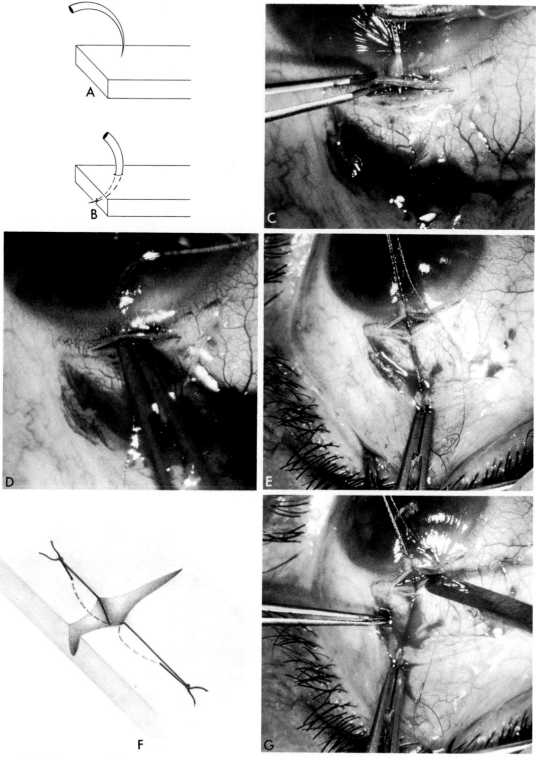

FIGURE 4–43. Method of placement of preplaced suture. The suture is placed more superficially than the depth of the incision and then retracted from the incision to form two loops that may be used to provide gentle retraction and excellent visualization of the depth of the incision.

TABLE 4–19. Uses for Paracentesis

A. *In Glaucoma Surgery*
 1. Formation of anterior chamber and bleb after every filtering surgical procedure
 2. Re-formation of shallow or flat anterior chamber postoperatively
 3. To maintain chamber depth during goniotomy or anterior vitrectomy
 4. Chamber-deepening gonioscopy
 5. Washout of blood from anterior chamber
 6. Rapid re-formation of anterior chamber and restoration of intraocular pressure to above-normal limits after cyclodialysis
B. *With Cataract Extraction*
 1. Re-formation of the anterior chamber after cataract extraction and at close of procedure
 2. Discission and aspiration
 3. Sweeping incision clear at end of surgery
 4. Separation of iris from vitreous face in aphakic pupillary block
C. *With Choroidal Detachment*
 1. Re-formation of anterior chamber
 2. Testing for filtration wound or cyclodialysis
D. *With Trauma*
 1. Irrigation and re-formation of anterior chamber
 2. Placement of air bubble into anterior chamber
 3. Fixation of intracorneal foreign body
E. *With Retinal Detachment*
 1. Lowering of intraocular pressure
 2. Lowering of intraocular pressure to gain space
 3. Re-formation of globe to normal firmness
F. *In Diagnosis*
 1. Differentiation between intraocular infection and inflammation
 2. Identification of epithelial downgrowth, phakolytic glaucoma, or ghost-cell glaucoma
 3. Chamber-deepening gonioscopy
G. *To Lower Intraocular Pressure*
 1. Before surgery
 2. After cycloablative procedures
 3. As temporizing procedure

and the benefits of the procedure are so considerable that it should probably be part of virtually every anterior segment intraocular operation.

A sharp and appropriate instrument must be used when performing a paracentesis. The Wheeler knife, a sharp disposable such as the Beaver #75, and a needle such as a 25-gauge are all thin enough to easily penetrate the cornea and wide enough to provide easy access with an irrigating instrument such as a blunt 30-gauge needle. Some of the knife-needles, such as those manufactured by Grieshaber, are sharper and may actually penetrate more easily. However, they may leave a track too small for introduction at a later time of a larger instrument. The best method to choose depends to some extent on the intended use for the paracentesis opening. I prefer to use a sharp disposable 25-gauge needle. This easily admits a #30 or even a #27 irrigating tip.

The surgeon should always inspect the instrument to be used before performing the paracentesis. The tip must be sharp, without bends or burrs. Deposits on the blade or material used to protect the blade during storage should be carefully removed.

Excellent visualization helps to assure a safe and successful paracentesis. The placement of the needle should be made under magnification of at least 8×, and preferably more, so that the passage of the knife through the cornea can be precisely monitored.

The globe must be fixated firmly. This is usually accomplished relatively easily if bare sclera is available. A forceps with 0.1-mm teeth and with relatively husky handles is useful for fixation. The 0.12-mm-toothed Castroviejo forceps is an example. The tips are held less than 2 mm apart and pushed firmly against the sclera, so as to engage firmly a small bite of stable tissue. Where the conjunctiva is intact, fixation is more difficult. Conjunctiva and Tenon's capsule do not provide a firm enough hold by themselves. If the surgeon chooses to fixate through the intact conjunctiva, the fixation forceps must be pushed against the globe firmly enough so that the dense episcleral tissue is engaged. When the surgeon wants to be certain that the conjunctiva is not damaged, as may be the case in an eye with a flat anterior chamber after a glaucoma procedure, an incision in the peripheral cornea approximately one-third the thickness of the cornea can be made with a sharp instrument such as a razor blade knife. The cut edge of this incision provides an edge, allowing firm fixation.

The position of fixation is important. The basic principle is to grasp the tissue in a location so that the knife or needle used for the paracentesis pushes in a direction around 180 degrees away from the point of fixation. For example, if the point of fixation is at 2 o'clock superotemporally on the right globe, the needle should enter the cornea at the 2 o'clock position on the cornea and be directed inferiorly (Fig. 4–44A). The point of engagement on the cornea is usually approximately 2 mm from the limbus. If the cornea is entered nearer the limbus, the entrance into the track may later be covered by overhanging conjunctiva or may be in a position where the surgeon would want to place a corneoscleral suture.

Once the globe has been securely fixated and the point of entry selected, the needle is held in a plane parallel to the iris surface and the tip engaged in the superficial cornea (Fig. 4–44A). The hand holding the fixation forceps then pulls

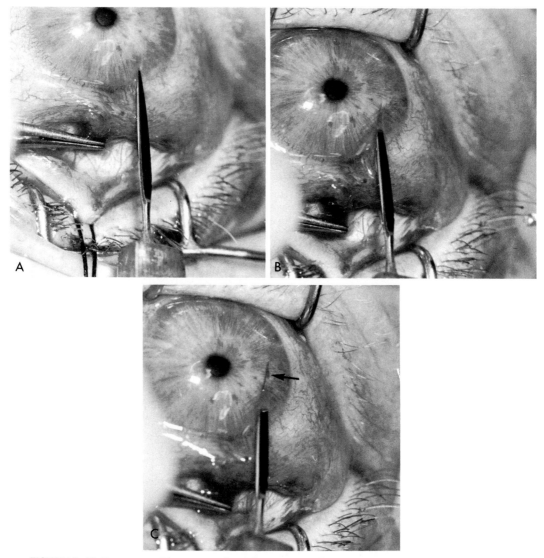

FIGURE 4–44. Paracentesis. The eyes are shown from a surgeon's position. *A*, The globe is firmly fixated on the posterior edge of the incompletely developed trabeculectomy flap, or a similar good holding surface. The needle and syringe are held in a plane parallel to the surface of the iris. *B*, The globe is pulled superiorly by the forceps while the needle is cautiously advanced. The needle never points toward the lens or iris. The globe is pulled toward the needle with the fixating hand. If a long paracentesis track is desired, the needle can be extended intracorneally for a longer distance before penetrating the endothelium. *C*, Penetration is achieved by first depressing the entire needle and syringe in the direction of the iris, which indents the cornea, and then pushing the needle inferiorly slowly or pulling the globe superiorly slowly. The needle must NEVER be pointed toward the iris; it must ALWAYS be held parallel to the plane of the iris. Direct visualization assures that the needle penetrated into the anterior chamber. A change in the appearance of the needle is a helpful clue. A short disposable 25-gauge needle is an excellent instrument to use for performing paracentesis.

the globe toward the needle; the needle is gently advanced at the same time, and gently eased through the cornea (Fig. 4–44*B*). The intracorneal portion of the track should be at least 2 mm long. This provides a seal that will prevent aqueous from leaking; the higher the intraocular pressure, the firmer the seal will

be. As the tip penetrates the corneal endothelium, a change in the color is noted. This color change can be a helpful clue that penetration into the anterior chamber is complete. If there is a question about this, the needle can be advanced further until the tip cautiously touches the iris surface. The needle is then slowly withdrawn. A blunt-tipped irrigator of appropriate size can then be placed through the track in order to be sure that such an instrument can be passed with ease into the anterior chamber.

A dull or damaged paracentesis knife is more than a bother to the surgeon; it can be a hazard to the patient. Handled properly, paracentesis knives should retain their sharpness for years. Immediately after use, the knife should be placed in a protective container and handed to the instrument nurse. After proper packaging the knife should preferably be sterilized in ethylene oxide, although heat may also be used.

Use of Cautery

It is frequently necessary to apply heat to tissue. The surgeon may want to stop bleeding, cause the tissue to contract, or develop a deep irritation that predisposes to increased scarring. The manner in which the heat is applied determines the nature of the effect.

Heat can result from a spark jumping across a gap. This method of cautery provides coagulation of blood vessels with minimal damage to the surrounding tissue. If the cautery grasps the tissue between the tips, the spark will pass directly through the tissue, causing considerable destruction. If, on the other hand, the cautery is held on the surface of well-moistened tissue, then the spark will jump through the surface fluid, causing minimal destruction of underlying tissue. Therefore, the surgeon may vary the depth and extent of cauterization of tissue merely by changing the manner in which it is applied. Obviously the higher the power setting and the greater the spark, the greater will be the degree of cautery. But even when the setting on the wet-field cautery is kept constant, the effect of the cautery may be considerably altered.

The refinement of control that is possible with wet-field cauterization gives the surgeon a welcome degree of control. The fact that the cautery may be used in a wet field also is helpful when cauterizing areas that cannot be dried, or that are best left moist. Additionally, if an area in which bleeding is present is gently irrigated, the source of the bleeding can be precisely identified and cautery appropriately applied. This permits control of the bleeding with minimal trauma to the surrounding tissue. Several instruments are now available, such as the "eraser," which provide different degrees and extents of cautery. The simple type of instrument shown in Figure 4–45 is satisfactory for many purposes and is my preference.

The wet-field cautery is not a particularly good instrument for causing shrinkage of tissue, as is desirable in certain procedures, such as peripheral iridectomy with thermal sclerostomy. In such circumstances a heated tip is preferable. When cautery with a heated tip is used it is important to test the cautery in an area in which cauterization of the tissue would not be expected to cause significant damage. The precise temperature of the tip of the setting on the instrument does not provide a reliable estimate of actual heat delivered. It is possible to modify the type of burn produced by the manner in which the tip is applied. If the instrument is heated first and then applied to the tissue, the burn will mainly be on the surface. If, in contrast, the tip is applied to the tissue first, after which the power is turned on, the burn will be more diffuse, extending deeper into the tissue.

The Seidel Test for Leakage

There are a number of instances in which the surgeon may want to determine whether aqueous is leaking from the eye. For example, is hypotony after a cataract extraction caused by lack of aqueous production or by an incisional leak? Is hypotony after a trabeculectomy caused by leakage through the cut edges of the conjunctival flap, leakage through a hole in the conjunctival flap, or "ciliary body shutdown"? These are not merely academic questions; their answers will determine the nature of therapy.

The Seidel test is the most useful method of determining whether a leak is present.

The patient is seated comfortably at the slit lamp. The eye is well anesthetized with several instillations of proparacaine or a similar topical agent. The binoculars are placed on low power, and the patient is positioned at the slit lamp so that the area under consideration can be easily viewed. The slit lamp light is turned on, using full power and the dark blue filter. The examining room is darkened, preferably totally. A fluorescein-impregnated strip is slightly moistened with proparacaine or saline solution. The wet fluorescein strip is applied to the area to be examined, densely covering it with fluorescein. With the blue filter in place the eye is examined.

The stained area should appear dark metallic brown. A leak can be noticed by the appearance of a brilliant green spot that gradually increases

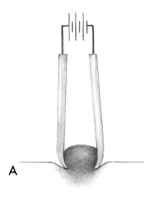

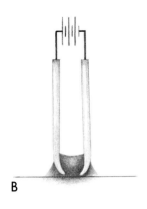

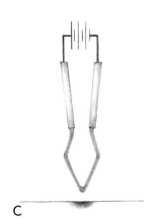

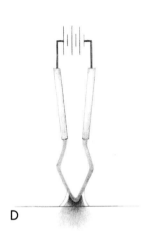

A

B

C

D

FIGURE 4–45. The effect of cautery will vary, depending on how it is used. *A,* A wet-field cautery is used to cause extensive deep burning of tissue. *B,* A wet-field cautery is used to cause superficial burning, as would be appropriate in cauterizing a superficial blood vessel. *C,* The cautery is heated before touching the tissue, resulting in a superficial burn. *D,* The cautery is turned on only after it has touched the tissue; this results in a deeper, more diffuse burn.

in size. There may be a trickle of brilliant green running down from the leaking area. The edges of the trickle fluoresce brightly, and the center may become clear.

If no leak is seen, the eye is pressed firmly in order to try to force aqueous out the suspected hole. The amount of pressure is roughly equal to that placed on the eye when massaging the globe in order to enhance a filtering bleb. Obviously the general condition of the eye will affect how much pressure the surgeon considers it wise to use.

The Seidel test should not be considered negative unless the preceding or a similar technique has been followed. A negative test does not prove the absence of a leak. The hole may be temporarily blocked by fibrin or other debris, or there may not be sufficient aqueous present when the test is performed. However, in eyes that do not have totally flat chambers,

a negative Seidel test is strongly indicative that a leak is not present.

On the other hand, a positive Seidel test does not necessarily indicate the presence of disease. For example, many normal filtering blebs cause positive Seidel tests, especially those blebs that form after corneoscleral trephination or sclerectomies.

REFERENCES

1. Troutman, R. C.: Microsurgery of the Anterior Segment of the Eye, Vol. 1. St. Louis, C. V. Mosby Co., 1974.
2. Eisner, G.: Augenchirurgie. Einführung in die operative Technik. Berlin and Heidelberg, Springer-Verlag, 1978.
3. Jakobiec, F. A., Sigelman, J.: Advanced Techniques in Ocular Surgery. Philadelphia, W. B. Saunders Co., 1984.
4. Spaeth, G. L., Katz, L. J.: Current Therapy in

Ophthalmic Surgery. Philadelphia, B. C. Decker, Inc, 1989.

5. Waltman, S. R., Kestes, R. H., Hoyt, C. S. et al: Surgery of the Eye. New York, Churchill Livingstone, 1988.

5a. Blankenship, G., et al (eds.): Basic and Advanced in Vitreous Surgery. New York, Springer-Verlag, 1986.

5b. Charles, S.: Vitreous Microsurgery. 2nd ed. Baltimore, Williams & Wilkins, 1987.

5c. Hornblass, A.: Oculolastic, Orbital and Reconstructive Surgery. Vol. 1. Eyelids. Baltimore, Williams & Wilkins, 1988.

5d. Jaffe, N. S., (ed.): Atlas of Ophthalmic Surgery. Philadelphia, J. B. Lippincott, 1988.

5e. Stark, W. J.: Anterior Segment Surgery: Intraocular Lenses, Lasers and Refractive Keratoplasty. Baltimore, Williams & Wilkins, 1986.

5f. Waring, G.: Radial Keratotomy. St. Louis, C. V. Mosby, 1989.

5g. Weinstein, G. W., Spaeth, G.: Cataract Surgery Perspectives from Ophthalmic Surgery. Thorofare, NJ, Slack Inc., 1987.

5h. Williams, B. Ophthalmic Surgical Assisting. Wolfe, C. (ed.), Thorofare, NJ, Slack Inc., 1988.

6. Heilmann, K., Paton, D.: Atlas of Ophthalmic Surgery. New York, Thieme Medical Publishers, 1987. (Three volumes)

7. Jaffe, N. S.: Cataract Surgery and Its Complications. St. Louis, C. V. Mosby Co., (4th ed) 1984.

8. Unterman, S. R., Rowsey, J. J.: Diamond knife corneal incisions. Ophthalmic Surg., 15:199, 1984.

9. Galbavy, E. J.: Use of diamond knives in ocular surgery. Ophthalmic Surg., 15:203, 1984.

10. Sternberg, I., Gassner, S., Sternberg, N.: A new concept of a needle holder. Ocular Ther. Surg., 2:23, 1983.

11. Rizzuti, A. B.: Clinical Evaluation of Suture Materials and Needles in Surgery of the Cornea and Lens. New York, International Eye Foundation, 1968.

12. Paton, D.: A selection of current cataract incision and wound closure techniques. Highlights Ophthalmol., 13:1, 1971.

13. White, R. H., Jr., Parks, M. M.: Polyglycolic acid sutures in ophthalmic surgery. Trans. Am. Acad. Ophthalmol. Otolaryngol., 78:632, 1974.

14. Helveston, E. M., Meyers, S. F.: Synthetic absorbable suture. Ophthalmic Surg., 5:63, 1974.

15. Munton, C. G. F., Phillips, C. I., Martin, B., et al.: Vicryl® (polyglactin 910): A new synthetic absorbable suture in ophthalmic surgery. A preliminary study. Br. J. Ophthalmol., 58:941, 1974.

16. Wille, C. R., McPherson, S. D., Jr.: Evaluation of 8–0 chromic collagen suture material. South. Med. J., 67:54, 1974.

17. Blayden, J. E.: The evaluation of 7–0 polyglactin 910 suture in cataract surgery. Ophthalmic Surg., 6:99, 1975.

18. Chatterjee, S.: Comparative trial of Dexon (polyglycolic acid), collagen, and silk sutures in ophthalmic surgery. Br. J. Ophthalmol., 59:736, 1975.

19. Williamson, D. E.: The use of polyglycolic acid sutures in outpatient cataract surgery. Ann. Ophthalmol., 8:333, 1976.

20. Adams, I. W., Bell, M. S., Driver, R. M., Fry, W. G.: Hospital practice: A comparative trial of polyglycolic acid and silk as suture material for accidental wounds. Lancet, 2:1216, 1977.

21. Ullerich, K., Muxfeld, H.: Physikalische Untersuchungen an augenärztlichem Nahtmaterial, Einfluss der Mikrochirurgie auf die Verfeinerung des Nahtmaterials. Ber. Dtsch. Ophthalmol. Ges., 70:331, 1970.

22. Henriquez, A. S., Robertson, D. M., Rosen, D. A.: Tolerance of the cornea and eyelid to polyglycolic acid and rat-tail tendon sutures. Canad. J. Ophthalmol., 9:89, 1974.

23. Harnisch, J.-P., Loschau, G.: Scanning electron microscopic investigations of synthetic suture material. Klin. Monatsbl. Augenheilkd., 166:131, 1975.

24. Faulborn, J., Theopold, H.: Experimentelle Studien über Prolene 10–0 und Vicryl 11–0 Nahtmaterial im Vergleich zur Nylon 10–0 an der Kaninchenhornhaut. Klin. Monatsbl. Augenheilkd., 170:605, 1977.

25. Blaydes, J. E., Berry, J.: A comparative evaluation of 9–0 monofilament and a 9–0 braid polyglactin 910 in cataract surgery. Ophthalmic Surg., 10:49, 1979.

26. Cowden, J. W.: The clinical evaluation of 9.0 and 10.0 monofilament polyglactin 910 absorbable suture for corneal surgery. Ophthalmic Surg., 10:50, 1979.

27. Sugar, A.: Evaluation of 9–0 polyglycolic acid and polyglactin suture in rabbit limbal wounds. Ophthalmic Surg., 11:335, 1980.

28. Blaydes, J. E., Werblin, T. P.: 9–0 monofilament polydioxanone (PDS): A new investigational synthetic absorbable suture for cataract wound closure. Ophthalmic Surg., 13:644, 1982.

29. Faulborn, J., Gülececk, O.: Über die Eignung resorbierbarer Fäden (PDS) zur Versorgung von Hornhaut Wunden. Klin. Monatsbl. Augenheilkd., 183:464, 1983.

30. Clayman, H. M.: Polypropylene. Ophthalmology, 88:959, 1981.

31. Cohan, B. E., Leenslag, J. W., Miles, J., et al.: An evaluation of ultrastrong suture and refractive status. Arch. Ophthalmol., 103:1816, 1985.

32. Gaskin, E. R., Childers, M. D.: Increased granuloma formation from absorbable sutures. J.A.M.A., 185:212, 1963.

33. Apt, L., Costenbader, F. D., Parks, M. M., Albert, D. G.: Catgut allergy in eye muscle surgery. Arch. Ophthalmol., 65:474, 1961.

34. Klemetti, A.: Late complications of 7–0 polyglycolic (Dexon) sutures in cataract surgery. Acta Ophthalmol., 57:33, 1979.

35. Cox, A. G., Simpson, J. E. P.: Polyglycolic-acid suture material in skin closure (letter). Lancet, 1:452, 1975.

36. Boruchoff, S. A., Donshik, P. C.: Degradation of "non-absorbable" sutures. Ophthalmic Surg., 8:42, 1977.

37. Kronenthal, R. L.: Intraocular degradation of non-absorbable sutures. Am. Intraocular Implant Soc. J., 3:222, 1977.

38. Aronson, S. B., Moore, T. E., Jr.: Suture reaction in the rabbit cornea. Arch. Ophthalmol., 82:531, 1969.

39. Moore, T. E., Jr., Aronson, S. B.: Suture reaction in the human cornea. Arch. Ophthalmol., 82:575, 1969.

40. Stewart, R. H., Kimbrough, R. L.: Complications of 10–0 nylon sutures. Ophthalmic Surg., 10:19, 1979.

41. Olson, R. J.: Complications associated with running 11–0 nylon suture in penetrating keratoplasty. Ophthalmic Surg., 13:558, 1982.

42. Kronenthal, R. L.: Nylon in the anterior chamber. Ophthalmology, 88:965, 1981.

43. Soong, H. K., Kenyon, K. R.: Adverse reactions to virgin silk sutures in cataract surgery. Ophthalmology, 91:479, 1984.

44. Rea, R. L.: The parallel cornea-scleral suture in cataract operations. Trans. Ophthalmol. Soc. U.K., 60:300, 1935.

45. Jolson, A. S.: The adjustable slipknot. J Occup. Ther. Surg., 3:187, 1984.

46. Postlethwait, R. W., Schauble, J. F., Dillon, M. L., Morgan, J.: Wound healing. II. An evaluation of surgical suture material. Surg. Gynec. Obstet., 108:555, 1959.

47. Fischbein, F. I.: Comparative evaluation of 10–0 monofilament nylon versus 7–0 chromic suture in cataract surgery. Ophthalmic Surg., 4:31, 1973.

48. Jones, S. M., Shorey, B. A.: Polyglycolic-acid suture and scar hypertrophy. Lancet, 2:775, 1975.

49. Cravy, T. V.: A modified suture placement technique to avoid suture drag or "cheese wire" effect. Ophthalmic Surg., 11:338, 1980.

50. Ryan, S., Maumenee, A. E.: The running interlocking suture in cataract surgery. Arch. Ophthalmol., 85:302, 1971.

51. McNeill, J. I., Kaufman, H. E.: A double running suture technique for keratoplasty: earlier visual rehabilitation. Ophthalmic Surg., 8:58, 1977.

52. Binder, P. S.: Evaluation of through-and-through corneal sutures. Arch. Ophthalmol., 96:1886, 1978.

53. Metz, D., Ackerman, J., Kanarek, I.: Use of argon laser in suture removal after cataract surgery. Am. J. Ophthalmol., 97:393, 1984.

54. Bendel, L., Reynolds, E., Stoffel, F.: Ophthalmic needles: An engineering analysis. Ophthalmology, 93:61, 1986.

5

ANESTHESIA

by Richard P. Wilson

Anesthetic requirements for intraocular surgery differ from those for most other kinds of surgery. Proper anesthetic technique is of major importance for the successful outcome of surgery as well as for the continued well-being of the patient. Both intraoperative and postoperative complications can seriously affect the patient's health. This is especially true for the young and the elderly, the two groups that constitute the majority of ophthalmic surgical practice.

REQUIREMENTS FOR OPHTHALMIC ANESTHESIA

The following objectives should be met to assure optimal surgical results with intraocular procedures:

1. Akinesia of the globe and lids
2. Anesthesia of the globe and adnexa
3. Control of intraocular pressure
4. Control of systemic blood pressure
5. Relaxation of the patient undergoing local anesthesia
6. Absence of untoward episodes during the induction or maintenance of anesthesia (e.g., oculocardiac reflex, malignant hyperthermia)
7. Smooth emergence from the anesthetic state without vomiting, blood pressure fluctuations, coughing, or respiratory depression
8. Adequate postoperative analgesia

The priority of these criteria depends on the health of the patient, the nature of the eye disease, and the surgical procedure. As an example, for a healthy young patient undergoing penetrating keratoplasty, the major requirement is complete akinesia of the eye. For an elderly individual with far-advanced glaucoma undergoing combined cataract–glaucoma surgery, close control of both intraocular pressure and systemic blood pressure is crucial; a hypotensive episode could cause wipe-out of the small remaining field.

Close cooperation and communication between the anesthesiologist and the surgeon are essential if each patient's requirements are to be satisfied. The surgeon must ensure that the patient is in optimum physical condition, consulting the patient's private physician and subspecialists as necessary to achieve this. He must inform the anesthesiologist of any medications the patient may have been taking that would affect anesthesia (e.g., echothiophate, systemic steroids). He must also take from the patient a history regarding possible bleeding diatheses (e.g., easy bruising, hemorrhaging during previous surgical procedures or dental extractions, obstetrical problems).

The anesthesiologist should determine the patient's physical status and ability to undergo anesthesia. Useful questions include the following: Have you had anesthesia before? How much physical exercise do you get? Do you routinely take any drugs? Have you ever had any adverse reactions to medications? Are you allergic to any drugs? Have you any capped, loose, or broken teeth? Is there any family history of problems with anesthesia?[1]

During the operation all of the surgeon's attention is focused on the surgical field. This leaves the anesthetist the responsibilities of administering the sedation or anesthesia and monitoring the patient.[2] Pending legislation in Congress may strip the ophthalmologist of this assistance in Medicare patients who require local anesthesia for cataract surgery. Even with an anesthetist monitoring the patient, the surgeon, as leader of the surgical team, may be legally responsible for patient care in its entirety. In this role he must be capable of recognizing anesthetic-related complications at an early stage, developing a differential diagnosis to include the common causes, and carrying out necessary treatment with or without the assistance of the anesthetist.

LOCAL ANESTHESIA

Topical Anesthesia

Proparacaine and tetracaine are the most widely used topical anesthetics (Table 5–1). Butacaine, dibucaine, phenacaine, and piperocaine have lost favor, owing to problems with irritation, allergy, and toxicity.[3] Proparacaine is a benzoic acid ester and tetracaine, a para-aminobenzoic acid ester. Proparacaine and benoxinate have a rapid onset of action, and little irritation is associated with their application, making them good choices for tonometry. Tetracaine penetrates tissue more deeply than the other two, but produces a stinging sensation that may last for up to 30 seconds. Along with proparacaine and lidocaine, tetracaine is among the topical anesthetics that are least toxic to the epithelium. All of these agents, however, in a dose-related manner,[4] delay the healing of epithelial defects by inhibiting cell division and migration, and should seldom be used except for surgery or diagnostic tests.[5, 6] When used repeatedly, as during surgery, the toxicity is cumulative, and care should be taken to keep the cornea moist and to minimize trauma. When used in conjunction with a facial nerve block, the eye should be patched postoperatively to prevent corneal drying and epithelial slough.

Patients who are most susceptible to postoperative superficial corneal problems are those with dry eyes. Corneal erosion and massive superficial punctate keratitis may follow exposure to the operating microscope or extended contact with gonioscopic solution, as during a panretinal photocoagulation or laser trabeculoplasty. Liberal use of ocular lubricants for weeks or, in rare cases, months may be required to return the cornea to its normal state.

Except for cocaine, serious systemic reactions to topical anesthetics are almost nonexistent. Localized hypersensitivity may develop either to the agent itself or to preservatives in the vehicle. However, cocaine (Fig. 5–1), the first local anesthetic to be clinically used,[7] affords excellent surface anesthesia with 1% to 4% solution as well as scleral and conjunctival vasoconstriction. However, it has a greater frequency of adverse reactions. These include mydriasis without cycloplegia,[3] potentially more of a problem with occludable angles than when cycloplegia deepens the anterior chamber, and a marked loosening of the corneal epithelium, which may lead to large erosions. Because it

TABLE 5–1. Topical Anesthetic Agents*

AGENT	TRADE NAME	CONCENTRATION
Benoxinate HCl (combined with fluorescein sodium 0.25%	Fluress	0.4%
Cocaine HCl		1%–4%
Proparacaine HCl	Ak-taine	0.5%
	Alcaine	0.5%
	Ophthaine	0.5%
	Ophthetic	0.5%
Tetracaine HCl	Anacel	0.5%
	Pontocaine	0.5%
Onset within 1 minute Duration of action 10 to 20 minutes		

*Only currently marketed topical anesthetics in United States. (From Physicians' Desk Reference for Ophthalmology. Oradell, NJ, Medical Economics Co, 1987.)

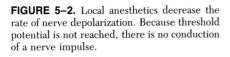

FIGURE 5–1. Chemical structure of cocaine.

acts systemically to block the reuptake of nor-epinephrine at the neuron level, cocaine may produce hypertensive crisis in patients who are also on reserpine, guanethidine, methyldopa, or monoamine oxidase inhibitors.[8]

Regional Anesthesia

Most local anesthetics belong to one of two groups, determined by structural differences. The amino esters, which include cocaine, pro-caine, chloroprocaine, and tetracaine, contain an ester linkage between the benzene ring and the intermediate chain. They have low toxicity and a rapid onset of action, but are infrequently used in ophthalmic surgery because of a very short duration of action.[9] The amino amides, including bupivacaine, etidocaine, lidocaine, mepivacaine, and prilocaine, have an amide link between the benzene ring and the intermediate chain. These agents have a longer duration of action, but are more toxic.[10]

Structural differences also determine the rate and route of metabolism of the agents. The ester-linked anesthetics are hydrolyzed in the plasma by the enzyme pseudocholinesterase. The amino amides undergo enzymatic degradation in liver microsomes.

Pharmacology

Local anesthetics produce their effects by preventing the resting potential in nerve endings from reaching threshold potential (i.e.,

firing level) (Fig. 5–2). The normal resting potential, a polarization across the cell wall, is -60 to -90 mV. When stimulated, the membrane slowly depolarizes until threshold potential is reached; a rapid depolarization then occurs as the nerve fires. After the depolarization phase is complete, the resting potential of the nerve membrane is reestablished by a slow repolarization.

The potential produced across the nerve cell membrane is the result of different concentrations of ions, mainly potassium and sodium, in the cell versus the extracellular fluid. The nerve membrane at rest is quite permeable to potassium ions, but only minimally so to sodium ions. Stimulation increases the permeability to sodium ions and depolarizes the cell membrane. At $+40$ mV, the action potential peak, sodium permeability decreases and potassium ions move into the extracellular fluid. Repolarization continues until the resting potential is reached.

The effect of local anesthetic agents on this process is to block the movement of sodium across the nerve membrane. Without the rapid flux of sodium ions, depolarization never reaches threshold potential, and nerve conduction is blocked. Therefore, local anesthetics produce a nonpolarizing block. The smaller fibers, autonomic in nature, are blocked first, followed by the sensory fibers, until finally the largest fibers, motor and proprioceptive, are blocked.[11] Low concentrations of anesthetic (e.g., bupivacaine 0.25% versus 0.75%) may give a sensory block without paralysis.[12, 13]

The effectiveness of the different anesthetic agents is determined by physical chemical properties such as lipid solubility, protein binding, and pKa.* Because the nerve membrane is mostly lipid, the intrinsic activity of the different agents depends on their lipid solubility; for

---

*The pKa value is the pH of a half neutralized solution of acid. Weak acids have high pKa values and strong acids low pKa values.

FIGURE 5–2. Local anesthetics decrease the rate of nerve depolarization. Because threshold potential is not reached, there is no conduction of a nerve impulse.

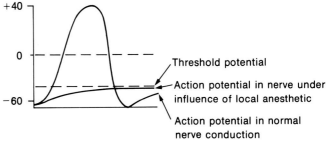

example, in the amide group, a butyl group added to the amide of mepivacaine forms bupivacaine, which is 35 times more lipid soluble and 4 times more potent than mepivacaine.

The duration of anesthesia seems to depend on the binding affinity of the agent for the proteins in the nerve membrane. The greater the protein binding, the longer the anesthesia will endure. Tetracaine has 10 times more protein binding capacity than procaine and lasts 3 to 4 times longer.[14]

The rapidity of onset for each local anesthetic is a function of its pH and pKa. The agent exists in solution in both a charged ion and an uncharged base; the proportion of each depends on the pKa of the drug and the pH of the tissue. The proportion of the agent in the base form determines the onset of action, since the uncharged form diffuses more quickly across the nerve sheath.[12]

At tissue pH of 7.4, lidocaine and mepivacaine, each with a relatively low pKa, are approximately 35 per cent in the base form and possess a rapid onset of action. Tetracaine and procaine have a much higher pKa and are primarily in the ionic state (80 to 95 per cent) at pH 7.4. They therefore have a slower onset of action.[12]

Regional anesthetics produce peripheral vasodilation by a direct relaxant effect on vascular smooth muscle; the stronger the agent, the greater the vasodilation. This effect encourages vascular absorption, so that less drug is available and the agent is thus less effective. Epinephrine added to the anesthetic solution in dilute concentrations (1:200,000)[15, 16] will counter the vasodilation of the local anesthetic, producing a longer-acting block and reducing peak blood levels. This allows a greater amount of anesthetic to be administered without systemic toxicity. The increased duration depends on the agent used. Lidocaine has a much longer duration of action in combination with epinephrine. The action of prilocaine and mepivacaine is prolonged, but to a lesser extent, and bupivacaine and etidocaine are not prolonged at all.[17, 18] The added epinephrine also decreases bleeding and counteracts the depressing effects of local anesthetics on the cardiovascular system. Epinephrine, however, introduces risks of its own. It is not needed with ophthalmic anesthesia other than for oculoplastic procedures, and it is not recommended. Patients with hypertension, diabetes, cardiovascular disease, or thyrotoxicosis are especially prone to the serious side effects of epinephrine, and patients under

halothane anesthesia are subject to an increased risk of cardiac fibrillation with its use.[3] Glaucoma may be a contraindication to the use of epinephrine, as a significant decrease in ophthalmic artery pulse pressure has been reported when epinephrine was added to the local anesthetic.[19]

Hyaluronic acid, a viscous polysaccharide found in the extracellular space, inhibits diffusion of injected solutions. The addition of hyaluronidase, an enzyme that hydrolyzes hyaluronic acid, to the anesthetic solution enhances rapid diffusion through tissue. A greater area is thus anesthetized, and the induction time of anesthesia is markedly lowered (e.g., from 10 minutes to 3 minutes for retrobulbar mepivacaine[20]), but the rapid absorption of the anesthetic agent may increase the chances of toxicity. The enzyme is measured in turbidity reducing units (TRU), the usual ophthalmic solution being 7.5 to 15.0 TRU per 1 ml of anesthetic solution.

The choice of the local anesthetic agent for each procedure is a matter of personal preference. The onset of action, duration of action, and safe dosage for each of the various regional anesthetic agents are given in Table 5–2. The agent used most commonly for retrobulbar, facial, and plastic surgery blocks at the Wills Eye Hospital in Philadelphia is mepivacaine, which has a duration of action of up to 2 hours. For surgical procedures expected to last for 1½ hours or more, bupivacaine or etidocaine is preferable.[7, 21–26] The duration of anesthesia they afford is significantly longer than with any other commonly used agent, and a period of analgesia remains after return of motor function and tactile sensation, thus extending the length of time before postoperative analgesics are needed.[27] This also makes it an ideal agent for cryopexy and cyclocryotherapy, procedures that often produce a considerable amount of pain after the local anesthetic wears off. If bupivacaine or etidocaine is also used for the facial block, however, appropriate steps must be taken to protect the cornea during the long duration of akinesia.

When added to local anesthetic solutions, hyaluronidase allows rapid and consistent blocks. In patients for cataract surgery the extent of the block and its effect on intraocular pressure can be evaluated with minimal waiting. Hyaluronidase also helps to limit the rise of intraocular pressure that may occur transiently with retrobulbar injection. Similarly, tissue distortion from local anesthetics is ame-

TABLE 5–2. Regional Anesthetic Agents

AGENT (TRADE NAME)	CHEMICAL STRUCTURE	CHEMICAL CLASS	CONCENTRATION	MAXIMUM DOSE (mg)	RELATIVE POTENCY	ONSET OF ACTION	DURATION OF ACTION
Procaine (Novocaine)	$H_2N-\langle\rangle-COOCH_2CH_2-N\langle^{C_2H_5}_{C_2H_5}$	Ester	1%–4%	500	1	7–8 min	30–45 min
Chloroprocaine (Nesacaine)	$H_2N-\langle\rangle(Cl)-COOCH_2CH_2-N\langle^{C_2H_5}_{C_2H_5}$	Ester	1%–3%	800	1	6–12 min	60 min
Mepivacaine (Carbocaine)	NHCO / ring with CH₃, N-CH₃	Amide	1%–2%	500	2	3–5 min	120 min
Lidocaine (Xylocaine, Dalcaine)	$NHCOCH_2-N\langle^{C_2H_5}_{C_2H_5}$, CH₃/CH₃	Amide	1%–2%	500	2	4–6 min	40–60 min
Bupivacaine (Marcaine, Sensorcaine)	NHCO / ring N–C₄H₉, CH₃/CH₃	Amide	0.25%–0.75%	175	8	5–11 min	4–12 hr
Etidocaine (Duranest)	$NHCOCH\langle^{C_2H_5}... -N\langle^{C_2H_5}_{C_3H_7}$, CH₃/CH₃	Amide	1%–1.5%	400	8	3–5 min	5–10 hr

Modified from Raj PP: Handbook of Regional Anesthesia. New York: Churchill Livingstone, 1985; Physicians' Desk Reference for Ophthalmology. Oradell, NJ: Medical Economics Co, 1987; Crandall DC: Pharmacology of ocular anesthetics. In Duane TD, Jaeger EA (eds): Biomedical Foundations of Ophthalmology. Philadelphia, Harper & Row, 1986) liorated for oculoplastic surgery when the enzyme is added to the anesthetic solution.[28]

Because of its systemic effects, most anesthesiologists discourage the use of epinephrine in local anesthetic solutions for retrobulbar anesthesia. One study has suggested that the use of hyaluronidase in combination with the local anesthetic does not shorten its duration of action as previously thought.[11, 29] Therefore, the addition of epinephrine to local anesthetic solutions whenever hyaluronidase is used may be neither necessary nor desirable. If a longer-acting block is needed, bupivacaine or etidocaine should be used. The major indication for the adjunct use of epinephrine is to inhibit bleeding in vascular areas.

The admixture of a short-acting anesthetic to bupivacaine might seem to overcome the main criticism to its use, the longer and more variable onset. However, studies have shown this to be unnecessary as long as hyaluronidase was used to potentiate the action of bupivacaine or etidocaine.[30] If such a mixture is chosen, however, it appears that the combination of mepivacaine–bupivacaine is superior to that of lidocaine–bupivacaine.[31]

Toxicity

The major systemic effects of local anesthetics are excitation of the central nervous system and depression of the cardiovascular system (Table 5–3). The seriousness of these reactions is underlined by reports of death occurring in young, healthy patients during minor operations. Preferably, all patients have an intravenous infusion started before administration of local anesthetic, along with monitoring of their electrocardiogram, blood pressure, and pulse. Oxygen is administered by way of nasal cannula throughout the procedure.

Toxic effects of local anesthetics are dose related. Because the concentration sufficient to cause a neural blockade is nearly 600 times that required to cause serious systemic effects,[10, 13] toxicity is directly related to systemic absorption. This in turn is related to the amount of drug used, rate of injection, vascularity of the area injected and vasoactive properties of the drug, toxicity of the drug, and its rate of deactivation and excretion. Neurological effects result from passage of the anesthetic through the blood–brain barrier with blockage of inhibitory pathways and secondary central nervous system excitation. Cardiac effects stem from the stabilizing effects of local anesthetics on the cell membranes of the myocardium. The drugs cause a drop in conduction rate, contraction force, and excitability.

Exaggerated central nervous system and cardiac side effects, from either overdose, unintentional intravascular injection of a usual dose, or extraordinarily quick absorption from a very vascular tissue, produce a typical pattern. A common prodrome is garrulousness, perioral numbness and tingling, diplopia, and tinnitus. Tremors and muscle twitching may progress to generalized myoclonic seizure with depression of the nervous system if blood levels are high. Along with loss of consciousness and respiratory depression, circulatory collapse may develop as a result of the depressant effect on the myocardium and peripheral vasodilation. Hypoxia and acidosis accompany these changes.[32] Respiratory arrest and grand mal seizures have followed retrobulbar injection of bupivacaine and bupivacaine combined with lidocaine or mepivacaine.[33, 34] Direct injection of anesthetic into the subdural space surrounding the optic nerve allows a small amount of anesthetic agent direct access into the subdural space surrounding the pons and midbrain.[35, 36] This would result in respiratory arrest without prior cardiovascular symptoms.[37] Supporting this is the report of three cases of reversible contralateral amaurosis after retrobulbar anesthesia. The only plausible explanation for this occurrence is the dissection of anesthetic solution along the subdural space of the optic nerve back to the chiasm and the contralateral nerve.[38, 39]

Another proposed explanation is the rupture of an arterial wall in the presence of a large volume of anesthetic under sufficient pressure to allow the drug to enter the arterial system and flow in a retrograde manner to the cerebral circulation.[40] Several studies support this possibility.[41, 42] Injection of anesthetic into the venous system is an unlikely cause, as the total

TABLE 5–3. Signs of Local Anesthetic Toxicity

CENTRAL NERVOUS SYSTEM	
Mild	Severe
Tingling	Muscle twitching
Tinnitus	Generalized myoclonic
Diplopia	seizure
Drowsiness	Respiratory depression
Disorientation	Unconsciousness
CARDIOVASCULAR SYSTEM	
Decreased heart rate	Sinus bradycardia
Decreased cardiac output	Cardiac failure
Falling blood pressure	Hypotension
	Asystole

dose given with retrobulbar anesthesia is less than the toxic intravenous dose.

Postoperative diplopia can be ascribed not only to gross intraorbital hemorrhage, and isolated intramuscular hemorrhage, both mechanical causes, but also to the myotoxicity of local anesthetics. Lidocaine and, to a lesser extent, bupivacaine have been shown to cause a toxic degeneration of muscle fibers with later regeneration. This effect can lead to transient diplopia in the postoperative period.[43]

The incidence of the side effects mentioned above is low, but significant. In one study[44] 9 of 1000 patients for cataract surgery developed a complication with local anesthesia. Eight had hypotension that required intervention with pressor agents or other intravenous drugs. One case of respiratory arrest occurred within 5 minutes of a retrobulbar block using 0.75% bupivicaine and 2% lidocaine. In another study[35] respiratory arrest occurred on three occasions in 1500 consecutive cases.

Prevention of these serious side effects should be in the mind of anyone using local anesthetics. The most common cause of toxicity is overdosage. The smallest effective volume of the lowest concentration should be used, and the dose adjusted to the patient's weight. To avoid intravascular injection, aspiration before injection and, when possible, movement of the needle during injection should be practiced. Lidocaine and mepivacaine, nonester anesthetics that are degraded in the liver at a slower rate than the ester anesthetics are hydrolyzed, should be used with caution when large doses are required.[45, 46] When symptoms of toxicity appear, injection of the drug should be stopped. Oxygen should be given at a high flow rate to raise the patient's oxygen reserve if convulsions should follow. If convulsions—or even tremors and muscle twitching—occur, intravenous diazepam (5–10 mg) or rapid-onset barbiturates (thiopental sodium, 50–100 mg) should be administered. If the seizure cannot be controlled, succinylcholine, intubation, and 100% oxygen are required. Intravenous infusions and vasopressors are used as needed for hypotension. Cardiac arrest, if it occurs, is treated in the usual manner.[47]

Regional Blocks

Anatomy. Sensation in the eye, orbit, and periorbital tissues is mediated by the first two divisions of cranial nerve V, the trigeminal nerve (Fig. 5–3). The first division, the ophthalmic nerve, divides into the frontal, nasociliary, and lacrimal nerves, all of which enter the orbit through the superior orbital fissure. The frontal nerve, while still in the orbit, further divides into the supratrochlear and supraorbital nerves. The supratrochlear nerve exists from the orbit above the trochlea, supplying the medial part of the lid. A needle inserted along the medial wall of the orbit to a depth of ½ inch with a small amount of anesthetic will block this area (Fig. 5–4).

The supraorbital branch of the frontal nerve innervates the central upper lid, the superior

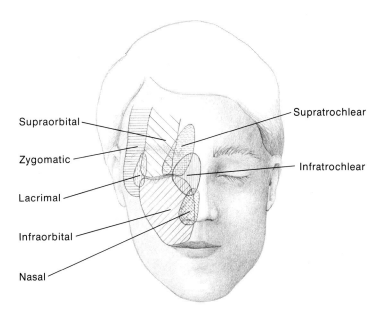

FIGURE 5–3. Sites for regional anesthesia blocks. The anatomy of this region, including the location of the nerves, is detailed in Figure 16–1B.

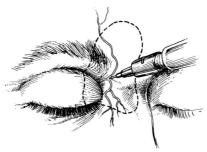

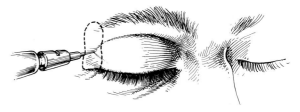

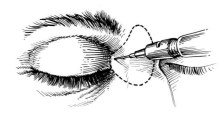

FIGURE 5–6. The lacrimal nerve is blocked by an injection along the outer wall of the orbit to a depth of 1 inch. The area of anesthesia produced is outlined.

FIGURE 5–4. The supratrochlear nerve is blocked by injection of anesthetic just above the trochlea to a depth of ½ inch. The area of expected anesthesia is outlined.

conjunctiva, and the supraorbital portion of the forehead. After running just inferior to the orbital roof from the superior fissure, the nerve emerges over the orbital rim at the supraorbital notch, an easily palpable landmark. Injection here provides an effective block. If the needle is inserted posteriorly along the roof of the orbit 1¼ inches deep to a point just lateral to the supraorbital notch, a block encompassing both branches of the frontal nerve can be obtained, and bleeding from the vessel in the supraorbital notch avoided (Fig. 5–5).

The lacrimal nerve supplies the lacrimal gland and lateral upper lid; it can be blocked with an injection along the upper outer wall of the orbit to a depth of 1 inch (Fig. 5–6).

The nasociliary nerve, a branch of the first division, divides into the anterior and posterior ethmoidal nerves and the infratrochlear nerve, which supplies the inner canthus and lacrimal sac plus the adjacent nasal skin. By injecting anesthetic just superior to the medial canthal ligament along the inner wall of the orbit 1 in.

posterior to the orbital rim, one can provide an effective block of these structures (Fig. 5–7).

The maxillary or second division of the trigeminal nerve enters the orbit through the infraorbital fissure, where it becomes the infraorbital nerve. It passes through the infraorbital canal and out the infraorbital foramen, which is palpable as a small depression in the maxilla, two-thirds of an inch inferior to the midpoint of the lower lid. This nerve supplies sensory fibers to the greatest part of the lower lid and cheek as well as to part of the inner canthus and lacrimal sac. The infraorbital nerve can be blocked as it enters the canal by an injection along the floor of the orbit ½ inch deep to the rim. This will also anesthetize the nasolacrimal duct and the floor of the nose.[10, 48] To block only the skin distribution, the needle may be placed at the external opening of the foramen and, after aspiration, 2 ml of anesthetic injected (Fig. 5–8).

The blocks described so far are used largely for plastic procedures. Intraocular surgery, however, requires complete akinesia of the lids and extraocular muscles. Traditional approaches are those described by O'Brien, Atkinson, and Van Lint, accompanied by a retrobulbar block.

Van Lint Block. Van Lint first described an infiltrative block with local anesthetic for cataract extraction.[49] First a small skin wheal is made at the lateral orbit rim and then the needle is inserted along the inferotemporal rim

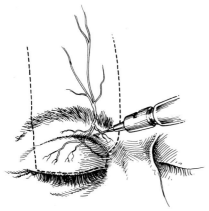

FIGURE 5–5. A block of the supraorbital branch of the frontal nerve is obtained by injection of anesthetic just lateral to the supraorbital notch to a depth of 1¼ inches along the roof of the orbit. Anesthesia of the outlined area will result.

FIGURE 5–7. An injection of anesthesia just above the medial canthal ligament to a depth of 1 inch will block the branches of the nasociliary nerve. These supply the area outlined.

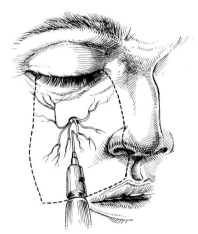

FIGURE 5–8. The lower lid and much of the cheek (outlined area) can be blocked by injection of anesthesia at the mouth of the infraorbital foramen. The nerve can also be blocked as it enters the canal on the floor of the orbit ½ inch deep to the rim.

for an inch or more and 3 to 5 milliliters of anesthetic is injected as the needle is withdrawn. Through the same wheal a similar injection is carried out along the superotemporal orbital rim. This produces an excellent block, especially if pressure is applied to the area to help the diffusion of anesthetic. A side effect of this method is variable swelling of the lids. The Van Lint block can be modified by placing the injections more laterally over the lateral wall of the orbit, catching the facial nerve as it crosses the periosteum, yet avoiding the lid edema (Fig. 5–9).

O'Brien Block. To avoid periorbital edema, O'Brien developed a method to block the facial nerve over the condyle of the mandible inferior to the posterior zygomatic process. Two milliliters of anesthetic are injected anterior to the tragus of the ear over the head of the condyle. The head of the condyle in the area of the temporomandibular joint can be identified by

asking the patient to open and close his mouth while feeling the condyle move anteriorly out from under the zygomatic process. Because the course of the facial nerve is not always predictable, and the O'Brien block does not always achieve complete akinesia, further modification is often necessary. After the classic O'Brien injection, the needle is withdrawn to just beneath the skin and directed inferiorly along the posterior edge of the ramus of the mandible for about 1 inch. Three milliliters of anesthetic is injected as the needle is withdrawn. The same procedure is followed with another injection anteriorly along the zygomatic arch for 1 inch. Pressure is applied to increase diffusion of the anesthetic (Fig. 5–10).

Atkinson Block. In the Atkinson method the facial nerve is blocked midway between its emergence from the stylomastoid foramen and the orbicularis muscle. The needle is introduced through a skin wheal at the inferior border of the zygoma directly inferior to the lateral orbital rim. The needle is directed first along the inferior edge of the zygomatic bone and then superiorly across the zygomatic arch, aiming at the top of the ear. About 3 ml of the drug is injected as the needle is advanced, and care is taken to stop before the superficial temporal vessels just anterior to the ear are encountered (Fig. 5–11).[50]

Spaeth Block. A block by Spaeth aims at avoiding the inconsistencies of the O'Brien block. This method involves making the injection proximal to the classic approach of O'Brien over the mandibular condyle, thereby catching the facial nerve before it divides (Fig. 5–12).

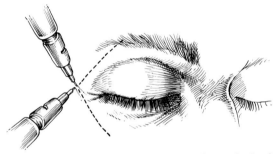

FIGURE 5–9. The Van Lint block can anesthetize the facial nerve branches to the orbicular muscle as they run over the periosteum just lateral to the orbit.

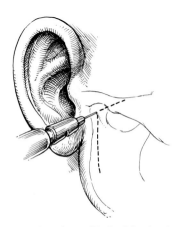

FIGURE 5–10. The O'Brien block of the facial nerve with its anterior and inferior extensions will provide paralysis of the orbicular muscle. It can be combined with the Van Lint block to ensure complete paralysis.

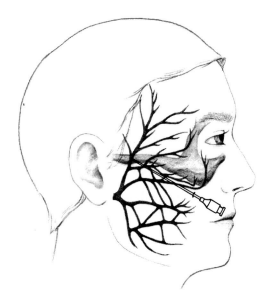

Atkinson akinesia

FIGURE 5–11. An alternative method of providing paralysis of the orbicular muscle proposed by Atkinson intercepts the facial nerve fibers as they cross the zygomatic arch.

The O'Brien block chiefly anesthetizes the superiormost branches of the facial nerve, the upper, lower, and zygomatic. These branches themselves may swing inferior to the point at which O'Brien's block begins to act, and peripheral branches of the facial nerve intercommunicate distal to this area. Rami communicantes spread up from the buccal and even the mandibular branches to the zygomatic branches that innervate the orbicularis oculi. Therefore, if the inferior branches of the facial nerve are not blocked, akinesia of the orbicularis may be incomplete. To perform the block described by Spaeth, the fingers are placed along the posterior border of the mandible as superiorly as possible. The needle is placed just anterior to the most superior finger; bone should be felt quickly. If not, the needle is withdrawn and landmarks rechecked before a second attempt is made. After the bone is reached, suction assures that a vessel has not been punctured. Then 5 ml of anesthetic is injected. Although usually not necessary, the needle can be pulled back until it rests under the skin and then directed slightly superiorly to the outer canthus for a distance of 1½ inches, where an additional 5 ml is injected. An almost complete unilateral facial palsy should be evidenced by 30 seconds.[51]

Nadbath Block. The Nadbath block also produces a complete facial block. It uses an injection into the concavity between the mastoid process and the posterior border of the mandibular ramus (Fig. 5–13). The injection starts with a skin wheal 1 to 2 mm anterior to the mastoid process and inferior to the external auditory canal. A 12-mm, 26-gauge needle is used, and injection of anesthetic extends from the skin wheal, passing through a taunt membrane midway down, to the full depth of the needle. A total of approximately 3 ml provides good results, and intermittent aspiration prevents inadvertent intravascular injection.

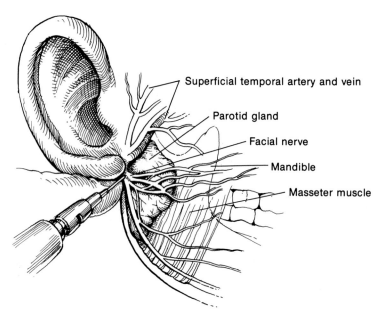

Superficial temporal artery and vein

Parotid gland

Facial nerve

Mandible

Masseter muscle

FIGURE 5–12. In the Spaeth modification of the O'Brien technique, the facial nerve is blocked where it crosses the posterior edge of the mandible, thus catching the nerve before it divides. This provides more complete paralysis of the inferior orbicular muscle.

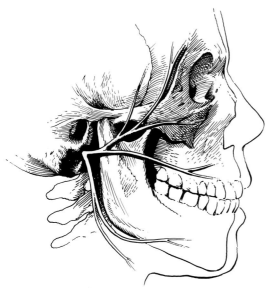

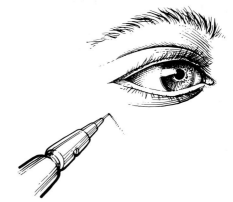

FIGURE 5–14. The needle during a retrobulbar injection should pass midway between the lateral and inferior recti with the eye elevated and adducted.

FIGURE 5–13. The Nadbath block catches the trunk of the facial nerve after its emergence from the stylomastoid foramen before it passes into the parotid gland.

The advantages of the Nadbath block are the ease of performance and the paucity of complaints concerning not only the original injection, but also jaw movement postoperatively.[52] Side effects include a bitter taste in the mouth as the parotid gland secretes the anesthetic.[53] Dysphonia, swallowing difficulty, and respiratory distress have been reported in 3 out of 300 blocks in one study and by several other authors. In the cases cited, 5 ml of anesthetic was used rather than the 3 ml recommended by Nadbath, and in the cases where it was reported, a 16-mm needle was used rather than a 12-mm needle, as recommended. Because this complication is predominantly seen in very thin patients and seems to stem from the spread of anesthetic to the jugular foramen 1 cm deeper than the stylomastoid foramen, the length of the needle and the depth of injection are crucial. The Nadbath block should never be done bilaterally or in patients with preexisting unilateral oropharyngeal or vocal cord dysfunction to avoid bilateral vocal cord paralysis. If signs of dysphonia or difficulty with swallowing or respiration occur, lateral positioning will allow for a clear airway.[54–56]

Retrobulbar Block. Retrobulbar injection of local anesthetic, if done properly, will provide akinesia of the extraocular muscles by blocking cranial nerves III, IV, and VI, and anesthesia to the conjunctiva, cornea, and uvea by blocking the ciliary nerves. The patient is instructed to look either straight ahead or upward and nasally at the surgeon's discretion (see below). A 1¼-inch or 23- or 25-gauge needle with a blunted tip is inserted through the lower lid midway between the lateral and inferior rectus muscles (Fig. 5–14). After the needle penetrates the orbital septum, and passes the equatorial region of the globe, it is directed upward toward the apex of the orbit. The bevel of the needle faces the globe, allowing the best possibility of a glancing rather than penetrating injury if contact with the globe is made (Fig. 5–15). A small amount of anesthetic may be injected as the needle progresses, pushing vessels out of its path, it is hoped. The operator can often feel the resistance offered by the orbital septum and the intermuscular septum. He can also usually judge when the tip of the needle is resting within the muscle cone and further penetration is unnecessary (Fig. 5–16). Aspiration before injection is appropriate whenever the needle is stationary. One to 3 ml of anesthetic is injected, and firm pressure is immediately applied for 10 seconds.

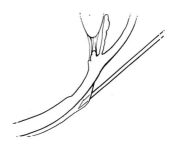

FIGURE 5–15. With the bevel of the needle facing the globe, there is more chance of a glancing rather than penetrating contact if the globe is encountered during a retrobulbar or sub-Tenon's injection.

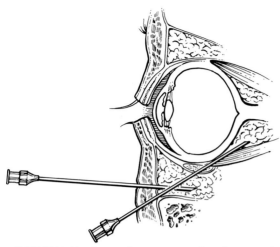

FIGURE 5–16. The anesthetic agent need not be injected deep in the orbit. Injection within the muscle cone is all that is necessary.

A less frequently used technique is to pull down the lower lid, with the patient looking up and nasally, inserting the needle through the inferior cul-de-sac. The direction and injection then proceed as described. For a quicker, more complete block hyaluronidase may be added to the local anesthetic.

Pressure is then intermittently applied to produce a soft eye with the greatest distribution of local anesthetic. The pressure is firm, applied for 10 to 20 seconds on and 5 to 10 seconds off, so that retinal circulation is not critically compromised. Alternative techniques such as the Honan balloon, the super-pinkie, or a mercury bag may be used to achieve the correct intraocular pressure.

After 5 to 10 minutes of pressure has been applied, the eye should be soft and almost immobile. The superior oblique muscle, outside the annulus of Zinn, will not be paralyzed after a retrobulbar block, and the eye may intort when the patient is instructed to look down. If significant movement persists, a supplemental retrobulbar injection and additional pressure may be required. Any nonparalyzed muscle may be injected separately.

Intraocular pressure should be checked either digitally or with a sterile tonometer before commencement of surgery. Surgery should ordinarily not be initiated until the eye becomes hypotonic.

COMPLICATIONS. Retrobulbar hemorrhage is an infrequent but unfortunate complication of retrobulbar injection. The globe becomes increasingly proptotic, and subconjunctival blood may become evident as the hemorrhage extends anteriorly. Blood may not become visible until the next day. Bleeding in a closed space raises the pressure and limits further hemorrhage, but intraocular pressure is elevated and surgery must usually be postponed. In most instances surgery can be performed 2 to 3 days later, preferably under general anesthesia. In cases in which the presence of blood in the episcleral tissues will interfere with the surgery, as with glaucoma filtering operations, the procedure should usually be deferred for at least 1 week.

In some instances the anesthetic is injected into the space between Tenon's capsule and the globe. The intraocular pressure rises dramatically, to 50 mm Hg or higher. However, there is no proptosis, ecchymosis, or other sign of retrobulbar hemorrhage. In cases in which the surgeon is sure that sub-Tenon's injection of anesthetic is the problem, he may choose to wait 5 to 10 minutes, by which time the agent will have diffused into the tissues and the pressure will have fallen to a satisfactorily low level. At that point it is usually safe to proceed with surgery, although the adequacy of akinesia and anesthesia of the globe should be checked and additional anesthetic given if needed.

Although retrobulbar injection with or without retrobulbar hemorrhage is usually not associated with sequelae, it has rarely been associated with total permanent loss of vision and optic atrophy. This is thought to be due to direct injury to the nerve by the needle, damage to its blood supply, or injection into the optic canal with compressive ischemia of the optic nerve. Disc and retinal edema and intraretinal, preretinal, and vitreous hemorrhage are usually seen on examination. Combined central retinal artery and vein occlusions have been described as a consequence of hemorrhage in the optic nerve sheath. Occasionally this hemorrhage can evolve slowly over several days. If diagnosed with computerized tomography or B-scan ultrasonography, optic nerve sheath decompression can improve the prognosis.[57–60]

When the toxic manifestations of presumed intraoptic nerve sheath injection are added to the complications above, it becomes clear that problems with retrobulbar injection are significant. Multiple authors have proposed modifications in technique to avoid side effects. Several advocate a change in the traditional Atkinson ocular position with the patient looking upward and inward at the time of retrobulbar block. Atkinson recommended positioning the globe in this manner "to move the inferior oblique muscle and the fascia between the lateral and inferior rectus muscles forward and upward, out of the way."[61] Computerized scanning of a cadaver orbit as a retrobulbar needle is introduced, however, has shown that this maneuver moves the optic nerve, the ophthalmic artery, the superior orbital vein, and the posterior pole of the globe adjacent to the needle tip, and places the optic nerve on stretch so that it is more easily pierced. The authors of that study[62] recommend that the patient's gaze be directed straight ahead or slightly downward and outward, and that the needle be directed toward the inferior part of the superior orbital fissure rather than toward the orbital apex, as recommended by Atkinson.

Other authors have suggested directing the needle through the inferior orbit in the sagittal plane of the lateral limbus and remaining in that plane at all times. This leaves the needle within the muscle cone but inferior to the globe and just nasal to the lateral rectus, well away from the optic nerve.[37] I and others believe that the traditional approach is acceptable as long as needle insertion is stopped and injection completed as soon as the surgeon feels the pop of the needle tip as it punctures the muscle cone. A 1.3-cm needle can be used to assure that the needle tip will not penetrate far enough to endanger the optic nerve.[63] With the eye looking down and out, the muscle cone is relaxed and the surgeon may have a more difficult time ascertaining when the needle tip is within the cone.

Posterior Peribulbar Block. Another alternative that appears safer than a retrobulbar block and provides adequate orbicularis akinesia without resorting to a facial block is the posterior peribulbar block (Figs. 5–17 and 5–18). This technique, introduced by Kelman and modified by others (Table 5–4), uses two stepped injections, one above the inferior orbital rim 1 cm medial to the lateral canthus and one just below the supraorbital notch, that

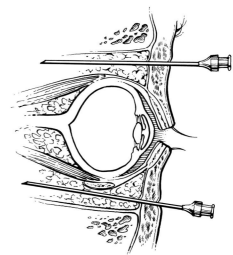

FIGURE 5–18. Lateral view of needle position for posterior peribulbar anesthesia.

deposit anesthetic at the level of the skin, the orbicularis muscle, just beneath the muscle, and in the posterior orbit. The advantages of this block include safety, less pain on injection and during the postoperative period, no postoperative loss of vision in one-eyed patients, and the ease of teaching the technique. The chief disadvantage is the wait for the block to be effective, variously described as 12 to 25 minutes often in conjunction with the "super pinkie" or other compression methods.[64]

Preoperative Preparation

Patients who undergo surgery using local anesthesia require careful preoperative preparation. This includes an explanation of the anesthetic technique, and the assurance that their preoperative medications will make them comfortable and allay their apprehension. They should be aware that an anesthetist will be with them to monitor their vital signs and give them additional intravenous analgesia or sedation as necessary. A short period in the preoperative room that allows the anesthetist to develop rapport with the patient and reassure him will go far to ensure a relaxed and cooperative patient.

Preoperative medications are individualized according to the type of surgery and the nature of the patient. When pain is probable, for example, in the case of a reoperation that cannot be done under general anesthesia because of the patient's poor health, a narcotic will supply helpful analgesia. When patient anxiety is a factor, an agent such as diazepam is often help-

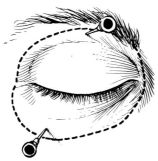

FIGURE 5–17. Anteroposterior view of needle position for posterior peribulbar anesthesia.

TABLE 5–4. Procedure for Posterior Peribulbar Block

With I.V. going or heparin lock in and after desired sedation and eyelid prep:

1. Make small skin wheal in lower eyelid 1 cm medial to lateral canthus over inferior orbital rim.
2. Make small skin wheal in upper eyelid in the skin fold directly inferior to the supraorbital foramen.
3. Through inferior skin wheal with 27-gauge needle inject 0.5 ml lidocaine 1% in orbicular muscle and inject 1 ml just deep to the muscle.
4. Through upper lid skin wheal repeat as in step 3.
5. Through lower lid skin wheal inject 1 ml lidocaine 1% with bupivacaine ¾% and hyaluronidase solution in the orbicular muscle and 1 ml immediately deep to it. Advance along the floor of the orbit to the equator of the eye; aspirate and inject 1 ml; aiming slightly superomedially, advance the needle to its full depth and inject 1.0 to 1.5 ml.
6. Pushing globe inferiorly with free index finger, enter through upper lid skin wheal and inject 1 ml 1/2 inch deep to the orbicular muscle and slightly nearer the canthus than is the original skin wheal; direct needle along orbital roof without engaging periosteum to the equator, where 1 ml is injected, and then to the superior orbital fissure, where a final 1 ml of solution is injected.
7. Pressure on the globe/orbit and time are essential to a good block; after 8 minutes if incomplete akinesia remains, 3 to 4 ml of additional anesthetic solution is injected by the lower approach if lateral or inferior movement is seen, by the superior approach if superior or medial movement is seen (always perform lower lid injections before upper lid injections).

Adapted from Nugent CC: Peribulbar anesthesia a safe, simple, effective, and relatively painless technique. Obtained from the author at Medical-Surgical Eye Center, 1237 B St., Hayward, CA 94541.

ful. This is currently the most frequently used agent at the Wills Eye Hospital. Barbiturates provide sedation and minimize toxic reaction to local anesthetics. The undesirable effects of each of these medications, such as nausea, hypotension, and respiratory depression, must also be considered. For example, anticholinergic drugs such as atropine and scopolamine, which limit upper airway secretions, are seldom used before local anesthesia because the dry mouth that results can be uncomfortable. An exception is the patient with chronic bronchitis, cough, or postnasal drip, who may be helped to minimize coughing with these agents.[65] A drug should not be used routinely, but rather because it fulfills a specific need.

The pain associated with the local anesthetic injections and its memory can be totally abolished if desired with an intravenous injection of thiopental sodium (50–100 mg) or ketamine (10–25 mg), or the use of 70% nitrous oxide inhalation. For less anxious patients the amnesic effect of intravenous diazepam will usually suffice.

GENERAL ANESTHESIA

General anesthesia has changed markedly in the past 20 years. The improvements in available drugs and anesthetic practice have resulted in a reduction of operative and postoperative complications, which in turn have generated a new popularity for general anesthesia with the physician and the patient. Current techniques allow a smooth and rapid induction, an uneventful anesthetic course, a quiet emergence from anesthesia, and few adverse drug reactions. Operating conditions are excellent, since the anesthetist has complete control of the patient. Nervous or confused patients are more easily handled under general than under local anesthesia. The surgeon and operating room personnel can be more relaxed, with freer flow of communication. The risks of retrobulbar hemorrhage, intrabulbar injection, and toxic reactions to the local anesthetic are avoided. Finally, many patients prefer general to local anesthesia. These advantages must be balanced against the greater risks inherent in using a potentially lethal drug to produce unconsciousness, as well as against the ease of administration and relatively small number of physiological alterations that characterize local anesthesia with sedation. The postoperative period after local anesthesia is much pleasanter with less nausea and residual malaise, and there is often a prolonged period of pain relief, depending on the local anesthetic agent chosen.

Most ophthalmic patients are either young (under 10 years) or older than 55 years, a factor that increases the chance of problems with any kind of anesthesia. The majority of patients in a Manhattan Eye, Ear, Nose and Throat Hospital study[66] had some form of cardiovascular disease: hypertension, ischemic heart disease with a history of myocardial infarction, atrial fibrillation, or past cerebrovascular accidents. Diabetes mellitus, chronic bronchitis, and psychiatric disorders are also frequently seen in conjunction with ophthalmic problems.

Medical Conditions That Affect the Use of General Anesthesia

Diabetes. Diabetes is more than a disease of high blood sugars and ketoacidosis. It is associated with a multisystem disease complex including microangiopathy manifested in both the kidneys and the retina, peripheral neuropathy, autonomic dysfunction (e.g., postural hypotension and gastroparesis), infections, atherosclerosis, and cardiovascular disease with ischemic episodes to myocardium, which are often painless. The diabetic patient, whether the young, brittle juvenile diabetic or the older adult-onset diabetic, requires complete medical evaluation preoperatively to identify problems and optimize his or her physical condition before surgery. Blood sugar levels are measured before, during, and after surgery, and an internist should be available to follow the patient if complications should ensue.

Those controlled on oral hypoglycemic drugs do not take the medication on the day of surgery until after the operation is finished and they are restarting their normal diet.[67, 68]

There are a variety of ways to manage insulin-dependent diabetics. One proven regimen is to discontinue the routine dose of insulin on the day of surgery. A blood sugar is drawn and an intravenous drip of dextrose 5% in normal saline solution started. Regular insulin is administered subcutaneously to cover the amount of glucose given (10–15 U/1000 ml D_5NS), and additional amounts are given as indicated by dextrose sticks on blood samples before surgery and every hour during surgery, and then by blood sugars from the laboratory when the patient is back in his or her room. As soon as the patient resumes an oral diet, the usual insulin regimen is restarted. Patients with diabetes that is difficult to control are best operated on under local anesthesia, if possible.[69]

Hypertension. Hypertensive patients should be well controlled if possible,[70, 71] and should not stop their medications preoperatively. Every effort should be made to keep blood pressure in the normal range. Hypertension on intubation can usually be prevented by giving an adequate induction dose of anesthetic agent along with laryngotracheal lidocaine (2 mg/kg of a 4% solution).[68, 72, 73]

Pulmonary Disorders. Determination of the degree of pulmonary disability is important if general anesthesia is planned. The most valuable laboratory tests are arterial blood gases while breathing room air, vital capacity, and forced expiratory volume in 1 second.[74] Of even more value is the degree of physical activity of patients—for example, if they are short of breath walking on flat ground, or only become so on climbing two flights of stairs.

Although many patients with pulmonary disease are often safer having local anesthesia, patients with chronic bronchitis are often best treated surgically under general anesthesia. Good control of the patient by the anesthetist can eliminate coughing during the operation. Preoperative preparation of the patient is still necessary. If the patient is producing much sputum, a course of intermittent positive pressure breathing with bronchodilator drugs and, if needed, postural drainage and physiotherapy is used. Infected patients should be treated with specific antibiotic therapy. The patient should enter the operating room in the best condition possible for him or her, and an anesthetic technique that provides a high oxygen availability and minimal postanesthetic respiratory depression should be used.

Control of Intraocular Pressure

Average intraocular pressure ranges from 10 to 22 mm Hg, the highest extravascular tissue pressure in the body. This pressure is maintained by the active secretion of aqueous humor in the ciliary body, and the diffusion and ultrafiltration of serum into the posterior chamber of the eye.[75, 76] These processes depend on the difference in solute concentration between the plasma and aqueous. A small increase in the plasma solute concentration can greatly decrease the intraocular pressure; conversely, a small decrease in the plasma solute concentration can greatly increase intraocular pressure as well. Systemic arterial pressure, however, has much less effect on intraocular pressure. Arterial pressure can double and still only raise intraocular pressure a few millimeters of mercury. Venous pressure, on the other hand, has a major effect. Probably two-thirds or more of the aqueous humor leaves the eye by way of the trabecular meshwork to the canal of Schlemm, then out through the aqueous veins to the collecting venous system, and eventually back to the right side of the heart. Elevation of pressure within the episcleral veins results from any blockage of venous return (e.g., retrobulbar hemorrhage) or any cause of elevated central venous pressure (e.g., coughing). Any rise in episcleral venous pressure results in not only a 1:1 rise in intraocular pressure, but also an expansion of the venous volume in the choroid.

Thus straining, coughing, or vomiting can produce sudden increases in intraocular pressure and choroidal volume, predisposing to positive pressure and expulsive hemorrhage. Hypoventilation with consequent increase in P_{CO_2} also raises the intraocular pressure; conversely, hyperventilation and hypocapnia reduce it.[68]

Effect of Drugs on Intraocular Pressure

Constant control of intraocular pressure is obviously important, since even a momentary elevation when the globe is open can result in bleeding and prolapse of the ocular contents. Fortunately most general anesthetics cause a fall in intraocular pressure unless there is carbon dioxide retention or hypoxemia to counteract the fall. Most narcotics, tranquilizers, neuroleptics, hypnotics, and barbiturates also decrease intraocular pressure 10 to 15 per cent, again, provided there are no counterbalancing influences.[68] Nitrous oxide also lowers pressure, but when it is used alone, patients may become overly sensitive to airway manipulation. Intratracheal intubation can cause a transient rise of pressure that may be as great as 40 mm Hg.

Unlike most general anesthetic agents, ketamine (Ketalar) tends to elevate intraocular pressure. This rise is of the same magnitude as the drop caused by other anesthetics. Its effect is thought to be secondary to an increase in extraocular muscle tone. The age of the patient and the depth of anesthesia have no bearing on the extent of intraocular pressure rise. When mixed with another anesthetic, the pressure-elevating effect of the ketamine is balanced to some extent by the decreasing effect of the other drug, often providing a more accurate assessment of awake intraocular pressure.[77]

Effect of Muscle Relaxants on Intraocular Pressure

Muscle relaxants can have a variable, but often profound effect on intraocular pressure. Nondepolarizing muscle relaxants either lower intraocular pressure by blocking extraocular muscle tone, or have no effect on it.[78–82] However, endotracheal intubation in a lightly anesthetized but paralyzed patient can still lead to a sudden rise in intraocular pressure. This pressure rise can be minimized with the use of topical tracheal anesthesia, a well-anesthetized patient (relaxed with obtunded reflexes), and, if necessary, intravenous lidocaine.[68, 83]

Succinylcholine and, to a lesser extent, decamethonium can cause a transient increase in intraocular pressure. This rise is related to the amount of drug administered, averages about 10 mm Hg, and lasts for 1 to 10 minutes after injection with a peak at 2 to 4 minutes.[84, 85] Special muscle fibers known as Felderstruktur and found only in extraocular muscles react to depolarizing muscle relaxants with a slow tonic contraction that may be the cause of the pressure rise. The deeper the general anesthesia at the time of administration, the less marked the rise in intraocular pressure.

Because the rise in pressure is short-lived and seems related to the fasciculations induced by succinylcholine, it may follow that drugs that abolish these fasciculations would eliminate the secondary pressure increase. The studies, however, are controversial.[86–90] It has been reported, however, that prior treatment with acetazolamide and propranolol can prevent a succinylcholine-induced intraocular pressure rise.[91]

Drug Interactions

Atropine. It was formerly believed that atropine should not be given as a premedication to patients with occludable angles, for fear of risking an acute angle-closure attack. These fears are probably groundless.[92] If 0.4 mg of atropine is distributed evenly in a 70-kg patient, the amount of drug reaching the eye would be only about 0.0001 mg, far less than the 0.6 mg found there after one drop of 1% solution placed in the conjunctival sac. If a concern exists, pilocarpine 1% instilled twice in the eye 1 hour before administration of the atropine is adequate to prevent pupillary dilation.

Psychiatric Drugs. Most psychiatric drugs do not complicate anesthesia. Monoamine oxidase (MAO) inhibitors, tricyclic antidepressants, and lithium are exceptions. MAO inhibitors augment the effects of meperidine and may give rise to dangerous hypertensive attacks if sympathomimetics are used during anesthesia. Monoamine oxidase inhibitors should be stopped 2 weeks before surgery.

Tricyclic antidepressant drugs block the reuptake of neurotransmitters and can cause fatal dysrhythmias in combination with halothane and pancuronium.[93, 94] Lithium carbonate decreases the release of neurotransmitters centrally and peripherally, and may prolong neuromuscular blockade. Because it blocks brain stem release of norepinephrine, epinephrine, and dopamine, it may decrease anesthetic requirements.[95–97]

Cholinesterase Inhibitors. The long-acting anticholinesterase agents such as echothiophate and demecarium, when used as eye drops, are absorbed systemically in sufficient quantity to cause a marked decrease in pseudocholinesterase, up to 95 per cent after 4 to 6 weeks of use. This effect may last up to 8 weeks after the drug is discontinued. Modest doses of succinylcholine used to facilitate anesthesia are not rapidly inactivated in patients with low pseudocholinesterase. The usually transient apnea produced by succinylcholine may last up to 5 hours in patients treated with echothiophate. Thus, in cases in which general anesthesia is to be used and surgery is elective, the drug should be stopped at least 1 month before surgery and the anesthetist informed. If this is not feasible, and general anesthesia should be required, another muscle relaxant may be chosen. Adequate intravenous atropine should be given preoperatively to block muscarinic effects and prevent vagal responses.[68]

Steroids. Steroid production in the adrenals is suppressed for 6 months or more after a prolonged course of oral steroids. If surgery occurs during this period, supplemental steroids should be given preoperatively and postoperatively.

Propranolol. Sudden discontinuation of propranolol may precipitate unstable angina or even myocardial infarction. Modest doses of up to 180 mg total per 24 hours may be given up to the time of surgery. Higher doses should be tapered to the minimum therapeutic level, and the morning dosage may be omitted the day of surgery.[98]

Technique

Preoperative medication usually consists of an anticholinergic, either atropine or scopolamine, and either a narcotic, a tranquilizer, or a barbiturate. Atropine has a greater effect on cardiac function, and scopolamine on secretions. Scopolamine may induce a helpful amnesia for the procedure, but it may also produce irrational behavior. Therefore, atropine is generally the drug of choice.

Narcotics provide analgesia, sedation, and, in some cases, a slight euphoria. The analgesic effect allows the use of smaller amounts of anesthetic agents. This is part of the balanced anesthesia principle that small doses of several drugs may act synergistically to give adequate anesthesia with few side effects, since the total amount of drugs used is much smaller.[2] On the other hand, narcotics may cause nausea and vomiting and tend to depress respiration.

Tranquilizers offer an antiemetic effect but may produce extrapyramidal tract symptoms or cause hypotension. Neither tranquilizers nor barbiturates contribute analgesia, but barbiturates produce more sedation.

Most sources agree that 0.4 to 0.6 mg of atropine is recommended. Few sources agree on the sedative. One suggested regimen for a healthy 70-kg adult is secobarbital (Seconal), 100 mg, plus meperidine hydrochloride (Demerol), 12.5 to 50 mg.[51] Another suggestion is to use a moderate dose of narcotic without added tranquilizers.[2] A third authority claims that narcotics cause too much nausea and respiratory depression, barbiturates too much postoperative restlessness, and that therefore tranquilizing drugs (e.g., diazepam, 5 mg) are preferred. At the Wills Eye Hospital the most frequently used regimen includes 5 to 10 mg of oral diazepam with a sip of water 2 hours preoperatively; this may be supplemented when necessary with an intravenously administered agent such as midazolam hydrochloride (Versed) or fentanyl (Sublimaze), or, less frequently, nalbuphine hydrochloride (Nubain), or pentazocine hydrochloride (Talwin). Day surgery patients are usually given no oral premedications, since they must be ready to leave soon after surgery, and the duration of action is unpredictable. However, fentanyl (25–50 mg) and diazepam (2–3 mg) are given intravenously.[69]

Adequate monitoring is vital to the successful administration of a general anesthesia. Before induction, patients have a blood pressure cuff, a temperature probe, electrocardiographic monitoring equipment, and a precordial stethoscope applied. The vital signs are continuously watched and recorded throughout the operative procedure. Pulse oximetry is used to monitor oxygen saturation, and end tidal carbon dioxide to determine the efficiency of ventilation.[99–101]

Because most patients find breathing gas anesthetics through a mask disagreeable, induction is often best accomplished by intravenous injection of an anesthetic agent. At the time of the injection, the patient is breathing oxygen through the mask to reduce the partial pressure of nitrogen in his blood. Succinylcholine is then administered to paralyze the patient, and intubation accomplished.

General anesthesia is usually maintained with inhalation agents, since hyperventilating the patient can hasten removal of the drug. In contrast, intravenous agents must be metabolized or excreted, a much longer process.

Thiopental sodium (Pentothal), a very short-acting barbiturate, is the mainstay of intravenous induction. The usual dose for adults is 4 to 6 mg/kg, given at the rate of 50 mg every 30 seconds. If given quickly, it causes apnea; but given slowly, only mild respiratory depression may result. It is given in dilute solution to prevent phlebitis. Thiopental is contraindicated in patients with porphyria, which it may reactivate.[2]

Nitrous oxide and isoflurane or, to a lesser extent, halothane are the most commonly used inhalation agents. Nitrous oxide is the least toxic and least potent of general anesthetic agents. Even used in concentrations of up to 70% it requires the use of a complementary intravenous or additional inhalation agent.

Isoflurane is the most recently introduced and the most slowly metabolized of the fluorinated inhaled anesthetics.[102–104] Because of the very limited metabolism of isoflurane, hepatitis is not a problem. It does not sensitize the myocardium to catecholamines. With the rapid emergence from anesthesia and the minimal postoperative nausea and vomiting, these qualities have made isoflurane the most popular of the inhalation agents.[102, 105]

Halothane may be used as an adjunct in concentrations of 2% or less, to ensure a deep level of anesthesia. It provides a rapid, easy emergence from anesthesia, is nonexplosive, and can be used alone if desired. On the negative side, it sensitizes the heart to catecholamines, limiting the use of epinephrine during surgery.[106] Repeated employment of halothane may also produce liver damage in those thought to have an allergy to it.[2] Patients should be screened with liver enzymes and serum bilirubin before being administered halothane anesthesia. In children, however, liver changes are extremely rare, and therefore it is ordinarily not necessary to wait the 2 to 3 months recommended for adults before an additional procedure using halothane anesthesia may be done.

Two other anesthetics need to be mentioned, Innovar and ketamine. Innovar is a combination of a powerful narcotic, fentanyl (Sublimaze), and a long-acting tranquilizer, droperidol (Inapsine). It is used as a premedication, as a supplement to local anesthesia, or as part of a balanced generalized anesthetic.

Ketamine is a rapid-acting, nonbarbiturate general anesthetic that can be used for induction, especially in unmanageable children, or

for maintenance of anesthesia. Its disadvantages are significant, especially for eye surgery. Hypertonus and involuntary movements are common during sleep and are not lessened by increased dosages. Nystagmus often occurs during induction and recovery. Some elevation of blood pressure is usual, and emergence delirium is common in adults, especially women, and especially if the patient is disturbed during recovery. Administration of 5 mg of diazepam seems to be effective in decreasing the incidence of unpleasant dreams.[107] Two cases of lasting psychosis in children after examinations under ketamine anesthesia have been reported.[108] Ketamine can no longer be recommended for routine use. In rare instances it is the anesthetic of choice, for example, the mentally retarded patient who will not cooperate for the placement of an intravenous line. Ketamine given intramuscularly in the preoperative or operating room will calm the patient and allow the administration of a general anesthetic with a minimum of trauma to the patient and operating room personnel.[109]

Muscle Relaxants

These drugs have changed anesthesia to the extent that currently few people undergoing general surgery require deep anesthesia. A small dose of general anesthesia and a muscle relaxant can keep the patient unconscious and motionless. These agents fall into two classes: nondepolarizing and depolarizing. Curare, gallamine, pancuronium, and the newer atracurium and vecuronium are all nondepolarizing drugs. Depending on the dosage and agent, paralysis will last for 20 minutes to an hour. Bronchospasm and hypotension may occur with curare, and tachycardia is common with gallamine and pancuronium. On the other hand, atracurium and vecuronium have few side effects and minimal cardiovascular effects. They provide a shorter, more predictable duration of action, and the ability to use the drugs in patients with kidney failure (both agents) and liver failure (atracurium). These advantages have outmoded the older agents.[110, 111]

The antidote for the nondepolarizing relaxant is a combination of neostigmine and atropine. Although not always successful, its use at the end of a procedure usually permits rapid return to the preanesthetic condition.

Succinylcholine is a depolarizing muscle relaxant whose only virtues over newer agents are its rapid onset and short (4 to 5 minutes) duration. The paralysis is preceded by fasciculations thought to be the cause of postoperative muscle aches and pains in many patients. The fasciculations may be avoided by the use of a deeper anesthesia or a small dose of a nondepolarizing muscle relaxant before the administration of succinylcholine.[112]

There is no antidote for succinylcholine, and administration of neostigmine may worsen the condition. The only treatment for prolonged paralysis is continued artificial respiration.

In some patients succinylcholine or even halothane can trigger malignant hyperthermia (Table 5–5), a reaction in which a familial defect in muscle metabolism generates more heat than the body can dissipate. If not controlled, temperatures may rise to 110° F (43° C), with a fatal outcome. This problem is said to be more common in children, especially those with strabismus and myotonia. At Wills Eye Hospital in the last 40,000 cases there have been 3 cases of malignant hyperthermia. These involved a 17-year-old male having retinal detachment surgery and two adults undergoing penetrating keratoplasty.

The clinical findings include increased temperature, sweating, unstable blood pressure, a lack of response to succinylcholine, muscle rigidity, tachypnea and tachycardia, cardiac arrhythmias, mottling of the skin, cyanosis, respiratory and metabolic acidosis, and remarkable oxygen consumption. Treatment must begin before body temperature has reached 105° F (40° C) or success is unlikely. Anesthesia and surgery are immediately stopped, and the patient is hyperventilated with 100% oxygen.

TABLE 5–5. Malignant Hyperthermia

Symptoms
Increasing temperature, sweating
Unstable blood pressure
Muscle rigidity
Tachypnea and tachycardia
Cardiac arrhythmias
Respiratory and metabolic acidosis

Treatment
Stop anesthesia and surgery.
Hyperventilate with 100% oxygen.
Administer Dantrolene: 2 mg/kg initially and repeat prn symptoms q 5 minutes until 10 mg/kg total dosage.
Administer sodium bicarbonate: 100 mEq stat and up to 600 mEq as needed to maintain arterial pH.
Institute packing in ice, cold intravenous saline, and stomach and colon irrigation with ice water.
Administer 10 units of regular insulin.
Maintain urine output with mannitol and furosemide.
Administer procainamide for arrhythmia control.

Dantrolene should be given intravenously, 2 mg/kg as an initial dose and repeated every 5 minutes until 10 mg/kg total dose is reached or symptoms disappear. Sodium bicarbonate is administered (100 mEq immediately and up to 600 mEq as needed to maintain arterial pH). Maximal cooling may be achieved by administration of iced intravenous saline (not Ringer's lactated) solution, stomach and colon irrigation with ice water, and packing in ice or immersion in an ice water tank. Ten units of regular insulin in 10 ml of dextrose 50% in water may be given as a bolus to reduce potassium. This must be done slowly, as hypokalemia frequently follows the period of hyperkalemia. Urine output is maintained with mannitol and furosemide; procainamide is used to control arrhythmias. If the onset of treatment is not delayed, the survival rate with this regimen is excellent.[113–117] Dantrolene is the key, and attention should not be diverted to control of other systemic factors at the expense of delaying the dantrolene administration.

Clearly preoperative screening for susceptibility is important in the early recognition of malignant hyperthermia. A family history of anesthetic exposure going back two generations may be helpful. Measurement of blood creatine phosphokinase has been used in the past to screen for susceptibility, but a recent study has shown that there are too many false-positive and false-negative results for this to be a useful test.[118] *In vitro* contracture testing of muscle biopsy tissue is probably more than 90 per cent reliable and is the most valuable test.[116] Because this procedure is only done in 10 centers in the United States and four in Canada, it may be impossible to obtain. Patients with a suspicious history can be treated as if they have the disease. This entails pretreatment with intravenous (2 mg/kg) dantrolene just before induction of anesthesia, avoiding the uncertainty in blood levels associated with the oral route.[119] Anesthesia should consist of nitrous oxide, barbiturates, narcotics, opiates, tranquilizers, and nondepolarizing muscle relaxants. Potent volatile agents and depolarizing agents are avoided even in the presence of dantrolene.[116, 120, 121]

LOCAL VERSUS GENERAL ANESTHESIA

General anesthesia produces a more profound physiological disturbance than local anesthesia, and therefore should usually be used only if the

TABLE 5–6. Local Versus General Anesthesia

Advantages of Local Anesthesia
1. Is safer systemically
2. Produces residual postoperative analgesia
3. Requires less sophisticated anesthesia support
4. Requires less preoperative and postoperative anesthesia time, resulting in faster patient turnover in the operating room

Advantages of General Anesthesia
1. Is preferred by some patients
2. Permits better management of patients with psychiatric or mental retardation problems, frequent coughing, painful arthritis, epilepsy, etc.
3. Allows freer communication among operating staff
4. Is useful in longer or more painful procedures
5. Can be used after retrobulbar hemorrhage
6. Is safer for the eye in cases in which a rise in intraocular pressure, as could occur with retrobulbar hemorrhage, would be damaging (e.g., ruptured globe, iris prolapse, totally flat anterior chamber, etc.)

operation cannot be carried out safely and easily with a local anesthetic. Factors that favor general anesthesia include patient apprehension; difficulty with communication or cooperation as a result of language, hearing problems, or senility; and the necessity for prolonged, technically demanding surgery, such as that for retina repair (see Table 5–6).

Several independent studies have investigated the morbidity and mortality of local and general anesthesia for eye surgery and found no significant differences. However, since the patient's physical status frequently mandates local anesthesia, the health of the two groups may differ, confounding the results. Similarly, the incidence of complications such as vitreous loss, iris prolapse, and hyphema was nearly equal.[122–124] Nausea and vomiting, however, were more often seen with general anesthesia and in one study were considered to be due to the more frequent use of meperidine in these patients. Patients operated on under local anesthesia benefited by the pain-blocking effect of their anesthesia well into the immediate postoperative period. Because of today's finer sutures and strong wound closure, and the increased use of antiemetics, complications from vomiting were few. Table 5–6 lists the advantages of local anesthesia versus those of general anesthesia.

The decision of whether to use local or general anesthesia should be a collective one among the patient, the surgeon, and the anesthetist. The outcome usually depends primarily on the health of the patient, his psychological makeup, and the requirements of the surgery.

PEDIATRIC ANESTHESIA

Anesthesia for neonates and children is dissimilar in many ways from that for adults, and requires an understanding of the physiological and pharmacological differences. By way of example, the surface-volume ratio is 70 times greater for a neonate than for an adult, and the therapeutic range for drugs is much narrower in this age group.[125]

Psychological support and a careful presentation of technique by the anesthetist is important at any age, but doubly so in the child. Strong-arm tactics may ensure induction with the uncooperative child but leave a deep-seated fear of medical personnel and surgery. This can usually be avoided if the anesthetist can establish rapport before surgery, and instruct the child on what to expect. Allowing the parent to wait with the child in the preoperative room may supply additional reassurance.

The most frequent problem seen in pediatric anesthesia is the child with a low-grade fever. This can be the first sign of an oncoming illness, mild dehydration, or emotional stress and crying. Surgery for patients with obvious upper respiratory tract infections is postponed until they are free of symptoms for 2 weeks. This allows laryngeal edema to subside.

Infants are easily dehydrated, and therefore should be scheduled early in the day. Appropriate preoperative orders should allow solid food and milk until 8 hours preoperatively; clear liquids are encouraged until 6 hours before surgery.[69]

When surgery is required for infants of less than 44 weeks' gestation, oxygen concentrations greater than those in room air are relatively contraindicated unless required for life. Retinopathy of prematurity is a possible sequela.[126]

An enzymatic defect seen in children as well as in adults is congenital atypical pseudocholinesterase. Because pseudocholinesterase is responsible for hydrolyzing succinylcholine, these patients are subject to prolonged apnea if administered the drug. They also exhibit varying response to muscle relaxants and anesthetic agents.

The Oculocardiac Reflex

The oculocardiac reflex, which occurs markedly in children, is a slowing of the pulse in response to traction on the extraocular muscles or pressure on the eye. It often is associated with arrhythmias and even periods of asystole. In the absence of anesthesia these maneuvers have much less effect except in the presence of paroxysmal atrial tachycardia. However, because of the effect of anesthesia on the vagal sympathetic balance, most patients (85 per cent) will show a reflex bradycardia in response to pressure on the globe. The frequency of serious arrhythmias, on the other hand, is vastly lower. Traction on the medial rectus is the most common stimulus but even retrobulbar injections can cause enough compression to elicit the reflex in about half the patients.[127–130] The bradycardia persists for 10 to 15 seconds after traction is released. If traction is again initiated, the occurrence of bradycardia is less likely.[131] Children under 12 years of age and individuals with brown irides are more frequently affected. All anesthetics produce the reflex with approximately the same frequency. Hypercapnia may exacerbate this incidence.[132]

The pathway for the oculocardiac reflex consists of an afferent limb made up of fibers from the short and long ciliary nerves. These run in the ophthalmic division of the trigeminal nerve to the trigeminal ganglion and terminate in the main sensory nucleus of the trigeminal nerve in the fourth ventricle. The efferent limb is contained in the vagus nerve.[133]

Prevention and treatment have been aimed at both ends of this loop. A retrobulbar block cuts the incidence in half,[134–137] but the risk of complications caused by the retrobulbar block itself probably exceeds the slight risk from the arrhythmias caused by the oculocardiac reflex. Gallamine, by increasing the heart rate, is helpful in decreasing the oculocardiac reflex, but it is not consistently effective.[138] The use of atropine to prevent and treat the oculocardiac reflex is still controversial.[139, 140] Intravenous atropine given in 0.007-mg/kg increments is effective in preventing bradycardia associated with the oculocardiac reflex. Glycopyrrolate is probably equally effective with less tachycardia, but has a slower onset time.

Current recommended practice is to provide anticholinergic protection, and keep the patient well ventilated to avoid hypercapnia and under constant electrocardiographic surveillance. An adequate depth of anesthesia is helpful as well as encouragement to the surgeon to be gentle. If an arrhythmia develops and persists, the surgeon should halt manipulation until the heart beat is regular again. If severe bradycardia persists, atropine is titrated as above. Smaller doses of atropine may have no effect or, paradoxically, worsen the arrhythmia. If the reflex is still a problem, infiltration of the recti with local anesthesia may block the stimulus.[68]

Anesthetic Agents in Children

As with adult anesthesia, preoperative medications are as varied as the number of sources consulted. Morphine and a barbiturate are suggested, with meperidine sometimes used in place of morphine, and diazepam in place of the barbiturate. Innovar (droperidol and fentanyl in a 50-1 ratio) can also be used. Children done as outpatients usually receive no premedication, to avoid prolonged sedation. The use of atropine is especially important in infants, who are more subject to the bradycardia induced by halothane, succinylcholine, and laryngoscopy.

Children, whose surface area–body weight ratio is high, need warming blankets and temperature monitoring. The same general anesthetic agents as in adults are used. Induction in children, however, is often done with inhalation agents, allowing the anesthetist a still patient for inserting the intravenous line. Games may be used to get the patient to breathe the gas. If these fail, administration of ketamine intramuscularly or sodium pentothal rectally will provide the necessary cooperation to finish induction.[109]

Anesthesia may be maintained by mask insufflation or endotracheal intubation. Insufflation is used only for brief evaluations when the child is healthy and between 6 months and 10 years of age. By this method the patient is breathing spontaneously in a constant, deep plane of anesthesia and anesthetic gases are brought to him through an oropharyngeal airway or nasopharyngeal tube. Insufflation avoids the trauma of intubation and its main complications, croup and subglottic edema. On the other hand, it allows the anesthetist only minimal airway control, and both he and the surgeon must work in the same area.

ANESTHESIA IN OCULAR EMERGENCIES

The patient with a penetrating eye injury and a full stomach presents a special and distressingly frequent problem. Topical or local anesthesia is impossible with an open globe. In order to assure safe general anesthesia, it is optimal to have an 8-hour interval since food was ingested before starting surgery. If, from the ocular point of view, surgery cannot be safely postponed, the following technique may be used. Mannitol can be given intravenously 45 minutes before surgery. At the time of induction 3 to 6 mg of D-tubocurare or 10 to 20 mg of gallamine is given intravenously. The patient is then preoxygenated for 3 to 4 minutes. Sodium pentothal, 4 to 6 mg/kg, is given, followed immediately by succinylcholine, 80 to 120 mg. Lidocaine, 1 mg/kg I.V., or fentanyl, 1.0 to 1.5 μg/kg I.V., or both can be used at induction to lessen the possibility of cough on intubation. As soon as consciousness is lost, cricoid pressure is applied to prevent esophageal reflux and is maintained until placement of the endotracheal tube.[141] This allows a rapid intubation and prevents aspiration. The intraocular pressure-elevating effects of succinylcholine can be minimized by the combined use of preoperative mannitol, a defasciculating dose of curare or gallamine, and induction with sodium pentothal.[142]

CONCLUSION

Because opinions regarding anesthesia in ophthalmic surgery are diverse, current knowledge does not permit the choosing of one "best way." Therefore, a variety of techniques have been described in this chapter. In order to give some guidance, approaches proved safe and effective at a busy eye hospital have been indicated.

Combining optimal operating conditions for the surgeon with the greatest safety for the patient demands close cooperation between the anesthetist and the ophthalmologist. This is most easily achieved if each has an understanding of the other's task and problems.

REFERENCES

1. Leahy, J.: Notes on the preoperative interview (unpublished). 1979.
2. Jacoby, J.: General anesthesia. In Duane, T. (ed.): Clinical Ophthalmology, Vol. 5. Hagerstown, Md., Harper & Row, 1976, Ch. 1.
3. Havener, W. H.: Ocular Pharmacology. St. Louis, C. V. Mosby, 1978, Ch. 5.
4. Maurice, D. M., Singh, T.: The absence of corneal toxicity with low-level topical anesthesia. Am. J. Ophthalmol., 99:691, 1985.
5. Man, W. G., Wood, R., Senterfit, L., Sigelman, S.: Effect of topical anesthetics on regeneration of the corneal epithelium. Am. J. Ophthalmol., 43:606, 1957.
6. Duffin, R.M., Olson, R. J.: Tetracaine toxicity. Ann. Ophthalmol., 16/9:836–838, 1984.
7. Koller, K.: Uber die Verwendung des Cocain zur Anasthesierung am Auge. Wien Med. Bl., 7:1352, 1884.
8. Smith, R. B., Everett, W. G.: Physiology and pharmacology of local anesthetic agents (anesthesia in ophthalmology). Int. Ophthalmol. Clin., 13:56, 1973.
9. Ritchie, J. M., Cohen, P. J.: Cocaine, procaine and other synthetic local anesthetics. In Goodman, L. S., Gilman, A. (eds.): The Pharmacological Basis of Therapeutics. New York, Macmillan, 1975, Ch. 20.
10. Frayer, W. C.: Local anesthesia: Indications and techniques. In Duane, T. (ed.): Clinical Ophthalmology, Vol. 5. Philadelphia, Harper & Row, 1978, Ch. 2.
11. deJong, R. H.: Physiology and Pharmacology of Local Anesthesia. Springfield, IL., Charles C Thomas, 1970.
12. Crandall, D. C.: Pharmacology of ocular anesthetics. In Duane, T., Jaeger, E. A. (eds.): Biomedical Foundations of Ophthalmology, vol. 3. Philadelphia, Harper & Row, 1983, Ch. 35.
13. Carolan, J. A., Cerasoli, J. R., Houle, T. V.: Bupivacaine in retrobulbar anesthesia. Ann. Ophthalmol., 6:843, 1974.
14. Covino, B. G.: Pharmacology of local anesthetic agents. Surg. Rounds, July 1978, p. 44.
15. Adriani, J.: Newer anesthetics, sedatives, preoperative regimens. In Symposium on Ocular Pharmacology and Therapeutics: Transactions of the New Orleans Academy of Ophthalmology. St. Louis, C. V. Mosby, 1970, Ch. 20.
16. Bryant, J. A.: Local and topical anesthetics in ophthalmology. Surv. Ophthalmol., 13:263, 1969.
17. Löfstrom, B.: Aspects of the pharmacology of local anesthetic agents. Br. J. Anaesth., 42:194, 1970.
18. Löfstrom, B., Green, K., Jansson, O., McCarthy, G.: An evaluation of bupivacaine (Marcaine) without adrenaline. Acta Anaesth. Scand. [Suppl.], 37:282, 1970.
19. Hoven, I.: Ophthalmic artery pressure, retrobulbar anesthesia. Acta Ophthalmol., 56:574, 1978.
20. Mindel, J. S.: Value of hyaluronidase in ocular surgical akinesia. Am. J. Ophthalmol., 85:643, 1978.
21. Adriani, J.: The clinical pharmacology of local anesthetics. Clin. Pharmacol. Ther., 1:645, 1960.
22. Carolan, J. A., Cerasoli, J. R., Houle, T.V.: Bupivacaine in retrobulbar anesthesia. Ann. Ophthalmol., 6:843, 1974.
23. Smith, P. H., Kim, J. W.: Etidocaine used for retrobulbar block: A comparison with lidocaine. Ophthalmic Surg., 11(4):268, 1980.
24. Smith, P. H., Smith, E. R.: A comparison of etidocaine and lidocaine for retrobulbar anesthesia. Ophthalmic Surg., 14:569, 1983.
25. Thorburn, W., Thorn-Alquist, A. M., Edström, H: Etidocaine in retrobulbar anesthesia: a comparison with mepivacaine. Acta Ophthal., 54:591, 1976.
26. Holekamp, T. L. R., Arribas, N. P., Boniuk, I.: Bupivacaine anesthesia in retinal detachment surgery. Arch. Ophthalmol., 97:109, 1979.
27. Henkind, P., Friedman, A., Berger, A. W. (eds.): Physicians' Desk Reference for Ophthalmology. Oradell, NJ, Medical Economics Co., 1978.

28. Smith, R. B., Everett, W. G.: Physiology and pharmacology of local anesthetic agents. Int. Ophthalmol. Clin., 13(2):36, 1973.

29. Lyman, J., Swan, K. C.: Technique for evaluating effectiveness of anesthetic solution for orbicularis akinesia. Scientific poster, American Academy of Ophthalmology Meeting, San Francisco, November 1979.

30. Chin, G. N., Almquist, H. T.: Bupivacaine and lidocaine retrobulbar anesthesia. Ophthalmology, 90:369, 1983.

31. Gills, J. P., Rudisill, J. E. L.: Bupivacaine in cataract surgery. Ophthalmic Surg., 5(4):67, 1974.

32. Alper, M. H.: Toxicity of local anesthetics. N. Engl. J. Med., 295:1432, 1976.

33. Meyers, E. F., Ramirez, R. C., Boniuk, I.: Grand mal seizures after retrobulbar block. Arch. Ophthalmol., 98:847, 1978.

34. Smith, J. L.: Retrobulbar bupivacaine can cause respiratory arrest. Ann. Ophthalmol., 14:1005, 1982.

35. Drysdale, D. B.: Experimental subdural retrobulbar injection of anesthetic. Ann. Ophthalmol., 16:716, 1984.

36. Lombardi, G.: Radiology in Neuro-ophthalmology. Baltimore, Williams & Wilkins, 1967, p. 6.

37. Hamilton, R. C.: Brain stem anesthesia following retrobulbar blockade. Anesthesiology, 63:688, 1985.

38. Friedberg, H. L., Kline, O. R.: Contralateral amaurosis after retrobulbar injection. Am. J. Ophthalmol., 101:688, 1986.

39. Follette, J. W., LoCascio, J. A.: Bilateral amaurosis following unilateral retrobulbar block. Anesthesiology, 63:238, 1985.

40. Chang, J., Gonzalex-Abola, E., Larson, C. E., Lobes, L.: Brain stem anesthesia following retrobulbar block. Anesthesiology, 61:789, 1984.

41. Beltranena, H., Vega, M. J., Garcia, J. J., Blankenship, G.: Complications of retrobulbar marcaine injection. J. Clin. Neuro-ophthalmol., 2:159, 1982.

42. Wittpen, J. R., Rapoza, P., Sternberg, P., Jr., et al.: Respiratory arrest following retrobulbar anesthesia. Ophthalmology, 93:867, 1986.

43. Osher, R. H.: Is postop diplopia associated with retrobulbar anesthesia? Ophthalmol. Times, August 15, 1986, p. 1.

44. Fallor, M.K.: Ophthalmol. Times, November 1, 1984.

45. Chostain, G. M.: Acute blood levels of lidocaine following paracervical block. J. Med. Assoc. Ga., 158:426, 1969.

46. Keating, V.: Anesthetic Accidents, 2nd ed. Chicago, Year Book Publishers, 1961, p. 176.

47. Arimes, D. A., Cotes, W., Jr.: Deaths from paracervical anesthesia used for first-trimester abortion, 1972–1975. N. Engl. J. Med., 295:25, 1966.

48. Truex, R. C., Kellner, C. E.: Detailed Atlas of the Head and Neck. New York, Oxford University Press, 1948, p. 55.

49. Van Lint, A.: Paralysie palpebrale temporaire provoquee dans l'operation de la cataracte. Ann. Ocul. (Paris), 151:420, 1914.

50. King, J. H., Jr., Wadsworth, J. A. C.: An Atlas of Ophthalmic Surgery. Philadelphia, J. B. Lippincott Co., 1970, Ch. 2.

51. Spaeth, G. L.: A new method to achieve complete akinesia of the facial nerve muscles of the eyelids. Ophthalmic Surg., 7:105, 1976.

52. Nadbath, R. P., Rehman, I.: Facial nerve block. Am. J. Ophthalmol., 53:143, 1963.

53. Kaplan, L. J., Jaffe, N. S., Clayman, H. M.: Ptosis and cataract surgery, a multivariant computer analysis of a prospective study. Ophthalmology, 92:237, 1985.

54. Wilson, C. A., Ruiz, R.S.: Respiratory obstruction following the Nadbath facial nerve block. Arch. Ophthalmol., 103:1454, 1985.

55. Shoch, D.: Complications of the Nadbath facial nerve block. Arch. Ophthalmol., 104:1114, 1986.

56. Rabinowitz, L., Livingston, M., Schneider, H., Hall, A.: Respiratory obstruction following the Nadbath facial nerve block. Arch. Ophthalmol., 104:1115, 1986.

57. Sullivan, K.L., Brown, G. C., Forman, A. R., et al.: Retrobulbar anesthesia and retinal vascular obstruction. Ophthalmology, 90:373, 1983.

58. Pautler, S. E., Grizzard, W.S., Thompson, L.N., Wing, G. L.: Blindness from retrobulbar injection into the optic nerve. Ophthalmic Surg., 17:334, 1986.

59. Klein, M. L., Jampol, L. M., Concon, P. I., et al.: Central retinal artery occlusion without retrobulbar hemorrhage after retrobulbar anesthesia. Am. J. Ophthalmol., 93:573, 1982.

60. Bolder, P. M., Norton, M. L.: Retinal hemorrhage following anesthesia. Anesthesiology, 61:595, 1984.

61. Atkinson, W.S.: The development of ophthalmic anesthesia. Am. J. Ophthalmol., 51:1, 1961.

62. Unsöld, R., Stanley, J. A., DeGroot, J.: The CT-topography of retrobulbar anesthesia. Graefes Arch. Clin. Exp. Ophthalmol., 217:125, 1981.

63. Laval, J.: Retrobulbar block. Arch. Ophthalmol., 104:22, 1986.

64. Davis, D. B., II, Mandel, M. R.: Posterior peribulbar anesthesia: An alternative to retrobulbar anesthesia. J. Cataract Refract. Surg., 12:182. 1986.

65. Donlon, J. V., Jr.: Local anesthesia for ophthalmic surgery: Patient preparation and management. Ann. Ophthalmol., 12:1183, 1980.

66. Wolf, G. L., Lynch, S., Berlin, I.: Intraocular surgery with general anesthesia. Arch. Ophthalmol., 93:323, 1975.

67. Roizen, M. F.: Anesthetic implications of concurrent diseases. In Miller, R. D. (ed.): Anesthesia, Vol. 1. New York, Churchill Livingstone, 1986, Ch. 9.

68. Donlon, J. V., Jr.: Anesthesia for eye, ear, nose and throat. In Miller, R. D. (ed.): Anesthesia, Vol. 3. New York, Churchill Livingstone, 1986, Ch. 52.

69. Libonati, M. L.: Personal communication on standard practice. Wills Eye Hospital, Philadelphia, PA, 1986.

70. Prys-Roberts, C., Meloche, R., Foëx, P.: Studies of anesthesia in relation to hypertension. I. Cardiovascular responses of treated and untreated patients. Br. J. Anaesth., 43:122, 1971.

71. Goldman, L., Caldera, D. L.: Risks of general anesthesia and elective operation in the hypertensive patient. Anesthesiology, 50:285, 1979.

72. Adams, A., Fordham, R. M. M.: General anesthesia in adults. Int. Ophthalmol. Clin., 13:83, 1973.

73. Stoelting, R.K.: Endotracheal intubation. In Miller, R. D. (ed.): Anesthesia, Vol. 1. New York, Churchill Livingstone, 1986, Ch. 16.

74. Gal, T. J.: Pulmonary function testing. In Miller, R. D. (ed.): Anesthesia, Vol. 3. New York, Churchill Livingstone, 1986, Ch. 59.

75. Turndorf, H.: Anesthesia for eye surgery. Audio Digest Anesthesiol., 17, 1975.

76. Shields, M. B.: A study guide for glaucoma. Baltimore, Williams & Wilkins, 1982, p. 11.

77. Corssen, G., John, J. E.: A new parenteral anesthetic—CL-581: Its effect on intraocular pressure. J. Ped. Ophthalmol., 4:20, 1962.
78. Goldsmith, E.: An evaluation of succinylcholine and gallamine as muscle relaxants in relation to intraocular tension. Anaesth. Analg., 46:557, 1967.
79. Litwiller, R. W., DiFazio, C., Rushia, E. L.: Pancuronium and intraocular pressure. Anesthesiology, 42:750, 1975.
80. Balamoutos, N. G., Tsakona, H., et al.: Alcuronium and intraocular pressure. Anesth. Analg., 62:521, 1983.
81. Cunningham, A. J., Kelly, P. C., et al.: Effect of metocurine-pancuronium combination on IOP. Can. Anaesth. Soc. J., 29:617, 1982.
82. Agarwal, L. P., Mathur, S. P.: Curare in ocular surgery. Br. J. Ophthalmol., 36:603, 1952.
83. Van Aken, H.: Prevention of hypertension at intubation with intravenous lidocaine. Anaesthesia, 37:82, 1982.
84. Pandey, K., Badola, R. P., Kumar, S.: Time course of intraocular hypertension produced by suxamethonium. Br. J. Anaesth., 44:191, 1972.
85. Magora, F., Collins, V. J.: The influence of general anesthetic agents on intraocular pressure in man. Arch. Ophthalmol., 66:806, 1962.
86. Eakins, K. E., Katz, R. L.: The action of succinylcholine on the tension of extraocular muscle. Br. J. Pharmacol., 26:205, 1966.
87. Miller, R. D., Way, W.L., Hickey, R. F.: Inhibition of succinylcholine induced increased intraocular pressure by nondepolarizing muscle relaxants. Anesthesiology, 29:123, 1968.
88. Bowen, D. J., McGrand, J. C., Palmer, R. J.: Intraocular pressure after pretreatment with pancuronium. Br. J. Anaesth., 48:1201, 1975.
89. Meyers, E. F., Krupin, T., Johnson, M., et al.: Failure of nondepolarizing neuromuscular blockers to inhibit succinylcholine induced increased intraocular pressure. Anesthesiology, 48:1149, 1978.
90. Giala, M. M., Balamoutos, N. G., et al.: Failure of gallamine to inhibit succinylcholine induced increase in IOP. Anesthesiology, 51:578, 1979.
91. Carballo, A. S.: Succinylcholine and acetazolamide in anesthesia for ocular surgery. Can. Anaesth. Soc. J., 12:486, 1965.
92. Rosen, D. A.: Anesthesia in ophthalmology. Can. Anesth. Soc. J., 9:545, 1962.
93. Edwards, R. E., Miller, R. D., Roizen, M. F., et al.: Cardiac effects of imipramine and pancuronium during halothane and enflurane anesthesia. Anesthesiology, 50:421, 1979.
94. Kosanin, R.: Anesthetic considerations in patients on chronic tricyclic antidepressant therapy. Anesthesiol. Rev., 8:38, 1981.
95. Hill, G. E., Wong, K. C.: Lithium carbonate and neuromuscular blocking agents. Anesthesiology, 46:122, 1977.
96. Martin, B. A., Kramer, P. M.: Clinical significance of the interaction between lithium and a neuromuscular blocker. Am. J. Psychiatry, 139:1326, 1982.
97. Physicians' Desk Reference. Oradell, NJ, Medical Economics Co., Inc., 1989, p 2052.
98. Haidinzak, J. G., Didier, E. P.: Case history number 95: Anesthetics and propranolol, anesthesia and analgesia. Curr. Res., 56:283, 1977.
99. Swedlow, D. B.: Capnometry and capnography: The anesthesia disaster early warning system. Semin. Anesth., 5:194, 1986.
100. Paulus, D. A.: Oximetry as a warning of inadequate ventilation. Semin. Anesth., 5:188, 1986.
101. Brodsky, J. B.: Oxygen monitoring in the operating room. Semin. Anesth., 5:180, 1986.
102. Baden, J. M., Rice, S. A.: Metabolism and toxicity of inhaled anesthetics. In Miller, R. D. (ed.): Anesthesia, Vol. 1. New York, Churchill Livingstone, 1986, Ch. 22.
103. Holaday, D. A., Fiserova-Bergerova, V., Latto, I. P., et al.: Resistance of isoflurane to biotransformation in man. Anesthesiology, 54:383, 1981.
104. Mazze, R. I., Cousins, M. J., Barr, G. A.: Renal effects and metabolism of isoflurane in man. Anesthesiology, 40:536, 1974.
105. Shimosato, S., Carter, J. G., Kemmotsu, O., Takahashi, T.: Cardiocirculatory effects of prolonged administration of isoflurane in normocarbic human volunteers. Acta Anaesthesiol. Scand., 26:27, 1982.
106. Katz, R. L., Katz, G. J.: Surgical infiltration of pressor drugs and their interaction with volatile anesthetics. Br. J. Anaesth., 38:712, 1966.
107. Bovill, J. G., Coppel, D. L., Dundee, J. W., Moore, J.: Current status of ketamine anesthesia. Lancet, 1:1285, 1971.
108. Meyers, E. F., Charles, P.: Prolonged adverse reactions to ketamine in children. Anesthesiology, 49:39, 1978.
109. White, P. F.: Outpatient anesthesia. In Miller, R.D. (ed.): Anesthesia, Vol. 3. New York, Churchill Livingstone, 1986, Ch. 53.
110. Payne, J. P.: Atracurium. Semin. Anesth., 3:303, 1984.
111. Miller, R. D.: Vecuronium. Semin. Anesth., 3:312, 1984.
112. Lee, C.: Succinylcholine: Its past, present, and future. Semin. Anesth., 3:293, 1984.
113. Sedwick, L. A., Romano, P. E.: Malignant hyperthermia. Considerations for the ophthalmologist. Surv. Ophthalmol., 25:378, 1981.
114. Malignant hyperthermia: Nightmare for anesthesiologists—and patients. JAMA, 255:709, 1986.
115. Herschel, E. O. (ed.): Malignant Hyperthermia: Current Concepts. New York, Appleton-Century-Crofts, 1977.
116. Gronert, G. A.: Malignant hyperthermia. In Miller, R. D. (ed.): Anesthesia, Vol. 3. New York, Churchill Livingstone, 1986, Ch. 56.
117. Gronert, G. A.: Malignant hyperthermia. Semin. Anesth., 2:197, 1983.
118. Paasuke, R.T., Brownell, K. B.: Serum creatine kinase level as a screening test for susceptibility to malignant hyperthermia. JAMA, 255:769, 1986.
119. Flewellen, E. H., Nelson, T. E., Jones, W. P., et al.: Dantrolene dose response in awake man: Implications for management of malignant hyperthermia. Anesthesiology, 59:275, 1983.
120. Ruhland, G., Hinkle, A. F.: Malignant hyperthermia following preoperative oral administration of dantrolene. Anesthesiology, 60:159, 1984.
121. Fitzgibbons, D. C.: Malignant hyperthermia following preoperative oral administration of dantrolene. Anesthesiology, 54:73, 1981.
122. Petrusak, J., Smith, R. B., Breslin, P. P.: Mortality rate related to ophthalmological surgery. Arch. Ophthalmol., 89:106, 1973.
123. Snow, J. C., Sensel, S.: Review of cataract extraction under local and general anesthesia at MEEI. Anesth. Analg., 45:742, 1966.
124. Lynch, S., Wolf, G., Berlin, I.: 2200 cases of cataract

surgery under general anesthesia. Anesth. Analg., 53:909, 1974.

125. Gregory, G. A.: Pediatric anesthesia. *In* Miller, R. D. (ed.): Anesthesia, Vol. 3. New York, Churchill Livingstone, 1986, Ch. 49.

126. Betts, E., Downes, J. J., Shaeffer, D., Johns, R.: Retrolental fibroplasia and oxygen administration during general anesthesia. Anesthesiology, 47:518, 1977.

127. Pontinen, P. J.: The importance of the oculocardiac reflex during intraocular surgery. Acta Ophthalmol., 86:1, 1966.

128. Newell, F. W.: Current trends in ophthalmic anesthesia. Ophthalmic Surg., 6:15, 1975.

129. Alexander, J. P.: Reflex disturbance of cardiac rhythm during ophthalmic surgery. Br. J. Ophthalmol., 59:518, 1975.

130. Mirakhur, R. K., Jones, C. J., Dundee, J. W., et al.: Atropine or glycopyrrolate for the prevention of OCR children undergoing squint surgery. Br. J. Anaesth., 54:1059, 1982.

131. Blanc, V. F., Hardy, J. F., Milot, J., et al.: The OCR: A graphic and statistical analysis in infants and children. Can. Anaesth. Soc. J., 30:360, 1983.

132. Forestner, J. E., Imbrech, P.: Controlled respiration does not inhibit OCR during strabismus surgery. Anesthesiology, 59:A457, 1983.

133. Atkinson, W. S.: Anesthesia in Ophthalmology. Springfield, IL., Charles C Thomas, 1955, p. 42.

134. Monnie, G. T., Rees, D. I., Elton, D.: The oculocardiac reflex during strabismus surgery. Can. Anesth. Soc. J., 11:621, 1964.

135. Berler, D.: The oculocardiac reflex. Am. J. Ophthalmol., 56:954, 1963.

136. Mendelblatt, F., Kirsch, R. E., Lemberg, L.: A study comparing methods of preventing the oculocardiac reflex. Am. J. Ophthalmol., 53:506, 1962.

137. Alexander, J. P.: Reflex disturbances of cardiac rhythm during ophthalmic surgery. Br. J. Ophthalmol., 59:518, 1975.

138. Linn, J. G., Jr., Smith, R. B.: Intraoperative complications and their management. Int. Ophthalmol. Clin., 13:149, 1973.

139. Blanc, V. F.: The effect of anticholinergic premedication for infants and children on the OCR. Can. Anaesth. Soc. J., 30:683, 1983.

140. Steward, D.: The effect of anticholinergic premedication in infants and children on the OCR. Can. Anaesth. Soc. J., 30:684, 1983.

141. Sellick, B. A.: Cricoid pressure to control regurgitation of stomach contents during induction of anesthesia, preliminary communication. Lancet, 2:404, 1961.

142. Libonati, M. M., Leahy, J. J., Ellison, N.: The use of succinylcholine in open eye surgery. Anesthesiology, 62:637, 1985.

6

INTRAOCULAR INFECTIONS*

by Denis M. O'Day

Postoperative endophthalmitis is a dreaded complication of ocular surgery. Even with aggressive modern therapy and rapid diagnosis, many eyes thus infected fail to retain useful vision. In the past, efforts directed toward prevention of infection have been effective in lowering the incidence to 1 in 1280 cases, a level that has remained stable for several decades.[1] Despite this trend, the eye surgeon cannot be complacent. Intraocular infection continues to occur,[2] and occasionally the number of cases reaches epidemic proportions.[3-5] This chapter examines the causes, diagnosis, prophylaxis, and treatment of postoperative infections of the eye.

PROPHYLAXIS FOR OCULAR SURGICAL INFECTION

The surgical approach to the eye has to be made through a nonsterile field. Despite numerous suggested preoperative regimens for the cleansing of the lid and conjunctiva, the fact remains that it is probably impossible to completely sterilize these tissues.[6, 7] Thus a list of potential sources for microbial invasion of the eye during surgery must include the lids and conjunctiva. Indeed, the predominance of coagulase-negative staphylococci among isolates

from cases of endophthalmitis suggests that the external eye may be an important source. However, from previous experience we know that many cases are probably due to lapses in aseptic technique or contamination of instruments, fluids, or materials.

Lid and Conjunctival Sterility

The normal lids harbor both pathogenic and nonpathogenic bacteria. In the presence of active inflammatory disease of the lids, single species, such as *Staphylococcus, Pseudomonas, Streptococcus,* and *Diplococcus pneumoniae,* may become dominant. In the preoperative evaluation of patients for eye surgery, the lids should be carefully examined, looking for evidence of active inflammatory disease or permanent structural change that may indicate chronic bacterial invasion of the lids and lid glands. The nasolacrimal system also needs to be considered, since partial or complete obstruction may be present and act as a reservoir for contamination of the conjunctival sac.

More often neglected and of equal importance is an evaluation of the tear function. Patients who undergo intraocular surgery, and especially cataract surgery, frequently are in the older age group. In these patients it is not uncommon for lacrimal function to be depressed. Lack of an adequate tear film removes one of the defenses of the outer eye against infection, and thus increases the possibility of a post-operative infection.

Unfortunately, apart from a few broad general

*Preparation of this chapter was supported in part by NIH grant EY 01621, an unrestricted grant and a Senior Scientific Investigator Award from Research to Prevent Blindness.

principles, there is no consensus as to the appropriate way to minimize this risk. Certainly in those patients with active lid and lacrimal sac disease, surgery should be avoided until the infection is eliminated or under firm control. The question that remains is how to handle those patients with "normal" lids and conjunctiva who undoubtedly harbor potentially pathogenic organisms. Approaches range from the use of systemic antibiotics preoperatively to the avoidance of antibiotic therapy in any form.[8-10] Insofar as it is virtually impossible to sterilize the lids and conjunctiva, the goal of prophylactic therapy must necessarily be a less than ideal one: in the absence of acute infection to suppress the growth of bacteria for the period that the eye is open and exposed to the danger of infection. In light of this, the use of systemic antibiotics is difficult to justify because of the dangers of sensitization and toxicity, especially in older patients. Topical antibiotics, however, appear to be of value, especially if given within the three-day period immediately preceding surgery.[16] Various studies have shown a substantial reduction in the incidence of endophthalmitis when antibiotics were given over this period.[8] It would appear that most broad-spectrum topical antibiotics are effective, with the most desirable being those that cause a minimum of allergic reactions or toxicity. Neomycin, bacitracin, polymyxin, and chloramphenicol are likely to be the most useful. Jaffe and others, on the other hand, do not use routine prophylactic antibiotics, administering instead a subconjunctival injection of antibiotic, usually gentamicin, at the beginning of surgery.[11, 12] In one other series, in India, the use of intracameral gentamicin at the time of cataract extraction reduced the incidence of postoperative infection 10-fold.[13]

Most studies stress the need for antibiotics either immediately preoperatively or at the time of surgery as a means of reducing the incidence of intraocular infection.[14]

Contamination During Surgery

Intraocular surgery has entered a period of rapidly increasing complexity, a change that began more than 20 years ago with the introduction of the surgical microscope. More recently, miniaturized instrumentation has opened the way for ingenious techniques, and entirely new surgical subspecialties have developed within the realm of ocular surgery. Intraocular lenses, extracapsular cataract extraction, corneal preservation, vitreous surgical techniques, vitreous surgical instruments, and various infusion fluids have added a new dimension to the ophthalmic surgeon's responsibilities, and there now exists, in addition to the usual hazards from breakdown in aseptic technique, a whole new group of potential problems in which responsibility for maintaining asepsis is widely diffused. The incidence of endophthalmitis has remained low despite a few lapses that have led to the tragic loss of a number of eyes over a short period of time.[4, 5, 15]

There are five potential sources of infection owing to contamination at the time of surgery: air, tissues, fluids, instruments, and implants. Airborne infection is clearly of major concern in all operating rooms. Sources include the surgeon, the assistant, the operating room staff, visitors, and the patient. Measures designed to limit airborne infection are generally well understood and are subject to various rules and regulations and procedures in most operating rooms today. They will not be discussed further here.

Contaminated Tissues

There is no uniformity of opinion concerning the most appropriate way to cleanse the lids and conjunctiva before surgery. Because it is virtually impossible to sterilize the lids, the goal of skin preparation is to reduce the bacterial population to as low a level as possible, thus minimizing the risk of contamination of the eye while it is open during surgery. However, studies have shown that bacteria from the lids can be readily cultured from the wound during surgery without the patient subsequently developing endophthalmitis.[6, 16] In one study 23 per cent of lenses removed during a standard cataract extraction procedure were found to be contaminated with bacteria that could only have been acquired intraoperatively.[17]

Skin preparation for surgery includes cleansing of the eyelids, brows, and adjacent facial skin. The lashes may or may not be trimmed, depending largely on the preference of the surgeon. Although lash trimming may reduce the bacterial population to a degree, organisms are still present, and it is likely that trimming the lashes is more of a convenience to the surgeon than a hygienic maneuver.[16] Isenberg and his associates have shown in a series of elegantly executed experiments that it is possible to almost eliminate organisms from the surgical field, using a combination of a germicide (Betadine) and topical antibiotic therapy. Neosporin drops are instilled three times a day for three days preceding surgery. The skin of the lids, lid margins, and face is painted with Betadine solution in preparation for surgery. Several drops of half-strength Betadine solution are then instilled into the conjunctival sac and allowed to remain. Irrigation is not used. Silver nitrate is unnecessary. The diluted Betadine solution is well tolerated by the cornea. Iodophor solutions that contain detergent should not be used.[18]

When the skin preparation is complete, the patient is draped. Because a great many eye operations are performed under local anesthesia, draping presents some unique difficulties that have never been entirely solved. Ideally the purpose should be to completely seal off the eye from the skin of the eyelids and the patient's airway. Before the development of adhesive plastic drapes this was impossible, and air breathed by the patient was able to flow over the surgical site. This problem is partially solved by the use of adhesive drapes, but as surgery progresses the drapes frequently become wet and tend to separate from the skin, so that patient-respired air again gains access to the surgical field. In order to avoid this, a plastic adhesive drape may be prepared in such a way that it can be tucked over the lid margin and into the fornix, and be held in place by the speculum, effectively preventing contamination from the lids while denying access of patient-breathed air to the field. Despite its many advantages, this method has not gained universal acceptance, and most surgeons still do not cover the eyelashes with the plastic drape.

Contamination from the surgeon's gloved hands may also occur. Thin rubber is prone to perforation, and minute holes frequently go unnoticed, allowing the passage of organisms from the surgeon's hand onto the surgical field and instruments.[19]

Contaminated Fluids

The possibility of exposing the eye to contaminated solution has long been a major concern in ophthalmology.[20, 21] This concern has become more pressing with the almost universal acceptance of the extracapsular procedure and the development of closed vitreous surgery.[15] The modern ophthalmic surgeon is forced to use solutions prepared and packaged elsewhere, placing his faith in the standards of others and accepting a solution as sterile when he has no means of determining whether or not aseptic techniques have been breached. In addition to the usual breakdowns in procedure that may occur in any large manufacturing process, fine cracks may develop in the walls of glass containers, leading to contamination.

A recent outbreak of postoperative infection was traced to the use of an ocular irrigating solution contaminated with *Candida parapsilosis*.[3] Before the product was withdrawn, 23 proven and 15 possible cases of endophthalmitis were identified. Similar episodes are likely to occur in the future, since it is virtually impossible to guarantee the sterility of these products. One effective way to minimize the risk is to use a microbiological filter.[22] The 0.22-μm Millipore filter can be used with the manual aspiration technique, but it does not provide sufficient flow rates for mechanical systems. However, filters with a larger surface area and increased flow rates are now available. The risk is further reduced by using a fresh vial of fluid with each patient, rather than the unexpended volume from a previous procedure.

Contaminated Instruments and Surgical Materials

Contamination of the instruments and materials used in surgery is an ever-present possibility and may occur through faulty sterilization and improper techniques of autoclaving, failure of gas sterilizers, poor surgical technique, or inadvertent contamination through unrecognized defects in gloves. The increasing complexity of ocular surgery, the use of the surgical microscope, and complicated instrumentation make the possibility of breaks in technique more likely. The frequent manipulation of the microscope that is necessary during eye surgery increases the possibility of accidental contact with nonsterile surfaces. In addition, the microscope may shed airborne bacteria on the opened eye. The greatest hazard probably lies with the complexity of the new equipment that is crowding eye operating rooms. These instruments require tedious setup and breakdown procedures for which the sterile and nonsterile zones are frequently not clearly delineated. Operating room personnel, including the surgeon, may inadvertently contaminate lines or components that subsequently enter the surgical field.

In order to avoid these risks, it is essential for the surgeon to be familiar with all the operational aspects of each instrument that he must use, and for the operating room staff to set up procedures that monitor for possible transgressions of aseptic technique. A particularly hazardous situation is the combination of a surgeon operating under the microscope surrounded by new instruments and a number of visitors. It has always been prudent to limit the amount of movement within the operating room to that essential for support of the surgeon. This rule becomes even more important as instrumentation and procedures increase in complexity.

The epidemics of bacterial and fungal infections associated with the implantation of intraocular lenses dramatically demonstrate the reliance the ophthalmic surgeon has to place on others for maintenance of standards of sterility. Two major outbreaks of endophthalmitis have occurred with *Pseudomonas*, both resulting from breakdowns in sterilization technique and standards at the sites of manufacture of the lenses. The first outbreak of fungal infection is particularly illustrative of the hazard that may surround the introduction of new techniques into eye surgery. *Paecilomyces* is a common contaminant of sterile solutions and is extremely difficult to eradicate. It has been considered to be a harmless saprophytic organism, although an occasional case of endophthalmitis had been reported before the recent outbreak with intraocular lenses.[23]

The wet sterilization technique previously used with intraocular lenses failed to take into account the possibility that organisms of this nature may survive and be harmful to the eye. This has now been replaced by gas autoclaving and has, so far, been successful in preventing further outbreaks of this nature.

In corneal transplantation, techniques for short-term and medium-term preservation that use various specially modified tissue culture media have not been associated so far with any epidemics, although sporadic cases of infection owing to contamination of the tissue culture medium have been reported.

Leisengang and colleagues have shown that the introduction of an antibiotic to the tissue culture medium does not guarantee sterility.[24] It is, therefore, encumbent on the surgeon who uses preserved tissue for corneal transplantation to be aware of this hazard. No satisfactory method yet exists for checking the sterility of the medium at the time of surgery, but culture of the medium and the scleral rim should be performed routinely. When fresh donor material is used, contamination is also possible.[25, 26] Although no single method will eliminate all microorganisms, the most effective procedure is immersion of the globe in a mixture of gramicidin, neomycin, and polymyxin B.[25, 27] Irrigating antibiotic solution onto the surface of the eye appears to be less desirable. In addition,

direct cultures should be taken from the cut cornea margin of the donor eye after the button has been removed.[28]

In retinal detachment surgery the problems with infection are similar to those associated with intraocular surgery, although the implantation of foreign material and the prolonged duration of surgery may make the risk of postoperative infection somewhat higher.[6] However, the major problem is an infectious episcleritis rather than endophthalmitis. McMeel and Wapner demonstrated the presence of pathogenic bacteria in and around the surgical field, including the implant, in 85 per cent of cases by the end of surgery. This was despite preoperative antibiotic therapy and standard skin preparation and draping.[6] In another study of 1000 scleral buckling procedures McMeel demonstrated a 66 per cent incidence of contamination of the wound site by the termination of surgery.[29] In the first 500 patients in this study the incidence of subsequent overt infection was 2 per cent; in the second 500 this incidence dropped to 1.2 per cent, a significant change, possibly reflecting an increased awareness of the surgical team of the necessity for careful skin preparations and maintenance of sterile technique. The practice of soaking the implant material in an antibiotic before use is now fairly widespread.[30] Sub-Tenon's injection of gentamicin solution around the implant at the conclusion of the surgery as well as the use of prophylactic and intraoperative antibiotics have been advocated.[30, 31]

The choice of an antibiotic for treatment is a difficult one. It would appear that a majority of the infections are caused by *Staphylococcus aureus*. Fortunately many hospital laboratories now maintain a log of antibiotic sensitivities for hospital staphylococci that will enable the appropriate selection to be made. It is further recommended that this selection be periodically reviewed, since susceptibility to antibiotics will change from time to time.

Infections Acquired Postoperatively

Endophthalmitis may occur as a result of infection acquired during the postoperative phase. The infection may occur through an inadvertent filtering bleb, a suture track, or a vitreous wick, or as a complication of filtering surgery for glaucoma.[32] The use of cryosurgery for formal closure of filtering blebs is of some help in eliminating the potential for infection in these cases. With filtering surgery the use of long-term prophylactic antibiotic therapy is practiced by many surgeons. Fortunately the overall incidence of infection is not high.

The visual prognosis for culturally proven postoperative endophthalmitis has been poor.[33] Only in the case of *Staphylococcus epidermidis* infection has anything approaching reasonable vision been salvaged.[34] The generally unsatisfactory nature of conventional therapeutic approaches has spurred interest in a number of techniques that involve direct intervention with the infectious process. These include both the injection of antimicrobial agents into the vitreous cavity and therapeutic vitrectomy.

INFECTIOUS ENDOPHTHALMITIS

Signs and Symptoms

The clinical recognition of a suspected infectious endophthalmitis is the first step in treatment. Signs and symptoms may become apparent within 24 to 48 hours of surgery, or may be delayed for days or months. There is no sure way to distinguish clinically the infectious from the so-called sterile endophthalmitis.[35] The onset of pain postoperatively is a symptom that should always be viewed with grave suspicion, as it may be the first sign of a developing endophthalmitis. However, in an occasional case, pain may be absent. Swelling and redness of the upper eyelids develop; the lid is intensely inflamed and the bulbar conjunctiva may become chemotic. The development of intraocular signs of inflammation may be explosive, with corneal edema, anterior chamber hypopyon,

loss of the red reflex, and decrease in vision to light perception occurring (Figs. 6–1, 6–2, and 6–3). Alternatively, there may be a more insidious evolution of intraocular inflammation. Once initiated, the course is usually a relentless one. Mycotic infections tend to develop somewhat more slowly, usually 2 weeks or more after surgery. Floaters may be an early symptom before the development of an hypopyon (Fig. 6–4); focal infiltrates may be seen in the posterior vitreous followed by the development of membranes in the anterior vitreous, and, again, relentless progression of the inflammatory process.[4] Focal white infiltrative lesions may develop on the vitreous face or just behind it in the anterior vitreous.

A number of authors have recently described a later-occurring endophthalmitis caused by infection with anaerobic bacteria. Most commonly the organism isolated has been *Propionibacterium acnes*. The period of incubation may be weeks to months and the signs of infection extremely subtle in the early stages, so the infection is easily confused with a sterile inflammation.[36, 37] Evidence should always be sought for an exogenous route to endophthalmitis; for example, an abscess may be visible around an exposed suture (Fig. 6–5), or an infected filtering bleb may be apparent with the peculiar finding on occasion of a fluid level of inflammatory cells within the bleb (Fig. 6–6). All patients who undergo ocular surgery should undergo regular slit-lamp examination during the period of postoperative observation, as a careful notation of the signs of inflammation will help to detect the early case before structural change has become irreversible.

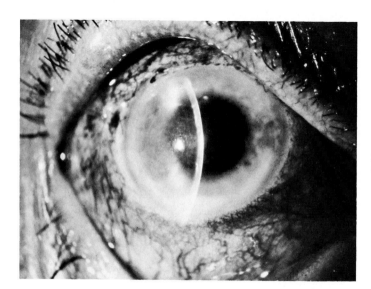

FIGURE 6–1. The development of hypopyon 5 days after an uncomplicated intracapsular cataract extraction.

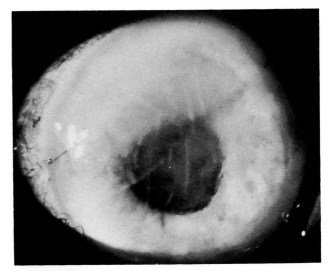

FIGURE 6–2. Same patient 3 days later. The cornea is now diffusely edematous. Vitreous tap yielded *Staphylococcus epidermidis*. →

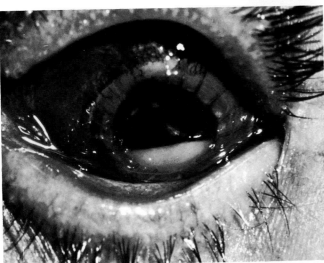

← **FIGURE 6–3.** A large hypopyon appeared 3 weeks after a penetrating keratoplasty was performed on an aphakic eye. *Candida albicans* was isolated from a vitreous tap.

FIGURE 6–4. Stringy infiltrations in the vitreous are characteristic of fungal endophthalmitis. →

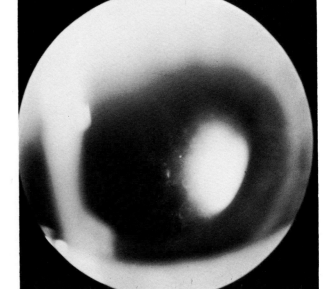

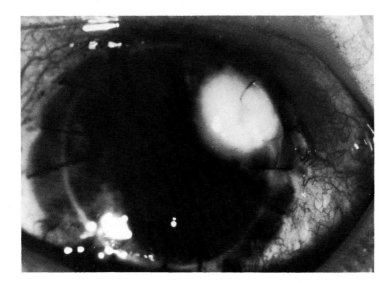

FIGURE 6–5. Suture abscess caused by *Staphylococcus aureus*.

Diagnosis

When a provisional clinical diagnosis of infective endophthalmitis has been made, an immediate attempt to establish an etiologic diagnosis is essential. There is no place for either a waiting period of observation or the use of blind antibiotic or steroid therapy in this situation. The crux of the problem in postoperative endophthalmitis is whether the inflammation is due to a replicating or nonreplicating stimulus, because the decision of whether or not to attempt recovery of an isolate rests on this provisional diagnosis. As already discussed, certain features of an infectious endophthalmitis, particularly the presence of pain and the timing of the inflammation, are helpful in making a provisional diagnosis. It is clear, however, that the features of a sterile endophthalmitis may be identical to those of an endophthalmitis caused by bacteria or fungi—at least in the early stages, when the diagnosis is crucial. The outcome of a microbial postoperative endophthalmitis depends on a number of important factors[33, 38, 39]: virulence of the organism in question, delay in diagnosis and its relation to permanent structural damage already engendered by the inflammation, severity of the host response, and efficacy of the specific antimicrobial and anti-inflammatory therapy. It is virtually impossible to analyze the impact of all these factors on the outcome, but it has recently become apparent that the type of organism isolated has a direct influence on the prognosis. As many as 50 per cent of all cases of endophthalmitis appear to be due to infection with coagulase-negative staphylococci. These infections have a good prognosis, with most patients achieving vision

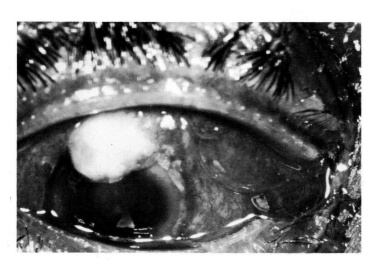

FIGURE 6–6. Endophthalmitis may develop from an infected filtering bleb.

in the 20/50 or better range. Anaerobic infections are also generally associated with a good visual prognosis.[40] In contrast, the outcome in the remaining cases made up of infections with *Streptococcus* sp., *S. aureus*, gram-negative rods, and other miscellaneous organisms is far less optimistic, a final visual acuity of 20/400 being considered a good outcome.

The time to diagnosis is also important, but experience shows that the inflammation is usually already well advanced when the diagnosis is made. Alertness to the possibility of an endophthalmitis in its early stage and a willingness to perform the whole range of isolation techniques offer the best chances of improving the diagnosis.

Diagnostic Techniques

The rate of isolate recovery from cases of endophthalmitis has improved in recent years.[38] Studies by Forster indicate that in the aphakic eye devoid of a posterior capsule, sampling of the vitreous offers the best chance of a positive culture.[33] In the eye with an intact posterior capsule the same appears to hold true despite the theoretical barrier present.[32, 38] In the phakic eye the inflammation is usually in the anterior segment, and an anterior chamber tap appears to be the logical approach.

Techniques to obtain an isolate are best approached as a formal procedure in the operating room with normal skin preparation and draping. Usually only a sterile plastic drape is necessary. Because of the dangers of wound dehiscence, there may be reluctance to use retrobulbar anesthesia in a very recently operated eye, so general anesthesia may be preferred. If local anesthesia is to be used, lid akinesia should also be used. Vitreous and anterior chamber aspiration are necessary as separate procedures, whether an intracapsular or extracapsular procedure has been performed. A pars plana approach to the vitreous through a prepared sclerotomy using a 22-gauge needle for aspiration can be performed in the aphakic eye under the operating microscope with accuracy. The aspirate should be inoculated directly on blood agar, Sabouraud's agar, chocolate agar, thioglycolate broth, and brain heart infusion media. Isolation of anaerobic organisms is best attempted on Brucella or Columbia agar–based medium with vitamin K and hemin.[41] The fluid should be placed on the center of the plate so as to identify any possible contamination that may have occurred during the procedure. In addition, it is helpful to mark the site of inoculation on the bottom of the plate with a wax pencil. An alternative approach is to use a vitreous suction cutter device, passing the fluid through a sterile filter. The anterior chamber tap should then be performed. A partially penetrating keratotomy, using a Bowman or Wheeler knife, is made at the limbus down to Descemet's membrane. The opening should be large enough to accommodate a 27-gauge needle. The needle is introduced on a syringe through Descemet's membrane, and aqueous contents are aspirated. This technique avoids any undue stress on the recent surgical wound. Care should be taken to introduce the needle through clear cornea at the limbus, to avoid contamination by the conjunctiva. Conjunctival cultures should also be taken. If a stitch abscess or infected bleb is present, the stitch abscess should be cultured with removal of the suture; aspiration directly into the bleb for culture is effective. While the patient is in the operating room, the diagnostic stains should be examined so that more material can be obtained if these are unsatisfactory. It is useful to have several unstained smears on hand in case special techniques are deemed advisable.

Diagnostic Criteria

The therapy of endophthalmitis is determined to some extent by the results of the diagnostic techniques and the need to eliminate or neutralize the inflammatory stimulus and to control the host response. There is some uncertainty regarding the criteria for diagnosis of microbial endophthalmitis. Logically, it would appear that the diagnosis must remain questionable in the presence of negative cultures despite a "typical" clinical course. Likewise, a contaminant may masquerade as a pathogen despite the most stringent precautions. Most series of microbial endophthalmitis that have been reported contain cases in which an etiologic diagnosis was not established, the cases being treated on a presumptive basis.[33, 38, 39, 42–44] In both Forster's and Peyman's series the patients in whom an isolate was not recovered fared far better visually than those in whom there was positive isolation from the vitreous or anterior chamber. This curious finding casts considerable doubt on the value of a clinical diagnosis of infectious endophthalmitis, since a number of these cases must almost certainly have been noninfectious in origin. It may be that negative cultures and smears, when appropriately performed, are of more value than has been heretofore recognized.

Treatment

In the face of the unreliability in clinical diagnosis, the physician is forced to make a presumptive diagnosis of infection and to treat accordingly. Although the diagnostic smears are useful if positive, too much weight should not be placed on positive identification at this stage, since it is prone to error even in the hands of the most experienced diagnostician.[42, 45] Similarly, if hyphal fragments or budding yeasts are seen on Giemsa stain, a preliminary diagnosis of fungal infection can be made, but positive identification of species is not possible until culture becomes positive.

How, then, should treatment be initiated until recovery of an isolate provides a firmer basis for therapy? Four components must be considered: route of administration, antibiotic selection, role of vitrectomy, and anti-inflammatory therapy. Although interrelated to a considerable degree, for clarity they are best considered separately.

Route of Administration. A major controversy has developed over the most effective ways to administer antibiotics in cases of endophthalmitis. Most authors subscribe to the principle of administering antibiotics by topical, subconjunctival, and systemic routes to all patients with endophthalmitis (Tables 6–1, 6–2, and 6–3), but there is some difference of opinion regarding the appropriate indications for intravitreal injection of antibiotics. The debate has recently been sharpened by the recognition of aminoglycoside toxicity as a hazard of intravitreal therapy.[46–48]

The issue is not an easy one to resolve, and there is clearly room for judgment. Behind the decision to inject antibiotics into the vitreous cavity lies the need to administer antibiotics in

TABLE 6–1. Antimicrobials for Subconjunctival and Retrobulbar Injection

AGENT	DOSAGE
Methicillin	100 mg
Oxacillin	100 mg
Ampicillin	100 mg
Carbenicillin	100 mg
Cefazolin (Ancef)	100 mg
Gentamicin	40 mg
Tobramycin	40 mg
Vancomycin	25 mg
Penicillin G	1.0 mega units
Miconazole (Monistat)	5 mg (undiluted Monistat)

TABLE 6–2. Antibiotics in Artificial Tears

ANTIBIOTIC	DOSAGE	DURATION OF ACCEPTABLE POTENCY AT ROOM TEMPERATURE
Penicillin	100,000 U/ml	3 days
Cephazolin	50 mg/ml	4 days
Bacitracin	10,000 U/ml	7 days
Carbenicillin	6.2 mg/ml	7 days
Gentamicin	14 mg/ml	7 days
Amikacin	10 mg/ml	7 days
Vancomycin	25 mg/ml	7 days

TABLE 6–3. Topical Preparations of Antifungal Agents

AGENT	CONCENTRATION
Natamycin	5% suspension
Flucytosine	10 mg/ml
Miconazole	10 mg/ml
Amphotericin B	1.5 mg/ml

effective concentrations as rapidly as possible to the site of infection. Because the penetration of antibiotics delivered by other routes is questionable, it is suggested that only injection into the vitreous can provide the levels needed to combat infection. It is also true, however, that not all infections require the same rigorous approach. In fact, for infections caused by *S. epidermidis*, despite the reportedly low levels achieved in the eye, the results in one series treated without recourse to intravitreal therapy were better than similar cases treated by intravitreal antibiotics and vitrectomy[34] (Fig. 6–7). On the other hand, infections with the more virulent organisms clearly require a more aggressive approach to save the eye, but even then the visual outlook is likely to be poor. Although most of these eyes are now saved, visual goals are modest, with results of 20/400 being reported as successful.

Antibiotic Selection. The selection of the appropriate antibiotics is predicated on the need (a) to achieve therapeutic intraocular concentrations as rapidly as possible; (b) to provide effective therapy against the organisms most likely to be encountered (coagulase-negative staphylococci, penicillinase-producing *S. aureus*, *Pseudomonas*, and other gram-negative rods); and (c) to provide as broad a spectrum of antibiotic cover as possible. These ideals are clearly impossible to attain with any single drug but are feasible using a combination of drugs. Modification of this regimen will be necessary

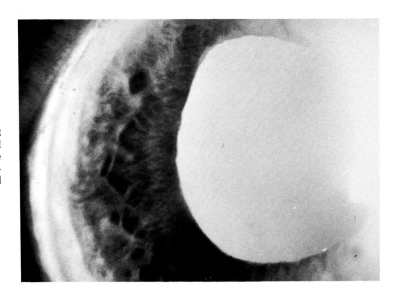

FIGURE 6–7. Appearance of eye 2 months after endophthalmitis caused by *Staphylococcus epidermidis*. The inflammation has resolved and the vitreous has cleared after intensive local antibiotic and corticosteroid therapy.

if other infectious organisms resistant to these drugs are suspected or later isolated.

Currently the agents most commonly advocated are cefazolin (a cephalosporin) and gentamicin (an aminoglycoside). Both can be administered by topical subconjunctival and systemic routes and, with appropriate safeguards, appear well tolerated. Both agents are used for intravitreal injection (Table 6–4), although, as noted above, toxicity with gentamicin, even in the doses currently recommended, remains a problem. In the event that allergy to penicillin is present and cross-allergenicity with the cephalosporin is a hazard, vancomycin may be substituted.

The administration of a single dose of an antibiotic selected without knowledge of the offending organism or its antibiotic sensitivities carries with it some aspects of a hit-or-miss approach. In order to broaden the spectrum of coverage, therefore, the injection of two antibiotics is now advocated—an aminoglycoside and a cephalosporin—usually gentamicin and cefazolin. Cefazolin, in the dose recommended, appears safe and well tolerated except in patients who are allergic to penicillin, but with

gentamicin the difference between the toxic and therapeutic dose is narrow. Studies have demonstrated the retinal toxicity of intravitreal gentamicin and have spurred interest in alternative, less toxic agents.[50]

During this period the patient should be under close observation, so that any changes that may represent response to therapy or a worsening in the process may be detected. It has to be admitted that these changes are extremely difficult to evaluate. Further deterioration in vision, increasing pain and chemosis, and enhancement of the inflammatory signs within the eye clearly indicate a deterioration, whereas a lessening of pain and a stabilization of ocular inflammation are grounds for optimism that the infection is responding to specific therapy. Sequential close observation is helpful in determining the direction of these early trends.

Once an organism has been identified, the diagnosis is on firmer ground, and susceptibility testing may dictate an alteration in antibiotic therapy. If, however, the infection appears to be responding to the current therapy, it is wise to maintain this approach.

In those cases in which fungal infection is strongly suspected, based on the results of the smear or proved through isolation, antifungal therapy should be used. The approach is best considered on the basis of the type of fungus identified. If budding yeasts are seen on Gram stain, the approach of combining flucytosine (5-FC) and amphotericin B is used. The agent flucytosine (Ancobon) is administered orally in a dosage of 150 mg/kg/day and can be injected subconjunctivally and administered topically,

TABLE 6–4. Intravitreal Antibiotics

ANTIBIOTIC	DOSE
Gentamicin	0.1 mg
Cefazolin sodium	2.25 mg
Vancomycin	1.0 mg
Lincomycin	1.5 mg
Amphotericin B	5 μg

although the intraocular penetration by these routes remains uncertain.[51] Amphotericin B is administered systemically, using the approach of Drutz and co-workers to minimize systemic toxicity of the drug.[52] Both periocular and topical administration of amphotericin B are associated with marked local toxicity and should be avoided. However, frequent topical application of dilute amphotericin B (0.05% to 0.15%) is well tolerated, and ocular penetration is enhanced if the cornea is debrided daily.[54] If a filamentous organism is demonstrated on smear or isolated, amphotericin B should be administered using the same technique. Miconazole, an excellent alternative, is now also available for systemic and periocular use.[53] Ketoconazole, a related imidazole, can be administered orally and should be considered for use in conjunction with amphotericin B. Intravitreal amphotericin B (5 μg) is indicated in all filamentous fungal infections. *Candida albicans* infections usually respond well to systemic amphotericin B, but other yeasts may not be so susceptible and may require intravitreal therapy.[55]

The therapeutic armamentarium for fungal endophthalmitis is extremely limited, and the agents are too toxic to entertain the possibility of intraocular administration. Some filamentous fungi, however, particularly *Cladosporium*, have been demonstrated to be sensitive to 5-FC, so that the combined use of 5-FC and amphotericin B may be advisable because the situation is so desperate. In addition, synergism has been demonstrated with these drugs for some organisms, particularly yeasts.

Anti-inflammatory Therapy. Corticosteroid administration is being increasingly advocated in the management of microbial endophthalmitis.[38, 42, 56] The severity of an ocular inflammatory reaction such as endophthalmitis is an indication of the intense interaction between the host and the offending stimulus. This is a complex process, with tissue damage resulting from the inflammatory response itself as well as direct tissue damage by enzymes and toxins that may be liberated by the microorganisms. Effective antimicrobial therapy is, therefore, a prime requisite for the treatment of endophthalmitis, although it will not immediately alter the clinical course of the inflammatory reaction. Anti-inflammatory therapy for the concomitant control of the host response is necessary in order to eliminate the inflammatory cells that are contributing to the tissue damage (see Fig. 6–2). The most frequently used and available anti-inflammatory agents are corticosteroids. These hormones produce an involution of those inflammatory cells that have invaded the eye, and suppress the migration of additional polymorphonuclear leukocytes to the site of injury. They inhibit the release of hydrolytic enzymes from inflammatory cells and also produce an involution of mature lymphocytes, thereby depressing cellular hypersensitivity. It must be emphasized that corticosteroid therapy is nonspecific.[57]

Ideally the administration of effective antimicrobial therapy is a prerequisite for the introduction of corticosteroid management of microbial endophthalmitis. This follows the concept of a combined approach to therapy in which control or elimination of both the stimulus to inflammation and the host response is the goal.[57] In endophthalmitis there is seldom sufficient time to allow evidence of a clinical response to be sought, since tissue destruction occurs so rapidly that the eye may be lost within a very short period. Therefore, it is necessary to initiate corticosteroids at an early stage of therapy. Baum and Rao[42] have suggested waiting 24 hours before initiating corticosteroid therapy; others introduce it somewhat later. We would suggest that the decision to introduce corticosteroid be influenced by (a) the degree of inflammatory response at the time of initiating antimicrobial therapy and (b) by the causative agent identified and its anticipated susceptibility to antimicrobial therapy.

Although experience has shown that combined therapy is effective for most of the agents involved in infectious endophthalmitis, for several classes of agents, particularly the gram-negative rods and fungi, speedy sterilization of the infection is less certain. In these cases caution in introducing corticosteroid is advised, despite the need to limit tissue damage induced by the inflammatory response.

An especial concern exists in patients who develop endophthalmitis from an infected filtering bleb after prior glaucoma surgery. Here the inflammatory response must be limited quickly and completely. Except in rare cases suppression and elimination of the infection is readily accomplished. But this achievement is of little solace to the patient whose vision has been ruined by the sequelae of inflammation itself. In such cases early, vigorous use of corticosteroids is mandatory. The situation is quite unlike most other types of endophthalmitis. No studies have been reported that provide any better guidelines for this therapy.

Corticosteroids should be administered periocularly by sub-Tenon's and retrobulbar injections. Higher levels within the eye can be achieved in the laboratory animal by this route than by systemic administration, with the advantage that the systemic effects of these compounds can thereby be minimized.[42] The value of supplementary topical corticosteroid has yet to be defined. Leibowitz and others have shown that prednisolone acetate appears to be the best topical preparation in terms of ocular penetration and anti-inflammatory potency, producing peak levels in the anterior chamber within 40 minutes of administration.[56, 58] Therefore, there seems adequate reason to combine the periocular and topical routes in the anti-inflammatory treatment of microbial endophthalmitis. Both dexamethasone, 4 mg/ml, and methylprednisolone sodium succinate (sodium Medrol), 40 mg/ml, have been advocated as the agents of choice. The anti-inflammatory effectiveness of dexamethasone is roughly equivalent to the methylprednisolone preparation, but there are three times more corticosteroid in the latter preparation.[59] There may be some advantage to using a combination of 4 mg of Decadron subconjunctivally (or retrobulbarly) with topical prednisolone acetate administered hourly.

Combined antimicrobial and corticosteroid therapy needs to be continued while the progress of the inflammation is carefully observed for signs of involution or exacerbation. The use of intraocular corticosteroids has also been recommended at the time of vitreous aspiration.[60] Little data are available on the efficacy of this procedure, and toxicity remains uncertain.

Therapeutic Vitrectomy. The appropriate indications for vitrectomy in infectious endophthalmitis are still controversial. The procedure itself is not without risk. Visualization is likely to be poor, reducing the effectiveness of the procedure, while at the same time increasing the risk of retinal damage or detachment. Given these problems and the excellent response to treatment without recourse to vitrectomy in patients with less fulminating infections, limiting immediate therapeutic vitrectomy to fulminant, rapidly progressive cases and cases unresponsive to initial therapy appears reasonable. Mandelbaum and Forster have listed their indications for therapeutic vitrectomy as follows: (a) patients presenting at an advanced stage of inflammation; (b) failure to improve within 36 to 48 hours on standard therapy (including intravitreal antibiotics); and (c) isolation of a highly virulent organism (i.e., gramnegative dipthroids, *Streptococcus* sp.).[61] To these may be added the isolation of a filamentous fungus. After the inflammation has resolved, the indications for vitrectomy are clearer, since removal of opacified vitreous and membranes may restore visual acuity and avoid the long-term complications of retinal detachment.

REFERENCES

1. Allen, H. F.: Postoperative endophthalmitis: Incidence and etiology. Ophthalmology, 85:317, 1978.
2. Katz, L. J., Cantor, L. B., Spaeth, G. L.: Complications of surgery in glaucoma. Early and late bacterial endophthalmitis following glaucoma filtering surgery. Ophthalmology, 92:959, 1985.
3. O'Day, D. M.: Value of a centralized surveillance system during a national epidemic of endophthalmitis. Ophthalmology, 92:309, 1985.
4. Mosier, M. S., Lusk, B., Pettit, T. H., et al.: Fungal endophthalmitis following intraocular lens implantation. Am. J. Ophthalmol., 83:1, 1977.
5. O'Day, D. M.: Fungal endophthalmitis caused by *Paecilomyces lilacinus* after intraocular lens implantation. Am. J. Ophthalmol., 83:130, 1977.
6. McMeel, J. W., Wapner, J. M.: Infections and retinal surgery. Arch. Ophthalmol., 74:42, 1965.
7. Anderson, K. F., Crompton, D. O., Lillie, S.: Contaminated ophthalmic ointments. Trans. Ophthalmol. Soc. Aust., 23:86, 1963.
8. Allen, H. F., Mangiaracine, A. B.: Bacterial endophthalmitis after cataract surgery. Arch. Ophthalmol., 72:454, 1964.
9. Kolker, A. E., Freeman, M. I., Pettit, T. H.: Prophylactic antibiotics and post-operative endophthalmitis. Am. J. Ophthalmol., 63:434, 1967.
10. Locatcher-Khorazo, D., Gutierrez, E.: Eye infections following cataract extraction, with special reference to the role of *Staphylococcus aureus*. Am. J. Ophthalmol., 41:981, 1956.
11. Jaffe, N. S.: Cataract Surgery and Its Implications. St. Louis, C. V. Mosby Co., 1972, p. 298.
12. Cassady, J. R.: Prophylactic subconjunctival antibiotics following cataract extraction. Am. J. Ophthalmol., 64:1081, 1967.
13. Peyman, G. A., Sathar, M. L., May, D. R.: Intraocular gentamicin as intraoperative prophylaxis in South India Eye Camps. Br. J. Ophthalmol., 61:260, 1977.
14. Post-operative Endophthalmitis. Symposium on Ocular Pharmacology and Therapeutics. P. P. Ellis, ed. Trans. New Orleans Acad. Ophthalmol., 1970.
15. Blankenship, G. W.: Endophthalmitis following pars plana vitrectomy. Am. J. Ophthalmol., 84:815, 1977.
16. Perry, L. D., Skaggs, C.: Preoperative topical antibiotics and lash trimming in cataract surgery. Ophthalmic Surg., 8:44, 1977.
17. Kohn, A. N.: Bacterial cultures of lenses removed during cataract surgery. Am. J. Ophthalmol., 86:162, 1978.
18. Isenberg, S. J., Apt, L., Yoshimori, R., Khwarg, S.: Chemical preparation of the eye in ophthalmic surgery. Arch. Ophthalmol., 103:1340, 1985.
19. Devinish, E. A., Miles, A. A.: Control of *Staphylococcus aureus* in an operating theatre. Lancet, 1:1088, 1939.
20. Theodore, F. H., Feinstein, R. R.: Preparation and maintenance of sterile ophthalmic solutions. J.A.M.A., 152:1631, 1953.
21. Theodore, F. H., Feinstein, R. R.: Practical suggestions for the preparation and maintenance of sterile

ophthalmic solutions. Am. J. Ophthalmol., 35:656, 1952.

22. Jaffe, N. S.: Elimination of contamination from ophthalmic solutions for intraocular surgery. Trans. Am. Acad. Ophthalmol. Otolaryngol., 74:406, 1970.

23. Rodrigues, M. M., McLeod, D.: Exogenous fungal endophthalmitis caused by *Paecilomyces*. Am. J. Ophthalmol., 79:687, 1975.

24. Leisengang, T., Robinson, N., Jones, D. B.: Effect of temperature and antibiotics on the replication of bacteria in McCarey-Kaufman modified tissue culture medium. Presented at the Association for Research in Vision and Ophthalmology, Sarasota, Florida, 1977.

25. Polack, F. M., Locatcher-Khorazo, D., Gutierrez, E.: Bacteriologic study of donor eyes. Arch. Ophthalmol., 78:219, 1967.

26. Buxton, J. N., Brownstein, S.: Bacterial cultures from donor corneas. Arch. Ophthalmol., 84:148, 1970.

27. Capella, J. A., Edelhauser, H. F., Van Horn, D. C. (eds.): Corneal Preservation. Springfield, Ill., Charles C Thomas, 1973.

28. Shaw, E. L., Aquavella, J. V.: Pneumococcal endophthalmitis following grafting of corneal tissue from a cadaver kidney donor. Ann. Ophthalmol., 9:435, 1977.

29. McMeel, J. W.: Infections and retinal surgery, II. Arch. Ophthalmol., 74:45, 1965.

30. Lean, J. S., Chignell, A. H.: Infection following retinal detachment surgery. Br. J. Ophthalmol., 61:593, 1977.

31. McMeel, J. W.: Acute and subacute infection following scleral buckle operations. Ophthalmology, 85:341, 1978.

32. Driebe, W. T., Mandelbaum, S., Forster, R. K., et al.: Pseudophakic endophthalmitis. Ophthalmology, 93:442, 1986.

33. Forster, R. K.: Endophthalmitis. Diagnostic cultures and visual results. Arch. Ophthalmol., 92:387, 1974.

34. O'Day, D. M., Jones, D. B., Patrinely, J., Elliott, J. H.: *Staphylococcus epidermidis* endophthalmitis. Ophthalmology, 89:354, 1982.

35. Aronson, S. B.: Starch endophthalmitis. Am. J. Ophthalmol., 73:570, 1972.

36. Jones, D. B., Robinson, N. M.: Anaerobic ocular infections. Trans. Am. Acad. Ophthalmol. Otolaryngol., 83:309, 1977.

37. Beatty, R. F., Robin, J. B., Trousdale, M. D., Smith, R. E.: Anaerobic endophthalmitis caused by *Propionibacterium acnes*. Am. J. Ophthalmol., 101:114, 1986.

38. Forster, R. K., Zachary, I. G., Cottingham, A. J., Jr., et al.: Further observations on the diagnosis, cause, and treatment of endophthalmitis. Am. J. Ophthalmol., 81:52, 1976.

39. Peyman, G. A.: Antibiotic administration in the treatment of bacterial endophthalmitis, II. Intravitreal injection. Survey Ophthalmol., 21:332, 1977.

40. Omerod, L. D., Topping, T. M., Paton, B. G., et al.: Anaerobic bacterial endophthalmitis. Ophthalmology (Aug Suppl), 93:78, 1986.

41. Sutter, V. L., Citron, D. M., Edelstein, M. A. C., Finegold, S. M. (eds.): Anaerobic Bacteriology Manual. Belmont, Calif., Star Publishing Co., 1985.

42. Baum, J. L., Rao, G.: Treatment of post cataract bacterial endophthalmitis with periocular and sys-temic antibiotics and corticosteroids. Trans. Am. Acad. Ophthalmol. Otolaryngol., 81:OP151, 1976.

43. Kanski, J. J.: The prevention and management of postoperative bacterial endophthalmitis. Trans. Ophthalmol. Soc. U.K., 94:19, 1974.

44. Fahmy, J. A.: Endophthalmitis following cataract extraction. Acta Ophthalmol., 53:522, 1975.

45. Jones, D. B.: Initial therapy of suspected microbial corneal ulcers. Survey Ophthalmol., 24:97, 1979.

46. Conway, B. P., Campochiaro, P. A.: Macular infarction after endophthalmitis treated with vitrectomy and intravitreal gentamicin. Arch. Ophthalmol., 104:367, 1986.

47. Talamo, J. H., D'Amico, D. J., Hanninen, L. A., et al.: The influence of aphakia and vitrectomy on experimental retinal toxicity of aminoglycoside antibiotics. Am. J. Ophthalmol., 100:840, 1985.

48. D'Amico, D. J., Libert, J., Kenyon, K. R., et al.: Retinal toxicity of intravitreal gentamicin. Invest. Ophthalmol. Vis. Sci., 25:564, 1984.

49. Baum, J. L.: Antibiotic administration in the treatment of bacterial endophthalmitis. I. Periocular injections. Survey Ophthalmol., 21:332, 1977.

50. Talamo, J. H., D'Amico, D. J., Kenyon, K. R.: Intravitreal amikacin in the treatment of bacterial endophthalmitis. Arch. Ophthalmol., 104:1483, 1986.

51. Richards, A. B., Jones, B. R., Whitewell, J., Clayton, Y.: Corneal and intraocular infections by *Candida albicans* treated with 5-fluorocytosine. Trans. Ophthalmol. Soc. U.K., 89:867, 1969.

52. Drutz, D. J., Spickard, A., Rogers, D. E., Koenig, M. G.: Treatment of disseminated mycotic infection: A new approach to amphotericin B. Am. J. Med., 45:405, 1968.

53. Foster, C. S., Stetanyszyn, M.: Intraocular penetration of miconazole in rabbits. Arch. Ophthalmol., 97:1703, 1979.

54. O'Day, D. M., Head, W. S., Robinson, R. D., Clanton, J.: Bioavailability and penetration of topical amphotericin B in the anterior chamber of the rabbit eye. J. Ocular Pharmacol., 2:371, 1986.

55. Stern, W. H., Tamura, E., Jacobs, R. A., et al.: Epidemic postsurgical *Candida parapsilosis* endophthalmitis. Ophthalmology, 92:1701, 1985.

56. Aronson, S. B., Moore, T. E., Jr., Williams, F. C., Goodner, E. K.: Corticosteroids in infectious ocular disease. *In* Kaufman, H. E. (ed.): Anti-inflammatory Ocular Therapy. St. Louis, C. V. Mosby Co., 1970, p. 14.

57. Aronson, S. B., Elliott, J. H.: Ocular Inflammation. St. Louis, C. V. Mosby Co., 1972.

58. Leibowitz, H. M., Berrospi, A. R., Kupferman, A., et al.: Penetration of topically applied prednisolone acetate into the human aqueous. Am. J. Ophthalmol., 83:402, 1977.

59. Leibowitz, H. M., Kupferman, A.: Periocular injection of corticosteroids. Arch. Ophthalmol., 95:311, 1977.

60. Peyman, G. A., Sanders, D. R.: Advances in Uveal Surgery, Vitreous Surgery, and the Treatment of Endophthalmitis. New York, Appleton-Century-Crofts, 1975, p. 207.

61. Mandelbaum, S., Forster, R. K.: Module 9: Infectious endophthalmitis. *In* Focal Points: Clinical Modules for Ophthalmologists. Am. Acad. Ophthalmol., Basic and Clinical Science Course, Sect. 3, 1983.

7

OPHTHALMIC LASERS: CURRENT STATUS

by Francis A. L'Esperance, Jr.

The development of the laser in 1960 made available to the world for the first time an extremely bright, monochromatic, highly directional beam that operated in the visible portion of the spectrum. It quickly became apparent to ophthalmic investigators that the potential use of the laser principle in photocoagulation was enormous. The increased predictability of absorption of laser radiation by the ocular structures, the precise focusing capabilities of the monochromatic, coherent beam, and the high photon energy density were attractive facets of the principle. The first actual laser photocoagulation trials in 1961[1] and 1963[2] supported these contentions, and in addition showed that laser photocoagulation was efficient and highly effective and required no anesthesia or akinesia.

The lasers available for photocoagulation have increased during the past several years, with the result that various monochromatic beams can produce selective histopathologic alterations of ocular tissue. The lasers currently used therapeutically or in ocular research are discussed briefly here.[3]

The lasers that are now commercially available as photocoagulation or photovaporization instruments are listed in Table 7–1, along with the year that each laser was introduced clinically in ophthalmology and the wavelengths emitted by each particular laser source. The outstanding advantages and disadvantages of each ophthalmic laser system are individually listed and then more extensively discussed. Certain background information, some clinical uses, and an

TABLE 7–1. Therapeutic Photon Sources in Ophthalmology

SYSTEMS	DATE OF CLINICAL INTRODUCTION	WAVELENGTHS
Xenon-arc system	1959[4]	400.0–1600.0 nm
Ruby laser	1963[2]	694.3 nm
Argon laser	1968[5]	457.3–524.7 nm
Neodymium-YAG laser—frequency-doubled	1971[6]	532.0 nm
Krypton laser	1972[7]	647.1 nm (red)
Carbon dioxide laser	1972[3(p63)]	10,600.0 nm
Dye laser		Multiple
Pulsed	1979[8]	
CW	1981[3(pp53, 343)]	
Neodymium-YAG laser—Q-switched or mode-locked	1980[9]	1064.0 nm
Excimer laser (ArF)	1985[10]	193.0 nm

overall appraisal of each laser modality are presented to familiarize the reader with the various attributes of each system.

ARGON LASER

Advantages

The advantages of the argon laser are as follows:

1. Highly absorbed by hemoglobin and melanin
2. Extremely large coagulation range possible
3. Large range of exposures available
4. High-power density available
5. Negligible ocular media absorption
6. Excellent variable delivery system

The argon laser is extremely well absorbed by oxyhemoglobin and reduced hemoglobin as well as by melanin; therefore, it can be used advantageously with both vascular abnormalities and structural problems of the retina and choroid. The variability of power density and spot size and the excellence of the delivery systems now developed make the argon laser the primary photocoagulation system for both anterior and posterior segment defects.[5]

Argon laser photocoagulation systems operate in the continuous-wave (CW) mode or the quasi-CW (burst) mode. The latter configuration is represented by the Britt laser photocoagulator; all other lasers produce radiation continuously. With the "cool" Britt laser the energy is delivered in multiple spikes or bursts of energy. The total energy produced can be varied by adjusting the power of each individual pulse as well as by changing the number of pulses produced per second. With this instrument various parameters such as peak power, average power, and laser pulse repetition rate must be considered for each diverse clinical application. Proponents of this type of laser emphasize that less energy is required for certain applications, particularly in the anterior segment of the eye.

The most common photocoagulation systems for ophthalmic surgery use argon lasers with a total power output ranging from 3 to 5 W. These wattages are sufficient for all photocoagulation efforts, even in cases where the 514.5-nm (green) wavelength has been split off from the 488.0-nm (blue) wavelength for foveal coagulations. Relatively compact argon lasers exceeding 20 W can be used for various aspects of photocoagulation or laser surgery, but these high powers are seldom required.

Argon laser endophotocoagulation has been advantageous for the intravitreal photocoagulation of retinal tears, abnormal vascular complexes, and other chorioretinal defects at the time of pars plana vitrectomy.[11, 12] The argon laser endophotocoagulator can be positioned farther away from the retina during photocoagulation and can be used in an air or gas medium such as the vitreous cavity after gas-fluid interchange. This instrument provides additional flexibility with various vitreoretinal surgical approaches.

Although the total argon laser beam consists of nine separate wavelengths, the beam is almost entirely composed of the blue (488.0-nm) and green (514.5-nm) wavelengths. At very low powers the beam is predominantly composed of the blue wavelength. If the beams are separated into the blue and green components by the appropriate prismatic or filter attachment, the absorption and optical characteristics of each portion of the argon beam (as well as the krypton and dye laser beams) become important for the most efficient coagulation of different ocular defects (Table 7–2).

Disadvantages

The disadvantages associated with the use of the argon laser are as follows:

1. Treatment of diffuse hemorrhagic retinopathies contraindicated (central retinal vein occlusion, branch retinal vein occlusion, and the like.)
2. Blue-green foveal coagulation contraindicated because of xanthophyll
3. Penetration of large vascular abnormalities usually minimal (capping)

TABLE 7–2. Treatment Effectiveness

Disease	Argon	Red Laser Wavelengths (610–750 nm)
Inner retinal vascular diseases	Excellent	Poor
Outer retinal structural diseases	Excellent	Good; excellent in fovea
Inner retinal structural diseases	Poor	Poor
Outer retinal structural diseases	Excellent	Excellent

The argon laser cannot be used effectively with advanced hemorrhagic retinopathies, especially with superficial retinal hemorrhages, because of the heat produced and the potential damage to the nerve fiber layer. Foveal coagulations at the pigment epithelial level are difficult because of the high absorption of the blue component (488.0 nm) of the argon laser beam by the xanthophyll pigment in this area of the retina. The red or yellow krypton laser, the yellow or orange dye laser, or the green argon laser beam has been shown to be more advantageous in the coagulation of subpigment epithelial neovascularization in the foveal region.

Irradiation from the blue portion, green portion, or total argon laser beam is highly scattered by particulate matter in the cornea, anterior chamber, lens, or vitreous. Considerable scatter can be produced by the aging lens, flare or cells in the anterior chamber, and blood or pigment in the vitreous body. This scatter is considerably more than that produced by the longer wavelengths in the yellow or red portion of the visible spectrum. In addition, the yellow discoloration common in the aging lens acts as a selective filter, absorbing a significant proportion of the shorter blue and green laser wavelengths (argon laser), while absorbing little of the longer laser emissions (yellow and red krypton or dye lasers). All of these factors should be considered when selecting the appropriate laser wavelength to treat a specific ocular disease entity.

RED KRYPTON LASER

Advantages

Using the red krypton laser has the following advantages:

1. Excellent foveolar avascular zone coagulations
2. Effective panretinal photocoagulation with hemorrhagic retinopathies
3. Good production of adhesive chorioretinitis with structural defects
4. Excellent subpigment epithelium neovascularization therapy

The red (647.1-nm) krypton beam can be used advantageously for panretinal photocoagulation when confronted with moderate retinal hemorrhagic activity secondary to diabetic retinopathy, and for central or branch retinal vein occlusions, or any vaso-obliterative hemorrhagic

retinal disease. The red krypton beam is excellent in the foveolar region for the photocoagulation and obliteration of subpigment epithelial neovascularization because of minimal absorption by the central xanthophyll pigment and good absorption by the pigment epithelial and choroidal membrane. Structural retinal defects (e.g., retinal tears) can also be treated effectively (see Table 7–2).

Histopathologically, the red krypton laser beam is transmitted through the inner layers of the retina, including the deep and superficial vascular plexi, with little absorption. Approximately 45 per cent of the light striking the pigment epithelium and 55 per cent of the light incident on the choroid is absorbed and practically converted to heat. Therefore, the coagulation has been noted to be located at the level of the inner portion of the choroid–Bruch's membrane–pigment epithelium junction and to penetrate deeper into the choroid than an argon laser beam of similar power. This deeper and more extensive choroidal coagulation was demonstrated in our investigations[7, 13] and more recently by Bird and Grey[14] and Marshall and Bird.[15] It has been postulated that the deeper choroidal coagulation results from more energy being transmitted through the pigment epithelium into the choroid for choroidal absorption and transformation to heat. It is also possible that the choroid contains a higher percentage of reduced hemoglobin when the choroidal blood flow is decreased by pressure exerted on the neutralizing contact lens, creating a much higher absorption potential for the red krypton laser beam (27 per cent of incident light).[16]

Landers and Wolbarsht[17] have noted that only 4 per cent of the oxygen carried by hemoglobin in the choroid is removed by the tissues surrounding the choroid under normal conditions. Thus choroidal venous oxygen concentration is almost as high as arterial concentration, with most of the oxygen in the retina consumed by the rods and cones, because more than 90 per cent of mitochondria are located in this region between the pigment epithelium and the external plexiform layer. Despite this fact, it may be possible that sufficient pressure is exerted on the contact lens by the surgeon to restrict the choroidal blood flow during photocoagulation, with a concurrent increase in the proportion of reduced hemoglobin.

As noted in Table 7–3, the red (647.1-nm) krypton laser photocoagulation beam can be highly advantageous in the treatment of minimal to moderately hemorrhagic central retinal vein occlusions, branch vein occlusions, dia-

TABLE 7–3. Advantages of Red Laser Photocoagulation Wavelengths (610–750 nm)

DISEASE OR DISORDER	ADVANTAGES OF PHOTOCOAGULATION
Retinal hemorrhagic diseases (panretinal photocoagulation treatment)	Less absorption by hemoglobin
Central retinal vein occlusion	
Branch retinal vein occlusion	
Hemorrhagic diabetic retinopathy	
Hypertensive retinopathy	
Retinal edematous diseases	Less scatter
Diffuse diabetic maculopathy	
Early diabetic renal retinopathy	
Retinal structural diseases	Less absorption by hemoglobin or xanthophyll
Retinal tears	
Peripheral retinal degenerations	
Pigment epithelial abnormalities	
Serous detachment of pigment epithelium	
Chronic pigment epitheliopathy	
Central serous choroidopathy	
Serous detachment of sensory retina	
Vitreous opacifications	Less scatter, less absorption
Diffuse vitreous hemorrhage	
Diffuse vitreous cells or veils	
Corneal or lenticular haze	Less scatter, less absorption

betic retinopathy, hypertensive retinopathy, or any of the vaso-obliterative hemorrhagic retinal diseases. This is because the decreased amount of absorption by hemoglobin in the retina or the preretinal space allows effective panretinal photocoagulation to be produced at the level of the pigment epithelium and outer retinal layers. Retinal edematous diseases such as diffuse diabetic maculopathy and early diabetic retinopathy respond somewhat better to treatment with the red krypton laser beam because of the minimal amount of scatter produced by the edematous retina, allowing more incident energy to reach the pigment epithelium for coagulation. In many of these particular cases the pigment epithelium has been badly damaged and atrophied, so that photocoagulation with any laser wavelength is not effective.

As noted previously, the red krypton laser wavelength is highly effective with structural abnormalities, such as retinal tears or peripheral retinal degenerations, as well as with pigment epithelial abnormalities in the macular region, including serous detachments of the pigment epithelium, chronic pigment epitheliopathy, central serous choroidopathy, and serous detachment of the sensory retina. These and other chorioretinal defects can be treated through moderately diffuse vitreal hemorrhages, diffuse vitreous accumulations of cells or veils, and minimal to moderate corneal or lenticular haze. This is because there is minimal scatter and decreased absorption of the red krypton laser beam as it is transmitted through these refractive tissues toward the retinal surface (see Table 7–3).

Disadvantages

There are also certain disadvantages to using the red krypton laser. These are as follows:

1. Inadequate absorption for focal retinovitreal neovascular coagulation
2. Possible power density inadequacy
3. Limited retinal layer application
4. Coagulation effect owing to melanin concentration only

The red krypton laser beam is minimally absorbed by retinovitreal, surface, or papillovitreal neovascularization and, therefore, has little effect on abnormalities or structures in the inner retina, especially vascular abnormalities. Similarly, any structural defects such as cysts or partial-thickness tears would not be affected in any way by the red krypton laser beam, which would be transmitted through the abnormality. The red krypton laser beam could be used to create an adhesive chorioretinitis because the pigment epithelium would be sufficiently irritated for an adhesion to develop between it and the sensory retina. In addition, areas of neovascularization beneath the pigment epithelium or on the inner surface of the pigment epithelium could conceivably be coagulated by virtue of the heat produced by the nearby pigment granules enveloping the subretinal neovascularization in a large coagulum.

In some cases the overall power of the krypton emission in the red (647.1-nm) portion of the spectrum is inadequate for photocoagulation of the chorioretinal structures. The maximal power currently available with conventional krypton lasers is 1.5 W at the red wavelength, and this may not be sufficient to produce an adequate power density at the retina if vitreous blood, lenticular haze, or other refractive media obstruction is present in sufficient quantities to obstruct the laser beam. These power limitations can prove frustrating in some cases, although advancing laser technology will allow this problem to be circumvented.

DYE LASER

Advantages

The advantages of the dye laser are as follows:

1. Production of any wavelength (360 to 960 nm)
2. High relative power levels

The dye laser is able to produce any wavelength in the visible portion of the spectrum at high powers. It requires a high-powered argon (or excimer) laser to "pump" it into full CW or quasi-CW operation; this particular system only recently has been adapted for ophthalmic photocoagulation use. Ultimately the dye laser can function as the instrument for the photocoagulation treatment of all ocular lesions directly or as a catalyst for photodynamic therapy with certain photosensitizing substances.

Because the wavelengths, generated by the various dyes contained in the dye lasers, are in the visible portion of the spectrum, it is not difficult to transport or channel the laser energy through a fiberoptic cable to the optics of a slit lamp in the manner now conventionally used. In other instances the laser exit beam or the beam from a primary fiberoptic bundle can be split into multiple laser beams of lesser power, which can be introduced into separate fiberoptic cables and relayed to different portions of the eye. The power, versatility of delivery systems, and multitude of wavelengths and colors available make this laser ideal for all photic functions now conceived.

Disadvantages

Certain disadvantages are associated with using the dye laser. These are as follows:

1. Minor technical problems (e.g., filters) exist
2. Changing dyes (and available wavelengths) difficult

The potential for the dye laser is extraordinary, and the dye laser has been simplified and is available for ophthalmologists. The difficulties of maintaining the laser in proper alignment, changing the fluid dyes and regulating the pumping mechanism, and servicing the argon laser required to produce lasing action in the dye laser are all problems that have been solved, so that the ordinary "nonphysicist" ophthalmologist can operate the dye laser without difficulty.

CARBON DIOXIDE LASER

The carbon dioxide (CO_2) laser is a continuous-action laser of great power with an emission located in the far infrared. This laser has characteristics that differ significantly from those of the pulsed ruby laser or other CW lasers, such as the argon or krypton laser, more familiar to clinical ophthalmologists. The very long wavelength of its emission (10,600 nm) means that its radiation is outside the visible region and that its absorption and transmission characteristics are significantly different from those generally encountered at shorter wavelengths, particularly in the visible portion of the spectrum.[3]

Surgical Advantages

1. Operations in which the anticipated blood loss would be significant. In ophthalmology the use of the CO_2 laser for orbitotomies, blepharoplasties, removal of orbital tumors, and excision of lid and conjunctival tumors is apparent. Intraocular procedures, including penetration of the globe for sclerostomies with neovascular glaucoma and full-thickness ocular wall resections for intraocular tumors, are obvious uses for this highly hemostatic laser beam.
2. Surgery on patients with bleeding tendencies. In the eye any surgery involving the lids, conjunctiva, or intraocular contents would yield to this highly advantageous form of therapy.
3. Surgery for malignant disease. It has been universally accepted by surgeons that surgery for cancer should be performed with minimal transection of blood vessels and lymphatics, and manipulation of tissue, together with maximal visualization. Because the CO_2 laser seals blood vessels and lymphatics during surgery and concurrently permits an almost nontouch extirpation of the tumor while enabling the surgeon to distinguish between pathologic and normal tissue, its application in cancer surgery is obvious. Many surgeons are using the CO_2 laser for the incision of accessible malignant tissue because the laser beam exerts a cauterization and obstructive effect on the lymphatic and blood circulation. During ocular surgery the encirclement of the tumor by the laser beam interrupts to and from the tumor the blood supply that

could carry malignant cells away from the tumor to the surrounding circulation.

4. Vaporization surgery. The use of the CO_2 laser with its microscopic attachments and its other advantages over other modalities has been well established as a result of the pioneering work by otolaryngologists in which tumors of the vocal cords such as papillomata and nodules have been vaporized directly. Direct vaporization of tumors of the bronchi has also been performed and has been highly advantageous in many instances. Perhaps the most highly successful surgery has been cauterization of the uterine cervix in cases of carcinoma *in situ*, in which the outer layers of the cervix have been vaporized down to the stromal layers. Vaporization of cranial tumors in neurosurgery has also been accomplished, and this has become a highly practical and useful adjunct to regular neurological procedures in many centers throughout the world.[18]

When one considers the extirpative surgery performed with a CO_2 laser on a clinical basis within the past decade, it is apparent that its application in general surgery, as well as in ocular surgery, will become more universal as more surgeons introduce this modality into their armamentarium.

NEODYMIUM-YAG LASER—FREQUENCY-DOUBLED

Advantages

There are several advantages to using the frequency-doubled neodymium-YAG laser. These are as follows:

1. Extremely compact, simply operated laser
2. Very high absorption by hemoglobin and melanin

This type of neodymium-YAG laser (532.0 nm) is extremely compact and has the capability of high power. It also operates with all the advantages of the argon and certain wavelengths of the krypton laser.

Disadvantages

In addition to this laser's having all the disadvantages of the argon laser, its nonlinear crystal, which doubles the frequency and halves the wavelength of the infrared beam, has only recently been reproducible commercially. The basic wavelength of the neodymium-YAG laser in the near infrared portion (1064.0 nm) of the spectrum is highly absorbed by the ocular media and must be halved (532.0 nm) into the visible region (pea green) to reach the retina. The production of a reliable frequency-doubling (KTP, potassium titanium phosphate) crystal will establish this laser as one of the more useful instruments in the photocoagulation armamentarium.

NEODYMIUM-YAG LASER—Q-SWITCHED OR MODE-LOCKED

Advantages

The advantages of this type of neodymium-YAG laser are as follows:

1. High-power density (1 to 1.6×10^{12} W/cm²)—high photon flux (3.0 to 6.0 mJ); small coagulations (50 μm)
2. Negligible thermal diffusion
3. Short exposure times (12 ns or 20 ps)
4. Cutting and lysis of transparent tissue

This laser is operated in a Q-switched mode or mode-locked configuration, and tremendous power (gigawatts) can be developed in extremely short periods of time (nanoseconds[19] or picoseconds[9, 20, 21]). It can transect the anterior and posterior capsule as well as certain transpupillary and vitreal strands.

The ophthalmologic operative neodymium-YAG laser delivers infrared light impulses that last for less than 10^{-8} sec, completely precluding any thermal effects; the impulses act in a purely mechanical way through the process of optical strain. The technique works according to the following principle:

1. Low energy of ultrashort duration with fine focalization produces
2. a power density greater than 10^{12} W/cm², which creates
3. optical strain and plasma formation, leading to
4. an opaque plasma that provides a protective screen for the retina and
5. shock wave formation.

The disruptive radius in the plane perpendicular to the beam axis is 100 to 150 μm, while the extent of action, depending on beam axis, is 0.5 mm on either side of the focal point.

Laser Design and Application

The neodymium-YAG laser emits extremely short pulses of light energy in the nanosecond or picosecond range at an infrared wavelength of 1064.5 nm and a frequency of one pulse per second. The modulating pulses in the mode-locked laser have a gaussian temporal envelope in which the duration of the pulse at the l/e is less than 30 nsec. Because the neodymium-YAG laser beam is invisible, a helium-neon laser beam is used in a coaxial manner and is coincident with the neodymium-YAG laser beam. Therefore, the position and focus of the neodymium-YAG laser beam are indicated rather precisely by the focus of the He-Ne target laser beam. Using an absorptive filter that attenuates any backward reflection, it has been shown that the maximal irradiation to be received by the surgeon lies under the accepted safety level by a factor of 10^6.

According to the calculations of Aron-Rosa and others,[9] the laser beam energy at the point of corneal contact is typically between 3.0 and 4.5 mJ per impact or less. The diameter of the beam's impact area is maintained at 50 μm (in air) because of the mechanical configuration of the optical system of the laser; the peak power density that can be generated lies between 1.0 and 1.6×10^{12} W/cm^2. It has been postulated by these authors that the laser irradiation ionizes the target tissue, thereby causing plasma formation.

According to these authors, preliminary experiments have shown that the target tissue can be transected in the region of the human lens and vitreous without injury to the cornea, retina, or iris tissues. There has been no significant change in corneal endothelial cell counts, intraocular pressure, visual acuity, or appearance of the cornea on slit-lamp evaluation, done immediately before and after laser treatment, using this particular laser. However, other authors seriously disagree with these findings. Pathology of the corneal endothelium and other tissues has been documented. Nevertheless, the potential use of this laser appears to be considerable, and many innovative techniques will most assuredly be forthcoming.

REFERENCES

1. Zaret, M. M., Breinin, G. M., Schmidt, H., et al.: Ocular lesions produced by an optical laser. Science, 134:1525, 1961.
2. Campbell, C. J., Rittler, M. C., Koester, C. J.: The optical laser as a retinal coagulator: An evaluation. Trans. Am. Acad. Ophthalmol., 67:58, 1963.
3. L'Esperance, F. A.: Ophthalmic Lasers: Photocoagulation, Photoradiation, and Surgery. St. Louis: C. V. Mosby, 1983.
4. Meyer-Schwickerath, G.: Light Coagulation. Trans. S. M. Drance. St. Louis: C. V. Mosby, 1960.
5. L'Esperance, F. A.: An ophthalmic argon laser photocoagulation system: Design, construction, and laboratory investigations. Trans. Am. Ophthalmol. Soc., 66:827, 1968.
6. L'Esperance, F. A.: Clinical applications of the frequency-doubled neodymium-YAG laser. Arch. Ophthalmol., 47:77, 1971.
7. L'Esperance, F. A.: Clinical applications of the krypton laser. Arch. Ophthalmol., 15:225, 1972.
8. Bass, M. S., Cleary, C. V., Perkins, E. S., Wheeler, C. B.: Single treatment laser iridotomy. Br. J. Ophthalmol., 63:29, 1979.
9. Aron-Rosa, D. S., et al.: Use of the neodymium-YAG laser to open the posterior capsule after lens implant surgery: A preliminary report. Am. Intra-ocular Implant Soc. J., 6:352, 1980.
10. Seiler, T.: Personal communication, 1985.
11. Landers, M. B.: Argon endophotocoagulation. Personal communication, 1985.
12. Peyman, G. A., Grisolano, J. M., Palacio, M. N., et al.: Intraocular photocoagulation with the argon-krypton laser. Arch. Ophthalmol., 98:2062, 1980.
13. L'Esperance, F. A.: The ocular histopathologic effect of krypton and argon laser radiation. Am. J. Ophthalmol., 68:263, 1969.
14. Bird, A. C., Grey, R. H.: Photocoagulation of disciform macular lesions with the krypton laser. Br. J. Ophthalmol., 63:669, 1979.
15. Marshall, J., Bird, A. C.: A comparative histopathological study of argon and krypton laser irradiations of the human retina. Br. J. Ophthalmol., 63:657, 1979.
16. Yannuzzi, L. A.: Personal communication, 1982.
17. Landers, M. B., Wolbarsht, M. L.: Laser eye instrumentation: Diagnostic and surgical. In Goldman, L., ed.: The Biomedical Laser. New York: Springer-Verlag, 1981, p. 126.
18. Stellar, S., et al.: Lasers in surgery. In Wolbarsht, M. L., ed.: Laser Applications in Medicine and Biology, vol. 2. New York: Plenum Press, 1974, p. 241.
19. Fankhauser, F., et al.: Use of neodymium-YAG laser to open posterior capsule after lens implant surgery. J. Fr. Ophthalmol., 41:279, 1980.
20. Aron-Rosa, D.: Use of a pulsed neodymium-YAG laser for anterior capsulotomy before extracapsular extraction. Am. Intra-ocular Implant Soc. J., 7:332, 1981.
21. Aron-Rosa, D. S., Griesemann, J.: Use of the mechanical effects of YAG lasers by neutralization of their thermal effects: Applications-section of neoformed intraocular membranes. Clin. Ophthalmol., 3:47, 1980.

II

SURGICAL DISORDERS

8

CATARACT SURGERY

by George W. Weinstein

INTRODUCTION

Surgery of the lens has been practiced for at least several thousand years. However, until relatively recent times, cataract was believed to be the coagulum of a humor anterior to the crystalline lens. This was thought to block the emanation of the visual spirit from the eye, thereby interfering with sight. Couching for cataract involved inserting a sharp instrument near the limbus and using the point of entry as a fulcrum to dislodge the cataract inferiorly. This improved vision somewhat by dislocating the cataractous lens. However, the fact that cataract is an opacified lens was not appreciated until hard-won information about the anatomy and pathology of the eye was acquired during the 17th and 18th centuries.

Extraction of the cataractous lens was first formally proposed by Daviel in the middle of the 18th century. His technique remained essentially unchanged for nearly two centuries. However, in the early years of this century, increasing attention was paid to the intracapsular method for cataract extraction. That technique has continued to dominate the scene until this day, although newer methods for extracapsular surgery are rapidly gaining more adherents.

Nearly every ophthalmologist is more familiar with cataract extraction than with any other aspect of ophthalmic surgery. However, even experienced ophthalmic surgeons have been forced to critically reevaluate their carefully evolved favorite techniques. Although many of the current generation of ophthalmologists were trained while the field was still undergoing a relatively quiet process of evolution, the pace has quickened to the point where ophthalmic surgery, and particularly cataract surgery, has undergone a revolution.

Because cataract is a common disorder, and one that is economically important, in that the visual disability it causes results in a loss of work productivity, the public, individually and collectively, has shown increasing interest in this subject. Even the attempts to expand knowledge and improve care have brought with them increasing public involvement. The surgeon who is interested in developing innovations must understand his increasing responsibility to individuals and to society as a whole in ensuring their rights and safety. In return, society should be sympathetic with the problems of surgeons who are attempting to work creatively in order to improve health, and protect them from unnecessary legal and bureaucratic harassment. The relationship between patient and surgeon—as well as that between society and the medical profession—should be a cooperative and not an adversarial one.[10, 17]

GENERAL CONSIDERATIONS—PATIENT PREPARATION

In many respects, the preparation for surgery is more demanding of both patient and surgeon than the operation itself. The surgeon must recognize the patient's right to understand, at least in general terms, the goals of the proposed surgery, as well as the more common and important risks. The patient should also be told about the alternatives, together with the risks these alternatives might entail. In fact, many patients have preferred, and probably will continue to prefer, to keep their cataracts because of their fear of surgery.

The ethical responsibilities of the surgeon to the patient have never changed through the long history of the medical profession. How-ever, the surgeon's *legal* responsibilities to the patient *have* changed, and indeed are different in various locales. Many factors have made today's medicolegal climate a stringent one, requiring that the surgeon be explicit in informing the patient about all aspects of the coming surgery. Most legal experts emphasize the importance of careful explanation and thorough documentation. However, authorities also agree that the most significant factor in the prevention of legal action against the surgeon is the establishment of a sound surgeon-patient relationship at this time, a factor even more effective than even the most elaborately conceived consent form.[34, 50, 54]

Certainly the patient is entitled to learn about each of the following when cataract surgery is contemplated:

1. The need for the operation
2. The alternatives to surgery
3. Surgical morbidity and duration of hospitalization
4. The role of preexisting medical disorders
5. Possible risks and complications, including anesthetic, operative, and postoperative difficulties
6. The types of optical correction available and the reason for the surgeon's choice in this case. When will the final correction be given? Will spectacles be needed in addition to contact lenses? What alternatives exist if the patient is unable to tolerate the proposed method of optical correction, or if the surgeon finds it injudicious to implant an intraocular lens if one had been planned?
7. The nature of adjustment and the limitations of aphakic vision, both uncorrected and as corrected with the proposed optical device[42]
8. The probable ultimate visual outcome if there are no complications
9. Surgical fees and insurance coverage

Often much of the information above can be provided with preprinted material, or by an office assistant. However, there is nothing more valuable to a patient than having the surgeon take the time to go over this with him.

Usually the patient does not want to have an elaborate explanation of the anatomical details, nor does he want to hear a litany of all the possible complications that might detract from a good result. Nevertheless, the surgeon must provide at least general information about both of these areas, and offer to provide more specific details if desired by the patient. There is an ethical as well as a legal imperative to obtain the patient's informed consent, although studies indicate that truly informed consent is an impossible goal.[54]

It is easy to forget that the patient does not go to the doctor to have a cataract removed, but in order to see again. The patient literally places his future sight in the hands of the surgeon. Not only must the surgeon perform the best surgical procedure possible, but he should also try to ease the pain and anxiety of his patient before, during, and after the operation.

Although almost every ophthalmic surgeon places the best interest of the patient foremost, unfortunately this is not always the case. A new breed of entreprenurial ophthalmologist, "the buccaneer eye surgeon," has emerged in recent years. Working under the protection of regulations that permit tasteless, and even false and deceptive advertising, this individual has been able to exploit the patient by espousing the latest developments as his own inventions, using nonmedical practitioners to take over "bothersome" postoperative care, and, in the process, acquiring a huge and lucrative practice. Ophthalmology and the medical profession as a whole are being forced to confront some of their own members in courts of law. The outcome will be worthwhile, however, if the one overriding principle of medical ethics can be reaffirmed: the patient's welfare is foremost.[78]

SURGICAL ANATOMY

Relevant Extraocular Structures

The surgeon should be familiar with the normal anatomy of the orbit and eyelids as well as with the normal variations and abnormalities of these structures that might influence the operative procedure. A prominent brow, a relatively enophthalmic globe, or a small eyelid fissure might make surgical exposure of the globe difficult. Sometimes this problem is eased with the retrobulbar injection of anesthetic, which makes the eye somewhat more proptotic. A bridle suture beneath the superior rectus, which inserts an average of 7.9 mm from the superior limbus (ranging, however, between 7.7 and 8.1 mm), may help this situation further. In addition, a bridle suture placed beneath the inferior rectus muscle may aid surgical exposure even more. However, it is not safe to place too much traction on the bridle suture, and certainly, before an incision is made into the globe,

traction should be markedly reduced or eliminated.[19]

Cornea and Limbus

The anatomical relations of the structures in the superior limbal area are shown in Figure 8–1. Note that the conjunctiva inserts onto the cornea, whereas Tenon's capsule terminates approximately 1 mm posteriorly, inserting near the posterior limbal border. The corneoscleral limbus lies between these structures, and represents the zone of transition from the more steeply curved cornea to the gentler curvature of the sclera. Variably, strands of tissue continuous with the episclera may fill the space between the termination of Tenon's capsule and the insertion of conjunctiva. Therefore, in order to prepare the limbal area for an incision it might be necessary to cut this tissue by knife or scissors, or to push it away with a sharp or semisharp instrument.[19]

The limbus is the zone of tissue overlying the anterior chamber angle, bordered anteriorly by the cornea and posteriorly by the sclera. Its width varies from 1 to 2 mm, being wider above and below, and narrower horizontally.[30, 34] The relative locations of Schwalbe's ring, Schlemm's canal, the trabecular meshwork, and the angle recess are shown in Figure 8–1. However, it is important to appreciate that the positions of these structures vary with relation to external limbal landmarks. The midlimbal portion, for example, can be located anterior to the trabecular area in the myope and posterior to the scleral spur in the hyperope.[30]

Except for its posterior extent, and usually only superficially even there, the limbal zone is relatively avascular. The exact position as well as the extent and angle (bevel) of the incision have long been the subject of controversy in ophthalmology. Ideally, one would choose a location for the incision that is relatively avascular, but where wound healing may still proceed quickly. The incision should lend itself to closure by sutures that produce a minimal amount of wound distortion and postoperative astigmatism. The extent of the incision should be adequate to permit the introduction of needed instruments, as well as the extraction of the lens without difficulty, but small enough to require only minimal wound healing and rapid rehabilitation. The angle of the incision should be such that there is relatively little risk of lamellar splitting of the cornea or stripping of Descemet's membrane, but with enough

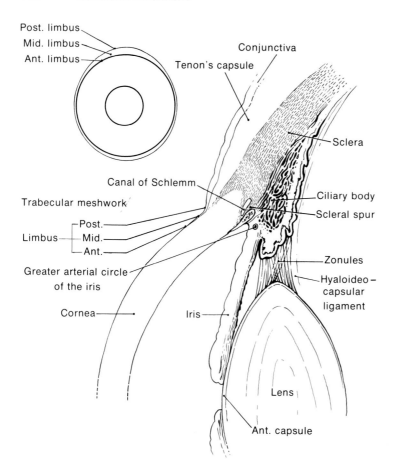

FIGURE 8–1. Anatomy of anterior segment of the eye. Note limbal relations.

bevel to permit a self-sealing effect on the internal lips of the wound by the normal intraocular pressure. Many of these goals seem mutually contradictory. Still, the choice of the incision site must be based on knowledge of the anatomy of the limbus.[34]

Note also in Figure 8–1 the relative position of the iris root, ciliary body, and greater arterial circle of the iris with respect to the external limbal landmarks. Often the cataract incision begins posterior to these structures, but the internal aspect of the wound is anterior to each of these.[11]

Lens and Attachments

The relative position and dimensions of the normal crystalline lens are shown in Figure 8–1. Of course, the cataract operation does not involve a normal lens, although it may or may not be normal in dimensions. Often the lens is somewhat swollen, sometimes considerably when an intumescent cataract is present. With hypermature cataract, the lens is often shrunken and amorphous.

The lens capsule is thickest on its anterior surface, mid-peripherally. The posterior capsule is quite thin uniformly. If the lens is to be removed with a grasping instrument (capsule forceps), it is ordinarily grasped in the thickest zone. This feature is less important for cryoextraction of the lens.[30]

The zonules attach to the lens at its equator, and anterior and posterior to it as well. The zonular ligament originates from the ciliary body between the ciliary processes, with occasional fibers originating even more posteriorly from the pars plana of the ciliary body.[30] The zonular attachments generally weaken with age, permitting intracapsular extraction of the cataract more easily in the older person. The dynamics of the zonular ligament are such that once a few of the fibers are ruptured, the process tends to propagate much like an "unzippering" effect.[34]

Because some of the zonular fibers insert fairly anteriorly, one should avoid making the anterior capsulotomy too large. An anterior capsulotomy of 6 to 7 mm in diameter is probably optimal.

In younger people, a firm attachment exists between the anterior portion of the vitreous and the posterior capsule of the lens. This is the ligamentum hyaloideocapsularium (Weigert's ligament), present as a circular adhesion between vitreous and lens (see Fig. 8–1). In children this attachment is so strong that the entire vitreous body can be extracted along with the lens if intracapsular extraction is attempted. In addition, because in children there are attachments of formed vitreous to the retinal surface as well, the possibility of retinal tear and later detachment is significant. Later in life the attachment to the lens weakens, and if desired, intracapsular extraction can ordinarily be performed without complication after the patient is 35 years of age or older.[30]

DIAGNOSTIC PROCEDURES

Examination

History

As in most areas of medical practice, the patient's history is all-important. It is on the basis of the history that the correct decision as to whether or not surgery is indicated can be made. The history might also indicate the need for specific modifications of the surgical techniques to be used, as well as special precautions that should be taken. The time and place for careful history taking should be when surgery is first contemplated, in the ophthalmologist's office, rather than on the day before the scheduled operation, when the patient is already in the hospital. This approach tends to minimize the need for the cancellation of elective surgery, a trying experience for both patient and surgeon.

The important points to be noted in the history include the following:

1. *Previous ocular disease*—such as trauma, amblyopia, glaucoma, infections, inflammatory episodes—and information regarding any topical medications that have been or are being applied by the patient

2. *Similar surgery (especially cataract surgery) on the fellow eye.* There is a remarkable symmetry characteristic of certain complications that may be due to host factors, such as poor wound healing, hemorrhage, vitreous loss, capsular rupture, and infection.

3. *Vocational or other needs.* Because cataract extraction is only a means to an end, the surgeon should clearly understand the visual requirements of each patient as an individual.

In modern society one frequently assumes that every individual needs vision good enough to permit reading, driving, television viewing, and similar visual tasks. However, for those whose visual requirements are not so demanding, the indications for cataract surgery might be less compelling.

4. *Medical history.* It has often been said that poor general health is in itself no contraindication to cataract surgery. Nevertheless, various systemic illnesses might well influence the need for improved vision, or, conversely, might make surgery riskier or the postoperative period more prolonged. Sometimes debilitating illnesses may make it more difficult for a patient to lie comfortably in a supine position long enough for the surgical procedure, or might make postoperative office appointments difficult to keep.

The following medical factors should be considered in determining whether or not to perform surgery:

1. The patient's life expectancy
2. Diabetes—its control together with the presence of retinopathy and systemic complications
3. Systemic hypertension—its control as well as its importance as a predisposing factor in operative hemorrhage
4. Obstructive urinary tract—particularly if osmotic agents are to be used before or during surgery
5. Chronic pulmonary disease with coughing spells during and after surgery
6. Obesity with elevated intraocular pressure at surgery
7. Medications taken, such as anticoagulants, which might produce intraoperative hemorrhage, and corticosteroids requiring adrenocorticotropic hormone and postoperative maintenance
8. Ischemic heart disease
9. History of renal disease, especially the presence of urinary calculi—particularly if carbonic anhydrase inhibitors are to be used postoperatively
10. Senility with mental confusion. Frequently this is aggravated when the patient is placed in the hospital, where the unfamiliar surroundings together with the administration of medications that affect the psyche, such as tranquilizers and sedatives, as well as occlusion of one eye, cause considerable disturbance.[24, 34]

Visual Acuity

The aspect of visual function that receives the most attention with regard to cataract is that of visual acuity. However, ophthalmologists must be aware that other aspects of visual function, such as the visual field, color vision, adaptation, and depth perception, are affected by cataract as well. Because cataract often coexists with a degree of macular dysfunction in older people, one would not expect that the patient's eyesight invariably will be "like new again" when the cataract is removed.[34, 79]

The preoperative evaluation of visual acuity should be performed under conditions that are as comparable as possible to real life visual situations. Distance vision should be tested in a lighted room as well as in a dimly lit room. Near vision should be checked as well, as it is not uncommon for a discrepancy to exist between the near and distance visual acuity in cataract patients. (For example, patients with posterior subcapsular cataracts frequently have better distance than near acuity, whereas those with nuclear sclerosis tend to have better near than distance acuity.) Naturally, a careful refraction with pinhole and lenses should be performed. Experienced ophthalmologists know how appreciative many patients are when cataract surgery can be deferred for a while if desirable, merely by making a change of eyeglasses, as in cases in which the patient wants to take a trip, spend holidays with family, or tend to other personal matters that would be disrupted by insistence on immediate surgery.

When subjective visual acuity cannot be tested, as with the elderly uncooperative patient or with an infant, the retinoscope or direct ophthalmoscope held at a distance of 1½-feet gives the examiner some appreciation of the effect the cataract has on retinal imagery. Although this method is inexact, it is generally superior to the use of the slit lamp, with which lens opacities tend to appear more significant visually than they actually are.[60]

Pupil

The pupillary response to light should be brisk even in the presence of a mature cataract. If this is not the case, one should suspect optic neuropathy.

The degree of pupillary dilation in response to mydriatics and cycloplegic solutions should be noted. Unless the pupil will not dilate widely, some forms of cataract surgery, such as phacoemulsification, should not be performed. If the patient has previously been on miotic solutions for the treatment of glaucoma, or if he has an Argyll Robertson pupil or atonic pupil, a sector iridectomy might be indicated.[34]

Adnexa

One should carefully evaluate the eyelids and lacrimal apparatus for the possibility of problems that might be associated with infection, keratitis, or faulty wound healing. One should be aware of even minor degrees of blepharitis, ectropion, entropion, lagophthalmos, keratoconjunctivitis sicca, and dacryocystitis. Appropriate measures, including prophylactic medical treatment or even surgical correction, should be undertaken before performing the cataract surgery.

Slit-Lamp Examination

The following features are significant if discovered during the preoperative evaluation.

Cornea guttata. These indicate early corneal endothelial dysfunction that might result in clinically significant corneal decompensation. One should take extra care to prevent corneal damage during surgery by avoiding corneal bending, insertion of instruments into the anterior chamber, excessive irrigation of the anterior chamber, or phacoemulsification. Some surgeons believe that a more posterior limbal or scleral incision is indicated in this situation.

Specular microscopy has emerged as an important technique in the evaluation of corneal endothelium. It should be recognized that this technique provides information about only the morphology of endothelial cells, not their function. However, a low cell density implies compromised function, and specular microscopy is now widely used to detect impending corneal decompensation. This method can be supplemented with corneal pachymetry. The measurement of corneal thickness can serve as another parameter of endothelial cell function.[45, 69, 71]

Very shallow anterior chamber. One should take care to prevent iridodialysis when enlarging the incision with scissors, as well as inadvertent rupture of what one might expect to be fragile capsule surrounding a swollen lens. Phacoemulsification is probably contraindicated.

Dense posterior synechiae. One should look for preexisting complications of uveitis, such as glaucoma and retinal scarring, as well as for the possibility of recurrent uveitis in the postoperative period.

Iridodonesis. This is the sign of a dislocated or subluxated lens, possibly in conjunction with vitreous in the anterior chamber. One might have to use mechanical support of the sclera with ring or expander, and be prepared to perform vitrectomy for anticipated vitreous presentation or loss.

Coexisting Glaucoma and Cataract
(See Chapter 11)

As a general rule, one may perform routine cataract extraction if the glaucoma has been well controlled. In most cases control will be no more difficult and may be more easily achieved postoperatively. When control of the glaucoma is poor and unrelated to the lens itself, such as in chronic open-angle glaucoma, then a combined cataract-glaucoma procedure should be considered.[46, 62] Currently most surgeons favor trabeculectomy combined with cataract extraction. However, the complications after such surgery can be serious, including flat anterior chamber and hemorrhage.[70]

In cases of glaucoma secondary to lens pathology, such as in phacolytic glaucoma or with an intumescent lens and secondary angle-closure glaucoma, cataract extraction alone may control the glaucoma if this is done before optic nerve function is destroyed.[44, 68]

A major concern in our current era of careful wound closure is the marked rise of intraocular pressure that is frequently present during the first several days after surgery. Intraocular pressure may rise to 60 mm Hg or more. Ordinarily, in eyes with healthy vasculature and with healthy optic nerves this does not constitute a serious threat. However, central retinal vein or central retinal artery occlusion can develop. Also, the rise of intraocular pressure often leads to significant discomfort or pain. Finally, wound leak, iris prolapse, filtering blebs, choroidal detachment, and hypotony may follow a transient period of elevation of intraocular pressure. It is wise to measure intraocular pressure at least once during the immediate postoperative period because pressure elevation may occur silently. Treatment is usually medical, and includes topical preparations such as timolol, or oral or systemic osmotic agents such as glycerol or mannitol, together with carbonic anhydrase inhibitors. Although the period of pressure elevation usually is over within a few days, it is not uncommon for it to extend for several weeks.

Several causative factors may be associated with postoperative pressure elevation. When alpha-chymotrypsin is used in intracapsular extraction, the particulate matter resulting from enzymatic zonulysis may block the pores of the trabecular meshwork, producing this phenomenon. However, transient elevation of intraocular pressure certainly occurs even when alpha-chymotrypsin is not used. Lens particulate matter, particularly cortical material resulting from inadvertent or planned extracapsular cataract surgery, may produce the same effect. The use of sodium hyaluronate (Healon) may also lead to pressure elevation, even when efforts are made to remove it. Many surgeons use carbonic anhydrase inhibitors or timolol routinely in the early postoperative period in order to avoid or minimize this problem.

Evaluation of Visual Function in an Eye with Mature Cataract

One should not assume that the fundus cannot be visualized when a cataract is present. Often, even in the presence of advanced cataract changes, the fundus can be seen through a widely dilated pupil by use of the indirect ophthalmoscope. One should attempt to evaluate the macula, the optic disc, and the fundus periphery, particularly for evidence of retinal tears, detachments, or tumors.[34, 79]

Nevertheless, many patients present with cataracts that do not permit ophthalmoscopic observation. For these patients the following techniques might be used.

Pupillary response. No cataract is truly opaque. As described above, pupillary responses should appear normal, and if an afferent defect is present, it should be taken as presumptive evidence of an optic nerve lesion.

Light projection and two-light discrimination. These are crude forms of visual field testing and give important information about a visual function (the light sense) that is fundamentally different than that provided by testing of visual acuity. Color vision can also be tested by asking the patient to identify which color filter is being used in front of a test light. The tests in this group give indications of retinal function, and should not be interpreted as being due solely to macular function.

Entoptic phenomena. A small light illuminating the interior of the globe through the eyelids and sclera produces for many people the sensation of seeing a pattern of branches or cracks. This is the result of self-visualization of the retinal vessels. When it can be elicited, it can be a useful indicator of the presence of retinal function, but unfortunately this is a highly variable phenomenon. The blue field entoptic phenomenon also relies on a subjective response, that of seeing one's own white corpuscles. It is also a distressingly variable effect.

Potential Acuity Meter (PAM).[53] This device attaches to a slit lamp and permits projection of Snellen optotypes onto the patient's retina through a 0.2-mm^2 aperture in the lens opacity, if one can be found. It is generally reliable, but its accuracy is decreased if the patient has advanced glaucoma.[5]

Laser Interferometry. The coherent light of a low-power laser can be used to produce grid (grating) patterns of various widths, and these patterns are little affected by lens opacities. There is a tendency for this test to overestimate acuity, especially in patients with coexisting amblyopia.[22]

Ultrasonography. A "view" of the interior of the globe can be obtained with sound waves rather than light waves producing an acoustical picture of the interior of the eye. Patterns of vitreous hemorrhage, retinal detachment, and intraocular tumors are well known. Compared with ophthalmoscopy, this technique is less precise for visualizing the ocular fundus. However, when direct examination is impossible, ultrasonography is a useful adjunct.

Another important use of ultrasonography is the measurement of the axial length of the eye. This value is an important calculation of intraocular lens power. Unfortunately another important value, the anterior chamber depth, can only be estimated, since it refers to the ultimate position that the intraocular lens implant will take. For this purpose, values of approximately 3.0 mm for anterior chamber implants, 3.5 mm for iris-fixated implants, and 4.0 mm for posterior chamber implants are most often used.

Computerized tomography. This x-ray method is in its infancy with relation to evaluation of visual function in an eye with opaque media.

However, it has been shown to be of some use in patients with cataract and retinoblastoma, and it is conceivable that further technical developments will result in improved resolution and specificity.

Visual electrophysiology. Electroretinography (ERG) records the electrical response of the entire retina to light stimulation. However, in a patient with opaque media, it is not possible to determine whether macular function is intact using this technique. The visually evoked potential (VEP) is the averaged electrical response from the visual cortex to repeated light stimulation. Because the macular area of the retina is much more heavily represented centrally than is the retinal periphery, the electrical response that is recorded is closely related to visual acuity. Any abnormality coexisting with a cataract, such as macular degeneration, optic atrophy, or amblyopia, will produce an abnormal VEP, whereas a patient with cataract alone, but otherwise normal visual pathways, will show an intact VEP response (Fig. 8–2). Accordingly, the VEP is much more closely related to a good visual prognosis than is the ERG in a patient with cataract or other opacities of the ocular media.[74, 76]

Coexisting Cataract and Corneal Opacity

Many patients with corneal opacities as well as cataracts can have an excellent visual result if cataract surgery alone is done, particularly if the opacity is paracentral and is not associated

V E P

10/sec.

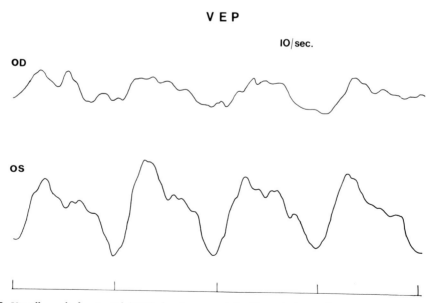

FIGURE 8–2. Visually evoked potential (VEP) showing normal double-peaked waveform in a patient with cataract OS, indicating good prognosis after surgery. Subnormal responses from OD with cataract indicate poor prognosis.

with irregularities of the corneal surface. However, when surgery is indicated for the corneal lesion, the question arises as to which procedure to do first, or whether to do both simultaneously. Before the advent of vitreous surgery, the presence of the lens at the time of keratoplasty was regarded as favorable as a way of keeping the vitreous away from the graft. However, with the advent of anterior vitrectomy, the problem of graft failure secondary to vitreous touch has lessened. The concern of trauma to the graft by subsequent cataract extraction has been judged as the more important factor, and improved techniques of corneal surgery have influenced this question in favor of doing the cataract extraction first. However, many surgeons now favor simultaneous cataract extraction with keratoplasty, often combined with anterior vitrectomy, as the ideal way of managing this situation with the shortest rehabilitation time for the patient. Finally, the addition of intraocular lens implantation has led to the development of the dramatic "triple procedure" of combined cataract extraction with keratoplasty and lens implantation. Remarkably favorable results have been achieved in some patients.[34, 49, 59]

Types of Cataract

Senile Cataract

The most important aspect of the cataract to the patient is its ability to interfere with the visual function. This in fact depends more on the light-scattering effects of the lens changes than on the "blocking out" of the light rays from the eye (Fig. 8–3). Diffuse increase in lens pigmentation, or a gradual increase in the index of refraction of the lens nucleus, results in less degradation of the image than does posterior subcapsular cataract. The peripheral spokelike cortical opacities seen in many older people have scarcely any visual significance.

Many patients still ask whether their cataracts are "ripe enough" for surgery, recalling the first incarnation of extracapsular cataract surgery when cortical lens material could be moved adequately by irrigation only if enough liquefaction of the lens fibers had occurred. This problem was overcome with the development of the intracapsular cataract operation, in which the entire lens may be removed regardless of the degree of maturity of the cataract. Also, in the latest forms of extracapsular cataract surgery virtually all lens material, except for the capsular "bag," is removed. For posterior subcap-

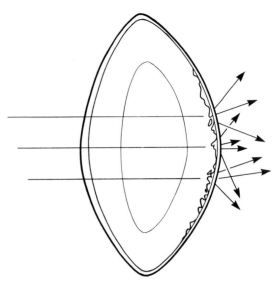

FIGURE 8–3. Light scatter from posterior or subcapsular cataract.

sular opacities "polishing" of the posterior capsule may be required.[20]

Secondary Cataracts

There are numerous types of secondary cataracts, and in most cases the cause has little to do with the technique of extraction. However, awareness of systemic disease, drug toxicity, and other ocular abnormalities associated with the cataract are important in the management of both the patient and the lens itself. Occasionally the appearance of the cataract is so distinctive that the ophthalmologist is able to provide important diagnostic information about the patient's systemic problem.[20]

The following are some specific disorders associated with cataract:

1. Rheumatoid arthritis (particularly of the juvenile variety) associated with corticosteroid therapy
2. Tetany secondary to hypocalcemia, as may be found in hypoparathyroidism. This is occasionally seen after thyroidectomy.
3. Myotonic dystrophy
4. Atopic dermatitis
5. Sarcoidosis with uveitis
6. Traumatic glaucoma

INDICATIONS FOR SURGERY

Reduced Visual Function

Usually the indication for cataract extraction is reduced visual function owing to the presence of cataract. When visual impairment is severe the decision is easy because there is much to gain and little to lose. However, for lesser degrees of visual impairment the risk-benefit ratio changes. Eventually each surgeon must decide for the individual patient when cataract surgery is indicated for visual purposes. Into the decision-making process must go factors such as near and distance visual acuity, coexistent ocular and systemic disorders, and vocational and avocational factors. No matter how much some might wish it, indications for cataract surgery can never be simplified into a few simple quantifiable numbers such as visual acuity or age. Unfortunately for those who would like to refashion the practice of medicine and surgery into a "health care industry," the physician still works one-on-one with the patient.

Visual function is a subjective phenomenon. The patient who says "I see just fine" should not be encouraged to have cataract extraction no matter what the actual visual acuity might be. Cataract surgery for that patient would be meddlesome.

A more difficult clinical situation is the patient with moderately reduced visual function who might still perform well at some tasks while being hampered in other important areas. The librarian with posterior subcapsular cataracts might need surgery when the distance visual acuity is 20/25. The farmer with severe nuclear sclerosis may need surgery when the near acuity is still Jaeger 1. On the other hand, the elderly patient with distance vision of 20/200 but near acuity of Jaeger 2 may be content with that visual function. Also, it may be difficult to assess the relative degree of visual loss caused by the cataract itself when there is associated disease such as senile macular degeneration or corneal dystrophy. Some of the diagnostic methods described above might be useful here. However, often the only way to resolve this matter is through "trial by fire," that is, by removing the cataract and learning what the outcome will be. Naturally the prognosis must be guarded in such a situation. Ordinarily when cataracts are present in both eyes, the worse eye is operated on first. If the patient has a good visual result, the need to have cataract surgery for the second eye is lessened. However, most patients will want to have the second eye operated on because they want to regain binocular vision, if they ever had it. An interval of 3 to 6 months is customary. Occasionally, for a debilitated patient or a patient with bilateral mature cataracts, both eyes are operated on during the same hospitalization, several days apart. Except for unusual circumstances, simultaneous surgery is not performed.[34]

Medical Indications

In addition to the restoration of visual acuity, there are "medical indications" for cataract surgery as well. Actually almost all of the "medical indications" have secondary visual indications. These include the leaking lens, causing phacolytic glaucoma; the swollen lens, producing angle-closure glaucoma; the opaque lens that obscures the view of the fundus, thus preventing necessary treatment such as photocoagulation; and various types of dislocated or subluxated lenses, such as when a lens is trapped in the anterior chamber and causes glaucoma. Cataract extraction is indicated in none of these, however, unless there is some expectation of improving visual acuity. This may occur rarely in the absence of light perception, such as with phacolytic glaucoma, but otherwise, a blind eye with cataract should not be subjected to lens extraction.

In many cases noncataractous subluxated lenses do not need removal. Optical iridectomy may be the procedure of choice if the lens is causing reduced visual acuity, and peripheral iridectomy is usually the correct operation if there is a pupillary block.[13] If the lens is dislocated into the vitreous, it may be left there unless it becomes hypermature and induces a phacolytic reaction.[44]

Indications for surgery for a second eye with cataract may be modified by the type of result achieved for the first eye. If the result is favorable, the surgeon might consider recommending that the operation be performed on the second eye at a somewhat earlier stage than if the result had been less satisfactory. Conversely, if the result is unfavorable, one might expect the development of aphakic glaucoma, hemorrhage, or cystoid macular edema in the second eye, and this would tend to defer surgery. Certain exceptions to this general rule must be recognized; an example would be the discovery in the fellow eye of a retinal detachment secondary to a preexisting lesion such as lattice degeneration of the retina, which perhaps could be evaluated and treated better if cataract surgery were to be done sooner rather than later.[33]

In a patient with bilateral cataracts, even though most patients will prefer to regain binocular vision, a good surgical result on the first eye may provide the patient with all the visual ability needed. The second surgical procedure may then be regarded as unnecessary. Conversely, if the first surgical result is unfavorable, the patient's visual needs might demand surgery on the second eye, perhaps even sooner than one had planned despite a more guarded prognosis. One might hope that experience with the first eye would guide the surgeon in a way so as to avoid the same complications with the second eye. Also, in some cases it might be advisable to perform surgery on the eye with the worst prognosis first, so that the experience gained can be of help in management of the second eye. For example, in a patient with bilateral cataracts and visual acuity reduced to the same level for each eye, but with macular degeneration worse in one eye, it would probably be wiser to operate first on the eye with the greater degree of macular degeneration. If successful, the surgeon might plan to go ahead with the second eye shortly thereafter. Both the surgeon and the patient should realize that the likelihood for achieving excellent central vision in the eye with the worse macular degeneration might not be good, but that useful information can be obtained by proceeding in this way.

PREOPERATIVE MANAGEMENT

Lowering the Intraocular Pressure

It is desirable to reduce intraocular pressure before cataract surgery so as to minimize the effects of several difficulties that can develop during the operative procedure. These events include bulging of the lens-iris diaphragm, vitreous presentation and vitreous loss, and expulsive choroidal hemorrhage. These events may occur even if introcular pressure is lowered substantially, but the risk of each is considerably lower.[26, 34]

Preoperative lowering of intraocular pressure may be accomplished in a number of ways, several of which are commonly used together as a routine by ophthalmic surgeons.

Preoperative Medications

These include the following:

1. Oral glycerol, usually given as a 50% solution in fruit juice, 75 to 150 ml, 1 to 2 hours before surgery.

2. Acetazolamide (Diamox), 250 to 1000 mg, administered orally or parenterally the evening before or the morning of the surgery.

3. Mannitol intravenously, 20% to 25% solution, administered rapidly over a 20- to 40-minute period, ½-to 2 hours before surgery.

All of these preparations may result in diuresis, and patients with obstructive uropathy may be subject to bladder distention.[26, 34]

Eyelid Akinesia and Retrobulbar Anesthesia or General Anesthesia

Elimination of the actions of the extraocular muscles as well as blockage of the ciliary ganglion results in lowered intraocular pressure. The pressure-lowering effect of general anesthesia may include an additional factor of elimination of central pressure regulatory mechanisms.[34]

Preoperative and Intraoperative Tranquilization

Many modern tranquilizers, such as diazepam (Valium), induce not only a state of well-being, but have sedative and antiemetic effects as well. Unfortunately occasional patients, particularly the elderly, will manifest idiosyncratic responses, ranging from restlessness and mental confusion to agitation, delirium, coma, and even death. The depression of the central nervous system with these medications can be potentiated by narcotic substances.

Accordingly, there is a growing tendency when using local anesthesia to provide only minimal amounts of tranquilizers, such as administering 2.5 to 5.0 mg of diazepam orally or intramuscularly 1 hour before surgery, and supplementing this with 1.25 to 2.5 mg of diazepam intravenously at the time of surgery, which is generally enough to induce an anxiety-free, relaxed, but not somnolent patient. In order to achieve this, as well as to provide continuous monitoring of the patient, it is best to have an anesthesiologist or nurse-anesthetist in the operating room throughout the surgical procedure.[26, 34]

Pressure on the Globe

Immediately after administration of a retrobulbar block, some pressure should be put on the globe through the closed eyelids. The aim is to compress any vessel that might be nicked by the needle. This firm steady pressure (*not massage*) should be maintained for about 20 seconds and then completely released in order to assure adequate vascular perfusion of the intraocular contents. Pressure may then be administered again several times (no longer than 15 to 20 seconds at a time) over a 3- to 5- or even 10-minute period until the intraocular pressure has fallen further and the vitreous volume has been significantly reduced. Central retinal artery occlusion and decreased final vision have occurred after the production of excessive pressure. Some surgeons use a rubber ball held continuously in place over the globe by an elastic band for an hour or even more before surgery, in order to achieve marked hypotony before surgery. There have been sporadic reports of vascular occlusions in association with this method as well.

Honan's balloon is another device that allows for continuous pressure on the globe for 10 to 60 minutes. This sphygmomanometer-like instrument is placed over the closed eyelids with an intervening gauze square, and inflated to 35 mm Hg. It has gained wide acceptance as an effective means for lowering intraocular pressure.[38]

Local versus General Anesthesia

Local anesthesia remains the favorite method of most ophthalmic surgeons for cataract surgery. The increased popularity of longer-acting substances such as bupivacaine (Marcaine), which extend the duration of anesthesia from approximately 1 hour to several hours or more, eliminates the occasional uncomfortable situation when the retrobulbar block begins to "wear off" prematurely.

On the other hand, general anesthesia is favored by many ophthalmic surgeons, especially for procedures that are likely to last for 1 to 2 hours, such as phacoemulsification and intraocular lens implantation. With general anesthesia, it should be possible to achieve virtually complete immobility of the globe except for occasionally annoying movements with respiration. However, the demands on the anesthesiologist are increased, requiring smooth induction and extubation, so as to avoid Valsalva maneuvers. Occasionally it is necessary to convert from local to general anesthesia. This may occur because of an unexpected development during the procedure requiring extended operating time, or because of patient restlessness (if this occurs in association with diazepam tranquilization, the central nervous system stimulation can be reversed with intravenous administration of physostigmine, 1.25 mg). In anticipation of this possibility, it is wise to prohibit all oral intake for at least 12 hours before surgery. This would proscribe the use of oral medications, including oral glycerol, mak-

ing intravenous mannitol the drug of choice of the osmotic agent group. Other medications should be administered parenterally as well.[6, 34]

Prophylaxis of Infection

The incidence of postoperative endophthalmitis has steadily declined during the past century. Despite the fact that this condition has become very uncommon, its seriousness influences the management of every patient undergoing cataract surgery. Sterility must be strictly observed during every aspect of the patient's intraoperative care. The use of the incise drape, which tends to isolate the bacteria-rich eyelid margins from the operative field, represents an important advance in ophthalmic surgery. Finally, there is evidence that the routine preoperative use of antibiotics such as topical gentamicin, together with subconjunctival administration of antibiotics and postoperative topical antibiotics, may reduce the incidence of operative infections even further. The incidence of infection has reached a point so low that individual surgeons will probably be unable to accurately judge the efficacy of these methods in their own practices unless they are so unfortunate as to have a cluster of several infections in a relatively short period, and these are likely to be due to factors such as contaminated lens implants or irrigating solutions.[1, 43]

Management of the Pupil

Wide dilation of the pupil preoperatively is desirable and even mandatory for certain procedures, such as phacoemulsification. A combination of an adrenergic substance such as phenylephrine 2.5% together with an anticholinergic preparation such as tropicamide (Mydriacil) 0.5% or 1% or cyclopentolate (Cyclogyl) 0.5% or 1% one to four times at 5- to 15- minute intervals 1 to 2 hours before surgery will achieve this effect.[18] One must be cautious, however, about the use of adrenergic substances in elderly patients, particularly those subject to cardiac arrhythmias, as significant amounts of these substances can be absorbed systemically even when administered topically. One should also note the decrease in effectiveness in dilating drops, particularly sympathetic-acting substances, on the pupil when their administration is repeated on subsequent days (tachyphylasix). In fact, for routine intracapsular cataract extraction, the prompt pupillary dilation achieved when retrobulbar injection is given is often sufficient to permit delivery of the lens.

ANESTHESIA*

It may be said that anesthesia is for the patient and akinesia is for the surgeon. Part of the dread of surgery that every patient harbors is the fear of pain during the actual operation. Modern anesthesia, both local and general, minimizes but does not eliminate this pain. There is an inevitable amount of pain associated with the various injections immediately before surgery, and many patients "hate getting stuck with needles" more than anything else. The compassionate anesthetist can infiltrate a small amount of subcutaneous anesthetic before making a venipuncture with the intravenous catheter. The ophthalmic surgeon can also lessen the patient's discomfort by using a 25-gauge 1½-inch disposable needle to administer the eyelid akinesia and retrobulbar anesthesia. Although one does not feel the definitive "pop" as this needle passes each tissue plane, the experienced surgeon soon becomes confident in the placement of the retrobulbar injection, and the incidence of retrobulbar hemorrhage is slight. A suitable anesthetic agent is an equal mixture of 2% lidocaine (Xylocaine) and 0.75% bupivacaine (Marcaine). A total of 20 ml of this mixture is drawn into a syringe, and 150 units of hyaluronidase (Wydase) is mixed with it. The same mixture is used for akinesia (a total of 5 to 8 ml is administered for this purpose) and retrobul-

*See also Chapter 5.

bar injection (3 to 4 ml for this purpose). This makes a total of 8 to 12 ml of anesthetic solution administered, an amount well below the toxic dose, even if all is inadvertently administered intravascularly.

The use of bupivacaine has made it unnecessary to add epinephrine to the mixture in order to prolong the effect. The elimination of epinephrine greatly reduces the risk of cardiovascular side effects. Some surgeons have found the use of bupivacaine alone to be sufficient for local anesthesia, while others prefer the lidocaine-bupivacaine mixture to assure the early onset of the anesthetic effect.

After administration of the anesthetic mixture, the surgeon should repeatedly test for residual motor function. Just as the patient hopes to feel not even a twinge of pain, the surgeon should beware of even the smallest residual eyelid or eye movement, as the possibility of vitreous loss is greatly increased if this occurs. In addition, one should carefully inspect the globe for the possibility of retrobulbar hemorrhage. This may occur shortly, within a few moments of administration of the retrobulbar anesthetic, or many minutes after. Although some degree of proptosis of the globe is an invariable concomitant of retrobulbar anesthesia, this should not progress. Indeed, as the anesthetic effect begins, it should be progressively easier to perform ballottement of the globe into the orbit. If proptosis becomes progressive, and if orbital pressure appears to increase, a retrobulbar hemorrhage may be in progress (Fig. 8–4). One should continue to apply intermittent pressure to the globe as described above. The hemorrhage may or may not dissect anteriorly to become visible under Tenon's capsule in the interpalpebral fissure.

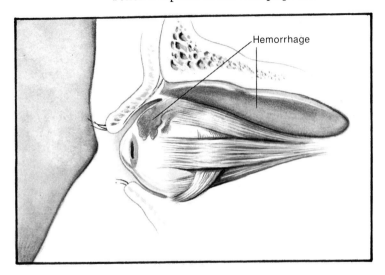

FIGURE 8–4. Retrobulbar hemorrhage with dissection anteriorly beneath Tenon's capsule.

Hemorrhage

If retrobulbar hemorrhage is suspected, the surgeon should perform tonometry, usually with the Schiötz tonometer. A scale reading of 10 to 15 (less than 3 mm Hg) should be achieved. Even without the signs of retrobulbar hemorrhage described above, the inability to lower intraocular pressure to this level should make the surgeon suspect that a small retrobulbar hemorrhage has occurred. Cancellation of the case at this time, even if there is doubt about the presence of retrobulbar hemorrhage, is wise.

The use of bupivacaine, or a bupivacaine-lidocaine mixture, appears to have a longer onset to complete akinesia, as compared with lidocaine alone. Time devoted to administering intermittent pressure, or even to injecting an additional amount of anesthetic mixture in order to achieve complete akinesia, is well spent.[26, 34]

OPERATIVE TECHNIQUE AND INTRAOPERATIVE COMPLICATIONS

Instrumentation

Magnification

Over the past quarter century there has been a growing trend toward the use of magnification in ocular surgery. In fact, ophthalmic surgery in general and cataract surgery in particular are very well suited for microsurgical techniques and instrumentation. The operating loupe, offering a modest amount of magnification (usually 1.5× to 2.5×) requires relatively little orientation in its use and provides the surgeon with a fairly large depth of field and excellent mobility around the operative field. However, the operating microscopes have been developed for even greater magnification (usually in the range of 6× to 15×, averaging 10×), permitting an order of visual control that cannot be achieved by other methods. Beginning with simple binocular devices incorporating coaxial illumination but little else, operating microscopes have evolved into complex instruments with every conceivable form of illumination, as well as photographic and television attachments, with motorized controls for changing position, focus, and magnification. There is virtually no end to the sophistication (and expense) of these devices, and the popularity of microsurgical techniques, particularly for cataract surgery, seems to be increasing. A good operating microscope with coaxial illumination is a prerequisite for

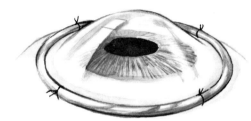

FIGURE 8–5. Scleral ring sutured in place, supporting anterior segment.

modern cataract surgery. Undoubtedly ophthalmic microsurgery has contributed much to the excellent results that may now be achieved almost routinely by even newly trained surgeons.[25]

Scleral Support

Various devices have been introduced for providing mechanical support of the sclera in order to prevent collapse of the globe during cataract surgery. The two most popular are the scleral ring described by Bonaccolto and Flieringa (Fig. 8–5) and the scleral expander of Girard. Both of these devices must be sutured to sclera, a step that requires some not inconsiderable skill. Unfortunately to date no device has been developed to deal with the most common site of scleral collapse, indentation of the globe by the rectus muscles. The problem of scleral collapse is greatest in children and in myopic patients, both of whom have especially thin and elastic scleral tissue.[34]

Forceps

During the cataract procedure several pairs of forceps are likely to be used. Larger-toothed forceps with teeth that are 0.3 or 0.5 mm long are used for grasping the superior rectus and placing the bridle suture. Finer-toothed forceps, with teeth 0.1 or 0.12 mm in length, are used during the remainder of the procedure for tissue fixation and may be used for grasping conjunctiva, cornea, and even iris (Fig. 8–6). Many surgeons consider the forceps (and other instruments manufactured by Grieshaber) the finest of their kind, and well worth their high cost. Some surgeons prefer using smooth forceps for conjunctiva, and fine-pointed jeweler's forceps for grasping iris. Neither type of forceps, smooth or toothed, is entirely atraumatic, and the surgeon must become accustomed to grasping tissue as few times as possible, and holding it firmly once grasped, to minimize crushing. Specialized forceps for uses such as grasping intraocular lenses (with or without

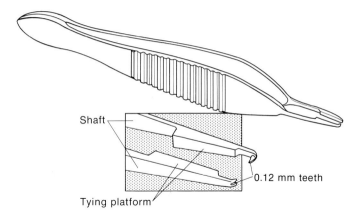

FIGURE 8–6. Fine-toothed forceps showing tying platform.

Shaft

Tying platform

0.12 mm teeth

attached irrigating cannulas), clot extraction, and suture tying are also available. For this last purpose, many surgeons prefer use of the tying platform, a 3-mm long flat surface behind each set of teeth on many models of tissue forceps, which allows the instrument to serve both purposes. Forceps that are particularly suitable for grasping fine monofilament nylon suture are the ones manufactured by Metico. These forceps, made of titanium steel, have a textured tungsten surface near the tips, providing a secure grasp of the fine suture material when closed.

The handle designs of various forceps provide the surgeon a wide choice. Most surgeons prefer the wide grip, nonslip grip models, either straight or curved. The miniature-handled colibri forceps (named for their resemblance to a hummingbird beak when held upside down) are grasped with the fingertips alone, and because of their angulation do not obstruct the surgeon's view through the operating microscope. Rounded handles of the Kirby design permit easy rotation of the instrument during use. The handle design selected is essentially a matter of personal choice on the part of the surgeon.

The delicacy and precision demanded by a good pair of fine-toothed forceps represents a high state of the surgical instrument maker's art. They should be handled, cleaned, and stored carefully. When passed to the surgeon, they should be grasped at the nonworking end between the nurse's thumb and forefinger so that they are ready for action by the surgeon. Forceps as well as other instruments should be handed off to the nurse carefully, and returned gently to the instrument tray.

Knives

At one time there was a saying "the incision is everything in cataract surgery." The incision remains a critical step with regard to its placement, angulation, extent, and closure. However, fewer of today's ophthalmic surgeons use the full Graefe section that was the pride of masterful eye surgeons of decades ago (and which may still be witnessed in many European eye clinics). However, the full Graefe section, which took many years to master, also could produce disastrous results. After the limbus is punctured, the blade is passed across the anterior chamber and the counterpuncture is made at approximately 180 degrees opposite. The knife is then drawn toward the superior limbus in one or two even strokes, producing an incision from within (*ab interno*). This maneuver requires an exquisitely sharp knife, a steady and practiced surgeon, and ambidexterity, since the knife is traditionally held in the right hand for the patient's right eye, and in the left hand for the patient's left eye. Today most surgeons prefer the safer external approach to creation of the incision (*ab externo*). This is usually accomplished with a knife that makes a small perforating incision in the globe, and the incision is then enlarged to the desired amount with curved-blade scissors. The knife (Fig. 8–7) used to make the initial entry into the anterior chamber may be pointed with a single cutting edge (razor blade), pointed with two cutting edges (keratome), or nonpointed, providing a cutting edge alone (scalpel, using a Bard-Parker or Beaver blade). It is important that the entire depth of the incision, including the internal aspect, be long enough to permit atraumatic insertion of the scissors for enlargement of the wound.

The most important attribute of any knife is the sharpness of its cutting edge. Modern disposable knives that fit into reusable handles have reduced the need for testing sharpness and resharpening. However, this is still necessary for some knives such as the needle knife (Ziegler) or the excellent, but expensive dia-

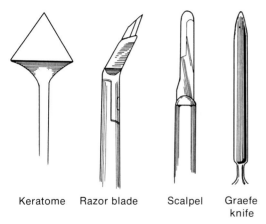

Keratome Razor blade Scalpel Graefe knife

FIGURE 8–7. Knives used in cataract surgery.

mond keratome knife. The diamond knife never loses its sharpness in cutting tissue. Synthetic rubies are also used for ophthalmic knives. They may lack some of the exquisite sharpness of diamonds, but they are far less expensive.[34]

Scissors

As with forceps, a variety of scissors (Fig. 8–8) are used during the cataract operation; these vary in design according to the delicacy required of them. Blunt-tipped, spring-bladed scissors (Stevens) are used for preparing the conjunctival flap, both because of their cutting action and for their spreading effect when undermining conjunctiva. They may also be used for cutting all but the finest sutures. Sharp-tipped spring-bladed scissors (Westcott) may be

used for incising the adherent Tenon's capsule from its insertion at the corneoscleral limbus, especially with limbus-based conjunctival flaps. Corneoscleral and corneal scissors are usually spring-bladed and come in many models with varying length blades, angulations, and curvatures. The most popular are the left- and right-hand models originally introduced by Castroviejo. The scissors designed by José Barraquer resemble the Stevens scissors, but are intended to produce a "two-plane" incision by their cutting action.

Cutting the iris is ordinarily done with very delicate scissors originally designed by De-Wecker and miniaturized further by Joaquin Barraquer. Their butterfly design permits grasping and activation with thumb and forefinger alone.

Because scissors work by shearing one blade against the other, tissues that are entrapped between the blades are first crushed to some degree and then cut. The crushing effect may promote hemostasis, but most scissors used in ophthalmic surgery are meant to be kept as sharp as possible to minimize this effect. As with forceps, the nurse should hand the surgeon the scissors from the nonworking end so they can be grasped without the necessity of repositioning the hand. They should be handed back to the nurse, never tossed back onto the instrument tray, and cared for meticulously.[34]

Cryoextraction

One of the great advances in intracapsular cataract extraction was the introduction of cryoextraction of the lens by Krawicz. With cryoextraction, not only is the lens grasped by its capsule, but the iceball incorporates lens cortical fibers as well. This wider and deeper attachment thereby reduces the possibility of inadvertent rupture of the lens capsule. Most cryoextraction instruments achieve the necessary low temperatures (-20 to $-40°$ C) by using the Joule-Thompson principle, in which a compressed gas (carbon dioxide, nitrous oxide, or Freon) is allowed to expand rapidly, thereby producing adiabatic lowering of temperature. Defrostable models permit flushing of the probe tip with room temperature gas for rapid thawing.

Auxiliary Methods of Intracapsular Lens Extraction

Because cryoextraction had proved itself to be the safest method of intracapsular cataract extraction, other techniques such as expression, capsule forceps, and erysiphake fell out of favor.

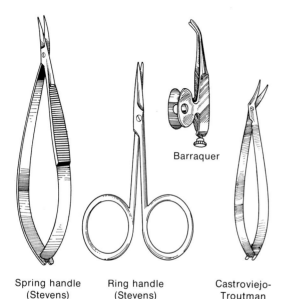

Barraquer

Spring handle (Stevens) Ring handle (Stevens) Castroviejo-Troutman

FIGURE 8–8. Scissors used in cataract surgery.

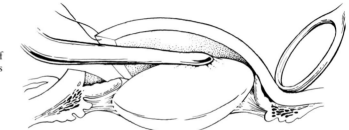

FIGURE 8–9. Capsule forceps extraction of cataract, showing counter-pressure with lens loop.

However, it is still a good idea to have some familiarity with one or more of these methods.

In the external expression technique perfected by Colonel Smith in India (the "Smith Indian technique") the entire lens is extruded from the eye by expression, beginning at the inferior limbus with a blunt instrument such as a muscle hook, and following the lens as it is delivered superiorly. This had the advantage of simplicity of instrumentation as well as the important feature of requiring no instrumentation within the anterior chamber. However, like the Graefe knife incision (with which it was traditionally coupled), it required more skill and practice than most ophthalmic surgeons were able to muster. Nevertheless, there are occasions when a lens is only partially delivered and a cryoextractor perversely thaws and loses its adhesion; when this happens the remainder of the lens delivery can be affected by gentle external pressure. External expression is still used to express the lens nucleus during extracapsular extraction. Naturally it is all too easy to force iris or vitreous from the eye as well, so this maneuver must be performed cautiously.

Capsule forceps, as mentioned above, are placed on the anterior capsule several millimeters peripheral to the anterior pole of the lens. For the tumbling maneuver, the capsule is grasped inferiorly (Fig. 8–9). Capsule forceps should not be used for an intumescent cataract because of the heightened danger of capsular rupture. The erysiphake uses a suction action

to obtain capsular adhesion by the use of an elastic rubber or silicone bulb, or a motor pump (Fig. 8–10).

Suture Types

Suture selection in cataract surgery remains the subject of intense controversy. Most eye surgeons have acquired some experience with many suture materials and have arrived at their current choice as much by default as by genuine satisfaction. The only area of general agreement has been the increasing tendency for sutures of smaller diameter. The standard of a decade or two ago was 6-0 material, silk or catgut, whereas now 7-0 suture material is virtually the largest used. Many surgeons prefer the smallest diameter material available, such as 22-μm diameter (10-0) nylon. However, one should avoid assuming that the finest gauge material is also the best for the purpose, since this is not necessarily the case.

Formerly, it was assumed that nonabsorbable suture material required removal. This is probably still true of 7-0 silk. However, 8-0 silk as well as 10-0 nylon and polypropylene need not necessarily be removed. Sizes 8-0 and 9-0 silk may be allowed to remain if covered by a flap, as it will be covered by epithelium, particularly if the suture is rotated so that the knot is buried and no ends protrude. Degradation of the suture material proceeds at various rates with the different forms of sutures that are available. Catgut, collagen, and synthetic absorbable su-

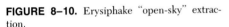

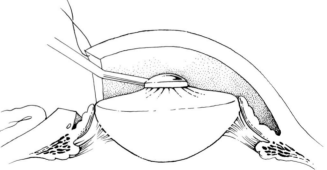

FIGURE 8–10. Erysiphake "open-sky" extraction.

tures such as polyglactin 910 (Vicryl) and polyglycolic acid (Dexon) all have their proponents. Various factors such as predictability of absorption time and loss of tensile strength, tissue reaction, ease of handling, and knot time have been subjected to critical analysis. At this time it would appear that the newer synthetic materials have an edge over the natural materials for the surgeon who prefers absorbable suture material. However, one would expect that suture manufacturers will continue to improve these products because in fact once the wound has healed, there is no longer any need for the suture.[55]

Materials that were formerly considered nonabsorbable may still undergo degradation within tissues. Silk is well known for exciting a foreign body response, and although nylon is associated with much less reaction, there is definite evidence that it, too, weakens with time when implanted in ocular tissues, including cornea and iris. Still, for practical purposes, both of these materials can be considered nonabsorbable in that they remain long after the wound is healed.

Probably the only truly nonabsorbable material available today—and even this may be subject to revision some years hence—is polypropylene (Prolene). It is available in 9-0 and 10-0 sizes, and many surgeons prefer it even though it is stiffer than nylon and doesn't snug down into tiny knots as well.

Sutures for ophthalmic surgery commonly are swaged on needles of varying sizes, shapes, and curvatures. Most attention has been paid to suturing the limbal incision, and the cross section of the needle is designed to allow it to pass through this tough tissue, with its lamellae of collagen fibers, with relative ease. The ideal needle has a sharp point and sharp edges and is flat ("spatula" needle). The curvature is round with a radius of 5 mm, and covers an arc of 160 degrees. These superbly crafted needles deserve a large measure of the credit for the excellent wound closure that is achievable by eye surgeons today.[34]

Phacoemulsification and Phacofragmentation

Basic Principles

Aspiration of a cataract through a small incision is an ancient technique that had been carried into modern times largely for the soft cataract of infants, or after trauma. Techniques for maintaining normal intraocular pressure during the aspiration, by a "two-needle technique," or by a two-way aspiration-irrigation system, have also been used successfully in these situations for many years. Kelman modified this method further by adding ultrasonic energy to the aspirating cannula, which allows the surgeon to break up harder lens material that could not otherwise be aspirated.

In fact, the phacoemulsification technique has incorporated a series of maneuvers that are quite unlike any formerly performed during intracapsular cataract extraction. First, a beveled limbal incision of 2.5 to 3.0 mm is made with a razor blade or keratome. With microsurgical control, a controlled anterior capsulotomy is performed by removing a 6- to 7-mm disc of capsular material (Fig. 8–11A). For this purpose, an irrigating cystotome is used. Small interconnecting triangular tears are made, each with the apex toward the periphery. Then the lens nucleus is delivered into the anterior chamber, by use of the same cystotome with which the capsulotomy was performed (Fig. 8–11B). Surgeons may find this the single most difficult maneuver of the procedure. With the lens nucleus in the anterior chamber, ultrasonic fragmentation is performed (Fig. 8–11C). Now phacoemulsification is usually performed with the nucleus in the posterior chamber, to prevent it from coming into contact with the corneal endothelium. This also minimizes the possibility of inadvertent contact between the sonic probe and the corneal endothelium.[48] For both anterior and posterior chamber phacoemulsification, a bimanual technique is used by many ophthalmic surgeons.[12] For this method, a small spatula is used for a variety of maneuvers, including manipulation of the lens nucleus toward the probe tip, and retraction of the iris during cortical aspiration. The instrument designed by Kelman permits simultaneous ultrasonic fragmentation, aspiration, and irrigation. The phacofragmentation instrument of Shock does not permit simultaneous aspiration; rather, the lens particles are simply irrigated out of the wound of entry. The instrument designed by Girard uses a two-needle technique for simultaneous irrigation and aspiration through incisions for 20-gauge cannulas.

Residual cortical lens material is aspirated with a different handle and tip attached to the same console (Fig. 8–11D), but the popularity of various extracapsular techniques has led to the development of freestanding aspiration-irrigation instruments. This technique of lens surgery may include polishing the capsule with the roughened shaft of a fine cannula until no

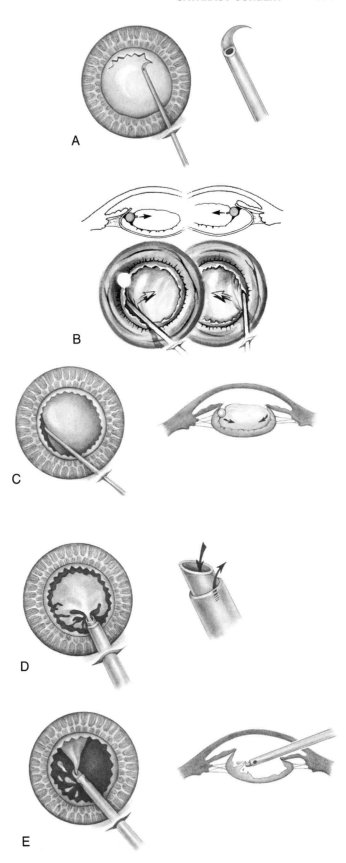

FIGURE 8–11. Phacoemulsification. *A*, Anterior capsulotomy with irigating cystotome—"beer can" technique. *B*, Prolapse of lens nucleus into anterior chamber with cystotome. *C*, Ultrasonic fragmentation of lens material. *D*, Aspiration of residual cortical lens material with simultaneous irrigation. *E*, Polishing of posterior lens capsule with rough-tipped cannula.

residual opacity remains (Fig. 8–11E). At this point the posterior capsule is usually left intact, although there is a growing tendency to perform a small capsulotomy in order to avoid having to do one at a later time, especially if the procedure is being performed on an infant or a child.[41, 48] A peripheral iridectomy is performed and the small incision is closed with one or two fine-gauge sutures.

History

As mentioned above, phacoemulsification and phacofragmentation represent evolutionary modifications of lens surgery, rather than a totally new approach. Nevertheless, cataract surgery has changed since their introduction. The most striking change is the marked reduction in the length of stay of the average hospitalized patient, dropping from 8 to 10 days to 0 to 2 days nationwide. In many locations it is only the exceptional patient who is hospitalized for cataract surgery. In addition, the advent of phacoemulsification forced ophthalmologists to become self-critical again about their surgical methods and outcomes. What had for many years become a self-satisfied approach to cataract surgery has become again a struggle for perfection.[40]

Instrumentation

The direct aim of phacoemulsification is to fragment the lens into particles small enough that they may be aspirated through a needle, or irrigated along the shaft of the cannula through the exit wound (Fig. 8–12). The technique of fragmentation varies from very rapid bombardment with ultrasonic energy to suction-

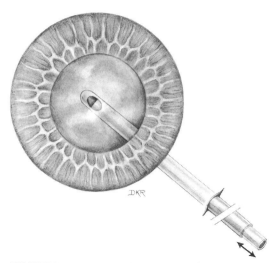

FIGURE 8–13. Ocutome that performs simultaneous aspiration, cutting, and irrigation.

cutting using a triple-bore instrument with a rotating blade in the innermost position (Fig. 8–13). Results may well differ depending on the technique used and the nature of the cataract attacked. The most expensive and complex instruments are those in which infusion and suction are automatically balanced to maintain a stable intraocular pressure, such as in the Kelman instrument. The simplest instruments use only an irrigating needle attached to the ultrasonic source, as in the Shock and Girard instruments. The latest generation of phacoemulsification instruments provides an array of control possibilities, including self-tuning of the ultrasonic generator by integrated microprocessors. As usual, with any instrument, complexity and automation cost more, and the current range of prices is from $15,000 to $50,000.

In patients with advanced nuclear sclerosis the techniques of phacoemulsification, phacofragmentation, and rotoextraction of the lens are not recommended, as the amount of energy required to fragment the lens material might damage ocular tissues, particularly the corneal epithelium. One cannot always predict when a nucleus too hard to emulsify will be encountered, and the surgeon must always be prepared to "convert" the procedure to a standard extracapsular lens extraction.[63]

Advantages and Disadvantages

The major advantage of phacoemulsification for most patients who need cataract extraction is rapid ambulation and return to work. Not all eye surgeons agree that this goal can be achieved only by phacoemulsification. However, any ophthalmic surgeon who has seen a

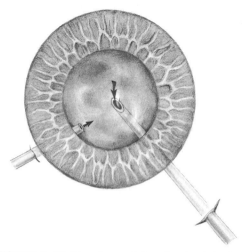

FIGURE 8–12. Phacofragmentation showing irrigation of lens particles out of eye along side shaft of cannula.

patient who has undergone phacoemulsification a day or two before by someone experienced in this technique has marveled at the quiet appearance of the operated eye. Also, for younger patients who are good candidates for extracapsular surgery of some form, phacoemulsification is the most refined technique available for this type of surgery. However, most of the estimated 900,000 cataract extractions performed yearly in the United States are for middle-aged or elderly patients for whom phacoemulsification is an alternative, but not necessarily preferable to the standard wide-incision extracapsular cataract operation.[27]

The second apparent advantage of phacoemulsification relates to the smaller incision required with this technique, which thus decreases corneal trauma and the likelihood of incisional problems such as dehiscence, astigmatism, localized edema, infiltration, and epithelial ingrowth. This advantage is undeniable. The absence of significant distortion of the cornea permits prompt fitting with a contact lens, significantly shortening the interval between the time of surgery and functionally useful recovery of vision.[57]

Disadvantages of phacoemulsification include complications related to the operative procedure, such as corneal injury from introduction of the emulsifier tip, irrigating solutions, or ultrasonic energy; trauma to the iris; dislocation of the lens nucleus into the vitreous; and loss of vitreous. Postoperative complications include persistent corneal edema, opacification of the posterior capsule, posterior synechia formation, cystoid macular edema, retinal detachment, persistent filtration from the site of the incision, and glaucoma. Obviously several of these complications are found with all forms of cataract extraction. It is recognized that this group of complications depends in large part on the skill and experience of the surgeon.

The other disadvantage is associated with the expense of the procedure, including the high initial equipment cost as well as the need for disposable packs for each procedure. Also, the effort and expense of training in this technique should be considered, although more and more phacoemulsification techniques have been incorporated into many major training centers.

However, if one takes into account shortened or eliminated hospitalization, as well as the more rapid return to prodcutive work that is possible when phacoemulsification is used, the expense of phacoemulsification to the patient and to society may not be higher than that for standard cataract surgery.

Indications and Contraindications

The best candidates for this procedure are younger patients, particularly those under 40 or 50 years of age, who merit cataract surgery for visual purposes. There should be an absence of corneal endothelial disease, normal anterior chamber depth, a pupil that dilates to at least 7 mm, and no more than moderate nuclear sclerosis. Except for the most experienced surgeon, the absence of one or more of these factors probably represents a contraindication to phacoemulsification. Subluxation or dislocation of the lens constitutes absolute contraindication to phacoemulsification, although phacofragmentation through the pars plana may be the technique of choice in these cases. As mentioned above, sometimes it is difficult to judge the degree of nuclear sclerosis on the basis of the preoperative evaluation. Often the hardness of the nucleus is related to the amount of brown pigmentation present, but this is not always the case. Sometimes a white nucleus may prove too difficult to emulsify, necessitating enlargement of the incision and expression of the nucleus.[16, 21, 28]

Technique of Phacofragmentation

The steps involved in phacofragmentation are outlined above and shown in Figure 8–11A to E. Each step of this procedure is quite dependent on the successful completion of each preceding step.

An operating microscope with coaxial illumination is essential during phacoemulsification because many of the maneuvers, including anterior capsulotomy, polishing of the posterior capsule, and posterior capsulotomy, are performed with visual control alone, using the silhouettes and highlights seen against the red fundus background with the coaxial illuminator of the operating microscope. Working with the posterior capsule can be done only with visual control, as there are no tactile clues to guide these maneuvers.

Phacofragmentation or ocutome removal of the lens (sometimes termed "lensectomy") is frequently performed in conjunction with vitrectomy procedure if cataract is present, or even if it is anticipated that cataract may develop later. This procedure may be done by way of the pars plana with a knife incision carried into the lens equator, and the ultrasonic phacofragmenter or the ocutome cutter/aspirator inserted into the knife tract for removal of lens material. Usually the entire nucleus and most of the cortical material are removed before the central portions of anterior and posterior capsule are excised with the ocutome.[34]

Phacoemulsification served to revolutionize cataract surgery, not so much because it became the predominant technique of cataract removal (fewer than 20 per cent of ophthalmic surgeons who perform cataract extraction now use this technique), but because it forced ophthalmologists to reevaluate the cataract procedure as a whole. What has evolved as the standard technique, wide-excision extracapsular extraction, is probably the combined result of phacoemulsification techniques and the introduction of the posterior chamber intraocular lens implant. The credit for these changes does not belong to one or two persons, but to scores, or even hundreds of innovative ophthalmologists who have striven to make cataract surgery the effective and relatively safe operation that it has now become.

Surgical Solutions

During cataract surgery it is useful to flush an irrigating solution over the surgical field intermittently or even continuously in order to maintain maximum visibility, and to prevent tissue drying. Certain solutions such as acetylcholine (Miochol) and sodium hyaluronate (Healon, AmVisc) are designed for intracameral injection. These solutions, as well as irrigating solutions to be injected into the eye, must undergo the most rigid control possible for sterility and removal of other particulate material. Bacterial organisms, dust particles, and undissolved medications may be removed by a disposable presterilized filter (Swinnex-13 Millipore filter). The composition of the irrigating solution itself deserves attention. It has been shown that a Ringer's-type solution (balanced salt solution) produces fewer corneal endothelial changes than does normal saline solution. By the addition of glutamate and bicarbonate, a solution that is essentially nontoxic to the endothelium (GBR solution; BSS+) has been developed. This more expensive solution is more justifiable for procedures that involve large volumes of irrigating solution, such as phacoemulsification or vitrectomy, whereas there probably is a negligible difference when standard cataract surgery is performed.[34] In either case, 0.5 ml of epinephrine can be added to the 500-ml bottle of irrigating solution to assist in maintaining pupillary dilation.

Stages of the Cataract Operation

All techniques for cataract extraction include six distinct stages during the operative phase.

These are as follows:

1. Akinesia and anesthesia, cleansing of the surgical field, and tonometry
2. Incision to enter the anterior chamber
3. Iridectomy and lens removal (sometimes performed in reverse order, as in the phacoemulsification operation)
4. Intraocular lens implantation
5. Incisional closure
6. Injection and/or instillation of medications; application of an eye patch or protective shield[26, 34]

Preparation and Exposure

Cleansing of the Surgical Field

Skin preparation is performed with a standard soap solution containing iodine. The area extending from the midline to well above the eyebrow and well below the cheek should be scrubbed for 3 to 5 minutes (Fig. 8–14A). One must take care to avoid getting any of the soapy material onto the eye itself, as this can damage the corneal epithelium. Next, the eyelid margins are carefully scrubbed with cotton-tipped applicators moistened with an iodinated soap solution (Fig. 8–14B). Again, one must take care to avoid getting this solution onto the eye itself. Finally, and perhaps most important, the eye and the conjunctival cul-de-sacs are irrigated thoroughly with copious quantities of body temperature saline solution to remove any mucous strands (Fig. 8–14C). The skin is then thoroughly dried with lint-free towels to permit adequate adherence of the adhesive drapes to the eyelids. With these drapes it is undesirable to trim the eyelashes, as these are everted with cotton-tipped applicators by the assistant as the surgeon applies the drapes over the parted eyelids. An incision is made through the drape ending ¼ cm beyond the inner and outer canthi. With a muscle hook, the free edges of the drape are inverted behind the upper and lower eyelids and an eyelid speculum is applied. A light-weight speculum such as the Barraquer colibri is favored. The eyelids and globe must be carefully inspected after insertion of the speculum, to assure that the eyelids are exerting no pressure on the globe (which may be caused by direct contact with a blade of the speculum or by folding of the tarsus).[26]

Additional Steps in the Preparation of the Patient

Other considerations in assuring low intraocular pressure have been described above and include the following:

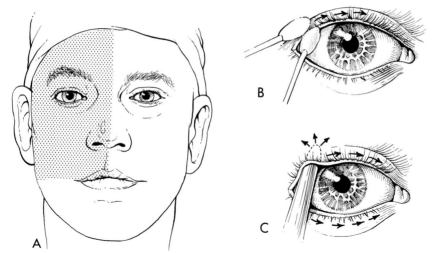

FIGURE 8–14. Cleansing of surgical field. *A*, Area of skin preparation (shaded). *B*, Eyelid margin scrubbing with cotton-tipped applicators. *C*, Irrigation of cul-de-sacs with tip of bulb syringe.

1. Adequate akinesia and anesthesia
2. Intermittent pressure on the globe
3. Proper retraction of the eyelids by the speculum
4. Anatomically adequate eyelid fissure opening
5. Proper traction on the superior rectus suture
6. Avoidance of Valsalva maneuvers such as grunting, straining, coughing, or gagging (one may need to provide the patient with urinal or bedpan, especially if diuretic or osmotic agents have been used)
7. Preoperative use of osmotic agents (proven value) and carbonic anhydrase inhibitors (doubtful value)[34]

Grasping the Superior Rectus Muscle

This maneuver is performed by gently sliding a closed pair of 0.3- or 0.5-mm toothed forceps under the upper lid while the forceps are held in a closed position. When the forceps are approximately 1 cm superior to the limbus, they are opened about a centimeter and pressed slightly downward into the globe. When the forceps are then squeezed shut, they will enclose the tendon of the superior rectus muscle. The globe is now rotated gently as the forceps with the enclosed muscle tendon are brought into the operative field. The needle with an attached 4-0 black silk suture is then placed through the conjunctiva beneath the muscle tendon, and on through the conjunctiva on the other side (Fig. 8–15). The needle is grasped with forceps and drawn through the tissues.

Gentle traction is obtained by looping the two ends through the open jaws of a hemostat, which is then clamped to the drapes. Some surgeons prefer to have an assistant rotate the globe downward by grasping the globe at the inferior limbus with fine smooth forceps or by placing a muscle hook into the inferior fornix, but this maneuver can dislodge the meticulously placed speculum and may be eliminated by the technique described.[26, 34]

Retesting Intraocular Pressure

Before incision into the globe, intraocular pressure should be tested again. This can be done by palpating the globe with an instrument such as a forceps or muscle hook, although some surgeons prefer to have a sterilized tonometer available for this procedure.[34]

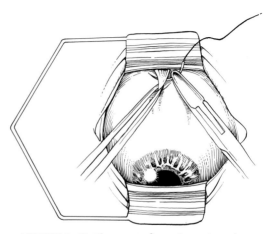

FIGURE 8–15. Placement of superior rectus suture.

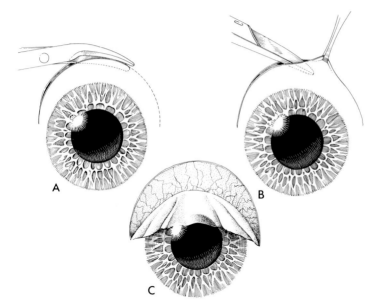

FIGURE 8–16. Preparation of limbus-based conjunctival flap, showing (A) incision, (B) undermining, and (C) reflection.

Specific Techniques

Incision

Conjunctival Flap.* Healing of the limbal wound proceeds more rapidly and more comfortably if it is covered by a conjunctival flap. In the limbus-based flap, and incision is made 3 to 5 mm posterior and parallel to the limbus, and the flap is reflected downward as the sub-conjunctival tissues are dissected with scissors (Fig. 8–16). Because the conjunctiva is extremely thin near its insertion, it is easy to tear the flap when it is used for traction. Nevertheless, a limbus-based conjunctival flap provides a convenient way to elevate the cornea during maneuvers such as iridectomy and lens extraction. This type of flap does have the disadvantage of partially obscuring visualization of the anterior chamber, so the surgeon must frequently manipulate it in order to see the relation of instruments, such as the posterior blade of corneoscleral scissors, during the preparation of the incision. The flap is sutured at the end of the procedure with a fine silk or an absorbable suture, either interrupted or running style, or it may be sealed by electrocoaptation, using the bipolar cautery.

A fornix-based flap is easier to prepare, requiring only a peritomy with blunt scissors, to separate the conjunctiva from its insertion into the peripheral cornea, followed by a blunt dissection toward the fornix for 5 to 7 mm (Fig. 8–17). Sometimes a relaxing incision is needed at the horizontal ends of the flap, in order to allow it to retract neatly away from the field. Some surgeons prefer waiting until this flap is prepared before placing the superior rectus

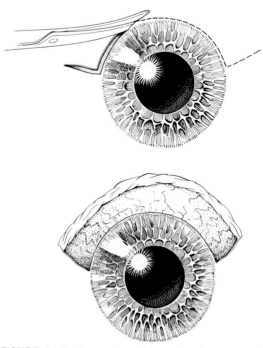

FIGURE 8–17. Preparation of fornix-based conjunctival flap, showing peritomy and relaxing incisions at horizontal ends.

---

*See Chapter 11, p. 262.

suture, using it to retract the flap away from the wound. This type of flap does have the advantage of interfering less with visualization of the anterior chamber than the limbus-based flap. However, at the end of the procedure the flap is pulled down hood-like over the limbal wound, and left unsutured.

In either type of conjunctival surgery it is necessary to incise the insertion of Tenon's capsule, 2 to 3 mm posterior to the conjunctival insertion. Hemostasis is then achieved with the bipolar cautery

Wound leaks may develop with either type of flap, since they result from inadequate closure of the limbal wound regardless of the nature of the conjunctival surgery performed. However, a wound leak with a limbus-based flap is more likely to produce a filtering bleb than is one with a fornix-based flap. Also, in case of wound leak, the Seidel test is more likely to be positive with a fornix-based flap. There is no evidence that the type of flap used influences the development of epithelial downgrowth.[26, 34]

Some surgeons prefer to dispense with a flap altogether, either making the incision entirely within the cornea or simply cutting through the conjunctival insertion. This certainly is acceptable so long as suture material such as 9-0 or 10-0 nylon or polypropylene is used, and care is taken to bury the knots and suture ends within the tissue.

Corneoscleral Incision. The corneoscleral incision has four aspects: size, location, entry of anterior chamber, and enlargement of incision (Fig. 8–18).

The *size* of the incision for intracapsular cataract extraction must be adequate to permit good surgical exposure, and ease of delivery of the lens. A 90-degree incision (3 "clock hours") is the smallest one that will allow the lens to be delivered, and even so, there must be some "molding" of the lens through the incision for this to be done. A 180-degree incision (6 "clock hours," usually from 3 to 9 o'clock) is more than adequate, and because one might encounter branches of the anterior ciliary vessels in the horizontal meridian, it is best to foreshorten the incision somewhat to approximately 160 degrees.[26, 34]

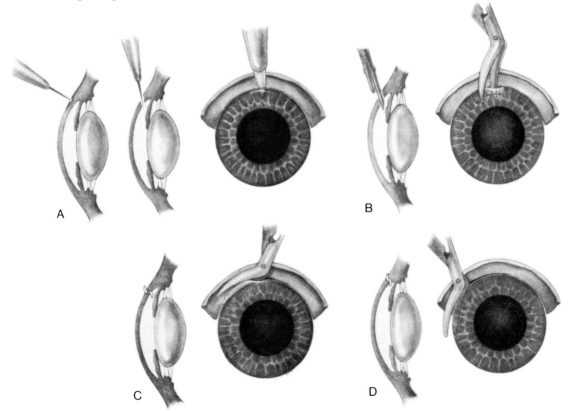

FIGURE 8–18. Corneoscleral incision, side and front view. *A,* Razor-blade entry, showing perpendicular (left) and beveled (middle) incisions. *B,* Introduction of posterior blade of scissors. *C,* Positioning of scissor blades along limbus and beginning of extension of incision. *D,* Further extension of incision. Note angulation of scissors, permitting correct bevel of incision along full extent of wound.

The *location* of the incision in terms of the anterior and posterior boundaries of the limbus has received much attention, but there is little agreement among ophthalmic surgeons as to the ideal location. Generally speaking, the more anterior the incision, the less problem encountered with operative or postoperative hemorrhage. More posterior incisions have a relative advantage with regard to resultant astigmatism and more rapid healing. Many surgeons prefer a compromise mid-limbal position for the incision. Because the cornea is not infinitely thin, the angle at which the incision is made is also important. A more posterior incision must be a longer one in order to produce the same size internal wound as that produced by an anterior incision. This effect is increased if the incision is greatly beveled. At the same time, a highly beveled incision produces a larger surface area of the wound, promoting better healing as well as providing a "self-sealing" effect, caused by compression of the internal lips of the wound when intraocular pressure is restored.[34]

A two-planed incision (Fig. 8–19) increases the wound surface area, and therefore the potential improved wound strength when healed, even further. This is ordinarily done by making a perpendicular incision toward the posterior aspect of the limbus with a knife such as a rounded miniature scalpel (Beaver blade #64). However, it is somewhat difficult technically to produce a single continuous groove of the proper depth with one sweep of the knife around the limbus. Maintaining adequate fixation during this maneuver is also a problem. Ideally, the globe should be fixated at two points, one being the superior rectus suture.

The horizontal rectus may be grasped with forceps, or forceps may be used to grasp the sclera or episcleral tissues. Scleral pics (two-pronged or twist-pic type) are favored by some. With completion of the groove, one may pre-place one or two sutures so that the needle bite goes through nearly the full depth of the groove, which may be as much as two-thirds the thickness of the limbus. The suture is then looped out of the wound so as to stay out of the way until it is ready to be tied.

The second step in the two-plane incision begins with *entry* into the anterior chamber, with a knife held for a more beveled incision. The initial entry should be 1 mm in length, to permit both introduction of the capsulotomy instrument and later easy placement of the posterior blade of the corneoscleral scissors (Fig. 8–18A). If the surgeon withdraws the knife at the first gush of aqueous, there may be only a pinpoint opening in the anterior chamber, and attempts to push the posterior blade of the scissors into the entry wound may end with lamellar dissection of the cornea, or stripping of Descemet's membrane.[26, 34]

Another variation of the two-planed incision is the "scleral groove." This incision is initiated as a 7-mm long incision, 2 or 3 mm posterior to the limbus. Lamellar dissection of the sclera is then carried toward the limbus as for trabeculectomy, except that the radial incisions toward the limbus are omitted. The anterior chamber is entered at the limbus with a small knife, in capsulotomy, and then phacoemulsification can be performed through this port. The incision is then enlarged to the full 7-mm length of the pocket for insertion of an intraocular lens.

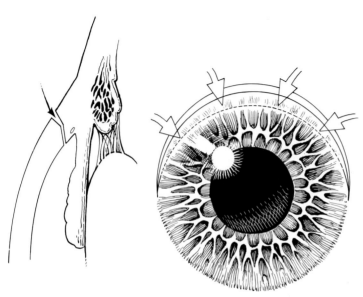

FIGURE 8–19. Two-planed incision, side and front views.

Whether or not a groove is used to create the incision, *enlargement* of the wound with scissors should produce a beveled incision. Care must be taken to avoid engaging the peripheral iris before the cut is made with the scissors. In order to do this, a three-step maneuver is used. First, the posterior blade of the scissors is directed toward the center of the cornea until the surgeon can ascertain that it is definitely within the anterior chamber and beyond Descemet's membrane for a millimeter or two (Fig. 8–18*B*). Then the scissors' handle is repositioned slightly so the blade is parallel to the limbus, and free of entanglement with the peripheral iris (Fig. 8–18*C*). Finally the desired bevel is achieved by angulating the scissors' handle, and the cut is made by closing the scissors' handle with gentle traction on the posterior blade of the scissors. If the handle is not closed completely, a partial cut will be made, and the scissors' blades opened wider, the scissors advanced, and the cut continued until the full extent desired has been achieved before the scissors are removed (Fig. 8–18*D*). This continuous maneuver is less traumatic than repeated insertion of the posterior blade of the scissors for each portion of the cut. To facilitate this, some surgeons prefer a "stop" that is built onto the scissors' handle and manipulated with the thumb. With the stop in position, the scissors' blades do not close entirely, and as the last portion of the incision is to be made, the thumb slides the stop out of the way to complete the cut.

Some surgeons prefer making the point of entry at one of the horizontal extents of the wound, using a single scissors pair for the entire length of the incision. Most surgeons, however, favor making the point of entry into the anterior chamber one and a half "clock hours" to the right of the 12 o'clock position (if right-handed; to the left if left-handed) and using two separate scissors pairs for the left- and right-hand portions of the wound.

As the incision is made, there is nearly always some bleeding, usually from superficial vessels, even if there has been some prior attempt at their cauterization. The introduction of the bipolar cautery (Codman Wetfield cautery) permits precise hemostasis by allowing the surgeon to observe the exact bleeding points under a film of irrigating solution (Fig. 8–20). With this device, there is a minimum amount of thermal cauterization effect, with its attendant shrinkage of collagen that can distort the wound and lead to later wound leakage. Furthermore, with the finest bipolar tips, even deeper vessels at the

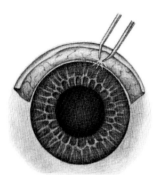

FIGURE 8–20. Bipolar cauterization of limbal vessels.

wound edge or the iris or ciliary body may be cauterized. For these sites the minimal current flow for effective hemostasis should be used, and cauterization must be done only under direct visualization.

Because bleeding ordinarily occurs only during preparation of the conjunctival flap and the limbal incision, and because this can be controlled so effectively by electrocautery, there is no need to make special plans for patients taking anticoagulants such as aspirin or sodium warfarin (Coumadin).

If a significant area of Descemet's membrane is stripped during creation of the incision, it may be repositioned at the end of the procedure with a large air bubble, causing the scroll of attached membrane to uncurl and adhere permanently to the stromal bed.[20]

During the process of extending the incision with the corneoscleral scissors, the ciliary body may be accidentally detached from the scleral spur. Such an inadvertent cyclodialysis may lead to persistent hypotony, requiring techniques such as that described by Stark and Maumenee (penetrating cyclodiathermy) for repair.[52]

Inadvertent puncture of the lens capsule during entry of the anterior chamber is a special problem when the keratome is used. If this is recognized, one may be able to incorporate the puncture site into the iceball by applying the cryoprobe directly over the area of the puncture, permitting total lens extraction as usual.

A potentially ominous sign that may occur during the limbal incision is iris prolapse (Fig. 8–21). The surgeon must decide whether the operation should be terminated or continued. If iris prolapse is the result of retrobulbar or choroidal hemorrhage, it is most important to avoid extending the incision further, and to proceed with securing closure of the wound by

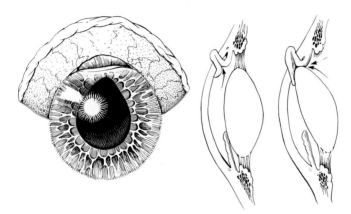

FIGURE 8–21. Iris prolapse (front and side views) owing to entrapped aqueous (center) or "positive vitreous pressure" with forward displacement of superior pole of lens (right).

tying preplaced sutures, or by postplacing sutures. Before proceeding further, it is important to carefully check the surgical field for possible external causes of increased vitreous pressure. The bridle suture should be released, the eyelid speculum should be checked to be sure that the eyelids are not putting any pressure on the globe, and the adequacy of the eyelid akinesia should be tested. The patient's general status should also be checked, to make sure that no Valsalva maneuvers are occurring, and the position of the operating table may have to be adjusted if it appears that the head is in too dependent a position, particularly for an obese patient. Although all of these items should have been checked to the surgeon's satisfaction before the beginning of the operation, some factors may have changed during the intervening minutes.[34]

The prolapse may be a result of a delayed retrobulbar hemorrhage, and evidence of proptosis of the globe as well as hemorrhage under the conjunctiva or Tenon's capsule should be sought. If the iris prolapse appears to be expanding, particularly if the lens-iris diaphragm appears to have moved anteriorly, the possibility of a choroidal hemorrhage should be considered. Most often the iris prolapse does not increase, and is simply the result of aqueous entrapped in the posterior chamber. This can be relieved by gently stroking the iris with a blunt-tipped irrigator or by performing a peripheral iridotomy or iridectomy; if desired, the anterior chamber can be re-formed with a small amount of irrigating solution (Fig. 8–22).[26, 34]

If "positive vitreous pressure" appears to be increasing with persistent uncontrolled prolapse of the iris and impending prolapse of the lens, bleeding into the choroidal or suprachoroidal space is likely. Rapid closure of the incision should be the first step. Then a sclerotomy may be performed with a sharp knife 9 mm posterior

to the limbus in any quadrant (Fig. 8–23). This will decompress the globe spontaneously, although aspiration through a needle or cannula might be helpful in addition.[34]

When the iris-lens diaphragm appears to be bulging from increased vitreous pressure, but this is not progressive and is unrelieved by iridectomy, some surgeons choose to do an aspiration of the fluid vitreous by way of the pars plana. A small incision is made with a Ziegler knife or razor blade knife through sclera and uvea, 4 mm posterior to the limbus, and an 18- or 20-gauge needle is inserted into the wound for about 5 to 8 mm, directed toward the center of the globe. Fluid, but not formed vitreous, is easily aspirated (Fig. 8–24). As this occurs, the globe becomes soft, and the iris and lens diaphragm should drop back significantly.

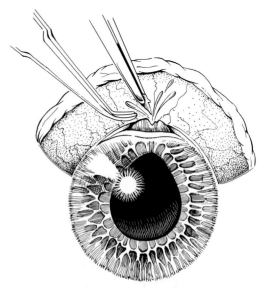

FIGURE 8–22. Peripheral iridectomy releasing entrapped aqueous.

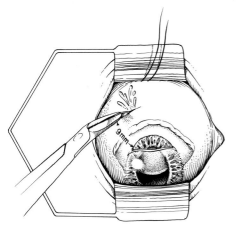

FIGURE 8–23. Sclerotomy with razor blade knife for choroidal hemorrhage.

Sutures

Secure and accurate wound closure is the key to an early and safe period of recuperation as well as full visual rehabilitation for the patient. Microsurgical techniques have probably been more helpful in this phase of cataract surgery than in any other. Because precise visual control can be achieved with the operation microscope, the advantages of track sutures and sutures placed within a groove but before penetration (preplaced sutures) have been diminished. Even surgeons who use preplaced sutures must become skilled at the postplacement of sutures, since it has become customary to use 5 to 10 or more bites with the needle for either the interrupted or the running suture technique.[26, 51]

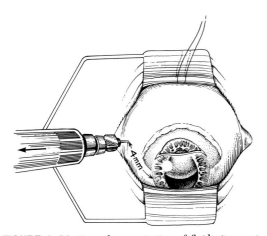

FIGURE 8–24. Pars plana aspiration of fluid vitreous to decompress globe.

Preplacement of sutures favors improved security in the face of prolapse of intraocular contents, and minimizes suture effects on astigmatism. However, postplaced sutures increase the speed of the operation, reduce the tangling of sutures during incision, iridectomy, and lens extraction, and, with microsurgical control, can result in excellent wound alignment with relatively minimal postoperative astigmatism.

Suture placement demands the use of an excellent pair of tissue forceps, usually with 0.12-mm teeth, and a needle holder whose jaws are delicate enough to grasp the fine curved needle near its middle, but strong enough to hold the needle firmly, preventing it from rocking or rotating while it is passed through the limbal tissues. A needle holder that fills these criteria well is the Troutman-Barraquer model, with curved jaws and without a lock. The needle holder should be demagnetized at regular intervals, to eliminate inadvertent repositioning of the needle as the jaws of the needle holder are opened. The needle with attached suture may be passed to the surgeon in working position by the nurse if the instrument is grasped by pinching the springs together. In this way the surgeon need not reposition the needle holder, and the needle and suture are ready for use.

The first essential step of proper suture placement is firm and accurate fixation of the tissue to be sutured. When beginning the suture placement, one jaw of the forceps is placed on the corneal surface, the other with its teeth on the wound surface (Fig. 8–25A). An adequate grasp will assure that the tissue will not tear away while the needle is being placed. The needle then enters the tissue approximately 0.5 mm from the edge of the wound, is directed downward, and then rotated deeper in the tissues until it reaches a depth of two-thirds to three-fourths of the tissue thickness before the tip emerges in the wound. At that moment the corneal side of the wound is released and the opposing scleral aspect of the wound is grasped similarly with the forceps (Fig. 8–25B). A frequent mistake at this point is to make too superficial a grasp of the scleral tissues. However, when the tissues have been firmly fixated, the surgeon judges the correct wound alignment, both side to side and with regard to depth, and then continues to pass the needle through the scleral tissues. The surgeon should take advantage of the curvature of the needle, and can best control the needle's passage if this is done with gradual force, allowing the needle to work its way through the tissues rather than

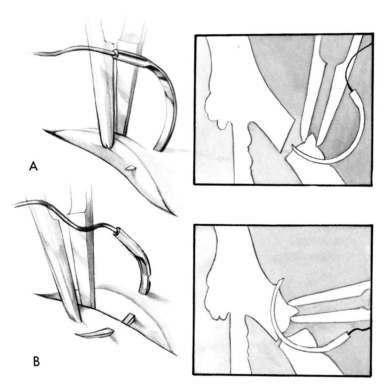

A

B

FIGURE 8–25. Postplaced suture, side and front views. *A*, Corneal side of wound firmly fixated with forceps as needle tip emerges at two-thirds the wound depth. *B*, Scleral side of wound fixated as needle continues passage through tissue.

to pop unexpectedly to the surface. When the needle does emerge through the surface on the scleral aspect of the wound, it should be pushed a bit further until 2 or 3 mm of it is through the tissue before the grasp of the middle of the needle is released. This eliminates the necessity of grabbing the needle near its point end, which risks damaging it for later use. The tissue forceps must not be released until the needle has been moved on from the tissue completely and an adequate length of suture material has been pulled through.

Knowing the correct amount of tension to be placed on each suture requires a certain amount of experience. Ideally, the tissues should simply be brought into approximation, but excessive tissue compression should be avoided, as this can lead to cutting through of sutures, as well as post-operative astigmatism. A suture that is tied too loosely does not achieve the desired effect of wound closure. Also, the tension on individual sutures can change as additional sutures are placed, and it is important to recheck all suture tensions when suturing seems complete and to remove and replace those that appear too tight or too loose. Nylon and, to some extent, polypropylene are somewhat elastic materials, and this must be taken into account when adjusting their tension. Most other suture materials are essentially inelastic. In any case, tension on the suture may very well

change as the knot is being tied, sometimes loosening and sometimes tightening as various throws are completed. Surgeons should take time to practice with various suture materials in order to become accustomed to their "feel" before committing them to an actual operation.

A general surgical principle in wound closure is that the suture must be placed perpendicular to the wound. In the case of closing a limbal wound in ophthalmic surgery, perpendicular is equivalent to radial placement. Before each suture is placed the surgeons should position both hands in order to achieve radial placement, thereby ensuring optimal wound apposition (Fig. 8–26).

In the past some surgeons have advocated through-and-through suture placement with material such as 10-0 nylon or 10-0 polypropylene. This type of placement was thought to provide optimal apposition through the full depth of the wound, eliminating the gaping on the posterior aspect of the wound that is said to occur with even deeply placed sutures. However, it has been shown that immediately after creation of the incision, the corneal stroma swells on the internal aspect of the wound, producing a ridge rather than a gap, the ridge then persisting for several months. Thus, even without deep suture placement, there is ample wound contact to permit healing even in the deepest aspects of the wound. Certainly suture

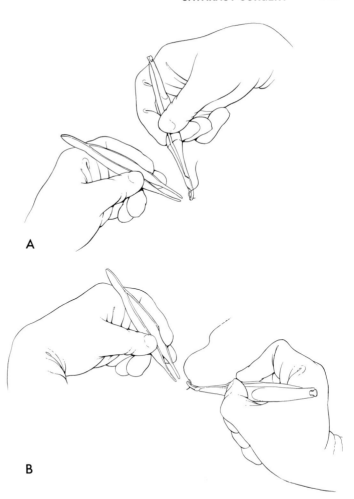

FIGURE 8–26. Hand position for forceps and needle holder to achieve radial suture placement. *A*, For suture on right side of wound. *B*, For suture on left side of wound.

A

B

material of large diameter should not penetrate the full thickness of the wound, as wound leak, possibly together with epithelialization of the suture track, may develop.[26, 34]

Iris Surgery

Iridectomy has long been incorporated into cataract extraction to prevent pupillary block in the aphakic eye; even with iridectomy, however, this may still occur. Any type of iris opening, such as sector iridectomy (Fig. 8–27), peripheral iridectomy (Fig. 8–28), or peripheral iridotomy, will serve this purpose, and the choice among these usually depends on other factors. There is no evidence that there is better postoperative acuity or improved visual comfort with any one of these forms of iris surgery. There certainly are indications for sector iridectomy, most of which have to do with the inability to dilate the pupil adequately to permit lens extraction during the operative procedure, or with the desire to allow maximum visibility of the ocular fundus postoperatively, such as in a patient with proliferative diabetic retinopathy

or other retinal disorders that require photocoagulation treatment. However, if intraocular lens implantation is contemplated, sector iridectomy would be undesirable if an iris-fixated lens is to be used. For this purpose, if the pupil will not dilate to a size adequate to permit lens delivery, a peripheral iridectomy together with radial iridotomy can be performed to communicate with the pupillary space (Fig. 8–29). After lens delivery the iris can be sutured with one or two 10-0 polypropylene sutures.[26, 34]

In performing sector iridectomy the iris is usually grasped near the root and excised with one or two cuts of the Barraquer scissors, producing a large boat-shaped pupil (Fig. 8–29). Sector iridectomy performed at the mid-iris, or closer to the pupillary border, will produce an inverted keyhole-shaped pupil. Performing a basal iridectomy, by making a radial iridotomy and cutting or tearing the iris from its insertion on the ciliary body, was thought to be of some advantage in patients subject to secondary glaucoma caused by angle closure. However, there is danger of hemorrhage from this maneuver,

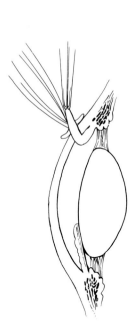

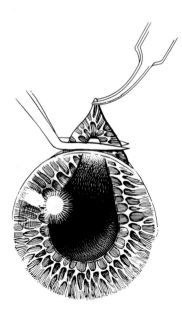

FIGURE 8–27. Sector iridectomy, side and front views.

and it is probably best to avoid this. An alternative to performing a large sector iridectomy is to perform a sphincterotomy, in which a small cut is made, usually at the 6 o'clock position, with the Barraquer scissors (Fig. 8–30). This alone or together with one or more sphincterotomies may permit delivery of the lens through a relatively round pupil. Care must be taken to avoid tearing the anterior lens capsule during this maneuver.[34]

For a peripheral iridectomy, the iris should be grasped near its periphery (Fig. 8–28), using a shallow bite with fine-toothed (0.12-mm) forceps, or with blunt or jeweler's forceps. The "tent" of iris is excised with scissors. One should carefully inspect the iridectomy to be sure that a full-thickness iridectomy has been performed. During the maneuvers of iris surgery, several complications may be encountered. As mentioned above, one should avoid too much trac-

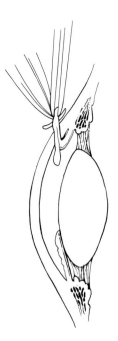

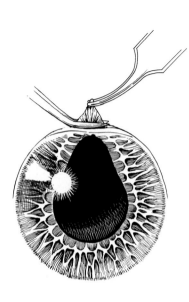

FIGURE 8–28. Peripheral iridectomy, side and front views.

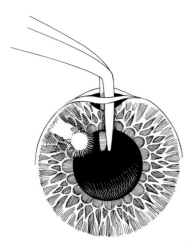

FIGURE 8–29. Peripheral iridectomy with radial iridotomy.

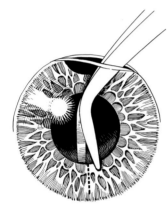

FIGURE 8–30. Inferior sphincterotomy.

tion on the iris root, which might result in excessive hemorrhage. If the posterior pigment layer remains, it is often possible to irrigate through this with irrigating solution. Also, one should take care to control the size of the iridectomy—whether it is a peripheral or a sector iridectomy—during excision with the

scissors.[26, 34, 40] Iris surgery should be performed in as deliberate a manner as possible.

Lens Surgery

Intracapsular Cataract Extraction. It is difficult to believe that the elegant procedure of intracapsular cataract extraction has been largely supplanted by the extracapsular method, but this is exactly what has happened. Nevertheless, there are occasions when intracapsular extraction is appropriate even today, and for that reason the technique is discussed here.

Some day cataract formation will be prevented or reversed by medical means. Until that time the extraction of the lens by whatever means remains at the heart of the management of cataract.

To facilitate lens extraction, enzymatic zonulolysis with alpha-chymotrypsin is used virtually routinely by many eye surgeons. Because of the secondary elevation of intraocular pressure associated with this procedure, it is not entirely without hazards. However, there is ample documentation that this medication has no adverse effect on wound healing. A fresh solution, 1:10,000 concentration, is irrigated into the posterior chamber through the peripheral iridectomy for the superior zonules and through the pupil for the inferior zonules through an olive-tipped cannula (Troutman) (Fig. 8–31). It is not necessary to push the tip of the cannula too far underneath the iris for this purpose. Usually 0.25 to 0.50 ml of solution are used. Before lens extraction, it is helpful to irrigate the anterior chamber thoroughly with balanced salt solution in order to minimize the number of zonular fragments that remain.[7, 83]

Cryoextraction (Fig. 8–32) is most easily performed with an assistant who gently retracts the cornea with the attached limbal-based conjunctival flap, or a suture loop. The assistant should

FIGURE 8–31. Enzymatic zonulolysis with olive-tipped cannula, showing irrigation of superior zonules through peripheral iridectomy (left) and inferior zonules through pupil (right).

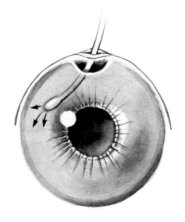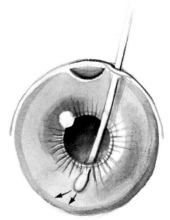

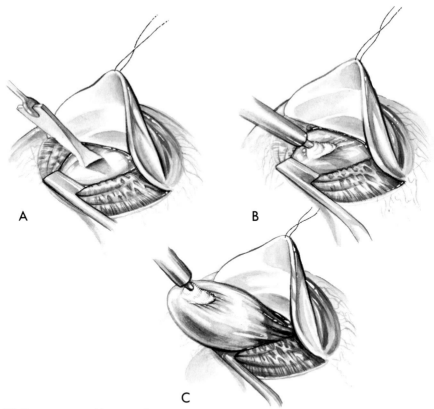

FIGURE 8–32. Cryoextraction of lens. *A,* Elevation of cornea, retraction of iris, and removal of excess fluid with cellulose sponge. *B,* Application of cryoprobe. *C,* Sliding extraction of lens.

also be on the lookout for adhesion of the cryoprobe to sutures, cornea, or iris, and must be prepared to defrost with irrigating solution if the cryoextractor is not self-defrosting. As the cornea is retracted, one should avoid excessive bending of it, which might result in endothelial damage as manifested by striate keratopathy, possibly together with corneal edema. However, adequate retraction of the cornea must be obtained to avoid incorporation of the endothelial surface of the cornea into the iceball.

The iris must be retracted adequately so that the cryoextractor can be applied to the anterior and superior mid-periphery of the lens. This is most easily done with an angulated Teflon iris retractor (Rosenbaum-Drews), available in both left- and right-handed models (Fig. 8–32A). A right-handed surgeon uses the left-handed model for both left and right eyes. With both cornea and iris retracted, excessive fluid on the lens surface should be removed by touching a cellulose sponge to the fluid (Fig. 8–32A). However, a thin film of fluid should remain on the lens surface to produce optimal adhesion when the cryoextractor is activated (Fig. 8–32B). When a sector iridectomy has been done, a

cellulose sponge may be used to retract the iris pillars, as the plastic iris retractor is ineffective in this situation. Some surgeons prefer to use the cellulose sponge to retract the iris in every case.[26]

If 2 or more minutes have been allowed to elapse after irrigation with alpha-chymotrypsin, the strength of the zonular membrane is usually much reduced. The remaining zonules are usually broken by gentle traction as the lens extraction is initiated (Fig. 8–32C), and remaining zonules break by an "unzippering" action (Fig. 8–33). Occasionally direct stripping with a blunt instrument such as a vitreous sweeper or muscle hook is necessary. The vitreous usually spontaneously peels from the posterior aspect of the lens during the extraction, but occasionally, especially in younger patients, in whom this adhesion is firmer, the vitreous might have to be wiped from the posterior surface with a vitreous sweeper, to prevent rupture of the anterior hyaloid face.[26, 34]

Various techniques have been devised for eye surgeons who find themselves without assistance. Retraction of the cornea can be achieved by attaching a suture to the lower post

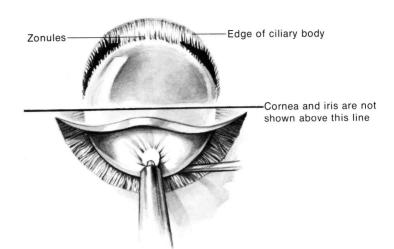

Zonules⸺

⸺Edge of ciliary body

⸺Cornea and iris are not shown above this line

FIGURE 8–33. Rupture of inferior zonules by "unzippering" action.

of an eyelid speculum. Plastic iris retractors have been incorporated into the sleeves of cryoprobes so that both maneuvers can be accomplished with one hand. However, for the surgeon who is unassisted, capsule forceps delivery is probably still a better solution.

During lens extraction vitreous may present itself at the incision without actually prolapsing from the globe. In order to prevent vitreous loss the surgeon should slow down the rate of lens extraction. Direct stripping of the hyalo-ideocapsular ligament can be performed as described above with an instrument or by sliding the lens over the pupil edge to close the gaps. An assistant can help by lifting the globe gently with forceps, especially if a Flieringa ring is in place. Finally, one can attempt to pull down sutures as the lens is delivered, to block the vitreous prolapse. This last maneuver requires the efforts of a well-coordinated team, and is one of the many maneuvers that demand nearly as high a level of technical skill from assistant as from surgeon.

Certainly one of the most important advances in cataract surgery has been the introduction of anterior vitrectomy for vitreous prolapse. It is now recognized that vitreous loss may impair the visual outcome whether the amount of vitreous is small or large. If strands of formed vitreous remain adherent to the wound, the traction effects may lead to retinal detachment, chronic inflammation, and cystoid macular edema. Anterior vitrectomy has markedly reduced these complications. Other methods for management of prolapsed vitreous, such as air injection and sweeping with a spatula, are ineffective.

The technique of anterior vitrectomy at its simplest requires only the use of small trian-

gular cellulose sponges such as those supplied by Weck. When the sponge tip touches formed vitreous, the fibrils adhere to it, and when gentle traction is applied, a glob of formed vitreous may be excised by scissors (e.g., sharp Westcott scissors) with a single clean cut (Fig. 8–34). This is usually done repeatedly until it can be clearly demonstrated that no formed vitreous remains adherent to the wound, and preferably until formed vitreous had been excised to the plane of the iris. At this time there is usually a partial collapse of the globe as manifested by indentations along the horizontal and vertical meridians made by the rectus muscles. Most ophthalmic surgeons rely on more elaborate instruments for the same purpose, such as the SITE (Federman) and the ocutome (O'Malley), which, by means of a chopping action together with the use of an aspirated syringe operated by the assistant, permits formed vitreous to be nibbled away from the wound and the anterior chamber (Fig. 8–35).

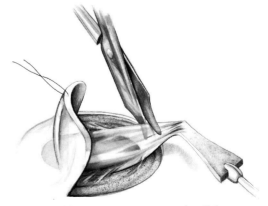

FIGURE 8–34. Anterior vitrectomy with cellulose sponge and scissors.

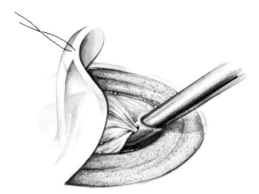

FIGURE 8–35. Anterior vitrectomy with aspiration-cutting device such as an ocutome.

However, again, cellulose sponges should be used to ascertain that there are no vitreous strands remaining adherent to the wound or on the iris surface.[26, 34]

Extracapsular Cataract Extraction. As mentioned earlier, extracapsular cataract extraction has been part of ophthalmology longer than intracapsular cataract surgery. Along with the newer forms of extracapsular surgery such as phacoemulsification and phacofragmentation, older (but updated and modified) techniques for extracapsular extraction have been received with great enthusiasm. There is good evidence for reduced incidence of cystoid macular edema and retinal detachment with extracapsular surgery.[58] Another factor in the revived popularity of extracapsular surgery is the interest in posterior chamber fixation of intraocular lens implants. The "standard" operation for cataract extraction is now extracapsular extraction. Most ophthalmic surgeons trained in intracapsular

extraction (including me) have converted to extracapsular surgery as the preferred method of cataract extraction.[17] The enormous interest in lens implantation has obviated one of the supposed advantages of phacoemulsification by requiring that the 3-mm incision be opened at least large enough to permit implantation of the 6-mm pseudophakos.

For extracapsular cataract extraction with a large 160-degree incision (Fig. 8–36), the procedure is much the same as for intracapsular surgery except that enzymatic zonulolysis is not performed. The pupil should be dilated as fully as possible. An anterior capsulotomy may be performed with toothed forceps (Schweigger) (Fig. 8–36A), but usually the anterior capsulotomy is performed as for phacoemulsification, using an irrigating cystitome or a bent 27-gauge needle. The neodymium:YAG laser may also be used for anterior capsulotomy, although transient elevations in intraocular pressure commonly occur with this technique. The bulk of the lens material (the nucleus) is removed by the curved, blunt nucleus expresser, providing external pressure beginning at the 6 o'clock position and following the lens toward the 12 o'clock position as it is delivered (Fig. 8–36B). The lens loop may be modified into an irrigating instrument (the lens vectus) to be slipped between the nucleus and the posterior lens cortex to aid in nuclear delivery. If the nucleus is being delivered by expression, fine-toothed forceps are held in the surgeon's other hand and the scleral lip of the wound is grasped at the 12 o'clock position. Slight posterior pressure is exerted as the nucleus is delivered through the wound. Three sutures are placed and tied,

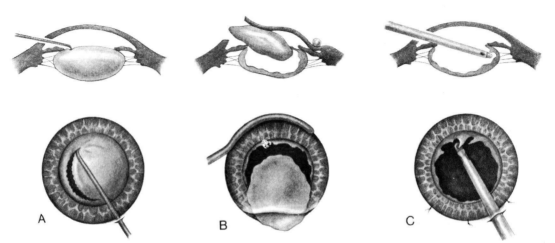

FIGURE 8–36. Extracapsular cataract extraction, side and front views. *A*, Anterior capsulotomy with toothed forceps. *B*, Expression of lens nucleus with lens loop. *C*, Irrigation of residual cortical material with use of flat cannula.

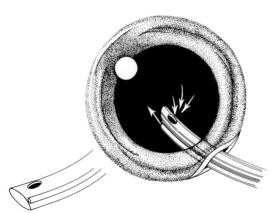

FIGURE 8–37. Simultaneous irrigation and aspiration performed with the Fink-Weinstein two-way cannula.

leaving 3-mm "ports" through which the aspiration-irrigation cannula may be introduced. Some surgeons have taken to fashioning their own aspiration-irrigation systems with readily available materials. Automated aspiration-irrigation devices are even more commonly used. The surgeon must remove most of the cortical lens material, including that which must be stripped from the fornices of the capsular bag. Automated instruments give the surgeon the option of irrigation only, thereby expanding the capsular bag and giving the aspiration port direct access to peripheral cortical material, or irrigation together with aspiration, permitting rapid removal of all material impacted into the aspiration port. The multiposition foot pedal allows the surgeon instantaneous control over the procedure.

In younger patients the entire lens may be aspirated, and this may even be performed in a subluxated lens. The aspiration-irrigation technique is preferred, with use of either a double (side-by-side or coaxial) cannula (Fig. 8–37) or the two-needle method. One may choose to rely on an assistant to operate the aspiration control, or do this oneself, aided by an automated instrument for maintaining intraocular pressure as described above (Fig. 8–38). The ocutome, together with an infusion cannula, is also useful for a soft cataract. Lenses with harder nuclei may be aspirated easily after phacoemulsification or fragmentation with the Girard ultrasonic unit in conjunction with the ocutome.

The other forms of extracapsular cataract extraction, phacoemulsification and phacofragmentation, have already been discussed. Generally it can be said that extracapsular surgery can be used for patients in all age groups, and intracapsular surgery is reserved for older patients (those over 40 years of age). The indications for intracapsular extraction have now been reduced to a relatively few and unusual situations, such as subluxation or dislocation of the lens, or hypermature or calcitic cataract.

Even when intracapsular extraction is planned, inadvertent rupture of the capsule may occur. The single most important consideration when this happens is to attempt delivery of the lens nucleus as atraumatically as possible. Dislocation of the lens nucleus into the vitreous almost invariably leads to severe uveitis, and attempts at removing it with instruments such as the phacofragmenter or ocutome are not always successful. However, one must avoid expressing the lens nucleus as described above for planned extracapsular cataract extraction, since the zonular membrane has been broken at least in part, and vitreous loss may result. Sometimes it is possible to perform cryoextrac-

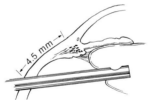

FIGURE 8–38. Pars plana lensectomy performed with the ocutome.

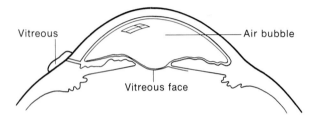

FIGURE 8–39. Air bubble is used in order to re-form the anterior chamber.

tion of the lens nucleus after inadvertent capsular rupture.[21, 31, 34, 40, 73]

Incisional Closure

After removal of the lens material, the wound edges should be carefully inspected to see if iris or vitreous is caught in the incision. Usually this situation can be corrected by gentle irrigation of the wound edge and into the anterior chamber across the iris face. Even when only a single suture at the 12 o'clock position is tied, the anterior chamber can be partially formed, helping intraocular tissues to resume a normal position. An air bubble can usually be retained more easily than solution, and this can be injected by placing the tip of a bent 30-gauge cannula into the anterior chamber, across the iris face, avoiding the site of the iridectomy. The air bubble should extend into the superior angle, peripheral to the incision (Fig. 8–39). If it does not, iris may be adherent peripherally, and this may lead later to peripheral anterior synechia.[26, 34] Even more effective than air, the viscoelastic substance sodium hyaluronate (Healon, AmVisc) may be used to re-form the anterior chamber as well as to expand the capsular bag so as to ready it to receive a posterior chamber lens implant.[23]

When interrupted sutures are used, an average of 7 or 8 sutures are usually needed, ranging from 5 to 10 sutures. The exact number is not important, but at the end of the procedure the wound should be secure without evidence of leakage when the intraocular pressure has been restored with balanced salt solution.[26] The field should remain dry even when gentle pressure is applied to the scleral side of the wound between each pair of sutures with the tip of the sponge.

Virtually all ophthalmic sutures for cataract surgery should be handled only with instruments, never with fingers. The suture is usually grasped about 2 cm from the wound on the scleral side and is wrapped around the needle holder for a triple-throw surgeon's knot. The first throw should have two turns if silk or catgut is used, three turns for synthetic absorbable sutures, and three or four turns with nylon or polypropylene. The position of the hands is reversed as the first throw is tightened, and without releasing the suture end being held by forceps, the second throw is applied by looping the suture over the needle or the jaws in the direction opposite to the first. A third throw is completed in a similar way. Judging the correct tension to be applied to the suture knot requires practice (Fig. 8–40), and must take into account the relative elasticity of nylon and polypropylene as compared with other suture material. The suture must be cut so that the ends are 1 to 2 mm long for chromic and silk, but on the knot for nylon and polypropylene. For synthetic absorbable sutures, the ends may be most comfortable when left 3 to 4 mm long. The knot

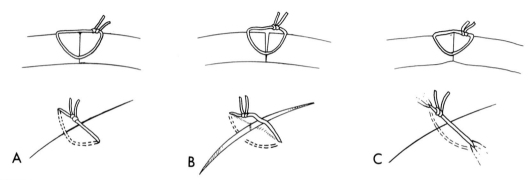

FIGURE 8–40. Interrupted sutures shown illustrating *(A)* correct wound apposition, *(B)* improper apposition with too loosely tied suture, and *(C)* improper apposition with too tightly tied suture.

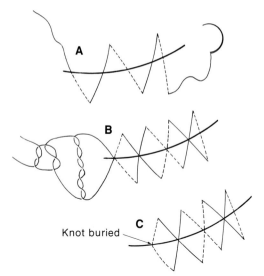

FIGURE 8–41. Wound closure using double running suture technique. Suturing begins on the left, continues to the right *(A)*, returns to the left for tying *(B)*, and is completed after knot is buried in the incision *(C)*.

can remain on the surface for chromic, silk, and synthetic absorbable materials, but must be buried for nylon and polypropylene.

Some surgeons prefer running sutures to interrupted sutures (Fig. 8–41). Some time is saved by using running sutures, since there are fewer knots to be tied and fewer sutures to be cut. However, nothing can match the security provided by independently acting interrupted sutures. Also, it is somewhat more difficult technically to place a running suture symmetrically, as well as to make final adjustments of suture tension so that this is equal throughout the wound.

A suture that is tied too tightly can produce distortion of the cornea with resultant astigmatism (Fig. 8–42). The astigmatism tends to be correctable by a plus cylinder in the axis of the offending suture. This can be explained by likening the effect of the tight suture to a bow string that, when shortened, increases the curvature of the bow. During the postoperative period when high astigmatism is judged to be the result of a suture that has been tied too tightly, the suture may be cut with a knife, scissors, or the tip of a disposable needle (Fig. 8–43), with the patient seated at the slit lamp and with only topical anesthesia. The argon laser photocoagulator may also be used for this purpose. Often a correction of as much as 5 diopters of astigmatism, which tends to be "with the rule," is possible by dividing a single suture.

After closure of the limbal incision the conjunctival flap is secured. Topical as well as subconjunctival antibiotics and cortical steroids may be used as prophylaxis against infection and inflammation, respectively. However, these are not essential in most cases, even though many ophthalmic surgeons make this routine.

Although it has been customary to dilate the pupil with a cycloplegic solution at the end of the case, this step is omitted if a posterior chamber lens implant is used, as it can lead to "pupillary capture" of the lens. Usually, if no medication is used, the pupil tends to become miotic within a few hours, unless repeated attempts to dilate the pupil have been made during the surgery, in which case the pupil may redilate even if acetylcholene was used.[26, 34]

Placement of Intraocular Lens (Pseudophakos)

Although removal of the opaque crystalline lens eliminates the problem of cataract, management of the aphakic patient is incomplete without optical correction. The spectacle correction of aphakia (Fig. 8–44A) results in a distorted form of vision with various problems

FIGURE 8–42. Shortening effect on corneal curvature created by tying sutures too tightly. The effect is likened to shortening a bowstring on the curvature of the bow.

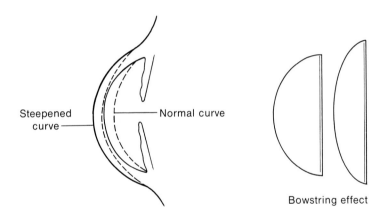

Steepened curve — Normal curve

Bowstring effect

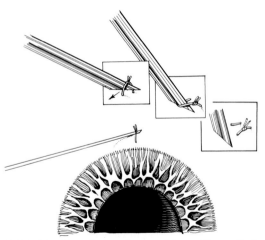

FIGURE 8–43. Technique for use of disposable needle for cutting tight corneoscleral suture. The needle is inserted with the bevel down, and the sharp edge of the bevel is used to cut the suture.

owing to spherical aberrations, magnification effects, and prismatic distortions.

Although many aphakic patients, particularly those who are bilaterally aphakic, are able to make a satisfactory adjustment to spectacle correction, the correction of aphakia with contact lenses, both of the hard and soft types, in both daily- and extended-wear varieties, represents an improved visual result in many respects (Fig. 8–44B). Not only is there less spherical aberration, but there are fewer distortions owing to magnification, since the correcting lens is closer to the principal planes of the original crystalline lens. Furthermore, because the contact lens moves as the eye rotates, there are fewer prismatic effects as well. The improvement in contact lens technology has greatly improved the optical correction of aphakia. However, not every patient is a suitable candidate for contact lens correction. Many patients simply are unwilling to make this attempt, and most ophthalmologists have had the disappointing experience of being unable to adequately motivate otherwise suitable candidates for contact lens wear into trying them, or continuing with their use. Also, many patients are anxious about the thought of touching their eyes with a contact lens, and patients with disorders such as dry eyes and allergic conditions, or those with glaucoma filtering blebs, may not be able to tolerate the lens. Also, many elderly patients have lax eyelids, and although a contact lens can be fashioned to the eye, poor eyelid function may interfere with its use.

The concept of intraocular lens implantation (Fig. 8–44C) is attractive for a number of reasons. First and foremost in this "bionic" age,

there is definite appeal to the idea of replacing a defective organ with an artificial one. Many patients also are attracted to the idea that once the lens is implanted, they need never "bother" with it again (and of course the surgeon hopes that he won't have to either). Of course, the major theoretical advantage to the intraocular lens implant is that its principal planes are much closer (but seldom coincident) with the principal planes of the crystalline lens that has just been removed. Thus magnification effects leading to faulty spatial localization (aniseikonia) are markedly diminished.

Intraocular lens implantation began in England about 40 years ago and then spread through Europe before being performed for the first time in this country in 1952. However, many problems developed during the first decade of lens implantation, and the procedure was discontinued by all but a few surgeons, primarily Binkhorst of the Netherlands and Choyce of England. The revival of interest in lens implantation has far exceeded the initial experience, and by now several million lens implantations have been done worldwide. In many respects, clinical experience has outstripped fundamental knowledge, so that many aspects of the optics, physiology, and tissue effects are only now being revealed. Nevertheless, it is certain that the clinical effectiveness of this adjunct to cataract surgery has been firmly established. Many of the principles of the design, manufacture and optical characteristics of lenses, as well as their insertion and fixation, have now been well established.[9, 61, 64]

Perhaps the most important information derived from clinical experience to date relates to patient selection for lens implantation. Although there are no firm indications for intraocular lens implantation, certain patients can be regarded as optimal candidates. These are individuals who are elderly (older than 60 or 65 years of age), with no significant ocular disorder other than cataract, and who would not be expected to do well with spectacle or contact lens correction. As favorable experience with lens implants grows, younger and younger patients are being considered as suitable candidates as well.[8, 56, 67, 77]

Coexisting macular disease is regarded by some surgeons as a relatively favorable factor, since peripheral vision is more likely to be normal with this method of correction than with spectacle correction, even though central visual acuity is not benefited as much.

Some surgeons believe that unilateral trauma leading to aphakia in young children is a relative

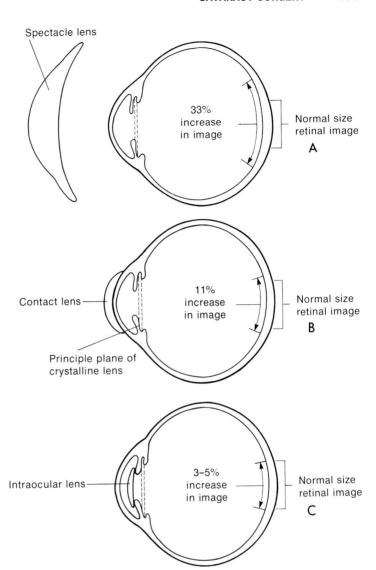

Spectacle lens

33%
increase
in image

Normal size
retinal image

A

FIGURE 8–44. Effect on retinal image size by optical correction by using (A) spectacle lens, (B) contact lens, and (C) intraocular lens.

Contact lens

11%
increase
in image

Normal size
retinal image

B

Principle plane of
crystalline lens

Intraocular lens

3–5%
increase
in image

Normal size
retinal image

C

indication for lens implantation, in view of the notoriously poor results obtained with occlusion therapy and contact lens correction. However, definitive information supporting this contention has not yet been developed.

During the first wave of lens implantation several decades ago, an unacceptably high percentage of patients developed serious complications, including corneal edema, chronic uveitis, and dislocation of the lens implant. Many surgeons who lived through that experience are unwilling to reconsider lens implantation, especially since some of the poor results did not develop for several years after surgery. Much credit must be given to Jaffe in this country for his cautious reintroduction of lens implantation and for his efforts to maintain a conservative attitude about this procedure.

There is a growing concern about several contraindications to lens implantation. Factors militating against this procedure include previous or active uveitis, predilection to retinal detachment, rubeosis iridis, iris atrophy, proliferative diabetic retinopathy, small anterior segment with shallow anterior chamber, and corneal endothelial disease. Lens implantation should be considered with great care in patients with high myopia (more than 10 diopters) or with only one useful eye. Operative problems such as intraocular bleeding, dilated fixed pupil, and bulging of the iris and vitreous face after lens extraction should make the surgeon consider abandonment of implantation. Vitreous loss is considered a relative contraindication, although some surgeons believe that when meticulous anterior vitrectomy can be performed, implantation may proceed as planned. Medically controlled glaucoma, somewhat surprisingly, has not proved to be a negative factor, although the postoperative care of the glaucoma patient with an intraocular lens may be difficult.

The complications associated with lens implantation vary with the technique and the surgeon. Implantation of the lens beneath a cushioning air bubble or a bolus of sodium hyaluronate has been associated with relatively little corneal morbidity, even though the endothelial cell population as evaluated with specular microscopy may be reduced (as it may after the cataract procedure itself as compared with the preoperative state). Improvements in the design of rigid lenses fixated in the anterior chamber angle, such as the Choyce lens modified by Tennant, have attracted a great deal of interest, as have flexible anterior chamber lenses, such as the one-piece C-loop lens designed by Simcoe.[72] This lens design is quite versatile in that it may be implanted at the time of cataract surgery, or at a later date in patients unable to tolerate contact lenses (primary and secondary implantation, respectively). This lens type may be used after either intracapsular or extracapsular surgery, and the technique for its insertion is relatively simple and atraumatic. Unlike the case with lenses that are fixated to the iris or through the pupil, dislocation or subluxation is a rare problem. This lens can be used regardless of the type of iris surgery used, and full dilation of the pupil can be performed postoperatively. This last problem occurs with all types of iris-fixated lenses, with or without transiridial or transiridectomy anchoring sutures.[8, 9]

The technique for intraocular lens implantation varies considerably, in large part because of individual lens design. Nevertheless, the starting point for each intraocular lens in every case is a meticulously performed and atraumatic extraction of the cataract, whether by intracapsular or planned extracapsular technique.

The rigid anterior chamber angle-supported lenses, such as the Choyce lens and its modification by Tennant, or the flexible anterior chamber lens of Simcoe may be inserted at the time of cataract surgery through the superior limbal incision or, secondarily, through a horizontal limbal incision (Fig. 8–45). Because fixation is created by mild pressure of the lens haptics in the anterior chamber angle, the exact sizing of the lens relative to the eye is critical, with an allowable error of $\pm$ 0.5 mm. First, approximation to the correct lens size is obtained by careful measurement of the horizontal

diameter of the cornea, adding 0.5 to 1.0 mm to the "white-to-white" measurement. After extraction of the cataract the incision is partially closed with two interrupted sutures placed 6 to 8 mm apart, straddling the 12 o'clock limbal position. The pupil is constricted with acetylcholine or bolus of sodium hyaluronate, and a moderate-sized air bubble is introduced into the anterior chamber. As with every type of lens implant, the pseudophakos is carefully inspected with the highest power of the operation microscope, thoroughly irrigated, and polished with a moistened cellulose sponge. The implant is then grasped with forceps such as the curved tantalum-tipped titanium forceps manufactured by Metico, and is introduced through the lips of the incision until the haptics reach to the inferior angle (Fig. 8–45B). Careful positioning of the lens in the plane of the iris is then performed, but care is taken to avoid pushing the lens into the inferior angle. Final placement of the lens is accomplished by grasping the sclera just posterior to one of the superior haptics and then "popping" the haptic into position by pressing the anterior surface of the haptic in a posterior direction. This maneuver is repeated with the other haptic, and the superior haptics are then carefully inspected to assure correct positioning of the lens. A blunt instrument such as a vitreous sweeper may then be introduced between the two superior haptics, and an attempt made to rotate the lens within the anterior chamber. A lens of correct size should resist rotation, whereas a lens that is too small will rotate easily. A lens that is too small should be removed by slipping the vitreous sweeper posterior to the superior haptics and displacing each of these forward until they can be grasped in the wound and the lens extracted. Once the correct size lens has been placed, the wound is closed with additional interrupted nonabsorbable sutures.

Manipulation of the haptics of flexible anterior chamber lenses is best performed with the Sinskey hook, by inserting the tip of the instrument into the appropriate positioning holes of the implant (Fig. 8–45C).

Although each of the lenses above may be used after either intracapsular or extracapsular cataract extraction, the posterior chamber lens is specifically designed for use after extracapsular surgery only, particularly phacoemulsification. A lens of great current popularity is designed by Shearing; its round optical portion has embedded in it two springy J-shaped haptics curved in opposite directions, giving the implant an **S** shape. The springs are partially

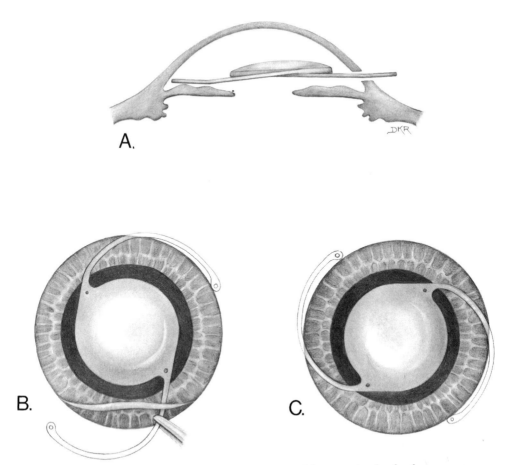

FIGURE 8–45. Insertion technique for Simcoe C-loop anterior chamber lens.

clasped with the insertion forceps and the implant is slipped into place into the "capsular bag" (Fig. 8–46). With the springs released, the lens is fixated into the "ciliary sulcus," where adhesions between the recesses of the capsule are fixated securely into place. This lens may also be fixated in the ciliary sulcus anterior to the capsular bag. The implant so secured may be quite difficult to visualize, even with slit-lamp examination. A variation of this lens designed by Simcoe is preferred by many, including me. That lens implant has broadly curved C-shaped loops designed to distribute pressure over a larger area.[65]

The complications associated with implantation of intraocular lenses include all of the problems attendant to cataract surgery alone. However, in addition, there are certain complications unique to lens implantation, such as dislocation or subluxation of the implant; excessive motion of the implant, resulting in inflammation, hemorrhage, or corneal edema; and the deposition of inflammatory cells and debris on lens surfaces.[2]

Extracapsular cataract surgery carries with it the definite possibility that the posterior capsule will become opaque if left intact. This occurred in between one-third and one-half of patients studied in one series.[80] Other series, though, have had opacification rates as low as 8 or 9 per cent.[58] Although discussion of the posterior capsule is not a difficult procedure, it may be associated with complications, including the vitreous wick syndrome, cystoid macular edema, and retinal tears and detachment.

It has been suggested that secondary cataract is an unavoidable consequence whenever the posterior capsule is intact. A secondary procedure might then be considered inevitable. The introduction of the neodymium:YAG laser for posterior capsulotomy has met this problem with great safety and efficacy (Fig. 8–47).[3, 4]

The management of these complications may include everything from conservative medical

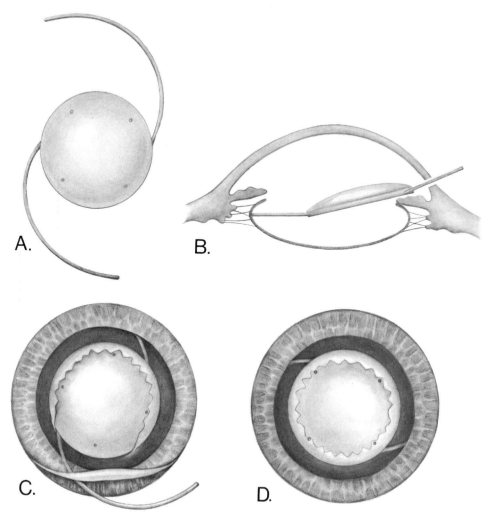

FIGURE 8–46. Simcoe C-loop posterior chamber lens (*A*) with "in the bag" insertion technique (*B–D*).

measures to a repositioning or even removal of the lens implant. The prime indication for removal of the lens implant has become a recurrent hemorrhage and/or inflammation, especially if this can be directly attributed to the presence of the implant. The anterior chamber implants are by far the easiest to remove, since there tend to be a few adhesions between intraocular tissues and the lens implants. Other types of implants might require careful dissection of the implant from the iris and/or vitreous, in addition to the possible necessity of severing (and leaving in place) their haptics. The instrument designed by Scimeca easily permits this last maneuver.

A partially dislocated posterior chamber implant ("sunset" or "sunrise" syndromes) may be "dialed" forward into the anterior chamber by inserting a Sinskey hook through a 1-mm limbal incision after injection of sodium hyaluronate.

Retinal detachment in pseudophakic patients presents a special problem, since the retinal surgeon may find it extremely difficult to obtain adequate visualization of the fundus in appreciation of all possible retinal tears. One recent large series of extracapsular cataract extractions shows a retinal detachment rate of 1.4 per cent.[14] Reports of retinal detachment after phacoemulsification show retinal detachment rates ranging from 1.3 to 3.6 per cent.[32, 81] There is some suggestion that posterior chamber lenses may be associated with an even lower incidence of retinal detachment.[47] In the best hands, the cure rate for pseudophakic retinal detachments has been comparable to that obtained in aphakic detachments. If given the choice, however,

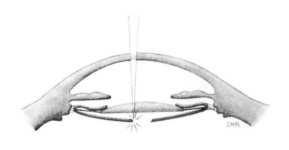

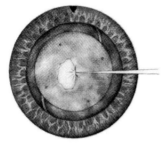

FIGURE 8–47. Neodymium: YAG posterior capsulotomy.

most retinal surgeons would prefer to deal with pseudophakic patients whose implants permit full pupillary dilation, such as anterior or posterior chamber implants.

One of the complications that has received the most attention recently is that of cystoid macular edema. More than half of all patients who undergo intracapsular cataract extraction develop this condition to at least a subclinical degree, as manifested by characteristic changes on fluorescein angiography. Significant reduction of visual acuity occurs in approximately 10 per cent of these cases. In extracapsular techniques it appears that the incidence of clinically significant cystoid macular edema is reduced to only 2 or 3 per cent. Most studies comparing the incidence of cystoid macular edema in intracapsular versus extracapsular techniques show two to four times greater incidence in the former.[36, 37] Usually this condition is self-limited and lasts for only several months, but occasionally permanent macular changes do occur. The incidence of this complication must be weighed against the drop in visual acuity associated with opacification of the posterior lens capsule, which appears to occur at the rate of 20 per cent per year of patients operated on by any extracapsular technique. When lens implantation is superimposed on cataract extraction, the incidence of cystoid macular edema is at least

as great as in intracapsular and extracapsular cataract extraction, respectively, and it may be higher. Lens designs that are associated with broad iris contact and synechia formation, such as iris-fixated lenses of the iris plane or medallion type, are more frequently associated with cystoid macular edema than are anterior chamber lenses. Posterior chamber lenses have the lowest association with this complication of all types. The common denominator in the development of cystoid macular edema appears to be that of persistent uveitis. It appears likely that direct mechanical irritation of the iris by the lens implant, or traction on vitreous strands at their attachments to the pars plana and peripheral retina when the vitreous body has shifted anteriorly at the time of vitreous loss, produces this condition. For some currently inexplicable reason, these chronic inflammatory changes lead to abnormal leakage of the perifoveal capillaries, resulting in cystoid macular edema. Attempts at using various anti-inflammatory preparations, including corticosteroids and indomethacin, have not been definitely effective in treating or preventing this condition. In some patients whose cystoid macular edema is obviously associated with vitreous adhesions to the wound or to the lens implant, pars plana vitrectomy of the adherent strands has produced dramatic improvement of the condition. Unfortunately it may be difficult to visualize the macular when a lens implant is in place.[8]

Recent developments in both medium and high water content soft contact lenses for aphakic patients have added a new dimension to contact lens technology. Although "permanent" contact lenses are still a thing of the future, "extended wear" lenses are currently available and appear to be useful for some patients especially those for whom lens implantation is contraindicated. Their usefulness is still limited by the accumulation of deposits on surfaces and the occasional development of overwear symptoms. Of greatest concern is the development of corneal abscess and ulcer. Also, the long-term expense of contact lenses is significantly greater than that of lens implants. Developments in this field, however, have been rapid in the past several years. The availability of these lenses provides yet another important alternative for the aphakic patient.

Therefore, despite persistent problems and with much room for improvement in design and surgical technique, it would be accurate to consider this the "Age of the Implant." This "Age" will not end unless nearly universally acceptable and permanent wear contact lenses can be developed, or until cataracts themselves can be treated or prevented from forming.

POSTOPERATIVE CARE

Course

Critical evaluation of the operated eye during the immediate postoperative period (several hours to several days after surgery) is extremely important. The appearance of the eye and its inflammatory response are the products of both surgeon and patient. Successful attempts at minimizing operative trauma will generally be evident at this time. One must take into account, however, host factors because there is certainly a variability in the tendency to hemorrhage, the inflammatory response, the susceptibility of the cornea to become edematous, and so on, from one person to the next. Nevertheless, the surgeon, remembering "if the case went well," should be able to determine whether the eye appears as expected.

There is always some degree of lid edema and ptosis, conjunctival hemorrhage and injection, corneal edema and Descemet's folds, "flare and cells" in the anterior chamber, and operative hyphema, even though some of these findings may be quite minimal indeed in ideal cases. Subjectively, many patients are amazed that they have no pain whatsoever, or only mild discomfort. Deep ocular pain in fact is rare, and if present should lead one to suspect the existence of corneal abrasion, corneal edema, elevated intraocular pressure, or intraocular infection. Some of these subjective findings may be partially masked by a patient who has had retrobulbar anesthesia including bupivacaine, which might last as long as 1 or 2 days postoperatively.

The gradual recovery of the eye to a more normal appearance usually is dramatic over the first several days and then proceeds much more slowly over the subsequent weeks after surgery. It has become customary to perform cataract surgery on an outpatient basis, making it necessary for patients to return for office evaluation. One should remember that certain complications, such as significant hemorrhage or intraocular infection, may not develop for several days or longer, and one should not be lulled into complacency.

Steroids and antibiotic preparations are often used routinely in postoperative care, although this need not be the case. For patients with posterior chamber lens implants, pupillary dilation may lead to pupillary capture. Appropriate treatment should be administered to patients with the more intense inflammatory response seen after extracapsular cataract extraction if a large amount of cortical material is retained as well as after vitreous loss and vitrectomy. One should also be aware of the possibility of pupillary block with secondary glaucoma. Medical treatment including carbonic anhydrase inhibitors, timolol, and osmotic therapy should be used if this should occur.

Healing of the cataract wound has come a long way since the days (not really so long ago) when corneoscleral sutures were not commonplace, and patients were put at bedrest with their heads immobilized by sandbags. Now one can rely on a securely sutured wound to bear the brunt of most of the ordinary activities of the patient. Corneoscleral wound healing actually proceeds quite slowly except for the corneal epithelium, which heals within a few days. In fact, there is good evidence that the weakest part of an eye that has undergone cataract extraction remains the site of the old wound, and there have been instances of even minor trauma leading to wound rupture many years after surgery.[34]

Surgeons who use 7-0 or 8-0 nonburied silk sutures generally remove these after 2 or 3 weeks. However, the limbal stromal tissue is still undergoing active healing at this stage, and the eye is definitely vulnerable for several months longer. The strength of the stromal wound develops more rapidly for posteriorly placed incisions than for anteriorly placed incisions, since the sclera heals more quickly than the avascular cornea.

The operated eye may be patched for a day or two after surgery, since most patients find this more comfortable. Otherwise, patients often complain of a scratchy sensation with eye and eyelid movements while the conjunctiva is still inflamed and healing. However, patching has been shown to raise the temperature of the conjunctival cul-de-sacs and increase the bacterial flora, so this should not be unnecessarily prolonged. Patients should be encouraged to discontinue wearing of the patch as soon as they feel comfortable without it. However, with a patch or without, some form of protective shield is advisable during the first week or two after surgery. In the daytime the patient can simply wear his own glasses, or a pair of sunglasses for this purpose. However, when glasses are not being worn, a plastic or metal shield (such as the Fox perforated aluminum shield) should be taped in place to prevent accidental trauma to the eye.

The patient should be encouraged to get "up and around" as soon as possible, even on the day of surgery. Because the patient may be confused and ataxic from the unfamiliar environment, as well as from operative medications, a nurse or relative should be on hand to prevent accidents. Most often patients will prefer to rest and doze in bed during the first day or two, but patients generally appreciate the privilege of going to the bathroom instead of having to use a bedpan. Gradual return to fuller activity, including sitting, standing, or strolls down the hospital corridor, should be encouraged but not forced. Certainly every effort should be made to avoid making an elderly patient bedridden. The popularity of cataract surgery on an outpatient basis has obviated many of these concerns.

Complications

Choroidal Detachment

Detachment of the choroid, often including the pars plana of the ciliary body, may follow a wound leak (Fig. 8–48). The wound leak cannot always be demonstrated, but the shallowing of the anterior chamber that is associated with this condition cannot be explained on the basis of the choroidal detachment serving as a "space-occupying lesion." This complication is quite uncommon now that secure wound closure has become a routine procedure. In those cases in which it occurs, the wound leak usually heals spontaneously, and with it choroidal detachment, hypotony, and shallowing of the anterior chamber disappear. The onset of choroidal detachment usually is a week or two after surgery, and the entire course usually is no longer than 1 to 2 weeks.[34] (See page 376 for further discussion of choroidal detachment.)

Flat Anterior Chamber

Flat anterior chamber is associated with wound leak, but is usually noted earlier in the postoperative course. Again, the intraocular pressure is usually quite low, sometimes immeasurably so. As for choroidal detachment, initial management is conservative, consisting of patching and repeated observation. Carbonic anhydrase inhibitors are believed to be helpful, but their beneficial effect may simply be a function of time. If the anterior chamber reforms spontaneously in a few days, it may not be necessary to do anything further. However, flat anterior chamber associated with hypotony may require exploration and resuturing of the limbal incision. The surgeon may be surprised to find one or two untied sutures. The anterior chamber may be re-formed with an air bubble or sodium hyaluronate at this time, and sclerotomy over the pars plana with the evacuation of 0.5 to 1.0 ml of serous fluid from the suprachoroidal space is a helpful adjunct (Fig. 8–49). A flat anterior chamber is a particularly serious problem in patients with intraocular lens implantation, and re-formation of the anterior chamber should be done without delay in these

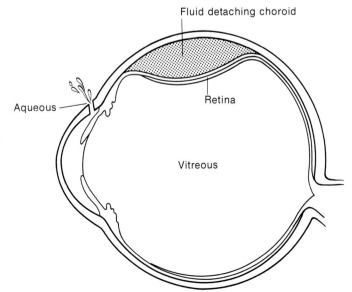

FIGURE 8–48. Aphakia, with shallow anterior chamber and choroidal detachment, associated with leaking corneosclera incision.

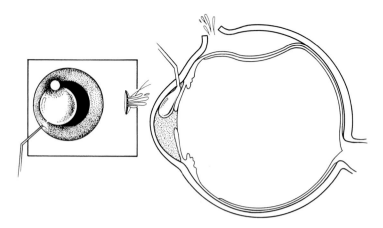

FIGURE 8–49. Surgical correction of shallow anterior chamber with air injection into anterior chamber and posterior sclerotomy for drainage of choroidal detachment.

cases. Ironically, modern techniques for tight wound closure may be associated with high elevation of intraocular pressure in the early postoperative period, which may then lead to wound rupture and flat anterior chamber.[15, 34] (The differential diagnosis and management of flat anterior chamber are discussed further on pp. 337–343.)

Aphakic Pupillary Block

Aphakic pupillary block is another cause of flat anterior chamber in the early postoperative period, but in this case, unlike flat anterior chamber associated with wound leak, intraocular pressure is usually elevated. Commonly the intact anterior hyaloid face of the vitreous plugs the pupillary opening as well as iridectomy openings (Fig. 8–50). Medical management is

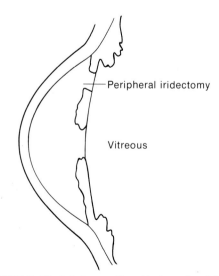

Peripheral iridectomy

Vitreous

FIGURE 8–50. Aphakic pupillary block produced by anterior hyaloid face adherent to posterior iris surface, occluding pupil and peripheral iridectomy.

initiated with carbonic anhydrase inhibitors and osmotic agents. Also, vigorous attempts at dilating the pupil should be made, using atropine and phenylephrine solutions applied repeatedly. If this is not effective, other methods should be considered. Sometimes one can ascertain that the iridectomy has not been made through the full thickness of the iris. In this case it is easy to complete the iridectomy with laser photocoagulation. Otherwise, reoperation is necessary, usually under general anesthesia. A sclerotomy can be made in the pars plana region and aspiration of fluid vitreous attempted followed by injection of air into the anterior chamber. Perhaps the most definitive approach to this condition is by pars plana vitrectomy using an instrument such as the rotoextractor or ocutome.[15, 34] (Pupillary block is discussed in detail beginning on page 248.)

Aphakic Bullous Keratopathy

Aphakic bullous keratopathy is commonly seen to a mild degree in the early postoperative period. Corneal edema is frequently seen adjacent to the limbal incision, but this usually resolves spontaneously. Central corneal edema may be due to preexisting endothelial corneal disease, surgical trauma, and elevated intraocular pressure. Later in the postoperative course vitreous adhesion to the cornea may produce progressively severe corneal edema.

The prevention of trauma to the corneal endothelium has been discussed above. Once this condition has occurred, attention should be directed at medical therapy for elevated intraocular pressure, if this is judged to be its cause. If corneal edema is unassociated with elevated intraocular pressure, one can use topical osmotic therapy with anhydrous glycerin after topical anesthesia has been achieved with proparacaine (Ophthaine). This treatment may be necessary two or three times a day for several days or longer until corneal metabolism begins to function more adequately.[16, 34]

Cystoid Macular Edema

Described earlier in relation to intraocular lens implant, cystoid macular edema remains one of the most frustrating situations of all for both patient and ophthalmologist. Usually the patient's spirits have been lifted by a seemingly good result for several months after surgery when, unexplainably, central visual acuity drops, often to the level of 20/200. Although sometimes this condition is associated with vitreous loss, it occurs frequently enough in uncomplicated cases. Usually the ophthalmologist has little choice other than to advocate patience and forbearance until the macular edema resolves. Blessedly, this is its usual course.[34] For persistent cystoid macular edema, especially when associated with vitreous abnormalities, anterior vitrectomy including lysis of vitreous adhesions may be warranted.[36, 37]

Hemorrhage

Some hemorrhage may remain after the operative procedure, but occasionally new hemorrhage accumulates in the anterior chamber after surgery. It often originates from superficial vessels, although it is somewhat puzzling that such hemorrhage can enter the eye in the presence of tight wound closure. Nevertheless, postoperative hemorrhage usually resolves spontaneously without treatment. If the anterior hyaloid face of the vitreous is broken, blood can become enmeshed in the vitreous body and take longer to clear.[75]

Occasionally choroidal hemorrhage (rarely even as an expulsive hemorrhage) develops during the postoperative period, sometimes several weeks after surgery. It is more likely to occur in elderly patients with arteriosclerosis, especially those patients who have been engaging in Valsalva maneuvers such as straining at stool or coughing. It is not possible to prevent this entirely, but patients should be warned about excessive straining during the early postoperative period.[34]

Endophthalmitis

Inflammation of intraocular tissues can occur after surgical trauma, in response to inadvertent instillation of irritating substances into the eye, and secondary to the introduction of microorganisms at the time of surgery. As stated earlier, prevention is all-important, but once this process has started, it is important to determine whether endophthalmitis is sterile or due to bacterial (or other) microorganisms. The classic findings include severe ocular pain, eyelid swelling, hyperemia, chemosis of the conjunctiva, and hypopyon. It is essential that the surgeon act as early as possible in the course of endophthalmitis (preferably as soon as it is discovered), rather than wait until the full-blown picture has developed. The key to diagnosis is paracentesis with aspiration of both aqueous and vitreous. A smear and Gram stain of the specimen may give a presumptive diagnosis. The limulus lysate test is a rapid method for the detection of gram-negative infection. Definitive microbiological studies, including culture for identification of the organism, should be initiated, but antibiotic therapy must be begun even before all of the data have been assembled. The course of bacterial endophthalmitis often runs over a period of only 1 or 2 days before visual function is destroyed, so prompt action is absolutely essential if anything useful is to be salvaged.[34] (The diagnosis and management of endophthalmitis are fully discussed in Chapter 6.)

Iris Prolapse

Iris prolapse is a manifestation of wound failure. If it occurs early in the postoperative course, the patient should be reoperated on under general anesthesia, the wound explored, and resuturing performed. The late occurrence of iris prolapse does not necessarily require surgical repair, and indeed this may be difficult to perform if attempted.[34]

Epithelial Invasion of the Anterior Chamber

Epithelial invasion of the anterior chamber is another manifestation of inadequate wound closure. Epithelium has a tendency to cover unopposed raw wound surfaces in a few days. Once the epithelium enters the anterior chamber, it may spread as a sheet on the posterior corneal surface, or on the iris or vitreous surface. Also, sometimes the epithelium tends to develop cystic structures filled with mucinous material. These structures have been incorrectly termed "iris cysts," but they should be recognized for what they are: epithelial inclusion cysts (see Fig. 8–51). Once this condition has developed, it tends to be progressive, and fairly radical techniques for eradication of the epithelial tissue are necessary to prevent loss of the eye. The extent of the epithelialization may be outlined by preoperative photocoagu-

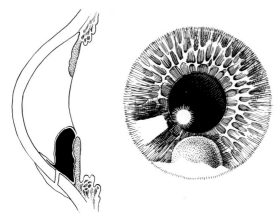

FIGURE 8–51. Epithelial inclusion cyst of the anterior chamber subsequent to wound dehiscence.

lation, and the epithelial tissue may be destroyed by curettage, cauterization with alcohol solution, direct cryotherapy of the epithelial tissue, or *en bloc* excision. As the epithelium proceeds to line the angle of the anterior chamber, intractable glaucoma may develop. In such cases, even when managed by the most experienced surgeon, the prognosis for the recovery of vision is not good.[34]

Retinal Detachment

Retinal detachment after cataract surgery occurs in 1 to 2 per cent of cases in most series that have been reported. Most often the detachment occurs within the first 2 years after surgery, particularly within the first 6 months. Naturally, patients predisposed to retinal detachment, such as those having lattice degeneration, myopia, or retinal detachment in the fellow eye, are at a higher risk than patients without these factors. Vitreous loss is an impor-

tant factor in aphakic retinal detachment, although it is hoped that the development of anterior vitrectomy may affect this favorably. The pathogenesis of retinal detachment in aphakia, particularly in eyes that have suffered vitreous loss, is related to the associated forward shift of the vitreous body. Characteristically, aphakic retinal detachments manifest a series of small retinal breaks at the posterior border of the vitreous base. Adequate visualization of the fundus and localization of the retinal breaks are important considerations. Intraocular lens implants, particularly iris-fixated types, which prevent full dilation of the pupil, may hamper the retinal surgeon's efforts to fully evaluate the fundus abnormalities.[14, 29]

Secondary Membrane ("After-Cataract") Associated with Extracapsular Cataract Surgery

The development of pupillary membranes is a common sequel to extracapsular cataract extraction. Usually this involves opacification of the posterior capsule as a result of persistent lens fibers adherent to the capsule, or metaplasia of the remaining lens fibers. In addition, persistent subcapsular lens epithelium may undergo aberrant attempts at regeneration of lens fibers, producing the "fish egg" appearance of Elschnig's pearls.

For the milder degrees of secondary membrane formation, a small capsulotomy may be performed by cutting open the posterior capsule with a needle knife (Ziegler; Fig. 8–52A). Alternatively, an intentionally barbed 27-gauge disposable needle may be used to engage and then tear a small opening in this membrane (Fig. 8–52B). When the capsulotomy instru-

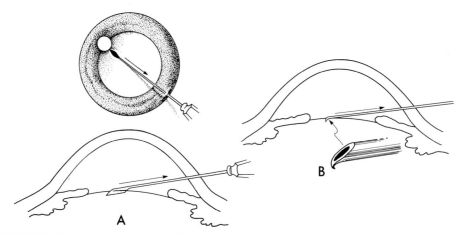

FIGURE 8–52. Posterior sclerotomy performed with (A) Ziegler knife, and (B) barbed disposable needle.

ment is held parallel to the plane of the membrane, it is possible to produce an opening in the posterior capsule without damaging the anterior hyaloid face.[26, 34]

Because of the high incidence of secondary membrane after extracapsular surgery, some surgeons used to elect to do this at the conclusion of the primary procedure. Other surgeons performed capsulotomy at a later time as an office procedure.

Now the YAG laser is widely available for posterior capsulotomy, and although complications such as transient intraocular pressure rise, retinal detachment, and cystoid macular edema have been reported, it has largely supplanted traditional knife surgery of the posterior capsule (Fig. 8–52).[39, 66, 82]

Rehabilitation of Patients

Once the operative procedure has been completed, and the brief hospital stay is over, the patient should be encouraged to return to usual preoperative activities as soon as possible. Usually the patient is seen within several days after discharge from the hospital (or the day after surgery if this was done on an outpatient basis) and then again at weekly intervals for several weeks. Office visits can be spaced further apart to first two weekly intervals and then monthly intervals for the first 6 months. During this time the patient may have to rely on temporary aphakic spectacles if an intraocular implant has not been used, in order to allow normal functioning. Many patients are delighted to find that, so soon after surgery, they see better than they did preoperatively.

The ophthalmic examination at each visit should include a brief refraction with determination of best corrected visual acuity, external examination, a slit-lamp examination, tonometry, and ophthalmoscopy. Medications should be adjusted according to the needs of the individual patient. Often it is possible to discontinue the use of carbonic anhydrase inhibitors after 1 week, and topical solutions including cycloplegics, corticosteroids, and antibiotics after 2 or 3 weeks if healing is progressing satisfactorily.

When a stable refraction has been obtained, and no further improvement in visual function appears to be forthcoming (usually between 6 and 8 weeks postoperatively), final prescription for aphakic spectacles can be given. Several types of aspheric plastic lenses for aphakic patients are available, and these are preferable to the heavier glass spherical lenses that are somewhat less expensive. These should be fitted as close to the eye as possible, and the vertex distance carefully noted for the optician. Usually a round-top bifocal segment is incorporated with an add of +2.75 diopters. Patients who are candidates for contact lenses may also be fitted at this time, although it is sometimes possible to do this even earlier after phacoemulsification or phacofragmentation procedures.[34]

Postoperative care of the cataract patient need take only a few minutes of the ophthalmologist's time for each visit, in the hospital as well as in the office. However, the psychological support that the surgeon can give at this time is crucial to the rehabilitation of the patient. He should be encouraged to use his "new vision" to the fullest extent possible but at the same time urged to be patient until full recovery is achieved. Even when results are not perfect, the rapport developed at this time may be quite useful in helping a patient accept the outcome contentedly.

Because postoperative care for the patient who has had cataract surgery is generally a routine matter, requiring only a short time for each visit, there has been a broad movement to shift the entire event to an outpatient setting, often in a facility near or even part of the surgeon's office. Although there appear to be some important advantages to this trend, including lower cost and reduced apprehension on the part of the patient, serious concerns remain. Surgeons have traditionally functioned best when working under the scrutiny of their colleagues, when mutual criticism and discussion can promote an optimal pattern of patient care. If outpatient surgery for the cataract patient is to work most effectively, it must incorporate a peer review mechanism that will guarantee the patient the same kind of safeguards that are present in our hospitals.

REFERENCES

1. Allen, H. F., Mangiaracine, A. B.: Bacterial endophthalmitis after cataract extraction. Arch. Ophthalmol., 72:454, 1964.
2. Apple, D. J., Mamalis, N., Loftfield, K., et al.: Complications of intraocular lenses. A historical and histopathological review. Surv. Ophthalmol., 29:1, 1984.
3. Aron-Rosa, D., Aron, J. J., Griesemann, M., et al.: Use of the neodymium-YAG laser to open the posterior capsule after lens implant surgery: A prelimi-

nary report. Am. Intraocular Implant Soc., 6:354, 1980.

4. Aron-Rosa, D., Griesemann, J. C., Aron, J. J.: Use of a pulsed neodymium YAG laser (picosecond) to open the posterior lens capsule in traumatic cataract: A preliminary report. Ophthalmic Surg., 12:496, 1981.

5. Asbell, P. A., Chiang, B., Amin, A., Podos, S. M.: Retinal acuity evaluation with the potential acuity meter in glaucoma patients. Ophthalmology, 92:764, 1985.

6. Atkinson, W. S.: Anesthesia in Ophthalmology. 2d ed. Springfield, Ill, Charles C. Thomas, 1965.

7. Barraquer, J.: Surgery of the dislocated lens. Trans. Am. Acad. Opthalmol. Otolaryngol., 76:44, 1972.

8. Binkhorst, C. D.: The iridocapsular (two-loop) lens and the iris-clip (four-loop) lens in pseudophakia. Trans. Am. Acad. Ophthalmol. Otolaryngol., 77:OP589, 1973.

9. Binkhorst, C. D., Kats, A., Leonard, P. A. M.: Extracapsular pseudophakia. Am. J. Ophthalmol., 73:625, 1972.

10. Cairns, L., Sommer, A.: Changing indications for cataract surgery. Trans. Am. Ophthalmol. Soc., 82:166, 1984.

11. Christensen, R. E., Rundle, H. L.: Filtering conjunctival blebs as a complication of cataract extraction. Trans. Pac. Coast Otoophthalmol. Soc., 51:137, 1970.

12. Cleasby, G. W.: Bimanual phacoemulsification. Ophthalmic Surg., 11:348, 1980.

13. Cohen, J. S., Osher, R. H., Weber, P., Faulkner, J. D.: Complications of extracapsular cataract surgery. The indications and risks of peripheral iridectomy. Ophthalmology, 91:826, 1984.

14. Coonan, P., Fung, W. E., Webster, R. G., et al.: The incidence of retinal detachment following extracapsular cataract extraction: A ten-year study. Ophthalmology, 92:1096, 1985.

15. Cotlier, E.: Aphakic flat anterior chamber. I. Incidence among 8,533 cataract extractions. Arch. Ophthalmol., 87:119, 1972. II. Effect of spontaneous reformation and medical therapy. Arch. Ophthalmol., 87:124, 1972. III. Effect of inflation of the anterior chamber and drainage of choroidal detachments. Arch. Ophthalmol., 88:16, 1972. IV. Treatment of pupillary block by iridectomy. Arch. Ophthalmol., 88:22, 1972.

16. Dohlman, C.: Round table discussion. In Symposium on the Cornea. Transactions of the New Orleans Academy of Ophthalmology. St. Louis, C. V. Mosby Co., 1972, p. 257.

17. Dowling, J. L., Jr., Bahr, R. L.: A survey of current cataract surgical techniques. Am. J. Ophthalmol., 99:35, 1985.

18. Duffin, R. M., Pettit, T. H., Straatsma, B. R.: Maintenance of mydriasis with epinephrine during cataract surgery. Ophthalmic Surg., 14:41, 1983.

19. Duke-Elder, W. S., Wybar, K. C. (eds.): Sytem of Ophthalmology, Vol. II: The Anatomy of the Visual System. St. Louis, C. V. Mosby Co., 1961.

20. Duke-Elder, W. S., Jay, B. (eds.): System of Ophthalmology, Vol. XI: Diseases of the Lens and Vitreous: Glaucoma and Hypotony. St. Louis, C. V. Mosby Co., 1969, pp. 324–329, 339–355.

21. Emery, J. M., Paton, D.: Phacoemulsification: A survey of 2,875 cases. Trans. Am. Acad. Ophthalmol. Otolaryngol., 78:OP31, 1974.

22. Faulkner, W.: Laser interferometric prediction of postoperative visual acuity in patients with cataracts. Am. J. Ophthalmol., 95:626, 1983.

23. Fisher, Y. L., Turtz, A. I., Gold, M., et al.: Use of sodium hyaluronate in reformation and reconstruction of the persistent flat anterior chamber in the presence of severe hypotony. Ophthalmic Surg., 13:819, 1982.

24. Goldberg, M. (ed.): Diagnostic and surgical techniques. Surv. Opthalmol., 29:55, 1984.

25. Harms, H., Mackensen, G.: Ocular Surgery Under the Microscope. Chicago, Year Book Medical Publishers, 1967.

26. Havener, W. H., Gloeckner, S. L.: Atlas of Cataract Surgery. St. Louis, C. V. Mosby Co., 1972.

27. Heslin, K. B., Guerriero, P. N.: Clinical retrospective study comparing planned extracapsular cataract extraction and phakoemulsification with and without lens implantation. Ann. Ophthalmol., 16:956, 1984.

28. Hiles, D. A., Wallar, P. H.: Phacoemulsification versus aspiration in infantile cataract surgery. Ophthalmic Surg., 5:13, 1974.

29. Ho, P. C., Tolentino, F. I.: Retinal detachment following extracapsular cataract extraction and posterior chamber intraocular lens implantation. Br. J. Ophthalmol., 69:650, 1985.

30. Hogan, M. J., Alvarado, J. A., Weddell, J. E.: Histology of the Human Eye. Philadelphia, W. B. Saunders Co., 1971.

31. Hurite, F. G.: The contraindications to phacoemulsification and summary of personal experience. Trans. Am. Acad. Ophthalmol. Otolaryngol., 78:OP14, 1974.

32. Hurite, F. G., Sorr, E. M., Everett, W. G.: The incidence of retinal detachment following phacoemulsification. Ophthalmology, 86:2004, 1979.

33. Irvine, A. R., Bresky, R., Crowder, B. M., et al.: Macular edema after cataract extraction. Ann. Ophthalmol., 3:1234, 1971.

34. Jaffe, N. S.: Cataract Surgery and Its Complications. 4th ed. Philadelphia, J. B. Lippincott Co., 1984.

35. Jaffe, N. S.: The lens. Arch. Ophthalmol., 90:136, 1973.

36. Jaffe, N. S., Clayman, H. M., Jaffe, M. S.: Cystoid macular edema after intracapsular and extracapsular cataract extraction with and without an intraocular lens. Ophthalmology, 89:25, 1982.

37. Jampol, L. M., Sanders, D. R., Kraff, M. C.: Prophylaxis and therapy of aphakic cystoid macular edema. Surv. Ophthalmol., 28(Suppl.):535, 1984.

38. Jay, W. M., Carter, H., Williams, B., Green, K.: Effect of applying the Honan intraocular pressure reducer before cataract surgery. Am. J. Ophthalmol., 100:523, 1985.

39. Keates, R. H., Steinert, R. F., Puliafito, C. A., Maxwell, S. K.: Long-term follow-up of Nd:YAG laser posterior capsulotomy. J. Am. Intraocul. Implant Soc., 10:164, 1984.

40. Kelman, C. D.: History of emulsification and aspiration of senile cataracts. Trans. Am. Acad. Ophthalmol. Otolaryngol., 78:OP5, 1974.

41. Kelman, C. D.: Phacoemulsification in the anterior chamber. Ophthalmology, 86:1980, 1979.

42. Kirby, D. B.: Advanced Surgery of Cataract. Philadelphia, J. B. Lippincott Co., 1955.

43. Kolker, A. E., Freeman, M. I., Pettit, T. H.: Prophylactic antibiotics and postoperative endophthalmitis. Am. J. Ophthalmol., 63:434, 1967.

44. Kolker, A. E., Hetherington, J., Jr.: Becker-Shaffer's Diagnosis and Therapy of the Glaucomas. 4th ed. St. Louis, C. V. Mosby Co., 1976.

45. Kraff, M. D., Sanders, D. R., Lieberman, L.: Specular

microscopy in cataract and intraocular lens patients. Arch. Ophthalmol., 98:1782, 1980.

46. Kramer, S. G.: Penetrating keratoplasty combined with extracapsular cataract extraction. Am. J. Ophthalmol., 100:129, 1985.

47. Kratz, R. P.: Complications associated with posterior chamber lenses. Ophthalmology, 86:659, 1979.

48. Kratz, R. P., Colvard, D. M.: Kelman phacoemulsification in the posterior chamber. Ophthalmology, 86:1983, 1979.

49. Layden, W. E.: Pseudophakia and glaucoma. Ophthalmology, 89:875, 1982.

50. Leydhecker, W., Gramer, E., Kriegstein, G. K.: Patient information before cataract surgery. Ophthalmologica, 180:241, 1980.

51. Marmor, M. F.: Transient accommodative paralysis and hyperopia in diabetes. Arch. Ophthalmol., 89:419, 1973.

52. Maumenee, A. E., Stark, W. J.: Management of persistent hypotony after planned or inadvertent cyclodialysis. Am. J. Ophthalmol., 71:320, 1971.

53. Minkowski, J. S., Palese, M., Guyton, D. L.: Potential acuity meter using a minute aerial pinhole aperture. Ophthalmology, 90:1360, 1983.

54. Morgan, L. W., Schwab, I. R.: Informed consent in senile cataract extraction. Arch. Ophthalmol., 104:42, 1986.

55. Nielsen, N. V., Holbjerg, J. C., Westerlund, E.: Absorbable sutures (Dexon and Vicryl) in the corneolimbal incision. Uses in lens implantation surgery. Acta Ophthalmol. (Copenh.), 58:48, 1980.

56. Noble, M., Cheng, H., Jacobs, P., et al.: Long-term follow-up of intraocular lens implants: The first 127 compared with the latest 100 of the same style in a span of 9 years. Br. J. Ophthalmol., 68:373, 1984.

57. Paton, D.: A selection of current cataract incision and wound closure techniques. Highlights Ophthalmol., 13:3, 1970.

58. Pearce, J. L.: Modern simple extracapsular surgery. Trans. Ophthalmol. Soc. U.K., 99:176, 1979.

59. Raju, V. K., Weinstein, G. W.: Open-sky irrigation and aspiration of cataract during triple procedure. Ophthalmic Surg., 13:1004, 1982.

60. Rubin, M. L.: The woman who saw too much. Surv. Ophthalmol., 16:382, 1972.

61. Shearing, S. P.: Posterior chamber lens implantation. Int. Ophthalmol. Clin., 22:135, 1982.

62. Shields, M. B.: Combined cataract extraction and glaucoma surgery. Ophthalmology, 89:231, 1982.

63. Shock, J. P.: Phacofragmentation and irrigation of cataracts. Am. J. Ophthalmol., 74:187, 1972.

64. Simcoe, C. W.: Mechanical and design considerations in lens implantation. Int. Ophthalmol. Clin., 22:203, 1982.

65. Simcoe, C. W.: Simcoe posterior chamber lens: Theory, techniques and results. J. Am. Intraocul Implant Soc., 7:154, 1981.

66. Slomovic, A. R., Parish, R. K. II: Acute elevations of intraocular pressure following Nd:YAG laser posterior capsulotomy. Ophthalmology, 92:973, 1985.

67. Southwick, P. C., Olson, R. J.: Shearing posterior chamber intraocular lenses: Five-year postoperative results. J. Am. Intraocul. Implant Soc., 10:318, 1984.

68. Spaeth, G. L.: The management of cataract in patients with glaucoma: A comparative study. Trans. Ophthalmol. Soc. U.K., 100:195, 1980.

69. Stanley, J. A., Shearing, S. P., Anderson, R. R., et al.: Endothelial cell density after posterior chamber lens implantation. Ophthalmology, 87:381, 1980.

70. Stark, W. J., Maumenee, A. E.: Cataract extraction after successful penetrating keratoplasty. Am. J. Ophthalmol., 75:751, 1973.

71. Sugar, A.: Diagnostic and surgical techniques—clinical specular microscopy. Surv. Ophthalmol., 24:21, 1979.

72. Tennent, J. L.: Results of primary and secondary implants using Choyce Mark VIII lenses. In Weinstein, G. W., Drews, R. C. (eds.): The Surgery of Intraocular Lenses. Thorofare, N.J., Charles B. Slack, 1977.

73. Troutman, R. C., Callahan, A. C., Emery, J. M., et al.: Cataract survey of the cataract-phacoemulsification committee. Trans. Am. Acad. Ophthalmol. Otolaryngol., 79:OP178, 1975.

74. Vrijland, H. R., van Lith, G. H.: The value of preoperative electro-ophthalmological examination before cataract extraction. Doc. Ophthalmol., 55:153, 1983.

75. Watzke, R. C.: Intraocular hemorrhage from vascularization of the cataract incision. Ophthalmology, 87:19, 1980.

76. Weinstein, G. W.: Clinical aspects of the visually evoked potential. Ophthalmic Surg., 9:56, 1978.

77. Weinstein, G. W.: Implantation of the C-loop Simcoe posterior chamber lens. Ophthalmic Surg., 15:25, 1984.

78. Weinstein, G. W.: The buccaneer eye surgeon. Ophthalmic Surg., 11:831, 1980.

79. Weinstein, G. W., Odom, J. V., Hobson, R. R.: Visual acuity and cataract surgery. In Reinecke, R. D. (ed.): Ophthalmology Annual 1987. Norwalk, Conn., Appleton-Century-Crofts, 1987.

80. Wilhelmus, K. R., Emery, J. M.: Posterior capsule opacification following phacoemulsification. Ophthalmic Surg., 11:264, 1980.

81. Wilkinson, C. P.: Retinal detachment following phacoemulsification. Mod. Probl. Ophthalmol., 20:339, 1979.

82. Winslow, R. L., Taylor, B. C.: Retinal complications following YAG laser capsulotomy. Ophthalmology, 92:785, 1985.

83. Worthen, D. M.: Scanning electron microscopy after alpha chymotrypsin perfusion in man. Am. J. Ophthalmol., 73:637, 1972.

9

CORNEAL SURGERY

*by S. Arthur Boruchoff
and Gary N. Foulks*

INSTRUMENTATION

Surgery of the anterior segment of the eye is best performed with magnification and requires specialized instruments and sutures. Although the magnification obtainable with most loupes ($2\times-4\times$) suffices for many surgical procedures, it is not optimal for most anterior segment surgery, which usually requires some type of operating microscope. The operating microscope permits much more accurate assessment of any pathological changes, especially in a traumatized eye. Although at first somewhat cumbersome and limiting to the surgeon's mobility, the microscope, when mastered, allows more precise excision of tissue and control of wound apposition, as well as greater accuracy in suture placement. Most corneal surgeons perform the majority of each surgical procedure using the microscope, although some specific steps (e.g., Flieringa ring attachment, centering of a trephine, insertion of a rectus bridle suture) may be done under loupe magnification.

Suture Material. Suturing of the ocular surface requires special suture material of fine caliber. In general, absorbable sutures may be considered for scleral or conjunctival tissue, but nonabsorbable sutures are used for corneal tissue. Despite the fact that both silk and nylon undergo gradual fragmentation and biodegradation *in situ*, they are here considered "non-

absorbable." As absorbable sutures, polyglycolic (Dexon) or polyglactin (Vicryl) sutures have, for the most part, replaced plain and chromic surgical gut, by virtue of their better tolerance and less variable resorption. Of the nonabsorbable materials, 9-0 virgin silk with swaged needles is easy to handle yet is fine enough to cause little reaction in the ocular tissue. Although more difficult to handle because of its wispy character, 10-0 ($22\text{-}\mu\text{m}$) monofilament nylon is even finer and virtually nonreactive, and becomes regularly buried by surface epithelium. Wound healing is slower with the 10-0 nylon suture, which must be left in place longer than 9-0 silk. Polypropylene (Prolene, $16\text{-}\mu\text{m}$) suture is now commercially available on a swaged needle. Although this material is well tolerated and provokes little reaction, care must be taken not to apply excess suture tension, since its elasticity exceeds that of nylon and taut sutures may migrate in corneal tissue or produce striae at the suture bend. Discomfort, irritation, and vascular ingrowth in corneal tissue are usually due to exposed knots rather than to the suture material per se.

Wounds closed with a running suture or those closed with buried knots take longer to heal than wounds closed with interrupted sutures and exposed knots. Some studies have suggested that wound strength is initially greater with interrupted sutures. In many instances the

176

use of the interrupted suture allows greater control of wound healing by stimulating vessel ingrowth to the wound while allowing selected sequential suture removal without jeopardizing the entire wound apposition.

The choice between an interrupted suture and a running suture depends not only on the status of the host tissue, but also on a thorough knowledge of the different requirements in postoperative management necessitated by the overall status of the eye. For example, the presence of blood vessels in the host, particularly if they vary in density and location, is an indication for interrupted sutures so that sutures may be removed whenever healing is apparent. The running suture leads more rapidly to a quieter eye but is perhaps less secure; loosening of one loop of the suture often permits the inherent elasticity of the suture to allow loops on either side to loosen, thus leading to possible wound disruption.

Needles. The choice of needle is best made according to the depth of desired suture placement. Lamellar or superficial surgery is more easily done using a needle with a flatter curve (e.g., 137-degree, ⅜ curve), whereas penetrating or deeper suture position is achieved using a needle with a steeper curve (e.g., 160-degree, half circle). Modified-curve (J-curve) needles also allow placement of small, deep suture tracks with little tissue distortion.

A wide variety of microsurgical instruments that are both strong and durable is available for facilitating precise surgery without damage to tissue. To assure proper fixation and control of tissue less than a millimeter thick, instrumentation must be well designed and accurately aligned.

WOUND HEALING

The need for thorough knowledge of wound healing in corneal surgery is obvious. Healing of a normally avascular cornea depends on the response of all three layers—epithelium, stroma, and endothelium—and their interaction. Although review of the abundant experimental work on wound healing is beyond the scope of this chapter, several important observations deserve mention.

1. Epithelial response to injury is rapid, occurring within the first hour after insult. The initial sliding phase responsible for resurfacing of the cornea is followed by mitosis of the cellular layer to full thickness. The restoration of normal adhesion of epithelium to stroma depends on formation of an intact basement membrane, and may require weeks.

2. Stromal healing is variable and depends on the state of vascularization of the cornea. Healing is more rapid near the limbus or near areas of stromal vascularization. Polymorphonuclear infiltration occurs by the 5th hour after insult, and stromal healing begins by 96 hours, with transformation of keratocytes to fibroblasts and elaboration of a coarsely fibrillar chondroitin sulfate–rich matrix taking place by the end of the 1st week. Stromal healing is enhanced by an intact epithelial covering; indeed, if the epithelium is consistently absent, the stroma may heal hardly at all. Healing cells are derived from both donor and host tissue in the case of corneal transplant.

3. Endothelial healing occurs mostly by amitotic spreading and metaplasia, but some mitotic activity can occur, especially in the corneas of younger patients. The regenerated endothelium will produce a Descemet's membrane that is initially thinner than normal.

4. As previously mentioned, wound strength is influenced by the type and tension of the suture. Silk sutures are larger and produce more tissue reaction than 10-0 monofilament nylon; hence wound strength is achieved more slowly with nylon sutures. The relatively inelastic silk suture can more easily be adjusted to provide wound apposition without undue wound tension, whereas the more elastic nylon suture, when tightened, may induce greater wound compression, particularly when the continuous technique is used.

5. Topical medications commonly used after corneal surgery also affect wound healing. Corticosteroids, although not inhibitory to epithelial healing, decrease stromal wound strength when used in the 1st postoperative week. Idoxuridine, possibly by competing with thymidine incorporation, can diminish wound healing. The modern nonemulsive ointment medications do not adversely affect epithelial or stromal healing.

6. The clinical evaluation of the degree of wound healing is most critical when the surgeon considers suture removal. The interplay of many factors determines the optimal time for suture removal. Most important is the vascularity of the tissue. The loss of wound edema and contracture of the scar permit the suture to loosen. If a suture has loosened, particularly in the presence of vessel growth into the wound, it should be removed. Loose sutures are disadvantageous, since they may erode epithelium

and provoke inflammation or ulceration. Obviously sutures should not be removed before adequate wound healing, but it is often clinically impossible to assess wound strength by simple inspection. A gray opacity in the wound interface is a reasonably reliable sign of adequate healing and suggests a safe time for suture removal. In general, a nonvascularized corneal wound sutured with interrupted monofilament nylon sutures requires 6 to 8 months for healing adequate to prevent spontaneous wound slippage, while a running suture is best left in place a year or more. Vascularized cornea, on the other hand, often permits suture removal within a few weeks and is usually more resistant to shifting or rupture of the wound. The frequent or long-term use of steroids in the postoperative period prolongs the healing process, and sutures are prudently left in place up to 12 months or more under such circumstances, provided they are not producing unacceptable astigmatism.

OCULAR SURFACE INJURIES

Rational treatment of ocular surface injuries must take into account the time at which the injury occurred and the interval that has elapsed before initiation of treatment. Any emergency measures, medications, or manipulation administered before definitive treatment must be recorded. Knowledge of the patient's tetanus immunization status is important, and appropriate treatment should be instituted to reinforce immunity if needed. The functional and structural status of the eye before injury must be determined as accurately as possible, so that reasonable guidelines may be provided for restoration of function and realistic evaluation of potential rehabilitation.

Objective evaluation of the damage must be obtained and recorded by detailed examination. Protection of the injured eye with a shield, especially if ocular penetration is suspected, is mandatory, and pressure on orbital contents must be avoided. The examination should be as thorough as possible *without exerting force that might aggravate the injury.* If significant associated injury to facial structures has occurred, examination is often best deferred until general anesthesia is obtained. Facial nerve block may be necessary in evaluating some cases in which eyelid spasm could aggravate the injury. Visual acuity must be recorded. Photographic documentation is desirable for the medical record

and for medicolegal verification. Perforating injury to the globe must be considered, particularly if the history suggests access of fragments to the eye or if subconjunctival hemorrhage and edema interfere with examination. The possibility of the presence of an intraocular foreign body must be considered when ocular perforation has (or may have) occurred, and appropriate x-rays, ultrasonic examination, or computerized tomography should be performed to exclude any intraocular foreign body that cannot be visualized. Computerized tomography currently is the best procedure for accurate localization of an intraocular foreign body. Topical anesthetic must be used judiciously, if at all, and ointment medication should be avoided in initial treatment. Topical anesthetics should never be prescribed for or used by a patient. Delayed wound healing or severe toxic keratopathy can occur.

Contusion Injuries

Minor contusion about the eye can cause subconjunctival hemorrhage, for which no specific therapy is needed. Conjunctival and corneal edema may result from contusive trauma, but frequently this also resolves without specific therapy. Severer contusions can result in rupture of the globe, which is discussed in more detail in the following sections.

Abrasive Injuries

Tangential or shear injuries to the ocular surface can produce conjunctival and corneal abrasions. Conjunctival abrasions usually heal rapidly and need only prophylactic antibiotics, with lid patching for comfort as needed. Although most corneal abrasions heal well with firm patching and topical antibiotic, the possibility of traumatic recurrent epithelial erosion needs to be considered and closely followed up, especially in the case of a sweeping injury, such as that caused by paper, fingernail, or tree twig. The patient should be informed of the need for adequate follow-up to rule out superinfection and the possible recurrence of erosion. A topical short-acting cycloplegic is indicated if significant ciliary spasm and patient discomfort persists, or if traumatic iritis is present. Topical corticosteroids should be avoided in the presence of an epithelial defect, since they may predispose to superinfection. Treatment goals that must be observed are to prevent infection, to promote reepithelization, and to relieve pain. Topical anesthetics should never be given or prescribed for the patient to self-administer.

Foreign Bodies—Superficial and Embedded

One of the most common problems encountered in practice is the superficial conjunctival or corneal foreign body. Conjunctival foreign bodies are often located in the cul-de-sac, affixed to the upper tarsal conjunctiva, or embedded in the bulbar conjunctiva. Linear epithelial corneal abrasions vertically oriented are often the sign of an embedded tarsal foreign body, and eversion of the upper lid should be routinely performed in all cases of anterior segment foreign body. Often simple irrigation of the cul-de-sac or traction of the upper lid over the lower lid will release such a foreign body. Forceps will usually effectively remove those foreign bodies not readily irrigated from the eye (Fig. 9–1).

Corneal foreign bodies can be more difficult to remove. The degree of damage often depends on the composition of the foreign body. Metallic foreign bodies often erode superficially and, if ferrous, can deposit a rust ring in the corneal stroma. Vegetable matter often provokes considerable reaction, and may provide a source of superinfection from bacteria or fungi. Topical anesthesia is usually adequate for removal of these foreign bodies. If irrigation is unsuccessful, a cotton-tipped applicator may effect removal. Often, however, the tip of a fine needle, a hockey stick spud, or fine forceps are needed for removal. If there is a significant rust ring,

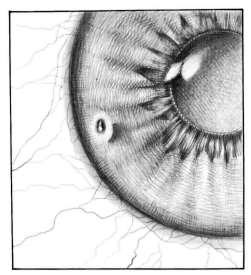

FIGURE 9–2. Corneal foreign body and rust ring.

the dental burr or a commercially available motorized burr can be used to remove it. Often it is easier to remove the residual rust ring after a day or two of patching and antibiotic treatment (Fig. 9–2), by which time the surrounding tissue has softened and can be gently curetted.

After removal of foreign bodies from the ocular surface, topical antibiotics and frequent follow-up are necessary until the ocular integrity has been reestablished.

Penetrating Foreign Bodies

Penetrating foreign bodies of the globe pose unique problems for the surgeon. A high index of suspicion for such injury must be maintained. The entrance wound can be so minor that it may go unnoticed or be obscured by conjunctival edema or hemorrhage. Even if no foreign material is visible in the anterior chamber, the cornea should be meticulously inspected under magnification to check for the presence of a full-thickness corneal wound or shallow anterior chamber that would signal the presence of perforating injury and prompt a search for an intraocular foreign body. Perforation of the iris or a break in the lens capsule alerts the examiner to the probability that a projectile has passed into the posterior segment. An intraocular foreign body in the anterior chamber angle can provoke focal or segmental corneal edema near the adjacent limbus; such foreign bodies usually settle inferiorly. All patients with uniocular corneal edema should be examined carefully with the gonioscope to check for the pres-

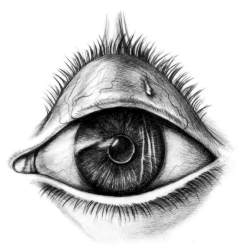

FIGURE 9–1. Corneal abrasions and foreign body under lid.

ence of a foreign body. It should be kept in mind that finding one foreign body does not preclude the possibility of multiple foreign bodies, and a complete search should be made.

The circumstances of the injury are especially important in determining the nature of the foreign body material. Rapid opacification of the anterior segment structures or anterior chamber hemorrhage obligates the surgeon to perform a complete slit-lamp and gonioscopic examination as soon as possible. Indirect ophthalmoscopy should be performed before the media opacify. Anterior segment foreign bodies represent approximately 23 per cent of all foreign body injuries to the eye and are usually visible; ultrasonography, routine orbital radiography, bone-free dental film x-rays of the globe, Sweet's localization, or computerized tomography may be needed if visibility is impaired. If visible, anterior segment foreign bodies are usually readily removed, but the location and magnetizability are important determinants of the method of surgical removal. Often the foreign body can be removed from the initial port of entry at the time of primary repair. A foreign body displaced into the angle or irregular in shape may require removal through a separate corneal incision directly opposite the foreign body or through a limbal incision overlying the foreign body. Metallic foreign bodies such as copper and iron are best removed expeditiously because of the known deleterious effects of those metals on the eye. Multiple fine inert foreign bodies such as plastic or glass embedded in the iris or lens or deep in the cornea may be managed conservatively without surgical excision if they cause no reaction and there are no complicating aspects to the presence of the foreign body. Organic material should be removed because of the greater possibility of bacterial or fungal infection.

The taking of smears and cultures from the affected surface before surgery may speed the detection of potential sources of infection. Antibiotic sensitivities to any culture growth will determine the appropriate antibiotics to be used. Placement of the foreign body in a culture medium followed by prompt incubation and analysis by the bacteriology laboratory is the best method of determining whether any potential infectious agents are present. Blood agar plates at room temperature should be used if fungus is suspected. Postoperatively, appropriate antibiotics are used: broad-spectrum antibiotics systemically and locally if there is not yet a positive culture, or the specific antibiotic if a culture has proved positive.

Corneoscleral Lacerations

Although most corneoscleral lacerations may be repaired by primary closure, donor corneal or scleral tissue should be available for possible use in repair of extensive injuries with tissue loss. Infection after laceration or perforation of the cornea is relatively uncommon, but because it is a disastrous occurrence, the use of prophylactic antibiotics is prudent. A combination of antibiotics providing a broad spectrum should be given at the termination of surgery (for example, methicillin and gentamicin or cephalothin and gentamicin); both subconjunctival injection and topical drops should be used. Ointment medication should not be used before operative repair. Repair of corneoscleral lacerations is best performed under general anesthesia, to avoid pressure on the globe from the manipulation and from the volume of the retrobulbar anesthetic itself. Traumatic induction of anesthesia or excessive manipulation during intubation must be avoided, as well as the spasm induced by depolarizing muscle relaxants. Repair should be performed as soon as possible to avoid wound edema, prolapse of ocular contents, hemorrhage, or late infection. The goals

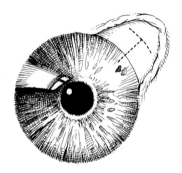 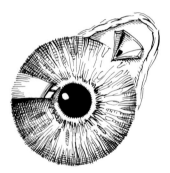

FIGURE 9–3. Removal of foreign body from anterior chamber.

should be accurate wound closure (including removal of all incarcerated tissue from the wound) and complete re-formation of the anterior chamber to prevent synechia formation. While some beveled, self-sealing lacerations may need only protection or reinforcement with a soft contact lens, most wounds require sutures to ensure accurate apposition. The Seidel test (2% fluorescein solution dropped onto the suspected wound site) aids in the diagnosis of a wound leak.

Surgical Technique

After adequate akinesia has been obtained, lid sutures or wire lid retractors are placed. These provide better exposure with less pressure on the globe than a bladed lid speculum. Wound irrigation is then possible. A preplaced knife puncture incision in clear cornea allows access to the anterior chamber for lysis of synechiae, injection of fluid or air, and later re-formation of the anterior chamber (Fig. 9–4). Exploration of the wound should be complete, including incision of the conjunctiva to expose the full extent of any scleral laceration extending from the limbus. Use of direct interrupted sutures is best. Attention must be paid to the position of these sutures, to ensure that they are not placed in the optical axis (Fig. 9–5). Size 10-0 nylon is most appropriate. Irregularities of the wound serve as landmarks for optimal tissue reapproximation. Corneal tissue should not be excised unless replacement by donor tissue is available.

Any incarcerated iris should be swept free, and clean, nonmacerated, prolapsed iris may be

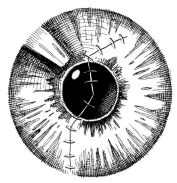

FIGURE 9–5. Wound approximation and suture placement to avoid visual axis.

reposited. If the iris has been prolapsed for more than 12 hours, if it exits through an unclean wound with foreign matter contamination, or if it has become macerated, then it should be excised. Spatulation of the iris through a clear corneal incision, followed by temporary inflation of the anterior chamber with air or a viscoelastic substance, is an effective method of preventing anterior synechiae (Fig. 9–6). Peripheral iridectomy by way of an external incision helps to prevent postoperative pupillary block and should be routinely used in an inflamed or severely damaged eye. Extensive iridodialysis is effectively corrected by incarceration of the posterior dialysis edge in a limbal wound (Fig. 9–7), which is then covered by a flap of conjunctiva.

Prolapsed ciliary body should not be excised unless grossly contaminated or severely traumatized. Transscleral diathermy to minimize

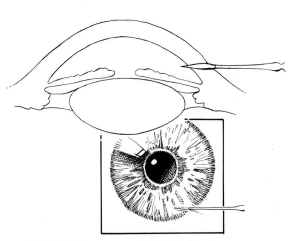

FIGURE 9–4. Anterior chamber knife stab-puncture.

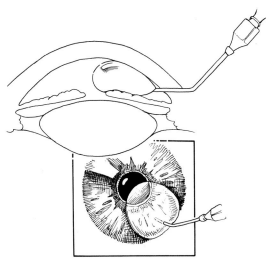

FIGURE 9–6. Inflation of anterior chamber with air to reposit iris.

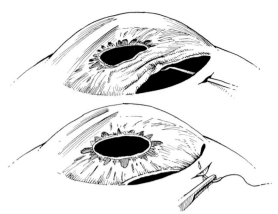

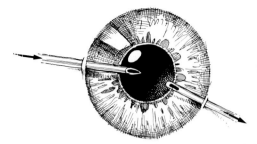

FIGURE 9–8. Infusion cutting and suction instruments in anterior chamber.

FIGURE 9–7. Incarceration of iris to repair iridodialysis.

ciliary body detachment and bleeding should precede excision of damaged ciliary body. If excised, the tissue should be submitted for histopathologic identification.

If the lens suffers a small (e.g., 1 mm) puncture and there is no flocculation of the tissue, it may be left alone. If there is enough flocculation that the chamber is likely to become shallow or tissue is likely to touch the corneal endothelium, primary lensectomy should be considered.

Often in extensive injuries involving the lens there is concurrent prolapse of the vitreous into the anterior chamber. Because fibrosis and contracture of vitreous after trauma are important causes of retinal detachment and subsequent loss of useful vision in the affected eye, an attempt should be made to remove prolapsed vitreous and perform an anterior vitrectomy if necessary through a separate limbal incision. The use of the motorized vitreous cutting and suction instruments either through the wound or through a limbal incision can facilitate the vitrectomy. After adequate closure of any corneoscleral laceration, a scleratome passed through the peripheral cornea at the limbus or beneath a small conjunctival flap allows access of a vitreous suction-cutting tip that can be manipulated to remove vitreous, lens fragments, blood clots, or iris. Although infusion through the instrument tip is often adequate to maintain anterior chamber depth, irrigation through a 27-gauge scalp vein needle placed in a second peripheral corneal site may also be used. A foreign body entrapped in fibrin or iris can be released by the use of Neubauer scissors with subsequent removal by vitrectomy forceps. The corneal wounds can then be secured with an interrupted 10-0 nylon suture. If a significant amount of lens material or debris is present

posterior to the iris, sometimes it is advantageous to enter the eye through a pars plana incision 3.5 mm posterior to the limbus. Such a portal of entry can be closed with an interrupted 7-0 Vicryl or 9-0 nylon suture. It is important to maintain adequate visualization of the vitreous suction-cutting tip at all times, removing vitreous in small bites with as little suction pressure as possible. The wound should be free of vitreous or vitreous strands at the end of the repair.

THE THIN CORNEA

Thinning of the cornea frequently follows episodes of chronic epithelial defect, particularly in patients with prior herpetic infection or in patients with dry eyes, such as those with rheumatoid arthritis. Prevention of perforation can often be achieved by a soft contact lens or tarsorrhaphy. Recalcitrant cases of indolent superficial ulceration may respond to a conjunctival flap. Lamellar keratoplasty or, for impending perforation, penetrating keratoplasty can be advantageous, but these procedures are usually not indicated in an inflamed eye.

THE PERFORATED CORNEA

Perforation of the cornea demands early treatment to restore the integrity of the eye. A small, pinpoint perforation, particularly if some anterior chamber remains formed, can often be managed successfully with simple patching or a soft contact lens. Conjunctival flaps alone usually fail; aqueous may percolate beneath the flap and perpetuate the leak. Lamellar keratoplasty is technically difficult in these situations. Butylcyanoacrylate (Histoacryl), although not yet FDA-approved, has, in our experience,

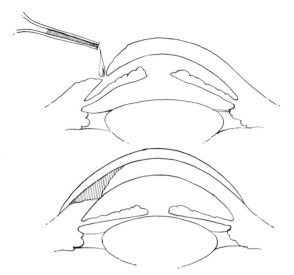

FIGURE 9–9. Corneal gluing. Soft contact lens covers glue.

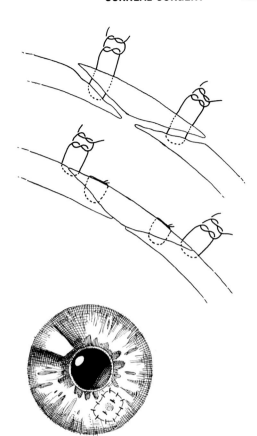

FIGURE 9–10. Patch graft.

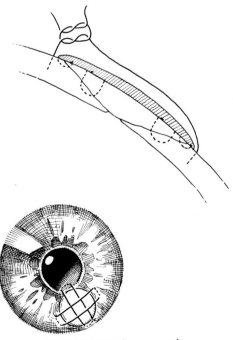

FIGURE 9–11. Blow-out patch.

been very effective in sealing perforations up to 1 mm. After application to an area of cornea free of epithelium or necrotic stroma, the fluid glue polymerizes and usually adheres well. Removal of necrotic tissue and epithelium can be by direct scraping or iodine cautery. A soft contact lens is applied after the glue has polymerized, to increase patient comfort and decrease the tendency toward mechanical dislodgment of the glue by the lid (Fig. 9–9). Corneal stroma regrows beneath the glue, which often sloughs spontaneously. If not, the glue can be removed after several weeks or months. Larger areas of necrotic stroma can be treated by a glued-on hard contact lens that acts as a splint as well as a barrier to future ulceration.

Perforations that have a relatively healthy margin of cornea remaining can be effectively sealed with a corneal "blow-out patch" (Figs. 9–10, 9–11). A thin lamellar button of fresh, frozen, or lyophilized donor corneal tissue is shaped to fit the greatest dimension of the perforation. A diamond or sapphire knife is useful to dissect a discrete wound edge in a soft eye. Sutures are placed through the base of the ulcer and brought through the donor to approximate the two tissues. The edges are shaped to fit the defect and then apposed with 9-0 or 10-0 silk or nylon. This technique closely approximates the patch graft with the patient's own tissue and usually prevents accumulation of aqueous between the patch and the base of the ulcer. It also minimizes swelling of the patch, which often occurs after this procedure. An alternate method of reinforcement is to introduce overlying mattress sutures of 7-0 silk, which secures a silicone disc that has been placed over the patch. After 2 weeks the silicone disc and 7-0 silk sutures can be removed.

If a perforated cornea is not infected or actively inflamed, penetrating keratoplasty can be effective treatment. A partially penetrating trephine mark delimits the keratoplasty site. A needle-knife incision through the partial penetration permits entrance into the anterior chamber, and the excision is completed with corneal scissors. A donor button 0.5 mm larger than the host is often used. Meticulous attention to prevention of synechiae by iridectomy and reformation of the anterior chamber is necessary. In case of inflammation, intraoperative intravenous steroids and postoperative topical steroids will usually control the inflammatory reaction. Steroids should be tapered as rapidly as possible, since cataracts secondary to steroids occur in a significant number of patients. The primary purpose of the initial treatment of the perforated cornea is to restore the ocular integrity. Visual impairment from corneal scarring and opacification may be treated subsequently when the globe is re-formed and quiet. In any case, the method of repair should be fashioned so that there is minimal disruption of the visual axis.

CONJUNCTIVAL FLAP

Greater success in the use of soft contact lenses and keratoplasty has decreased the frequency of conjunctival flap surgery, but the technique remains a valuable procedure when proper indications are observed. Patients with chronic, noninfected, indolent corneal ulcers that have failed to respond to the usual medical measures are candidates for the conjunctival flap procedure. The flap provides a vascular supply and a protective barrier for nonhealing ulcers. A conjunctival flap is not indicated for perforated or leaking wounds. Indeed, perforation of an ulcer beneath a flap is a possible complication of the procedure. Some surgeons recommend a flap for treatment of chronic fungal ulcers that are nonresponsive to antifungal medication; however, persistence of viable fungus beneath the conjunctival flap has been noted. For bullous keratopathy, flaps have been replaced for the most part by soft contact lenses to relieve pain or by penetrating keratoplasty to restore vision.

The disadvantages of the conjunctival flap are

decreased visibility of the anterior chamber, compromise of conjunctival mobility, and impaired ability to assess the intraocular pressure accurately. Topical drug penetration is also retarded.

The purse-string type of conjunctival flap tends to retract more readily and is thus less effective than the thin hood flap of Gundersen and the partial (vertical bridge) flap. The success of a conjunctival flap hinges on complete removal of corneal epithelium and necrotic corneal tissue and the dissection of a flap that is loose and free of adherence to underlying tissue. The flap should consist of conjunctiva alone and should not incorporate Tenon's capsule; it should not have perforations or be under traction from the lateral margins.

Anesthesia may be general, or a combined facial block and retrobulbar anesthetic may be used. A traction suture placed in clear cornea just inside the superior limbus allows downward rotation of the globe during flap dissection. The superior bulbar conjunctiva is ballooned with 2 ml of lidocaine and epinephrine introduced from the lateral margin of the flap to avoid perforation (Fig. 9–12). A 3-cm superior horizontal incision is made, with care taken to ensure that only conjunctiva and not Tenon's capsule is incised. The conjunctiva is dissected from Tenon's capsule with scissors (Fig. 9–12A). The flap is undermined to the limbus, where the inferior marginal incision is made (Fig. 9–12B). Then a 360-degree peritomy is completed (Fig. 9–12C), and the flap is undermined to relieve all tension and traction. Corneal epithelium and necrotic stoma are debrided by scraping with a rounded blade (e.g., Bard-Parker #15, Beaver #64). Topical 10% cocaine softens the epithelium to facilitate removal. The conjunctival edges are sutured (Fig. 9–12D and E) after the flap has been positioned over the debrided and de-epithelialized corneal stroma. Interrupted fine silk horizontal sutures placed just inside both the superior and inferior wound margins help to relieve traction on the flap, while the conjunctival edges are secured to Tenon's capsule superiorly and to conjunctiva inferiorly. Perforation of the flap is the most common operative complication, and care should be taken to avoid it. If it does occur, the perforation sites should be closed with fine nonabsorbable suture material.

Postoperative complications include retraction of the flap, fluid accumulation beneath the flap, cyst formation, and perforation of the cornea beneath the flap. Ptosis has also been reported, but is usually not a problem. The flap

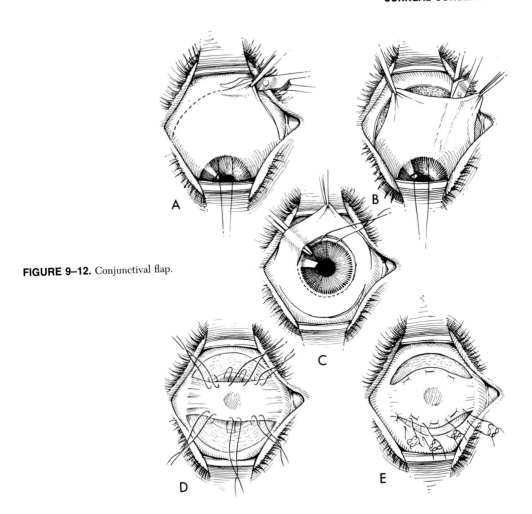

FIGURE 9–12. Conjunctival flap.

may be taken down after a year or when the underlying process has stabilized. Removal of the flap may be done in conjunction with a penetrating keratoplasty. In some instances, penetrating keratoplasty can be performed through the flap.

PTERYGIUM

A pterygium is a growth of fibrovascular tissue that extends from the conjunctiva onto the cornea. Pterygia occur much more frequently in people living near the equator, the incidence decreasing with increasing latitude; thus it is highly unusual to find them in people living above or below 40 degrees of latitude. The fact that they occur much more frequently in people exposed to sunlight and wind (fishermen and farmers, for example) also suggests that environmental factors such as ultraviolet exposure play a major role.

True pterygium occurs in the interpalpebral zone, particularly on the medial aspect of the globe. A pseudopterygium may have a similar appearance, but usually follows trauma or corneal ulcerations. A probe cannot be passed under the body of a true pterygium, but can be passed under the body of a pseudopterygium.

All ptyergia need not be removed. The major indications for removal of a pterygium are a significantly inflamed eye that does not respond to topical medication; relentless progression and documented growth of the pterygium so that it is reasonable to expect that it might approach the visual axis; keratometric documentation of change in corneal astigmatism associated with progressive growth of the pterygium; or physical appearance of the eye that the patient considers intolerable. In general, a conservative approach should be taken to the removal of pterygia, since the surgery is not without potential serious complications. The recurrence rate of pterygia is significant irrespective of the mode of excision, and recurrences are frequently far more exuberant in their regrowth than the original pterygium.

The goals of pterygium surgery are to remove the fibrovascular tissue, to restore the normal anatomical configuration at the limbus, and to prevent recurrences. The fact that there are so many proposed techniques for pterygium removal attests to the lack of uniformity of excellent results with any one technique.

Adequate anesthesia may be achieved by topical 10% cocaine, subconjunctival injection of lidocaine, or retrobulbar injection of lidocaine or a similar anesthetic. After insertion of a speculum the head of the pterygium is outlined by superficial dissection just beyond the farthest extension onto the cornea (Fig. 9–13). The head may then be dissected from the cornea and undermined toward the sclera by superficial stripping or from sclera to cornea (Fig. 9–14). Alternatively, an incision may be made above or below the body of the pterygium, a 4-0 silk suture may be passed under the body of the pterygium, and with a sawing motion of the thread the pterygium may be stripped from the cornea as the thread is pulled medially. The corneoscleral limbus should be left as smooth as possible, and, if rough, can be smoothed

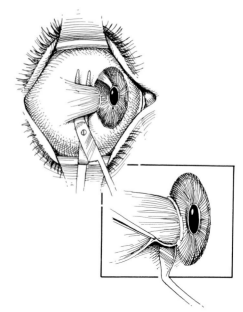

FIGURE 9–14. Pterygium. Dissection from body to head.

with a curved dissecting blade (e.g., Beaver #64 or Bard-Parker #15). The dissection itself should be as superficial as is consistent with removing the bulk of the adventitious tissue. In recurrent or large and fleshy ptyergia there is frequently a marked extension of the fibrovascular tissue under the conjunctiva that may extend to the insertion of the rectus muscles or even as far as the fornices. All this tissue must be carefully dissected or the rate of recurrence will be increased.

Some surgeons prefer to excise the undermined tissue totally. Others choose to transplant the pterygium into a tunnel directed either superiorly or inferiorly under the conjunctiva. A 4-0 silk suture passed through the head of the pterygium and then through the conjunctiva will secure the tissue until the suture is removed about 10 days later. The sclera may be left bare. Alternatively, the normal conjunctiva may be undermined, pulled together, and sutured over the raw surface. Careful dissection under the microscope, cautery of bleeding points, and making the dissected surface as smooth as possible are probably helpful in avoiding postoperative complications. Particular care must be exercised to avoid injury to the rectus muscles.

Various techniques have been advocated to reduce the incidence of recurrences. Some surgeons use topical steroids (e.g., hydrocortisone ointment every 3 hours for several weeks). Beta-radiation is recommended by some surgeons for

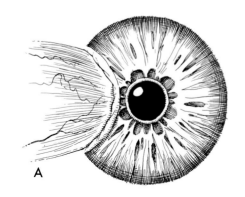

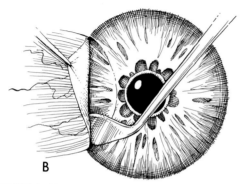

FIGURE 9–13. Pterygium. Superficial outlining and dissection of head toward sclera.

recurrent pterygia; other surgeons use beta-radiation routinely for all ptyergia. It is usually administered by use of a strontium-90 applicator. A radiotherapist should advise the correct dosage, and an ophthalmologist should apply the applicator immediately after excision of the pterygium. Thiotepa (1:2000) every 3 hours for 6 weeks postoperatively has also been advocated, but allergy to this drug and depigmentation of the skin surrounding the eye are potential complications of this method of treatment.

Despite the attention to technique and postoperative care, recurrences remain a significant problem. All patients should be cautioned before removal of a pterygium that there may be a recurrence, and that this may be worse than the initial lesion. Severe recurrences may require not only excision, but also lamellar keratoplasty; in these circumstances the results may be disappointing. Postoperative dellen formation may also predispose to recurrence; the best way to avoid this is to keep the transition zone from cornea to sclera as smooth as possible after the initial dissection. Recurrences may be so advanced as to extend onto the area of the rectus muscles, causing limitation of motion of the globe. Unfortunately surgery at this advanced stage of recurrent pterygium has disappointing results.

Fine recommends the use of buccal mucous membrane grafts for recurrent pterygium. All vascular conjunctival and subconjunctival tissue is removed over the nasal side. The mucous membrane graft is very thin, 0.2 mm, taken with a Castroviejo keratotome. The sclera must be clean and hemostasis complete. The graft is sutured to the sclera with slight tension to avoid wrinkling, using 8 or 10 mattress sutures of 7-0 silk; it is sutured to the cut edge of the conjunctiva with interrupted sutures. A corneoscleral contact lens (with the corneal portion cut out) is then placed as a conformer and left in place for 5 to 7 days. A free graft of conjunctiva from an uninvolved area of the patient's eye may be used in a similar manner.

KERATOPLASTY

The word keratoplasty is by common usage interchangeable with corneal transplantation. Lamellar keratoplasty refers to the replacement of a partial-thickness area of the cornea, whereas penetrating keratoplasty refers to the full-thickness replacement of corneal tissue. A total keratoplasty implies replacement of the entire area (limbus to limbus) of the cornea, whereas partial keratoplasty implies a less than total replacement of the corneal area. In practice, keratoplasty is seldom total in extent. In recent years, with the advent of finer suture materials, better knowledge of the physiology, and an increasingly good prognosis, most corneal transplants currently performed are penetrating, and lamellar keratoplasties are used relatively infrequently.

Donor Material

Table 9–1 outlines the criteria for donor material accepted in 1986 by the Eye Bank Association of America. These standards are intended to provide guidelines based on what is generally accepted and will undoubtedly be modified periodically as our technical knowledge increases.

LAMELLAR KERATOPLASTY

Although this technique is relatively infrequently performed, it is useful for treating localized irregularities of the corneal surface. It may also be used for superficial stromal opacities, which can be removed and replaced by a partial-thickness corneal graft. Obviously the cause of the condition must be something other than endothelial dysfunction; otherwise, recurrence of disease is certain. Among the clinical indications for lamellar keratoplasty, therefore, are superficial ulcers, anterior stromal dystrophies, posttraumatic or postinfectious surface irregularities, or stromal scarring that does not extend to the posterior limiting layers of the cornea. In general, the visual results with lamellar keratoplasty are less gratifying than those with penetrating keratoplasty, but serious complications are less frequent with lamellar as compared with penetrating keratoplasty.

Surgical Technique

After induction of anesthesia and routine preparation and draping of the patient, the first step is the preparation of the host bed. Because the original size and depth of the bed may be modified as the surgery proceeds, it is wise to prepare the bed fully so that an appropriate donor can be selected.

TABLE 9–1. Criteria for Donor Material for Corneal Transplants*

I. *Screening of tissue must be conducted for the following:*
  A. Penetrating keratoplasty
    The basis for rejection of donor corneal material is divided into two categories.
    1. Tissue that must represent a *health-threatening* condition for the recipient or be contraindicated because of endothelial dysfunction and that should not be offered for surgical purposes:
      (a) Cause of death unknown
      (b) Death caused by central nervous system diseases of unknown etiology
      (c) Creutzfeldt-Jakob disease
      (d) Subacute sclerosing panencephalitis
      (e) Congenital rubella
      (f) Progressive multifocal leukoencephalopathy
      (g) Reye's syndrome
      (h) Subacute encephalitis, cytomegalovirus brain infection
      (i) Septicemia   (j) Hepatitis   (k) Rabies
      (l) Intrinsic eye disease—retinoblastoma, conjunctivitis, iritis, glaucoma, corneal disease (e.g., keratoconus or pterygium), and malignant tumors of the anterior segment
      (m) Blast-form leukemia
      (n) Hodgkin's disease
      (o) Lymphosarcoma
      (p) Acquired immunodeficiency syndrome (AIDS)
      (q) High risk for AIDS groups, including known or suspected intravenous drug abusers, known or suspected male homosexuals or bisexuals, prostitutes, hemophiliacs, infants of mothers with AIDS, sexual contacts of high-risk groups
      (r) Human immunodeficiency virus (HIV)– seropositive donors
    2. Tissue that may require caution with regard to utilization:
      (a) Multiple sclerosis
      (b) Parkinson's disease
      (c) Amyotrophic lateral sclerosis
      (d) Jaundice (rule out hepatitis)
      (e) Chronic lymphocytic leukemia
      (f) Diabetes
      (g) Surgically induced eye abnormality (e.g., aphakia)
      (h) Syphilis
  B. Lamellar or patch grafts
    Criteria are the same as listed for penetrating keratoplasty except local eye disease that affects corneal endothelium (e.g., aphakia, iritis) is acceptable for use.
II. *Age of donor*
  The lower limit is full-term birth. There is no absolute upper limit.† It is recognized, however, that endothelial abnormalities and decreased cell density increase with age. The interval between donor death and enucleation should be as short as possible.† Cooling the body and/or placing ice packs over the closed lids is helpful. However, it is generally recommended that enucleation occur within 6 hours of death.
III. *Corneal retrieval procedures*
  The enucleation should be performed by sterile technique, after which the globe should be irrigated with sterile solution and placed in a sterile glass container, which is then put into a shipping container. The contents should be kept cool, but must not be frozen.

As soon as possible after arrival at the eye bank laboratory, the whole eye should be vigorously irrigated with sterile saline solution and immersed or irrigated with broad-spectrum antibiotics. The eyes should then be stored at 4° C until further evaluated.
The Eye Bank should report the following information to the surgeon:
  A. Gross appearance (e.g., presence of gross scars) of the eye, jaundice, etc.
  B. Microscopic appearance of the eye, including:
    1. State of the epithelium
    2. Gross thickness of the stroma
    3. Presence of folds in deep layers
    4. Presence of guttata (if possible)
    5. Evidence of ocular surgery, injury, or inflammation
IV. *Methods of preservation of donor material*
  A. The whole eye is placed in a closed, sterile, moist chamber, cooled at 4° C.
  B. The cornea with a rim of sclera is excised, using sterile technique, and placed into a sterile solution consisting of tissue culture medium (TC 199), dextran, and antibiotics (M-K [McCarey-Kaufman] technique).
  C. Cryopreserved tissue is still available in some eye banks.
  D. Organ-cultured tissue is available in only a few centers and is not generally available to the surgeon.
  E. Tissue stored in glycerin or frozen at −80° C is useful for lamellar grafts and, rarely, as an emergency patch-graft for a perforation.
V. *Time interval between death and surgery*
  A. Whole or refrigerated eyes may be used up to 48 hours after the death of the donor. Surgery is advisable as soon as possible.
  B. Tissue preserved by the M-K technique may be used up to 4 days after the death of the donor.
  C. Cryopreserved tissue may be used up to at least 1 year after the death of the donor.
VI. *Responsibility of surgeon and eye bank*
  The decision to accept a given donor rests with the operating surgeon. The eye bank's responsibility lies in furnishing as full and accurate data as possible to the surgeon, including:
  A. Age of donor   E. Time of enucleation
  B. Cause of death   F. Method of preservation
  C. Associated diseases   G. Results of examination
  D. Time of death   in eye bank
VII. *Miscellaneous*
  A. Culturing of eye bank donor eyes should be performed despite the recognition that bacteriological contamination of donor eyes does not necessarily lead to infection. Cultures may be performed either presurgically or at the time of surgery.
  B. All member eye banks must have operational an HIV screening program for all donors of surgically designated tissue. Any seropositive test must be retested in duplicate (for a total of three tests). Any repeatedly positive test should be further confirmed by a Western blot test.
  C. Emergency situations may arise in which it is necessary to use donor tissue that does not meet all the criteria. In such cases the urgency of the situation must be balanced against the overall quality of the donor.

*The decision to use a given donor resides with the surgeon.
†Left to discretion of medical director of the local eye bank.
Adapted from the criteria of the Eye Bank Association of America, revision of 6/28/86.

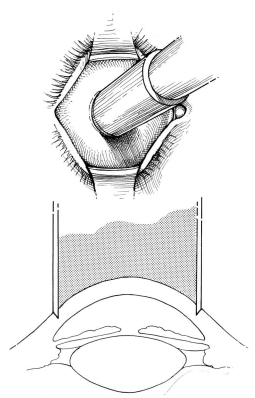

FIGURE 9–15. Trephine host.

A trephine is selected that is adequate in diameter to encompass most of the pathology, and the deepness guard is set at approximately 0.5 mm. The trephine is then applied to the host tissue concentric with the limbus, pressed uniformly against the host eye, and rotated so that a uniformly deep partial penetration of the stroma is made (Fig. 9–15). The dissection of the host pathologic button is then initiated at the depth of the penetration, the host bed is dissected with a Paufique knife or Desmarres scarifier, and the pathological button is removed

(Fig. 9–16). If the depth should prove inadequate, it can be increased by a reapplication of the trephine set at a lesser depth. The bed ultimately should be dissected smooth and as free as possible from scar or vascular tissue. After removal of the button, undermining of the peripheral host cornea for about 0.5 mm toward the limbus permits better suture apposition.

The donor button may be prepared in a variety of ways. Perhaps the easiest is to perform a partial-thickness cutdown at the limbus (Fig. 9–17) with a sharp Bard-Parker knife blade to the appropriate depth and, after establishing the correct plane of dissection, using a blunt double-ended Martinez dissector to sweep at the desired level all the way to the limbus, effectively separating the donor cornea into two layers attached at the limbus (Fig. 9–18). The trephine previously used for the host is then set deep and pressed against the donor button (Fig. 9–19). Many surgeons use a donor button 0.25 mm larger than the host bed. This encompasses the entire thickness of the donor, which can then be released from the trephine blade. The button is then placed into the host bed and sutured in place (Fig. 9–20); either interrupted fine sutures (usually 16 to 20) or a running nylon suture may be used. The sutures should anchor the button well and are left in place for 2 to 4 weeks, depending on the adequacy of wound healing (see section on wound healing).

Alternate methods of taking the donor button are a free hand dissection with a Desmarres scarifier or removal by an electrokeratome. In any case, the smoother the dissection, the less likely the occurrence of fibrovascular tissue at the junction of host and donor, which, particularly if accompanied by blood vessels, diminishes the visual prognosis.

Postoperatively, antibiotics are administered

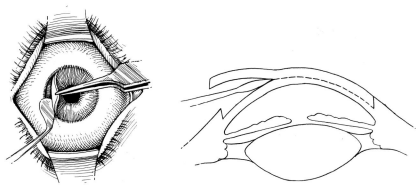

FIGURE 9–16. Dissection of host bed.

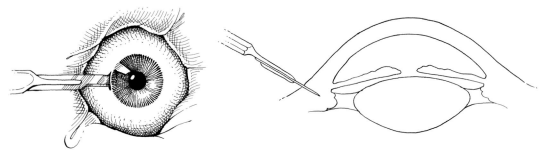

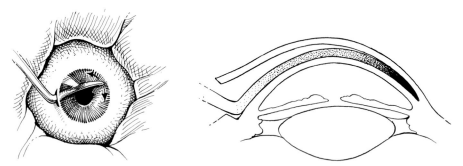

FIGURE 9–17. Donor limbal cutdown.

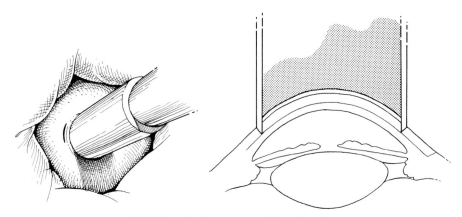

FIGURE 9–18. Dissection of donor lamella.

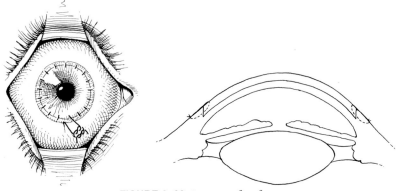

FIGURE 9–19. Trephination of donor lamella.

FIGURE 9–20. Suturing of graft.

topically, as long as sutures remain in place. Steroids are also used topically, the dose depending on the degree of vascularization and inflammation. Surgical judgment determines the amount of steroid to be used. The surgeon must balance the necessity to control inflammation against the potential side effects of the drug. Steroids may interfere with stromal wound healing, potentiate infection, and cause postoperative glaucoma or cataracts.

Operative and postoperative complications are generally caused by mishaps during surgery—such as irregular cutting of the donor or host bed, or inadvertent penetration of the anterior chamber—or by postoperative infection. The major complication is inadvertent penetration into the anterior chamber during dissection of the host bed; this may be repaired primarily or it may be necessary to convert a lamellar keratoplasty into a penetrating keratoplasty. The risk of this complication is all the more reason to withhold dissection of the donor button until the host bed is adequately prepared.

PENETRATING KERATOPLASTY

Penetrating keratoplasty has been more frequently performed and has had an increasingly good prognosis in recent years. A better understanding of the prognostic determinants, improved instrumentation, and more rational use of corticosteroids and antibiotics have all added to the improved prognosis. The spectrum of diseases for which penetrating keratoplasty now offers hope and even cure has expanded as knowledge of the basic pathophysiology has increased.

The prognosis for an avascular corneal disease process with a surrounding normal conjunctiva free of active inflammation in an otherwise uncompromised globe is now considered to be good to excellent. Among these disease categories are the corneal dystrophies, localized inactive corneal scars, keratoconus, and endothelial diseases with corneal edema.

There are, however, factors that limit the prognosis. Perhaps the gravest of these is diffuse and deep stromal vascularization. Sooner or later, most grafts implanted into a densely vascularized bed will succumb to graft rejection. Localized vascularization, particularly if relatively superficial, does permit a reasonably good prognosis if steroids are judiciously used in the postoperative period. Active inflammatory disease that cannot be completely excised, such as viral keratitis, keratouveitis, or bacterial ulceration, may also significantly limit the prognosis of a graft. If possible, disease processes should be inactive at the time of actual surgery. Disease processes that seriously interfere with tear function (e.g., postinflammatory conjunctival scarring, scarring after chemical burns of the anterior segment, pemphigoid, and the dry eye syndromes) all significantly limit the prognosis for penetrating keratoplasty. Likewise, lid abnormalities such as lid notching, malpositions, and incomplete lid closure may also interfere with adequate tear function after surgery, and thereby adversely affect the chances for complete recovery. Although preoperative glaucoma should be controlled medically or surgically before keratoplasty, the opposite condition, hypotony, probably carries an even worse prognosis. Although other abnormalities of the anterior segment, such as synechiae, absence of the iris, rubeosis, vitreous abnormalities, and the necessity for extensive repair of the anterior segment at the time of keratoplasty, limit the prognosis to some extent, they are not absolute contraindications, and increasingly keratoplasty may be successfully combined with significant reconstruction of other anterior segment abnormalities.

Penetrating keratoplasty is carried out for either tectonic or visual reasons. Tectonic keratoplasty is carried out to remove a disease process that alters the structure of the cornea (e.g., ulcerations, perforations, irregularities in thickness) or disease processes that do not yield to medical therapy, such as active infections. The other main purpose for keratoplasty is the removal of a corneal disease that interferes with vision. There are four major factors that prevent the cornea from acting as a clear optical medium:

1. Irregular surface contour (e.g., in keratoconus)
2. An irregular corneal surface (e.g., corneal edema from endothelial dystrophy)
3. Increased stromal thickness (e.g., corneal edema greater than 150 per cent of normal)
4. Opacities of the cornea (e.g., postinflammatory scarring)

In general, all disease processes that cause corneal blindness fall into one of these four pathophysiological categories. Surgeons tend to overestimate the degree to which stromal scarring interferes with vision and underestimate the extent to which corneal epithelial irregularity or edema interferes with vision. For this reason, all patients should undergo a careful contact lens refraction before keratoplasty.

Preoperative Preparation

Because penetrating keratoplasty is frequently performed on an emergent basis, it is important that the patient have had a thorough ocular evaluation and documentation as well as medical and anesthesia evaluation and clearance before the actual admission to the hospital. If there was active inflammation or uncontrolled intraocular tension, these should preferably be controlled before the time of the keratoplasty.

Frequent instillation of topical steroids should be undertaken in an inflamed eye, preferably for 12 to 24 hours just before the surgery itself. Although local anesthesia may be used, general anesthesia is frequently used, particularly in patients who are also undergoing vitrectomy or concurrent cataract extraction. In these latter cases, in addition to the use of general anesthesia, intravenous mannitol and the use of a ring for scleral support are helpful.

The size of the graft can be determined either preoperatively or at the time of surgery by actual application of trephines of various sizes to the eye. It must be emphasized that it is not necessary that all the diseased cornea be removed, the exception being that in cases of active inflammation or infection every attempt should be made to remove all of the diseased tissue. In general, grafts should be centrally placed and eccentric grafts should be avoided if at all possible. Most penetrating grafts vary in size from 6.5 to 8.5 mm, the larger grafts being recommended in cases of diseased endothelium. Grafts smaller than 6.5 mm may prove to be optically deficient, particularly if the graft is somewhat eccentrically placed. On the other hand, grafts larger than 8.5 mm have an increased tendency to cause anterior synechia formation and glaucoma.

Surgical Technique

After the trephine size has been chosen, but before excision of the host cornea, the donor button should be prepared. If the donor has been prepared by the excision of a cornea with scleral rim and placed in M-K (McCarey-Kaufman) medium, the cornea with the scleral rim is removed under sterile technique from the bottle in which it has been transported to the operating room, placed into a Teflon block, and

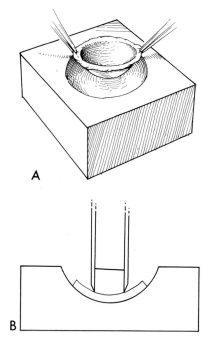

FIGURE 9–21. Punching of graft from behind. *A*, Teflon block. *B*, Trephine punch.

the button punched from behind, using a disposable trephine (Fig. 9–21). The trephine used for the donor button is often 0.5 mm larger than the host trephine. It is applied to the endothelial surface, and uniform pressure is applied against the donor tissue until the entire button has been cleanly punched through. The donor is then held in a double-pronged forceps, and a single suture of 9-0 or 10-0 silk or nylon is placed through the cut edge of the button. The donor button can then be set aside in M-K medium until used.

If, on the other hand, a whole eye is used for the donor, the button can be trephined from the anterior surface by use of a trephine either the same size as or 0.5 mm larger than that to be used on the recipient. The epithelium may either be left in place (if it is of excellent quality), or it may be removed by gentle scraping with a #15 Bard-Parker blade. The depth of the trephine blade is set at 1.5 mm and it is then placed against the anterior surface of the cornea. With a rotating motion the globe may be entered with the trephine. The button may be removed *in toto* by the trephine if the trephine is set deep, rotated in a uniform motion, and the button removed without losing the anterior chamber (Fig. 9–22). On the other hand, as soon as the anterior chamber is noted to become shallow and aqueous escapes, it is safest to remove the trephine and complete the

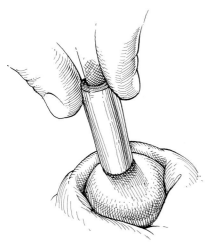

FIGURE 9–22. Trephination of donor.

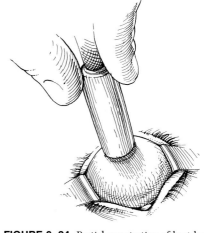

FIGURE 9–24. Partial penetration of host bed.

excision with scissors. Alternatively, a partial penetration using the trephine may be made. The anterior chamber may then be entered with a sharp knife and the excision completed with scissors. In either case, it is wise to place a single suture through the excised button (Fig. 9–23) and then place it onto a previously moistened gauze pad, with the epithelial surface against the pad and fluid immediately placed on the endothelial surface to prevent drying.

Attention is then directed toward the host cornea. The appropriate trephine is placed against the cornea, and a partial penetration, approximately 0.4 mm deep, is made (Fig. 9–24). Entrance into the anterior chamber is then achieved with a sharp knife, such as a Haab, or a broken razor blade (Fig. 9–25). Viscoelastic material may be introduced into the anterior chamber at this point to facilitate excision of the button and to minimize trauma to adjacent tissue. It is our preference that the entrance into the chamber be made in a slanting manner

and the excision of the button completed with the scissors (Fig. 9–26) at an angle so that a "skirt" of posterior host stroma is left in place to act as a gasket, and thus assure tight posterior apposition when the donor button is placed into position. Before placing the button into the host bed, careful attention should be paid to removing any adventitious tissue.

Any other procedures such as lens extraction, vitrectomy, synechiolysis, or other necessary maneuvers should now be performed. The triple procedure of penetrating keratoplasty, cataract extraction, and implantation of an intraocular lens is indicated when it is apparent that straightforward penetrating keratoplasty will not effectively improve the patient's vision because of current or imminent lens changes.

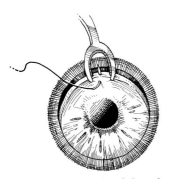

FIGURE 9–23. Suture is placed through donor.

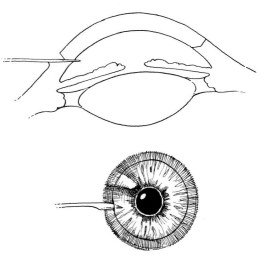

FIGURE 9–25. Anterior chamber is entered with Haab knife.

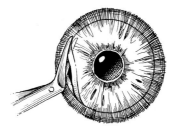

FIGURE 9–26. Beveled incision is made with scissors.

Under those circumstances, we prefer to use general anesthesia, preoperative lowering of intraocular pressure by an externally placed balloon, intraoperative use of intravenous mannitol, a Flieringa ring, and intraoperative use of muscle-relaxing agents. After the cornea has been removed, an anterior capsulotomy is performed, the nucleus is removed, residual cortex is removed by irrigation-aspiration, and a posterior chamber intraocular lens is placed. The calculation of appropriate intraocular lens power is best determined by the surgeon's studying his own previous keratoplasties to know the average keratometer readings based on his own experience. The donor button is then placed into the host bed and the previously placed suture tied at 12 o'clock. Additional sutures should be placed at the 6, 3, and 9 o'clock positions, and then final fixation of the graft may be undertaken (Fig. 9–27). Interrupted sutures of 9-0 or 10-0 silk or nylon may be used and are advisable in cases of vascularized, boggy, or inflamed corneas or if there is anticipation of problems with postoperative glaucoma. A running suture of 10-0 nylon may be used in avascular or edematous corneas that are free of the above-mentioned factors. In either case, the sutures or bites should number approximately four to five per quadrant, and the sutures should be placed approximately halfway through the thickness of donor and host and extend approximately 0.75 mm into the donor and almost to the limbus in the host. In either case, at the end of the suturing procedure each individual loop should be tested for accurate and equal tensile strength, remembering that nylon has approximately 20 per cent inherent elasticity. At the end of the procedure the anterior chamber should be re-formed to normal depth; this is perhaps best done by injection, through adjacent suture loops, of balanced salt solution through a #30 blunt irrigating tip attached to a 2-ml syringe. The wound should be watertight at the end of the procedure, and any leaking or weak areas should be repaired at that time.

Postoperatively, antibiotics are instilled topically several times a day and steroids are used topically, depending on the degree of vascularization and the amount of surgical trauma or postoperative inflammation. The frequency may vary from no or only occasional use in the completely uninflamed eye up to instillation as often as every hour in the presence of severe uveitis or inflammation. Occasionally pulsed doses of systemic prednisone (e.g., 80 mg every morning by mouth) may be administered if there is severe anterior segment inflammation.

Complications of Surgery

Most surgical complications occur at one of the following three phases:

1. During the operation
2. In the immediate postoperative period
3. In the late postoperative period

Graft rejection will be considered separately (see section on corneal graft failure, below).

Intraoperative complications are better prevented than treated. Such technical problems as poor excision of the donor button, inadvertent contact of instruments such as trephine or scissors to iris or lens, eccentric trephination, or leaving behind Descemet's membrane are examples of complications preventable by meticulous technique. In aphakic grafts undesired loss of vitreous may be minimized by use of general anesthesia, hyperosmotic agents, and the Flieringa ring, or the aspiration of 0.5 ml of fluid vitreous by way of the pars plana before opening the eye. Some complications, such as bleeding from the anterior segment, are unavoidable, but modern instrumentation such as

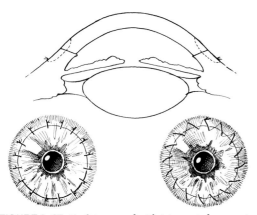

FIGURE 9–27. Graft is secured with interrupted or running suture.

bipolar coagulation permits more ready solution of the problem compared with previous years.

Immediate postoperative complications are often related to problems in wound healing or inadvertent apposition of anterior segment components. Inability to form the chamber at the time of surgery or the presence of a shallow or flat anterior chamber postoperatively is usually due to a wound leak, pupillary block, or both. The Seidel test may show an area of wound leakage even in the presence of a flat anterior chamber. Pressure patching or binocular bandaging may be all that is necessary to permit the wound to reappose and heal adequately. Sometimes soft contact lenses are helpful. If the pressure remains normal, bandaging may be tried for a day or two, but persistent wound leaks or major dehiscences must almost always be resutured in the operating room. Minor anterior wound dehiscences without leakage are best left alone, since they will frequently heal. If the wound leak is accompanied by prolapse of the iris, surgery is usually necessary. If the iris appears healthy and prolapse is of short duration (i.e., a day or less), the sutures may be removed around the iris prolapse, the iris reposited, and the wound resutured. Excision of the iris is probably indicated if the prolapse is of longer standing or if the iris appears macerated or devitalized.

Pupillary block should be suspected even in the presence of a normal pressure if the anterior chamber is shallow and the pupil not well dilated. Sometimes simply dilating the pupil vigorously with cyclopentolate and phenylephrine relieves the block and permits the chamber to deepen rapidly. Another mechanism that either causes or perpetuates a flat or shallow anterior chamber is that of a choroidal detachment. If this can be demonstrated either by direct observation or by ultrasonography, watchful waiting may be all that is indicated. If synechiae do form from the iris to the graft border, they are usually no major problem, and if they are small in extent, they are probably best left alone, since those that do not respond to dilation of the pupil usually do not lead to significant problems later. The risks of surgical separation of synechiae from the wound are probably greater than the risks the synechiae pose to the integrity and clarity of the graft.

Late complications are those that occur a few weeks or more after the operation. Premature loosening of sutures may lead to wound separation. One loose interrupted suture is usually sufficiently close to two intact sutures that separation of the wound is unlikely. With the running suture, however, especially if it is placed under tension, if one suture loop does pull through, the elasticity of the suture may permit several loops on either side to loosen and may indeed lead to a significant wound dehiscence. If the chamber does not re-form on patching, surgical repair becomes mandatory. Wound healing is much slower, particularly in the avascular graft, with a running buried nylon suture than with interrupted sutures. The wound is often not fully secure even a year after keratoplasty, and removal of sutures may cause an unpredictable shift in astigmatism, or even wound dehiscence. On the other hand, sutures can and should be removed as soon as the wound is strong enough (as manifested by the typical gray appearance of the wound margin, vessels that come to and along the wound margin, and loosening of the suture). Leaving sutures in place after the wound is healed, particularly if the sutures are exposed, does increase the risk of postoperative infection or suture abscess. This may lead to postoperative endophthalmitis, and therefore loose sutures should be removed. Postoperative infection *per se* is fortunately rare, but this dread complication must always be borne in mind as a possibility whenever a keratoplasty patient suddenly appears with an inflamed and irritated eye and intraocular inflammation.

CORNEAL GRAFT FAILURE

There are a variety of causes of graft failure. The common denominator in all of them is endothelial damage leading to corneal edema. Many of the failures are due to the technical factors mentioned under *Intraoperative Complications* above, as a result of which the endothelium becomes irreversibly damaged and the graft becomes edematous. In addition, however, there are certain specific causes of graft endothelial failure that should be mentioned.

Defects in donor material cannot always be ascertained before grafting, despite strict adherence to recommended standards for the use of donor tissue. If the donor endothelium is faulty, the graft, even from the first postoperative day, appears unduly thickened, and there may be deep folds in the posterior limiting layers. This is a grave sign but is sometimes reversible; therefore, a period of time should be permitted to elapse before the graft is considered irreversibly doomed. The only rational treatment is high doses of topical steroids, and these should be instituted immediately. The beneficial effect of systemic steroids is controversial and unproved. In addition to primary donor failure, there is always the possibility of severe damage to the endothelium during the course of surgery, against which attention to technique is the best preventive.

In the immediate postoperative period the graft may fail because of adherence of adventitious tissue. Iris rubbing on the endothelium, vitreous in contact with and adherent to the endothelium, and excessive manipulation and irrigation of the anterior chamber may all be mechanical causes of graft failure. Any intraocular inflammation, therefore, should be vigorously treated with topical steroids. Postoperative glaucoma should be controlled by medical means, particularly carbonic anhydrase inhibitors, timolol, and, if necessary, cyclocryotherapy. Sometimes vitreous adherence may be reversed by medical means such as systemic hyperosmotic agents and vigorous dilation of the pupil. Vitrectomy should be reserved for those cases in which it can be noted that the cornea is edematous where the vitreous is adherent and compact elsewhere. The vitreous touch *per se* does not necessarily lead to corneal edema, and widespread edema cannot be ascribed to localized touch.

The term *graft rejection* is reserved for cases of graft failure that follow a period during which there is a clear graft and then there is the sudden onset of inflammatory signs and graft edema. The edema usually occurs in one of two

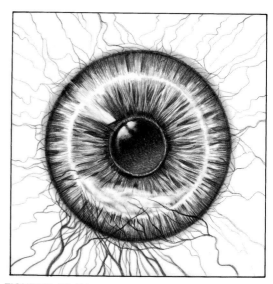

FIGURE 9–29. Edema at junction owing to graft rejection.

locations. Either there is the sudden onset of central edema associated with keratic precipitates and inflammatory cells in the anterior chamber (Fig. 9–28), or there is the onset of edema at the graft-host margin (Fig. 9–29). In the latter case, there is usually engorgement of blood vessels adjacent to the area where the edema occurs, and fine keratic precipitates are seen in that locality. All graft patients should be cautioned that any pain, redness, tearing, diminution in vision, or discomfort that appears suddenly and persists for more than 12 hours should *immediately* be brought to the attention of the operating surgeon. The graft rejection must be recognized at its earliest stage, so that prompt treatment can be instituted, in which case most graft rejection episodes can be reversed. The surgeon, therefore, should consider that in any grafted patient, the sudden onset of tearing, redness, segmental engorgement of vessels, edema of any part of the graft, keratic precipitates on the donor endothelium, or flare and cells in the anterior chambers are signs of graft rejection unless proved otherwise. The treatment consists of the prompt and vigorous instillation of topical steroids, used every hour around the clock at the beginning and gradually tapered as the inflammatory reaction becomes controlled. The tapering may take weeks or even months. The role of systemic or subconjunctival steroids is controversial, and there is no evidence that they add materially to improvement in the prognosis of a corneal graft rejection.

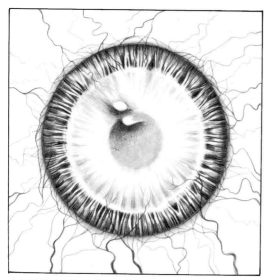

FIGURE 9–28. Diffuse edema owing to graft rejection.

10

RADIAL KERATOTOMY: Principles and Practice*

by J. James Rowsey

INTRODUCTION

Lans[1] noted the early effects of corneal relaxing incisions in rabbits in 1898, and Sato[2, 3] described a 1.5- to 7.0-diopter correction of myopia in 1950 and 1953. Sato's radial incisions into the anterior and posterior cornea were associated with bullous keratopathy approximately 20 years after the surgery, however, causing justifiable reservations about these experimental techniques. Durnev and others[4–6] reevaluated Sato's technique in the early 1970's and obtained 2.65 diopters of correction ± 0.2 diopters utilizing a 3-mm optical zone. This potential correction of myopia encouraged numerous U.S. investigators to evaluate radial keratotomy. Hoffer and colleagues reported 3.4 diopters of myopic reduction in 1981,[7] and Cowden and Bores reported 1.18 diopters of correction with a 16-incision radial keratotomy in 1982.[8, 9] Our results of 5.2 diopters of correction with an 8-incision procedure have encouraged our further investigation.[10] The procedure has progressed from a 16-incision to an 8-incision and finally to a 4-incision procedure,[11–13] with sufficiently satisfactory results to encourage further investigation.

The Prospective Evaluation of Radial Keratotomy (PERK)[14–16] collaborative study and careful follow-up of other authors demonstrated the range of potential efficacy of this procedure, predictive variables of importance, and numerous unsuspected complications.[16–20]

This chapter discusses the fundamental principles of refractive surgery, corneal topography, preoperative preparation of the patient for radial keratotomy, necessary operative instrumentation, surgical technique, postoperative care, and methods of minimizing complications in radial keratotomy.

PRINCIPLES OF REFRACTIVE SURGERY

The basic caveats in keratorefractive surgery are important for an understanding of the effects anticipated with surgical procedures.[20]

1. *The normal cornea flattens over any incision.* A traumatic or surgical incision in the cornea produces flattening of the corneal tissue adjacent to the incision. As the incision fills with collagen and epithelium during wound healing, the surface area of the cornea is increased. A longer radius of curvature is produced in this area, thus providing permanent corneal flattening. Corneal flattening decreases the refractive power of the cornea, a valuable asset to the myopic patient. Figure 10–1 is an eye bank eye with 16 radial incisions in the cornea, each filled with tattoo dye to demonstrate the flattening of the cornea along each

*Research for this chapter was supported by The Gustavus and Louise Pfeiffer Foundation, an unrestricted grant from Research to Prevent Blindness, Inc., and the private philanthropy of the citizens of Oklahoma.

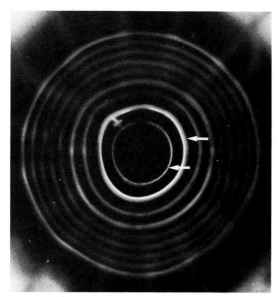

FIGURE 10–1. Kera corneascope photographs of a 16-incision eye bank eye radial keratotomy with tattoo in each incision, demonstrating marked corneal flattening over the incisions as shown by a wide separation of the central corneal rings (arrows).

incision. Figure 10–2 is a corneascope photograph of a patient eye 1 year after an eight-incision radial keratotomy, demonstrating an unusual, but persistent irregular ring pattern. Epithelium and collagen have filled each incision, flattening the center of the cornea.

2. *Radial corneal incisions flatten the adjacent cornea and the cornea 90 degrees away.* Incisions that traverse the cornea from the periphery to the center produce corneal flattening as described, but simultaneously flatten the dome of the cornea 90 degrees from the actual incision site. This provides a unique corneal symmetrizing from radial incisions. A four-incision radial keratotomy uses this propensity for flattening in two meridians. A single incision produces marked corneal flattening over the corneal dome by expansion in the center of the incision site.

3. *The corneal flattening effect increases as incisions approach the visual axis.* One of the major variables in radial keratotomy is the size of the optical zone. Smaller optical zones produce a larger magnitude of corneal flattening.[10, 15] Traumatic corneal lacerations that traverse the visual axis may produce 20 diopters or more of corneal flattening when repaired. Figure 10–3 shows that the magnitude of corneal flattening with corneal incisions is greatest in the center of the cornea and diminishes as incisions approach the limbus.

4. *The cornea flattens directly over any sutured incision.* The sutured corneal incision produces an indentation vector of corneal flattening. For this reason perforations that may require suturing are avoided in radial keratotomy. Suturing reverses the effect of the radial keratotomy and accentuates any induced corneal astigmatism.

5. *The limbal cornea flattens adjacent to loose sutures.* Circumferential limbal corneal inci-

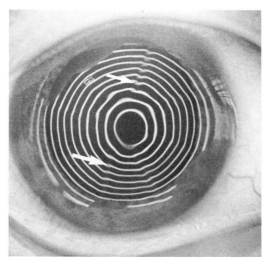

FIGURE 10–2. One year postoperatively, two incision sites are still visible in some patients as an uneven break in the rings on Kera corneascopy (arrows).

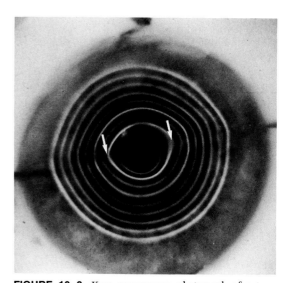

FIGURE 10–3. Kera corneascope photograph of a two-incision radial keratotomy in an eye bank eye, demonstrating flattening along the incisions of approximately 6 diopters and flattening 90 degrees away of approximately 3 diopters. A 3-mm optical zone is used. The central ellipse confirms flattening of the cornea along the incisions (arrows).

sions or cataract incisions produce wound gaping analogous to any other incision of the cornea. However, the circumferential or limbal corneal incision flattens the cornea directly over the incision and 180 degrees away while *steepening* the cornea 90 degrees away. Movement of the circumferential incision onto the clear cornea away from the limbus produces the astigmatic relaxing effect of tangential keratotomies. The effect of the circumferential incision should be distinguished from that of the radial corneal incision. The latter flattens the cornea both along the incision and 90 degrees away. The circumferential incision flattens the cornea in the axis of the incision and steepens the cornea 90 degrees away. The combination of radial and circumferential corneal incisions, therefore, have marked astigmatic correction potential.

6. *The limbal cornea steepens adjacent to tight sutures and steepens 180 degrees away; the cornea flattens 90 degrees away from tight sutures.* This description of the classic balloon model of Troutman[21] is easily visualized with a tight limbal compressive suture producing a vector of indentation of the cornea under the suture or flattening in this area (Fig. 10–4A). The cornea is steepened (Fig. 10–4B) anterior to the tight suture over the corneal apex and is flattened 90 degrees away. This steepening of the corneal apex anterior to limbal sutures produces "with the rule" astigmatism (plus cylinder at cylinder axis *90 degrees*) with routine 12 o'clock incisions.

7. *The cornea flattens overlying wedge resections.* Removal of corneal tissue in a microwedge allows for greater posterior vector compression from the sutures, and marked

FIGURE 10–4. *A,* A limbal suture produces an indentation vector at 12 o'clock (arrow), with flattening of the cornea directly beneath the suture, steepening of the cornea anterior to the suture, and flattening of the cornea 90 degrees away from the suture. (From Rowsey JJ: Corneal topography. Corneascope. Arch. Ophthalmol., 99:1093, 1981.) *B,* The sagittal view of the cornea after cataract surgery shows the vector of compression under the suture, shortening the radius of curvature (R) and displacing the corneal apex inferiorly. A ring reflection of increasing "with the rule" astigmatism is drawn below the cornea.

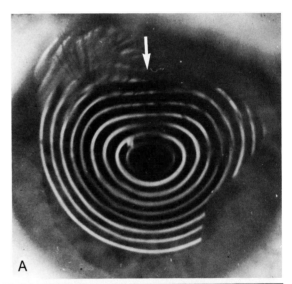

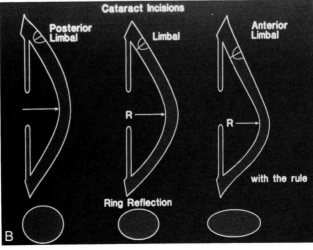

flattening of the cornea in the area of the wedge is observed.

8. *The cornea steepens anterior to wedge resections or tucks.* A limbal wedge resection or tuck produces apical corneal steepening. The steepened corneal apex moves away from the area of the wedge resection (Fig. 10–4B).

9. *Tissue removal produces corneal flattening over the site of tissue removal.* This insight is true for wedge resections regardless of their cause, both in surgery and in trauma. Therefore, during repair of traumatic corneal lacerations all possible tissue is preserved, with a conscious effort to remove as little tissue as possible.

10. *The cornea flattens adjacent to areas of full-thickness tissue additions to the cornea.* Wedge additions to the cornea accentuate the flattening effect seen in caveat number 1 by increasing the surface area over which the epithelium may heal. The microwedge addition technique, therefore, provides the potential for marked corneal flattening.

A basic understanding of these topographic insights is useful before radial keratotomy, relaxing incisions, or wedge resections are attempted, for the modulation of these caveats is under the control of the surgeon.

CORNEAL TOPOGRAPHY

The corneal shape, or surface topography, has been compared to a prolate ellipse,[22–25] with a short radius of curvature at the apex and flattening in all meridians (Fig. 10–5A). We have analyzed the corneal topography preoperatively and postoperatively in the PERK study and with the Humphrey keratometer, to determine the correlative factors in corneal shape that would allow for effective refractive change. Figure 10–5B and C present a sagittal view of the cornea compared to an ellipse. The steep central cornea flattens in the periphery. Henslee and Rowsey[25] have previously demonstrated the reversal of this topographic shape to a flat central cornea and steepening in the midperiphery after effective radial keratotomy surgery (Fig. 10–6A and B). The relation between the central radius of curvature and the peripheral radius of curvature appears to be a significant predictive factor in radial keratotomy. Corneas that are flat in the center and flatten more toward the periphery have the greatest potential for corneal flattening in radial keratotomy. Corneas that are steep in the cen-

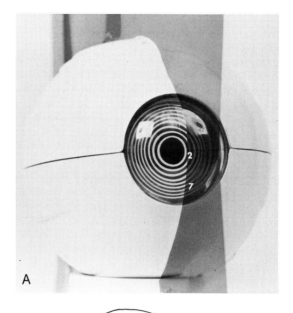

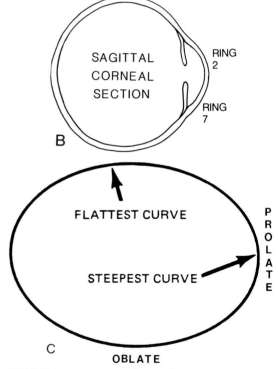

FIGURE 10–5. *A*, A sagittal corneal section approximates an ellipse with a steep central cornea (ring 2) and flattening toward ring 7. *B*, A sagittal plane through the cornea demonstrates the anterior-posterior relation of the central corneal rings (ring 2) and the peripheral rings of corneascopy (rings 7–9). *C*, The cornea shape approximates an ellipse. The prolate cornea is similar to an ellipse with a steep central curvature, the apices of the ellipse. The flat side of the ellipse is the oblate side.

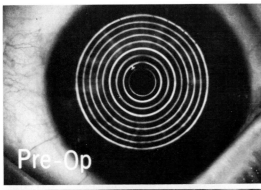

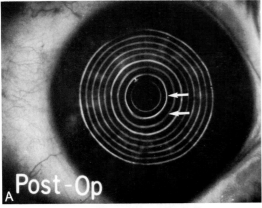

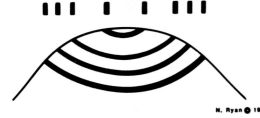

RADIAL KERATOTOMY =
FLAT CENTER &
B ## STEEP PERIPHERY

FIGURE 10–6. *A,* Preoperative Kera corneascope photograph of the cornea before radial keratotomy. Postoperative radial keratotomy photograph shows marked flattening of the cornea. Note the widening of the second and third rings, denoting central corneal flattening analogous to Figure 10–1. *B,* Schematic of the side view of the cornea, demonstrating marked corneal flattening after radial keratotomy.

ter and steepen toward the periphery have a resistance to the effect of radial keratotomy. The relation between the center and the periphery of these relative corneal shapes is a greater contributor to the effectiveness of the operation than either radius of curvature individually.[26] The prolate side of an ellipse (Fig.

10–5*A*) flattens toward the periphery, whereas the oblate side (Fig. 10–5*A*) of an ellipse steepens toward the periphery. The prolate corneal shape provides the ideal candidate for radial keratotomy, whereas the oblate corneal shape frequently seen after a radial keratotomy procedure resists further central corneal flattening, and therefore produces a diminished radial keratotomy effect. Figure 10–6*A* shows the preoperative and postoperative radial keratotomy corneascope photographs emphasizing the marked corneal flattening of the center of the cornea after this surgery.

PREOPERATIVE PATIENT SELECTION AND PREPARATION

Radial keratotomy is reasonably effective in the −2- to −8-diopter myopic patient, depending on the patient's age. Higher levels of myopia, between −8 and −15 diopters, may be satisfactorily repaired in the 50- to 60-year-old patient with a 16-incision technique. In general, patients should have a stable myopia that is nonprogressive and without signs of keratoconus. Slit-lamp examination should preclude significant external disease that may contribute to subsequent corneal infection. Collagen diseases or connective tissue diseases, uncontrolled lid infections, glaucoma, or uveitis should be avoided, since the operative results on these patients may be unpredictable and surgery may complicate their underlying ocular disease process. Patients who are satisfactorily corrected with glasses or contact lenses should not be encouraged to undergo radial keratotomy. "Medical, legal and ethical considerations can almost always be resolved by doing what is in the best interest of the patient without regard for finances, personal aggrandizement, or other possible benefits to the surgeon," as emphasized by Bettman.[27]

Adequate informed consent includes (a) detailed explanation of the proposed procedure; (b) explanation of the known risks and benefits; (c) discussion of the alternatives to surgery; (d) review of all questions provided by the patient and open discussion of risks and benefits; and (e) adequate time between the discussion and the surgical procedure so that the patient may review the information and withdraw his consent for the surgical intervention, awaiting further developments in the field.

It is especially important that patients realize that the results of the surgical procedure cannot be precisely predicted at this time. We have found it exceedingly important to explain presbyopic symptoms to patients, and this is our most difficult area of informed consent. The myopic patient realizes that he may read simply by removing his glasses; overcorrecting the prepresbyopic patient in the phoropter to demonstrate the incipient requirement for glasses is appropriate. A complete eye examination, including cycloplegic refraction, tonometry, external examination, slit-lamp examination, evaluation of the posterior pole and peripheral retina and muscle balance, is completed. An accurate measurement of the corneal thickness, along with endothelial evaluation, is necessary. Corneas that are thinner than 500 μm centrally and those that thin inferiorly may demonstrate early keratoconus, which should be avoided. Corneas that are thicker than 620 μm may be on the verge of corneal decompensation from endothelial dysfunction, and should be avoided.

A nomogram summarizing pertinent refractive results is shown in Figure 10–7A and B. The optical zone for each patient is reviewed. The greater the myopic refractive error, the greater the effect of a single operation, and the greater the patient's age, the greater the effect of the procedure. Male patients have a greater effect with a similar optical zone procedure than do females unless topical steroids are used postoperatively; topical steroids equalize the male and female effect for a given age and operation. The PERK patients summarized in Figure 10–7A did not use steroids, whereas the University of Oklahoma patients have all been placed on steroids. Three optical zones have been used in these two studies, a 3.0-, 3.5-, and 4.0-mm optical zone. The nomogram standard deviations of two of the procedures are outlined (Fig. 10–7B designates the regression formulas). The primary predictive factors emphasized in this nomogram are preoperative myopia and patient age. The higher the preoperative myopia and/or patient age, the greater the effect of the surgical procedure. The nomogram is used by determining the patient's myopia on the left and traversing horizontally until the patient's age is observed. The average refractive change observed for the studied population is presented as the sloping regression lines. If an undercorrection is desired, a fewer number of incisions are made or a larger optical zone is chosen. The primary surgical variables that may be altered include the optical zone and the depth and number of incisions. Refractions between the regression lines provided would infer that an intermediate optical zone

marker could be used at this position. However, the data to substantiate such a recommendation are not currently available.

SURGICAL TECHNIQUE

Topical anesthesia with 0.5% proparacaine is used in all patients. We initially used either retrobulbar anesthesia or topical anesthesia with cocaine, or both. Cocaine anesthesia was found to be too toxic to the corneal epithelium. Retrobulbar anesthesia, however, is excessively precarious in the elongated myopic eye. Topical anesthesia is initiated approximately 5 minutes before preparation of the patient. Deep conjunctival anesthesia is obtained with 2 drops of proparacaine every minute for 5 minutes until the visual axis is marked. The eye is draped in a sterile manner after alcohol and iodine anesthesia of the periocular skin has been accomplished. The visual axis marking (Fig. 10–8A and B,) is accomplished by observing the light reflex reflected from the corneal apex while the patient is viewing the reduced-intensity light filament of the microscope. The light must, of course, be coaxial with the viewing scope (Fig. 10–8A). Corneal displacement of the light reflex toward the observer's eye in a noncoaxial operating microscope (Fig. 10–8B) requires compensation during visual axis marking (Fig. 10–8B).[10] If the surgeon views the cornea with his own right eye, the left end of the corneal reflex is marked at the inferior edge of the light reflex (Fig. 10–8A). If the surgeon uses his own left eye, the right inferior end of the corneal reflex is marked. Fiberoptic light sources that attach to the operating microscope and produce a coaxial projection of light are also available. The patient is then directed to look away and subsequently refocus the light source to determine if a similar position is reflected from the cornea. Patients have a tendency to look away from the light source because of its irritation, and the visual axis determination should be confirmed. A Sinsky hook or 26-gauge needle may be used to lightly mark the epithelium, avoiding damage to the basement membrane or Bowman's membrane (Fig. 10–8A).

A trephine is selected between 3 and 5 mm (see Fig. 10–7), and the visual axis is circumscribed with the appropriate size optical zone (Fig. 10–9A and B). Trephines are typically calibrated by measuring inside edge to inside edge. Radial corneal incisions, therefore, must

THE UNIVERSITY OF OKLAHOMA
DEAN A. McGEE EYE INSTITUTE
J. JAMES ROWSEY, M.D. AND HAL D. BALYEAT, M.D.
RADIAL KERATOTOMY RECOMMENDATIONS
USE O.Z. INDICATED: Add 8 incisions with 2nd RK

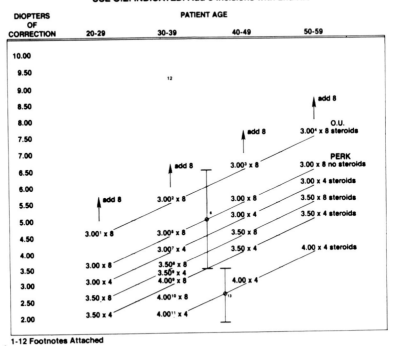

1-12 Footnotes Attached

A

FIGURE 10–7. *A,* Nomogram to determine the optical zone for radial keratotomy, depending on myopia and patient's age. *B,* Footnotes to *A.*

THE UNIVERSITY OF OKLAHOMA
DEAN A. McGEE EYE INSTITUTE
J. JAMES ROWSEY, M.D. AND HAL D. BALYEAT, M.D.
RADIAL KERATOTOMY RECOMMENDATIONS
USE O.Z. INDICATED: Add 8 more incisions with 2nd RK
page 2

1. O.U. calculated 2.53 diopters + 0.087 x 25 years = 4.70 diopters; use steroids.

2. O.U. 8 inc. 3.00mm oz = 5.36 diopters correction; Steroids subconjunctivally and four times a day; 36.5 years.

3. O.U. calculated 2.53 diopters +0.087 x 45 years = 6.44 diopters; use steroids.

4. O.U. calculated 2.53 diopters +0.087 x 55 yers = 7.31 diopters; use steroids.

5. PERK 8 inc. 3.00mm oz = 4.49 diopters correction; No steroids.

6. Standard deviation is larger for larger optical zones; see footnote 13.

7. O.U. 4 inc. 3.00mm oz. = 4.20 diopters correction; Steroids four times a day.

8. PERK 8 inc. 3.50mm oz = 3.41 diopters correction; No steroids.
   O.U. 8 inc. 3.50mm oz = 3.66 diopters correction; Steroids four times a day.

9. O.U. 4 inc. 3.50mm oz = 3.33 diopters correction; Steroids four times a day.
   O.U. 8 inc. 4.00mm oz = 2.77 diopters correction; Steroids four times a day.

10. PERK 8 inc. 4.00mm oz = 2.73 diopters correction; No steroids.

11. O.U. 2.33 diopters with 4.00mm oz and 4 inc.; Use steroids.

12. O.U. Δ C.R. refraction for myopic population beyond this chart. Δ C.R. = myopia x 0.46 + age x 0.071 + 0.0019 diopters. Thumb rule: Δ C.R. = 0.5 x myopia + 7% of age.

13. The effect, range of effect and standard deviation of effect is **LESS** with smaller optical zones, or fewer incisions. This greater safety, or greater predictability, would warrant consideration of fewer incisions to avoid over corrections, or a larger optical zone, or both. Be careful.

J. James Rowsey, M.D.

Hal D. Balyeat, M.D.

B

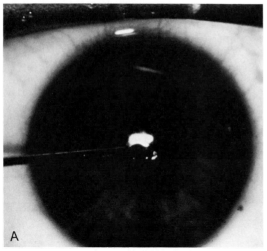

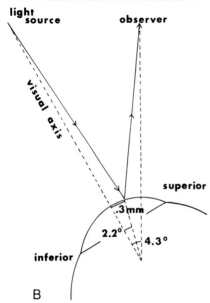

FIGURE 10–8. *A,* Marking the visual axis while the patient fixates on the operating microscope filament. The light reflex is marked, accounting for displacement of the light across the cornea. *B,* Displacement of the corneal reflection toward the observer eye requires compensation by the observer. Displacement of the light across the cornea requires compensatory marking of the visual axis. (From Rowsey, J.J., and Balyeat, H.D.: Radial keratotomy: Preliminary report of complications. Ophthalmic Surg., 13:27. 1982.)

begin on the inside edge of the corneal trephine mark, cutting across the trephine mark itself to maximize the effect of the procedure. A set of trephines is shown in Figure 10–9A, and the entire surgery tray in Figure 10–10 (diamond knife, coin gauge, Thornton fixation ring, ultrasonic pachymeter, irrigation canula [30-gauge], anesthetic, lid speculum, micro sponges, and syringe). We avoid a solid lid speculum, as the

diamond knife may be easily chipped on this device. The Thornton fixation ring allows performing the incisions by rotating the globe or rotating the knife around the cornea. It also simultaneously allows the pressure on the globe to increase, to maximize the depth of incisions.

Pachymetry (Fig. 10–11) is completed in the central cornea and at each of four positions along the trephine mark of the cornea. The pachymeter tip is set tangent to the trephine marks. The visual axis normally traverses the nasal cornea, and the geometric center of the cornea is, therefore, temporal to the visual axis (Fig. 10–11B). The geometric center of the cornea is thinner than any other cornea position, including the nasal visual axis. The thin geometric corneal center is routinely expected for the diamond knife setting. The diamond knife is extended to 100 per cent of the thinnest paracentral reading (Fig. 10–12A through C). Attention to the diamond is important to avoid chipping or overextending the blade. The current coin gauge allows the surgeon to set the diamond within 10 μm of the desired level (Fig. 10–12A and B). Variations in diamond knife length have been demonstrated with the new high-magnification gauges (Fig. 10–13A), which also allow inspection of the diamond for internal cleavage planes and chipping. The high magnification of the newer inspection tools demonstrates the unevenness of the platforms, the poor polishing frequently provided by the manufacturer, and the diamond defects provided in industrial-grade compared with gem-grade diamonds (Fig. 10–13A and B). The use of these inspection tools before surgery to calibrate the micrometer handles of the newer diamonds to greater precision avoids the need of the gauge block in surgery. The gauge blocks have been associated with trauma to the guard of the diamond, producing variable diamond extensions in subsequent surgery, and are best avoided. The diamond knife is provided with two advance mechanisms, coarse and fine. The coarse advance destabilizes the calibration. Only the fine advance and retraction are used, therefore, after the diamond micrometer handle has been calibrated.

The globe is fixed with the Thornton fixation ring (Fig. 10–14), and the intraocular pressure is increased to between 30 and 40 mm Hg. This higher intraocular pressure maximizes corneal sectility, or susceptibility to being incised. Improved sectility improves incision depth. The trephine mark must be excised (Fig. 10–15A). Vertical corneal incisions maximize the flattening of the cornea (Fig. 10–15B), according to

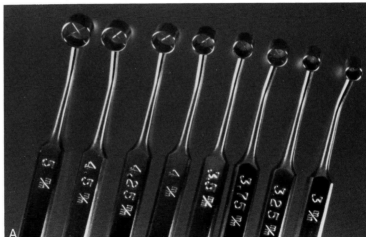

FIGURE 10–9. *A*, Blunt trephines are used to circumscribe the visual axis. *B*, A blunt trephine surrounds the visual axis, marking the optical zone.

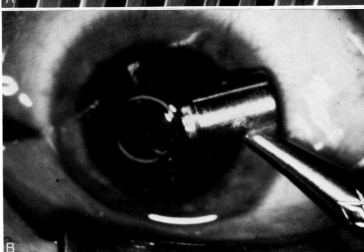

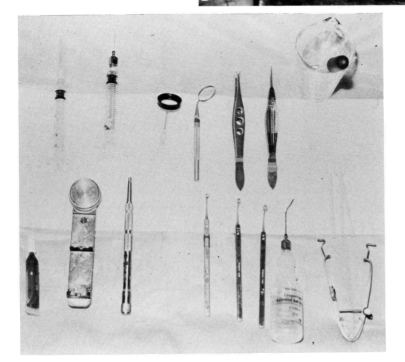

FIGURE 10–10. A radial keratotomy operative tray, showing the useful equipment.

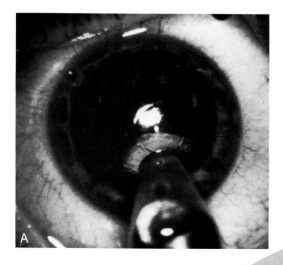

FIGURE 10–11. *A*, Ultrasonic pachymetry at each position surrounding the optical zone provides the thinnest corneal reading. *B*, The thinnest central cornea is temporal to the visual axis and is routinely the depth prescribed for radial keratotomy incisions.

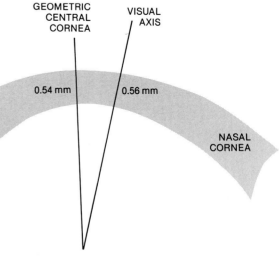

B

FIGURE 10–12. *A*, The diamond knife (arrow) and gauge block set at 560 µm. *B*, Tilting the gauge block away from the observer accentuates the appearance of the knife extension by the surgeon's vernier acuity. Tilting the knife toward the observer makes the knife appear too short.

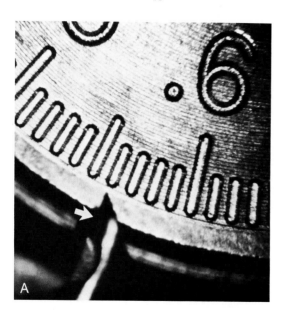

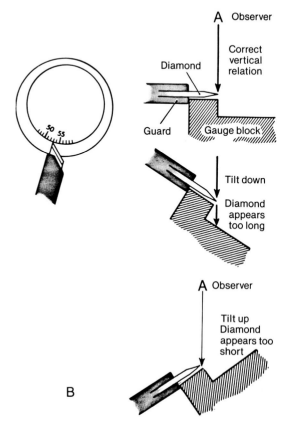

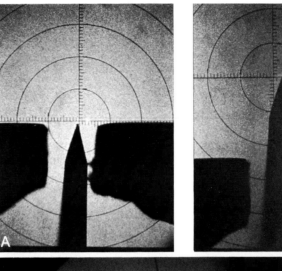

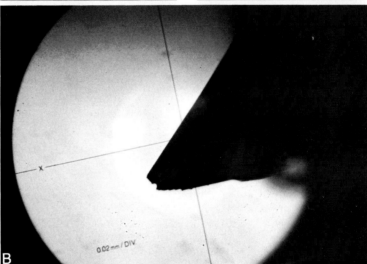

FIGURE 10–13. *A,* The diamond gauge evaluation shows correct diamond calibration. *B,* Diamond tip irregularities and edge defects are seen.

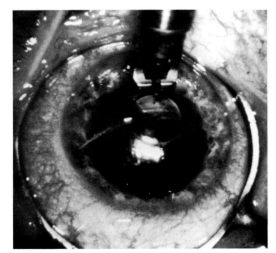

FIGURE 10–14. Radial corneal incisions maximize the corneal flattening effect. Adequate globe fixation is important. Thornton ring (arrow).

the valve rule of Eisner ("incisions through the wall of the globe produce valves whose margin of water tightness is proportional to the projection of the incision onto the wall of the globe").[28] Vertical corneal incisions, therefore, spontaneously open (see caveat number 1), whereas shelving corneal incisions spontaneously close, diminishing the effectiveness of radial keratotomy. The surgeon should, before surgery, practice producing a vertical radial corneal incision in all quadrants; this will accentuate the effect of the incisions. During the initiation of the incision the knife should be placed at full depth through the optical zone mark, and seated for a count of 1 to 2 seconds before the incision is initiated. If peripheral movement begins before complete seating of the diamond occurs, a diminished effect will be observed.

Meticulous irrigation of the incisions (Fig.

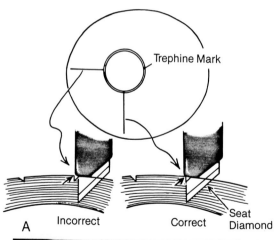

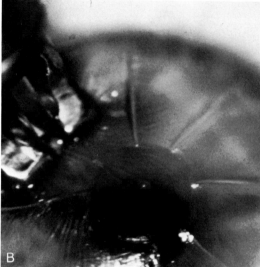

FIGURE 10–15. *A,* Incisions must incise the trephine mark after seating the blade (*B*) to full depth. *B,* Vertical corneal incisions maximize the corneal flattening. Oblique incisions produce shallow, self-closing valves.

harden and present as apparent dullness on subsequent surgical procedures. Inspection of the diamond knife under high magnification may demonstrate this epithelial or caked debris; this may be removed by wetting the blade with alcohol and making an incision through Styrofoam. The roughened incision edge of the Styrofoam will remove most debris.

AVOIDING COMPLICATIONS AT SURGERY

Good patient rapport is required to allow the patient to relax during surgery. After the visual axis is marked, we use 5 to 10 mg of intravenous diazepam. This medication is not used before

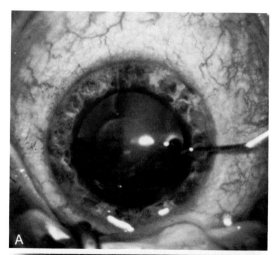

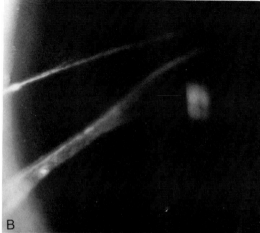

FIGURE 10–16. *A,* Irrigations of the incisions minimize epithelial debris. *B,* Epithelial debris (white dots) that remain in the incisions may produce glare and can be avoided by meticulous incision irrigation.

10–16*A*) at the end of the procedure precludes some of the major complications of excessive corneal scarring, epithelial ingrowth (Fig. 10–16*B*), and glare after the procedure. It is worthwhile to irrigate parallel to the incision, gently removing all epithelial debris. Descemet's membrane may be stripped from the posterior aspect of cornea if irrigation is too vigorous. The gentle use of intraoperative saline solution or balanced salt solution along the incisions with a 30-gauge needle is warranted.

The diamond knife should be carefully irrigated with saline solution and washed with alcohol or hydrogen peroxide to remove all epithelial debris before it is resterilized. If the diamond knife is steam sterilized with epithelial debris or serum on the tip, this material will marking the visual axis, as the patient may lose concentration. If the visual axis is mismarked, incisions may traverse the visual axis, producing marked glare and decreased vision. Excessive opening of the lids with the lid speculum when the lid is not blocked may produce lid spasm and conjunctival protrusion into the operative field during the surgical procedure. A gentle wire lid speculum avoids these complications. Ptosis has been reported after radial keratotomy, although there are other possible explanations. The ptosis may conceivably be related to the lid speculum. Topical anesthesia may be fortified with 0.1-ml injections of 2% lidocaine near the limbus to allow for adequate fixation with the Thornton ring or two-point fixation forceps.

The patient may find the light of the microscope the most uncomfortable portion of the procedure. It is important to diminish the light of the operating microscope from full illumination. This not only decreases discomfort, but also decreases the possibility of macular phototoxicity. It should be recalled that correct determination of the visual axis requires the patient to fixate the bulb of the microscope.

It is necessary to maintain good globe fixation pressure with the surgeon's nondominant hand to avoid complications. Inadequate globe pressure may allow the diamond to push the cornea posteriorly, engaging the iris or lens on the indented Descemet's membrane, thereby producing iris atrophy or a cataract.

Lack of irrigation of the incisions at the end of the procedure will produce epithelial debris and excessive corneal scarring, which is unacceptable.

If the anterior chamber is entered inadvertently, the chamber may collapse, engaging the iris or the lens on the diamond knife. Perforations are to be avoided. Microperforations, in an attempt to accentuate the effect of the operation, turn the procedure from an extraocular to an intraocular procedure, greatly increasing the risk to the patient without adding to the benefit.

POSTOPERATIVE CARE

Dexamethasone (4 mg) and gentamicin (20 mg) are injected subconjunctivally at the end of the procedure (along with 0.5 ml of 2% lidocaine mixed with this combination to decrease discomfort). The lidocaine also helps to alleviate the immediate operative discomfort. Depending on the patient's comfort, a light pressure patch may be affixed for 2 to 24 hours after the procedure. For the first 24 hours after surgery the patient may be irritated by the pressure patch, and find the eye more comfortable without a patch. Steroid eye drops, 0.10% dexamethasone phosphate, are initiated after 24 hours and are used four times a day for 4 weeks postoperatively. This maximizes the flattening effect of the procedure.

Patients are reevaluated 1 week postoperatively, 4 weeks, 3 months, 6 months, 1 year, 2 years, and 3 years after the surgery. No further surgery is initiated until 3 months after the initial surgical procedure.

COMPLICATIONS

The complications of radial keratotomy[10, 15, 29–33] should be thoroughly reviewed by the surgeon and the patient considering refractive surgery. The major problem is a *lack of predictability*.[31] We would consider a predictable operation one in which the residual ametropia misses a plano or zero refractive error by no more than 10 per cent of the original refractive error. For example, a desirable operative result in a −2.50 myope would be plano ± 0.25 of a diopter. A −10 myope would be reasonably pleased with a refractive error of plano ± 1 diopter. This expectation is being approached in radial keratotomy, but cannot be guaranteed. *Regression* of myopic flattening occurs with wound healing as corneal scarring ensues. The flat initial cornea gradually steepens, and the initially overcorrected patient will approach emmetropia. The patient who is undercorrected in the first 1 week postoperatively will seldom obtain an emmetropic state. More recent reports, however, demonstrate *progression*, or a hyperopic shift, 1 to 2 years after the surgery; this suggests that a slight undercorrection, instead of overcorrection, may be preferable. Clearly, further investigation is required to settle this matter.

Epithelial defects are observed in all patients postoperatively. The epithelium normally heals within 5 to 7 days after the surgery; in fact, it is frequently essentially healed within 24 hours with residual punctate epithelial staining remaining. *Recurrent erosions* may occur if Cogan's mapdot fingerprint corneal dystrophy precedes the radial keratotomy. Cogan's dystrophy is, therefore, a relative contraindication to the procedure. *Subepithelial fibrosis* indistinguishable from Cogan's dystrophy may occur after the procedure and may represent occult recurrent microepithelial erosions. *Moncreiff iron lines*[33] associated with corneal topography shift after the procedure are frequently observed, but are not associated with glare or patient complaints.

Residual blood in the incisions may be associated with subsequent *corneal vascularization* or excessive *glare* and should be avoided at the time of surgery. Vascular ingrowth with *contact lens wear* is associated with partial anoxia or decreased contact lens mobility. Contact lens–fitting problems may increase, and patients should be aware that if they have been contact lens failures, they will probably not subsequently succeed with a contact lens after radial keratotomy.

Perforation of the anterior chamber has been associated with localized *epithelial downgrowth, endophthalmitis,* and *cataract.*

Astigmatism is produced in a low magnitude, $+0.5$ to $+2.00$ diopters, as frequently as it is spontaneously eliminated by the symmetrization process of the procedure.

Incisional *epithelial ingrowth* can be avoided by meticulous irrigation of the incisions after the procedure. *Glare* is observed in all patients in the immediate postoperative period, and may persist for up to 5 years postoperatively. This glare is associated with decreased night vision potential. Rarely patients are unable to drive at night because of the glare of oncoming headlights through the corneal incisions.

Fluctuating vision is greatest in the early postoperative period. The cornea appears to be flattest in the morning and steepens throughout the day. The overcorrected patient is hyperopic in the morning and, as the cornea steepens throughout the day, approaches emmetropia. The patient barely corrected to emmetropia in the morning develops progressive corneal steepening from morning to evening associated with progressive myopia, requiring glasses by evening for the residual myopic correction. *Marked overcorrections* of 4 or 5 diopters may occur, but should be infrequent with the newer four-incision procedures. Precipitation of an *esotropia,* if the patient has a heterophoria before surgery and has a sudden anisometropia after the first operation, is possible, but infrequent.

Delayed bacterial keratitis may occur after the surgery, with or without the use of contact lenses. *Endothelial cell loss* appears to be between 7 per cent and 8 per cent with each operation, is nonprogressive, and has not been associated with endothelial decompensation with the current U.S. techniques.

SUMMARY

Radial keratotomy can reduce myopia in the -2- to -8-diopter range, depending on the patient's age. New instrumentation (including diamond knives, corneascopy, ultrasonic pachymetry, and globe fixation devices), control of incision depth and wound healing, and linear regression models of predictive variables may allow greater precision of this procedure in the future. The most common complications appear to be lack of predictability, glare, and fluctuating vision. The long-term complications of this procedure are not yet known.

Patients must be fully informed regarding the complications already known. In addition, they must be made aware that the long-term effects of radial keratotomy are unknown but could be harmful. The surgery may have a place in the treatment of myopia only in patients who have fully considered the risks and benefits of this new and still evolving procedure.

REFERENCES

1. Lans, R. J.: Experimentelle Untersuchungen uber Entstehung von Astigmatismus durch nicht-perforirende Corneawunden. Albrecht Von Graefes Arch. Ophthalmol., 45:117, 1898.
2. Sato, T.: Treatment of conical cornea (incision of Descemet's membrane). Acta Soc. Ophthalmol. Jpn., 43:544, 1939.
3. Sato, T., Akiyama, K., Shibata, H.: A new surgical approach to myopia. Am. J. Ophthalmol., 36:823, 1953.
4. Durnev, V. V.: Decrease of corneal refraction by anterior keratotomy method with the purpose of surgical correction of myopia of mild moderate degree. Proceedings of the First Congress of Ophthalmologists of Transcaucasia. Tbilisi, USSR, 1976, p 129.
5. Durnev, V. V., Ermoshin, A. S.: Determination of dependence between length of anterior radial non-perforating incisions and cornea and their effectiveness. Transactions of the Fifth All-Union Conference of Inventors and Rationalizers in Ophthalmology Field. Moscow, USSR, 1986, p 106.
6. Fyodorov, S. N., Durnev, V. V.: Operation of dosaged dissection of corneal circular ligament in cases of myopia of a mild degree. Ann. Ophthalmol., 11:1885, 1979.
7. Hoffer, K. J., Darin, J. J., Pettit, T. H., et al.: UCLA clinical trial of radial keratotomy: Preliminary report. Ophthalmology, 88:729, 1981.
8. Cowden, J. W., Bores, L. D.: A clinical investigation

of the surgical correction of myopia by the method of Fyodorov. Ophthalmology, 88:737, 1981.

9. Cowden, J. W.: Radial keratotomy: A retrospective study of cases observed at the Kresge Eye Institute for six months. Arch. Ophthalmol., 100:578, 1982.

10. Balyeat, H. D.: Radial keratotomy: Preliminary report of complications. Ophthalmic Surg., 13:27, 1982.

11. Bonham, R. D., Hays, J. C., Rowsey, J. J.: Efficacy of four incision radial keratotomy. ARVO Abstracts. Invest. Ophthalmol. Vis. Sci., 26(Suppl):202, 1985.

12. Salz, J. J., Villasenor, R. A., Elander, R., et al.: Four-incision radial keratotomy for low to moderate myopia. Ophthalmology, 93:727, 1986.

13. Vaughan, E. R.: The 4-cut radial keratotomy in low myopia. Refractive Surg., 2:164, 1986.

14. Waring, G. O., Moffitt, S. D., Gelender, H., et al.: Rationale for and design of the National Eye Institute Prospective Evaluation of Radial Keratotomy (PERK) Study. Ophthalmology, 90:40, 1983.

15. Waring, G. O., Lynn, M. J., Gelender, H., et al.: Results of the Prospective Evaluation of Radial Keratotomy (PERK) study one year after radial keratotomy. Ophthalmology, 92:177, 1985.

16. Waring, G. O., Laibson, P., Lindstrom, R., et al.: Changes in refraction, keratometry and visual acuity during the first year after radial keratotomy in the PERK study. Invest. Ophthalmol. Vis. Sci., 26(Suppl):202, 1985.

17. Rowsey, J. J., Balyeat, H. D., Rabinovitch, B., et al.: Predicting the results of radial keratotomy. Ophthalmology, 90:642, 1983.

18. Dietz, M. R., Sanders, D. R., Marks, R. G.: Radial keratotomy: An overview of the Kansas City study. Ophthalmology, 91:467, 1984.

19. Arrowsmith, P. N., Sanders, D. R., Marks, R. G.: Visual refractive, and keratometric results of radial keratotomy. Arch. Ophthalmol., 101:873, 1983.

20. Rowsey, J. J.: Ten caveats in keratorefractive surgery. Ophthalmology, 90:147, 1983.

21. Troutman, R. C.: Microsurgery of the Anterior Segment of the Eye. Vol. 2, The Cornea: Optics and Surgery. St. Louis, C. V. Mosby, 1977, p 268.

22. Smith, T. W.: Corneal topography. Doc. Ophthalmol., 43:249, 1977.

23. Mandell, R. B., St. Helen, R.: Mathematical model of the corneal contour. Br. J. Physiol. Optics, 26:183, 1977.

24. Humphrey Instruments, Model 410 Auto keratometer. Owner's manual by Humphrey Instruments, Inc. San Leandro, CA.

25. Henslee, S. L., Rowsey, J. J.: New corneal shapes in keratorefractive surgery. Ophthalmology, 90:245, 1983.

26. Au, Y-K, Rowsey, J. J.: Bending moment modeling in radial keratotomy. *In* Spaeth, G. L., Katz, J., Parker, K. W. (eds.): Current Therapy in Ophthalmic Surgery. Philadelphia, B. C. Decker, Inc., 1989, p. 47.

27. Bettman, J. W.: Refractive keratoplasty: Medicolegal aspects. *In* Sanders, D. R., Hofmann, R. F., Salz, J. J. (eds.): *Refractive Corneal Surgery*. Thoroughfare, N.J.: Slack Inc., 1985, p 17.

28. Eisner, G.: Eye Surgery: An Introduction to Operative Technique. Berlin, Springer-Verlag, 1980.

29. Hoffer, K. J., Darrin, J. J., Petit, T. H., et al.: Three years' experience with radial keratotomy: The UCLA study. Ophthalmology, 90:627, 1983.

30. Neumann, A. C., Osher, R. H., Fenzl, R. E.: Radial keratotomy: A comprehensive evaluation. Doc. Ophthalmol., 56:275, 1984.

31. Rowsey, J. J., Balyeat, H. D.: Radial keratotomy: Preliminary report of complications. Ophthalmic Surg., 13:27, 1982.

32. Rowsey, J. J., Hays, J. C.: Recent Advances in Ophthalmology, Radial Keratotomy, Vol. 7. Edinburgh, Churchill Livingstone, 1985.

33. Davis, R. M., Miller, R. A., Lindstrom, R. L., et al.: Corneal iron lines after radial keratotomy. J. Refractive Surg., 2:174, 1986.

11

GLAUCOMA SURGERY

by George L. Spaeth

FUNDAMENTAL PRINCIPLES OF GLAUCOMA SURGERY

The fundamental principles that apply to other surgical procedures also hold true for glaucoma. The success of the procedure is di-

rectly proportional to accuracy of preoperative diagnosis, appropriateness of the operative procedure, competence during the preoperative, operative, and postoperative periods, and ability of the surgeon to prevent, recognize, and correct, so far as possible, everything tending to divert the clinical course away from the desired conclusion. These principles have been considered in detail in the introductory chapter of this text.

---

*Laser iridotomy is considered separately later in this chapter.

In at least one important aspect, however, surgery on the eye of the glaucomatous patient is different from most other types of surgery, even ophthalmic surgery. With most conditions the patient who needs surgery knows that he has an abnormality. He has something noticeably "wrong": a pain, a mass indicating the presence of a tumor, or poor sight. Such is not ordinarily the case with the glaucoma patient, especially in the early stages of the disease, when surgery offers the best chance of a successful result. The patient with unrecognized glaucoma is often asymptomatic. Even a patient who has already been told that he has glaucoma may feel completely normal. He usually believes that he "sees just fine." Unlike most patients with a significant disease process, the glaucoma patient often comes to the doctor thinking he is well, only to be told that he is sick.

It is helpful if the surgeon can explain to the patient the findings that led to the diagnostic conclusion. Only after the surgeon has demonstrated charts documenting progressive loss of visual field, or has explained the nature and significance of a closed anterior chamber angle, can the patient start to understand the need for treatment. Consider the dilemma facing the patient who is told that the recommended surgery will probably make his vision worse and will not be curative, but will, at best, merely control the glaucoma. Under such circumstances the physician's and the patient's goals demand precise definition, full expression, and thorough discussion (Fig. 11–1). The patient must understand that he is already in trouble: the decision involves balancing *risk against risk and risk against benefit* (Table 11–1). In the patient with glaucoma, risk cannot be avoided. The possibility of short-term loss is usually balanced against long-term gain. The definitions of loss and gain are different for every patient. The decisions as to whether, when, and how to treat must be made only after the different factors that characterize the totality of the event have been scientifically and compassionately considered. Such consideration demands an understanding of the nature of the patient, the character of his disease, and the unique interaction of these two factors over a period of time. This becomes increasingly difficult in a DRG (diagnosis-related group) society, in which patients can easily become code numbers. It also requires the ability to communicate disturbing information in such a way that the patient is reassured rather than frightened. Most patients are scared of the unknown; once they know that

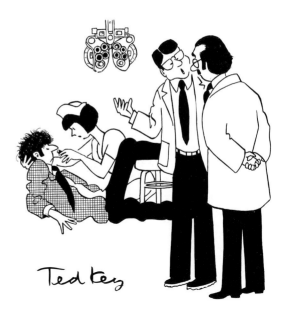

"HE THOUGHT HE JUST NEEDED NEW GLASSES, BUT WAS HE SURPRISED WHEN I TOLD HIM HE NEEDED SURGERY FOR GLAUCOMA!"

FIGURE 11–1. The perceptions and goals of the patient may differ from those of the physician. Communication between the two must be truthful, expressive, and sensitive.

their doctor understands what is wrong and will guide them through the hazardous waters of illness with skill and consistency, their anxiety usually disappears. The tone in which words are said is probably more important than the specific meanings of the words that are said.

Medical vs. Surgical Care

There are many types of glaucoma; it would be surprising if the same therapeutic principles could be applied to all. Even when considering the same type of glaucoma, there is still controversy regarding the best mode of treatment. This is partially due to incomplete knowledge about the natural history of glaucoma. The variance in the degree of competence that different physicians have in using medical and surgical modes of therapy is another factor; some are better with drugs and others, with surgery. Still other considerations are the philosophical approaches of both the ophthalmologist and the patient; some have a medical bent and others, a surgical.

In a few types of glaucoma, surgery is the treatment of choice (Table 11–2). Congenital

TABLE 11–1. Risks Versus Benefits of Glaucoma Surgery*

Immediate Purposes of Surgery

Preserve or enhance patient's quality of life	All cases
Control intraocular pressure	Most cases
Correct anterior chamber angle	Some cases
Correct anterior chamber angle and control pressure	Few cases

RISKS AND BENEFITS	INCIDENCE
A. *Trabeculectomy*	
Risks	
Immediate risks	
Sudden, permanent loss of central vision in otherwise uncomplicated procedure	5% of cases in which visual field loss has advanced into fixation; 2% of cases in which field loss is advanced and impinges on but does not involve fixation; very rare in others
Infection	Very rare, less than 0.1%
"Malignant glaucoma" (high pressure with collapse of anterior chamber)	Rare except in a few predisposed cases
Serious bleeding inside the eye	2% of cases with advanced disease
Excessive filtration with flat anterior chamber	10%
Need for second surgery related to the first	10%
Technical problem (tear of conjunctiva, etc.)	5%
Droopy lid (temporary)	Common (occasionally permanent)
Severe blurring of vision for weeks	Usual
Late risks	
Progression of glaucoma	15%
Progression of preexisting cataract	Usual
Droopy lid	Rare
Infection	Rare: less than 0.1%, though more frequent with full-thickness filtration procedures
Benefits	
Increased likelihood of maintaining vision	90%
No further progression of glaucoma	80%
Less need for medicines	80%
No need for medicines	40%
Improved vision	30%
B. *Surgical Iridectomy*	
Risks	
Immediate risks	
Decreased vision for 2 weeks	Usual
Technical problem (need for additional suture, etc.)	5%
Serious bleeding	Less than 1%
Infection	Less than 0.1%
"Malignant glaucoma"	Very rare
Late risks	
Progression of preexisting cataract	15%
Recurrent closure of angle	1%
Development of other type of glaucoma	5%
Continuing need for medication	(Depends on preoperative condition)
Benefits	
Eliminates future attacks of angle-closure glaucoma	95%
Returns anterior chamber angle toward normal	95%
Prevents "creeping angle closure"	90%
Reduces need for medicine	40%
Eliminates need for medicine	10%

glaucoma, acute primary angle-closure glaucoma, and progressive primary open-angle glaucoma are examples, and surgery should not be considered a "last resort" in these conditions. On the other hand, there are entities, such as neovascular glaucoma, in which the results of surgery are generally so poor that medical therapy is clearly preferable where feasible (Table 11–2; see also Tables 11–11 and 11–13).

Goals of Surgery in Glaucoma

The usual purpose for performing glaucoma surgery is to preserve or restore sight (Table 11–3). The major cause for reduced visual ability in patients with glaucoma is damage to the optic nerve. Although other conditions may be present, such as corneal edema and cataract, vision lost from these peripheral

TABLE 11–1. Risks Versus Benefits of Glaucoma Surgery* *Continued*

RISKS AND BENEFITS	INCIDENCE
B1. *Laser Iridotomy*	
Risks	
Immediate risks	
Rise of intraocular pressure	Frequent
Transient blurred vision	Usual
Bleeding of significance	Very rare
Inflammation	Very rare
Retinal burn	Very rare
Late risks	
Progressive cataract	15%
Closure of iridotomy	5%
Recurrent angle closure	5%
Development of other type of glaucoma	5%
Continuing need for medications (depends on preoperative condition)	(Variable)
Benefits	
Eliminates future attacks of angle-closure glaucoma	90%
Returns anterior chamber angle toward normal	95%
Prevents "creeping angle closure"	90%
Reduces need for medicine	20%
Eliminates need for medicine	10%
C. *Combined Cataract-Glaucoma Surgery*	
Risks	
Immediate risks	
Sudden, permanent reduction of vision	5%
Temporary reduction of vision	90%
Slow recovery of vision (6 months)	20%
Need for second surgery related to first	10%
Retinal edema	20%
As per trabeculectomy	
Late risks	
Retinal edema	5%
Trouble with intraocular lens	5%
Failure of pressure control	15%
As per trabeculectomy	
Benefits	
Improvement in visual function	90%
As per trabeculectomy	
D. *Cataract Extraction Following Filtration Procedure*	
Risks	
Immediate risks	
Infection or serious bleeding	Very rare, less than 0.1%
Need for second operation related to first	1%
Temporary reduction of vision	80%
Late risks	
Retinal edema and poor recovery of vision	3%
Trouble with intraocular lens	3%
Need for capsulotomy (laser)	30%
Benefits	
Improved visual function	95%

*Estimates of frequency are rough approximations based on my experience.

causes can usually be recovered. Thus *the physician's primary goal in caring for patients with glaucoma is to preserve the health of the optic nerve, and at the same time consider the well-being of the whole eye and the whole patient.*

There are two major ways to preserve or restore the visual ability of the patient with glaucoma: (1) *lowering intraocular pressure* and (2) *preventing a sudden rise of intraocular pressure.* The first method is usually achieved by correcting or circumventing blocked outflow of aqueous humor from the eye. Such blockage is the usual cause for elevated intraocular pressure, regardless of the type of glaucoma. The second technique usually involves restoration of the eye to a more normal anatomical state;

TABLE 11–2. Advisability of Surgical Treatment in Selected Types of Glaucoma

CONDITION	USUAL PROCEDURE OF CHOICE	ALTERNATIVE PROCEDURE
Surgery Almost Always Required		
Congenital glaucoma	Goniotomy	Trabeculotomy
Phakolytic glaucoma	Cataract extraction	
Acute primary angle-closure glaucoma	Peripheral iridectomy*	Trabeculectomy with tightly sutured scleral flap
Pupillary block glaucomas	Peripheral iridectomy*	Synechialysis
Fellow eye of patient with primary angle-closure glaucoma	Peripheral iridectomy*	
Progressive primary open-angle glaucoma	Trabeculectomy or laser trabeculoplasty	Laser trabeculoplasty or standard filtering procedure
Glaucoma with 8-ball hemorrhage	Removal of clot	
Glaucoma with intraocular tumor	Enucleation	Irradiation
Failed filtration surgery	Filtering procedure with 5-FU Molteno implant	Nd:YAG cyclophotocoagulation
Surgery Often Required		
Asymptomatic narrow anterior chamber angle	Peripheral iridectomy*	
Primary open-angle glaucoma (and its variants: pigmentary glaucoma, glaucoma with exfoliation syndrome, etc.)	Laser trabeculoplasty or trabeculectomy†	Standard filtering procedure, or trabeculotomy
Chronic primary angle-closure glaucoma	Trabeculectomy with tightly sutured scleral flap	Peripheral iridectomy* or synechialysis (chamber deepening)
Glaucoma owing to posterior misdirection of aqueous humor	Vitrectomy	Transpupillary rupture of vitreous or lens extraction with vitrectomy
Secondary angle-closure glaucoma	Iridectomy*	
Noninflammatory secondary angle-closure glaucomas (Chandler's syndrome, etc.)	Trabeculectomy	Cyclodialysis
Inflammatory secondary angle-closure glaucomas	Molteno implant	Nd:YAG cyclophotocoagulation
Developmental glaucomas other than congenital	Trabeculectomy	Standard filtering procedures
Glaucomatocyclitic crisis	Trabeculectomy	Standard filtering procedures
Glaucoma in aphakic patients	Trabeculectomy or nd:YAG cyclophotocoagulation	Molteno implant or cyclocryotherapy
Angle-cleavage glaucoma in quiet eye	Trabeculectomy	Standard filtering procedures
Glaucoma with traumatic hyphema	Drainage of blood	Drainage with trabeculectomy
Surgery Usually to Be Avoided But Not Contraindicated		
Aniridia	Trabeculectomy	Goniotomy
Uveitic glaucomas	Trabeculotomy	Anterior trabeculectomy
Neovascular glaucoma	Molteno implant or nd:YAG cyclophotocoagulation	Peripheral iridectomy with thermal sclerostomy or anterior trabeculectomy or cyclocryotherapy
Glaucoma with Sturge-Weber syndrome	Anterior trabeculectomy	Goniotomy in infants
Glaucoma secondary to scleritis or episcleritis	None good	Filtering procedure or nd:YAG
Ocular hypertension	Trabeculectomy	
Surgery Rarely Advisable		
Nanophthalmos	None good: occasionally laser iridotomy	Nd:YAG cyclophotocoagulation or cyclocryotherapy
Blind painful eye	Retrobulbar alcohol or enucleation	Evisceration

*Laser iridotomy is usually preferred over surgical iridectomy. (See Tables 11–19 and 11–37.)

†Laser trabeculoplasty is the procedure of choice for some cases of primary open-angle glaucoma. (See p. 330.)

the effect of peripheral iridectomy on the patient with narrow anterior chamber angles is an example.

A third goal in occasional patients is the relief of pain. Comfort usually follows restoration of pressure to a satisfactory level. In occasional cases in which the visual ability of the eye is so poor that it is no longer of benefit to the patient, the surgeon may choose to perform surgery solely to relieve discomfort. Because every glaucoma procedure that requires penetrating surgery has been associated with sympathetic ophthalmia, the usual treatment for such painful blind eyes is enucleation or evisceration (Table

TABLE 11–3. Goals in Glaucoma Surgery

PRIMARY GOAL (Improve Quality of Life)
1. Preserve or restore visual ability
   a. Maintain health of the optic nerve
   b. Avoid or correct other ocular abnormality

SECONDARY GOAL
2. Lower intraocular pressure
   a. Lower mean intraocular pressure*
   b. Eliminate intraocular pressure spikes
3. Correct abnormal structure†
   a. Narrow or closed anterior chamber angle
4. Relieve pain
5. Avoid or correct complications, such as:
   a. Flat anterior chamber
   b. Hypotony
   c. Bleeding
   d. Failure to filter
   e. Malignant glaucoma
   f. Cataract
   g. Cystic bleb

*The amount of intraocular pressure–lowering will vary from patient to patient.

†Other abnormal structures that need correction are pupillary block, dislocated lens, hypermature cataract, etc.

11–4). In some cases a retrobulbar injection of alcohol may be adequate (see p. 321). Cyclocryotherapy has been advised as a way to provide relief of pain and allow retention of the globe. If cyclocryotherapy is elected, it should preferably be combined with a retrobulbar injection of 100% alcohol.

The fourth goal of the surgeon is to avoid or correct complications. For example, the surgeon may want to perform surgery so that a high cystic bleb will be avoided, or to remedy an eye in which a complication is already present, such as a ruptured bleb.

It is essential that the surgeon realize that there is usually a series of goals to be accomplished in performing surgery. Furthermore, these goals are often quite independent of one another, and in some circumstances surgical decisions are complicated by the fact that the goals are mutually exclusive. For example, the surgeon may set as his primary goal marked lowering of intraocular pressure. But in order

TABLE 11–4. Glaucoma Procedures Known to Have Sympathetic Ophthalmia As a Complication

Iridencleisis
Iridectomy
Trephination
Sclerectomy
Thermal sclerostomy
Trabeculectomy
Cyclodialysis
Cyclodiathermy

to accomplish this he will need to develop a large fistula, which will lead to the development of a large cystic bleb. He may want to avoid creating a cystic bleb because the patient has another condition that would make such a bleb undesirable, such as a severe chronic blepharitis or the need to wear a contact lens.

Another example of conflicting goals would be the case of a 70-year-old patient with chronic angle-closure glaucoma, moderate damage to the optic nerve, and an immature cataract. In such a case the surgeon will want to lower intraocular pressure, correct the abnormal structure, and avoid the development of a progressive cataract. A trabeculectomy with a peripheral iridectomy would probably accomplish the first of these goals, but would predispose the patient to progressive development of cataracts. A surgical peripheral iridectomy would accomplish only the second goal—correction of the abnormal structure—but would not be expected to lower intraocular pressure or eliminate the surgical trauma leading to progressive cataract. A laser iridectomy might accomplish the latter two goals—specifically, correct the abnormal structure and avoid a procedure that would predispose to progressive cataract.

In considering every case the surgeon must assess the risks and benefits (Table 11–1), define all goals, and decide their priority (Table 11–3). *He must also be sure that his objectives and those of the patient coincide* (Fig. 11–1).

Surgical Anatomy

Accurate understanding of the anatomy of the limbal area is essential for the performance of correct glaucoma surgery. Important anatomical features are shown in Figures 9–1, 11–2, 11–3, and 17–1.[1–5]

An important landmark in glaucoma surgery is the corneoscleral sulcus. This groove results from the difference between the radius of curvature of the scleral shell and that of the cornea. Where these two curves meet a pronounced groove is formed. Because of the overlying conjunctiva this groove may not always be readily apparent until the conjunctiva has been reflected. This corneoscleral sulcus is of importance for two reasons. First, the conjunctiva usually terminates just anterior to this position; hence a limbus-based conjunctival flap cannot usually be dissected anterior to this point. Second, in most emmetropic eyes the corneoscleral sulcus usually lies anterior to the iris root; consequently a perpendicular incision made just

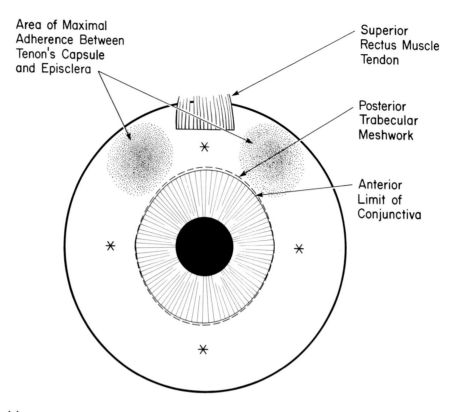

Area of Maximal Adherence Between Tenon's Capsule and Episclera

Superior Rectus Muscle Tendon

Posterior Trabecular Meshwork

Anterior Limit of Conjunctiva

✳ Approximate position at which anterior ciliary vessels penetrate sclera

FIGURE 11–2. Surgeon's view of the eye, showing points of major anatomical importance (see also Fig. 17–1).

posterior to the corneoscleral sulcus will ordinarily enter the anterior chamber. This is an important consideration, since most glaucoma procedures require an incision into the anterior chamber. If the incision does not enter the anterior chamber, but is mistakenly made into the posterior chamber or over the ciliary body, the operation will fail.

The positions of the iris insertion and the scleral spur in relation to the corneoscleral sulcus vary from eye to eye. They tend to be more anteriorly placed in patients with hyper-

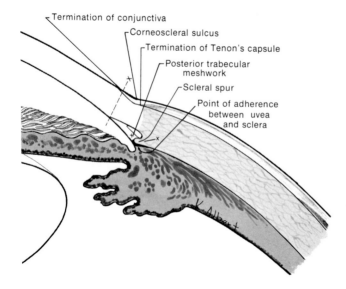

Termination of conjunctiva
Corneoscleral sulcus
Termination of Tenon's capsule
Posterior trabecular meshwork
Scleral spur
Point of adherence between uvea and sclera

K. Albert

FIGURE 11–3. Schematic cross section of limbal area at 12 o'clock position on the globe. The corneoscleral groove (sulcus), a landmark of paramount importance, is located posterior to the termination of conjunctiva and just anterior to termination of Tenon's capsule. A perpendicular incision (dashed line) at the corneoscleral sulcus should usually enter the anterior chamber just anterior to Schlemm's canal. Normally the uvea is adherent to the anterior uvea in only one area, a narrow ring just at the scleral spur. See also Figures 9–1 and 17–1.

opia and primary angle-closure glaucoma, especially when peripheral anterior synechias are present. In contrast, they are usually more posteriorly placed in myopes and in patients with congenital glaucoma. The relation between internal landmarks and the surgical limbus is even more variable, since the conjunctiva may terminate posterior to, at, or anterior to the corneoscleral sulcus.

Because external and internal landmarks do not correspond exactly, the surgeon should consciously inspect the eye before making an incision; he does this to determine where and how to make his incision so that he is sure to enter the anterior chamber. Usually the position of the iris root can be ascertained by simple inspection. Some surgeons recommend transillumination to help establish the actual location of the most peripheral portion of the angle recess. This technique works beautifully, but it is seldom necessary.

The position of the posterior trabecular meshwork and the point of adherence of the iris to the inner surface of the globe are two important considerations. Accurate determination of these landmarks may require gonioscopy before surgery. During surgery it may be necessary to repeat the gonioscopy if the surgeon needs to determine the exact position of the trabecular area, as is the case in goniotomy and trabeculotomy.

If the surgeon wants to avoid the trabecular area entirely, as he may want to do in performing an iridectomy, he must either make a perpendicular incision anterior to the corneoscleral sulcus or shelve the incision markedly anteriorly, as would be done in using a keratome.

The posterior trabecular meshwork and Schlemm's canal are, of course, anterior to the point at which the ciliary body adheres to the scleral spur. It is thus possible to excise trabecular meshwork without performing a cyclodialysis (without separating the ciliary body from the scleral spur) (Fig. 11–3).

Figures 9–1 and 11–2 show the difference in curvature between the line along which the conjunctiva blends into the anterior cornea, and that of the posterior trabecular meshwork. Because the latter has a steeper curve than the former, the area separating these two differs, depending on what point on the globe is being examined. For example, at the 12 o'clock position on the limbus the conjunctival termination is usually around 2 mm anterior to the posterior trabecular meshwork. In contrast, at the 3 and 9 o'clock positions it is less than 1 mm anterior to the posterior trabecular meshwork. There-

fore, it is difficult at the 3 and 9 o'clock positions to make an incision that is posterior to the surgical limbus and that the surgeon knows will enter the anterior chamber. It is even harder to be sure that such an incision will enter anterior to the posterior trabecular meshwork. The more eccentrically and the more perpendicularly the surgeon places his incision, the more likely that ciliary body will be found at its base.

Figure 11–3 shows the usual anterior termination of Tenon's capsule and episclera. This is ordinarily posterior to the point at which the conjunctiva inserts into the cornea. Consequently, by continuing the dissection of a limbus-based flap anteriorly, a flap can be developed that consists only of conjunctiva.

Tenon's capsule is most adherent to the episclera at the 10:30 and 1:30 positions on the globe.

The surgeon should be aware of the position of the termination of Descemet's membrane, the anterior and the posterior trabecular meshwork, the iris root, and the major arterial iris circle; the point of penetration of the anterior ciliary vessels in relation to both the limbus (Fig. 11–2) and the four rectus muscles (Fig. 11–3); and the point at which the ciliary body is adherent to the scleral spur (Fig. 11–2). It is important to recall that the anterior uvea is normally adherent to the overlying sclera only at the point at which the scleral spur and the ciliary body come in contact. Elsewhere there is no adherence between these tissues. The implications of this are important. For example, it is possible to excise posterior trabecular meshwork without unroofing the ciliary body. Furthermore, in order to perform a cyclodialysis one need make the incision only a very short distance posterior to the position of the scleral spur.

It is helpful to recall that the transition from the opaque white of the sclera to the clear gray of the cornea occurs more anteriorly (that is, closer to the corneoscleral sulcus) in both the most superficial and the deepest layers of the globe. Thus the relation of Schlemm's canal and the posterior trabecular meshwork to the transition between the opaque sclera and the clear cornea will vary, depending on the depth of the scleral flap. On the surface a line dropped perpendicularly from the area of the transition will usually pass anterior to Schlemm's canal. Approximately half the way through the sclera a similar line would catch the posterior edge of Schlemm's canal (Fig. 11–3).

Incisions need to be made differently, depending on the surgeon's intent and the position of the incision on the globe. For example, let us consider the incisions at 12 o'clock. A perpendicular incision for a peripheral iridectomy should be placed at or anterior to the termination of the conjunctiva. A shelved keratome incision for iridectomy should be started 1 mm posterior to the corneoscleral sulcus. The incision for a thermal sclerostomy or an anterior-lip sclerectomy cannot be correctly placed unless the conjunctiva is dissected to its anteriormost position on the globe; the incision should then be made approximately 1 mm posterior to the point of anterior dissection. If the surgeon chooses a trephine larger than 1 mm in diameter and wants to avoid the ciliary body, he may have to split the cornea slightly in order to be sure that the trephine is placed anteriorly enough. After having made a half-thickness scleral flap, the surgeon is most likely to find Schlemm's canal immediately anterior to the point of transition from the white sclera to the clear cornea. For the ciliary body to be frozen by performing a cyclocryotherapy, the tip should be placed about 2 mm posterior to the corneoscleral sulcus.

The surgeon should be familiar with the anatomical relation between conjunctiva, Tenon's capsule, and episclera. These are discussed in detail in the subsections dealing with the development of conjunctival flaps (Fig. 11–41, p. 266).

Definition of Glaucoma

Glaucoma is a group of conditions unified by a final common pathway: *damage to the optic nerve related to intraocular pressure higher than the optic nerve can tolerate*. The damage to the optic nerve manifests itself in different patterns, depending on the mechanisms of damage and the underlying physical makeup of the patient. The three classic signs of glaucoma are (1) elevation of intraocular pressure, (2) cupping and pallor of the optic disc, and (3) loss of visual field.

Pathogenesis of Optic Nerve Damage in Glaucoma

Intraocular pressure higher than the eye can tolerate is the most important of the many factors that contribute to the development of optic nerve damage in patients with glaucoma (Table 11–5).[6–10] The validity of this concept has been the cornerstone on which the entire management plan of glaucoma patients has been

TABLE 11–5. Factors That Influence Development of Glaucomatous Nerve Damage

I. Structural (ability of optic nerve to resist pressure damage)
  A. Heredity
  B. Race
  C. Myopia
  D. Preexisting damage to optic nerve (glaucomatous or other)
  E. Increasing age?
II. Acquired
  A. Direct effect of elevated intraocular pressure on neuron or supporting tissues
  B. Local factors
    1. Elevated episcleral venous pressure
    2. Vascular insufficiency or anomaly
    3. Vasospasm
  C. Systemic factors
    1. Cardiovascular
      a. Anemia
      b. Other factors that cause diminished oxygen-carrying capacity of blood
      c. Hypotension
      d. Low cardiac output
      e. Sedentary life-style
      f. Hematologic disorders associated with hyperviscosity
      g. Elevated episcleral venous pressure
      h. Vascular anomalies
    2. Metabolic
      a. Obesity
      b. Diabetes mellitus
      c. Vitamin deficiency
      d. Other
III. Behavioral
  A. Ability to manage one's life
  B. Ability to act in one's own best interest
  C. Accessibility to care
IV. Time*

*The duration of action and the degree of abnormality of the risk factor are of major importance. Thus a mild elevation of intraocular pressure acting for many years, or a severe elevation of intraocular pressure acting only for a few months, will both cause damage.

built during the past hundred years. The existence of other factors that also contribute to optic nerve damage and the marked individual variability of response to intraocular pressure must not obscure this fundamental concept, which still is the basis of treatment for glaucoma today (Figs. 11–4 and 11–5).[10–35]

If intraocular pressure higher than the eye can tolerate is the primary factor responsible for glaucomatous damage, then it would seem possible to study populations statistically, determine what is "normal intraocular pressure," and set a figure above which patients would develop damage. This concept has for many years been assumed to be valid. However, it is not.[6, 10, 35, 36] Populations can be studied and *average* intraocular pressure determined (Fig. 11–7). Indeed this has been done, and average intraocular pressure found to be about 15 to 16

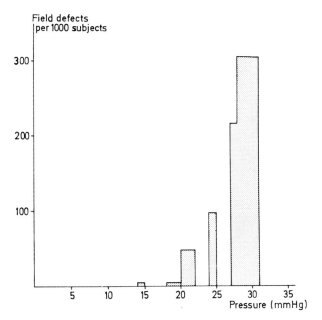

FIGURE 11–4. Frequency of glaucomatous optic nerve damage as manifested as a field defect in relation to intraocular pressure. There is a marked increase with rising pressure. (From Graham, P.: Epidemiology of chronic glaucoma. *In* Heilmann, K., Richardson, K. T. (eds.): Glaucoma: Conceptions of a Disease. Stuttgart, Georg Thieme, 1978.)

mm Hg, showing a slight rise with increasing age, especially in females. The standard deviation is about 3 mm Hg, suggesting that 95 per cent of the population would be expected to have intraocular pressures ranging between 10 and 21 mm Hg. Thus, statistically speaking, people with intraocular pressure above 21 mm Hg would be expected to be sufficiently different from normal that they are abnormal. In fact, they are abnormal in the sense of not being

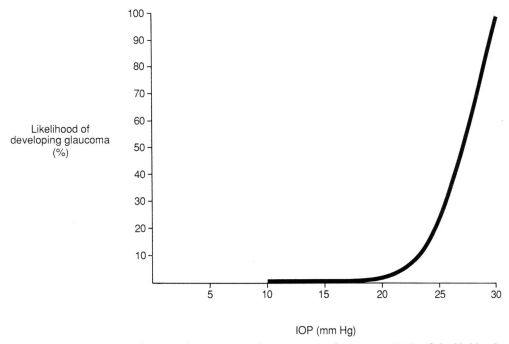

FIGURE 11–5. Hypothetical curve indicating relation between intraocular pressure (IOP) and the likelihood of development of glaucomatous nerve damage. The exact position of the curve of the abscissa is not certain; it should perhaps be displaced to the right or to the left. However, it is certain that the likelihood of developing glaucomatous damage increases greatly with increasing intraocular pressure, probably in a logarithmic manner. This particular hypothetical curve suggests that optic nerve damage can be anticipated in about 50 per cent of all people with intraocular pressure persistently above 27 mm Hg and in almost all people in whom intraocular pressure remains above 30 mm Hg.

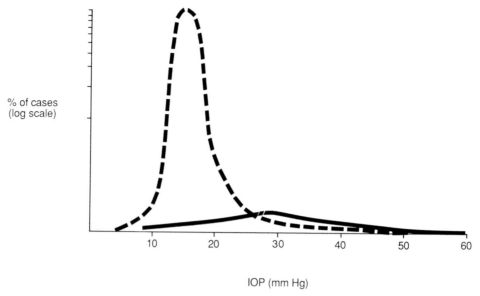

% of cases
(log scale)

IOP (mm Hg)

FIGURE 11–6. Distribution of intraocular pressure (IOP) in a large population including patients with and without glaucoma. Those with glaucoma are included in the lower curve.

average, but they are not necessarily abnormal in the sense of being diseased.

Careful examination of the curve of intraocular pressures shows a preponderance of people with elevated intraocular pressures. That is, the normal curve is skewed to the right (Fig. 11–7). What is relatively new information is the knowledge that has come from long-term studies that established that only a relatively small proportion of people with so-called elevated intraocular pressure, that is, intraocular pres-

sure above 21 mm Hg, actually develop glaucomatous damage.[3, 6, 34, 36–39] Although the precise figure is still unknown, it appears that only about 5 per cent to 10 per cent of those with intraocular pressures above 21 mm Hg will in fact ever develop "glaucoma," that is, glaucomatous damage to the optic nerve.[40] In the first place, the vast majority of people with intraocular pressures above 21 mm Hg have intraocular pressures that range between 21 and 24 mm Hg. Thus they are within three standard devia-

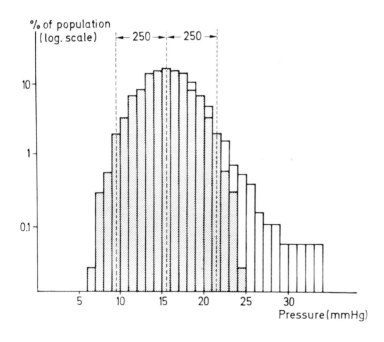

FIGURE 11–7. Distribution of intraocular pressures in population aged 40 to 75 years living in Ferndale, Wales, showing an excess of high intraocular pressures. A standard distribution is shown in the shaded bars. (From Graham, P.: Epidemiology of chronic glaucoma. *In* Heilmann, K., Richardson, K. T. (eds.): Glaucoma: Conceptions of a Disease. Stuttgart, Georg Thieme, 1978.)

tions of normal; it is not surprising that many such people would not have deterioration of the optic nerve. But even those with intraocular pressures above 24 mm Hg will not always develop damage. However, these patients are at much greater risk, and the higher their intraocular pressures, the more likely they are to develop glaucomatous nerve damage. Clearly, factors other than intraocular pressure determine who will develop glaucomatous disease. *Within the range of 10 to 40 mm Hg, the level of intraocular pressure per se cannot be used as a measure of presence or absence of disease.*

It appears that 27 mm Hg is a watershed line; most people with intraocular pressure consistently above 27 mm Hg can be expected eventually to develop glaucomatous nerve damage unless intraocular pressure is effectively lowered (Fig. 11–5).[40] Saying this, however, is not the same as saying that all patients with intraocular pressure above 27 mm Hg should be treated or that those with intraocular pressure below 27 mm Hg should not be treated. The decision whether or not to treat must be based on many factors other than intraocular pressure (these factors are discussed later in this chapter).

An additional and vitally important piece of information that must be considered in the pathogenesis of optic nerve damage in glaucoma is the frequency with which individuals with "low" intraocular pressures develop damage. Although the existence of "low-tension glaucoma" has been known for more than a hundred years, it has generally been considered to be rare. This assumption is wrong.[6, 10, 35] If an intraocular pressure two standard deviations above the mean is taken as the dividing line between "normal" and "elevated" intraocular pressures—specifically 21 mm Hg—then one-third of patients with glaucomatous nerve damage will fall in the group who have "normal" intraocular pressures (Fig. 11–8).[6] Obviously, a "normal" intraocular pressure does *not* guarantee safety from glaucoma.

In summary, then, when we recall that less than 10 per cent of people with intraocular pressures above 21 mm Hg develop glaucomatous damage and that about one-third of all people who actually have glaucomatous damage have intraocular pressures below 21 mm Hg, we see that arbitrary levels of intraocular pressure cannot be taken as adequate definitions of the presence or absence of glaucoma.

Other factors that may adversely affect the optic nerve include those listed in Table 11–5.

A simplified schema of the pathogenesis of nerve damage in glaucoma is shown in Figure 11–9. This stresses the role of intraocular pressure, which itself causes or exacerbates structural damage and predisposes to vascular insufficiency (see left and middle columns of figure).

Can it be said that progressive, glaucomatous-appearing damage to the optic nerve proves that intraocular pressure is too high, and that adequate lowering of the pressure would cause the progressive damage to cease? This question still cannot be answered. However, with important qualifications the answer that best serves patients is yes. That is, we should probably assume that *if the intraocular pressure is*

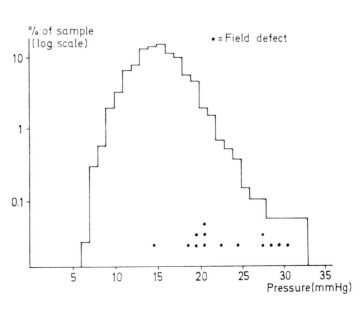

FIGURE 11–8. Newly discovered field defects in relation to intraocular pressure in the Ferndale (Wales) population (data of Graham and Hollows). Of the 14 patients with glaucomatous nerve damage, 7 had intraocular pressure below 22 mm Hg. (From Graham, P.: Epidemiology of chronic glaucoma. *In* Heilmann, K., Richardson, K. T. (eds.): Glaucoma: Conceptions of a Disease. Stuttgart, Georg Thieme, 1978.)

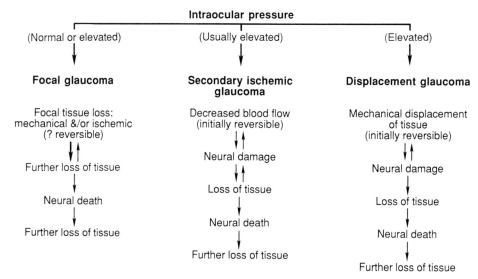

FIGURE 11–9. Simplified schema of the pathogenesis of optic nerve damage in glaucoma, stressing the roles of mechanical distortion of the optic nerve (displacement glaucoma) and ischemia, both caused by increased intraocular pressure.

adequately lowered, glaucomatous damage will no longer occur. Several caveats must be added to this statement (Table 11–6). In the first place, there will be instances in which the neurons have been so badly damaged by the glaucomatous process that even if intraocular pressure is lowered to a point that would previously have allowed preservation of the health of the neurons, such mortally damaged neurons will continue to deteriorate. Furthermore, associated factors may overwhelm the therapeutic benefit of lowering intraocular pressure. For example, lowering the intraocular pressure to 10 mm Hg may be adequate to preserve the health of the nerve in a person with definite glaucomatous nerve damage, but when trauma to the nerve is added because of an associated chiasmal tumor, glaucoma-like damage may continue. It is thus vitally important for the physician to be reasonably certain that causes other than intraocular pressure are not responsible for progressive nerve damage that mimics glaucoma.

TABLE 11–6. Causes for Progressive Optic Nerve Damage in the Patient Thought to Have Glaucoma

1. So much distortion of the optic nerve structure and so much damage to the optic neurons that the neurons are "mortally wounded"

2. A condition other than glaucoma

3. Intraocular pressure higher than the affected eye can tolerate

Anesthesia

The overwhelming majority of glaucoma procedures are best performed under local or topical anesthesia with an anesthetist in attendance. The reasons for this preference are listed in Table 11–7. In most cases sedation should be minimal or mild. The patient who understands what is to be done and has confidence in the surgeon may not need *any* systemic sedation. Especially in the elderly, who constitute a large percentage of patients who require glaucoma surgery, it is advisable to keep sedation as light as possible. Clearly the patient should not be overly anxious, apprehensive, or uncomfortable. Diazepam in small doses (4–6 mg) administered intravenously immediately before the onset of surgery provides sedation that can be accurately controlled and is usually well tolerated. In cases in which analgesia is also required, a narcotic agent may need to be added.

A retrobulbar injection is definitely not required in all cases. Under certain circumstances it is preferable to avoid this potentially complicating procedure and perform surgery using topical anesthesia alone (Tables 11–7 and 11–8). Proparacaine, 0.5%, is a suitable agent, and should be instilled in the eye every 30 seconds for 5 minutes before draping the patient, and again every 30 seconds for 2 minutes after preparation of the patient. Tetracaine and other agents may be used, but they are more likely to cause desquamation of the epithelium.

TABLE 11–7. Preferred Anesthesia for Glaucoma Procedures

LOCAL

Rapid mobilization
   Allows hyphema to settle inferiorly
   More rapid recuperation of patient
Less traumatic to patient
Permits use of oral osmotic agents preoperatively
Assures minimal chance of hypotensive or hypertensive
   episode
Minimizes untoward reactions to anesthetic agents
Eliminates need to catheterize patient when mannitol is
   used
Facilitates postoperative evaluation
Less expensive than general anesthesia
Less time-consuming than general anesthesia
Less personnel required than with general anesthesia
Facilitates discharge on same day as surgery

TOPICAL

Eliminates need for retrobulbar block
Eliminates possibility of retrobulbar hemorrhage
Allows maintenance of small pupil
Same advantages as for local anesthesia

GENERAL

Eliminates need for retrobulbar block
Assures most complete comfort of patient
Assures most complete and long-lasting patient
   cooperation
Assures most complete elimination of "positive-pressure
   eye"
Is usually required for infants and children, or retarded,
   senile, or psychotic patients

There are circumstances in which general anesthesia is preferred (Tables 11–7 and 11–8). For example, a retrobulbar block is inadvisable when repairing a wound dehiscence or when spread of infection may be a concern.

In all cases in which general anesthesia is not used, akinesia of the facial nerve must be obtained. A modified O'Brien block is most suitable, and should provide total paralysis of the facial muscles on the side requiring surgery.

The duration of the procedure and of the desired anesthetic effect will determine which anesthetic agent is chosen (Table 11–8).

Factors That Influence Which Eye Should Have Surgery First

Many patients will need glaucoma surgery on both eyes. Guidelines for determining which eye should be operated on first in such cases are included in Table 11–9. In most cases the more badly damaged eye should have surgery first, the main reason being that in the event of a bad surgical result, it is preferable to have operated on the eye of less importance to the patient. Furthermore, the general response of the patient's eyes to surgery may be learned from the first eye, enhancing the chances for

TABLE 11–8. Preferred Type of Anesthesia*

PROCEDURE	ROUTE	PREFERRED AGENT FOR LOCAL ANESTHESIA
Iridotomy—laser	Topical	Proparacaine drops
Reformation of anterior chamber	Topical	Proparacaine drops
Iridotomy—surgical	Topical	Proparacaine drops + mepivacaine facial block
Paracentesis	Topical	Proparacaine drops with or without mepivacaine facial block
Laser trabeculoplasty	Topical	Proparacaine drops
Trabeculectomy	Local	Mepivacaine facial and retrobulbar block
Standard filtration procedure	Local	Mepivacaine facial and retrobulbar block
Trabeculotomy	Local	Mepivacaine facial and retrobulbar block
Goniotomy	Local	Lidocaine or mepivacaine facial and retrobulbar block
Cyclodialysis	Local	Lidocaine or mepivacaine facial and retrobulbar block
Anterior chamber reformation	Topical	Proparacaine drops
Anterior chamber reformation and drainage of choroidal detachment	General	Bupivacaine facial and retrobulbar block
Drainage of hemorrhagic choroidal detachment	General	Bupivacaine facial and retrobulbar block
Revision of bleb	Local	Bupivacaine facial and retrobulbar block
Repair of scleral dehiscence	General	Bupivacaine facial and retrobulbar block
Anterior segment reconstruction	General	Bupivacaine facial and retrobulbar block
Cyclocryotherapy	Local	Bupivacaine facial and retrobulbar block
Nd:YAG laser cyclophotocoagulation	Local	Bupivacaine retrobulbar block
Enucleation	Local or general	Bupivacaine facial and retrobulbar block
Combined cataract extraction with glaucoma procedure	Local or general	Bupivacaine or mepivacaine facial and retrobulbar block
Cataract extraction after prior glaucoma operation	Local or general	Mepivacaine facial and retrobulbar block

*Other considerations may take precedence, such as age or general health of patient.

TABLE 11–9. Factors That Influence Which Eye Should Have Surgery First

Surgery should usually be performed first on the eye with:
  Worse visual acuity
  More damaged optic nerve head
  Poorer control of intraocular pressure
  Better visual field if field loss extends to 5 degrees of fixation
  Less inflammation
  Better chance of success, if there is little likelihood that patient will permit operation on other eye

success in the second eye. An additional reason for doing the more severely damaged eye first is that such an eye will tolerate higher pressures less satisfactorily than a less damaged eye. If surgery needs to be delayed for any reason, the less damaged eye can probably tolerate delay better than can the more damaged eye. Furthermore, if carbonic anhydrase inhibitors are used preoperatively, they are best stopped postoperatively, which will almost certainly allow the pressure to rise, further jeopardizing the more badly damaged eye.

There are some exceptions to operating on the worse eye first. Some patients may not be agreeable to having surgery on both eyes. In such cases the eye with the better visual potential should usually have surgery first, for the better eye is more important to the patient. There are also patients who are not likely to permit the second eye to have surgery if there is a poor result in the first eye. In such cases the surgeon should also usually decide to do the better eye first, as it is that eye in which he is more likely to obtain a good result.

The second eye should have surgery as soon as the quality of the result on the first eye can be predicted with reasonable validity. This varies with the type of surgery performed (Table 11–10).

TABLE 11–10. Intraoperative Interval When Both Eyes Need Same or Similar Procedure*

PROCEDURE	INTERVAL
Surgical iridectomy	1 day
Trabeculectomy	5 days
Standard filtration procedure	7 days
Combined cataract extraction with glaucoma procedure	28 days
Goniotomy†	3 days
Trabeculotomy†	3 days
Laser iridotomy	2 weeks
Laser trabeculoplasty	2 months

*Assumes that first procedure was uncomplicated.
†Bilateral simultaneous surgery often justified with this procedure when used as therapy for congenital glaucoma.

Preoperative Care: Basic Principles

A few principles are applicable to almost every patient in whom glaucoma surgery is to be done. Ideally, the intraocular pressure should be between 15 and 30 mm Hg and should be in that range for several days before surgery. If the pressure is below 10 mm Hg, the surgical technique is complicated by the softness of the eye. If it is excessively high, there tends to be more bleeding at the time of the surgery; also, rapid decompression when the globe is entered may predispose to an expulsive hemorrhage. Although lowering the intraocular pressure before surgery will not eliminate this latter possibility, allowing time for the pressure to equilibrate at a lower level before opening the eye seems like a sensible goal.

Ideally, the eye should be as quiet as feasible. Inflammation at the time of surgery predisposes to excessive bleeding and increased scarring after surgery.

The urgency with which surgery needs to be performed is primarily related to the vulnerability of the optic nerve, coupled with the rapidity with which the optic nerve is deteriorating. The vulnerability of the nerve is a function of the amount of nerve damage already present and the likelihood that the factors responsible for the damage will continue to take their toll; of these, intraocular pressure in a range that will cause continuing harm is of most concern (Table 11–5).

The absolute level of pressure is less important than the proximity to the level of pressure that caused harm in the past. For example, consider an eye with a healthy disc and with intraocular pressures consistently around 35 mm Hg; when the current intraocular pressure is 35 mm Hg there is no urgency for surgery. On the other hand, take the person whose far-advanced cupping has occurred at an intraocular pressure of about 20 mm Hg, but who now has an intraocular pressure of 35 mm Hg; in this patient surgery is urgent.

The rapidity with which damage occurs must not be underestimated. Primary open-angle glaucoma is a chronic disease, and it may have been present for many years before causing severe visual loss. Nevertheless, when vulnerability is high—as it is when field loss starts involving fixation, and pressure is rising above the level that caused the damage in the past—*sight can deteriorate rapidly*, within days or even hours. Thus the urgency with which surgery should be performed must be carefully considered. A good general rule is "Once the need for surgery has been agreed upon by the physician and the patient, it should be performed as soon as it can reasonably be done."

Intraocular pressures above 40 mm Hg can produce damage to the eye other than merely optic nerve compression. Intraocular pressure in this highly elevated range may predispose to acute anterior ischemic optic neuropathy, retinal vein occlusion, or even retinal artery occlusion.

Other factors that influence the timing of surgery are listed in Table 11–11.

Long-acting cholinesterase inhibitors should be stopped at least 2 weeks before the performance of standard filtering procedures, trabeculectomy, or iridectomy. These "irreversible" parasympathomimetics predispose to increased bleeding at the time of surgery, increased postoperative inflammation, and shallow postoperative anterior chamber.* Furthermore, they make dilation of the pupil difficult in the postoperative period. It is prudent to stop all miotics, such as pilocarpine, far enough in advance of surgery that their short-term effects will have worn off (unfortunately the long-term effects of the medication on vascularity and pupil rigidity will still be operative). Carbonic anhydrase inhibitors and topical beta blockers should also theoretically be stopped long enough before surgery designed to produce a filtering wound

*Because of their effect on blood pseudocholinesterase, they also may lead to complications in general anesthesia.

that their effects will have worn off; this requires 6 to 12 hours for the carbonic anhydrase inhibitors and around 2 to 4 weeks for the beta blockers. These agents suppress aqueous formation, and thus, at least theoretically, may slow the rate of complete reformation of the anterior chamber and the flow of aqueous through the fistula. Because aqueous flow appears to be essential to the development of a functioning fistula, suppression of flow may tend to predispose to surgical failure.

In actual practice, however, surgery is being performed because the intraocular pressure is too high; therefore, the theoretical advantages of stopping pilocarpine, beta blockers, and the carbonic anhydrase inhibitors preoperatively are often of less concern than preventing further pressure damage. What is done in each individual case, therefore, must be determined by the ability of the optic nerve to resist pressure and the degree of effect of the agents on the intraocular pressure. One method of proceeding, which is frequently helpful, is to add carbonic anhydrase inhibitors or increase the dose of carbonic anhydrase inhibitors 2 weeks before the surgery, stop the beta blocker 2 weeks before the surgery, stop echothiophate 2 weeks before the surgery, and stop pilocarpine 2 days before the surgery.

In extraordinary circumstances standard attempts to lower intraocular pressure may not succeed. For these cases, Table 11–12 describes a method that will provide maximum intraocular pressure–lowering potential.

TABLE 11–11. Factors That Influence the Timing of all Types of Glaucoma Surgery*

FACTOR	FAVORS DELAY OF SURGERY	FAVORS PROCEEDING WITH SURGERY PROMPTLY
Health of optic nerve	No apparent cupping	Advanced cupping
Visual field	Loss not approaching fixation	Loss approaching fixation†
Current level of intraocular pressure, in comparison to level at which nerve damage occurred	Lower	Higher
Absolute level of intraocular pressure	Less than 10 mm Hg	Greater than 40 mm Hg‡
Patient's ability to tolerate medications	Good	Poor
Degree of ocular inflammation	Marked	Minimal
Patient receiving long-acting cholinesterase inhibitors§	Yes	No
Patient receiving anticoagulant	Yes	No
Rapidity of rise of intraocular pressure	Slow	Sudden

*See other tables for specific indications for surgery of specific types of glaucoma.
†If field defect has reached to within 5 degrees of fixation, chance of wipe-out increases.
‡The closer the intraocular pressure to systolic central retinal artery pressure, the more urgent the surgery.
§The reason for delaying is to allow the effect of the agent to wear off; this is not necessary for cyclodialysis.

TABLE 11–12. Method of Lowering Intraocular Pressure Maximally Prior to Surgery*

AGENT	ROUTE	DOSE†	TIME BEFORE SURGERY TO ADMINISTER
Mannitol 20%	Intravenous	7 ml/kg	90 minutes
Glycerol, anhydrous‡	Oral	1 ml/kg	60 minutes
Timolol 0.5%	Eye drop	2 drops	60 minutes
Acetazolamide	Intravenous	7 mg/kg	30 minutes
Mepivacaine 0.75%	Retrobulbar block	2 ml	10 minutes
Pressure on globe	—	—	10 seconds on and 10 seconds off for 2 minutes

*This method is not advised for routine use, but should be used only in cases in which intraocular pressure is extraordinarily resistant to standard therapy.

†Dose is expressed in terms of amount per kilogram of body weight.

‡Glycerol is preferably administered in a 50% solution, in which case the dose given in this table should be doubled.

INDICATIONS FOR SURGERY

Primary Open-Angle Glaucoma

Surgery for open-angle glaucoma is indicated when there is documented or anticipated damage to the optic nerve or visual field owing to glaucoma, despite maximum tolerated medical therapy, that is developing at a rate that will diminish the patient's quality of life to the extent that the patient decides to undergo surgery in hopes that the disadvantages of surgery will be fewer than the advantages (see Tables 11–1 and 11–13).

The essential consideration in determining the need for treatment or for surgery is to determine the effect of the illness on the patient, that is to say, the clinical course of the disease. The intensity of intervention will vary, depending on the anticipated effect of the disease on the patient.

Condition of the Optic Nerve Head

The current management of glaucoma rests primarily on the observation of deterioration. It is hoped that in the future this system will be changed, so that management is determined primarily by lowering intraocular pressure to the level that causes an improvement in the optic disc or visual field. However, this new system of management by improvement demands more meticulous examination of the pa-

tient than is currently practiced, or in many areas currently available.

Because the optic disc will often show changes before the development of detectable deterioration of the visual field, especially in the early stages of disease, documentation of disc change is of paramount importance in management, especially in glaucoma suspects or in those with early or moderately advanced glaucoma.[41–47] Proper evaluation of the nerve head is thus an essential part of the diagnostic evaluation of every case. The disc should be drawn. When possible photographs should be obtained. Although still largely investigational, quantitative image analysis with an instrument such as those currently marketed by Topcon and Rodenstock will almost certainly provide the best documentation. The evaluations should be made often enough to be reasonably sure that changes are not missed. Alterations may occur rapidly, such as the cupping that can develop within weeks in patients with congenital glaucoma or in children with secondary glaucoma. Usually, however, the changes occur slowly; in most instances it is adequate to check the disc at about 6-month intervals and repeat the disc photographs every 2 to 3 years. The level of intraocular pressure will obviously influence the frequency with which the optic nerve head needs to be evaluated: the higher the pressure, the more frequent the examination.

The appearance of the optic disc in some patients with glaucoma is so characteristic that the examiner is almost surely correct in making this diagnosis (Fig. 11–10). However, this is not invariably the case.[48] It is generally believed that discs with large central cups, such as those with a cup-disc ratio greater than 0.8, are more sensitive to the damaging effects of elevated intraocular pressure. Some physicians also believe that myopic nerve heads or those with a posteriorly bowed lamina cribrosa are predisposed to damage.[22, 72]

TABLE 11–13. Treatment Preferences

CONDITION	TREATMENT
Progressing disease	Surgery
Progressive disease	Usually surgery
Definite disease but undetermined course	Medical with surgery possible
Abnormal findings but not established disease	Observation or medical

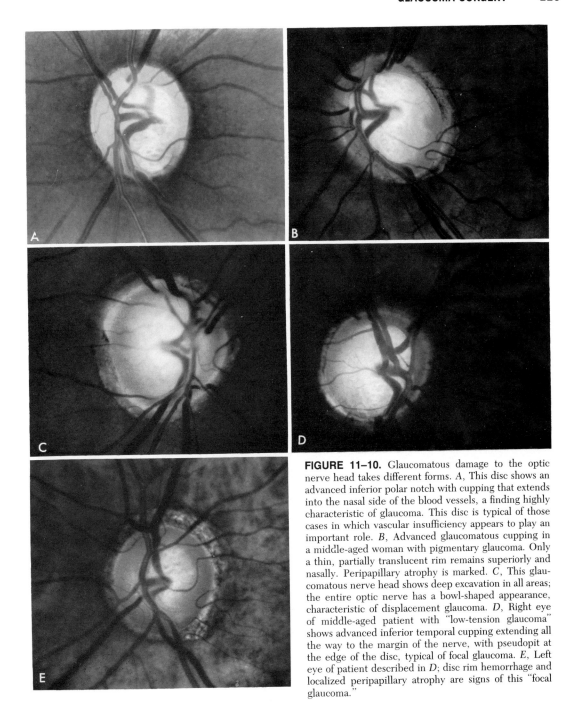

FIGURE 11–10. Glaucomatous damage to the optic nerve head takes different forms. *A*, This disc shows an advanced inferior polar notch with cupping that extends into the nasal side of the blood vessels, a finding highly characteristic of glaucoma. This disc is typical of those cases in which vascular insufficiency appears to play an important role. *B*, Advanced glaucomatous cupping in a middle-aged woman with pigmentary glaucoma. Only a thin, partially translucent rim remains superiorly and nasally. Peripapillary atrophy is marked. *C*, This glaucomatous nerve head shows deep excavation in all areas; the entire optic nerve has a bowl-shaped appearance, characteristic of displacement glaucoma. *D*, Right eye of middle-aged patient with "low-tension glaucoma" shows advanced inferior temporal cupping extending all the way to the margin of the nerve, with pseudopit at the edge of the disc, typical of focal glaucoma. *E*, Left eye of patient described in *D*; disc rim hemorrhage and localized peripapillary atrophy are signs of this "focal glaucoma."

Progressive narrowing of the neural rim of the optic nerve head in a patient with glaucoma is virtual proof that the glaucoma is not adequately controlled. If the cup is enlarging, the physician must assume that the glaucoma is getting worse, or that there is a different or additional cause for progressive cupping.[41] Although there do appear to be cases in which optic nerve damage is so marked that the neu-

rons are "mortally wounded" (and will die no matter how low the intraocular pressure), a good working rule is to assume that the cause for progressive deterioration is intraocular pressure higher than the eye can tolerate (Table 11–6). This approach demands reasonable certainty that the deterioration is not due to causes other than glaucoma, such as compression of the chiasm by a pituitary adenoma. It also demands that the ophthalmologist and the patient be prudent in ruling out other causes of optic nerve damage, and use appropriate diagnostic tests, for example, a sedimentation rate, measurements of optic blood flow, where appropriate, and, most important, studies such as computed tomography and magnetic resonance imaging. In the simplest terms, if the glaucoma is getting worse, this is an indication that the intraocular pressure is too high, regardless of its absolute level. Progressive deterioration of the optic nerve head must be expected unless the intraocular pressure is lowered further. Such progressive cupping may occur despite intraocular pressures in the range that has been considered normal; such was the case in the person whose optic disc is shown in Figure 11–11B. This middle-aged woman was never observed to have intraocular pressures above 15 mm Hg. However, during the three years the patient was followed on no treatment with intraocular pressures between 13 and 15 mm Hg, there was progressive cupping and visual field loss. After the intraocular pressure had been lowered to the range of 10 to 12 mm Hg, deterioration stopped; there has been no further damage observed in the past 10 years.

Progressive cupping may occur without detectable visual field loss. One clue that this is occurring is the presence of significant asym-

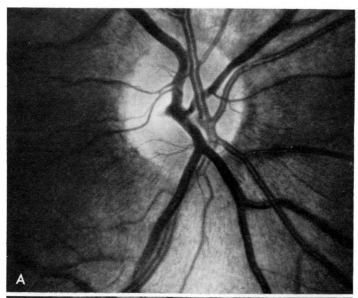

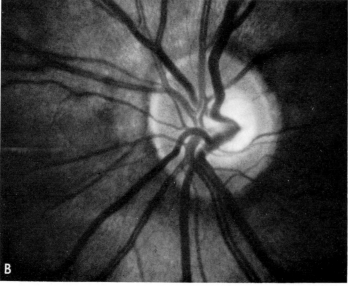

FIGURE 11–11. *A*, Optic disc of patient with an apparently normal right eye. *B*, Optic disc of glaucomatous left eye of same patient, showing markedly enlarged cup caused by elevation of intraocular pressure. The only clue that this disc is abnormal is asymmetry. The underlying diagnosis is glaucoma secondary to essential iris atrophy, left eye. Despite the acquired cupping, visual field loss was not detectable.

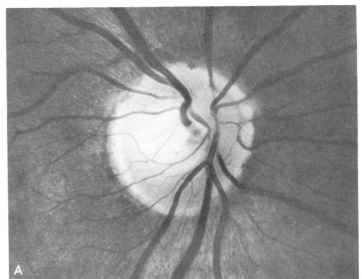

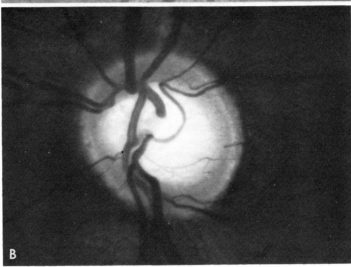

FIGURE 11–12. The left eye *(B)* of this young man shows a cup that is unmistakably larger than the cup in the right eye *(A)*. Furthermore, there is cupping on the nasal side of the blood vessels *(B)*. Note, however, that the entire disc in *B* is larger than the disc in *A*. The total rim area in *A* and *B* is, thus, similar. The larger cup in *B* is more a reflection of difference in disc size than of loss of tissue.

metry between the optic discs, as seen in Figure 11–12. The left optic disc of this young adult with essential iris atrophy appears entirely normal when considered by itself. However, an obvious difference between the two eyes is observable when the left optic disc is compared with the right optic nerve head of the same patient. The narrowing of the optic rim of this person with persistently elevated intraocular pressure represents an acquired change.

Changes in the appearance of the optic disc need not be marked to be highly significant. Note the narrowing of the rim, the enlargement of the cup, and the deviation of the blood vessels that occurred in the 3 years separating Figure 11–13A and 11–13B. The intraocular pressure was approaching 40 mm Hg during this time. After the disc deterioration was recognized, a trabeculectomy was performed, after

which the disc showed a significant improvement (Fig. 11–13C).

Cupping is definitely reversible, especially in infants or young children.[43, 44, 49] A permanent improvement in the appearance of the optic nerve head is to be expected after successful treatment of early congenital glaucoma. Improvement in adults also occurs far more frequently than previously believed.[49, 49a–49c] In one study one-third of surgically treated patients showed reversible change.[49c] Temporary filling-in of the optic nerve has been observed. This is presumably the result of edema and should not be confused with real improvement.

Nature of the Visual Field

Visual field loss may occur in the absence of apparent deterioration of the optic nerve head.[7, 50, 51] This is uncommon in early glau-

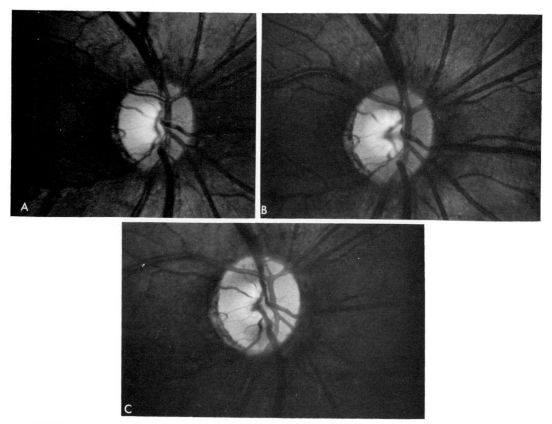

FIGURE 11–13. *A*, Right optic nerve head of a young woman with persistent elevation of intraocular pressure to 30 mm Hg or slightly higher; there is no detectable visual field loss and an apparently normal-appearing optic nerve head. *B*, Three years later the rim had become narrower and the cup deeper, despite maximum medical treatment. It is unlikely that the slight change that occurred could have been noticed if photographs had not been taken. No visual field loss was demonstrable. *C*, After surgery the cupping unquestionably regressed, as seen in this postoperative photograph. This improvement has persisted for 8 years.

coma. But in cases with advanced cupping, progressive visual loss often occurs without the ophthalmologist's being able to note further deterioration of the optic nerve head. Consequently satisfactory management of glaucoma requires careful and frequent documentation of the visual field (Fig. 11–14).

Visual field loss in glaucoma may take various forms.[50-54] It most commonly first expresses itself as an isolated scotomatous loss in the Bjerrum area, that is, within a zone approximately 10 degrees wide extending from the blind spot, becoming wider as it sweeps toward the nasal side (Fig. 11–15). The superior field is more often involved. Unless the visual field examination includes a specific search for such scotomas, abnormalities will be missed.[7, 55] Static perimetry is of great assistance in this regard. Instruments that examine the field using computer-controlled static perimetry offer the physician the most satisfactory method of documenting the nature of the visual field and observing deterioration (Fig. 11–16).[56, 57]

Artifacts that affect the visual field must be considered in interpreting repeat visual fields. Change in the pupil size, clarity of the media, intensity of the testing light, cooperation of the patient, speed with which the object is presented, and many other factors affect the apparent visual field. It is essential that these artifacts be considered when comparing visual fields (Table 11–14). The surgeon is attempting to determine whether the visual field has become worse owing to progressive damage to the optic nerve. When this is the case, and when other organic causes have been ruled out, then the progressive field loss must be assumed to be glaucomatous, and by definition, the glaucoma is out of control, regardless of the level of intraocular pressure (see p. 228).

When visual field loss is so extensive that it cuts close to fixation, there is a possibility that

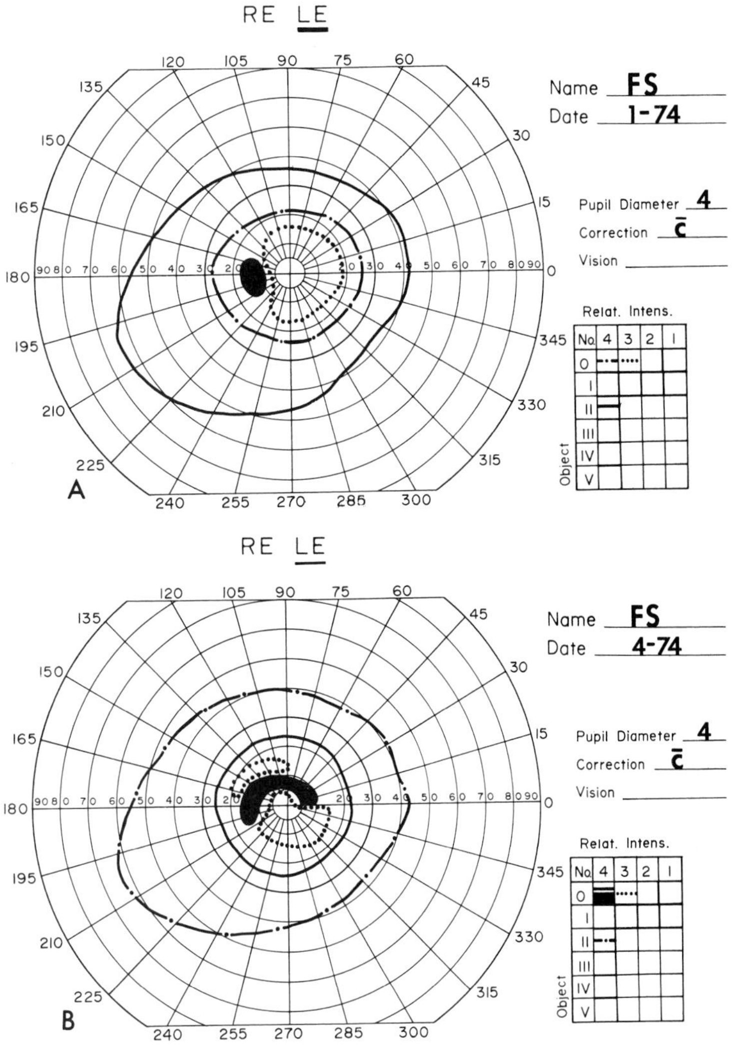

FIGURE 11–14. Within 3 months this middle-aged woman, who had an inferior polar notch of the left eye, progressed from having a normal visual field *(A)* to having a pathological field in which a complete arcuate scotoma developed *(B)*. This type of change is typical of "focal glaucoma." It occurred in this patient despite her intraocular pressure's consistently being around 15 mm Hg. (Modified from Spaeth, G. L.: The Pathogenesis of Visual Loss in Glaucoma; The Contribution of and Indications for Fluorescein Angiography. New York, Grune & Stratton, 1977.)

central visual acuity will deteriorate suddenly after surgery. This phenomenon of "wipe-out" is rare but real (Fig. 11–17).[57, 58] The risk must be included in the assessment as to whether or not surgery is warranted (see Table 11–1). Completely satisfactory figures are not available, but patients must be given an estimate of the likelihood that their vision will be made immediately much worse by the surgery. If central acuity is already affected (fixation is already involved), I tell them that they have about a 10 per cent chance of sudden visual loss; if loss cuts within 5 degrees of fixation but does not actually involve central acuity, then I tell them that the likelihood of loss is about 5 per cent. If the visual field is tubular, not cutting into fixation, the likelihood of "wipe-out" appears to be much less. For evaluation of the visual field to be clinically meaningful, the method of examination must be sufficiently sensitive that changes that are occurring can be detected (Fig. 11–18).[56]

Intraocular Pressure

The *control* of open-angle glaucoma is defined by what is happening to the optic disc and field. It is *not* defined by the level of intraocular pressure. Consequently intraocular pressure *per se* is rarely an indication for surgery in open-angle glaucoma (see p. 228).

Intraocular pressure, on the other hand, is important in deciding whether or not surgery should be undertaken. The reason for this is that the level of intraocular pressure helps to indicate whether or not disc and field changes can be anticipated. That is, intraocular pressure is a predictive indicator.

For intraocular pressure to be a valid predic-

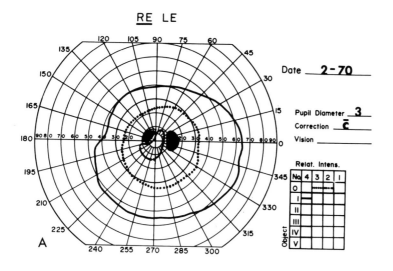

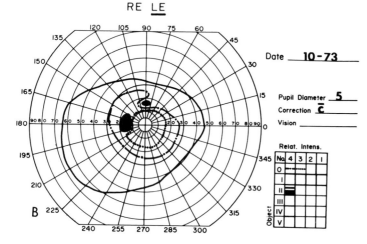

FIGURE 11–15. Early to moderate visual field defects. In *A* a relative scotoma was present, resulting in a superior nasal step. No absolute defect could be found. Though the isopters in *B* are quite full, a tiny but dense scotoma at 12 o'clock was detected. More advanced loss is shown in *C*, the optic disc of a young woman with a large inferior polar notch (similar to that shown in Fig. 11–10A). (Modified from Spaeth, G. L.: The Pathogenesis of Visual Loss in Glaucoma; The Contribution of and Indications for Fluorescein Angiography. New York, Grune & Stratton, 1977.)

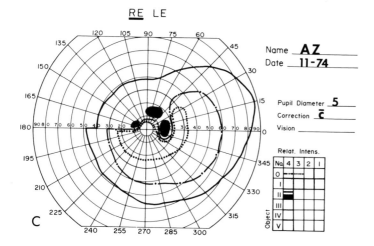

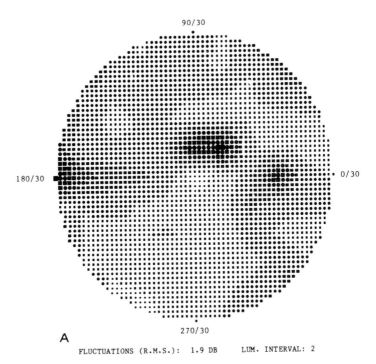

90/30

180/30

0/30

270/30

A

FLUCTUATIONS (R.M.S.): 1.9 DB   LUM. INTERVAL: 2

FIGURE 11–16. A small but clinically significant progression of the superior nasal step *(B* compared with *A)* was documented by Octopus computerized perimeter in this middle-aged chemist with low-tension glaucoma. Such lesser degrees of change need to be confirmed by repeated field examinations before being considered valid.

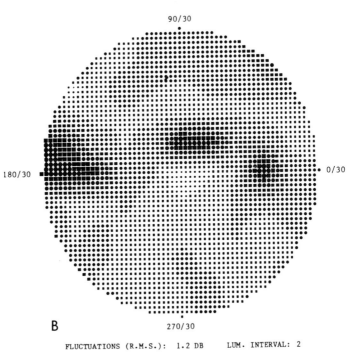

90/30

180/30

0/30

B

270/30

FLUCTUATIONS (R.M.S.): 1.2 DB   LUM. INTERVAL: 2

TABLE 11–14. Factors That May Make the Visual Field Deteriorate*

1. **Decreasing Brightness or Clarity of Image on Retina**
   a. Smaller pupil
   b. Opacities in media
   c. Inaccurate refractive correction
   d. Lower light intensity of object
   e. Brighter background illumination
   f. Smaller test object
   g. Greater distance of patient from screen

2. **Methods of Testing**
   a. Shorter exposure of object
   b. More rapid motion of object
   c. Excessively long test
   d. Technical errors
   e. Improper positioning of patient

3. **Patient Factors**
   a. Lack of alertness or understanding
   b. Fatigue or illness
   c. Changed anatomic factors (e.g., lid droop)

4. **Deterioration of Visual Receptors, Pathways, or Centers**

*Of the four factors listed, only the last is an indication of actual worsening of the patient's disease. Furthermore, even this situation may be caused by many factors other than glaucoma.

tive indicator, the level harmful to the patient under consideration must be established: this cannot be determined *a priori*. For although it is possible to accurately predict that in a population of 100 patients who have intraocular pressure of X mm Hg, a certain percentage will eventually develop disc and field change, one cannot predict with certainty *which* of the 100 will deteriorate and which will remain stable. Therefore, until a track record for the individual patient has been established, intraocular pressure provides nothing more than a rough guideline. With adequate evaluation and with time it is usually possible to determine what general level of intraocular pressure is tolerated by the patient under consideration. Only after this determination has been made does intraocular pressure itself become a valid predictive indicator.

Consider individual A, whose intraocular pressure with medical treatment has ranged between 20 and 25 mm Hg for a period of 5 years, during which time there is no suggestion of deterioration of the disc or field. Patient A can be presumed to be under control (although it is not possible to say with 100 per cent certainty that disc or field damage will not develop 5 to 10 years later even if the intraocular pressures stay in the same range). On the other hand, consider patient B, whose intraocular pressure also ranged between 20 and 25 mm

Hg for 5 years, during which time there has been progressive deterioration of the optic disc or visual field. It is now established that the intraocular pressure in patient B must be lowered, and appropriate steps are taken to achieve this. The physician now sets a new level that he believes may be satisfactory, perhaps 13 to 18 mm Hg. If it is possible to achieve such a pressure level on medication, this course is followed and the patient is then watched to determine if deterioration occurs at that new level. *If, after pressure lowering, the disc or field improves, the new level of intraocular pressure can, with great confidence, be considered satisfactory. Such improvement in disc or field must, however, be real, and not merely a reflection of testing techniques (e.g., larger pupil, better acuity) or incorrect interpretation* (see Figs. 11–13 and 11–19). Merely because surgery has been "successful" and has lowered intraocular pressure to a range that the surgeon may have considered *a priori* to be satisfactory does not mean that the surgery will be truly successful. Achieving an intraocular pressure of, for example, 15 mm Hg after surgery may not be achieving control. Control is defined only in terms of the health of the optic nerve. A recent study has shown that almost 50 per cent of patients who had surgery that was considered successful for glaucoma, and in whom the intraocular pressure had been lowered to an average of 19 mm Hg, had progressive visual field loss 5 years later; in contrast, in the same population, having surgery performed by the same surgeons with the same indications, those patients in whom the mean intraocular pressure was 14 mm Hg fared far better, with only 6 per cent showing progressive visual loss.

Another vitally important limitation of the value of intraocular pressure in managing glaucoma is the inability to monitor intraocular pressure in more than the most rudimentary manner. A physician sees a patient for isolated, planned, brief moments of the patient's life, and often concludes that such a moment is representative of the vast period of time over which the patient is not being monitored. It is true that more information can be provided by "home tonometry," the practice of measuring the patient's intraocular pressure at more frequent intervals during his ordinary day. However, home tonometry by no means provides a full description of what is truly happening to the patient's pressure. Paradoxically, it may make it even more difficult for the patient and physician to keep clearly in mind the truth that

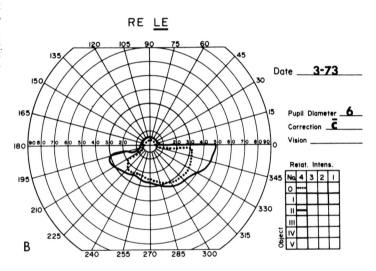

FIGURE 11-17. Although the extent of visual field loss in *A* is greater than in *B*, the risk for deterioration of vision after surgery is just as great, if not greater, in *B* as in *A* because of the closeness with which the field loss approaches fixation. "Wipe-out" occurs in roughly 5 per cent of cases in which field loss reaches into fixation preoperatively. (Modified from Spaeth, G. L.: The Pathogenesis of Visual Loss in Glaucoma; The Contribution of and Indications for Fluorescein Angiography. New York, Grune & Stratton, 1977.)

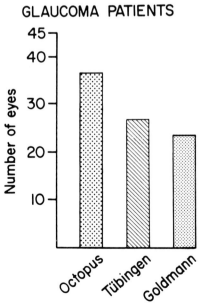

FIGURE 11-18. The management of glaucoma depends on the documentation of stability or change. Obviously, then, the quality of the management will depend on the ability to detect change. This graph depicts the superior ability of the Octopus computerized perimeter to detect visual field loss in patients with glaucoma using program 31 with the Octopus, two cuts with the Tübingen perimeter, and the Armaly-Drance screening method with a Goldmann perimeter. Both forms of static perimetry were superior to this kinetic method. The Octopus was superior to the Tübingen perimeter despite the fact that the time required to examine a field was approximately half as long with the Octopus as with the Tübingen perimeter. Computerized perimetry provides not only increased *sensitivity*, but increased *specificity* as well.

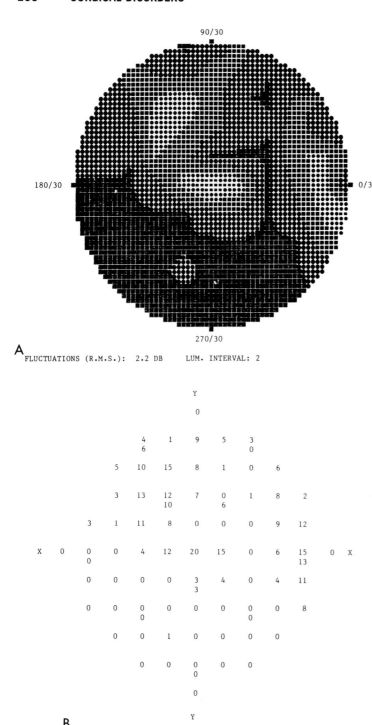

90/30

180/30

0/30

A
FLUCTUATIONS (R.M.S.):   2.2 DB   LUM. INTERVAL: 2

270/30

Y

0

			4	1	9	5	3				
			6				0				
		5	10	15	8	1	0	6			
		3	13	12	7	0	1	8	2		
				10		6					
	3	1	11	8	0	0	0	9	12		
X	0	0	0	4	12	20	15	0	6	15	0	X
		0								13	
	0	0	0	0	3	4	0	4	11		
					3						
	0	0	0	0	0	0	0	0	8		
			0				0				
		0	0	1	0	0	0	0			
			0	0	0	0	0				
					0						

0

Y

B
FLUCTUATIONS (R.M.S.):   2.2 DB   LUM. INTERVAL: 2

FIGURE 11–19. *A* and *B* represent the visual field of a woman who had demonstrated progressive glaucomatous visual field loss. The visual field, determined just before glaucoma surgery, is shown in both the gray scale and the digital mode.

the matter of real concern is the patient's health, most specifically the patient's optic nerve.

It is generally accepted that when glaucoma surgery is successful it is because the mean intraocular pressure has been adequately lowered. But it may be that an additional important function of glaucoma surgery is to eliminate pressure spikes. Such a hypothesis is consistent with the observation that the patient may, before surgery, show progressive deterioration of disc and field at pressure **X**, and yet after surgery not show further deterioration at the same pressure level.

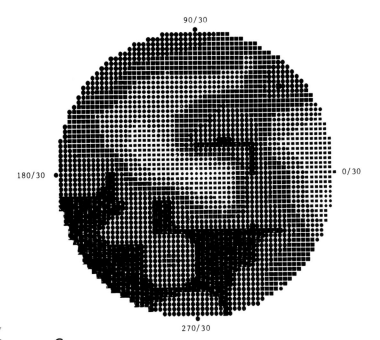

90/30

180/30 •   • 0/30

270/30

C   FLUCTUATIONS (R.M.S.):   1.7 DB   LUM. INTERVAL: 2

FIGURE 11–19 *Continued C* and *D* show the same patient approximately 1 year after successful surgical lowering of intraocular pressure. Despite the advanced nature of the visual field loss, there is a significant improvement. This improvement is not the result of change in pupil size or other artifact of testing technique.

```
                                            Y

                                            2


                          3      6      8      9      12
                          7                            11

                  5      12     15     12     12     10      0


          8     13      15     11      9      2      6     11     14
                               12             3

          8     11      20     15      0      0      0     16     19


  X    2     5      0     14     18     25     20      0      7     18     18   X
             1                                               16

             0      0      1      0     12     16      3      7     16
                                       10

             0      1      2      0      0      0      0      0     10
                    0                                 0

             0      0      7      0      0      0      8


                    0      0      0      0      3
                                  0

                                  5

                                  Y
```

D   FLUCTUATIONS (R.M.S.)   1.7 DB   LUM INTERVAL   2

Summary

A semiquantitative approach to the management of primary open-angle glaucoma is shown in Figure 11–20. Clearly the figures are not absolute indicators, but serve only as guidelines. However, the surgeon who considers carefully the factors listed will probably come to a logical conclusion.

Shown in Figure 11–20*B* is the traditional concept of the course of glaucoma and the effect

FACTORS AFFECTING CHOICE OF SURGERY IN OPEN-ANGLE GLAUCOMA

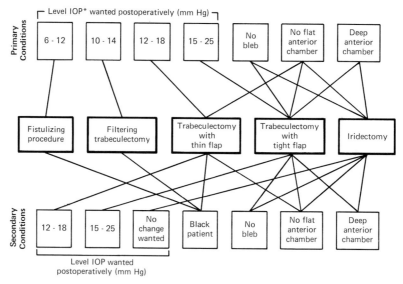

A   *Intraocular pressure

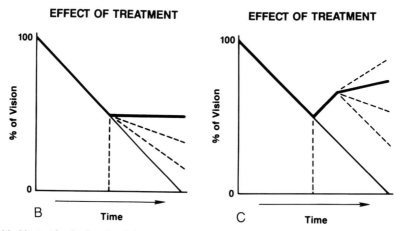

B   Time   C   Time

FIGURE 11–20. *A,* The final goals of the surgery combine with the nature of the case to determine which glaucoma surgical procedure is preferable. For example, if the goals are a postoperative intraocular pressure of around 15 mm Hg, with the least likelihood of a postoperative flat chamber, a trabeculectomy with a tight or a thin scleral flap is appropriate; if, on the other hand, the goal is to deepen the anterior chamber and no pressure lowering is required, then an iridectomy is indicated. *B,* Traditional concept of the effect of treatment on the clinical course of glaucoma. Treatment in some cases can make glaucoma worse, can slow the course, or can stabilize the condition, as indicated by the change in the slopes of the graph. *C,* New conception of management of glaucoma based on determination of clinical improvement in response to treatment.

or lack of effect of treatment. Figure 11–20C depicts the "new" method of management, based on lowering intraocular pressure enough to cause an improvement in the course of the disease.

The general approach to the timing of surgery in the patient with primary open-angle glaucoma has been far too aggressive in many patients and far too conservative in even more patients. Many patients will never lose functional damage, even though they have definite

glaucoma. Others will rapidly become seriously handicapped. The former group do not deserve the risks of treatment. In the latter group, while we wait for definite signs of deterioration, the patient is getting worse. Especially in the early stages, when cupping can progress without detectable loss of visual field, surgery is too often delayed. When progressive disease is present, that is, when it is known that the patient's optic nerve is worsening because of glaucoma and the patient's anticipated life span is such that it is probable that visual function will be significantly affected, the best choice of treatment is usually surgery (Table 11–13). When the disease has progressed, but it is not known to be actually *progressing*, medical therapy should usually be tried, with the realization that surgery will usually be needed. In those cases who have definite glaucoma, but no definite or anticipated loss, medical treatment is preferred initially. When *findings* are abnormal, such as a high intraocular pressure, medical treatment may or may not be appropriate, depending on a variety of factors (Tables 11–1 and 11–5).

Primary Angle-Closure Glaucoma

Indications for surgery in patients with narrow anterior chamber angles or with primary angle-closure glaucoma are still not entirely clear-cut. The reason for this uncertainty is the inability to accurately predict the future clinical course of these patients. When nerve damage is due to open-angle glaucoma, it is virtually certain that progressive deterioration will continue unless intraocular pressure is adequately lowered. However, there is little precision in prognosticating the future of many patients with narrow or partially closed anterior chamber angles. I present here an approach to the diagnosis and management of such cases that recognizes these uncertainties, but that has proved relatively satisfactory from a clinical point of view. As more knowledge is gained this approach will need revision and perhaps even major change.

The nature of the anterior chamber angle is clearly an important aspect in understanding angle-closure glaucoma. Meaningful examination of the angle by an informed person is essential. The use of gonioscopy must be mastered by anyone who wants to give patients with glaucoma satisfactory care.[59]

Nature of the Anterior Chamber Angle

The anterior chamber angle may be examined directly with the Koeppe lens or indirectly with a mirrored lens. Each system has disadvantages and advantages. Direct gonioscopy is easy to learn and provides a panoramic view of the angle. With the patient supine the anterior chamber becomes slightly deeper. Indirect gonioscopy is harder to learn and has more artifacts associated with it, predisposing to misinterpretation of the appearance of the angle unless the observer is fully aware of the accompanying problems. The advantages of indirect gonios-

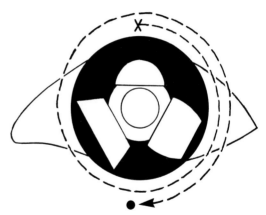

FIGURE 11–21. Schematic view of the Goldmann three-mirrored lens. Looking into the mirror at 12 o'clock permits good visualization of the angle at 6 o'clock. The mirror is rotated 360 degrees while the angle is viewed through the smallest mirror, permitting visualization of the entire angle.

copy, however, are the remarkable ease and rapidity with which it may be done (once learned), its wide range of magnifications and illuminations, and the ability to perform indentation gonioscopy.[60] These advantages are so overwhelming that I strongly believe that gonioscopy with a lens able to be used to perform indentation gonioscopy is, by far, the examination method of choice.

One of the standard lenses used in indirect gonioscopy is the Goldmann three-mirrored lens. This requires a viscous substance to maintain contact between the surface of the lens and the cornea. The examiner views the angle through the smallest mirror, and rotates the lens so that the entire angle can easily be examined (Fig. 11–21). The Zeiss four-mirror lens has a smaller surface with a convexity that more accurately mimics that of the cornea. Tears provide an adequate contact material and lubrication for the lens, greatly facilitating use and eliminating the blurring effect of the viscous gonioscopic fluids (Fig. 11–22). The Zeiss lens is difficult to use because the positioning must be precise in order to obtain a satisfactory view. The lens must be held very gently against the corneal surface so that it does not distort the cornea or displace aqueous humor, which would cause distortion of the angle. Firm support for the hand holding the lens is essential. Another problem with the four-mirror lens is the fragmentation of the view of the angle; the observer must reconstruct the angle panorama in his own mind (Fig. 11–23).

The advantages of the four-mirror lens are so great that its use is strongly recommended. Anyone with the dexterity required to perform

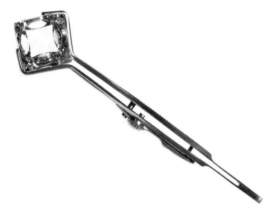

FIGURE 11–22. The Zeiss four-mirrored goniolens with the Ungen handle.

ophthalmic surgery can certainly master the technique of Zeiss four-mirror gonioscopy.

The unique advantage of indirect gonioscopy with a lens having a small area of contact is the ability to perform Forbes' indentation gonioscopy. This is the only method available for the ophthalmologist in his office to distinguish between mere contact of the iris with the cornea and actual adhesion of the iris to the cornea. In this technique the goniolens is placed centrally on the cornea and pushed posteriorly, so that it displaces aqueous into the periphery of the anterior chamber, forcing the iris posteriorly, where it is unsupported by the lens (Fig. 11–24). If the iris is adherent to the cornea, the iris will not fall posteriorly (Fig. 11–24C). In contrast, when the iris is not adherent it will

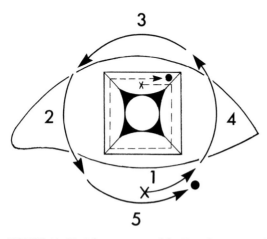

FIGURE 11–23. Schematic view of the Zeiss four-mirrored lens. When used with the handle shown in Figure 11–22, the mirror is not rotated; rather, the four quadrants of the angle are examined by moving the direction of gaze. If this is done in a regular clockwise manner, a fragmented view of the angle is obtained that must be reconstructed in the mind.

be displaced posteriorly, allowing visualization of the deeper angle recess (Fig. 11–24B).

Proper evaluation of the configuration of the anterior chamber angle requires the use of at least three descriptors: the point at which the iris is adherent to the cornea or uvea, the depth of the anterior chamber, and the curvature of the peripheral iris.[94] The Wills Eye Hospital system of grading the anterior chamber angle takes into account all three of these attributes, and has proved highly satisfactory.

The most important landmark is the posterior trabecular meshwork (Fig. 11–25). Visibility of this structure is what determines whether an anterior chamber angle is functionally open or closed, as it is through this region that the aqueous humor exits. Peripheral anterior synechias can develop posterior to the trabecular meshwork, indicating the occurrence of an angle-closure attack. Such synechias have no functional effect, but are a definite sign of disease.

The point of contact between the iris and the inner wall of the globe should be noted (Fig. 11–26). In the majority of eyes the iris is adherent to the anterior ciliary body, permitting visualization of all structures anterior to this. In younger people, especially those with brown eyes and most notably black patients, the iris may normally insert more anteriorly, so that it is adherent just posterior to the scleral spur (C in Fig. 11–26). In myopes the anterior chamber may be extraordinarily deep and the iris may insert more posteriorly than usual (E in Fig. 11–26). Figure 11–27 shows an eye with secondary angle closure and adherence of the iris anterior to the posterior trabecular meshwork. The angle is optically and functionally closed. Pressure gonioscopy would show that no matter how hard the central cornea is depressed, the iris cannot be displaced posteriorly beyond its current point of contact at the trabecular meshwork (Fig. 11–27).

The angle should also be graded in terms of depth of the anterior chamber. This can be measured directly in millimeters by several techniques. An easier, less exact, but clinically adequate method is to approximate anterior chamber depth in terms of angular approach to the recess (Fig. 11–28).

The third characteristic that needs description is the peripheral curvature of the angle (Fig. 11–29). In most people there is little anterior or posterior curvature; that is, the peripheral iris is flat (r, for regular). In others, especially the elderly, the peripheral iris bends sharply and steeply anteriorly, making the angle recess shallower than one would expect on the

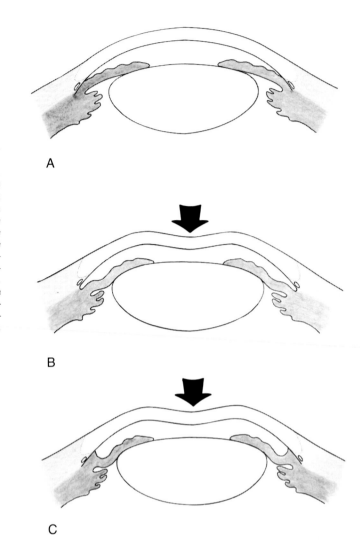

A

B

C

FIGURE 11–24. Indentation gonioscopy. Note that in *A* the angle appears closed. However, the observer cannot determine whether this is due merely to contact between the iris and cornea or to actual adhesion. In *B* the goniolens has been pressed against the central cornea, displacing aqueous into the periphery, which demonstrates that the angle is open. In *C*, indentation gonioscopy displaces the iris posteriorly, revealing peripheral anterior synechias. (From Schwartz, L. W.: Diagnostic evaluation of the patient. *In* Spaeth, G. L. (ed.): Early Primary Open-Angle Galucoma: Diagnosis and Management. Boston, Little, Brown & Co., 1979, p. 60.)

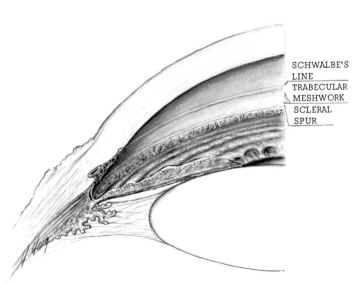

SCHWALBE'S
LINE
TRABECULAR
MESHWORK
SCLERAL
SPUR

FIGURE 11–25. Major landmarks of the anterior chamber angle. Iris processes are fairly prominent and reach up to the scleral spur. The trabecular meshwork is not pigmented. Schwalbe's line is prominent. The angle is wide open and normal. (From Spaeth, G. L.: The normal development of the human anterior chamber angle. A new system of descriptive grading. Trans. Ophthalmol. Soc. UK, 91:709, 1971.)

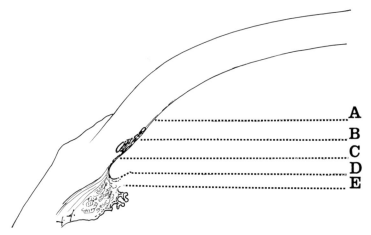

FIGURE 11–26. Schematic drawing of five possible locations where the iris may contact the inner portion of the globe. A = iris insertion into or anterior to Schwalbe's line (A = anterior); B = iris adherent to the globe just anterior to the posterior trabecular meshwork (B = behind Schwalbe's line); C = iris arising from scleral spur; D = iris inserts into the anterior portion of the ciliary body (D = deep); E = iris arises from posterior portion of the ciliary body (E = extremely deep). A and B insertions are certainly pathologic. C insertion may be pathologic or normal. (From Spaeth, G. L.: The normal development of the human anterior chamber angle. A new system of descriptive grading. Trans. Ophthalmol Soc. UK, 91:709, 1971.)

basis of the central or even peripheral depth of the chamber (s, for *steep*). It is this s-type curvature that limits the value of the Van Herrick system of angle grading using a slit lamp without a gonioprism. The only *sure* way to tell about the nature of the angle recess is to visualize it. In myopes, patients with dislocated lenses, or aphakics the iris falls backward, assuming a q configuration.

Figure 11–30 shows an anterior chamber angle that is clearly narrow; it is probably occludable. Without pressure gonioscopy one cannot see past the curve of peripheral iris to

determine whether or not the iris and cornea are merely close to each other, whether they touch each other (as they do in Fig. 11–24A), or whether they are actually adherent (Fig. 11–24B). With pressure gonioscopy it is possible to see that the insertion of the iris is at the anterior ciliary body; there are no adhesions. Thus the anterior chamber angle in Figure 11–30 would be graded D-30-s; this is a shorthand way of saying that the angle is open, the anterior chamber depth is average, and there is marked anterior convexity of the iris periphery, making the angle occludable. The angle in Figure 11–

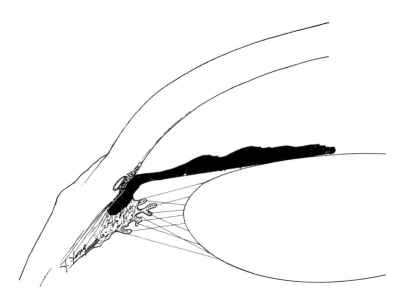

FIGURE 11–27. Anterior chamber angle with peripheral anterior synechia extending anterior to the posterior trabecular meshwork. This is a B insertion (see Fig. 11–26). (From Spaeth, G. L.: The normal development of the human anterior chamber angle. A new system of descriptive grading. Trans. Ophthalmol. Soc. UK, 91:709, 1971.)

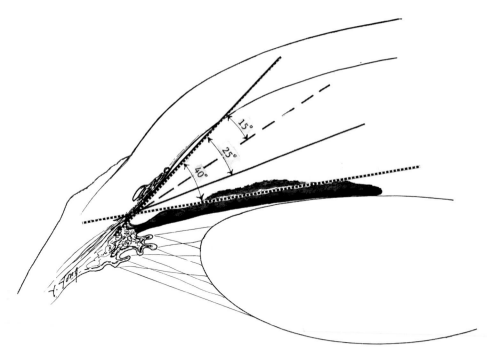

FIGURE 11–28. The angular width or depth of the anterior chamber recess may be estimated by constructing a tangent to the anterior surface of the iris about one-third of the distance from the most peripheral portion of the iris. The angle shown has an approach of about 40 degrees. (From Spaeth, G. L.: The normal development of the human anterior chamber angle. A new system of descriptive grading. Trans. Ophthalmol. Soc. UK, 91:709, 1971.)

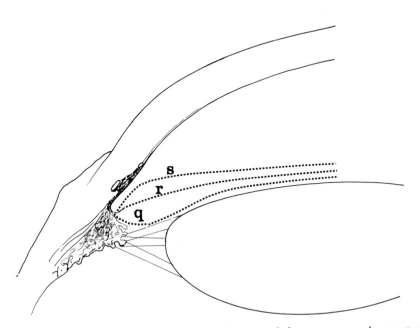

FIGURE 11–29. Description of the anterior chamber angle must include a comment on the curvature of the peripheral portion of the iris. It may bow steeply anteriorly (s). In a more regular case there is little curvature (r). In cases in which the iris has little support for the lens there may be a q configuration. (From Spaeth, G. L.: The normal development of the human anterior chamber angle. A new system of descriptive grading. Trans. Ophthalmol. Soc. UK, 91:709, 1971.)

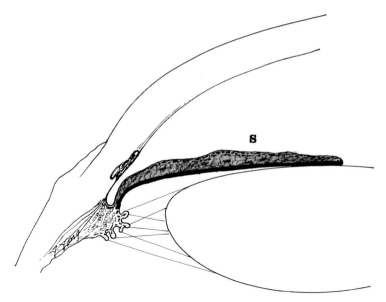

FIGURE 11–30. The exact nature of this angle would be difficult to determine without pressure gonioscopy. In actuality the angle is open, although the marked s-type of configuration makes visualization of the point at which the iris arises impossible. Pressure gonioscopy permits viewing of the entire angle, which would be graded D-30-s. (From Spaeth, G. L.: The normal development of the human anterior chamber angle. A new system of descriptive grading. Trans. Ophthalmol. Soc. UK, 91:709, 1971.)

27 would be a B-40-r—closed, with a deep chamber and a flat iris.

At the time of gonioscopy other aspects of the angle should be observed in addition to its configuration: such as amount, location, and nature of pigmentation; presence of inflammatory, exfoliated, or other debris; and location of any angle cleavage or cyclodialysis cleft.

History and Symptoms

The ophthalmologist should not treat "glaucoma." He or she should treat "a patient with glaucoma." It is the effect of the disease on the patient that is of concern, not the disease itself. It is the patient's "dis-ease" that is the important consideration. Therefore, because the way the ophthalmologist learns about the patient is through history taking, the history is the single most important part of the evaluation and treatment of the patient with glaucoma.

Accurate diagnosis is important if care is to be satisfactory, and events noted in the patient's history help to establish the correct diagnosis. For example, merely because an eye has suddenly become hard and painful does not mean that the diagnosis is primary angle-closure glaucoma. It could be a sudden onset of a neovascular glaucoma, or final decompensation after chronic angle-closure glaucoma, or an acute episode of a secondary angle-closure glaucoma. Thus, when confronted with a patient with an acute glaucoma, the physician should raise the following questions: Have there been previous attacks? Is there a family history of a similar condition? What was the quality of the vision before the attack? Exactly when did the symp-

toms begin? What were they? Is there diabetes in the family? Is the patient a diabetic? Was there trauma to the eye? The answers to these and other questions will help the surgeon come to a better understanding of the severity of the condition, the chronicity or acuteness of the glaucoma, and the possibility of causes other than primary angle-closure glaucoma.

Of course it is well known that halos may be a sign of an angle-closure attack. Halos, however, are not diagnostic of raised intraocular pressure, but rather are highly indicative of corneal epithelial edema. Because rapid elevation of intraocular pressure is a common cause for edema of the corneal epithelium, halos do suggest the probability of angle closure and are an indication for careful gonioscopy. The halos that occur with epithelial edema are quite typical. A diffuse, hazy ring surrounds a point source of light. This hazy ring is frequently faintly colored, so that it resembles a rainbow. The halos caused by corneal epithelial edema should be distinguished from the radiating, spoke-like rays of light that are characteristic of cataract or incorrect refraction.

Severe pain in the eye is a frequent accompaniment of any condition in which there is rapid rise of intraocular pressure. It is not the level of intraocular pressure that is responsible for the pain, but the rapidity of the increase. Thus a person can have an intraocular pressure of 80 mm Hg and be asymptomatic, or a pressure of 40 and be in extreme pain. The great majority of patients with angle-closure glaucoma do not have the fulminating attack that many have come to think of as characteristic of the

TABLE 11–15. Symptoms of Primary Angle-Closure Glaucoma*

SYMPTOM	FREQUENCY OF SYMPTOM
No symptoms	One-third of cases
Occasional headache	One-half of cases
Episodes of smoky vision	One-fourth of cases
Episodes of eyeache	Occasional
Attacks of severe pain associated with visual loss	Occasional
Episodes of visual loss	Rare
Awareness of loss of field	Rare

*Includes any conditions that cause sudden elevation of intraocular pressure, especially those that are recurrent: acute primary angle-closure glaucoma, chronic primary angle-closure glaucoma, uveitic glaucoma, the Posner-Schlossman syndrome, etc.

disease. Quite to the contrary, primary angle-closure glaucoma is asymptomatic in at least one-third of cases; in the majority of the other two-thirds the symptoms are mild (Table 11–15). In cases in which episodes of angle-closure are recurrent, they tend to become less and less symptomatic. It is common to see a patient with chronic angle-closure glaucoma who has *no* ocular symptoms, and yet has an intraocular pressure of 40 mm Hg and a cupped optic disc.

Signs

Physical findings may be prominent or almost normal in the primary angle-closure glaucomas. Elevations of intraocular pressure may be mild and transient, so that when the patient is seen in a doctor's office the eyes appear normal (although in fact they are not). Gonioscopy reveals an anterior chamber angle that was narrow enough to occlude spontaneously, or that perhaps already contained peripheral anterior synechias. Because most primary angle-closure cases are of the intermittent or chronic variety, it is more common for the eye of a patient with primary angle-closure glaucoma to appear grossly normal most of the time than for signs to be obvious.

In the case of acute fulminating primary angle-closure glaucoma physical findings are conspicuous: the patient is obviously having pain, the eye is bright red, the cornea is hazy, and the pupil is dilated and fixed (Table 11–16). Should the intraocular pressure spontaneously fall to normal, which is not rare, the eye will retain the signs of acute congestion and the cornea may become thicker and more edematous, but the intraocular pressure will be normal. To the inexperienced physician this may present a confusing picture (Table 11–16).

TABLE 11–16. Signs of Primary Angle-Closure Glaucoma*

SIGN	FREQUENCY
At Time of Acute Attack	
High intraocular pressure (above 40 mm Hg)	Always
Closed anterior chamber angle	Always
Signs that patient is having pain	Usual
Reduced vision	Usual
Red eye	Usual
Corneal epithelial edema	Usual
Dilated pupil	Usual
Abnormal optic disc	
Hyperemic and edematous	Usual
Blanched	Rare
Retinal hemorrhages	Common
One Day After Acute Attack Has Abated	
Low intraocular pressure (below 20 mm Hg)	Usual
Occludable anterior chamber angle	Always
Red eye	Often
Corneal epithelial edema	Occasional
Corneal thickening	Usual
Anterior uveitis	Usual
Oval, less reactive pupil	Usual
Anterior capsular lens opacity	Usual
Disc hyperemia and edema	Usual
Two Months or More After Acute Attack	
Normal intraocular pressure	Usual
Occludable anterior chamber angle	Always
Peripheral anterior synechias	Often
Pupil irregularity	Usual
Localized iris atrophy	Frequent
Flat pallor of the disc	Often
Increased pigmentation of posterior trabecular meshwork	Often
Peripheral visual field contraction	Often
At Time of Recurrent, Mildly Symptomatic or Asymptomatic Attack	
High intraocular pressure (above 30 mm Hg)	Always
Closed anterior chamber angle	Always
Peripheral anterior synechias	Often
Pupillary irregularity	Usual
Corneal epithelial edema	Occasional
Cupped optic nerve	Often
Iris atrophy	Occasional
Glaukomflecken	Occasional
Between Episodes of Recurrent Angle Closure	
Mild elevation of intraocular pressure (20–40 mm Hg)	Usual
Occludable anterior chamber angle	Always
Peripheral anterior synechias	Often
Pupillary irregularities	Usual
Optic nerve cupping	Often
Ireis atrophy	Occasional

*Includes other causes for acute or intermittent elevation of intraocular pressure. If the cornea is hazy, anhydrous glycerin should be instilled topically so that the angle and the fundus can be examined adequately.

The signs of recurrent or mild attacks are quite different (Table 11–16).

It is important to examine the fundus at the time the patient is first seen. The cornea can usually be cleared by instillation of topical anhydrous glycerin. Some patients will be treated with miotics after the attack and not come to iridectomy; there will be an understandable reluctance to dilate the pupil in these cases after the attack has quieted. The physician usually has the best chance to examine the fundus, then, at the time the patient is first seen.

Mechanisms of Angle Closure

There appear to be five mechanisms by which angle closure develops: (1) pupillary block, (2) angle jamming, (3) anterior displacement of the iris, (4) aqueous misdirection, and (5) blocking tissue (Table 11–17). Pupillary block is the mechanism in the overwhelming majority of cases of primary angle-closure glaucoma. It is enhanced by atrophy and flaccidity of the iris in the elderly, allowing the higher pressure in the posterior chamber to bulge the periphery of the iris anteriorly, which leads to angle closure. Factors such as partial dilatation of the pupil and anterior position of the lens increase the degree of pupillary block and predispose to the development of primary angle closure (Fig. 11–31A and B). Other causes of aqueous obstruction at the plane of the iris lead to secondary angle-closure glaucoma (Fig. 11–31C and D).

Wide dilatation of the pupil may jam the iris into the angle even in cases in which pupillary block does not play a role (Fig. 11–32). This is most frequently seen in patients with anterior insertion of the iris (C insertion in the Wills Eye Hospital grading system; see Fig. 11–26).

Ocular inflammation can cause the ciliary body to swell, with consequent rotation of the root of the iris anteriorly (Fig. 11–33). The inflamed tissue under such circumstances is more likely to be sticky, predisposing to the adherence of the tissue should swelling be so marked that angle closure actually develops. Anterior displacement of the peripheral iris may also occur in other conditions that move the ciliary body anteriorly: the use of miotics, ciliary body or choroidal "detachment," interference with outflow of the vortex veins, and compression of the globe by a tumor or encircling band.

In some instances the anterior surface of the iris is pulled anteriorly into the angle, covering the recess. This occurs in neovascular glaucoma, in which neovascular membrane "zippers up" the angle (Fig. 11–34). In the iris atrophy group

TABLE 11–17. Classification and Therapy of Glaucomas in Which Narrowness or Closure of the Angle Is a Factor

TYPE OF GLAUCOMA	THERAPY
1. Pupillary block	
Narrow, occludable, but open angle	
Asymptomatic	None, weak pilocarpine, or nd:YAG laser iridotomy*
Symptomatic	Pilocarpine or nd:YAG laser iridotomy*
Primary angle-closure glaucoma	
Acute	Nd:YAG laser iridectomy, nd:YAG laser iridotomy, surgical iridectomy, chamber-deepening iridectomy or trabeculectomy
Chronic	Trabeculectomy
Fellow eye of patient with angle-closure glaucoma in other eye	Nd:YAG laser iridotomy
Secondary pupillary block	Nd:YAG laser iridotomy or surgical iridectomy
2. Plateau iris glaucoma (angle jamming)	Weak pilocarpine or argon laser iridoplasty
3. Anterior displacement of iris	
Miotic-induced	Stop miotic and give cycloplegic
Ciliary body swelling	Steroids
Compression	
Scleral band	Cut band
Tumor	Irradiation
4. Secondary angle-closure glaucomas (other than those above)	
Malignant glaucoma	Atropine, phenylephrine, acetazolamide; vitrectomy if needed
Tumor	Irradiation or enucleation
Neovascular	Panretinal photocoagulation, atropine, steroids, and later trabeculectomy if eye quiets; Molteno implant or nd:YAG cyclophotocoagulation if unable to quiet eye

*See Tables 11–27 and 11–37.

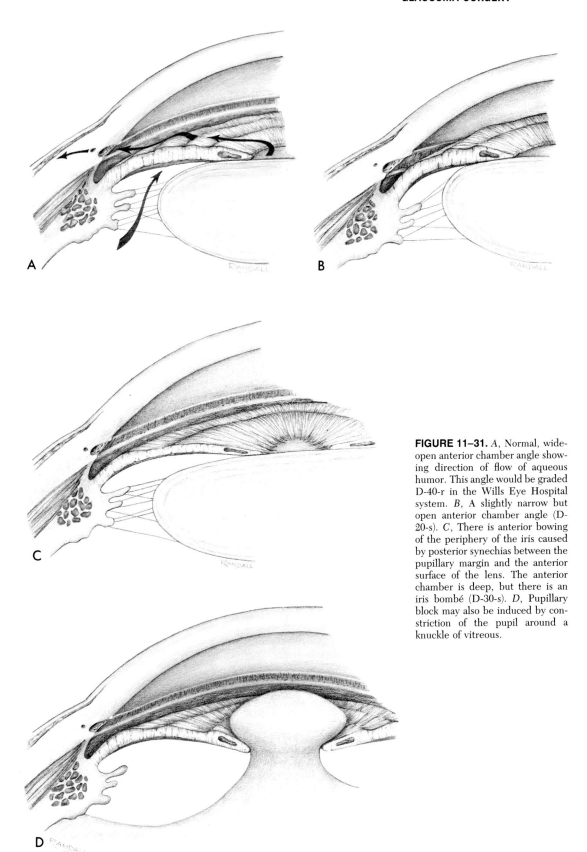

FIGURE 11–31. *A*, Normal, wide-open anterior chamber angle showing direction of flow of aqueous humor. This angle would be graded D-40-r in the Wills Eye Hospital system. *B*, A slightly narrow but open anterior chamber angle (D-20-s). *C*, There is anterior bowing of the periphery of the iris caused by posterior synechias between the pupillary margin and the anterior surface of the lens. The anterior chamber is deep, but there is an iris bombé (D-30-s). *D*, Pupillary block may also be induced by constriction of the pupil around a knuckle of vitreous.

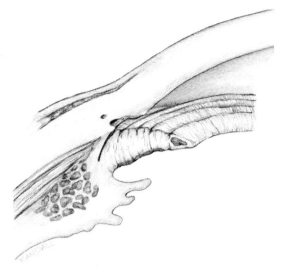

FIGURE 11–32. Wide dilatation of the pupil may cause the iris to become jammed into the angle recess in a predisposed patient. This is not a common mechanism for angle closure. It is more common in those with an anteriorly inserted iris root and those with a flaccid iris.

of glaucomas, all of which appear to have secondary angle closure as the cause for pressure elevation, a similar mechanism is at work.

Each of these three types of angle closure must be treated differently. Pupillary block is cured by creating a communication between the anterior and posterior chambers (Fig. 11–35A and B); angle jamming is corrected by contracting the pupil; and ciliary body swelling is relieved by suppressing the inflammation or eliminating the mechanical cause for the anterior displacement of the iris diaphragm.

Provocative Tests

The anterior chamber becomes shallower with increasing age. About 10 per cent of people over 80 years of age have anterior chamber angles that appear narrow enough to occlude.[32] However, angle-closure glaucoma is an uncommon disease; certainly 10 per cent of people over 80 years of age do not develop it. The ophthalmologist is thus left with a dilemma; how can one distinguish between the eye (with a narrow anterior chamber angle) that is going to proceed to angle closure and the eye (that has a similar narrow anterior chamber angle) that will *not* develop angle-closure glaucoma in the future? A variety of "provocative tests" have been developed in an effort to answer this question. Unfortunately, with the exception of the darkroom test, they are of little or no value.

The fact that one can cause intraocular pressure to rise and the angle to close in response to instillation of a cycloplegic or a mydriatic agent does not provide the ophthalmologist with information of much value, for the changes that occur spontaneously in the eye are not mimicked by those caused by cycloplegics or mydriatics. Cycloplegics not only dilate the pupil, but also cause a deepening of the anterior chamber (the opposite of the case shown in Fig. 11–33). Thus false-negative results are common; that is, that the angle does not close or the intraocular pressure rise in response to dilatation of the pupil by a cycloplegic agent cannot be taken as an indication that a person with a narrow anterior chamber angle will not spontaneously develop an angle-closure glaucoma. Nor does a rise in pressure secondary to use of a cycloplegic signal angle closure; cycloplegics cause increased pressure by interfering with aqueous outflow even in wide-open angles. In a patient with unstable open-angle glaucoma cycloplegics can induce a pressure increase of 20 mm Hg or more *without* causing angle

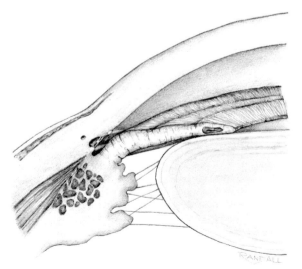

FIGURE 11–33. Inflammation of the ciliary body and the root of the iris may cause the iris to rotate anteriorly toward the angle recess, predisposing to peripheral anterior synechia and a secondary angle-closure glaucoma.

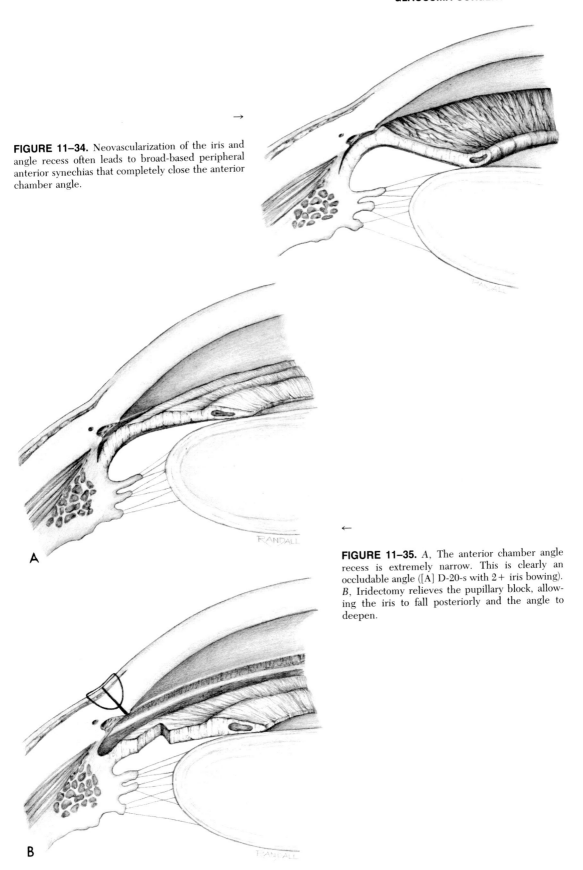

FIGURE 11–34. Neovascularization of the iris and angle recess often leads to broad-based peripheral anterior synechias that completely close the anterior chamber angle.

FIGURE 11–35. *A*, The anterior chamber angle recess is extremely narrow. This is clearly an occludable angle ([A] D-20-s with 2+ iris bowing). *B*, Iridectomy relieves the pupillary block, allowing the iris to fall posteriorly and the angle to deepen.

A

B

closure. Thus a rise in intraocular pressure in response to administration of a cycloplegic such as tropicamide (Mydriacyl) is *not* proof of angle closure (false-positive test).

Nor does the instillation of a mydriatic agent such as phenylephrine mimic normal physiology. Under normal circumstances, when the dilator muscle of the iris contracts, the sphincter muscle relaxes, permitting dilation of the pupil. However, when a mydriatic agent is instilled the dilator muscle is stimulated to contract at the same time that the sphincter muscle is still contracting; this causes an increase in the degree of pupillary block and, consequently, predisposes the subject to angle-closure glaucoma (Fig. 11–36). Thus, although it is clear that one can induce angle-closure glaucoma by dilating the pupil with a mydriatic agent, such an occurrence does not mimic an episode of spontaneous angle-closure glaucoma. In addition, most mydriatic agents cause such wide dilation of the pupil that they induce a second mechanism of angle closure, specifically angle jamming (Fig. 11–32). Such extreme dilatation of the pupil is rare in a physiological setting.

Some authors have recommended that patients be tested by combined administration of a miotic and a mydriatic, with simultaneous water drinking. Unquestionably this will increase the yield of positive provocative tests. It will also increase the number of people in whom surgery is unnecessarily performed. It will probably *not* increase the ability to detect those in whom angle closure will *spontaneously* develop.

The darkroom provocative test can provide useful information. It mimics a normal occurrence. One is not, however, trying to determine whether intraocular pressure becomes elevated after a person has been sequestered in a dark room for an hour, but whether there is an elevation of intraocular pressure *caused by angle closure*. Thus, when performing a darkroom test, the essential element is not the rise of pressure, but a rise of pressure occurring in conjunction with angle closure.

The darkroom test is performed as follows:

1. Intraocular pressure is determined in both eyes.

2. Gonioscopy is performed, noting the nature of the anterior chamber angle in both eyes.

3. The patient remains seated by the slit lamp, but the slit-lamp table is changed from its usual location so that the patient assumes a comfortable position with the arms lying crossed on the slit-lamp table, and the forehead resting against the crossed arms.

4. The patient is asked to close the eyes, keep the eyes closed, and to avoid falling asleep.

5. The room is darkened.

6. The patient is checked at 15-minute intervals, with no examination being done then.

7. After 1 hour the intraocular pressure is measured, as quickly as possible and with the introduction into the eye of as little light as feasible.

8. If there has been a rise of pressure greater than 5 mm Hg, slit-lamp gonioscopy is performed immediately.

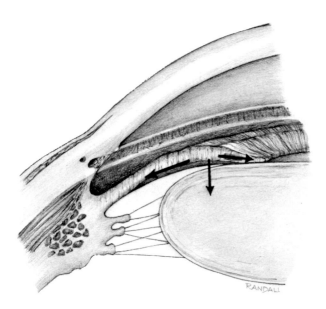

FIGURE 11–36. The arrow pointing to the right indicates the direction of pull of the iris sphincter; the arrow pointing to the left is the direction of force exerted by the iris dilator. The resultant vector of force is posterior. Thus simultaneous stimulation of the dilator and the sphincter muscle causes the iris to be apposed more tightly against the anterior surface of the lens.

9. A rise in pressure greater than 5 mm Hg in association with closure of the anterior chamber angle strongly suggests that the patient may be having episodes of spontaneous angle-closure glaucoma.

Classification

The mechanisms of angle-closure glaucoma have been discussed. Classification can be helpful in deciding on a logical therapeutic approach; both are given in Table 11–17.

Treatment

A plan of management is shown in Table 11–18.

The initial step in treatment is diagnosis. The next consideration is the urgency of treatment. Important factors are (a) the absolute level of intraocular pressure; (b) the rapidity with which the intraocular pressure has risen; (c) additional considerations that describe the health of the eye itself, such as degree of inflammation, appearance of the optic disc, and state of the retinal vessels; and (d) the general condition of the patient (Fig. 11–37).

If the intraocular pressure exceeds the systolic pressure in the arteries that supply the retina, blindness can develop in minutes. As systolic pressure is often around 70 mm Hg, intraocular pressures above this constitute a dire emergency. If the retinal arteries are collapsed and the disc pale, the pressure must be

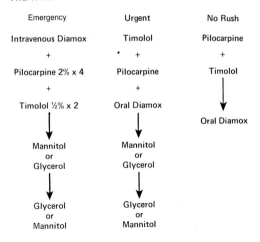

TREATMENT OF PRIMARY ANGLE-CLOSURE GLAUCOMA

Urgency is a factor of:
1) level of intraocular pressure;
2) rapidity of rise of intraocular pressure;
3) nature of the eye (visual acuity, amount of inflammation, healthiness of the optic disc, state of the retinal blood vessels).

FIGURE 11–37. Flowsheet for treatment of primary angle-closure glaucoma, depending on relative urgency of treatment.

lowered immediately. If the retinal vessels pulsate, indicating that the pressure is between the diastolic and the systolic levels, there is more urgency than if the retinal vessels appear unaffected. If the disc shows advanced glaucom-

TABLE 11–18. A Management Plan for Narrow or Closed Anterior Chamber Angles

FACTORS THAT PREDISPOSE TO MEDICAL MANAGEMENT	FACTORS THAT PREDISPOSE TO IRIDECTOMY	FACTORS THAT PREDISPOSE TO TRABECULECTOMY
Absence of peripheral anterior synechias	Documented attack of acute elevation of intraocular pressure in association with closure of the anterior chamber angle	Cupping of the optic disc or visual field loss
Absence of development of new anterior synechias	Patient less than 50 years old or with anticipated long life expectancy	Elevated intraocular pressure on therapy in association with an open anterior chamber angle
Complete 360-degree closure of angle with synechias	Recurrent attacks of angle closure	Progressive deterioration of the optic disc or visual field
Deepening of the anterior chamber in response to topical pilocarpine	Peripheral anterior synechias	Poor access to care
Short anticipated longevity of patient	Positive family history of visual loss associated with documented angle closure	Patient unable to care for himself or herself
Patient frightened by aspect of surgery	Poor access to care	
Patient comfortable with possibility of developing angle closure attack	Patient unable to deal with the uncertainty of possible angle closure attack in the future	
Patient good at caring for himself or herself	Lack of deepening of the anterior chamber angle in response to topical pilocarpine	
Nanophthalmos or hyperopia greater than 4 diopters	Progressive development of peripheral anterior synechias	
	Rising trend of intraocular pressure	
	Healthy disc and field	

atous cupping, it is unlikely that the eye will tolerate pressure as satisfactorily as it would if the disc were healthy.

If treatment is urgent, such as in the eye with an intraocular pressure of 80 mm Hg and collapsed retinal arteries, a paracentesis may be performed. If pressure is markedly elevated but not above systolic blood pressure, a suitable mode of therapy is to apply a drop of topical timolol 0.5% and give acetazolamide, 500 mg, intravenously (Fig. 11–37). Pilocarpine 2% is instilled and repeated every 5 minutes for four doses. Intraocular pressure should be checked 30 to 60 minutes later, and if pressure has not already started to fall markedly, an osmotic agent should probably be given. If the patient has a history of prostatic or cardiovascular disease, the treatment of choice is probably glycerol, 1 ml/kg body weight. If the patient is nauseated or already in the hospital, or if it is convenient to administer medications intravenously, mannitol 20% in an intravenous drip (7 ml/kg body weight) is appropriate. The infusion should be completed within 45 to 60 minutes.

If after 2 hours intraocular pressure has still not fallen, it may be necessary to combine timolol, acetazolamide, glycerol, and mannitol and be prepared to go ahead with surgery when the pressure has fallen. The medications are given so that the peak effect of each occurs simultaneously. It is rare that the intraocular pressure cannot be lowered satisfactorily. Topical timolol is instilled and a mannitol drip started; one-half hour later the glycerol is administered orally and a half hour after that the intravenous acetazolamide; all drugs are administered in full doses (see Table 11–12).

In cases of less urgency, such as when the eye is painful and inflamed but the intraocular pressure is only 40 mm Hg, it is probably adequate to administer timolol 0.5% once and pilocarpine 1% four times, and monitor the effect. If the pressure has not fallen within an hour, oral acetazolamide may need to be used as well.

When there are signs that an angle-closure attack has occurred but the intraocular pressure has fallen, treatment needs to be directed at maintaining a small pupil and eliminating inflammation. Thus topical steroids and weak pilocarpine are the agents of choice.

The next decision is whether or not surgery needs to be done. The factors entering into this decision include the level of intraocular pressure achieved with medical treatment, the percentage of the anterior chamber angle involved with peripheral anterior synechias, the response of the angle to the administration of pilocarpine, the status of the disc and visual field, the patient's ease of access to medical care, the personality and life expectancy of the patient, and the wishes of the patient. A semiquantitative schema can help to put these factors into perspective (Fig. 11–38A).

In the simplest terms three major considerations need to be considered: (1) the possible risk to the patient's eye should another attack occur, (2) the psychological anxiety that is an inevitable component of knowing that a subsequent attack can occur, and (3) the cost, inconvenience, and risk of the surgery itself.

A variety of studies suggest that approximately 50 per cent of patients having had an attack of primary angle-closure glaucoma in one eye will have an attack in the other eye within 5 years.[61, 62] The damage that may be caused by the attack of primary angle-closure glaucoma should be recalled. Peripheral anterior synechias develop in most eyes in which an angle-closure attack persists for longer than 3 days. Of more concern, however, is the development of cataract and the damage to the optic nerve that may occur. If the pressure elevation is extreme and the rise rapid, the attack can leave a previously normal eye with little or no visual function. It is my clinical impression that recovery of vision after most attacks of acute angle-closure glaucoma is seldom complete. Considering these matters together allows us to conclude that approximately 50 per cent of patients who have had an attack of acute primary angle-closure glaucoma in one eye can expect to lose a significant amount of vision in the other eye within the next 5 years, unless intervention is effective.

Another factor is the psychological effect of knowing that sight might be lost at any time. Although some patients handle this uncertainty with equanimity, others are incapacitated by the anxiety. The extent of the psychological damage to patients faced with such a terrible prospect is difficult to evaluate, and may be overlooked by ophthalmologists, who tend to be more deeply involved with the health of their patients' eyes than with the health of the entire patient.

Finally, it should be kept in mind that the risks of surgery are still less than the risk of an attack of acute glaucoma.

In conclusion, then, surgery on the involved eye is indicated in almost all patients who have had an attack of acute primary angle-closure

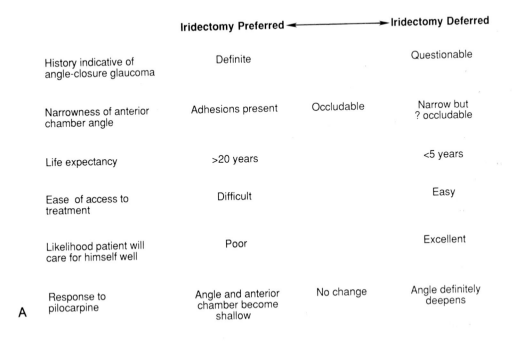

Factors Determining Choice of Treatment in Patients with Narrow Anterior Chamber Angles

Iridectomy Preferred ←——————→ Iridectomy Deferred

History indicative of angle-closure glaucoma	Definite		Questionable
Narrowness of anterior chamber angle	Adhesions present	Occludable	Narrow but ? occludable
Life expectancy	>20 years		<5 years
Ease of access to treatment	Difficult		Easy
Likelihood patient will care for himself well	Poor		Excellent
Response to pilocarpine	Angle and anterior chamber become shallow	No change	Angle definitely deepens

A

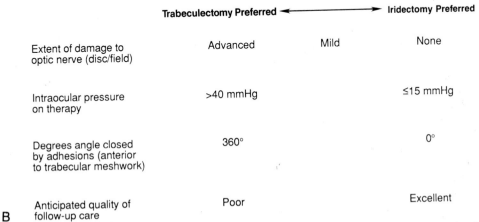

Factors Determining Choice of Surgical Procedure in Primary Angle-closure Glaucoma

Trabeculectomy Preferred ←——————→ Iridectomy Preferred

Extent of damage to optic nerve (disc/field)	Advanced	Mild	None
Intraocular pressure on therapy	>40 mmHg		≤15 mmHg
Degrees angle closed by adhesions (anterior to trabecular meshwork)	360°		0°
Anticipated quality of follow-up care	Poor		Excellent

B

FIGURE 11–38. *A*, Factors that determine the choice of treatment in patients with narrow anterior chamber angles. *B*, Factors that affect whether trabeculectomy or iridectomy should be performed in patients with primary angle-closure glaucoma.

glaucoma. Similarly, it is usually safer for the patient to have surgery on the fellow eye as well.

There are a few specific situations in which surgery appears to be either unnecessary or, at best, avoided. For example, in the patient who has had a devastating attack with massive iris atrophy as the result, a peripheral iridectomy may not need to be performed because the degree of atrophy may permit adequate communication between the posterior and the anterior chambers. If, after the attack, the pressure rapidly falls to normal and gonioscopy shows that the anterior chamber deepens remarkably in response to pilocarpine 1% twice daily, then the need for surgery decreases. In such a patient, should there be extenuating circumstances such as a morbid fear of surgery or far advanced visual field loss, then probably medical treatment is preferable. If one is considering surgery on the second eye, the experience on the first eye can be a valuable guide. If a significant complication occurred during the first procedure, and the cause could not be determined in order to prevent its occurring during a second operation, the surgeon must expect a similar complication to develop in the second eye.

The choice of procedure is the next decision. Before the development of trabeculectomy, the surgeon was best advised to perform an iridectomy in almost all cases of primary angle-closure glaucoma, whether acute or chronic.[63] For cases in which the pressure was not controlled by the iridectomy itself, the use of medical therapy postoperatively usually permitted control; further surgery for control of the intraocular pressure itself was occasionally needed. The reason for choosing an iridectomy over a filtering procedure was mainly the lower complication rate of the former. Especially in the angle-closure glaucomas, the standard filtering procedures too often led to serious problems, most notably flat anterior chamber and malignant glaucoma.

A trabeculectomy with a tightly sutured scleral flap, on the other hand, has a complication rate barely greater than that of an iridectomy. Consequently, in those cases in which it seems unlikely that an iridectomy alone will satisfactorily control the pressure, a trabeculectomy is the procedure of choice (Fig. 11–38B). I perform a trabeculectomy in most cases of primary angle-closure glaucoma with cupping and visual field loss, with 75 per cent or more of the angle closed with synechias, or with intraocular pressures that cannot be brought to a level lower than 30 mm Hg preoperatively.

Other factors that enter into the choice of surgery are the nature of the patient, the quality of follow-up care, the access to care, and the response to medical treatment (Fig. 11–38B).

When the surgeon is uncertain regarding the choice between iridectomy and trabeculectomy, he should consider an iridectomy through clear cornea. This is a satisfactory procedure with a complication rate higher than that of the standard iridectomy but lower than that of trabeculectomy.

The advent of laser iridotomy has, to some extent, altered the points just made. For example, whereas previously it was the policy to avoid surgery whenever possible in the fellow eye of a patient having had a malignant glaucoma, laser iridotomy permits the surgeon to go ahead with an iridectomy. (See p. 325 for further discussion of laser treatment.) There are times when laser iridotomy seems especially appropriate (Table 11–19).

Glaucoma in Infants

Glaucoma occurs only rarely in infants.[64] It will be dealt with here only briefly. The surgery and long-term management of glaucoma in infants is best accomplished in referral centers that have special facilities and personnel for caring for glaucoma in infants. Correct diagnosis is vital. None of the common diagnostic findings is, by itself, pathognomonic. The differential diagnosis of the most common symptoms and signs is given in Table 11–20. Despite the rarity of congenital glaucoma, infants with tearing and photophobia and cloudy or large eyes should be assumed to have congenital glaucoma and the appropriate diagnostic tests undertaken promptly.

Cupping of the optic disc develops rapidly in infants. Irreversible damage may occur in a period as short as 1 month. Thus, when infantile glaucoma is suspected, efforts should be made to reach a diagnosis within 1 week.

As with other types of glaucoma, the diagnosis is most certain when a constellation of findings is characteristic. As in adults, a variety

TABLE 11–19. Special Indications for Laser Iridotomy

Active external infection
Bleeding disorder (argon preferred)
Predisposition to malignant glaucoma
Complication at time of previous surgery
Nanophthalmos

TABLE 11–20. Glaucoma in Infants: Differential Diagnosis of Signs and Symptoms

Elevated intraocular pressure
   Spurious determination, owing to squeezing, ketamine, etc.
Corneal enlargement
   Megalocornea
Corneal haziness
   Trauma
   Mesodermal dysgenesis
   Keratitis
   Congenital hereditary corneal edema
   Congenital dystrophy of the cornea
   Cystinosis
   Familial plasma lecithin–cholesterol acyl transferase deficiency
   Generalized gangliosidosis
   Glycogenoses
   Hurler's syndrome
   Ichthyosis
   Maroteaux-Lamy syndrome
   Morquio's syndrome
   Mucolipidosis
   Osteogenesis imperfecta
   Scheie's syndrome
   Trisomy 18
Photophobia
   Albinism
   Cone dysfunction syndrome
   Cystinosis
   Down's syndrome
   Keratosis follicularis spinulosa decalvans
   Lowe's syndrome
   Menke's disease
   Phenylketonuria
   Porphyria
   Tryptophanemia
   Xeroderma pigmentosum
Tearing
   Congenital absence of lacrimal puncta
   Cystinosis
   Dacryocystitis
   Englemann's disease
   Porphyria

of types of glaucoma occur in infants (Table 11–21). Associated ocular or systemic abnormalities should be sought because the glaucoma may be part of a more global condition.

Congenital Glaucoma (Trabeculodysgenesis)

Congenital glaucoma is the traditional phrase applied to the glaucoma that occurs in infants in whom other systemic or ocular abnormalities are absent. That is, it is the "primary" glaucoma of infants. The adjective "congenital" is a poor one and probably should no longer be used. Although in some instances the condition is noted at birth, in most infants it does not become apparent until several months later. In some cases its onset may not occur until early adolescence.

The basic cause of the disease appears to be an anomaly of the angle structures that results in interference with aqueous outflow.[65, 66] In the great majority of cases a delicate incision into the covering of the angle recess (a goniotomy) is adequate to lower intraocular pressure.[18]

The diagnosis of congenital glaucoma is largely based on the same criteria used to diagnose other types of glaucoma: evidence of damage to the optic nerve caused by elevated intraocular pressure. Because an accurate assessment of intraocular pressure is difficult in infants, and visual field examination is obviously rudimentary at best, the appearance of the optic nerve takes on added importance.

TABLE 11–21. Classification of Glaucoma in Infants

I. Genetically related glaucoma
   A. Infantile or primary congenital glaucoma—trabeculodysgenesis
   B. Glaucoma with associated anomaly or disease
      1. Phakomatoses
         a. Encephalotrigeminal hemangioma (Sturge-Weber syndrome)
         b. Neurofibromatosis (von Recklinghausen's disease)
         c. Oculodermal melanocytosis (nevus of Ota)
         d. Retinocerebellar angiomatosis (von Hippel-Lindau disease)
         e. Tuberous sclerosis (Bourneville's disease)
      2. Mesodermal anomalies
         a. Axenfeld's syndrome
         b. Peter's anomaly
         c. Rieger's syndrome
      3. Metabolic disease or syndrome
         a. Amyloidosis
         b. Hallermann-Streiff syndrome
         c. Homocystinuria
         d. Hurler's syndrome
         e. Lawford's syndrome
         f. Lowe's syndrome
         g. Marfan's syndrome
         h. Pierre Robin's syndrome
         i. Refsum's disease
         j. Rubenstein's syndrome
         k. Weill-Marchesani syndrome
      4. Iris anomalies
         a. Aniridia
         b. Aniridia with Wilms' tumor

II. Nongenetic glaucoma
   A. Secondary glaucoma
      1. Trauma
      2. Inflammations
      3. Tumors
      4. Vascular problems
   B. Embryopathies
      1. Rubella syndrome
      2. Trisomy 13
      3. Trisomy 18
      4. Chromosome 18 deletion

Modified from Shaffer, R. N., Weiss, D. I.: Congenital and Pediatric Glaucomas. St. Louis, C. V. Mosby Co., 1970, pp. 8–9.

The intraocular pressure of the anesthetized infant may be misleading. If taken in the early stages of anesthesia or when the infant is in a light plane, the intraocular pressure tends to be spuriously high. If determined when the infant is fully anesthetized, the intraocular pressure is lower than it would be in the unanesthetized subject. Occasional agents, such as ketamine, cause an elevation of pressure even when the child is deeply anesthetized. This effect of sedation or incomplete relaxation must be recalled when intraocular pressure is measured in the infant. The small size of the infant cornea also makes measurement with a Schiøtz tonometer imprecise. The hand-held applanation tonometers are recommended; I prefer that of Draeger or Perkins. If intraocular pressure is 4 mm Hg or higher in one eye than in the other, or if the level when determined with the infant in a deeply sedated, intubated condition is above 25 mm Hg, it is likely that the intraocular pressure is abnormal.

The optic nerve heads of the infant's two eyes should be symmetrical and normal in appearance.[68] Asymmetry is highly suggestive of glaucoma. Cupping occurs rapidly and resembles that seen in the "hyperbaric" type of primary open-angle glaucoma; that is, there is progressive enlargement of the cup, usually in a concentric manner but occasionally in a pattern of increasingly large ovals. The appearance of the discs should be drawn at each examination.

Corneal changes, when present, are strong indicators of pathology, but they occur only in the later stages of the disease. Thus corneal enlargement, edema, and tears in Descemet's membrane should be looked for, but their absence does not mean absence of glaucoma. Their presence does not necessarily mean a glaucoma, either (Table 11–20).

Gonioscopy in the infant is of little diagnostic value. In the first place, because this type of examination is so rarely done in infants and there is no standard for determining what is "normal," most ophthalmologists have never seen a normal infant angle; consequently they cannot distinguish between the normal and the pathological. Second, the angle of the infant with congenital glaucoma does not present a pathognomonic picture. For example, although an apparently imperforate sheet spreading over the whole angle recess is typical of congenital glaucoma, this so-called Barkan's membrane is present in almost all infant angles, though to a lesser extent.[32]

When the question of congenital glaucoma arises, an attempt should be made to obtain an adequate examination of the unanesthetized infant. The use of Richardson's infant diagnostic Koeppe lens is helpful, more for fundus examination than for the less essential gonioscopy. After this, an examination under full anesthesia is usually required promptly. Infants tend to tolerate the inhalation anesthetic agents well, without developing liver damage. Therefore, in centers properly equipped and staffed to provide care for infants, there is little risk from the anesthesia itself.

Accurate determination of the axial length of the eye with A-scan ultrasound will help in both diagnosis and management. Globes that are longer than normal, especially when different from the other eye, are highly suspicious. Globes that elongate more rapidly than normal are almost certainly actively glaucomatous.

If intraocular pressure is marginal and the disc changes are suspicious but not definite, repeat anesthesia examination 2 to 4 weeks later should usually make the diagnosis clear. If corneal diameters and axial lengths remain unchanged, intraocular pressure is roughly the same, and, most important, the discs have not changed for the worse, usually it is best to defer any surgery and reexamine the infant again 1 month later. A third examination without change is strongly indicative that glaucoma is not present. Nevertheless, close follow-up is in order, as marginal cases can become frankly glaucomatous many months later.

If the initial examination is diagnostic, or if on subsequent examination an enlargement of the cup is noted or the intraocular pressure is unquestionably high, surgery should be performed during the same anesthetic experience. If the angle can be well seen, goniotomy is the procedure of choice. If the surgeon is not a skilled gonioscopist and is not fully familiar with the technique of goniotomy, a trabeculotomy should be done.

Repeat anesthetic examinations should be made 1 month after surgery, at which time goniotomy or trabeculotomy can be repeated if necessary.

If further surgery is required, the infant should again be reexamined 1 month later. If three goniotomies or two trabeculotomies have failed, then a peripheral iridectomy with thermal sclerostomy (or as a second choice a trabeculectomy) is usually the treatment of choice. Filtering procedures are not the initial choice because they are more traumatizing, have no higher success rate than that with goniotomy or trabeculotomy, and predispose to scleral staphyloma.

In most children with congenital glaucoma it is now possible, with modern surgical techniques, to control the intraocular pressure satisfactorily. However, visual results are still poor. The proper management of these infants includes early refraction and appropriate correction to prevent the amblyopia that is a routine part of the condition. Contact lenses have been tried in some centers with moderate success. A pediatric ophthalmologist should be part of the team that provides the ongoing management of these cases.

Secondary Glaucomas

The secondary glaucomas constitute a heterogeneous group of conditions in which intraocular pressure is elevated owing to a mechanism different from that in either primary angle-closure or primary open-angle glaucoma. In almost all instances the basic mechanism is interference with outflow.

Obstruction of aqueous flow in the secondary glaucomas occurs in different locations. A classification of the secondary glaucomas is given in Table 11–22.

The goal of medical and surgical therapy in the treatment of the secondary glaucomas is the same as in the primary glaucomas: to preserve the sight of the eye by preventing damage to the optic nerve caused by intraocular pressure

TABLE 11–22. Classification of Secondary Glaucomas

I. Aqueous block
  A. In vitreous (malignant glaucoma)
  B. At anterior face of vitreous (malignant glaucoma)
  C. At pupil
    1. Iris adhesions to lens, pseudophakos, vitreous, or any membrane; "air block"
  D. At angle recess
    1. Epithelial ingrowth
    2. Fibrinous membrane
    3. Neovascular membrane
    4. Iris
    5. Angle cleavage
    6. Extension of Descemet's membrane
    7. Tumor or cyst
  E. In trabeculum
    1. Pigment
    2. Inflammatory debris
    3. Exfoliated material
    4. Red blood cells or ghost cells
    5. Mucopolysaccharide (due to steroids?)
  F. In sclera
    1. Episcleritis
    2. Obstruction of extraocular veins

II. Aqueous hypersecretion
  A. Iridocyclitis

higher than the eye can tolerate (see p. 214). However, several aspects of the secondary glaucomas are so different from the primary glaucomas that the specifics of management differ markedly. In the primary glaucomas intraocular pressure rises progressively, causing progressive deterioration of the optic nerve, whereas in the secondary glaucomas the cause for pressure elevation is often transient. A second major difference is the reaction to surgery. In contrast to the primary glaucomas, in which surgery is usually successful, in many of the secondary glaucomas operative procedures have a discouragingly poor outcome, often resulting in further complications such as neovascular glaucoma, the Sturge-Weber syndrome, and uveitis.

As the clinical course of a secondary glaucoma evolves, the cause for the elevated intraocular pressure may change. This often complicates therapy significantly. For example, a patient with uveitis may initially have a rise in pressure because of a trabeculopathy; as the uveitis clears through treatment with corticosteroids, the pressure may remain elevated because of the topical steroids themselves, even though the trabecular meshwork is no longer inflamed; later, inflammatory synechias may close the angle so that the patient develops a secondary angle-closure glaucoma. Thus, in this particular patient, the treatment in the early stages of the disease would be corticosteroids, in the secondary stages elimination of the corticosteroids, and in the third stage aqueous suppressants or surgery designed to increase aqueous outflow. Some of these problems are shown in the therapeutic flowsheet in Figure 11–39.

The surgeon confronted with a patient with secondary glaucoma should proceed as follows in planning therapy:

1. Properly diagnose the underlying entity.
2. Determine the mechanism for elevation of the intraocular pressure.
3. Direct therapy first at the primary condition and then at the secondary elevation of intraocular pressure.
4. Recall that preservation of the health of the optic nerve is paramount and that proper monitoring demands repeated evaluation of the disc and field.

The only diagnostic test that will be mentioned here is the use of intravenous fluorescein to define the location of aqueous block. This simple test can provide invaluable information. Sodium fluorescein for injection (2.5 to 5.0 ml) is injected intravenously into the arm. The room should be dark. The eye is observed, using the

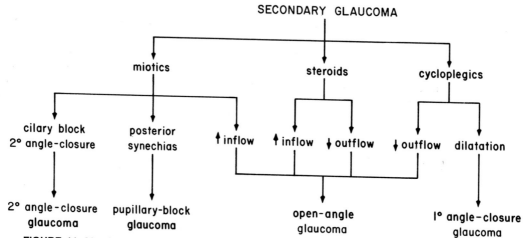

FIGURE 11–39. This flowsheet demonstrates how a patient with a secondary glaucoma may change from having one mechanism responsible for the pressure elevation to having another in response to treatment.

finely focused, maximally intense beam of the slit lamp, noting the pattern of entry of fluorescein. Fluorescein should seep around the pupil gradually, first being visible about 30 seconds after injection. No fluorescein should be seen posterior to the posterior chamber; that is, fluorescein should not be noted behind the lens or anterior vitreous face. In many instances this simple test will establish whether a secondary glaucoma is caused by aqueous misdirection into the vitreous cavity or aqueous sequestration in the posterior chamber. When the eye is markedly inflamed the iris vessels become permeable to fluorescein and the leakage that occurs must be distinguished from flow that originates in the ciliary body.

The appropriate surgical procedure for every type of secondary glaucoma can be established logically by thoughtful consideration of the patient (Table 11–22).

In summary, surgery to control intraocular pressure in patients with secondary glaucoma is indicated when, despite medical therapy, the intraocular pressure is sufficiently elevated that it is causing or is anticipated to cause damage to the optic nerve at a rate that will interfere with the patient's way of life. The surgery is directed toward the elimination of the cause for the elevated intraocular pressure. The risk of the surgery should be balanced not only against the potential benefit, but also against the risk of not performing surgery. This latter point should not be forgotten. Thus, for instance, although there is a moderate risk associated with cyclophotocoagulation in a diabetic whose intraocular pressure is 50 mm Hg owing to a complete closure of the anterior chamber by

peripheral anterior synechias related to a neovascular glaucoma, the risk of *not* performing a cyclophotocoagulation is higher.

Coexisting Cataract and Glaucoma

The occurrence of cataract and glaucoma together in one patient presents difficult management problems. There is still lack of unanimity regarding the best approach.

It was previously believed that cataract extraction alone would result in better control of glaucoma.[69, 70] This was, and still is, true when considering the long-term effect of cataract extraction. Especially with posterior chamber intraocular lens implantation, the intraocular pressure 6 months postoperatively seems to be lower than the intraocular pressure preoperatively. This beneficial effect, however, is not present immediately after surgery. The previous methods of surgery, with few "large" sutures, were probably often associated with temporary leaking wounds, and hence temporary low postoperative pressures. This is no longer the case.

Microsurgical technique permits a tight incision closure; incisions do not leak in the immediate postoperative period. We must change our thinking regarding the course of intraocular pressure that follows cataract extraction. In patients with glaucoma it is routine for the intraocular pressure to rise after uncomplicated cataract extraction. This increase is often marked, and not infrequently will reach a level of 50 to 60 mm Hg, even in the patient whose glaucoma appears to have been satisfactorily controlled

TABLE 11–23. Indications for Combining Glaucoma Surgery with Cataract Extraction

GLAUCOMA SURGERY NEEDED	GLAUCOMA SURGERY USUALLY APPROPRIATE	GLAUCOMA SURGERY USUALLY NOT ADVISABLE
Badly damaged optic disc	Unstable intraocular pressure	Healthy optic disc
Advanced visual field loss	Filtering fistula not entirely	Normal visual field
Inability to take medications and need anticipated	functional	Well-functioning fistula already present and disc damage only slight or
Deterioration of disc or field owing to glaucoma despite therapy	Filtering fistula satisfactory, but disc damage advanced	moderate
Poor access to continuing care	"Unreliable" patient	Patient takes medications well
Little chance for performing 2nd surgical procedure		No progressive damage on treatment Good access to continuing care

TABLE 11–24. Choice of Procedure in Patients Who Need Glaucoma Surgery at Time of Cataract Extraction

PATIENT'S CONDITION	PROCEDURE OF CHOICE	PATIENTS WHO ARE POOR CANDIDATES FOR THIS PROCEDURE
Routine cases	Extracapsular cataract extraction with trabeculectomy and posterior chamber intraocular lens	Patients who are good candidates for other procedures listed below
Marginal control after previous filtering procedure or dissection, or excessively thin bleb	Extracapsular cataract extraction with revision of fistula and implantation of a posterior chamber intraocular lens	Patients with well-functioning fistula with good optic nerve or large scleral opening from previous filtering procedure
Dislocated cataract or a loose lens, as may occur with the exfoliation syndrome or a hypermature cataract	Intracapsular cataract extraction with cyclodialysis	Patients with previous retinal detachment or retinal tears, or high myopia, or inability to take strong miotics, or bleeding diathesis

before the cataract extraction.[71, 72] Such an increase in intraocular pressure is usually not damaging in a patient with a healthy optic nerve. Thus, in the great majority of patients with cataract extraction, this postoperative rise in intraocular pressure is of little clinical consequence. Such is not the case in patients with glaucoma, especially those with advanced cupping of the optic disc, in whom the optic nerve can be rapidly and permanently damaged by increases in intraocular pressure, even if only mild or transient.

Because of the rise in intraocular pressure that follows the newer methods of performing cataract extraction, and because of the susceptibility of the damaged optic nerve to become more seriously injured by such an increase in intraocular pressure, the approach to the management of the patient with cataract and glaucoma must differ significantly from the concepts that govern cataract extraction in a nonglaucomatous eye.[73–76]

The general principles that guide surgery in patients who have both cataract and glaucoma are listed in Tables 11–23 to 11–25.

TABLE 11–25. Factors That Influence Choice of Procedure in Patients Having Cataract and Glaucoma

I. Need to improve visual acuity
   A. Type of cataract
   B. Stage of cataract

II. Stage of glaucoma (susceptibility of nerve head to damage)

III. Need to lower intraocular pressure
   A. Adequacy of glaucoma control
   B. Type of glaucoma

IV. Long-term considerations
   A. Need to fit contact lens
   B. Patient compliance considerations
   C. Availability of care
   D. Likelihood of endophthalmitis

V. Health of eye
   A. Condition of corneal endothelium and epithelium
   B. Presence of inflammation
   C. Presence of exfoliation syndrome
   D. Size and status of the pupil
   E. Nature of the anterior chamber angle

VI. Likelihood that the patient will be willing to have sequential procedures

VII. Experience with the other eye

From Spaeth, G. L.: Ophthalmic Surg., 11:780, 1980.

In the simplest terms, there are three major indications for combining a glaucoma procedure with a cataract extraction: (1) a visually significant cataract that warrants removal in a patient with uncontrolled glaucoma; (2) a visually significant cataract that warrants removal in a patient with severely glaucomatous optic nerve damage that would progress were there a postoperative rise of intraocular pressure; and (3) a cataract that is marginally significant from a visual point of view, but that would be expected to progress and become visually significant after glaucoma surgery.

Cataract Extraction in Patients Who Have Had Previous Glaucoma Surgery. With newer microsurgical techniques cataract extraction in patients who have had previous glaucoma surgery has a higher success rate than the older literature suggests. There are still cases in which failure of the bleb occurs, but less than the 50 per cent reported previously.[77]

If there is a cystic filtering bleb responsible for adequate control of intraocular pressure, the preferred mode of cataract extraction is often to leave the filtering area alone and go elsewhere to remove the cataract (Fig. 11–40*B–D*). I prefer to make the corneoscleral incision temporally or inferiorly; it may be helpful to convert the superior iridectomy to a "sector," especially when extracting the cataract extracapsularly. An alternative approach is to remove the cataract through an incision made in clear cornea anterior to the bleb (Fig. 11–40*A*). This often results in less satisfactory visual acuity in the immediate postoperative period because of the greater amount of postoperative corneal astigmatism. These sutures usually cannot be released for 6 months.

If the previous surgery was a filtering procedure that no longer controls the intraocular pressure adequately, or controls the intraocular pressure only with the use of medications, or is associated with severe optic nerve damage, it is usually appropriate to perform a glaucoma procedure again at the time of the cataract extraction (Fig. 11–40*E*). This can be done by revising the previous glaucoma procedure or performing a new one. The surgeon can raise the conjunctiva flap superiorly where the previous surgery had been performed and then proceed with the cataract extraction. If the prior surgery was a trabeculectomy, the corneoscleral incision can be made through the site of the previous trabeculectomy. This tends to encourage filtration through the area of thin sclera and, after closure of the conjunctiva, to predispose to formation of a filtering bleb and better control of intraocular pressure in the postoperative period. If there is a large sclerectomy, the closure of the incision may be difficult; in such cases it is usually advisable to perform a fresh filtration procedure elsewhere. In almost every instance the conjunctival flap should be fornix-based. Limbus-based flaps are more difficult and do not appear to have any better success rate.

Indications for surgery and the management of glaucoma in aphakic patients are discussed in the section on secondary glaucomas (p. 259).

SURGICAL TECHNIQUES

Conjunctival Flaps

The development of a conjunctival flap is an integral part of many glaucoma procedures. Even techniques that are designed to lower intraocular pressure without gross filtration require cutting the conjunctiva to reach the sclera. A conjunctival flap can be raised from either the limbus or the fornix (Table 11–26).

Limbus-Based Flaps

When filtration of aqueous humor through the sclera is intended, a conjunctival flap needs to be developed. The incision should preferably be made as high in the cul-de-sac as can be reasonably achieved, hinging the tissue at the limbus. This limbus-based flap is one of the most important parts of many glaucoma filtering procedures.

The following descriptions apply to conjunctival flaps developed at the 12 o'clock position of the eye. The anatomical considerations are shown in Figures 11–2 and 11–3. The presence of separate layers of conjunctiva, Tenon's capsule, and episclera should be recalled. I prefer to incise each independently, as this permits the best exposure and the most complete closure: The locations of these separate incisions in conjunctiva (1), Tenon's capsule (2), and episclera (3) are shown in Figure 10–41.

A superior rectus bridle suture is placed, using 4–0 braided black silk (see Fig. 11–81).

The conjunctiva is grasped with dressing or Pierse-Hoskins forceps and pulled inferiorly, using the superior rectus for countertraction (Fig. 11–42). The direction of traction is 180 degrees opposed to the pull of the bridle suture. This puts the conjunctiva on stretch. A blunt-tipped Westcott scissors incises the conjunctiva

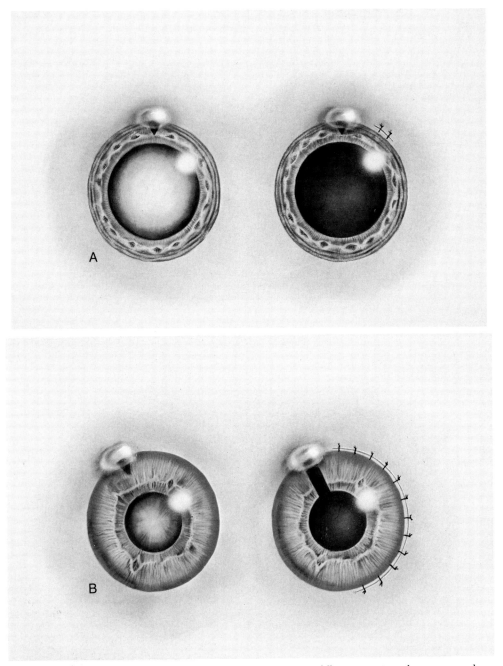

FIGURE 11–40. Different methods of performing cataract extraction following previous glaucoma procedure that has resulted in the presence of a filtering bleb. *A,* When the bleb is functional and the pupil can be dilated, a phakoemulsification may be performed. *B,* When the bleb is functional but the pupil cannot be widely dilated, extraction from the temporal aspect is usually preferable. Surgery is facilitated by converting the peripheral iridectomy to a sector iridectomy. *C,* When the pupil is extremely miotic, the iridectomy should be converted to a sector iridectomy, and a sphincterotomy performed. *D,* When the bleb is adequately functional and the disc is healthy, the cataract can be extracted by an incision in clear cornea or at the corneoscleral junction. *E,* In patients in whom the previous filtration procedure has failed, the cataract extraction should be combined with a new filtration procedure, using a fornix-based or a limbus-based flap. For the routine case, the fornix-based flap is to be preferred. If 5-fluorouracil is to be used postoperatively, a limbus-based flap is preferred.

Illustration continued on following page

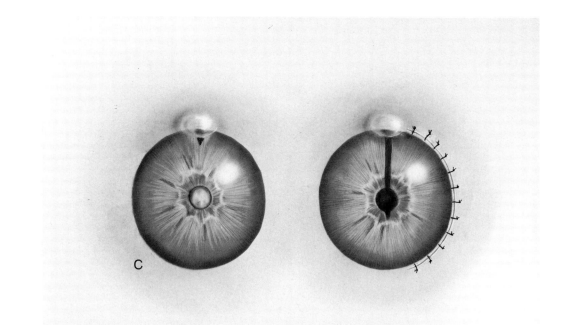

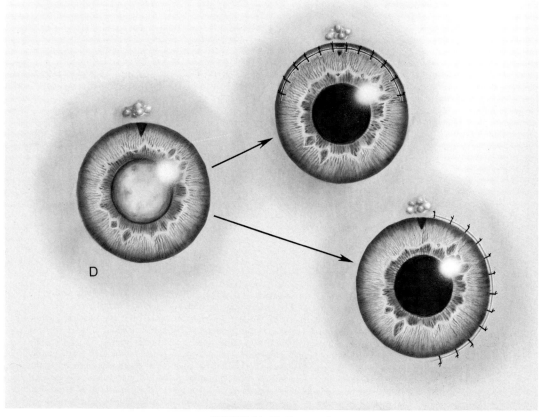

FIGURE 11–40 *Continued*

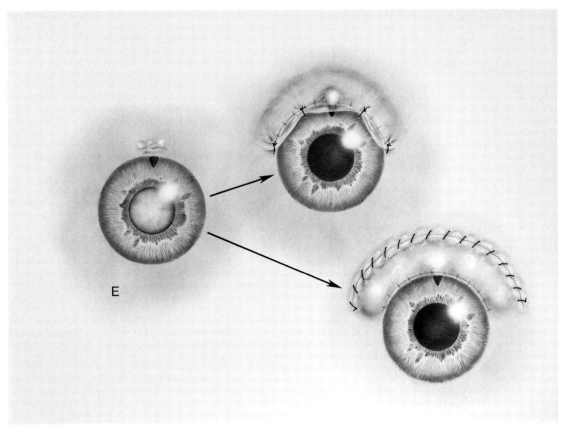

E

FIGURE 11–40 *Continued*

**TABLE 11–26. Indications for the Various Types of Counjunctival Flaps
in Glaucoma Surgery**

TYPE OF PROCEDURE OR DIAGNOSIS	PREFERRED APPROACH	ALTERNATIVE APPROACH
Peripheral iridectomy for neglected primary angle-closure, chronic angle-closure, or combined mechanism glaucoma	Clear cornea	Trabeculectomy with tightly sutured scleral flap
Peripheral iridectomy for primary angle-closure glaucoma	Small fornix-based flap	Clear cornea
Peripheral iridectomy for the fellow eye	Small fornix-based flap	Clear cornea
Trabeculectomy with a tightly sutured scleral flap	High limbus-based flap	Large fornix-based flap
Trabeculectomy with scleral flap intended to leak	High limbus-based flap	—
All standard filtration procedures	High limbus-based flap	—
All reoperations of standard filtration procedures and trabeculectomy	High limbus-based flap*	—
Cataract extraction without combined glaucoma procedure†	Clear cornea	Small fornix-based flap
Cataract extraction with cyclodialysis	Fornix-based flap	Clear cornea
Cataract extraction with trabeculectomy or other filtration procedure	Fornix-based flap	Large limbus-based flap

*Incision should usually be made at the same site as the primary incision.
†Patient under consideration has definite glaucoma, but glaucoma procedure not considered necessary at the time of cataract extraction.

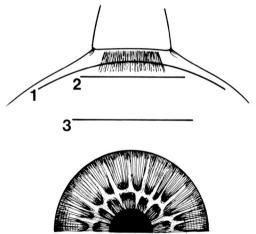

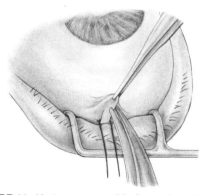

FIGURE 11–41. Schematic representation of the layers important in developing a conjunctival flap. The conjunctiva, Tenon's capsule, and episclera should be handled as separate layers. A three-stage development of the flap can be quickly and readily performed, leading to good exposure of the corneoscleral sulcus with minimum bleeding and minimum trauma to tissue. The conjunctiva (1) is incised over the superior rectus muscle. Tenon's capsule (2) is sectioned anterior to the insertion of the superior rectus tendon. The episclera (3) is button-holed 3 to 4 mm posterior to the corneoscleral sulcus.

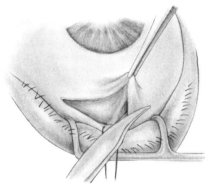

FIGURE 11–44. The conjunctival incision is extended temporally.

FIGURE 11–42. Conjunctiva is lifted away from the globe, put on stretch, and incised adjacent to the superior rectus muscle bridle suture.

immediately anterior to the superior rectus suture (Fig. 11–43). The incision is extended approximately 8 mm nasally and temporally, keeping it as high in the cul-de-sac as possible, and exposing the thicker, more opaque Tenon's capsule (Fig. 11–44). Tenon's capsule is grasped approximately 2 mm anterior to the conjunctival incision; this should be anterior to the superior rectus insertion. Tenon's capsule is then lifted up toward the microscope away from the globe and put on stretch by being pulled anteriorly as well (Fig. 11–45). The Westcott spring scissors is held at an oblique angle, shelved toward the limbus, so that the Tenon's capsule is buttonholed without the underlying tissue being cut. The scissors are then held vertically with the tips closed and inserted into the buttonhole; the tips are opened to spread the tissue further (Fig. 11–46). A sheath of blood vessels surrounding the insertion of the superior rectus muscle becomes visible (Fig. 11–47). If the incision is incomplete, blunt spreading and cautious cutting are continued until the episclera

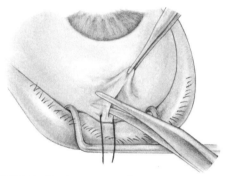

FIGURE 11–43. The incision in the conjunctiva is extended nasally.

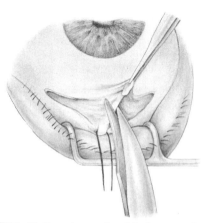

FIGURE 11–45. Tenon's capsule is lifted up away from the globe and incised with the scissors held obliquely, to avoid cutting into the underlying superior rectus.

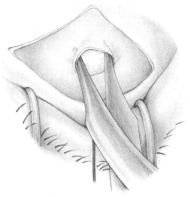

FIGURE 11–46. The incision in Tenon's capsule is spread bluntly.

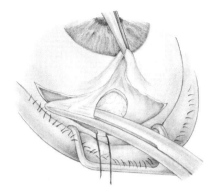

FIGURE 11–48. Tenon's capsule is incised nasally and temporally.

is clearly visible. The incision in Tenon's capsule is extended temporally and nasally to the same extent as for the conjunctival incision (Fig. 11–48). The superior rectus muscle is now clearly visible (Fig. 11–47).

The conjunctiva is retracted inferiorly over the cornea, so that the episclera is clearly exposed. The episclera is firmly grasped with a Pierse-Hoskins forceps or other similar forceps with very fine tips, retracted firmly away from the globe, and buttonholed (Figs. 11–49 and 11–50). The scissors are held so that the blades are parallel to the surface of the globe, and one tip is meticulously introduced through the buttonhole and pushed forward, bluntly dissecting the episclera from the underlying sclera (Fig. 11–51). The episclera is usually firmly adherent.

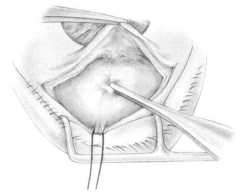

FIGURE 11–49. The connective tissue overlying the superior rectus is easily seen after Tenon's has been incised. This tissue is usually highly vascular in the area directly at the base of the superior rectus muscle.

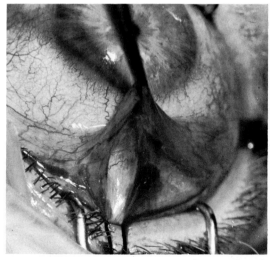

FIGURE 11–47. The superior rectus can be seen through the buttonhole in Tenon's capsule. Bleeding should be minimal; if it occurs, it should be controlled promptly with cautery.

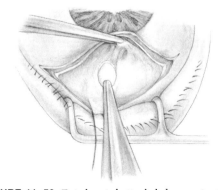

FIGURE 11–50. Episclera is buttonholed approximately 4 mm posterior to the limbus, revealing the underlying sclera.

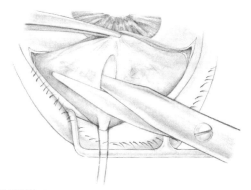

FIGURE 11–51. One blade of the scissors is insinuated between the sclera and the episclera, and the episclera is incised nasally.

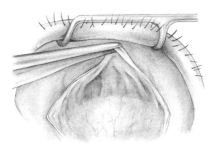

FIGURE 11–53. The episclera is grasped with a nontoothed forceps and pulled bluntly inferiorly.

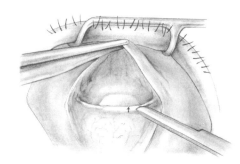

FIGURE 11–54. Remaining adhesions between the episclera and sclera are dissected in a semisharp manner, using the #67 Beaver blade, and pushing the blade at right angles to its cutting axis.

For this maneuver to be performed properly, the blade must be introduced gently, making sure that it hugs the sclera. The tip is introduced approximately 5 mm before the blades are closed. This incision is then extended in a similar manner in the opposite direction (Fig. 11–52). At this point the bare sclera is clearly visible (Fig. 11–53).

In occasional instances it is possible to complete the limbus-based conjunctival flap merely by grasping Tenon's capsule near the limbus and pulling it rather forcibly inferiorly, bluntly tearing it off the underlying sclera. In other instances, especially if medications have been used for long periods before surgery, this tissue is too densely adherent to permit this type of dissection. One satisfactory way in which to proceed is to use a moderately sharp knife, such as a #67 Beaver blade, to scrape the conjunctiva-Tenon's-episcleral flap off the underlying sclera (Fig. 11–54). This maneuver is continued

until the limbal area is cleaned as adequately as is necessary for the procedure under consideration. With adequate magnification it is possible to see the episcleral fibers crossing the corneoscleral sulcus from the retracted episcleral tissue to the underlying sclera. For most glaucoma procedures in which limbus-based flaps are used, it is necessary to continue to clean the limbal region until the corneoscleral

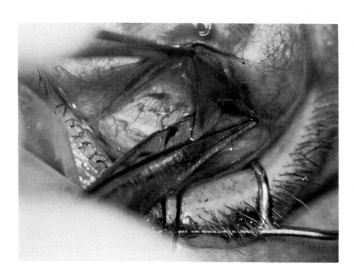

FIGURE 11–52. The episclera is incised temporally. Note that the plane of the scissors is flush with the sclera.

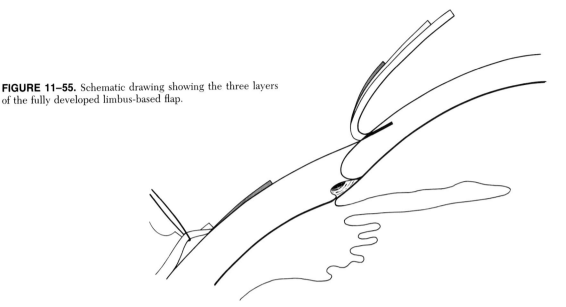

FIGURE 11–55. Schematic drawing showing the three layers of the fully developed limbus-based flap.

sulcus is clearly visible. Often the surgeon must use sharp dissection to finish cleaning the limbus. This is especially important—indeed it is essential—when performing a thermal sclerostomy or posterior sclerectomy, when operating on a hyperopic eye, or when raising a flap away from the 12 o'clock position. In most cases this means that there is an area of nonvascularized, nonopaque tissue visible for a distance of about 1 mm between the edge of the white sclera and the point at which the reflected conjunctiva inserts into the cornea. The corneoscleral sulcus should be present as an obvious groove.

The tissue that has been raised, then, consists of three separate layers: conjunctiva, Tenon's capsule, and episclera (Fig. 11–55).

I prefer to close a large limbus-based flap in two layers. This allows the best apposition of the tissue and restores the eye to a condition most similar to its preoperative state. Furthermore, the possibility of a leaking incision is virtually eliminated. The episclera is probably best left unsutured. Some surgeons prefer to remove episclera, or some or even all of Tenon's capsule. If the surgeon plans to release sutures in the scleral flap with an argon laser in the postoperative period, a tenonectomy may be necessary.

For a right-handed surgeon it is simplest to start at the right-hand edge of the incision, meticulously picking up Tenon's capsule on the corneal side and then finding the opposite side, which has usually retracted under the lid. It may take some searching to find the superior-most portion of Tenon's capsule. This can be

hooked over the tip of the needle and pulled inferiorly (Fig. 11–56). Once the initial suture has been placed and tied, the superior rectus bridle suture should be removed. This may make it more difficult to keep the lid elevated and the eye in a proper position, but if the superior rectus suture is not cut, the superior portion of Tenon's capsule cannot be retracted inferiorly, and proper closure is more difficult. After the first suture in Tenon's capsule has been secured, the cut end can be used for traction to keep the edges in view.

The suture to close Tenon's capsule should preferably be absorbable, 8–0 or 9–0 Vicryl or 8–0 chromic collagen. Collagen has the advantage of being a bit more comfortable, and is the suture I prefer. However, it is fragile and must be handled very delicately. Knots must be

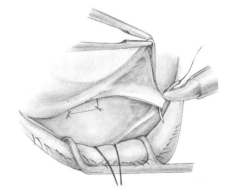

FIGURE 11–56. Tenon's capsule is closed in a separate layer with 8–0 chromic collagen sutures.

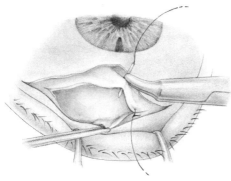

FIGURE 11–57. The superior edge of Tenon's capsule tends to retract up under the lid and must be looked for. It can be hooked over the needle and pulled inferiorly. Sutures are locked.

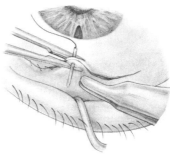

FIGURE 11–59. The conjunctiva is closed with closely spaced running, unlocked sutures. The final suture is securely tied.

placed squarely, and the suture cannot be kinked or it will break. Six to eight sutures, 2 to 3 mm apart, placed in a running, locked stitch will usually close Tenon's capsule securely (Fig. 11–57). It is important to make sure that the previously placed locked suture is pulled tight before proceeding to the next suture.

After the last suture has been placed the needle penetrates the conjunctiva from the episcleral side, exiting on the conjunctival side, thus exteriorizing the suture (Fig. 11–58). The conjunctiva is then closed, using the same suture material in a running stitch, going from the surgeon's left to the surgeon's right. These sutures are not locked, however. The conjunctival sutures should be closely placed, approximately 2 mm apart (Fig. 11–59).

After the needle has been placed through both edges of the tissue, it is lifted toward the

microscope firmly, with the tissue put on stretch. This allows the surgeon to reach underneath the needle with a blunt forceps, grasping the tissue and holding the needle securely in place (Fig. 11–60). When the needle is released, it remains firmly in place, permitting the surgeon to grasp it again so that it will be ready to be reintroduced into the tissue without having to change the position in the needle holder (Fig. 11–61).

Peritomy

The conjunctiva is grasped with fine forceps 1 mm posterior to its anterior attachment to the cornea. The tented-up conjunctiva is incised meridionally as close to the cornea as possible (Fig. 11–62). If a blade is used, it is important to cut tangentially to the globe, to avoid incising the scleral surface. I prefer the Westcott scissors with blunt tips. The forceps used to elevate the conjunctiva should have fine indentations (such

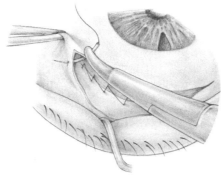

FIGURE 11–58. After Tenon's capsule is closed, the needle is placed from the underneath side to the superficial side of the conjunctiva, exteriorizing it so that it can be used to close the conjunctiva.

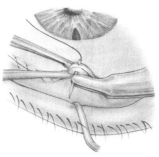

FIGURE 11–60. After the needle has passed through the tissue, it is lifted away from the globe rather firmly, with the underlying tissue put on stretch. A blunt forceps then grasps this underlying tissue firmly, as close to the needle as possible. This will hold the needle firmly in place, permitting the surgeon to release the end of the needle containing the suture without having to change the position of the needle.

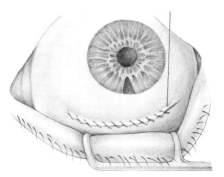

FIGURE 11–61. The closure of the conjunctiva should be watertight.

as the dressing or Pierse-Hoskins forceps), but should not have teeth. To widen the incision, the conjunctiva is pulled away from the conjunctival-corneal juncture and a single blade of the scissors is introduced through the buttonhole (Fig. 11–63). The blade's plane is tangential to the surface of the globe, with the cutting edge held as close as possible to the juncture of the conjunctiva and cornea. The tip of the blade is pushed bluntly forward, being kept flush with the scleral surface; care is taken that the tip does not push through the conjunctiva.

Pressure is exerted anteriorly so that the conjunctiva is cut close to the point of its adherence to the cornea. In this way no flap of residual conjunctiva remains.

Fornix-Based Flaps

A peritomy is made: the conjunctiva is grasped at its inferior cut edge and lifted up away from the globe so that good traction is placed on the episcleral fibers. Spring-type Westcott scissors are used to free the sclera from the overlying episclera. With the tips closed, the scissors are pushed radially against the taut episclera (Fig. 11–64). Once the episcleral tissue is penetrated, the blades are opened, spreading the tissue bluntly. This is continued until the desired amount of tissue is free (Fig. 11–65). Caution must be practiced when approaching the insertion of the rectus muscles. Although there is relatively little danger when using a blunt dissection technique, it is still possible to detach the rectus muscle from the globe. Special care must also be exercised when dissecting previously operated tissue. The

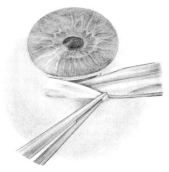

FIGURE 11–64. Tissue is separated from the globe by inserting the scissors with tips closed and then spreading them bluntly.

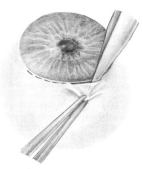

FIGURE 11–62. With a scissors or knife, conjunctiva is incised as close to the limbus as possible.

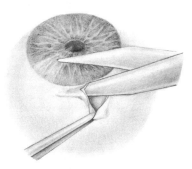

FIGURE 11–63. The incision is widened, with the surgeon making sure that the forceps puts the tissue on good stretch; the scissors cuts inferiorly so that there will be no remnant of conjunctiva left on the globe.

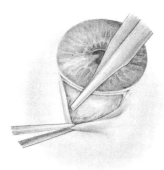

FIGURE 11–65. Blunt dissection is continued until the sclera is adequately cleaned. Bleeding from the cut conjunctival vessels is almost inevitable and usually exceeds that which occurs when raising a limbus-based flap.

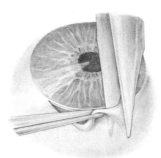

FIGURE 11–66. A radial cut at the edge of the peritomy will improve visualization of the sclera and permit a tidy closure of the conjunctiva.

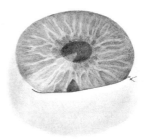

FIGURE 11–68. With large incisions it is usually necessary to suture both edges in order to ensure tight closure.

conjunctiva in such cases is usually adherent to the underlying sclera; sharp dissection may be necessary in such cases. A #67 Beaver blade is effective for this purpose. The surgeon tries to separate the episclera from the sclera, but the plane is not always easily developed. It is better to take off a bit of the scleral surface than to buttonhole the conjunctival Tenon's flap.

Radial relaxing incisions can be made at one or both ends of the cut edge of the conjunctiva (Fig. 11–66; see also Fig. 11–69). This facilitates retraction and closure, especially when the surgeon wants a neat, nonleaking adhesion to develop directly at the corneoscleral sulcus (Fig. 11–69).

A fornix-based flap need not always be closed. In cases in which leakage of aqueous is highly unlikely the flap can simply be pulled back to the limbus and left alone. I prefer to close the flap so that its cut edge is returned to the area of the cornea from which it was incised (Figs. 11–67 and 11–68). A 0.5-mm overlap is probably ideal (Fig. 11–69). The closure is accomplished by pulling the lateral edges of the flap away from the center of the incision so that the cut edge is opposed tautly against the limbus. This usually requires considerable overlap of the lateral conjunctiva. This may be excised if

too redundant. One fine suture placed at each edge is usually sufficient except with large flaps (Fig. 11–69). When a small flap (3 to 5 mm wide) has been developed there need be only one radial relaxing incision. This can be closed with one suture at the limbal edge (Fig. 11–68). The radial arm of the incision can be closed by running the suture from the limbus the length of the radial cut. This results in a beautiful closure after a peripheral iridectomy. An alternative and often preferred method is to coapt the flap with wet-field cautery rather than use a suture. To do this the edges of the tissue to be closed are firmly held between the jaws of a toothless forceps, cautery is applied and released, and *then* the nontoothed forceps releases the tissue.

The advantages of the fornix-based flap are the relative ease with which dissection is performed and the good visualization it gives of the anterior limbal area. It is the procedure of choice in patients who are having cataract extraction combined with a glaucoma procedure. There are disadvantages as well when used in conjunction with a filtering operation. The conjunctival vessels bleed as the conjunctiva is separated from the globe. The precise area where the cut edge of the conjunctiva will adhere to the globe during healing is neither certain nor within the surgeon's control, leakage of aqueous humor from under the cut edge of the conjunctival flap may occur, making the use of agents such as 5-FU inadvisable, and the surgeon cannot perform a Carlo Traverso maneuver in the immediate postoperative period (see Fig. 11–132), as it will cause continuing breakage of the adhesion developing between conjunctiva and cornea (see p. 132).

In some cases the development of a fornix-based flap results in loss of tissue at the cut limbal edge of the conjunctiva. It is usually possible to avoid such a loss of tissue. In some instances, however, such as when revising a previously made conjunctival bleb, tissue must

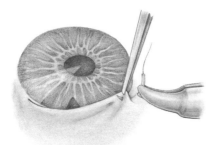

FIGURE 11–67. The cut edge of a fornix-based flap is pulled inferiorly and secured with a 10–0 nylon suture.

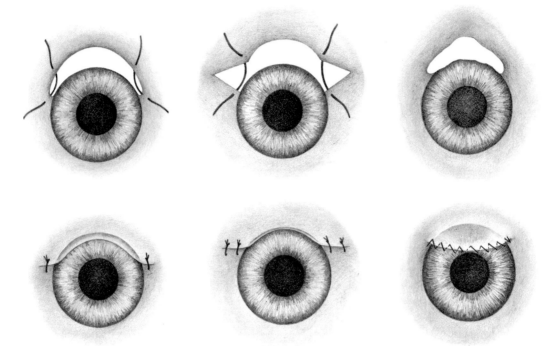

FIGURE 11–69. Methods of closing fornix-based flaps. *Left (top and bottom)*, Flap in which there is a small overlap of tissue. *Middle*, The use of relaxing incisions *(top)* has made it easier to approximate the conjunctiva back to its proper position *(bottom)*. *Right (top)*, Here tissue such as a failed bleb was excised. When this is done, the conjunctiva usually needs to be sutured into the cornea if the surgeon wants to cover the limbus tightly *(bottom)*.

be sacrificed (Fig. 11–69). In such cases the conjunctiva usually cannot be put back over the limbus using the techniques previously described. Rather, the conjunctiva must be sutured to the cornea; running 10–0 nylon works well to accomplish this (Fig. 11–69). This can be done directly at the limbus, or the conjunctiva can be pulled further inferiorly, as in Figure 11–69. The corneal epithelium in the area to be covered by the conjunctival flap must be removed. Otherwise, as soon as the sutures lose their holding capacity the tissue pulls through the sutures and retracts superiorly.

Iridectomy

Indications*

The purposes for which an iridectomy are performed are listed in Table 11–27. The primary indication for iridectomy is elimination of

*Indications for surgery, including timing of surgery and choice of procedure, have been discussed in detail earlier in this chapter, in the section dealing with primary angle-closure glaucoma. Especially see Tables 11–17 and 11–18 and Figure 11–38.

pupillary block. When this is the case one needs only to make a hole in the iris so that there will be constant communication between the posterior and anterior chambers. Other indications for iridectomy are related to the purpose for

TABLE 11–27. Reasons to Consider Performing Surgical Iridectomy

I. Removal of tissue
  A. Biopsy for diagnostic purposes
  B. Excision
    1. Tumor
    2. Necrotic or nonviable tissue
    3. Optical improvement
II. Elimination or prevention of block of aqueous by the iris
  A. Occludable angle
  B. Primary angle-closure glaucoma
  C. Secondary angle-closure glaucoma caused by pupillary block
    1. Dislocated lens
    2. Posterior synechias tolens or vitreous
  D. In association with other surgery
    1. Cataract extraction
    2. Keratoplasty
    3. Glaucoma filtering procedures
III. Contraindications to laser iridotomy
  A. Cloudy cornea
  B. Flat anterior chamber
IV. In association with chamber-deepening procedures and synechialysis

which the surgery is being performed. Neodymium:YAG laser iridotomy is now the usual procedure of choice when an "iridectomy" is indicated. However, there are still instances when laser iridotomy is inadvisable (as in eyes with flat anterior chambers) or impossible (as in eyes with cloudy corneas). Consequently surgical iridectomy is still an important procedure that ophthalmologists should be able to perform.

One should try to avoid an iridectomy when repairing a traumatized eye. If the iris is still viable, iridectomy should not ordinarily be performed, as any procedure that traumatizes the uvea may predispose to sympathetic ophthalmia.

Anesthesia

Most iridectomies can be performed with local anesthesia, with a facial nerve block and topical anesthesia being used. Retrobulbar anesthesia is usually not needed and should be avoided in many instances, especially if the intraocular pressure is high and the surgery is required on an emergency basis, as would be the case in an uncontrolled primary angle-closure glaucoma. Under such circumstances the development of a retrobulbar hemorrhage would cause the further problem of controlling intraocular pressure, and would almost certainly make it necessary to cancel surgery, resulting in a delay that could cause permanent loss of vision. In addition, a retrobulbar block may cause other complications of concern. Proparacaine 0.5% should be given topically for 10 minutes before the surgery. One drop every 30 seconds or so results in highly satisfactory anesthesia in virtually every case.

Preoperative Care

The eye should be as quiet as can feasibly be achieved. Ideally, the surgery should be done in the absence of any internal or external inflammatory reaction. However, it is not always possible to achieve a totally quiet eye. Furthermore, the need to lower intraocular pressure may be so urgent that one cannot wait for the eye to quiet. But the principle remains valid; surgical results are better in uninflamed eyes. (This argues for the performance of iridectomy early in the course of primary angle-closure glaucoma, ideally before an attack of acute congestive angle closure has occurred. It is also a reason for performing an iridectomy on the fellow eye at the time the eye that has had the attack of glaucoma is being brought into condition for surgery.)

The timing of the surgery, then, largely depends on the degree of inflammation and the degree of difficulty involved in controlling the intraocular pressure. The greater these two factors are, the longer the preparation for surgery; the lesser they are, the shorter the wait.

Topical corticosteroids such as prednisolone acetate 1% should be used as needed. These can be used as frequently as every hour. The steroids are used only during preparation for surgery and in the immediate postoperative period; the surgeon need not be concerned about the development of a steroid-induced glaucoma in these circumstances. However, should treatment lasting more than 2 weeks be required, the chance of this occurring should be kept in mind.

When the pupil is miotic it is easy to perform an iridectomy limited to the periphery. Consequently, if one is attempting to create such a cosmetically satisfactory iridectomy, the pupil should be small. In the quiet eye with a normal intraocular pressure, pilocarpine 1% instilled four times during the day before surgery and 2 hours before surgery is entirely adequate. More intensive treatment with pilocarpine is seldom necessary and may be counter-productive. If the pupil will not constrict to a satisfactory dimension with this treatment, it is unlikely that more vigorous therapy will accomplish anything more than increasing the degree of inflammation in the eye and inducing symptoms of parasympathomimetic overdosage in the patient.

Appropriate medication in the eye not receiving surgery should be ordered. If it is a "fellow eye" of a patient who has had an angle-closure attack in the first eye, probably pilocarpine 0.5% twice daily is adequate for a blue-eyed patient and 1% twice daily for a patient with a brown iris. Control of intraocular pressure before surgery has been discussed in detail (p. 226). The basic principles are to keep the pupil miotic with moderate amounts of pilocarpine and to control intraocular pressure with aqueous suppressants (beta blockers and carbonic anhydrase inhibitors) or osmotic agents.

Intraocular pressure should ideally be between 15 and 30 mm Hg at the time surgery is started. Pressure above 30 mm Hg may predispose to malignant glaucoma or expulsive hemorrhage. Pressure below 15 mm Hg makes spontaneous prolapse of the iris more difficult and complicates the surgery.

If all medical measures to lower intraocular pressure have failed (Table 11–12), a paracentesis immediately before the surgery may be required.

Patients should be told that after surgery their vision will be different. This is not the same as saying that their visual acuity will be worse. In the overwhelming majority of cases, especially when performing surgery on a quiet eye with a clear lens, a properly performed iridectomy will not result in a decrease in visual acuity. In fact, under such circumstances it may not even predispose to more rapid progression of cataract. However, the presence of the iridectomy itself may introduce symptoms, especially if it is not completely covered by the upper lid. When a cataract is already present, the patient should understand that surgery will probably hasten its development.

The patient should also understand the purpose of the surgery. In the secondary angle-closure glaucomas, such as aphakic pupillary block glaucoma, one purpose of an iridectomy is to lower intraocular pressure by eliminating the pupillary block. However, in the primary angle-closure glaucomas the purpose is quite different; it is to prevent or eliminate the cause for progressive closure of the anterior chamber angle. Thus patients should not be told that iridectomy will "control the glaucoma," as they will interpret this as meaning that the surgery will control intraocular pressure. Rather, the surgeon should explain that although the surgery is highly successful in preventing the progression of angle closure, medications for controlling intraocular pressure may still be needed in the postoperative period. Furthermore, although the iridectomy may cure the angle closure, it will not prevent the patient from developing elevated intraocular pressure owing to another mechanism, such as primary open-angle glaucoma.

Surgical Technique

Adherence to several principles will help to assure that an iridectomy is performed effectively and safely. An iridectomy consists of five steps: (1) incision into the eye, (2) exteriorization of a portion of the iris, (3) excision of a portion of the iris, (4) return of the remainder of the iris to its normal position within the eye, and (5) closure of the incision.

A superior rectus muscle bridle suture is placed as shown in Figures 11–79 and 11–80.

Incision. The nature of the incision will largely determine how the iris prolapses and how the incision heals. If the surgeon believes that surgery requiring development of a conjunctival flap may later be required, he may want to make the incision through the clear cornea, anterior to the insertion of the conjunctiva (Fig. 11–70). Other indications for clear corneal incision are extensive peripheral anterior synechias and the wish to minimize bleeding by avoiding incision through the sclera or conjunctiva.

In most cases, however, it is preferable to place the incision more posteriorly and use a conjunctival flap (Fig. 11–71). Such an incision traumatizes the corneal endothelium more peripherally, usually allows easier prolapse of the iris, and can be closed with a suture that is then covered with conjunctiva. Although leakage through the incision after an iridectomy is rare, it does occur in about 1 per cent of cases; if such a leak occurs underneath a conjunctival flap, the seriousness of the complication is less than it would be if such a flap were not present.[63]

The incision for a peripheral iridectomy being performed for primary angle-closure glaucoma should usually be at 12 o'clock, so that the iridectomy will be hidden under the upper lid. This will assure the best cosmetic and functional result. Other factors may make positioning the iridectomy elsewhere preferable. For example, an optical iridectomy should create an opening as close to the visual axis as possible.

The incision should be large enough to allow the iris to prolapse easily. This usually requires an incision that is about 2 mm wide at its base. It is better to have the incision slightly larger than required rather than smaller, as both prolapse and reposition of the iris are more easily accomplished with a large incision. It is simple to close an incision with fine suture, and the trauma to the eye will be less when the incision is slightly too large than when it is too small.

Before placement of a preplaced suture, and before entry into the anterior chamber, a paracentesis should be performed.

Preplacement of a suture after the incision has been made approximately one-half to the two-thirds of the way through the tissue facilitates both the completion of the incision in a safe manner and the prolapse of the iris. This technique is illustrated in Figures 4–43 and 11–72. The suture used should be strong enough to be used for traction; 8–0 white virgin silk and 9–0 nylon are both suitable.

A perpendicular incision will facilitate prolapse of the iris. However, such incisions are more likely to open in response to pressure on the globe or to increased intraocular pressure. Thus they should be closed with a fine suture, which may cause temporary astigmatism.

Incisions can also be shelved anteriorly or posteriorly. The major advantage of a shelved

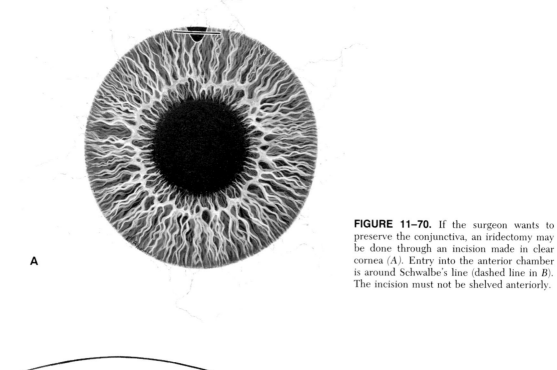

A

FIGURE 11–70. If the surgeon wants to preserve the conjunctiva, an iridectomy may be done through an incision made in clear cornea (A). Entry into the anterior chamber is around Schwalbe's line (dashed line in B). The incision must not be shelved anteriorly.

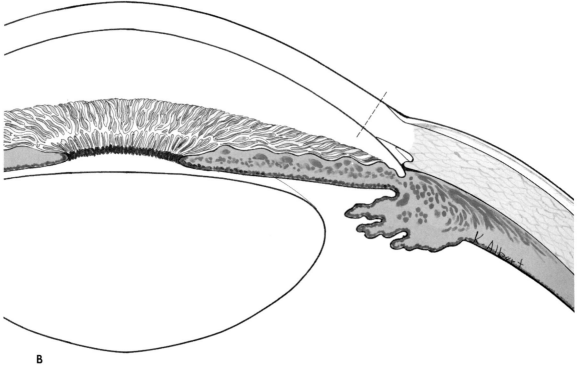

B

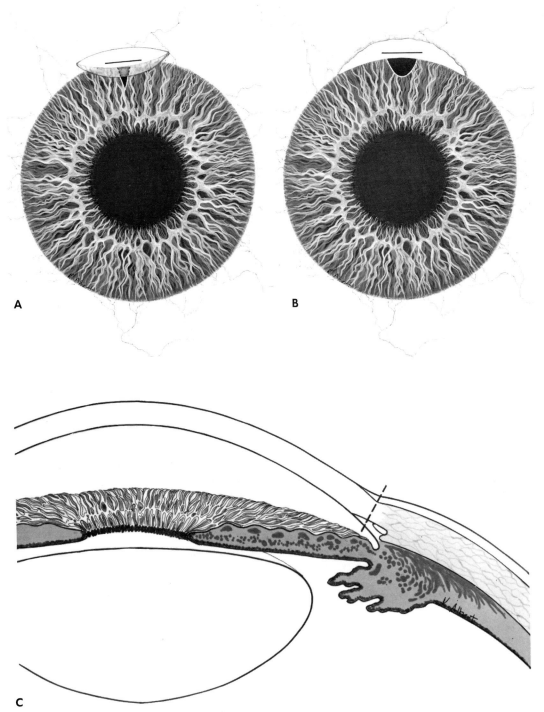

FIGURE 11–71. *A,* Usual location for placing the incision for a peripheral iridectomy. A small limbus-based incision has been developed. *B,* A peritomy provides adequate clearing of the conjunctiva, permitting proper placement of the incision for an iridectomy. *C,* A perpendicular incision through the corneoscleral sulcus usually enters the anterior chamber through the anterior trabecular meshwork.

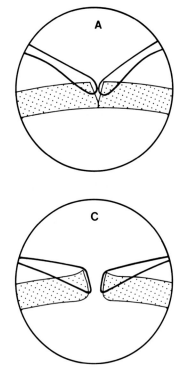

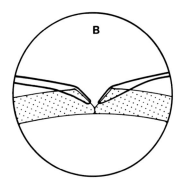

FIGURE 11–72. The use of a preplaced suture facilitates performance of an iridectomy. In *A* the sutures have been placed through an incision made in the cornea and looped to the sides. In *B* the traction on the sutures provides good visualization of the base of the incision. After the incision has been completed (*C*), traction pulls the edges of the incision apart, facilitating prolapse of the iris.

incision is the large overlap of the edges, which helps to assure tight closure. On the other hand, the iris is less likely to prolapse with such incisions, and closure is a bit more difficult in that the surfaces tend to slide on each other, complicating attempts to achieve exact apposition (Fig. 11–73).

Exteriorization of Iris. The iris prolapses from the anterior chamber through the incision because the pressure in the posterior chamber exceeds that in the anterior chamber. The surgeon, therefore, should be careful to assure maintenance of this pressure gradient (see Table 11–26). Before making the incision, the surgeon should have in mind exactly how he plans to perform the iridectomy, for once the anterior chamber has been opened no time should be wasted. The surgeon must not hesitate or debate because the gradient between the posterior and anterior chamber will be lost, as will the opportunity to achieve spontaneous iris prolapse. If the iris is penetrated, it will be far more difficult to prolapse. Such penetration can result from catching the iris on the tip of the knife at the time the incision is made. Factors that increase the likelihood of this complication include (1) the presence of peripheral synechias; (2) a peripherally placed incision; (3) an extremely shallow anterior chamber; and (4) use of an extraordinarily sharp knife, especially if the tip of the blade is pointed.

Other factors that affect how the iris prolapses include the size of the pupil and the texture of the iris, especially in its peripheral portions (Table 11–28). A small pupil assists prolapse of the iris. If the pupil has not been able to be reduced to a diameter of 2 mm before surgery, acetylcholine can be used after making the corneal incision. Clearly the iris cannot prolapse if the incision is made where the iris is adherent to the inner edge of the incision. Furthermore, the closer the incision is to the anterior extent of the adhesion, the less likely it is that spontaneous prolapse will occur. The ideal location for the incision is usually about 2 mm anterior to the base of the iris, or, if peripheral anterior synechias are present, 2 mm anterior to the point of contact between the iris and the corneal endothelium. The shallower the anterior chamber, the more corneal the incision should be, and the deeper the chamber, the more peripheral.

It is usually easier to prolapse the iris through a limbal than through a clear-corneal incision. However, a properly placed, swiftly performed corneal incision will be followed by satisfactory spontaneous prolapse of the iris in virtually every instance. Prolapse can be facilitated by gentle traction on the two loops of the preplaced suture.

Excision of Iris. Within a few seconds after the iris has appeared in the depths of the

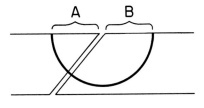

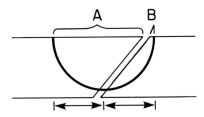

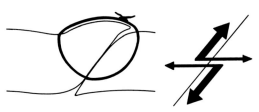

FIGURE 11–73. A shelved incision must be closed precisely if the tissue is not to be distorted. (Redrawn after Eisner, G., Augenchiurugie. Springer-Verlag, Berlin, 1978.)

incision, it should be grasped by a smooth or fine-toothed forceps; I prefer the Barraquer colibri 0.12-mm toothed forceps. If the iris prolapses only slightly, remaining in the depths of the incision, the forceps should be held so that it opens and closes in an axis parallel to the axis of the incision. Once the iris has been grasped, there is no longer a need to proceed rapidly.

TABLE 11–28. Factors That Predispose to Failure of Iris to Prolapse

1. Loss of posterior chamber pressure gradient
   a. Intraocular pressure below 15 mm Hg preoperatively
   b. Surgery performed too slowly
   c. Large pupil
   d. Penetration of iris
2. Anterior position of incision
3. Shelved incision
4. Peripheral anterior synechias
5. Fibrosed iris

With a limbal incision the iris is grasped as anteriorly as possible and lifted posteriorly (Fig. 11–74A). When the incision has been more anteriorly placed, the surgeon grasps the iris more posteriorly, lifting it anteriorly (Fig. 11–74B). These motions are designed to keep the iridectomy as basal as possible *without* tearing it from its root. The former goal is desirable for cosmetic reasons, and the latter, to prevent unnecessary bleeding.

After the iris has been lifted high enough that the pigment epithelial layer is exteriorized, the excision is performed. I use the micro DeWecker scissors. The iridectomy will be wide and peripheral if the axis of the blade is held parallel to the incision (Figs. 11–75 and 11–76). It will be narrower and more pointed if the scissors are held at right angles to the incision. The blades should be flush with the cornea, and the iris tissue should be deep in the crotch of the V made by the blades, as shown in the inset of Figure 11–75. If the tissue is near the tips of the blades, it will often slip out, failing to be cleanly cut and leaving a ragged iridectomy quite different from the one planned.

The position of the pupillary margin should be checked before the actual excision of tissue. If the surgeon wants the iridectomy to be peripheral, he must be sure that the pupillary margin has not prolapsed. If, on the other hand, a sector iridectomy is the goal, the pupillary margin needs to be exteriorized. With a sector iridectomy the scissors should usually be held at right angles to the incision, to avoid removing an excessive amount of iris.

After the blades have been closed the surgeon cautiously lifts the forceps containing the iris. This is done slowly, with the remainder of the iris through the cornea being observed in order to be sure that the excision has been complete and that the iris is not pulled away with the forceps. The excised iris is inspected to determine if the posterior pigment epithelium has been included. A dark smudge should be produced when the iris is rubbed against the drapes.

Repositioning of Iris. Up to this point the anterior chamber should remain formed. The incision is presently blocked by iris. The tip of a #21 irrigator is placed into the incision, but not *through* the incision or through the iridectomy itself (Fig. 11–77A). A gentle stream of balanced salt solution flushes remaining pigment epithelium away; irrigation is continued as long as pigment continues to be seen. The

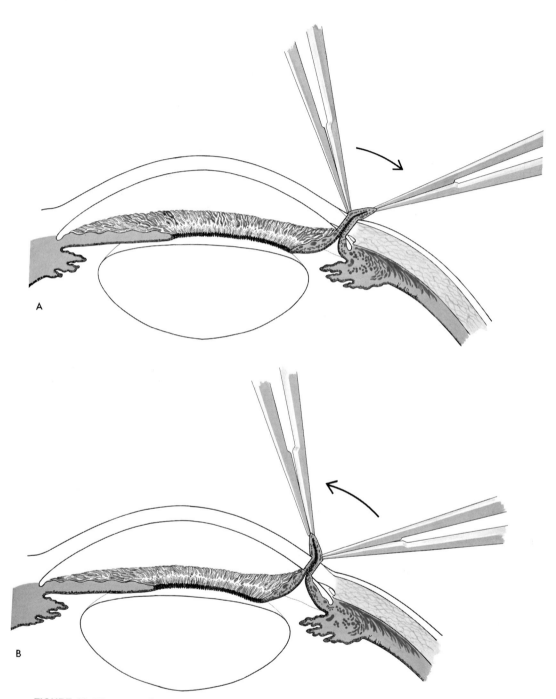

FIGURE 11–74. *A,* In order to avoid dialysis of the iris, after iridectomy done through a limbal incision the iris should be lifted slightly in a superior direction. *B,* With a corneal incision the iris should be pulled inferiorly in order to help avoid the sphincter and produce a more basal iridectomy.

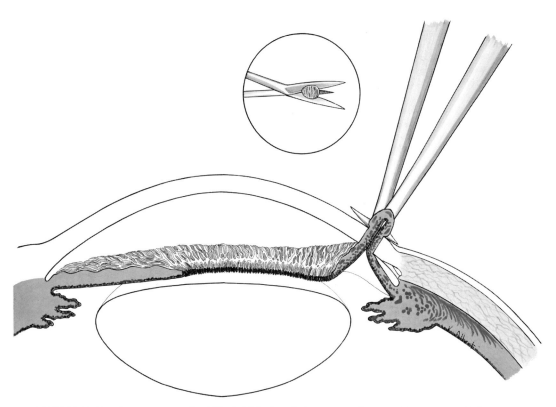

FIGURE 11–75. The iris scissors should be held flush with the cornea. The axis of the scissors will determine the shape of the iridectomy; if the goal is to keep the iridectomy as peripheral as possible, the axis should be held parallel to the incision (see Fig. 11–70). The inset shows how the iris should be cut in the crotch of the blades, not at the tips.

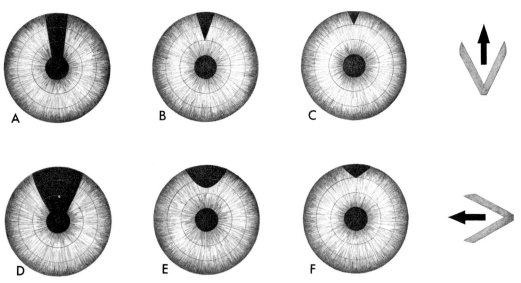

FIGURE 11–76. The position in which the scissors is held and the point at which the iris is grasped determine the final shape of the iridectomy performed. In A, B, and C, the scissors are held so that the cut is made at right angles to a tangent to the limbus. In D, E, and F, the axis of the scissors is meridional. To obtain iridectomies of the shape of those shown in A and D, the iris is grasped close to the pupillary margin (about 2 mm from the edge of the pupil). Iridectomies of the shape of those shown in B and E are a consequence of grasping the iris 2 mm anterior to its base. The most peripheral iridectomies (C and F) result from grasping the iris just anterior to its root.

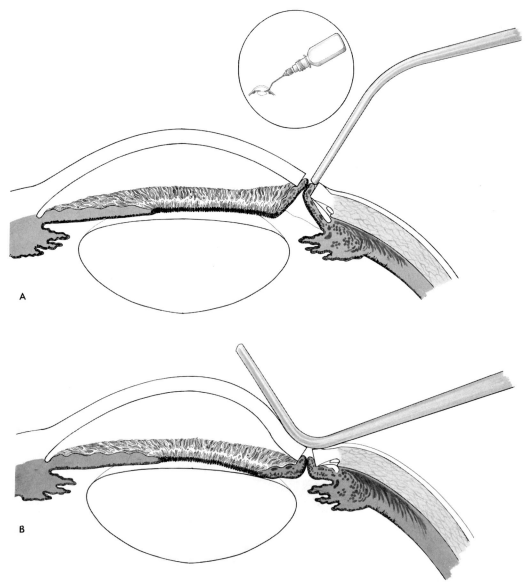

FIGURE 11–77. *A,* After iridectomy the iris may be repositioned by gentle irrigation. The tip of the irrigator should not be placed through the incision into the anterior chamber. *B,* Pressure on the incision causes the internal edges to gape, releasing the iris and facilitating its return to a normal position within the anterior chamber.

stream of balanced salt solution also flushes the iris back into the anterior chamber. If the irrigator is placed through the iridectomy itself, the fluid will enter the posterior chamber, forcing the iris out of the eye rather than aiding in its repositioning.

After the iris is released from the incision it can be returned to its proper position by the surgeon's gently stroking the cornea with a blunt instrument, thus "pulling" the apex of the iridectomy inferiorly (Fig. 11–78). If this ma-

neuver does not result in return of the iris to its preoperative condition, the internal edges of the incision can be made to gape by depressing the area of the incision with a blunt instrument, such as the heel of the irrigator tip or a muscle hook (Fig. 11–77B). This may release the iris when it is caught in the incision. If it does not, and if the iris sphincter is still functional, a small amount of acetylcholine can be introduced through the previously placed paracentesis track, caution being taken not to deepen the

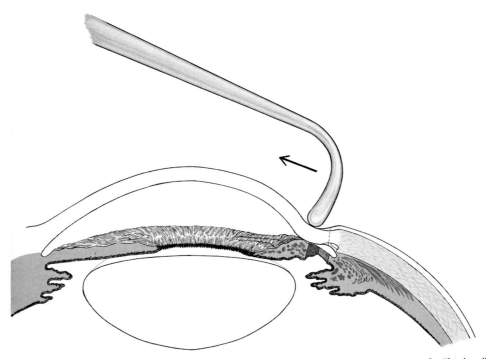

FIGURE 11–78. The iridectomy can be stroked open, returning the pupil to its proper position by "hooking" the inferior apex of the iridectomy tissue with the tip of a blunt instrument and pulling it inferiorly.

anterior chamber excessively. If the iris sphincter is dead, as is frequently the case after a severe attack of acute glaucoma, this maneuver will fail. Pressure on the posterior lip of the iris will release aqueous from the posterior chamber, almost certainly allowing the iris to fall back. The chamber will simultaneously collapse, which is of no concern when the surgeon has previously made a paracentesis, for the chamber can easily be re-formed at the end of the operation.

Closure of the Incision. At this point the preplaced suture can be tied tightly enough to close the incision but not so securely that it induces astigmatism. Additional sutures may be needed. If a conjunctival flap has been raised, it may be closed as described before, with a fine suture or with the wet-field cauter.

If the incision is corneal, its knot is buried.

After closure is completed the surgeon may want to re-form the anterior chamber so that it is deeper than preoperatively. This is done by introducing balanced salt solution through the previously placed paracentesis track. A finger should monitor the intraocular pressure so that it does not rise excessively. Forceful deepening of the chamber may open peripheral anterior synechias. Also, some have recommended mechanical separation of adhesions with an instrument such as a Barraquer sweep.

A small air bubble may be introduced and used as an internal probe to attempt to separate the iris from the cornea. The bubble is chased around the anterior chamber by applying external pressure on the cornea with a muscle hook or similar instrument; the eye must be soft for this maneuver to succeed.

At the end of the procedure the anterior chamber should be deep, the pupil round, the incision securely closed, and the intraocular pressure around 10 to 20 mm Hg. If a sector iridectomy has been performed, the pupil cannot be round, but the iris must have been returned to its proper plane.

A drop of pilocarpine 1% may be instilled, but this is usually unnecessary. In the routine case there is no reason to instill a cycloplegic at the time of surgery. Unless the patient is predisposed to a malignant glaucoma there is certainly no indication for atropine. The problem of the blur produced by the medication far exceeds the need for its use. If inflammation is unusually severe, periocular corticosteroids may be given. An example would be betamethasone (Celestone), 3 mg. An antibiotic-corticosteroid ointment is then instilled and a patch applied. The only purpose for the patch at this point is to protect the eye until the facial block has worn off. Figures 11–79 and 11–80 show the technique.

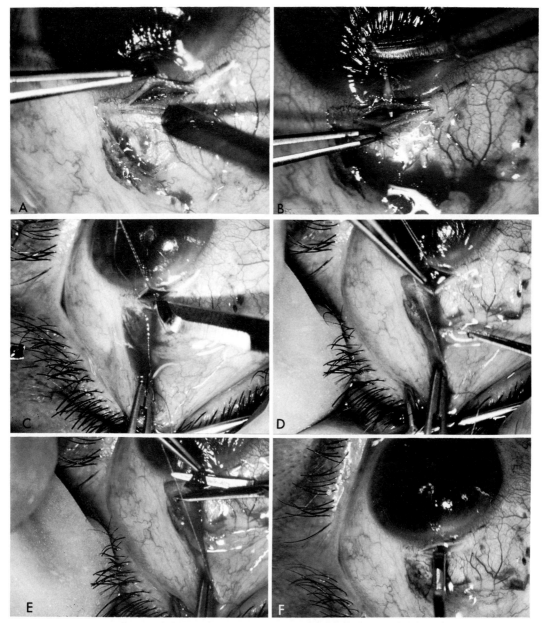

FIGURE 11–79. Peripheral iridectomy with a fornix-based flap and limbal incision. *A,* Incision is made through two-thirds the thickness of the sclera directly at the corneoscleral sulcus. *B,* An 9–0 white virgin silk suture is placed in such a way that it will be able to be retracted from the depths of the incision (see Fig. 11–72). *C,* The suture is looped and used to retract the edges of the incision superiorly and inferiorly. The incision is completed, permitting prolapse of a small knuckle of iris. *D,* The iris is grasped with a fine-toothed forceps. *E,* Iris is pulled over the blade of the DeWecker scissors; after the position of the iris is noted the blades are closed and the tissue is excised. *F,* The tip of an irrigator is placed just inside the incision, with care taken to ensure that it does not enter the anterior chamber. Remnants of the pigment epithelium are flushed away, and the iris is permitted to return to its proper position so that the pupil is completely round.

Postoperative Care

After the surgery there should be no limitation on the patient's activity other than the suitable precautions to be taken because of the sedation given. Attention should be paid to the general health of the patient, especially if extensive doses of carbonic anhydrase inhibitors and osmotic agents have been given. Serum electrolytes should be carefully monitored in

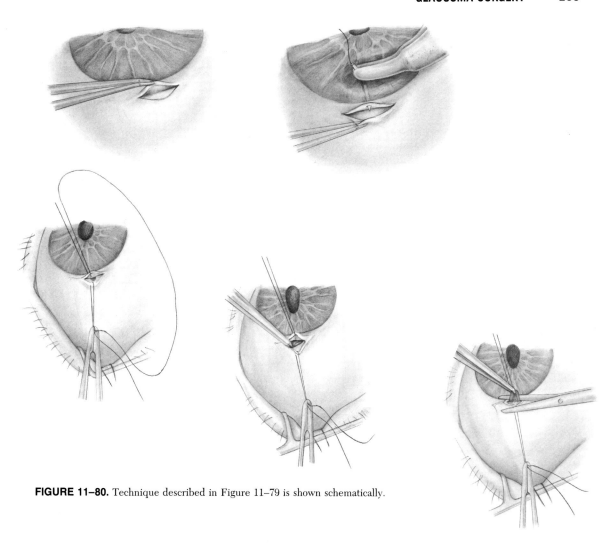

FIGURE 11–80. Technique described in Figure 11–79 is shown schematically.

such cases, and fluids encouraged to restore normal hydration.

The patch may be removed from the operated eye as soon as the facial block has worn off. An antibiotic-corticosteroid drop may be used for several days or a week.

A cycloplegic agent is routinely used to prevent posterior synechias and to assure adequacy of the iridectomy. Tropicamide 1% once or twice daily for 1 or 2 weeks is usually adequate. The intraocular pressure should be checked after dilatation. Topical corticosteroids may be used to control the inflammatory response. If the anterior chamber of an eye that has had an iridectomy for primary angle-closure glaucoma is not deeper than the unoperated eye, the possibility of malignant glaucoma must be kept in mind. If the chamber becomes shallower and intraocular pressure rises, atropine 1% and

phenylephrine 10% should be used in repeated doses until the pupil is maximally dilated; an osmotic agent should be given to shrink the vitreous and a carbonic anhydrase inhibitor administered to reduce the amount of aqueous that is being secreted into the vitreous cavity. When iridectomies are performed in the manner described in this chapter, the development of malignant glaucoma is extraordinarily rare.

Intraocular pressure may be measured with an applanation tonometer during the first few days, especially in patients in whom there has been a need to use medications to control the intraocular pressure preoperatively. Patients who have an iridectomy performed for longstanding chronic angle-closure glaucoma, or for a combined-mechanism glaucoma in which angle closure is superimposed on an open-angle glaucoma mechanism, will almost certainly have an elevated intraocular pressure after the surgery. This may not become apparent until the second or third day after the operation. In the immediate postoperative period the intraocular pressure should be controlled with the use of epinephrine and, if needed, a beta blocker or a carbonic anhydrase inhibitor. Miotics should be avoided, as their use predisposes to posterior synechias. Intraocular pressure should be carefully watched in the postoperative period, as optic nerve deterioration can occur if pressure remains high.

Postoperative evaluations should ordinarily be made 1 week and 1 month postoperatively. If all is in order at these visits, probably the patient should again be seen approximately 6 months later and then at yearly intervals. All patients should have baseline visual fields determined after the surgery. Photographs of the optic disc may also be taken, but are not essential.

Occasionally there is slight bleeding into the anterior chamber. This can be ignored unless it is so extensive that it causes pressure elevation; anterior chamber washout may be appropriate in such cases.

Trabeculectomy

Indications

Trabeculectomy is the surgical procedure of choice for primary open-angle glaucoma. Indications for surgery in this regard have been discussed in detail (p. 228). Trabeculectomy is also the procedure of choice for uncontrolled chronic primary angle-closure glaucoma and for acute primary angle-closure glaucoma in cases in which iridectomy is considered inadequate (see Fig. 11–38B). In addition, trabeculectomy is used as an alternative procedure in the treatment of infantile glaucoma, and several of the secondary glaucomas (see Table 11–2).

Anesthesia

Both local and general anesthesia are satisfactory (see Table 11–8). Local anesthesia is usually preferable, as it permits the patient a more rapid return to full activity. This is desirable because the patient should be in a sitting-up or standing position in order to allow any bleeding to settle inferiorly away from the site of the trabeculectomy.

Preoperative Care

Long-acting cholinesterase inhibitors should be stopped at least 2 weeks before surgery, as they predispose to bleeding, poor dilatation of the pupil in the postoperative period, and increased intraocular inflammation.

Carbonic anhydrase inhibitors should be stopped at least 6 hours before surgery so that aqueous inflow will not be suppressed in the postoperative period.[78] For the same reason, beta blockers should probably also be stopped preoperatively whenever possible. The exact duration of suppression of aqueous formation by these agents has not yet been determined, but it appears in many instances to be 2 weeks or longer.

When possible, photographs of the optic discs should be obtained before surgery.

Intraocular pressure should preferably range between 15 and 30 mm Hg, and the eye should be as uninflamed as possible.

In most cases surgery should first be performed on the eye with the more advanced disease (see p. 225). Patients should realize that it may be necessary to go ahead with surgery on the better eye quite promptly after the first procedure has been performed.

Patients should be informed that the likelihood of control of glaucoma in the average case is about 60 per cent without medications and 95 per cent with medications postoperatively.[79–82] If the lens is clear postoperatively, the patient can be reassured that the likelihood of a cataract developing as a result of the surgery itself is slim.[82] In cases in which a cataract is already present, the patient should be told preoperatively that the cataract will probably progress at a more rapid rate than it would if the surgery were not performed, and that cataract extraction may be required in the future if vision is to be restored. Patients in whom the visual field loss cuts through fixation should be informed that they have a small but significant chance of loss of central vision, a clinical estimate being around 5 per cent. If the field loss does not cut to within 5 degrees of fixation, the likelihood of central visual loss is so slight that it is negligible. The frequency with which reformation of the anterior chamber will be necessary depends on the method by which the surgery is performed.[82] In those cases in which gross filtration is the goal, so that the scleral flap is loosely closed, there is at least a 10 per cent likelihood of a flat anterior chamber postoperatively.[83] The surgeon will probably wish to tell the patient that bleeding into the eye occurs in almost every case, but that this usually clears up within 3 days. In about 10 per cent of patients it will last for as long as 1 week and in rare patients, slightly longer. The patient should also be informed that the lid may droop and the eye may tear.

Surgical Technique*

The intraocular pressure is checked before starting the anesthesia and immediately before proceeding with the surgery. If it is excessively

*Modified from references 84 and 85.

high, appropriate steps are taken to bring it into a satisfactory range.

A superior rectus muscle bridle suture of 4–0 black silk is placed. This technique has already been described in detail in Chapter 4. However, its successful performance is of such importance in trabeculectomy that it is again shown here (Fig. 11–81). It is essential to be sure that the conjunctiva between the superior

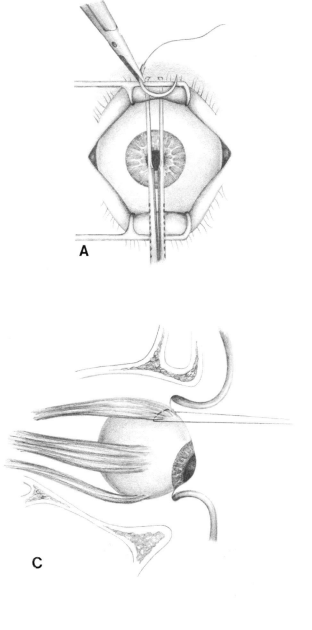

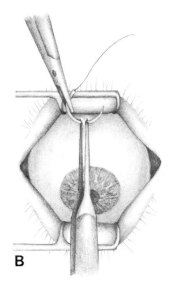

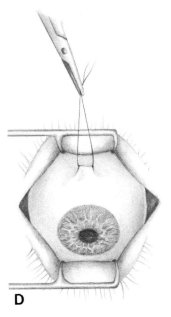

FIGURE 11–81. Placement of the superior bridle suture.

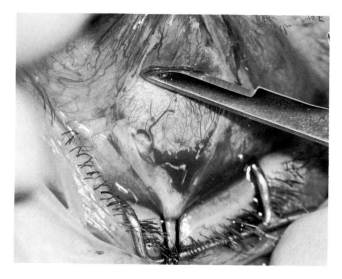

FIGURE 11–82. Episcleral tissue should be cleaned as far anteriorly as the corneoscleral sulcus.

rectus muscle and the limbus is not traumatized during the placement of this suture.

A limbus-based conjunctival flap is developed as described on page 262. I prefer to make the conjunctival incision at a point about 10 mm posterior to the limbus for a width of approximately 15 mm. The blade used to clean the limbal area should be pushed quite forcibly downward in the direction of the optic nerve so that as it is moved anteriorly toward the cornea, it falls into the corneoscleral sulcus and does not pass beyond this point (Fig. 11–82). In this manner the surgeon can avoid with complete certainty the serious complication of buttonholing the conjunctiva at the limbus.

A caliper may be used to measure the desired width of the flap (Fig. 11–83). Two millimeters is usually satisfactory, but the width will vary,

depending on the intent of the surgeon. If tight closure is desired, a larger flap should be used in order to create a larger area of overlap between the flap and the underlying sclera adjacent to the site of the trabeculectomy (Fig. 11–84).

Light cautery is used to outline the flap. The tissue should not be scarred. A setting of 15 or 20 with the Codman-Mentor wet-field cautery is appropriate. Light cautery is used to stop bleeding vessels; it is also applied surrounding the flap so that when sutures are later placed they will not initiate bleeding.

The shape of the flap is probably unimportant. I use a square flap.

A #67 Beaver blade is used to incise the sclera in the area outlined by the cautery to a depth of approximately two-thirds the thickness

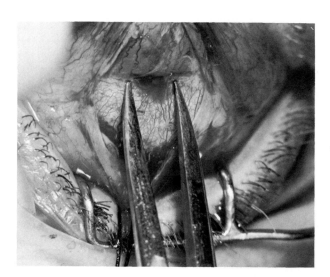

FIGURE 11–83. The width of the flap is decided on and a caliper used to measure this on the globe.

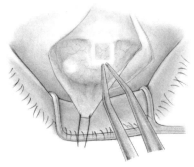

FIGURE 11–84. The sclera is cauterized lightly in the shape of the flap that is to be developed. All bleeding vessels elsewhere on the sclera are coagulated.

of the sclera (Fig. 11–85). It is important to make sure that the incision is deep enough and extended to the corners of the flap. Anteriorly, the surgeon must be careful not to penetrate the base of the conjunctival flap.

During this time the conjunctiva should be held out of the way with nontoothed forceps, such as the Pierse-Hoskins forceps or a dressing forceps. It should be kept constantly moist by irrigation with balanced salt solution. It should not be held with a desiccating sponge.

At this point the surgeon decides whether to start the administration of atropine eye drops. If the pupil is small and the patient has used miotics for many years, the pupil will be slow to dilate. The best chance of obtaining a dilated pupil, however, is at the time of surgery, before the onset of postoperative intraocular inflammation and simultaneous with paralysis of the sphincter muscle from the retrobulbar anesthetic block. The pupil should not be dilated prematurely, however, because this makes performance of a cosmetically satisfactory iridectomy more difficult. If the pupil is likely to dilate slowly, atropine drops should be started at this time and instilled at 1- to 2-minute intervals for the next 5 to 10 minutes.

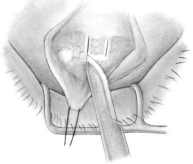

FIGURE 11–85. Following the lines of cautery, the sclera is incised to a depth of approximately two-thirds its thickness.

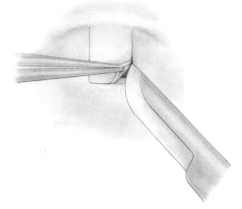

FIGURE 11–86. The edge of the scleral flap is firmly held and a flap is developed with a #67 Beaver blade. A nontoothed forceps is used.

One corner of the scleral flap is then grasped with a fine-toothed forceps such as a Barraquer colibri 0.12-mm forceps, and dissection of the scleral flap is started (Fig. 11–86). The thickness of this flap may vary between one-half and one-quarter the thickness of the sclera.* I prefer to use a thicker flap in patients in whom gross filtration is to be kept to a minimum, such as most of those with chronic primary angle-closure glaucoma, and a thinner flap when maximum filtration is desired, as in those with low-tension glaucoma. In all cases it is preferable to start with a thick flap and make it thinner as needed as one dissects anteriorly. In some cases a smooth plane is rapidly developed and easily continued up to the limbus. In others the scleral fibers appear to be at right angles, rather than parallel to the direction of dissection. The knife should be held as close to the brow as possible, so that the axis of the handle is almost parallel to the plane of the scleral bed. This permits the easiest dissection of the flap. Note in Figure 11–87 how the knife is lying against the speculum, and therefore cannot be used in a more horizontal plane. Some surgeons prefer an angled knife so that the goal of keeping the plane of the blade parallel to the plane of the scleral bed can be more easily accomplished. The thickness of the flap must be carefully monitored as it is developed, so that it becomes neither too thick nor too thin. The fibers of the sclera should be seen to part as the flap continues (Fig. 11–88). The scleral flap should be extended evenly to its edges, with the axis of the knife blade being changed in order to permit cutting with the tip of the blade, thus

*See page 299 for modification of this technique.

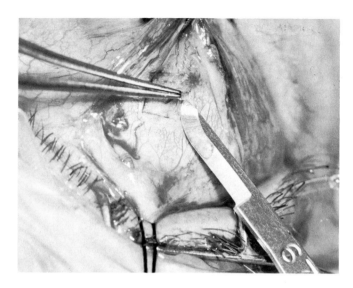

←

FIGURE 11–87. Note that the knife is held in a horizontal plane.

FIGURE 11–88. The dissection is carried well anteriorly, so that it reaches approximately 2 mm anterior to the junction between the sclera and the cornea. This exposes about 2 mm of clear cornea.

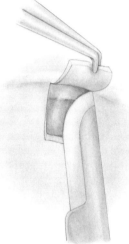

→

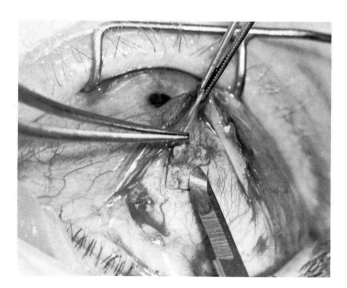

←

FIGURE 11–89. Magnification of at least 10× with the microscope is preferable when fastening the scleral flap. The blade should be parallel to the bed of the flap.

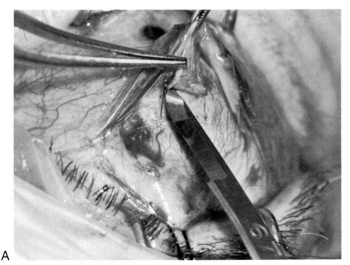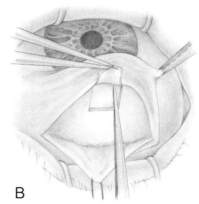

A   B

FIGURE 11–90. *A* and *B*, The tip of the blade is used to obtain precise cutting.

allowing better control (Fig. 11–89). The tip of the knife must always be visible. Rather firm traction should be placed on the scleral flap that is being developed. If a toothed forceps is used, the flap must be held at its extreme edge in order to avoid penetrating the flap with the teeth, which would produce leaking holes. Probably the Pierse-Hoskins forceps is ideal for this procedure.

The flap continues to be developed for a distance of at least 2 mm anterior to the junction of the white sclera and the clear cornea (Fig. 11–90). The anterior extent of the incision can be accurately determined by placing the knife under the scleral flap (Fig. 11–91) and retracting the conjunctival flap to allow visualization of the limbus (Fig. 11–92). In most cases the flap should be continued until the knife is visible *anterior* to the junction of the conjunctiva and the cornea (Fig. 11–92).

At this point a paracentesis track is placed into the anterior chamber, with the posterior edge of the scleral bed used for fixation (Figs. 11–93 through 11–96).

A radial incision is then made as anteriorly as possible. The knife should be held vertically so that cutting is done by the tip of the blade. A #75 Beaver blade or other very sharp blade can be used for this purpose, but if chosen, it must be used with great caution so as not to

FIGURE 11–91. The rounded edge of the blade is used to determine the anterior extent of the dissection.

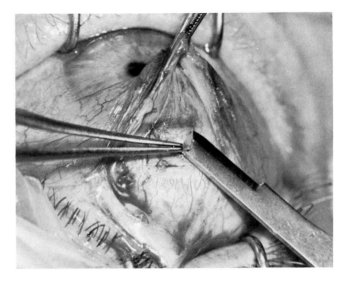

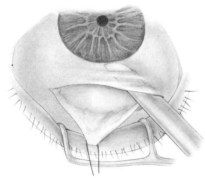

FIGURE 11–92. The anterior extent of the flap should be well anterior to the iris recess.

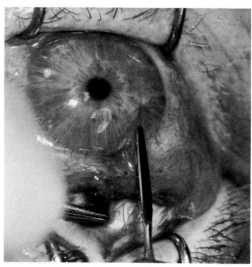

FIGURE 11–94. The blade is held in the plane parallel to the surface of the iris, to assure a long beveled track through the cornea and to avoid striking the iris or underlying lens.

damage the underlying iris and lens. I prefer to use a duller blade such as a #67 Beaver blade, and make multiple scratches. The knife should be held vertically so that cutting is done by the tip of the blade. Multiple scratches are made, usually about 0.5 mm inside the radial edge of the scleral flap (Fig. 11–97). This assures a small area of overlap between the underlying sclera and the external scleral flap. If the goal is to encourage gross filtration, the width of the ledge should be smaller; if the goal of the surgery is to encourage little filtration, as in patients with chronic angle closure, then the width of the ledge should be larger. The length of the radial incision is usually around 2 mm, but this is immaterial from the point of view of the final functioning, so long as the posterior edge of the excised tissue can be completely covered.[86a]

In many instances, as soon as this incision has been made, the iris will prolapse (Fig. 11–97). Creating a tiny iridotomy in the prolapsed iris with a Vannas scissors permits the iris to fall back into the anterior chamber (Fig. 11–98).

The Vannas scissors is then introduced into the anterior chamber through the radial incision. The tip of the scissors must be completely in the chamber and must not injure the iris or lens. This must be done under direct visualization. The blade of the scissors is advanced and pulled posteriorly until it is stopped by the junction between the scleral spur and the uvea. The width of this posterior incision varies with the purpose of the surgery, as already mentioned (Fig. 11–99). The tip of the Vannas scissors is held as horizontal to the surface of the globe as possible, in order to ensure that the tips do not dig into the uvea. It is helpful if the block to be excised is held firmly with a toothed forceps (Fig. 11–100). The other radial cut is then made, from the posterior edge anteriorly. The blade should be held firmly with a forceps, avoiding the underlying iris and lens (Fig. 11–101).

The block of tissue is cleanly excised at its anteriormost edge. The Vannas scissors should be inserted under direct visualization so that the position of the tip is always known (Fig. 11–102). After the scissors has been positioned, the handle is rotated so that the lower blade moves anteriorly and the upper blade poste-

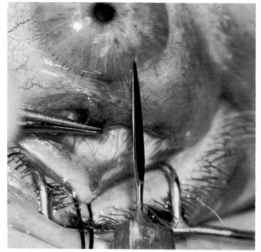

FIGURE 11–93. The sclera is fixated at the posterior edge of the bed of the scleral flap, and a Wheeler knife or similar sharp-tipped knife is introduced into the cornea 1 mm anterior to the limbus.

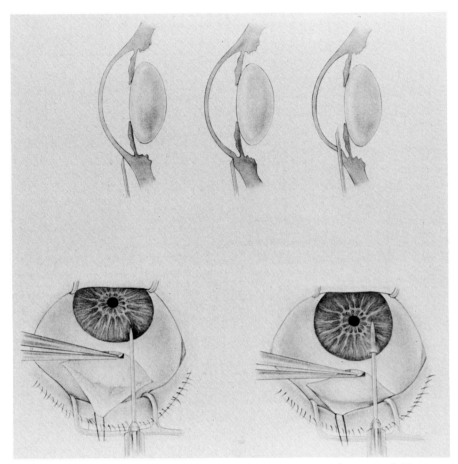

FIGURE 11–95. Schematic depiction of technique to perform a paracentesis (keratostomy). The instrument used here is a sharp, disposable 25-gauge needle. This is my preference. A second choice would be a disposable 27-gauge needle. Note, in the bottom illustrations, that the globe is pulled posteriorly with the left hand.

FIGURE 11–96. The width of the blade should be great enough to permit a #27 or #30 blunt irrigating tip to be introduced into the anterior chamber with ease. A magnification of at least 10× should be used so that the surgeon can be certain that the endothelial surface of the cornea has been penetrated and an adequately wide opening has been made into the anterior chamber. Change in the color of the knife blade helps to determine the point of entry into the anterior chamber.

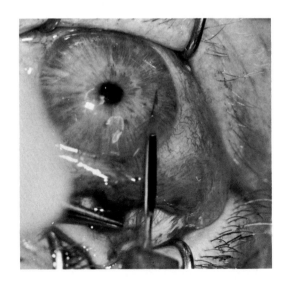

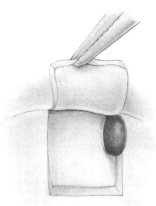

FIGURE 11–97. A radial incision is made in the base of the scleral flap in clear cornea. This is extended posteriorly to the junction between clear cornea and sclera. The iris often prolapses.

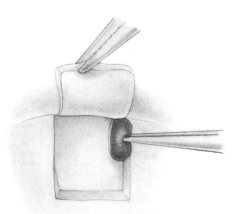

FIGURE 11–98. The prolapsed iris can be nicked with the scissors, allowing it to fall back into the globe.

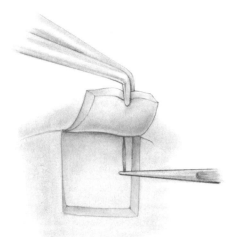

FIGURE 11–99. A Vannas scissors is placed into the anterior chamber and pulled toward the posterior aspect of the radial incision so that the posterior extent of the block to be excised will be anterior to scleral spur.

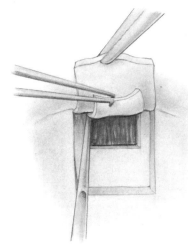

FIGURE 11–100. Using the Vannas scissors, the cornea is cut anteriorly. The colibri forceps pulls the cut edge of the block quite firmly posteriorly, and the Pierse-Hoskins forceps pulls the scleral flap quite vigorously anteriorly, permitting the radial incisions to be made as anteriorly as possible.

riorly, resulting in a cleaner section of the scleral block (Fig. 11–103). The surgeon should take care to ensure that the forceps used to hold the block does not traumatize the area of the trabecular meshwork. A specimen excised in this manner may provide important histopathologic information (Fig. 11–104).

The iris is grasped at approximately the midportion, preferably near the previous iridotomy (Fig. 11–105). The iris is then lifted up from the globe through the open blades of a De-

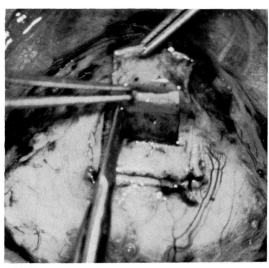

FIGURE 11–101. The radial incision should be carried into clear cornea.

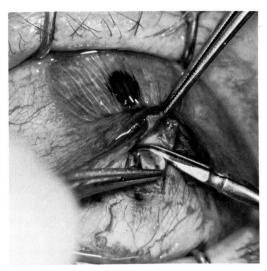

FIGURE 11-102. The block of scleral wall is amputated with a Vannas scissors. The tips are inserted under direct visualization.

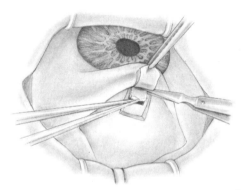

FIGURE 11-103. The handle of the scissors is rotated so as to avoid shelving the anterior incision.

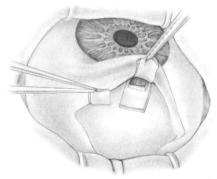

FIGURE 11-104. The removed specimen should be inspected. It should consist largely of cornea. The posterior trabecular meshwork may be included but need not be. Tissue posterior to the posterior trabecular meshwork should not be included.

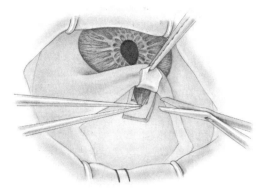

FIGURE 11-105. The iris is grasped, preferably near the previous iridotomy (see Fig. 11-98), and the tissue inspected making certain that it is iris and not ciliary body.

Wecker scissors (Fig. 11-106). The principles that underlie the technique of iridectomy are to achieve complete removal of the iris in the area in which the sclera and the cornea have been excised, to avoid the ciliary body and ciliary processes, and to keep the apex of the iridectomy as far from the sphincter as possible. When the iris has been sufficiently tented to achieve these aims, the blades are closed and the amputated tissue is slowly lifted away (Fig. 11-107).*

The scleral flap is sutured in place, usually with one suture in each of the two corners, and one between these in the center of the posterior edge of the flap. Care is taken not to penetrate the thickness of the sclera with the needle (Fig. 11-108). I prefer 10-0 nylon. If nylon is chosen, the suture must not be pulled too tightly or it may induce a permanent astigmatism (Figs. 11-109 to 11-111).

---

*See page 278 for further description of the technique of iridectomy.

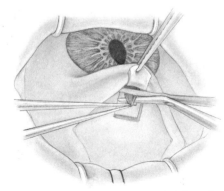

FIGURE 11-106. An iridectomy of the desired size is performed.

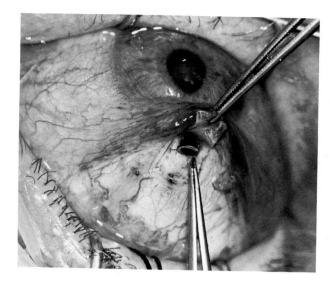

FIGURE 11–107. The iris tissue is carefully lifted away from the globe, making certain that the iridectomy is complete.

After three sutures have been placed the surgeon fills the anterior chamber with balanced salt solution through the previously placed paracentesis track and then inspects the area of the scleral flap. If the goal of the surgery is to avoid a leak, additional sutures near the limbus may be required. When trying to avoid leakage, it is especially important that the needle not penetrate the scleral flap. If, on the other hand, the surgeon hopes to obtain gross filtration, cautery may be applied to one or both of the radial edges of the scleral flap. Enough sutures are placed or sufficient cautery is applied to achieve the surgeon's goal.

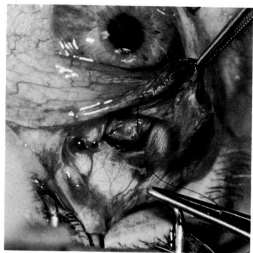

FIGURE 11–109. At least two throws are placed on the first tie to allow the tightness of this suture to be accurately adjusted.

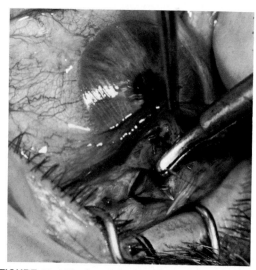

FIGURE 11–108. The scleral flap is closed with fine suture material; the needle must not penetrate the full thickness of the flap.

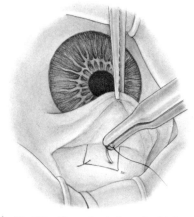

FIGURE 11–110. The scleral flap should be properly returned to its original position; it should not be sutured so tightly that astigmatism is produced.

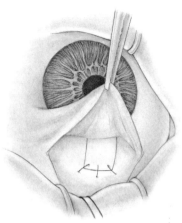

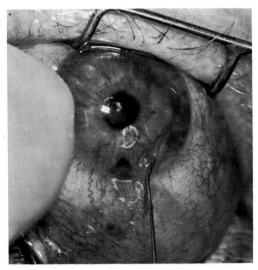

FIGURE 11–113. The anterior chamber is filled with balanced salt solution, with the intraocular pressure being carefully monitored with the tip of the finger.

FIGURE 11–111. At least three sutures are placed in the scleral flap. This permits releasing one or both of the sutures in the corners, to enhance aqueous filtration postoperatively, and yet assures that the scleral flap can remain in place by virtue of the suture placed in the middle of the posterior edge of the flap. If a "full-thickness" type of procedure is desired, all three sutures can be released postoperatively. Additional nonpenetrating sutures near the limbus may be required when filtration is excessive. A sufficient number of sutures should be placed to assure that the anterior chamber is well formed and that the pressure can be temporarily elevated.

The conjunctival flap is closed in two layers, as described on pages 269 and 270, using 8–0 chromic collagen suture.

During the procedure, atropine should have been given at appropriate times so that by this time the pupil is satisfactorily dilated and the ciliary body cycloplegic. If adequate pupillary dilatation has not been obtained, phenylephrine 2.5 or 10% is administered.

The eye is inspected. If there is no filtering bleb (Fig. 11–112), but the goal of the surgery is to develop one, then the anterior chamber is again filled with balanced salt solution (Fig. 11–113). The tip of the finger should monitor the pressure of the globe as the anterior chamber is filled, in order to avoid leaving the eye too soft (intraocular pressure below 5 mm Hg) or too firm (intraocular pressure above 20 mm Hg). In cases in which gross filtration has been allowed for, a conjunctival bleb will develop as the anterior chamber is formed (Figs. 11–114 and 11–115A–D). In all cases the anterior chamber should be well formed at the conclusion of the surgery. In fact, the anterior chamber should have been well formed before the closure of the conjunctival flap. If this goal cannot

FIGURE 11–112. After closure of the conjunctiva, a filtering bleb may not develop spontaneously.

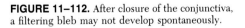

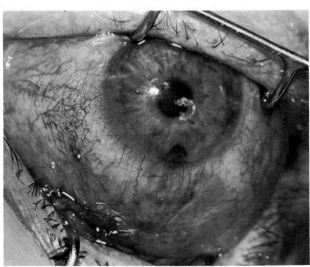

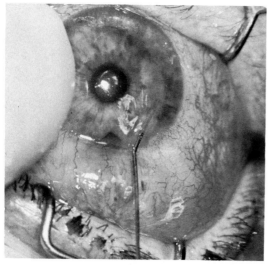

FIGURE 11–114. When filtration is desired postoperatively, a satisfactory bleb should be present at the close of the procedure.

be accomplished at this point, the conjunctival flap is taken down and additional sutures are placed in the scleral flap to achieve tighter closure. *Sutures can usually be easily cut with a laser postoperatively. It is my current practice to close most scleral flaps tightly, limiting hypotony and flat anterior chambers, planning to release sutures during the first few postoperative days.* If this cannot be accomplished, for instance, if the flap is excessively thin or technical errors have resulted in a tear in the flap, a graft of Tenon's capsule can be taken from the nasal or temporal edge of the conjunctival flap and secured tightly over the scleral flap.

It should be stressed that *at the conclusion of the procedure, the eye should appear as the surgeon wants it to: with a well-closed conjunctival flap without extruding Tenon's capsule, a totally formed anterior chamber, and an adequately dilated, round pupil, and either with or without a conjunctival bleb.* If the eye does

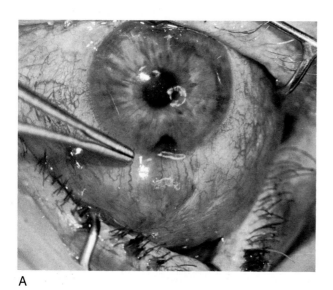

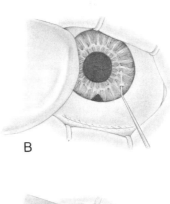

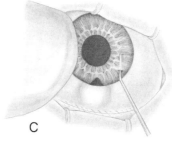

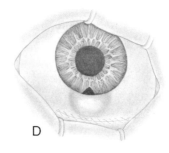

A

B

C

D

FIGURE 11–115. *A,* Here normal intraocular pressure has been restored, and a filtering bleb is readily visible. *B–D,* Schematic depiction of filling the anterior chamber through the keratotomy using a blunt 30-gauge cannula. *B,* The intraocular pressure is monitored as the balanced salt solution is injected. The chamber should form and the pressure should rise to around 25 mm Hg. *C,* A bleb is seen developing. The injection is stopped, and the finger monitors the intraocular pressure, which should fall spontaneously to around 10 mm Hg. *D,* The bleb shown here *is not* adequate in size. Additional balanced salt solution needs to be injected in order to extend the bleb so it reaches 180 degrees, covering the entire two superior quadrants.

not look right at the end of the surgery, it is unlikely that the result will be optimal.

In occasional instances in which trabeculectomy is performed in an inflamed eye, betamethasone (Celestone), 3 to 6 mg, may be indicated. This is administered deep in the inferior fornix, so that conjunctiva is not elevated.

Modifications of Surgical Technique. One of the major advantages of trabeculectomy is that it can be modified quite easily, so that the surgical result may be tailored to the surgeon's goals. For example, the thickness, shape, or size of the scleral flap can be altered. A small flap would involve less of the circumference of the eye, providing a greater area for repeat surgery should this become necessary. A larger flap allows excision of a larger block at the inner wall of sclera and cornea, which provides a better specimen for histopathologic examination. A larger scleral flap (e.g., 3 mm in a radial direction and 4 mm circumferentially) when combined with a small excision (e.g., 1 mm by 1 mm) permits construction of a wide ledge surrounding the excised block. This predisposes to firm healing of sclera to sclera, which tends to prevent gross filtration. This may be the surgeon's goal in performing surgery on the patient with acute primary angle-closure glaucoma: a poorly controlled intraocular pressure, but a completely healthy disc.

The thickness of the flap may also be varied. A thin flap appears to predispose to greater filtration with development of a more cystic bleb and a lower intraocular pressure. Instead of the flap being one-third the thickness of the sclera, it can be fashioned more thickly, leading to a tighter closure with less filtration.

The position of the excised block may also be varied considerably. Some surgeons prefer to use a trephine to remove the inner wall; although this has the advantage of producing an excision of standard size, it is not recommended; the tip of the instrument cannot be visualized, which violates a fundamental surgical principle, and the size and shape of the instrument puts limitations on the flexibility of the surgeon to modify the shape or position of the block to be excised.

Some of the early descriptions of trabeculectomy advised taking the block of tissue from the sclera and the trabecular area, the theory being that excision of the trabecular meshwork was necessary for surgery to work. Figure 11–116A shows this technique. As greater experience with this procedure was gained, it became apparent that it was not necessary to unroof the

ciliary body; intraocular pressure was just as satisfactorily lowered when the block was limited to tissue anterior to the scleral spur (Fig. 11–116B and C). Moreover, unroofing the ciliary body predisposed to complications such as increased bleeding from the large vessels of the ciliary body, formation of a cyclodialysis cleft with subsequent hypotony, and more inflammation than when the ciliary body was not traumatized. Consequently my preference is to keep the posterior edge of the inner block anterior to the scleral spur (Fig. 11–116C).

There is less likely to be bleeding after such a procedure, as Schlemm's canal has not been sectioned, so reflux of blood from the episcleral veins into the anterior chamber is less likely to occur.

In summary, then, the surgeon can modify the technique of trabeculectomy to fit the particular goals he has chosen for the individual case under consideration.

Trabeculectomy is a microsurgical procedure; magnification of $8\times$ is required.

Postoperative Care

Care after trabeculectomy is designed to encourage filtration and to keep the pupil adequately dilated, the ciliary body paralyzed, the eye as quiet as possible, and blood away from the trabeculectomy site. The usual orders are atropine 1% two to four times daily and a potent corticosteroid drop four times daily. It has been well established that topical corticosteroids result in better filtering blebs and markedly lower intraocular pressures postoperatively than when corticosteroids are not used topically. The corticosteroids also predispose to steroid-induced elevation of intraocular pressure and cataract, and should preferably not be used more than four times daily for 2 weeks, with rapid tapering after that. An antibiotic is often applied topically for a week or so. If the pupil is not adequately dilated, phenylephrine may be added. The patient should be encouraged to be in a head-up position, that is, to be sitting or standing, and to sleep on one side or the other so that blood does not settle in the area of the trabeculectomy. As soon as the intraocular pressure is 6 mm Hg or higher, there is no limitation placed on the patient's activities. When the intraocular pressure is below that level, the patient is vigorously cautioned to avoid straining, stooping, coughing, or other activities that would increase the venous pressure and predispose to expulsive choroidal hemorrhage.

The patient should be examined several hours after surgery to see if the desired goals have

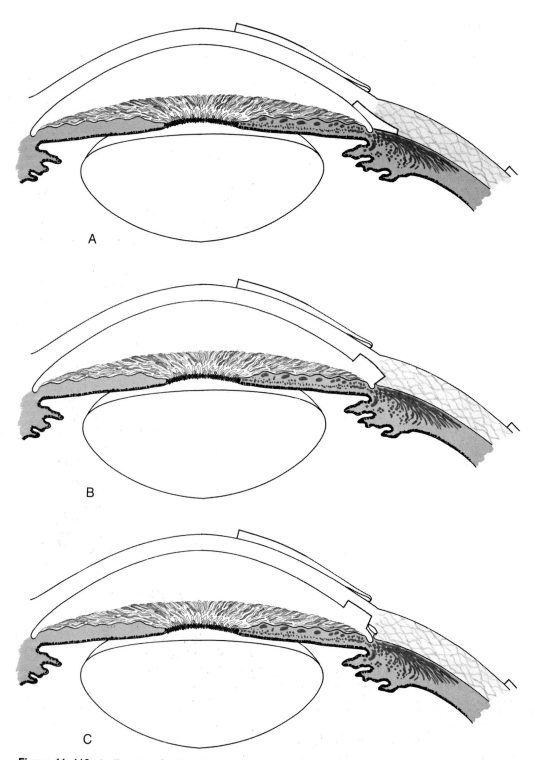

Figure 11–116. *A*, Excision of a thin block of cornea, posterior trabecular meshwork, and sclera. This technique is no longer recommended. *B*, The block of tissue excised here includes posterior trabecular meshwork and cornea and does not unroof the ciliary body. This eliminates the possibility of cyclodialysis and decreases the likelihood of bleeding. This technique is now preferred. *C*, A "trabeculectomy" will function even if trabecular meshwork is not removed. Some surgeons prefer to limit the excision of tissue to the anterior trabeculum and cornea.

been accomplished. If the intended outcome is a low intraocular pressure with gross filtration, the pressure should be low and the surgically created bleb raised to an adequate height, unless the sclera has been tightly sutured with intention of releasing the sutures postoperatively. If the anterior chamber is deep and the pressure above 15 mm Hg, the eye should be left unpatched after it is examined, drops started, and a Carlo Traverso maneuver performed (see page 345 and Fig. 11–132) and/or sutures in the scleral flap released with an argon laser in order to develop adequate filtration. If the chamber is shallow or even flat and the pressure below 5 mm Hg, probably the amount of filtration is excessive and a course of dilating drops should be given and the eye lightly repatched. This patch should not be firmly enough placed to cause pressure on the eye; a "pressure patch" is more likely to cause excessive hypotony than it is to be beneficial. On the other hand, if the surgeon's intended goal is to avoid filtration (as it may well be in patients with primary angle-closure glaucoma), and the pressure is above 15 mm Hg and the chamber deep, massage should *not* be given, though it may be advisable to leave the eye unpatched and to start routine drops. However, if the chamber is shallow and filtration is present in such an eye, then steps must be taken to rectify the situation: a course of atropine followed by phenylephrine is required, after which the patient should be given acetazolamide, 500 mg orally or intravenously, and have a firm pressure patch applied, with instructions not to unpatch the eye until rounds by the surgeon the next day.

It is not usual after trabeculectomy that the anterior chamber needs to be re-formed. The management of an excessively flat anterior chamber is discussed later.

Postoperatively, the eye should have a conjunctival suture line that is so high in the cul-de-sac that it is difficult to see. Tenon's capsule should be completely covered, the iridectomy should be under the overhanging upper lid if possible, and the eye should be quite quiet. In the immediate postoperative period there is usually an elevation of the conjunctiva over the trabeculectomy site; this is followed in some cases by the development of tiny cysts along the limbus that are highly indicative of a functioning filtering bleb (Figs. 11–117 to 11–119).

In about 10 per cent of cases intraocular pressure rises into a range higher than ideal; this usually occurs between 4 and 6 weeks postoperatively (Fig. 11–120). If the pressure rise is due to failure to filter, sutures in the scleral flap should be released, usually starting the second postoperative day. They should be released before 10 days postoperatively. Such rises are often transient and are usually best left alone if the surgeon believes that the optic disc will not be damaged; if necessary, they may be treated with topical epinephrine or other antiglaucoma medication. Carbonic anhydrase inhibitors and beta blockers are theoretically less preferable, as these drugs decrease aqueous inflow and may lead to failure of the procedure. From a practical point of view, however, there is little to support this theory, and beta blockers are frequently used to suppress postoperative intraocular pressure rises.

Gonioscopy should be performed postopera-

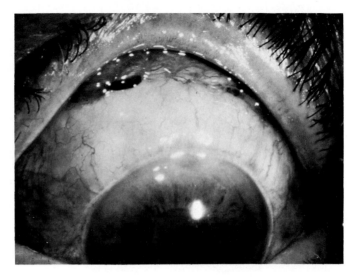

FIGURE 11–117. On the first postoperative day after a filtering trabeculectomy the conjunctiva-Tenon's flap should be elevated by aqueous leaking through or around the scleral flap. The conjunctival incision was correctly made near the insertion of the superior rectus muscle.

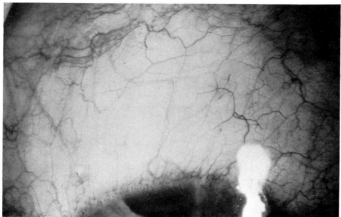

FIGURE 11–118. Though no apparent filtration is present here, intraocular pressure has fallen from 40 mm Hg preoperatively to 18 mm Hg postoperatively. The anterior chamber was wide open preoperatively, and the only reasonable explanation for the decreased postoperative intraocular pressure is transscleral filtration.

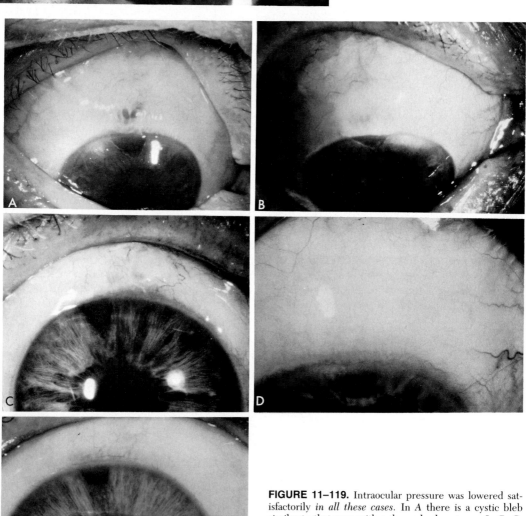

FIGURE 11–119. Intraocular pressure was lowered satisfactorily *in all these cases.* In *A* there is a cystic bleb similar to that seen with a thermal sclerostomy. In *B, C,* and *D* this is decreasingly apparent, and in *E* there is almost no detectable subconjunctival fluid.

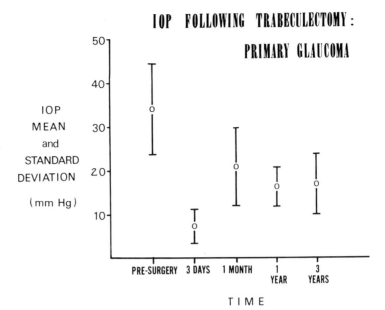

FIGURE 11-120. The course of intraocular pressure after trabeculectomy.

tively in order to evaluate the nature of the trabeculectomy (Fig. 11–121).

After surgery, even when apparently successful, the patient should again be followed closely. The discs and the fields should be meticulously monitored. Control can be defined only by determining the level of intraocular pressure at which disc and field deterioration no longer occurs. Ideally, there should be an improvement in the disc or field. Though the surgeon may have estimated before the operation that an intraocular pressure of a particular level would probably be satisfactory, the validity of his estimate can be determined only by redefining the adequacy of control after the surgery. Thus a statement that a surgical procedure was successful because the intraocular pressure was lowered below X mm Hg is meaningless. The only way a surgical procedure for glaucoma that is designed to lower intraocular pressure can be judged is by the health of the disc and field.

Peripheral Iridectomy with Thermal Sclerostomy

Indications

The indications for peripheral iridectomy with thermal sclerostomy are similar to those for trabeculectomy. However, as it is difficult to modify the procedure so that filtration is minimal, it is ordinarily not appropriate for conditions in which the surgeon believes gross filtration should be avoided. Thus a peripheral iridectomy with thermal sclerostomy is not the treatment of choice in patients with any type of primary angle-closure glaucoma. A trabeculectomy is not "merely another filtering procedure." Although it can be constructed to produce gross filtration, it can work satisfactorily in the absence of such filtration.

Some of the differences between trabeculectomy and peripheral iridectomy with thermal sclerostomy are shown in Figure 11–122. This information is taken from a study in which

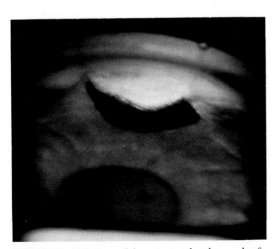

FIGURE 11-121. View of the anterior chamber angle after a trabeculectomy. The block of tissue excised included posterior trabecular meshwork, here lightly pigmented. The edge of the iridectomy is adherent to the cut edge of the sclera, a frequent occurrence when the iridectomy is too small. There is no cyclodialysis.

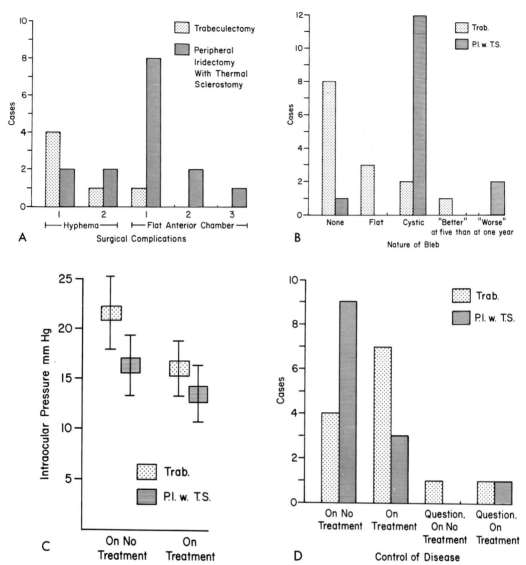

FIGURE 11–122. *A,* Frequency of complications in a controlled study in which patients had a trabeculectomy performed in one eye and a periperal iridectomy with thermal sclerostomy in the other, the basic indication being primary open-angle glaucoma. There were no intraoperative complications in any case. Slight shallowing of the anterior chamber occurred in two trabeculectomy cases and in eight of those having had peripheral iridectomy with thermal sclerostomy. In 1 of the 14 patients the anterior chamber needed to be reformed surgically in the eye that had had a peripheral iridectomy with thermal sclerostomy. *B,* The conjunctival bleb after trabeculectomy is flatter than that after peripheral iridectomy with thermal sclerostomy. This graph refers to the same 14 patients shown in *A. C,* The intraocular pressure was higher in the eye treated with trabeculectomy than in the eye treated with peripheral iridectomy with thermal sclerostomy. *D,* More patients required medical therapy to control their glaucomatous disease in the eye treated with trabeculectomy.

patients had a trabeculectomy performed on one eye and a peripheral iridectomy with thermal sclerostomy on the other. The incidence of collapse of the anterior chamber after surgery was markedly higher in the cases treated with peripheral iridectomy with thermal sclerostomy (Fig. 11–122A). This complication was of sufficient severity that reoperation was occasionally necessary for these patients. As would be expected, the patients treated with a procedure that produced gross filtration were left with cystic blebs, whereas those treated with trabeculectomy were not (Fig. 11–122B). Trabeculectomy was less effective in lowering intraocular pressure (Fig. 11–122C). Consequently more trabeculectomy patients required medical treatment for control of their disease postoperatively (Fig. 11–122D). However, in all instances the only drug required was epinephrine.

Although peripheral iridectomy with thermal sclerostomy produces a lower intraocular pressure than that noted after trabeculectomy, it does so at a greater risk to the patient. Furthermore, trabeculectomy may be modified to produce filtration and thus accomplish the goal of a gross filtering procedure, with less risk to the patient. For these reasons I have almost completely abandoned all surgical procedures designed to produce uncontrolled gross filtration. Trabeculectomy is almost invariably the procedure of choice.

In those patients for whom trabeculectomy has failed once or perhaps even twice, a peripheral iridectomy with thermal sclerostomy may be tried.

Anesthesia

The considerations for anesthesia are the same as those for trabeculectomy (p. 286).

Preoperative Care

Preparation of a patient for peripheral iridectomy with thermal sclerostomy is similar to that for trabeculectomy (p. 286).

Surgical Technique

The initial stages of the procedure are the same as for trabeculectomy. A limbus-based flap is preferred. However, an important difference is that it is necessary to clear more meticulously the corneoscleral sulcus, so that there is adequate room in which to place the cautery without danger of burning the conjunctival flap.

After development of the conjunctival flap a line of cautery 3 mm long is placed circumferentially 1 to 2 mm posterior to the corneoscleral sulcus. An incision one-third of the way through the sclera is made with a #67 Beaver blade directly in the line of cautery. Cautery is reapplied to the same area, making sure that the heat is sufficient to cause shrinkage of the tissue without producing charring. The tissue should not become brown. The tip of the cautery is placed into the depth of the incision and gently pushed anteriorly and posteriorly to fashion a trough-shaped depression in the sclera. The incision is deepened, again in a circumferential direction, making sure that the depth of the incision extends fully from one edge of the line of cautery to the other. This incision should now have extended to approximately two-thirds of the thickness of the sclera. Gentle cautery is again placed in the depth of the incision. By

this time the tissue should have retracted so that the superficial edges are about 1 mm apart. The surgeon again incises the depth of the trough, attempting to make the incision as deeply through the sclera as possible without entering the anterior chamber. Cautery is again applied. Further incision is made, so that the anterior chamber is entered for the full width of the line of cautery.

The remainder of the procedure is completed as has been described for a trabeculectomy (p. 296).

Atropine should be instilled throughout the procedure so that the pupil is widely dilated and the ciliary body as paralyzed as possible.

Postoperative Care

The patch and shield are left in place until the next day. At that point the patient should be examined with a slit lamp so that the depth of the anterior chamber may be estimated accurately. It is usual for this to be shallow and for there to be a high filtering bleb. Postoperative medications usually consist of atropine 1% four times daily, phenylephrine 10% four times daily, and an antibiotic-corticosteroid drop four times daily. The anterior chamber usually remains shallow for a week or two, gradually reforming at that time. If it becomes flat, or the eye hypotonous, treatment will probably need to be altered. Management of the flat anterior chamber is discussed in detail later in this chapter. If by the third postoperative day the chamber has remained formed over the central iris and lens, the prognosis for a satisfactory result is good.

Shunt Procedures

Important new methods to develop filtration are proving successful. These use a plastic shunt from the anterior chamber to a position well posterior to the limbus where the fluid leaks into the subtenon space, influenced by an additional plastic implant. The procedure that appears to hold the most promise is the Molteno implant. Other methods include the Schocket tube shunt to an encircling silicone band, the long tube version of the Krupin-Denver valve, and the one-piece valved tube and explant of Joseph and Hitchings. All of these devices use a small-diameter silicone rubber tube to carry aqueous to an equatorial filtration site developed around the explanted portion of the device.

The experience with all of these implants is relatively limited and the follow-up short. However, they appear to be more satisfactory solutions to certain types of case, as indicated in Table 11–2.

Surgical Technique. The surgery can be performed under local retrobulbar anesthesia, but general anesthesia is preferable. The Molteno implant can be placed in a one-stage or two-stage operation. With both procedures the anterior edge of the implant is positioned approximately 10 mm posterior to the limbus and secured in place firmly against the sclera with a heavy permanent suture.

This portion of the implant is connected to a thin silicone rubber tube that passes over the sclera, through a trabeculectomy-type flap, and into the anterior chamber through an opening made with a 23-gauge needle. The indications for the procedure are still relatively few and the technical aspects too complicated to deserve further description in this text devoted to general ophthalmic surgery. Patients who require this type of procedure are best referred to centers where such specialized surgery is being frequently performed.

Methods to Decrease Scar Formation Postoperatively

In order to prevent scarring of the Tenon's-conjunctival flap to the underlying sclera with consequent failure of a filtration procedure, agents designed to diminish the proliferation of capillaries and fibroblasts have been used. The most extensive experience has been with 5-fluorouracil (5-FU). As originally described, 5-FU was injected subconjunctivally into the quadrant opposite the site of filtration immediately after the surgery, using 5 mg of 5-FU (a 1-ml injection). This subconjunctival injection was then repeated twice daily for 1 week and once daily for 1 week. More recent experience with the agent suggests using the agent once daily in a much smaller dose (0.5 mg or 0.1 ml given once daily for 1 week). Whether smaller doses will be as effective has not been established. It appears that the original dosage schedule does indeed alter the clinical course of filtering procedures, resulting in a higher success rate in cases ordinarily not expected to do well, such as inflammatory glaucomas, aphakic glaucomas, and glaucoma in the very young patient.

The administration of 5-FU, however, is not without problems. Not only are the episcleral fibroblasts that are involved in the scarring of the filtration site affected by antimetabolites. These agents also damage rapidly proliferating corneal and conjunctival epithelium. Conse-

quently a major complication of subconjunctivally injected 5-FU is a leaking incision, with leaks along the suture tracks, or along the site of the injection itself. Additionally, conjunctival and corneal epithelial defects were frequent with the initial dosage. Moreover, because healing of the anterior margin of a fornix-based flap depends on adhesion between the conjunctiva and the underlying cornea, 5-FU is not appropriate for use with fornix-based flaps.

One method of avoiding the complications is to keep the eye well covered with ointment. Instead of using atropine and corticosteroid drops, the patient should be treated with atropine and corticosteroid ointments. Additionally, the ointment should be instilled in the eye immediately before subconjunctival administration of the 5-FU. Further, a tiny needle, such as a 30-gauge needle, should be used for the injection.

Other chemotherapeutic agents that act at different points along the path of cellular proliferation have also been used: beta-aminopropionitrile and cis-hydroxyproline.

The long-term effects of administration of the antimetabolites have not been established. If indeed it is correct that they result in thinner, more cystic conjunctival blebs, the long-term outcome may not be as pleasant as hoped. It is important to recall that one of the major reasons the full-thickness procedures were abandoned in favor of guarded procedures was the high rate of endophthalmitis that developed in such eyes. By using 5-FU, could we be predisposing patients to the complications of excessively thin blebs in the future?

Cyclodialysis

Indications

Cyclodialysis is indicated when medical control of glaucoma is inadequate and other procedures designed to lower intraocular pressure are not considered to be appropriate. Cyclodialysis has been most frequently used in surgical management of aphakic glaucoma, and has been relatively contraindicated in phakic patients, as it is thought to predispose to the development of cataract. However, the success rate appears to be higher in the phakic patient than in the aphakic patient, and I use cyclodialysis in some phakic patients in whom filtration procedures have failed. Noninflammatory open- or closed-angle glaucomas, such as Chandler's syndrome, appear to respond best.

The procedure is seldom successful in eyes with uveitis, or in those that cannot tolerate long-term administration of strong parasympathomimetic agents.

Anesthesia

A cyclodialysis should take only 10 to 15 minutes to perform. However, because the uvea is traumatized, the procedure can be painful, and topical anesthesia is usually not adequate. Local anesthesia with a short-acting agent for a facial and retrobulbar block is advised (see Tables 5–2 and 11–8).

Preoperative Care

The eye should be as quiet as possible. The long-acting cholinesterase inhibitors do not need to be stopped before surgery. On the other hand, atropine should not have been used for at least 1 week before cyclodialysis is performed. The angle should be examined so that blood vessels can be avoided if possible. Other principles of the preparation of the patient for surgery are essentially the same as those described in Chapter 2.

The patient should be told that vision will be severely blurred for at least 1 week because of intraocular bleeding or hypotony, or both. Patients should also be informed that there is a low likelihood of success, the rate being less than 50 per cent in even the most favorable case. Additionally, it is important to mention that the procedure will not eliminate the need for medications; a long-acting cholinesterase inhibitor will often be necessary indefinitely after the surgery.

Mechanism of Action

Cyclodialysis is thought by some to succeed because it allows aqueous humor to leave the anterior chamber through a cleft between the ciliary body and the sclera; the aqueous is then absorbed from the suprachoroidal space. Others believe that the mechanism of action is decreased inflow resulting from the presence of a ciliary body detachment. It is still not known which of these, if either or both, is the cause for the lowering of intraocular pressure produced by a successful cyclodialysis. However, unless a patent cyclodialysis cleft can be seen, the procedure will probably not have a beneficial effect on intraocular pressure.

Surgical Technique

The first decision to be made is where on the globe the cyclodialysis cleft should be made. The factors that enter into this are listed in

TABLE 11–29. Factors That Influence Location of Cyclodialysis Incision

Ease of performance
Avoidance of previous iridectomy
Avoidance of large blood vessels (12, 3, 6, and 9 o'clock positions)
Ease of keeping blood out of cleft
Avoidance of scleral staphyloma
Avoidance of area of previous cyclocryotherapy

Table 11–29. It is technically easiest to perform a cyclodialysis in the temporal quadrants. The area in which an iridectomy has been previously performed should be avoided, as the cyclodialysis spatula may penetrate the iridectomy, damaging the underlying lens or vitreous. The point at which the anterior ciliary vessels penetrate the globe *must* also be avoided, as tearing these may cause serious hemorrhage (see Fig. 11–2). If the cleft is developed superiorly, it is easier to keep blood from blocking the cyclodialysis in the immediate postoperative period. When performing cyclodialysis in conjunction with a cataract extraction, some authors have found a higher success rate when the cleft is placed infratemporally. The validity of this has not been established. It is unlikely that there is any advantage to performing a cyclodialysis in the area of existing posterior synechias.

Cyclodialysis does not produce an external fistula; consequently the state of the overlying conjunctiva is not a consideration.

After selection of the area in which the cyclodialysis is to be performed, the conjunctiva is incised for a distance of approximately a centimeter, 5 to 6 mm posterior to the limbus (Fig. 11–123A). Cautery is applied to the sclera so that the vessels in the superficial sclera will be coagulated. The dimensions of the oval of cautery may be 4 to 5 mm meridionally and 2 to 3 mm radially (Fig. 11–123B).

An incision 3 to 4 mm long is made in the center of the oval, using a rounded knife such as the rounded portion of a #67 Beaver blade. After the incision is approximately one-half to two-thirds the thickness of the sclera, a preplaced suture may be inserted (see Fig. 11–72). Virtually any adequately strong suture material may be chosen, although silk should probably be avoided. It is not essential to preplace the suture, but it does simplify completion of the incision without injuring the underlying uvea.

In order to disinsert the ciliary body from the sclera, the incision *must* be posterior to the scleral spur. This is the only area in which there is normally an adhesion between these tissue layers. Placing the incision further posteriorly offers no advantage. The incision through sclera must be complete. In some instances the surgeon may be misled when, after having incised almost completely through the scleral wall, he notices dark tissue at the base and incorrectly assumes he has penetrated completely; when the sclera is extremely thin it becomes virtually transparent. Thus the surgeon must visualize this incision carefully so that no question remains. The uvea has a granular consistency completely different from that of the sclera.

The anterior edge of the incision is grasped with a fine-tipped forceps, such as a Barraquer colibri, and using the scleral incision as a point on which to fixate firmly, a paracentesis track is made into the anterior chamber. This is best positioned 180 degrees opposite from the scleral incision (Fig. 11–123D).

The anterior lip of the scleral incision is again fixated firmly with a fine-toothed forceps. A spatula, such as the Heine cyclodialysis spatula or, preferably, the Barraquer sweep, is used to create the cyclodialysis cleft. The tip of the

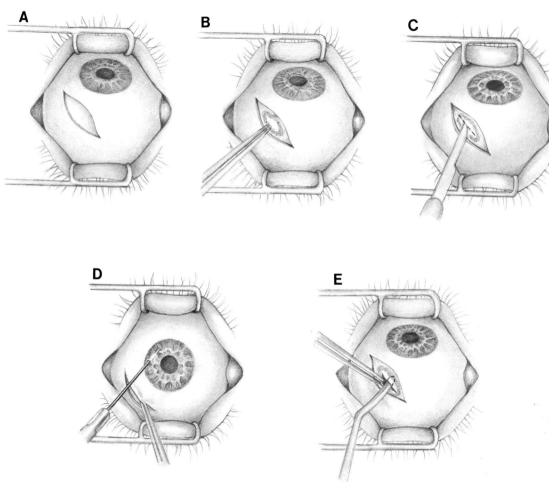

FIGURE 11–123. Cyclodialysis. *A*, Incision is made in conjunctiva approximately 5 to 6 mm posterior to the limbus. *B*, Cautery is applied in the shape of an oval donut 5 mm long and 3 mm wide. *C*, An incision 4 mm long is made in the center of the oval. A traction suture may now be placed. *D*, A paracentesis is made into the anterior chamber as described elsewhere. *E*, The tip of the cyclodialysis spatula is carefully introduced into the space between the cord and the sclera. *1.* As the tip is cautiously moved anteriorly, the heel of the spatula is depressed and the tip is lifted up toward the microscope, causing a small bulge in the sclera owing to the firm pressure used. *F, 1* and *2,* As soon as the tip is first seen in the anterior chamber it is retracted slightly and depressed posteriorly in order to avoid tearing Descemet's membrane. After the tip is in the anterior chamber it is advanced anteriorly in a plane parallel to the iris. *G,* The spatula is swept to both sides, with the pupil being carefully observed as the tip is moved posteriorly. The anterior ciliary vessels are meticulously avoided. *H,* An air bubble is introduced into the anterior chamber, raising the intraocular pressure to around 30 to 40 mm Hg.

instrument is carefully introduced into the incision in a radial direction (Fig. 11–123E). Immediately after the tip enters the space between the uvea and the sclera, the handle is rotated so that the heel of the spatula moves down toward the direction of the floor and the tip toward the ceiling (Fig. 11–123E).* The tip of the spatula is then pushed up toward the sclera; as this is done it is moved anteriorly, the sclera serving as a guide. Sufficient pressure should be made to produce a small bulge in the sclera; this can be seen as the tip moves anteriorly toward the limbus (Fig. 11–123E1). There should be no sense of resistance. If there is resistance, the spatula has probably been introduced into a layer within the sclera and is not in the space *between* the sclera and the uvea.

*This assumes, of course, that the patient is in a supine position.

A slight resistance should be felt when the spatula penetrates the adhesion between the ciliary body and the scleral spur.

The position of the tip can be monitored by observing the distortion of the sclera. As the cornea is reached, the pressure against the sclera should be reduced. As the spatula is moved further anteriorly, the tip becomes visible in the anterior chamber; the surgeon should at this point immediately stop further anterior motion (Fig. 11–123F). The spatula should then be retracted approximately half a millimeter posteriorly, to be certain that it has not disinserted Descemet's membrane.

After the surgeon is sure that the tip of the spatula is in the correct position, the handle of the spatula is tilted backward toward its original position, so that the heel is moved away from the floor and the tip of the spatula is depressed toward the surface of the iris, thus making the

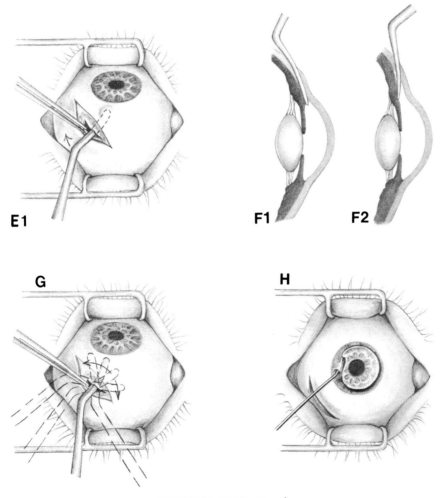

FIGURE 11–123 *Continued*

plane of the spatula parallel to the plane of the iris (Fig. 11–123F2).

The spatula is introduced until approximately 2 mm of the tip is visible. The handle of the spatula is then rotated about the axis of the handle so that the tip sweeps to the side toward the angle recess (Fig. 11–123G). As it does so, the tip is moved anteriorly once again, so it pushes up firmly against the sclera. The pupil is carefully observed. The iris will be pulled toward the angle recess by the spatula until the spatula has separated the uvea from the sclera. At that point the pupil will return to its previous round condition. As the spatula is swept into the angle *it must be kept tightly against the sclera*, so that it separates the iris from the sclera rather than tearing the peripheral iris root.

The process of dialysis requires mild force. If the resistance is excessive, attempts to dialyze the iris by sweeping should immediately be stopped. Under such circumstances it is better to withdraw the cyclodialysis spatula from the incision and reinsert it so that it enters in a meridional direction. The distance from the incision to the point at which the anterior ciliary vessels penetrate should be noted so that the tip of the spatula will not be introduced far enough to tear these vessels. This distance must be estimated, as the sweep is done blindly. It is better to err on the side of making a smaller sweep and being sure to avoid the anterior ciliary vessels. After having inserted the spatula to the proper length, usually around 4 to 5 mm, again making absolutely sure that the tip hugs the sclera, the surgeon then rotates the handle between the fingers so that the tip sweeps into the anterior chamber. The surgeon must be careful that the tip does not traumatize the posterior surface of the cornea by sweeping suddenly past the limbus. The scleral spur is then dialyzed in the opposite direction.

The spatula is withdrawn after it has dialyzed the ciliary body, to both the right and left sides of the incision, so that a cleft about one-fifth the circumference of the limbal area has been developed. Immediately the anterior chamber should be filled with air, using the previously placed paracentesis track, in order to increase the pressure within the globe to at least 30 mm Hg; this should tamponade any bleeding (Fig. 11–123H). Because this must be done *without delay*, the syringe containing the air with the appropriate blunt needle should be in readiness *before* performing the cyclodialysis. If bleeding is excessive, the blood is irrigated out through the scleral incision, saline being introduced through the keratostomy. The pupil should be miotic.

The previously placed scleral suture is then secured; if a preplaced suture was not used, a suture such as 7–0 polyglactin is placed and tied.

Postoperative Care

Postoperatively, the patient is positioned so that blood will settle away from the cyclodialysis cleft. If the cyclodialysis has been performed supratemporally on the right eye, the patient is asked to be up and around or in a sitting position during the day and to sleep on the left side at night.

A strong miotic is instilled in the operating room. This is an *essential* part of the procedure, especially for aphakic patients. I prefer echothiophate 0.125% in blue-eyed patients and in brown-eyed patients who have not previously been on strong miotics; echothiophate 0.25% is used in those with extremely dark irides or in those who have previously tolerated strong miotics well. These agents are used because of their stimulating effect on the sphincter of the ciliary body and, to a lesser extent, the sphincter of the iris. This assures that the uvea will be pulled away from the cyclodialysis cleft, enhancing the likelihood of success of the surgery.

The use of a strong miotic may be associated with considerable discomfort, browache, or even systemic parasympathetic symptoms. The patient should usually be advised of the expected discomfort. Miotics may also produce a greater postoperative inflammatory response; this can be partially limited by use of strong corticosteroids such as prednisolone acetate 1% every 2 to 3 hours for the first 3 or 4 days.

The intraocular pressure after successful cyclodialysis is usually below 15 mm Hg. It is not unusual for it to be in the range of 5 to 10 mm Hg for the first few days postoperatively. Pressures higher than this are often a sign that the surgical procedure will not work. In occasional instances, however, the cleft is, apparently, initially blocked with blood and becomes functional only after several days. Final decision regarding the success or failure of the procedure should be deferred until approximately 1 month after surgery. If at that point the pressure is below 15 mm Hg, the cyclodialysis cleft is open, and the eye has no inflammatory reaction, the prognosis for continuing low intraocular pressure is good.

Typically, the anterior chamber is shallow. This is usually a function of ciliary body detachment, but the possibility of pupillary block must be kept in mind. I routinely use strong mydriatics such as phenylephrine 2.5% or 10% four times daily for several weeks.

Complications

The intraoperative and postoperative complications of cyclodialysis are relatively few (Table 11–30). However, as continued success of the procedure usually requires continued use of a strong, long-acting cholinesterase inhibitor, the multiple complications of these agents must be added to those of the surgery itself.

Modifications of Technique

Phakic vs. Aphakic Patients. The technique, complications, and probably even the nature of the postoperative results of cyclodialysis will differ among patients, depending on whether they are with or without lenses. As the anterior chamber usually collapses at the time of surgery, the surgeon must be careful to avoid traumatizing the cornea or, in the phakic patient, the lens.

In contrast, the technique of dialyzing the iris in the aphakic patient is different. In the aphake the spatula is depressed down toward the floor (that is, in the direction of the optic nerve), so that the iris root is bluntly torn from the scleral spur by the downward pressure of the spatula. This method permits creation of a large cleft and at the same time assures that the cyclodialysis spatula does not inadvertently traumatize the cornea or peripheral iris.

In the postoperative period a strong miotic such as echothiophate iodide must be continued indefinitely in the aphakic patient. Whether or not this is necessary in the phakic patient is less clear. The pull of the lens zonules on the ciliary body may tend to keep the cyclodialysis cleft

TABLE 11–30. Complications of Cyclodialysis*

Intraocular bleeding
Hypotony
Stripping of Descemet's membrane
Late development of cataract
Rupture of lens capsule
Persistent uveitis

*As cyclodialysis requires continued use of long-acting cholinesterase inhibitors postoperatively, complications include the known effects of such agents: allergic conjunctivitis, blurring of vision, cataract, corneal bedewing, corneal endothelial change, dilatation of conjunctival vessels, frontal headaches, iris cysts, iritis, lid twitching, miotic-induced glaucoma, myopia, ocular pain, pseudopemphigoid, retinal detachment, rhinorrhea, abdominal pain, anorexia, bradycardia, bronchial constriction, cough, diarrhea, dyspnea, elevated blood pressure, excitability, generalized weakness, increased salivation, increased sweating, muscle cramps, muscle twitching, nausea and vomiting, paresthesia, restlessness.

open in the phakic patient, thus minimizing or perhaps even eliminating this need for the parasympathomimetic agent. Moreover, in the phakic patient it is desirable to avoid long-term use of strong cholinesterase inhibitors because of their known tendency to cause cataract.

Conclusions

The major problem with cyclodialysis is that too often it works either not at all or too well. Successful lowering of intraocular pressure is achieved in fewer than 50 per cent of patients. The success rate is higher in phakic patients and in those in whom cyclodialysis is combined with cataract extraction. When cyclodialysis does work it may lower the pressure to a range within which the eye is too soft to serve as a precise optical instrument. Because of the relatively low risk-benefit ratio, the procedure has not found many adherents.

Trabeculotomy

Indications

The major indication for trabeculotomy is infantile glaucoma, in which a cloudy cornea prevents an adequate view of the anterior chamber angle, thereby making goniotomy an unsatisfactory procedure. Trabeculotomy has also been used for primary open-angle glaucoma, but trabeculectomy is the preferred procedure in this condition. Other indications include secondary open-angle glaucomas, especially open-angle glaucoma associated with uveitis. In this condition trabeculotomy may be the procedure of choice.

Anesthesia

There are no special considerations regarding anesthesia for a trabeculotomy. Either a local or a general anesthetic may be used, depending on the requirements of the patient and the surgeon (see p. 224).

Preoperative Preparation

The same principles apply to the preparation of the patient for trabeculotomy as apply generally to other glaucoma procedures (p. 226).

Operative Technique

A superior rectus muscle bridle suture is placed. A paracentesis is performed, leaving a track that will allow injection into the anterior chamber.

If the pupil is dilated, it may be constricted

at this point by withdrawal of approximately 0.10 ml of aqueous from the anterior chamber by way of the paracentesis track (Fig. 11–95) and injection of acetylcholine 1% into the anterior chamber.

A limbus-based flap is raised superiorly (see p. 262). A 3 × 3 mm scleral flap is developed at the 12 o'clock position (Fig. 11–124A). The technique is similar to that used in performing trabeculectomy, although here the flap may be slightly thicker (see Figs. 11–85 to 11–87). The flap for trabeculotomy should be at least one-half as thick as the sclera; two-thirds thickness

is preferable. The surgeon notes carefully the zone of transition from opaque sclera to clear cornea. An incision is made starting 1 mm anterior to the center of the zone of transition and extending 1 mm posterior (Fig. 11–124B). Magnification must be adequate to visualize Schlemm's canal; this requires a minimum of 8× magnification and is most easily accomplished with a magnification of around 15×.

The incision into the bed of the flap is made tenderly, with the tissue being spread aside after each gentle cut so that Schlemm's canal can be searched for in the base of the incision.

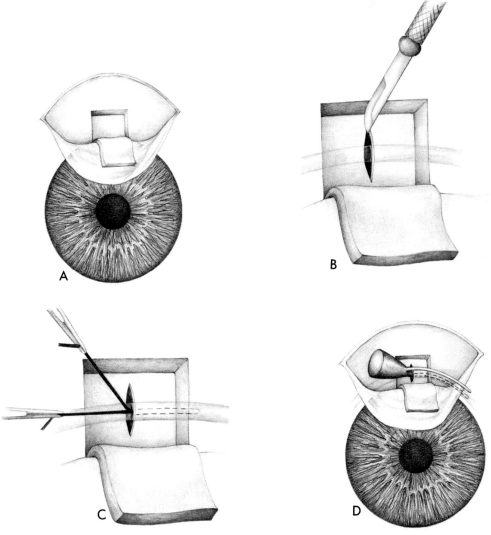

FIGURE 11–124. Trabeculotomy. *A,* After development of a limbus-based conjunctival flap, a small scleral flap approximately two-thirds the thickness of the sclera is made. *B,* The underlying sclera is cautiously incised, with care taken to watch for leakage of aqueous and search for Schlemm's canal. *C,* A suture is threaded into Schlemm's canal and its position is verified. *D,* The McPherson trabeculotome is gently threaded into Schlemm's canal.

When the outer wall of Schlemm's canal has been incised there may be a slight leakage of aqueous; this should be watched for, as it is a sign that the incision should not be deepened. This portion of the procedure should be carried out meticulously; penetration through the inner wall of Schlemm's canal will make completion of the trabeculotomy difficult or impossible.

After Schlemm's canal has been identified, a dark-colored 5–0 nylon suture is gently threaded into its cut edge. This firm suture should slide quite easily into the canal. After it has been introduced 1 cm the surgeon bends the extruding end of the suture posteriorly 45 to 90 degrees (Fig. 11–124C). This end is then released. If the suture has penetrated through the trabecular meshwork into the anterior chamber, the internal end, presumed to be in Schlemm's canal, will move anteriorly further into the anterior chamber, and the extruding end will not spring back when released. If the external end returns back to its former straight

position parallel with Schlemm's canal, it is a good sign that the suture is either in Schlemm's canal or in a manufactured canal in the sclera. In the latter case it is unlikely that the suture would have been introduced without considerable pressure. Proper placement of the suture can be confirmed by gonioscopy; this is neither simple nor necessary, however.

Once Schlemm's canal has been identified, a blunt-tipped trabeculotome is gently threaded into it. McPherson's modification of Harms' probe is a superior instrument for use in this procedure and facilitates proper performance (Fig. 11–124D). It has two probes, the distal one being the one introduced into Schlemm's canal and the proximal one serving as a visible guide, so that the position of the invisible probe is precisely known to the surgeon. There are both a left probe and a right probe, the curvature being similar to the curve of the limbus (Fig. 11–124D).

The probe is introduced into Schlemm's canal

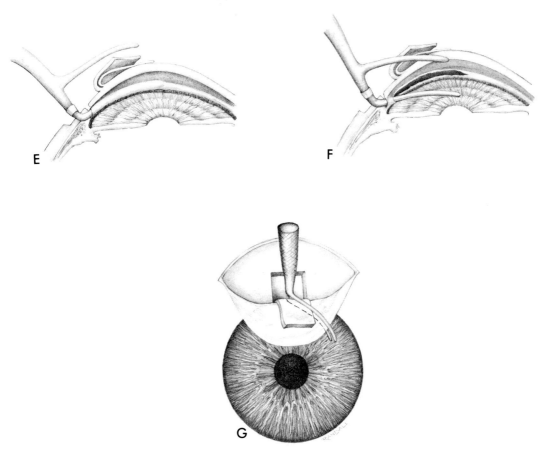

FIGURE 11–124 *Continued E,* Gonioscopic view showing trabeculotome in proper position. *F,* The plane of the trabeculotome must be parallel to the iris; the handle is rotated so that the tip is torn through the trabeculum into the anterior chamber. *G,* After the tip has entered the anterior chamber the trabeculotome is withdrawn and the chamber reformed.

for a distance of approximately 1 cm (Fig. 11–124E). It should meet with mild resistance. If one has to press firmly, probably the probe is not in Schlemm's canal, but rather in the sclera itself. If there is absolutely no resistance, it is likely that the inner wall of Schlemm's canal has been penetrated and the probe is in the anterior chamber.

The probe is rotated between the fingers so that it forces its way through the inner wall of Schlemm's canal and the trabecular meshwork into the anterior chamber (Fig. 11–124F and G). This requires mild force. The handle should be held so that the entering probe is in a plane parallel with the iris; care must be taken to avoid tearing off Descemet's membrane or digging into iris as the probe is swept anteriorly.

The probe is withdrawn; the opposite-handed probe is introduced and swept into the anterior chamber in the same manner. If the chamber has collapsed after the first sweep, it should be re-formed to its normal depth through the paracentesis track before introducing the second probe.

To prevent leakage of aqueous, the scleral flap is sutured firmly in place with 10–0 nylon (see pp. 295–296) and the limbus-based flap is closed in two layers with 8–0 chromic collagen (see pp. 269–270).

The anterior chamber is reformed with balanced salt solution through the previously placed paracentesis track. The intraocular pressure at the conclusion of the operation should be about 25 mm Hg.

An antibiotic-steroid ointment is instilled and the eye patched.

Postoperative Care

There is no limitation of activity after surgery. As bleeding is common, the patient should be kept in a head-up position, preferably either walking or sitting (Table 11–31). Intraocular pressure should be measured daily. If it rises in the postoperative period, pilocarpine 1% is probably the drug of choice to control it. During the period of time when the pressure may be

TABLE 11–31. Complications of Trabeculotomy

COMPLICATION	FREQUENCY
Hyphema	Frequent; occasionally requires drainage
Peripheral anterior synechias	Frequent
Corneal endothelial damage	Rare
Choroidal detachment	Rare
Cataract	Rare
Scleral staphyloma	Rare

elevated owing to intraocular bleeding, carbonic anhydrase inhibitors may be used in addition. Atropine should *not* be used. After several days tropicamide (Mydriacyl) can be used to dilate the pupil to prevent posterior synechias.

The long-term management of the infant with glaucoma has been discussed earlier (p. 258).

Simultaneous Cataract and Glaucoma Surgery

Indications

The basic indications for simultaneous glaucoma and cataract surgery are uncontrolled glaucoma that requires surgery for the glaucoma in a patient who needs cataract extraction to achieve satisfactory visual function, or the need for a cataract extraction in a patient with advanced or uncontrolled glaucoma. Further indications have been noted in detail in Table 11–23. The mere coexistence of glaucoma and cataract in itself is not an indication for combining cataract extraction with a glaucoma procedure.

Anesthesia

Combined cataract–glaucoma procedures are usually best performed under general anesthesia. The procedures are long and technically demanding. All reasonable steps should be taken to avoid a positive-pressure eye; having the patient in a condition of total immobility and deep anesthesia help to achieve this goal. If general anesthesia is elected, the anesthetist should use agents that are short-lived or that can be reversed, so that the patient returns to a fully active state as quickly as possible after the procedure. Most people on whom these procedures are performed are elderly and recover better if they are up and about the day of surgery. Prevention of nausea and vomiting after the operation is important, as the eye frequently has a scleral defect intentionally made by the surgeon, and a sudden decrease in venous pressure, caused by venous pressure or a Valsalva maneuver, may predispose to an expulsive hemorrhage.

The advantages of local anesthesia are that it (a) permits complete ambulation more rapidly after surgery, (b) does not produce nausea or vomiting, and (c) allows avoidance of a general anesthetic in patients who have many general medical illnesses, including the nonspecific deteriorations of old age. However, should the surgeon elect local anesthesia, it is important to make sure that the patient's sedation is

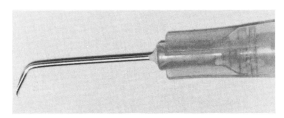

FIGURE 11–125. A bent 25-gauge needle makes an excellent hook with which to extract the nucleus atraumatically.

satisfactory. Elevations of blood pressure during the surgery predispose to expulsive hemorrhage, a complication that is especially common in patients with glaucoma who have cataract extraction. Therefore, in patients who are unduly apprehensive or in whom control of the blood pressure is a problem, general anesthesia is probably preferable to local anesthesia.

Immediately after the injection of retrobulbar anesthetic, the surgeon should, in most instances, apply firm pressure on the lids, closed over the eye, for a duration of approximately 30 seconds two or three times. This pressure serves two purposes: It helps to prevent bleeding into the retrobulbar space, and it softens the eye slightly, making the surgery safer.

If an osmotic agent has been given that will induce diuresis, it may be necessary to catheterize the patient before surgery, or to interrupt the procedure to permit the patient to void; otherwise, the bladder may become full and the patient uncomfortable, leading to a pro-

longed Valsalva maneuver and an elevation of venous and intraocular pressures.

Preoperative Care

The principles of preoperative care are the same as those used in preparation of the patient for trabeculectomy and cataract extraction.

Surgical Procedures

Combined Cataract Extraction and Trabeculectomy. A fornix-based conjunctival flap is developed. This is extended temporally and nasally 180 degrees so that it extends in a clockwise direction from 9 o'clock to 3 o'clock. Nontoothed forceps, such as a Pierse-Hoskins forceps, should be used. Some surgeons prefer a limbus-based flap for this combined cataract-glaucoma procedure. However, it is more difficult to perform and the results do not appear to be better than those obtained with a fornix-based flap (Figs. 11–126 and 11–127).

A rectangular scleral flap is outlined as if one were going to perform a standard trabeculectomy. This flap should be about 2 to 3 mm wide at the limbus and extended approximately 3 to 4 mm posterior to the limbus. A scleral flap is developed exactly as for a standard trabeculectomy. A groove, approximately one-half thickness in depth, is placed at the corneoscleral sulcus, extending a little less than 180 degrees (approximately 9:30 to 2:30 o'clock in a clockwise direction). Unless a phakoemulsification is performed, it is important not to make the

FIGURE 11–126. The conjunctival flap needs to be carried anteriorly into clear cornea 1 to 2 mm when performing a cataract extraction in conjunction with a trabeculectomy or filtering procedure.

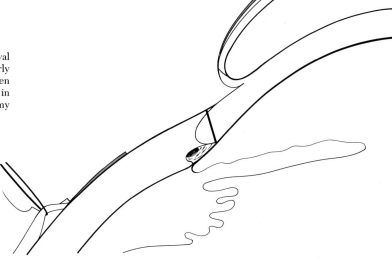

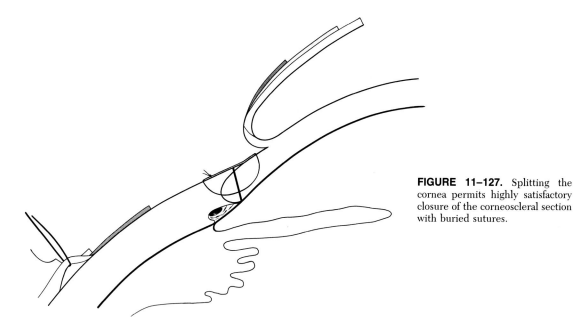

FIGURE 11–127. Splitting the cornea permits highly satisfactory closure of the corneoscleral section with buried sutures.

corneoscleral incision too small. The zonula and the capsule of patients with glaucoma are more fragile, and capsular or zonular rupture will occur at an unacceptably high rate if specific attention is not taken to avoid trauma to the capsule and zonula.

A paracentesis is made into the anterior chamber using a 25-gauge sharp needle. This should be placed approximately 5 mm anterior to the limbus in order to assure that it will not be covered by the conjunctiva after the fornix-based flap is closed at the conclusion of the procedure.

Preplaced "safety" sutures are positioned 7 mm apart, at approximately 10 and 2 o'clock. These must be placed as described earlier (see Fig. 11–72) in order to allow the sutures to be looped out of the incision so they will not be cut at the time the incision is extended. In a case at high risk for development of the suprachoroidal hemorrhage, such as the elderly, myopic patient with marked elevation of intraocular pressure (over 30 mm Hg) for many years, and with systemic hypertension, it is usually preferable to use a husky suture such as 8–0 black silk. In the patient whose only risk for developing an expulsive hemorrhage is the presence of glaucoma and the performance of a cataract extraction, it is usually satisfactory to employ 10–0 nylon as the safety suture.

Using a sharp blade such as a diamond knife or a #75 Beaver blade, a radial incision is made at the base of the scleral flap, extending from the anteriormost extent of the trabeculectomy flap back to the location of Schlemm's canal. As with a standard trabeculectomy, the block of tissue to be excised should comprise cornea with or without posterior trabecular meshwork, but should not include sclera.

An anterior capsulotomy is carefully performed by the surgeon's procedure of choice, being aware, however, that it must be modified so as to traumatize the zonula as minimally as possible.

If the pupil cannot be adequately dilated to perform a capsulotomy, a sector iridectomy is developed superiorly. A viscoelastic material such as sodium hyaluronate is placed under the iris anterior to the lens in order to lift the iris from the lens surface, permitting the capsulotomy to be performed with minimal trauma to the posterior surface of the iris. It may be helpful, in addition, to perform a sphincterotomy at the 4 and 6 o'clock positions in those eyes in which pilocarpine has been used for many years, when the pupil cannot be dilated.

A sharp corneoscleral scissors is placed into the radial incision at 12 o'clock and pulled posteriorly, and the corneoscleral incision made in a position that will constitute the posterior edge of the block to be removed later. This incision is continued approximately 90 degrees, being careful not to cut the previously placed safety suture. The corneoscleral scissors cutting in the other direction is then placed and the incision extended approximately 90 degrees in the opposite direction.

I prefer to perform the capsulotomy using a bent 25-gauge needle. This same needle is then bent again (Fig. 11–125), to produce a modified lens hook. The assistant elevates the cornea at 12 o'clock. Using a blunt lens loop, the surgeon gently retracts the iris and places the lens loop between the iris and the posterior surface of the lens nucleus. It may not be possible to accomplish this completely, in which case the lens loop is merely used to very gently depress the iris at the 12 o'clock position. The surgeon's other hand, holding an instrument such as a curved Pierse-Hoskins forceps, very gently depresses the sclera at the 6 o'clock position of the eye. The purpose of this pressure is not to express the lens nucleus; the goal is to tilt the lens nucleus slightly so that the superior pole comes into view. The lens hook is then used to hook onto the lens nucleus and the nucleus is gently rotated out of the eye. When the nucleus is fairly firm, the hook can actually hold onto the nucleus and the nucleus can be pulled out. When the nucleus is softer, it is necessary to rotate the nucleus frequently until it comes totally into the anterior chamber, where it can be easily lifted out with the hook. It is important to stress that at no time is the type of pressure ordinarily used in performing a lens expression in an extracapsular cataract extraction used.

After expression of the lens the safety sutures are rapidly secured. Additional sutures, 10–0 nylon, are placed to develop a relatively tight anterior chamber, permitting irrigation and aspiration of the remaining cortex in a highly controlled and gentle way.

A viscoelastic substance is placed into the eye and a posterior chamber lens implanted into the bag under careful direct visualization. Even in patients with the exfoliation syndrome it is probably preferable to place the posterior chamber lens into the bag.

Before removal of the sodium hyaluronate, the trabeculectomy block is excised at the 12 o'clock position. This is really more of a keratectomy than a trabeculectomy. The standard technique for excision of the corneal block is used.

The viscoelastic material is then removed completely with an irrigation-aspiration tip. Acetylcholine is injected into the anterior chamber. It is often helpful to place a small air bubble in the anterior chamber as well. After the pupil has become miotic a peripheral iridectomy is performed under the area of the keratectomy.

The corneoscleral incision is closed in a standard manner with interrupted 10–0 nylon sutures. The scleral flap is closed with one suture placed obliquely at each corner and one suture at the middle of the posterior edge.

Balanced salt solution is injected through the previously placed paracentesis track to test the patency of the incision and the amount of filtration that will occur through the cut edges of the scleral flap. If the pressure cannot be raised or the chamber adequately reformed, then additional sutures must be placed in the scleral flap in order to accomplish this. If the pressure becomes too high and adequate filtration is not present, cautery should be placed on one or both of the radial edges to encourage adequate filtration. The principle is the same as for standard trabeculectomy.

When the surgeon is assured that adequate filtration is present, the next step is closure of the conjunctival flap. The corneal epithelium between 3 and 9 o'clock superiorly should have been removed earlier in the procedure. If this was not done, the epithelium is removed at this point. The conjunctival flap will adhere more firmly to the cornea if the epithelium is not present.

The conjunctiva is sutured to the cornea 1 mm anterior to the anterior extent of the radial incisions in the sclera, using 10–0 nylon. The conjunctiva is tightly sutured to the cornea at this point. With a nontoothed forceps the cut edge of conjunctiva at 10 o'clock is pulled toward the 9 o'clock position and sutured into the cornea, putting the conjunctiva on extremely firm stretch, sufficiently tightly that the cornea is slightly indented owing to the taughtness of the tissue. There is usually some laxness of the remaining cut edge of the conjunctiva that requires placing one or two more sutures to close the conjunctiva over the sclera. A similar procedure is repeated at the opposite side. Usually five to seven sutures are necessary to firmly close the conjunctival flap.

Balanced salt solution is injected through the previously placed paracentesis, and a high bleb should develop. The cut edges of the conjunctiva are checked to determine if there is any leakage of saline. Usually when the conjunctiva has been pulled taughtly against the cornea, no leakage is present. A small amount of leakage at the more peripheral portion overlying the sclera is permissible, but it is to be avoided if possible. Additional sutures may need to be placed. There should be no buttonholes or leak through the conjunctiva itself.

An injection of betamethasone and an antibiotic such as gentamicin is given inferiorly deep in the cul-de-sac. This should be placed so that the material does not dissect up under the conjunctiva into the area of the filtering bleb. Were the antibiotic to reach into the area of the filtration, it may predispose to scarring, and were it to enter into the anterior chamber, it could cause intraocular damage.

The anterior chamber should resume normal depth and the intraocular pressure should rise to around 15 to 30 mm Hg. When the injection of balanced salt solution through the paracentesis track is stopped, the pressure should spontaneously fall to around 15 mm Hg.

POSTOPERATIVE CARE. Routine postoperative care consists of a fairly vigorous topical steroid medication such as prednisolone acetate 1% hourly and a topical antibiotic four times daily. The corticosteroids can be tapered rapidly, depending on the amount of postoperative inflammation. If the pupil is excessively miotic, atropine or a short-acting cycloplegic may be used. One does not want to dilate the pupil excessively, but one does not want the pupil to become bound down in a miotic state. If the intraocular pressure is elevated in the early postoperative period and there does not appear to be a satisfactory bleb, it is usually appropriate to release one of the sutures in the scleral flap. One corner is released using the argon laser. A Hoskins lens is helpful in this regard. A Zeiss four-mirror gonioscopic lens can also be used. If filtration does not occur when one corner suture is released, the other corner suture may also be released. Release of all three sutures is seldom necessary and is usually to be avoided. In some cases where more than three sutures have been placed, it is preferable to release one of the 10–0 nylon sutures placed in the radial aspect of the scleral flap first. At the time of surgery the surgeon should note which suture he plans to release first in the postoperative period if the pressure is excessively high.

The continuing postoperative care is a combination of the care appropriate for procedures to produce filtration and the normal care for an extracapsular cataract extraction.

Combined Cataract Extraction and Cyclodialysis*

INDICATIONS. The indications for a particular procedure in a patient with glaucoma and cataract have already been discussed (pp. 260 and 262). The combination of cyclodialysis and cataract extraction is especially appropriate in patients for whom maximum visual acuity is desirable postoperatively. It is not a preferred

*Adapted from references 91 and 92.

procedure for patients in whom long-term use of a strong miotic is undesirable.

ANESTHESIA. Anesthesia for this procedure is the same as that for combined cataract extraction–trabeculectomy (p. 314).

PREOPERATIVE CARE. Preoperative care is the same as that for cataract extraction–trabeculectomy, with the exception that it is not necessary to stop long-acting cholinesterase inhibitors before surgery.

SURGICAL TECHNIQUE. A fornix-based flap is developed from the 9 o'clock position clockwise to 3 o'clock. This is extended superiorly and temporally so that the sclera is exposed for a distance of 6 mm posterior to the limbus. A corneoscleral groove is made approximately half the depth of the tissue at the corneoscleral sulcus from 9 o'clock to 3 o'clock. Preplaced corneoscleral sutures may be used to ensure an optimum visual result. A paracentesis opening into the anterior chamber is made.

A standard cyclodialysis is performed supratemporally. Immediately after completion of the cyclodialysis the anterior chamber is filled with balanced salt solution so that the intraocular pressure is brought up to around 25 mm Hg. The scleral incision through which the cyclodialysis was performed is closed.

A standard cataract extraction is then performed, the only exception being that the iridectomy is done superonasally away from the area of the cyclodialysis, and that a long-acting cholinesterase inhibitor is instilled at the conclusion of the operation; I prefer echothiophate, 0.125% in blue-eyed patients and 0.25% in brown-eyed patients. Atropine is not used.

POSTOPERATIVE CARE. Postoperative care is similar to that after cataract extraction or cyclodialysis. Anti-inflammatory therapy should be used vigorously. Cycloplegic agents should *not* be used, but strong miotics are essential. If the anterior chamber becomes shallow owing to the development of a pupillary block associated with the use of the miotic, it may be necessary to stop the miotic temporarily and use phenylephrine 10% in order to dilate the pupil as adequately as possible. Phenylephrine will not compromise the result of the surgery, whereas a cycloplegic agent probably would; therefore, the latter should be avoided if possible. An osmotic agent may also be given to shrink the vitreous. Because of the need to use miotics in the postoperative period, it is important to perform an adequate iridectomy (or iridectomies) at the time of surgery. If the pupillary block persists and is demonstrated with fluorescein, use of the laser to perform a postoperative iridectomy may be helpful. If these steps are still not satisfactory in resolving the problem, cyloplegic agents may need to be used.

Most patients in whom a combined cataract extraction–cyclodialysis is performed will have more irritable eyes than is the rule for an ordinary cataract extraction by itself. Topical corticosteroids may need to be used for a longer period than is customary with simple cataract extraction. The strong miotic probably should be continued indefinitely.

Other Methods of Combined Cataract Extraction with Glaucoma Surgery. Several other methods of combining glaucoma surgery with cataract extraction have been suggested.[93–97] They offer few advantages, however, and the two techniques described in this chapter are suitable for almost all cases.

Cataract Extraction After Previous Glaucoma Surgery. There are definite theoretical and practical advantages to first developing an excellent filtering bleb and then 3 to 6 months later performing a cataract extraction. If the initial filtering procedure (trabeculectomy) is performed properly and the result is good, the patient need not use glaucoma medications for several months before the cataract extraction. This results in less operative and postoperative bleeding, a lower rate of postoperative complications, including pupillary capture, and a better final visual result in many patients. However, the inconvenience and the risk of performing two separate procedures frequently militate against this approach. Few patients who want to have better acuity are eager to postpone the achievement of that for a period of 6 to 8 months, as would be required in most cases in which the trabeculectomy is performed first and the cataract extraction later. Additionally, however, around 50 per cent of patients will have partial or complete failure of the filtering bleb after cataract extraction, even when the filtering bleb was working satisfactorily. Furthermore, the initial trabeculectomy must be performed in a way so that the pupil is widely dilated and that posterior synechias do not result, as these complicate the subsequent cataract extraction. To perform a trabeculectomy first and a cataract extraction later is my preferred way of proceeding in patients in whom the inconvenience and the delay are not a problem.

Theoretically, there are advantages to performing cataract extraction by an extracapsular method in an eye that has had a previous glaucoma filtering procedure. Presumably, the presence of the posterior capsule keeps the vitreous within the posterior cavity of the eye, away from the area of filtration. Most eyes that have had a glaucoma procedure are not easy ones in which to perform an extracapsular cataract extraction: the eyes are small and rigid, posterior synechias are frequently present, the iris is flaccid and atrophic, and the bleb interferes with the standard incision.

The cataract can be extracted by three routes: (1) through a corneoscleral incision superiorly (as in a usual cataract extraction), (2) through a limbal incision away from the area of the filtering bleb, or (3) through clear cornea (Fig. 11–40A–E).

1. In eyes in which there is an unsatisfactory filtering bleb, or inadequate control of intraocular pressure from the previous surgery, or a severely damaged optic nerve, I prefer the following technique. A fornix-based conjunctival flap is developed as for a standard cataract extraction–trabeculectomy. This must be done with meticulous care to avoid producing buttonholes. The previous bleb is often extremely friable and that tissue is usually excised. If filtration is present, a paracentesis should be performed before the development of the fornix flap, while the eye is still firm; when the sclera is uncovered, there will frequently be leakage of aqueous through the area of the previous filtration site, making the eye soft and complicating subsequent aspects of the surgery. When developing the fornix-based flap Tenon's capsule must be undermined extensively, usually up into the area of the superior rectus, in order to permit the conjunctival flap to be pulled down over the cornea at the conclusion of the procedure without placing the tissue on excessive stretch. If the previous trabeculectomy scleral flap was properly placed and fashioned, this is dissected free. The operation then proceeds as for a standard combined cataract extraction–trabeculectomy.

If the trabeculectomy flap is not proper, a new trabeculectomy is fashioned as close to the 12 o'clock position as possible. The scleral flap should be small (2 mm circumferentially and 3 mm radially) and thicker than usual (one-half thickness).

The surgeon may choose to extract the cataract through a round pupil, leaving the previous iridectomy unchanged, or to convert the previous iridectomy to a sector iridectomy. Removal of the lens is greatly facilitated by conversion to a sector iridectomy, and this procedure should be followed whenever there is a question. Sphincterotomies at 6 o'clock or at the 4 and 8 o'clock positions may be required to keep the iris away from the visual axis postoperatively. The less the iris is manipulated, however, the better, as it will stick to everything it contacts. Therefore, attempts should be made to protect the iris with a viscoelastic material and to traumatize it as little as possible. Maintenance of a reactive, round pupil allows better preservation of the normal anatomy of the anterior segment and better visual function, so that when possible I try to maintain a round pupil.

2. In eyes in which the previous glaucoma procedure resulted in a satisfactory control of intraocular pressure, or in which the filtering bleb is thin and cystic, the procedure of choice is extraction of the cataract through a limbal incision placed away from the filtering bleb. This is especially appropriate in eyes with relatively healthy discs, in which a postoperative rise of intraocular pressure would not be considered threatening to the health of the eye, and in eyes with large scleral defects caused by the previous glaucoma procedure. In these latter eyes the surgeon is best advised to avoid the previous filtration site, as closure of the "hole" will predispose to excessive astigmatism and failure to close the "hole" will predispose to excessive filtration and its unfortunate consequences.

The corneoscleral incision can be placed temporally, inferotemporally, or inferiorly. The technique used is that of a standard cataract extraction using a peritomy. A new iridectomy should not be performed. If the pupil cannot be dilated, the previous iridectomy superiorly may need to be converted to a sector iridectomy to facilitate removal of the nucleus. As mentioned earlier, the lens nucleus must not be expressed but must be lifted out.

3. An alternative technique in patients fulfilling the same criteria mentioned in the procedure just described (removal of the cataract from the temporal, inferotemporal, or inferior root) is to remove the cataract by placing an incision in clear cornea anterior to the filtering bleb. This incision is then enclosed with 10–0 nylon. This procedure results in a quiet eye and is technically the easiest of the three methods. The amount of astigmatism postoperatively is usually higher than with the other techniques, and because of the slow healing of the cornea, the 10–0 sutures cannot usually be removed until about six months postoperatively. At that point they should be removed to prevent vascularization of the incision.

Regardless of the technique chosen, efforts should be made to preserve the health of the filtering bleb by minimizing the amount of blood allowed to enter or remain in the anterior chamber. Furthermore, the eyes should not be left with viscoelastic material in the anterior chamber, as this will usually result in several days of severely elevated intraocular pressure. Moreover, the intraocular pressure should be raised to 15 to 20 mm Hg at the end of the procedure by filling the anterior chamber with balanced salt solution through the previously placed paracentesis track. The surgeon should consciously try to make sure that the previous bleb has been reinflated and is functioning. Betamethasone, 3 mg, or a similar agent, may be injected beneath Tenon's capsule at the end of the procedure to minimize inflammation, and topical steroids should be used vigorously. Lastly, the eye should not be patched for prolonged periods; probably the patch should be removed after around 4 hours to allow the blinking of the lids to produce mild intermittent pressure, helping to preserve the function of the previous filtering bleb.

A standard method of cataract extraction performed 90 to 180 degrees away from the area of a functioning filtering bleb is my procedure of choice. Around 25 to 50 per cent of blebs will fail postoperatively, regardless of the technique of cataract extraction used. A variety of techniques is shown in Figure 11–40A–E.

Cyclocryotherapy

Cyclocryotherapy causes necrosis of the secretory cells of the ciliary epithelium; this reduces inflow of aqueous humor and lowers intraocular pressure.[102–105] This destruction of tissue is also the explanation for the side effects and complications of cyclocryotherapy, as well as for its beneficial actions.

Indications

Cyclocryotherapy has played an important part in the management of patients with glaucoma in the past. However, since the advent of neodymium:YAG laser cyclophotocoagulation, cyclocryotherapy is seldom used. Where neodymium:YAG laser cyclophotocoagulation is not available, cyclocryotherapy still plays an important role in the management of patients with glaucoma.

The ideal candidate for cyclocryotherapy is an elderly patient (over 65 years of age) with an aphakic condition, advanced visual damage, previous failures with other glaucoma procedures, and poor likelihood of success with other procedures. Specific indications are the presence of neovascular glaucoma with secondary angle closure, other secondary angle-closure glaucoma, aphakic glaucomas, or inflammatory glaucomas. Cyclocryotherapy is not usually indicated in young people unless vision is seriously threatened by the glaucoma and other types of glaucoma surgery do not have a reasonable chance of succeeding.

Approximately 80 per cent of cases will have successful regulation of intraocular pressure; the incidence of serious complications is at least 5 per cent.

The presence of the crystalline lens within the eye is not an absolute contraindication to cyclocryotherapy. However, the likelihood of cataract developing is sufficiently high that I select cyclocryotherapy in phakic patients only when the likelihood of another procedure's succeeding is negligible.

In active neovascular glaucoma, cyclocryotherapy is a useful procedure when neodymium:YAG laser cyclophotocoagulation is not available.[109, 110]

When a patient wants to retain his eye despite an absolute glaucoma, cyclocryotherapy combined with a retrobulbar alcohol block may relieve pain yet preserve the globe.

Before performing a cyclocryotherapeutic procedure the surgeon should inform the patient that the procedure is a destructive one and that even when properly performed, it may result in loss of the eye in a small percentage of cases. The patient is also told that he can expect pain immediately after the procedure; this pain can vary from mild to excruciating, and is usually severe. In rare cases the pain persists for such a long time that the patient is unable to tolerate it. When this occurs, the cause is usually subchoroidal hemorrhage, which can be treated successfully. The cause for the persistent decrease in vision may be persistent uveitis, anterior chamber or vitreous hemorrhage, progressive cataract, or macular edema. Macular edema is probably rare except in cases in which excessive hypotony has developed.

Anesthesia

The conjunctiva is anesthetized with topical proparacaine 0.5% instilled several times over a period of 5 minutes. A retrobulbar block using 3 ml of a long-acting injectable anesthetic agent usually provides adequate anesthesia of the globe (see Table 5–2). In extremely apprehen-

sive patients or those likely to squeeze the lids shut tightly during the procedure, a block of the facial nerve may be helpful. General anesthesia is seldom necessary.

When the primary indication for performing cyclocryotherapy is relief of pain, retrobulbar alcohol should be used. In such circumstances 0.5 to 1.0 ml of anesthetic agent is injected first, followed by 1 ml of absolute alcohol, injected through the same needle. The alcohol should be injected slowly. The needle is then flushed with 0.25 ml of anesthetic.

Patients to be treated with retrobulbar alcohol should be warned of the potential complications (Table 11–32). When the goal of the cyclocryotherapy is to control intraocular pressure, but in addition the surgeon hopes to minimize pain in the immediate postoperative period, a reduced concentration of alcohol can be administered. In such circumstances administration of 2 ml of anesthetic agent followed by 0.5 ml of alcohol injected through the same needle will often be associated with decreased pain and will not necessarily have a deleterious effect on the postoperative vision. In patients in whom visual acuity is normal and the sole purpose of the cyclocryotherapy is to control intraocular pressure, the simultaneous use of alcohol with the retrobulbar injection is probably inadvisable.

Preoperative Treatment

Pretreatment with steroids and prostaglandin inhibitors may reduce the postoperative inflammation and rise in pressure. A potent topical steroid such as prednisolone acetate 1% may be used every hour for four doses, and aspirin, two 5-gr tablets (one 4 hours and one a half hour preoperatively), may be taken. Atropine may be given preoperatively.

The degree of pain after cyclocryotherapy may be severe. This may be associated with nausea, vomiting, or even shock. If these complications cannot be adequately managed in an outpatient setting, the patient is probably best hospitalized. The great majority of patients treated on the Glaucoma Service of the Wills Eye Hospital are hospitalized on the first day

TABLE 11–32. Complications of Retrobulbar Block with Absolute Alcohol

Pain
Swelling
Persistent anesthesia of periorbital region
Ptosis
Strabismus owing to extraocular muscle palsy
Failure to relieve pain

of treatment and are usually discharged from the hospital 2 days later. Cyclocryotherapy need not be performed in the operating room.

Surgical Technique

The use of a speculum to separate the lids facilitates the procedure slightly but is not essential.

Cryotherapy instruments are clearly not identical; even those designed to have a tip capable of reaching temperatures as low as $-70°$ or $-80°$ C have some variance. The size of the tip, the shape of the probe, the rapidity with which the cold temperature is achieved, the absolute level of temperature reached, and the rate of thaw all vary from instrument to instrument, and each of these factors influences the nature of the damage caused to the eye by the freezing. In the Glaucoma Service of the Wills Eye Hospital equal success has not been obtained with all instruments. The following technique refers to the portable Kryo-Med, manufactured by Cryomedics Inc. Other machines undoubtedly can be used with equal success. However, the program outlined here applies to the Kryo-Med instrument.

The valve is adjusted so that the pressure of nitrous oxide is 600 pounds per square inch. This results in a temperature of $-80°$ C at the tip of the probe. The machine is tested before giving the retrobulbar anesthetic block. After adequate anesthesia has been achieved the probe is applied to the conjunctiva 3 mm posterior to the limbus at the 12 o'clock position on the globe. The foot pedal is pressed to activate the freezing. The development of the iceball is watched. After approximately 45 seconds the first iceball will reach its maximum size. The probe is pushed moderately firmly against the globe so that the entire globe is depressed several millimeters into the orbit.

After the iceball has reached its maximum size, or starts to reach into the edge of the cornea the freezing is stopped. If the probe has been placed too close to the cornea, so that it appears that a larger iceball can be achieved, but only by having the iceball extend into the cornea further, then the freezing should be stopped and the probe placed more posteriorly, further away from the limbus. The freezing is then reactivated. After the iceball has reached its maximum, freezing is continued for an additional 15 seconds. The total freezing time, then, is usually between 45 seconds and 1 minute.

Eight applications are made. The initial site of application is at the 12 o'clock position. The second application is at 3 o'clock, the third application at 6 o'clock, the fourth at 9 o'clock, the fifth at 1:30, the sixth at 4:30, the seventh at 7:30, and the eighth and final application at the 10:30 position. The duration of freezing is approximately the same for each application. However, as subsequent applications are made, the rapidity with which the iceball is produced appears to increase. Consequently the last several applications may require less time than the first few.

The iceball that develops from the technique described is usually large enough to freeze almost the entire circumference of the globe posterior to the limbus. An area of approximately 2 mm between each application site will not be involved.

It is not usually necessary to irrigate the tip of the probe in order to hasten warming and permit more rapid removal of the probe from the globe. However, one must be certain that the probe is not adherent to the globe before it is pulled away.

Immediately after the freezing treatment the intraocular pressure of the globe should be determined, as a precipitous increase is not infrequent. If the intraocular pressure has increased to a level suggesting that the optic nerve will be damaged, immediate steps to lower the pressure need to be instituted. Intravenous acetazolamide, so helpful in patients with acute-angle glaucoma, is seldom adequate in these cases, and intraveneous mannitol or another osmotic agent in appropriate doses usually needs to be administered immediately. An even more rapidly effective technique is to perform a paracentesis. The effect of this is usually only temporary, but it relieves the urgent problem. Even if the intraocular pressure is not in a range suggesting that further optic nerve damage will occur, osmotic agents should almost always be given as a routine part of the postoperative care of patients with cyclocryotherapy.

Postoperative Care

The three major complications after cyclocryotherapy are pain, transient elevation of intraocular pressure, and late but persistent hypotony. The pain can be excruciating. Some patients have stated that the discomfort caused by cyclocryotherapy exceeds that associated with childbirth or the passage of a renal stone. Other patients have remarkably less pain. Pretreatment with steroids and aspirin appears to decrease the postoperative reaction, including the amount of discomfort. Aspirin, two tablets every 4 hours, is prescribed as a standing order.

For patients who suffer from gastrointestinal distress caused by aspirin, the buffered product may be used. A more potent analgesic such as propoxyphene (Darvon) every 4 hours is often required. Some patients may require a narcotic agent. The pain first becomes noticeable as the retrobulbar anesthesia wears off approximately 8 to 12 hours after the procedure. If a short-acting anesthetic agent is used, the pain will reach its peak about 6 hours postoperatively. It is for this reason that the long-acting agents bupivacaine and etidocaine are so strongly preferred (Table 5–2). By 18 hours postoperatively the pain usually starts to wane. In most cases the discomfort is mild 24 hours after the freezing, unless a complication has occurred. In about a fourth of the cases some pain will persist for up to 1 week in variable and unpredictable amounts. A dull ache may last for months. Most patients will have no significant persisting discomfort. Aspirin is usually continued for approximately 1 week, both for reduction of the inflammatory response caused by the freezing and for relief of pain.

In rare cases the pain caused by a cryotherapeutic procedure may be excruciating, and may continue to be intolerable. It is a mistake to assume that this severe discomfort is necessarily related to elevation of intraocular pressure. Rather, it is usually a sign of a suprachoroidal hemorrhage, which is apparently a response to the tissue destruction. Ultrasound examination should be performed to verify this. Drainage of the hemorrhage usually results in immediate relief of the severe pain, though a moderate ache usually persists (see pp. 343–346 for technique of posterior sclerotomy). When hemorrhage is suspected and pain persists the drainage should be done promptly; organization of a clot may have occurred, but even if it has, partial removal of the blood is still helpful.

Although the *intraocular pressure* may fall immediately in response to cyclocryotherapy, usually it rises several hours after the freezing. This is such a routine occurrence that a full dose of an osmotic agent such as mannitol 20%, 7 mm/kg body weight, is ordered routinely 1½ hours after performance of the cyclocryotherapy. The oral agents may be used, but tend to cause nausea at a time when the patient is already uncomfortable. Intraocular pressure is checked approximately 4 to 6 hours after the procedure, and osmotic agents are repeated as appropriate. In cases in which the optic nerve is already seriously damaged and the goal of the cyclocryotherapy is to preserve vision, attention

to this intraocular pressure rise must be especially vigilant.

Intraocular pressure usually remains elevated for approximately 24 hours. During this period it may also be helpful to use a carbonic anhydrase inhibitor in addition to the osmotic agent, in order to keep the intraocular pressure within a satisfactory level. The intraocular pressure should have started to fall by 36 hours after performance of the cyclocryotherapy. It often reaches its lowest point about 3 days after the procedure. This low pressure level will persist for 1 to 3 weeks before a gradual rise again occurs; the intraocular pressure stabilizes somewhere around 1 month after the cyclocryotherapy. The postoperative course and the intraocular pressure will be related to the extent of postoperative uveitis and choroidal detachment; the former is *always* present and the latter is seen in most cases,[111] and often persists for months or years.

Approximately 60 per cent of cases other than neovascular glaucoma will have a satisfactory reduction of intraocular pressure. Nevertheless, intraocular pressure must be carefully monitored during this period and appropriate medications ordered to regulate the intraocular pressure.

If intraocular pressure has not fallen by 48 hours postoperatively, it is unlikely that the response to the surgery will be adequate. Topical glaucoma medications are not usually used during the first few days, although timolol 0.5% every 12 hours may be added. After the second day, if it appears that control of intraocular pressure will not be satisfactory, osmotic agents should be stopped and the patient's pressure controlled if possible with tolerable doses of carbonic anhydrase inhibitors and topical timolol. Epinephrine hydrochloride twice daily may be added. Pilocarpine and other miotics should be avoided in the inflammatory glaucomas; even in the noninflammatory aphakic glaucomas pilocarpine usually has little beneficial effect on the intraocular pressure until the uveitic reaction produced by the freezing has abated.

If after 3 days the intraocular pressure is so high that the surgeon believes that permanent damage to the optic nerve is imminent, the cyclocryotherapy may be repeated, using four to eight applications. Preparation of the patient and postoperative care are essentially the same after a reoperation as for the first procedure.

If the intraocular pressure is not brought under control even after the second cyclocryotherapy, the situation is serious. The surgeon has few viable options. Standard filtration procedures are doomed to failure because of the extreme inflammatory response secondary to the tissue destruction. The likelihood of excessive bleeding and the certainty of failure for response to a standard cyclodialysis are so great as to contraindicate that procedure. The results of the third cyclocryotherapy are highly unpredictable, ranging from no effect on intraocular pressure to the condition of phthisis bulbi. Probably the best course is to pull out all the stops of medical therapy and try to regulate the intraocular pressure with drugs without making the patient too ill. If this is not possible, the patient is presented with the unpleasant choice of losing his vision as a result of the continued elevation of pressure, gambling with a repeat cyclocryotherapy, or, usually most appropriate, having a shunt procedure such as a Molteno implant.

Strong anti-inflammatory medications, such as atropine and prednisolone acetate, are given frequently in the immediately postoperative period and are continued in a four-times-a-day dosage for 2 to 3 weeks postoperatively. As the inflammation regresses, the dosages should be tapered. Because the inflammation persists for months, it may be necessary to continue anti-inflammatory therapy for a prolonged period. In such cases an agent less likely to cause elevation, such as fluorometholone, may be beneficial. Prednisolone acetate or fluorometholone with or without atropine may have to be continued for many months. The more inflamed the eye before the cryotherapy, the more likely it is that inflammation after the procedure will prove a problem. Systemic or periocular steroids may help in some cases.

Bleeding into the anterior chamber or the vitreous may occur. So long as the globe does not become hypotonous, this blood is usually absorbed rapidly from the anterior chamber and more gradually, but satisfactorily, from the vitreous. However, if the eye is hypotonous, this adjustment will not occur, and treatment is required. Treatment of the eye with hypotony is conservative, although anti-inflammatory compounds may need to be used for a longer period of time than when this complication has not occurred.

Total anterior segment necrosis may occur.[112] However, this is extremely rare, even in cases in which cyclocryotherapy has been applied over 360 degrees at one sitting. It is probably more common in patients in whom there is already an embarrassed circulation, such as diabetics. There is probably no effective treatment, although administration of topical corti-costeroids and antiprostaglandin inhibitors is logical therapy.

Cataract is an expected outcome of cyclocryotherapy in the phakic patient.

Hypotony is the most dreaded complication, as there is no effective treatment. Unfortunately performing "small" cryotherapies is not the solution to the problem. Inadequate treatment causes severe uveitis but inadequate decrease of inflow, with consequent elevation of pressure in some cases. We have found initial treatment of 360 degrees a satisfactory approach, with fewer complications and greater success than is achieved when treating only 180 degrees.

The success rate of cyclocryotherapy appears to be lower and the rate of complications higher in patients with neovascular glaucoma than in those with most other conditions, although literature provides disparate findings in this regard.[108-110] However, surgeon and patient alike should be aware that the success rate in these cases is probably only about 50 per cent. Nevertheless, the surgeon is encouraged to be aggressive in these cases. The health of the disc is difficult to evaluate because of the neovascularity. Blindness can occur rapidly as a result of the glaucoma, even when pressure elevation is moderate.

In summary, as with cyclodialysis, cyclocryotherapy often works either too poorly or too well. Although cyclocryotherapy does have some success, the high incidence of serious complications that develop as a result of the procedure is discouraging (Table 11–33).[113] I now almost never use cyclocryotherapy, preferring methods to develop filtration, or, when a cyclodestructive procedure is appropriate, a neodymium:YAG cyclophotocoagulation (Table 11–34). Cyclocryotherapy is included in this

TABLE 11–33. Complications of Cyclocryotherapy

1. Inflammation
2. Rise of intraocular pressure
3. Pain
   a. Secondary to uveitis
   b. Secondary to suprachoroidal hemorrhage
4. Reduced vision
   a. Secondary to uveitis
   b. Secondary to hypotony
   c. Secondary to intraocular hemorrhage
5. Intraocular bleeding
6. Cataract
7. Hypotony
   a. Secondary to excessive tissue destruction
   b. Secondary to ciliary and choroidal detachment
8. Scleral staphyloma
9. Anterior segment necrosis
10. Phthisis bulbi

TABLE 11-34. Comparison of Cyclodestructive Procedures

FACTOR	CYCLOCRYOTHERAPY	TRANSSCLERAL NEODYMIUM:YAG	THERAPEUTIC ULTRASOUND
Cost	Low	Moderate	High
Special equipment	No	Yes	Yes
Availability	Great	Good	Low
Portability of equipment	Easy	Easy	No
Experience in technique	Much	Moderate	Small
Morbidity	High	Low	Moderate
Ease of performance	Easy	Easy	Hard
Effectiveness	Good	Good	Fair
Serious complications	Frequent	Rare	Common
Postoperative inflammation			
External	Marked	Mild	Marked
Internal	Marked	Moderate	Mild

text because cyclophotocoagulation is not yet available everywhere.

Cyclophotocoagulation. This procedure is described in detail in the following section on laser surgery.

Laser Surgery

It is important for the patient and the surgeon to recall that treatment with a laser constitutes surgery. Occasionally the phrase "noninvasive" is used to describe laser surgery. This is seriously inappropriate. The laser is simply another method of altering the structure of tissue and is as invasive as a knife. Its advantage is that it is "relatively" invasive. That is, it may pass through some tissues without apparent damage on the way to affecting other tissues. Thus the eye does not need to be opened to perform a laser iridotomy. But this does not mean that the iridotomy is "noninvasive." When the surgeon is tempted to use the word noninvasive to describe laser surgery, or the patient wants to consider laser surgery in such a guise, it is prudent to recall that the same laser used to perform iridotomy is used to create atomic fusion, and a different type of laser is being prepared to blast distant missiles out of the sky.

It is essential that the observer and the instrument be exactly parfocal. This is true for all laser procedures, but especially when dealing with techniques such as Q-switched neodymium:YAG laser iridectomy, exact focus is of critical importance. Therefore, before performing laser surgery the surgeon should check the instrument to make sure that the oculars have been properly adjusted for his or her particular refractive error.

Laser Iridotomy (Iridectomy)

Iridotomy performed with a laser represents a major advance in ophthalmic surgery. The procedure is not, however, without complications (Table 11-35). Because of the relative ease with which laser iridotomy can be performed, there is a great temptation to overuse the procedure or to use it inappropriately. As with any surgical procedure—and laser iridotomy is surgery—the best results are obtained when performed most correctly in the most appropriate patients (Table 11-36). The indication for laser iridotomy is not merely a narrow angle. Properly performed, laser iridotomy is a remarkably safe and effective operation.

Several types of lasers are suitable for performing laser iridotomy (iridectomy).[114-121] There is no one type of laser light, however, to suit every case. For example, although the blue-green color of the argon laser is well absorbed by the dark or light brown iris, it is not the optimal color for the blue iris. Specific indications exist for specific types of iridotomy (Table

TABLE 11-35. Complications of Laser Iridotomy

Transient reduced visual acuity
Bleeding (nd:YAG)
Transient elevation of intraocular pressure
Transient corneal burns (argon)*
Inflammatory response (iritis)
Isolated permanent lens opacities (argon)*
Pigment dispersion
Late rise of intraocular pressure
Progressive cataract
Pain
Persistent corectopia (argon)
Cosmetic blemish (argon)
Closure of iridotomy†
Peripheral anterior synechias‡
Monocular diplopia‡
Retinal burns‡

*The complications are frequent with the argon laser but should not occur with nd:YAG iridotomy.
†Closure of the iridotomy is rare in properly selected cases using the nd:YAG laser. It is far more frequent (perhaps 40%) with the argon laser, especially when the eye is inflamed.
‡The complications usually denote a failure of technique; they generally are avoidable.

TABLE 11–36. Factors That Affect Success of Laser Iridotomy

FACTOR	FAVORS SUCCESS	LIMITS SUCCESS
Skill of surgeon	Great	Poor
Experience of surgeon	Great	Little
Inflammatory reaction in anterior chamber	Absent	Marked
Clarity of cornea	Clear	Hazy
Depth of anterior chamber	Deep	Shallow
Color of iris	Light brown	Light blue or very dark brown (with argon laser)
Presence of iris crypt	Yes	No
Thickness of iris	Thin	Thick
Race of patient	White	Black
Instrumental capability	Good	Poor

11–37). Regardless of the type of laser used, excellent visualization is necessary and requires a slit lamp. The delivery system from the laser source must permit sharp focusing of the beam; the more precise, the better. The focus must be accurate in all three dimensions. Thus both the position of the beam on the surface of the iris and the sharpness of focus of the beam at the correct depth of the iris are essential. With proper patient selection, correct use of the appropriate instrument, and proper preoperative and postoperative care, results are excellent (Table 11–38).

Preoperative Preparation. The pupil should be miotic. This is important. The cornea must be clear and the chamber sufficiently deep that the iridectomy can be performed without damaging the cornea. Anesthesia is produced by instilling a topical agent such as proparacaine several minutes before performing the laser iridotomy. Informed consent is obtained.

Operative Technique. The patient and the surgeon should be comfortably seated at the slit lamp used to deliver the laser beam. A contact lens is highly preferable; for the nd:YAG it is essential. The CGI 1.4 lens developed by Lasag is ideal for performing nd:YAG iridotomy. When using an argon laser the contact lens developed by Abraham specifically for laser

TABLE 11–37. Preferred Method of Performing iridotomy

Routine case	Nd:YAG
Pseudophakic pupillary block	Nd:YAG
Bleeding disorder	Argon
High hyperopia	Argon or nd:YAG
History of "malignant" glaucoma	Argon or nd:YAG
Cloudy cornea	Incisional
Definitive permanent iridectomy	Incisional
Chronic uveitis	Incisional

From Spaeth, G. L., and Katz, L. J., Current Therapy in Ophthalmic Surgery. Philadelphia, B. C. Decker Inc., 1989, p. 162.

iridotomy is preferred. The laser controls are adjusted, with the surgeon making certain that the activating switch is still in the "safe" position, that is, in a position in which the aiming beam is on but the full power of the laser itself cannot be activated.

NEODYMIUM:YAG LASER IRIDOTOMY. The surgeon must be familiar with the Q-switched neodymium:YAG laser system being used. The settings will vary, depending on the instrument used. With the Lasag instrument I prefer 6 millijoules with a run of three bursts. If the patient has difficulty fixating, the surgeon may prefer to use more power with a run of only one burst.

A contact lens is placed on the eye. The greater the power the better, so that the cone angle will be as great as possible. Because of the power of the instrument, a special lens may

TABLE 11–38. Postoperative Problems Associated with Iridotomy

PROBLEM	PREVENTION
Posterior synechias	Cycloplegics and steroids
Acute rise in intraocular pressure	Topical beta blocker therapy, oral or intravenous therapy with hyperosmotic drugs as needed; preoperative topical use of beta blockers and methazolamide, 50 mg orally, is often adequate
Cataract	Proper surgical technique
Continuing iritis	Proper case selection and steroids
Closure of iridectomy	Proper selection of method of performing iridectomy
Ghost image	Always performing iridectomy superiorly so as to be under upper lid
Retrobulbar hemorrhage	Avoid retrobulbar block; it is unnecessary even with incisional iridectomy

From Spaeth, G. L., and Katz, L. J., Current Therapy in Ophthalmic Surgery. Philadelphia, B. C. Decker Inc., 1989, p. 162.

be necessary, such as the CGI 1.4 lens used with the Lasag instrument.

Proper focus is absolutely essential. The aiming beam is focused so that it is exactly on the anterior surface of the iris. The neodymium:YAG laser beam is not retrofused, so that it will strike in exactly the same position as the aiming beam. This is such an essential aspect that the Q-switched neodymium:YAG laser must be properly aligned and properly calibrated. It is essential to check this periodically to be sure that the aiming beam and the power beam are exactly coincidental.

The contact lens should give a good view of the iris. The head must be in the proper position to permit visualization of the iris at the 12 o'clock position. The surgeon seeks a peripheral iris crypt, and the aiming beam is then focused in the depth of the crypt. The selection of the position for the iridotomy should be as peripheral as possible, so that the iris treated will be peripheral to the lens, minimizing the possibility of producing lens damage. It is best to choose a position just temporal or just nasal to the 12 o'clock position to avoid bubbles that may be produced at the time of the iridotomy, yet assuring that the iridotomy will be under the lid, to prevent later monocular diplopia. The iridotomy should be performed no further than 2 mm from the base of the iris, and preferably even more peripheral than that. Blood vessels should be avoided if possible.

The aiming beam should not be focused anterior to the iris. This will not increase the safety of the procedure, and will only result in shredding the anterior iris. The contact lens must be held so that the edge of the lens or the fingers do not obstruct the laser beam. The importance of accurate focusing cannot be overstressed.

Once everything appears to be ready, the joystick is advanced slightly so that the focus is now approximately 0.1 mm posterior to the anterior surface of the iris. That is, the most precise point of focus should be slightly in the iris stroma.

The patient is alerted that there will be a noise and a burst that he may feel, and the power is activated. If everything is proper and the focus is perfect, one application will usually result in an iridotomy of adequate size. The hole is too small to allow visualizing the anterior lens capsule through the opening of the iris. A transillumination defect, however, is not sufficient to be sure that the iridotomy is patent. The most valuable indicator of complete patency is seeing the posterior pigment epithe-

lium disrupted, and watching an immediate flow of posterior chamber aqueous humor gush through the patent iridotomy, carrying pigment with it into the anterior chamber, accompanied by immediate deepening of the peripheral portion of the anterior chamber.

If the iridotomy is not accomplished with one application of the laser beam, the surgeon may want to find another crypt close by and attempt to make an iridotomy in that crypt. It is not usually satisfactory to try to enlarge an iridotomy immediately, as the edges are shredded and further applications may only serve to develop a "sieve," rather than a discrete iridotomy. In some cases, however, if the iridotomy is not definitely patent, it can be enlarged by aiming just to the side of the previous iridotomy, avoiding the previous opening. Neodymium:YAG laser iridotomies are so likely to remain patent, even when tiny, that it is seldom necessary to enlarge the iridotomy, if indeed one is sure that the hole is completely penetrating through the iris (Fig. 11–128).

It is quite common to see bleeding immediately from the iridotomy site. This can be quite frightening because of the extreme magnification. This is usually easily controlled by pushing the contact lens firmly against the eye for 30 seconds, resulting in tamponade of the bleeding.

Postoperatively, a drop of topical corticosteroid is instilled and the intraocular pressure is measured about 1 hour later. If the surgeon expects a pressure spike, as in a patient with a combined mechanism glaucoma, the patient should have been pretreated with an osmotic agent or a carbonic anhydrase inhibitor in ad-

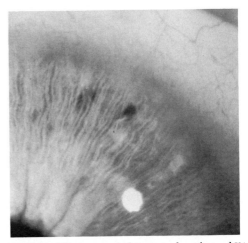

FIGURE 11–128. A patent iridotomy made with an nd:YAG laser should be placed far in the periphery of the iris.

dition to frequent instillations of pilocarpine. If no pressure rise has occurred at 1 hour, it is usually satisfactory to discharge the patient, ask him to return the next day if there is a concern regarding the health of the optic nerve, or 2 or 3 days later if this is not of concern. If the patient was taking glaucoma medications, these are continued. In addition, a topical corticosteroid is often appropriate four times daily for 1 week.

At the first postoperative visit, after it has been determined that the iridotomy is open, the pupils should be widely dilated. This not only tests the iridotomy, but also prevents posterior synechias. If the pupil is reactive and the eye completely uninflamed, it is not usually necessary to continue the dilatation. In eyes with small pupils secondary to long use of a miotic it is usually preferable to continue the dilatation with an agent such as tropicamide 1% at least once daily for 1 week or longer as appropriate.

If, after laser iridotomy, the intraocular pressure is in a range where treatment is necessary, pilocarpine should be avoided if possible, at least for the first month; pilocarpine in an eye that has had an iridotomy predisposes to posterior synechias.

ARGON LASER IRIDOTOMY. Performance of argon laser iridotomy is associated with more complications and less satisfactory results than iridotomy developed with a neodymium:YAG laser. Consequently, unless there is a specific indication for argon laser light (Table 11–37), I routinely perform all laser iridotomies using the neodymium:YAG laser. In patients who are predisposed to bleeding conditions, such as those receiving anticoagulates or with known blood-clotting disorders, the argon laser is preferable.

As laser iridotomy is frequently associated with a spike of intraocular pressure, the healthy optic nerve must be well understood before performing surgery. Intraocular pressure is determined. If the optic disc is in jeopardy, appropriate measures must be taken to monitor the intraocular pressure meticulously and medications such as pilocarpine, acetazolamide, and osmotic agents used.

The pupil should be miotic. Several drops of pilocarpine 1% or 2% should be instilled at least 1 hour before surgery.

For a brown-eyed patient, using the technique described below, appropriate settings on the argon laser would be exposure time 0.2 second, power 1000 mW, spot size 50 μm. Settings vary from instrument to instrument and must be determined by experience with the individual instrument being used. When using a pulse laser, such as the Britt, the mode is set to the pulsed or "cool" mode, the exposure time to 0.2 second, the spot size to 25 μm, and the power to 25 W (Fig. 11–129).

An appropriate site in the iris is selected, preferably a crypt just to one side of the 12 o'clock position, as near the iris root as can be visualized. The purpose of locating the iridotomy just to the side of 12 o'clock is to eliminate the presence of obstructing bubbles that form during the procedure.

The Abraham laser iridotomy contact lens is used. This contact lens has a strongly convex (high plus) lens cemented to the front in order to give higher magnification and a greater con-

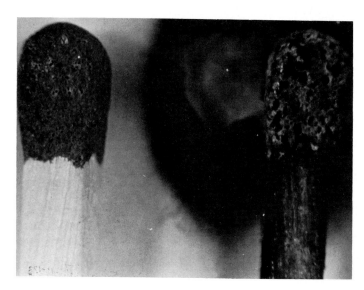

FIGURE 11–129. The pulsed laser produces such short bursts that it is able to pick away matter from the match head on the left, whereas the continuous wave laser produces more heat, causing the match on the right to become ignited. (Photograph courtesy of L. Schwattz.)

vergence angle of the argon laser beam. The previously chosen crypt is found and brought into meticulous focus.

The patient must *not* be looking toward the laser. The gaze can be either slightly up or in, or both, in order to ensure that when penetration of the iris occurs, the laser will not cause a burn on the posterior pole of the retina.

A test burn is placed in the depths of the crypt. An immediate pit in the iris surface should appear. Repeated applications are placed exactly in the same spot, deepening the pit until penetration occurs. If corneal endothelial haziness develops, the power is too high or the exposure too long.

When the laser beam actually penetrates the posterior pigment epithelium, the surgeon sees an immediate release of pigment. This pigment floats into the anterior chamber, resembling a smoke signal. Additional applications must be made to complete the destruction of the posterior pigment epithelial layer.

Complete penetration is suggested when transillumination of the iris is noted. However, a thin transparent layer may persist, giving the appearance of complete penetration when in fact this has not been achieved. Clearly the iridectomy will not be successful unless penetration is complete. Thus the surgeon should not be satisfied with transillumination, but must focus the slit lamp carefully in order to be sure that he can visualize the anterior surface of the lens or the vitreous cavity. The size of the penetration can be enlarged by chipping away at its edges until it is approximately 0.5 mm.

It may not be possible to penetrate at the first sitting. The cornea may lose its clarity, or there may be so much pigment released into the anterior chamber that the light beam is not intense enough to burn through the iris. In the latter circumstance the pigment may be allowed to settle over a period of approximately an hour, following which the laser treatment may be repeated.

With the method described, satisfactory penetration can be achieved in approximately 95 per cent of cases. Factors that influence the success rate are shown in Table 11–36. If penetration is not achieved, a repeat treatment approximately 2 weeks later will usually be successful.

In very light blue eyes, or in some other situations as well, an alternative method may be more successful. The exposure time is reduced to 0.01 second. The power may be reduced as well to around 500 mW. Two hundred to 500 applications are then placed, making

sure that they are in exactly the same position. This method of "chipping away" has the advantage of avoiding burns to the corneal endothelium.

Another method is to open the crypt by applying a "stretch" burn immediately adjacent to each side of the crypt before performing the iridotomy itself. This stretch burn is done using 500 mW, a large spot size, such as 500 μm, and a long exposure time, such as 0.5 second. The iridotomy is then performed in the depths of the crypt that has been put on stretch by the initial application; for this part of the procedure a spot size of 50 μm with an exposure time of 0.1 second is used.

Postoperative management is essentially the same as that described for neodymium:YAG laser iridotomy.

Immediately after laser iridotomy there may be a sudden marked rise in intraocular pressure. The mechanism for this does not appear to be angle closure, but rather interference with aqueous outflow owing to release of pigment and the presence of inflammatory debris. The intraocular pressure should routinely be checked about 1 hour after attempted laser iridotomy, whether or not the iridotomy is successfully completed.

Laser iridotomies may spontaneously close several months after surgery. This will usually occur only if the diameter of the penetration is less than 0.5 mm; it is most often noted in inflammatory types of glaucoma.

Potential complications of laser iridotomy are listed in Table 11–35. Of these, the two most serious are probably the late development of cataract and the late rise of intraocular pressure caused by blockage of the trabecular meshwork with debris, but experience has now demonstrated that these problems occur so seldom that they are of little real concern. As mentioned earlier, prevention of posterior synechias and relative proof of the effectiveness of the iridotomy are vital, and are accomplished by the same highly important maneuver: dilatation of the pupil.

Localized opacification of the lens under the iridotomy may occur, but there does not appear to be progression of this lens change. Several cases of late rise of intraocular pressure have been documented, but these are rare; nevertheless, the potential for a late rise in pressure after laser iridotomy should be recalled, and the intraocular pressure carefully monitored for the rest of the patient's life.

As with any other surgical procedure, the surgeon's ability to accomplish the goal of the surgery improves with experience; with increasing skill the frequency of complications also diminishes.

Argon Laser Iridoplasty

The major indication of argon laser iridoplasty is to deepen the anterior chamber periphery. When the anterior chamber angle is too shallow to permit the safe performance of a laser iridotomy, the deepening of the chamber with an iridoplasty may be helpful. Also, some angles may be deepened adequately with iridoplasty to permit a subsequent argon laser trabeculoplasty.

Iridoplasty does not cause permanent alteration in the configuration of the iris, however, and should not be used to replace iridotomy. Iridoplasty does not necessarily eliminate the possibility of angle closure, and should not be used as a substitute for iridotomy.

The basic principle of argon laser iridoplasty is to heat the peripheral portion of the iris so that the tissue shrinks, putting the iris on stretch and diminishing the peripheral anterior convexity of the iris. This lessening of the iris bowing deepens the anterior chamber. This is best accomplished with the laser in a thermal mode with a relatively low power intensity and large spot size. Suggested settings could be 200 to 500 mW, 500-μm spot size, and an exposure time of 1 second. The purpose is not to destroy tissue, but to shrink it. The beam is focused on the iris surface approximately 1 mm anterior to the insertion of the iris. As the laser burn is delivered, the iris flattens considerably. The degree of the burn should be modified depending on the response of the iris. Pigment release should be kept to a minimum. Repeated applications are administered to the iris periphery, moving slightly to one side or the other of the initial burn. It is helpful to observe the angle through a gonioprism as the applications are applied. Often the angle is so asymmetric that only one portion of the iris needs to be treated.

If inadequate flattening is achieved, an additional row of burns can be placed further from the angle root, but still well in the periphery. The distance between burns will be determined by the response of the iris to the laser, but usually one burn in each clock hour is adequate.

Complications of argon laser iridoplasty are similar to those of argon laser iridotomy (Table 11–35). Because an iridotomy is not made, the potential for development of an attack of primary angle closure is not eliminated by laser iridoplasty.

Argon Laser Trabeculoplasty

Principles of the Operation. Argon laser trabeculoplasty (ALT) is used to lower intraocular pressure in patients in whom this is required. It has the advantage of safety and the disadvantage of being only mildly effective. It is relatively simple to perform and causes minimal interference with the patient's life. However, it also lowers the intraocular pressure only mildly, and the risk of doing less than is actually required must be kept in mind.

In most instances ALT is used after medical therapy has failed, before filtration-type surgery. However, recent studies suggest that trabeculoplasty may, in certain instances, be used as primary therapy, or early in the treatment of disease after mild medical therapy has been found ineffective. The availability and effectiveness of ALT has resulted in many ophthalmologists proceeding with ALT in patients in whom medical treatment is effective but causes bothersome side effects. For example, an elderly patient with a cataract may be adequately controlled with pilocarpine but may be deeply bothered by the side effects; in such a patient an ALT may eliminate the need for pilocarpine, preserving the patient from the cataractogenic effects of filtering surgery.

The effectiveness of ALT is strongly related to the nature of the eye treated. ALT is more effective in the therapy of primary open-angle glaucoma than in any other diagnostic entity. The older the patient and the greater the pigmentation of the posterior trabecular meshwork, the more satisfactory the result. ALT is highly likely to lower the intraocular pressure in patients with the exfoliation syndrome and the pigment dispersion syndrome. It is less effective in the secondary glaucomas, especially those associated with inflammation or with structural abnormality of the angle. Indeed, ALT may produce a pressure increase in such cases. Some authors have reported success with the Sturge-Weber syndrome, but I have not found the procedure to be of value. Trabeculoplasty is of little or no use in the juvenile types of glaucoma. It is of value only in cases in which the anterior chamber is sufficiently deep and clear visualization of the posterior trabecular meshwork is possible. The anterior aspects of the eye must be sufficiently clear to permit excellent visualization of the posterior trabecular meshwork.

ALT may be repeated in some cases. In cases in which it has worked well it tends to be effective a second time. It may even be repeated a third time. However, the success rate decreases and the potential for pressure rise increases with repeat procedures.

The effectiveness and the duration of effectiveness of ALT have not been established with certainty. I generally tell patients that they have about a 50 per cent chance of obtaining a clinically significant benefit from ALT, and that the procedure usually lowers the pressure for about 2 years. It tends to be less lasting in patients with the exfoliation syndrome.

It normally takes about 4 weeks for the effect of ALT to become maximally apparent. In some patients it may take a bit longer—up to 6 or even 7 weeks. After that the intraocular pressure is usually fairly stable, with a decrease in the diurnal swings of intraocular pressure. It should be assumed that the beneficial effect on intraocular pressure of ALT will gradually diminish with increasing time. Patients with the exfoliation syndrome tend to have a greater initial success, but then a more rapid escape from the pressure-lowering effect of ALT. In many patients, including some with the exfoliation syndrome, the intraocular pressure can remain stable for many years after ALT. If the pressure has fallen adequately, medications may be cautiously withdrawn, one at a time, in order to determine whether or not they continue to be necessary.

Argon laser trabeculoplasty appears to be remarkably safe (Table 11–39). It is effective in lowering intraocular pressure somewhat in most patients with primary open-angle glaucoma. However, it is unusual that the intraocular pressure is lowered to the extent that it is possible to stop medical therapy entirely, and it is very unusual that the intraocular pressure is lowered as greatly as it is with filtration surgery. An average pressure decrease may be around 15 to 20 per cent. Patients should be instructed that they will probably need to continue medical therapy even after ALT has been performed, even when it is successful.

Patients whose intraocular pressures are initially low may have a small decrease in intraocular pressure caused by trabeculoplasty. However, this does not mean that the procedure is not indicated. Lowering intraocular pressure from 14 to 12 mm Hg may in some patients be sufficient to permit stabilization of visual field loss and may eliminate the need for filtering surgery, which in such cases might have a tendency to cause "wipe-out." Thus, although of limited value, ALT is not contraindicated in patients with low intraocular pressures. Similarly, in cases of far-advanced glaucoma, whether the pressure is low or high, ALT may be especially valuable because of its ability to lower intraocular pressure without the need to open the eye, thus eliminating the possibility of "wipe-out."

The major problem with trabeculoplasty has to do with the fact that the effect on intraocular pressure is frequently less than desired. In such cases it may be tempting to follow the patient on continued medical therapy, during which time progressive visual loss develops. To avoid this problem, *it is usually advisable to set a definite pressure-lowering goal that the surgeon and the patient want to achieve.* If the intraocular pressure after ALT fails to fall to the desired level, the surgeon and the patient will, in many instances, want to go ahead directly with the standard filtration procedure, rather than wait for further visual field loss. Surgeons may want to try ALT in conditions other than primary open-angle glaucoma, but the patient should be cautioned that the procedure is less likely to be successful.

An uncommon but important problem with ALT is the occasional patient in whom a spike of intraocular pressure occurs and persists. In patients with badly damaged optic discs this can result in further damage to the optic nerve, resulting in sudden and serious visual loss. Such pressure spikes can almost always be eliminated by pretreatment with pilocarpine every 5 minutes for four doses and administration of a carbonic anhydrase inhibitor or, in select cases in which the concern is greatest, an osmotic agent.

Trabeculoplasty lowers intraocular pressure by increasing aqueous outflow. The mechanism by which ALT does this is not known. Initially, Wise postulated that ALT caused "trabecular tightening," shrinking the trabecular tissue and producing traction on the scleral spur, mimicking the effect of pilocarpine. More recently it has been suggested that the effect is mediated by an increased number of endothelial cells, stimulated to reproduce by the laser light. It is

---

TABLE 11–39. Complications of Trabeculoplasty

1. Increased intraocular pressure (immediate or delayed)
2. Undetected progression of glaucomatous damage
3. May predispose to Tenon's capsule cysts after filtration surgery
4. Iridocyclitis (minimal)
5. Hemorrhage (extremely rare)
6. Peripheral anterior synechias*

*The development of peripheral anterior synechias usually denotes burns applied to foreign angle recess and/or with too much power.

known that trabeculoplasty does not work by producing holes in the trabecular meshwork.

Preparation for Surgery. The nature of the patient's glaucoma and the need for ALT must be determined preoperatively. The angle must be examined meticulously through 360 degrees. The cornea must also be evaluated to eliminate conditions that would make it unwise to proceed with ALT or that would require modification of the technique. If an anterior membrane dystrophy is present, the likelihood of significant corneal de-epithelialization must be considered; especially gentle technique, or perhaps a soft contact lens, may be necessary in such patients. If the cornea is edematous or unclear, the trabecular meshwork may not be able to be properly visualized, and the power of the laser beam will not be adequately delivered. Marked corneal endothelial dystrophy may make ALT unwise. The aqueous humor in the anterior chamber should be clear; the presence of significant flare or cells or even of significant amounts of fluorescein can limit the effectiveness and safety of ALT.

Preoperative Routine. The patient is seated at the laser; the cornea is anesthetized with proparacaine or a similar agent. A facial nerve block is unnecessary. The instrument is prepared for use. The exposure time is 0.1 second, spot size 50 μm, and power 700 mW; the mode is set at thermal for instruments that have both a "cool" and a "thermal" mode. The slit lamp is set for high power ($25\times$). The beam of the slit lamp is placed centrally between the oculars.

The laser beam is made parfocal with the viewer's gaze. With the patient seated comfortably, the eye is anesthetized, the instrument readied, and the gonioprism placed on the eye.

Surgical Technique. The trabecular meshwork is visualized through the appropriate mirror. It is essential that all landmarks be identified with certainty. The entire angle has been examined by the surgeon preoperatively, before deciding on trabeculoplasty. At this point the landmarks are again identified and the mirror is held at the 12 o'clock position so that the 6 o'clock portion of the angle is being examined.

The laser beam is meticulously focused by reflecting it from the mirror at 12 o'clock into the angle at 6 o'clock. The prism should be held so that the reflections from the viewing light shine directly back into the surgeon's eyes. This technique is entirely different from that used in standard gonioscopy. However, if the laser beam hits the mirror at an angle, as is the usual procedure with standard gonioscopy, it will be

reflected in an oval shape onto the surface of the trabecular meshwork, resulting in dissipation of energy and an inconsistent burn. Furthermore, if the energy is not perfectly focused, the power will be diffused, also resulting in inconsistent burns that are of larger size than the surgeon intends. The position of application of the burns is important. The more posterior the burn, the greater the reaction, the greater the tendency to peripheral anterior synechia formation, and the greater the likelihood of postoperative pressure rise. The more anterior the burn, the less the reaction, the less the likelihood of a pressure spike postoperatively, and the smaller the chance of producing posterior synechias. I prefer to place the burns just anterior to the pigmented portion of the posterior trabecular meshwork, so that the application is made posterior to Schwalbe's line in the area of the anterior trabecular meshwork. The application should certainly not be anterior to Schwalbe's line and should certainly not be posterior to the scleral spur.

A test burn is applied at 6 o'clock and the tissue reaction carefully observed. Sufficient power is present when a tiny, transient bubble appears. This bubble should be just faintly visible and requires constant observation with a properly focused instrument in order to be visualized. If the reaction appears too intense, the power is decreased and further test burns are applied until the appropriate response is obtained. If the reaction is inadequate, the power is increased until the appropriate reaction is obtained, or until the power reaches 1200 mW, above which the power is usually not increased. The more pigment in the angle, the less the power that is usually required.

Burns are then placed in the proper position, proceeding in a clockwise manner toward 12 o'clock, separating the burns by several degrees so that 25 equally spaced applications are made in each quadrant. The lens is turned after every two to three burns, in order to assure the clearest view and the best focus. If the lens is not frequently rotated, the applications will not be properly applied. The surgeon may elect to treat merely the right-hand 180 degrees of the angle (the patient's right) with 50 applications, or may prefer to treat 360 degrees with 100 applications. There are advantages and disadvantages to each technique.

Modifications. The position of the applications, the number of applications, and the intensity of power applied can be modified according to the surgeon's intent. According to the initial protocol of Wise and Witter, 100 burns for 360 degrees were applied in the posterior trabecular meshwork. Placing the burns more anteriorly appears to decrease the postoperative pressure spike without decreasing the effectiveness of the treatment and is recommended. Fewer burns have also been recommended, but appear to have less effect.

Surgeons will need to individualize the amount of treatment depending on the clinical characteristics of the patient under consideration and their experiences with the instrument being used.

If the anterior chamber angle is not sufficiently deep to permit a clear view of the trabecular meshwork, it may be possible to perform a trabeculoplasty by deepening the angle with an iridoplasty first (see p. 330).

Postoperative Management. Postoperatively, patients are continued on their same glaucoma therapy and, in addition, treated with a mild anti-inflammatory compound such as fluoromethalone 1% four times daily for 1 week. There is seldom a significant postoperative inflammatory response, and it is extremely rare that anti-inflammatory therapy must be continued for longer than a week. If so, a possibility of a steroid-induced glaucoma should be recalled. Other aspects of the postoperative management were discussed earlier.

Laser Pupillomydriasis

Light energy may effectively be used to enlarge the size of the pupil.[130] The continuous wave, or "thermal," mode of argon laser is especially appropriate.

Several drops of proparacaine are administered 5 minutes before the surgery. The spot size is set at 200 μm, power at 0.5 watt, exposure time at 0.2 second, and the mode at thermal in an instrument that has the ability to deliver both a continuous and a pulsed beam. A ring of burns is placed concentrically around the pupil, approximately 1 mm peripheral to the pupillary margin. As the procedure is being done, the iris tissue should contract, enlarging the pupil. A second concentric ring is placed outside the first ring. The laser burns should be adjacent to one another. The setting of the second, more peripheral, row should be 500 μm, 600 mW, and 0.2 second.

Postoperatively, the intraocular pressure must be carefully monitored. It is to be expected that there will be a temporary rise; there may even be a persisting rise in a small percentage of cases. Progressive iris atrophy will develop during the year after the laser treatment, leaving the iris discolored.

Topical corticosteroids may help to reduce the postoperative inflammation, but should not be continued for more than a week.

This procedure has not proved to be of much help to me and I rarely use it.

Cyclophotocoagulation

A substantial number of patients with glaucoma continue to get worse on medical therapy and yet do not do well with filtration surgery. One of the most attractive options currently available is neodymium:YAG laser cyclophotocoagulation. This appears to be the cyclodestructive procedure of choice. It works better and has fewer complications than is the case with therapeutic ultrasound. It works about as well, causes far less morbidity, and has fewer complications than cyclocryotherapy (see Table 11–34).

There are three methods of performing cyclophotocoagulation. The ciliary processes can be treated by direct application of laser light through the pupil or by endoscopic ablation, or the ciliary body can be treated by transscleral administration of neodymium:YAG laser light in the free-running mode. Transpupillary ablation is seldom indicated and is of limited usefulness. Endoscopic ablation requires expensive instrumentation and increases the hazard of the procedure. The treatment of choice, then, is transscleral cyclophotocoagulation.

The preparation of the patient is essentially the same as for cyclocryotherapy. The treatment requires deep anesthesia of the globe. I use a retrobulbar block with a long-acting agent. Some have reported successful ability to anesthetize the globe with topical cocaine 4%, but this has not been satisfactory in my experience.

A speculum is placed to separate the lids. The location of the ciliary body is determined by transillumination.

The laser must be taken out of the Q-switched mode and put into the free-running mode. A ruby laser has been used, but the current description refers to the Lasag neodymium:YAG laser. The power is set at around 6 joules (note, not millijoules). The dial of the retrofocus setting is placed at 9, which retrofocuses the neodymium:YAG laser beam 3.6 mm deeper than the level of focus of the aiming helium-neon beam.

Eight to ten applications are placed in each quadrant, aiming the beam so that the anterior portion of the ciliary body will be the site of the most intense focus. The helium-neon beam is carefully focused on the conjunctiva, and when the proper position is determined the

TABLE 11–40. Complications of Transscleral Neodymium:YAG Cyclophotocoagulation

COMPLICATION	FREQUENCY (%)
Flare	66–100
Iritis	52–100
Corneal edema	3–100
Air bubble in anterior chamber	38
Pain	33
Hyphema	3–29
Vitreous hemorrhage	3–13
Phthisis	0–21
Intraocular pressure spike after cyclophotocoagulation greater than 5 mm	2–9
Hypotony	5
Retinal detachment	2–7
Vitritis	2–7
Progressive cataract	3–4
Dellen	3–3
Choroidal detachment	3

Modified from Moster, M. R.: Neodymium:YAG Laser Transscleral Cyclophotocoagulation, in Spaeth, G. L., and Katz, L. J., Current Therapy in Ophthalmic Surgery. Philadelphia, B. C. Decker Inc., 1989, p. 176.

laser is activated. Eight to ten applications are placed in each quadrant, for a total of 32 to 40 applications over 360 degrees. The surgeon attempts to avoid the 3, 6, 9, and 12 o'clock positions in hopes of limiting trauma to the long ciliary arteries.

Applications may be limited to two quadrants if increased safety is the goal.

Postoperatively, the patient is given a subconjunctival injection of betamethasone, 3 mg. The intraocular pressure is measured.

The complications of neodymium:YAG laser cyclophotocoagulation (Table 11–40) are similar to those of cyclocryotherapy (Table 11–33). They are, however, much less marked and less severe.

The management of complications is similar to that described for complications of cyclocryotherapy.

COMPLICATIONS OF GLAUCOMA SURGERY

Various specific complications of glaucoma surgery have already been discussed briefly in this chapter in the subsections dealing with the individual procedures themselves. Additional, more general comment is needed. Table 11–41 provides a fairly comprehensive list of the complications that may follow glaucoma surgery. Clearly these will vary with the nature of the eye and the type of procedure performed.

A large number of glaucoma procedures are designed to make aqueous humor leave the eye more readily. The complication that occurs in all of these procedures is the flat anterior chamber.

TABLE 11–41. Complications of Glaucoma Surgery

1. Flat anterior chamber
   a. Excessive filtration
   b. Serous choroidal detachment
   c. Hemorrhagic choroidal detachment
   d. Diminished secretion of aqueous
   e. Pupillary block
   f. Malignant glaucoma
2. Intraocular bleeding
   a. Hyphema
   b. Subchoroidal hemorrhage
   c. Vitreous hemorrhage
3. Cataract
   a. Immediately postoperative
   b. Late
4. Hypotony
   a. Macular edema
   b. Pain
   c. Uveitis
   d. Choroidal detachment
   e. Decreased aqueous flow
5. Problems with conjunctival flap or bleb
   a. Immediately postoperative (leak, extrusion of Tenon's capsule, etc.)
   b. Excessively large bleb
      (1) Reduced visual acuity
      (2) Corneal dellen
      (3) Ptosis
   c. Late rupture or leak of bleb
   d. Recurrent endophthalmitis
6. Synechias (anterior or posterior)
7. Sudden rise of intraocular pressure
   a. From increased inflow
   b. From blockage of outflow channels
      (1) Filtering site
         (a) Iris
         (b) Ciliary processes
         (c) Blood
         (d) Inflammatory material
      (2) Trabecular meshwork
         (a) Blood
         (b) Inflammatory material
         (c) Ghost cells
8. "Wipe out" (sudden loss of visual acuity)
9. Corneal decompensation
   a. Secondary to flat chamber
   b. Secondary to stripping of Descemet's membrane
   c. Secondary to high intraocular pressure
10. Progressive optic nerve damage despite intraocular pressure below 10 mm Hg
11. Vitreous loss
12. Scleral staphyloma
13. Dislocation of lens
14. Retinal detachment

Flat Anterior Chamber

The term "flat anterior chamber" often suggests a precise diagnostic terminology. In actuality, however, interpretation of the phrase "flat anterior chamber" is very subjective; it may mean different things to different people.[131–133] Furthermore, the situations in which flat anterior chambers occur vary widely; a flat anterior chamber that may be relatively benign in one case may be destructive in another.

It is helpful to classify flat anterior chambers into three groups. In *type 1* there is contact between the peripheral iris and the corneal endothelium, with preservation of anterior chamber over the pupillary portion of the iris (Fig. 11–130). In *type 2* the iris touches the posterior surface of the cornea in all areas, but there is space between the anterior surface of the lens (or vitreous) and the corneal endothelium. In *type 3* the iris and cornea are in contact in all areas, and, in addition, the lens (or formed vitreous face) comes in contact with the posterior surface of the cornea. In type 1 flat anterior chambers there is usually preservation of chamber over the iris adjacent to any iridectomy that may be present, whereas in type 2 this is not usually the case, although there *is* space between the corneal endothelium and the anterior lens surface. In type 3 no chamber remains. The three types of flat anterior chambers tend to behave quite differently, and treatment, consequently, differs for each type.

Causes

There are five major causes for flat anterior chambers; these are listed in Table 11–42. These factors often operate simultaneously. Furthermore, there may be a variety of causes for any one individual factor. For example, anterior displacement of the lens-iris diaphragm has many causes. An additional complication that may prevent reformation of the anterior chamber, but that does not cause the problem itself, is adherence of the corneal endothelium to the deeper structures (iris, lens, vitreous). The determination of the responsible mechanism is based primarily on the nature of the filtering bleb, the intraocular pressure, and the depth of the anterior chamber, and how these factors change over time (Table 11–43).

Treatment of flat anterior chamber is based on an understanding of its pathogenesis. It is important to recall that the condition of the eye after surgery will be changing, and the pathogenesis for the flat anterior chamber one day

after surgery may be quite different from that on the 14th or 28th postoperative day. Examples of three possible clinical courses will illustrate the matter.

Case 1 is a 30-year-old healthy man with pigmentary glaucoma in its early stages. Treatment was a procedure designed to produce bulk flow of aqueous (such as trephination, Scheie procedure, and unsutured trabeculectomy). Intraocular pressure preoperatively was 40 mm Hg. On the first postoperative day the intraocular pressure is 6 mm Hg; there is an extremely high filtering bleb, no transconjunctival leakage of aqueous, and a type 1 flat anterior chamber. Four days later the intraocular pressure is 10 mm Hg, the bleb is still high, and the anterior chamber is formed in all areas except the periphery. One week later the pressure is 12 mm Hg and the anterior chamber is well formed everywhere.

Case 2 is the same patient with the same treatment and on the first postoperative day the same findings, with the exception that the intraocular pressure is 2 mm Hg. Three days later the appearance of the eye is essentially unchanged, although the intraocular pressure has fallen to zero. One week postoperatively the intraocular pressure continues to be zero, the bleb continues to be high, though less so than before, and the anterior chamber is a bit more shallow. Two days later the chamber shallows to within the type 2 range, so that there is now contact between the entire iris and the corneal endothelium; furthermore, the bleb is definitely lower. One week later the intraocular pressure is still zero, the anterior chamber continues to be type 2, and there is still chamber over the pupil and the iridectomy. However, filtration has apparently stopped. One week later the patient complains of sudden pain, at which time the intraocular pressure is found to be 50 mm Hg and the chamber well formed.

In the first instance described, the flatness of the anterior chamber was clearly caused by excessive filtration with too little resistance to the outflow of aqueous humor; as the Tenon's-conjunctival flap became scarred and adherent to the surrounding sclera, the resistance to outflow increased, and eventually the chamber reformed spontaneously. In the second instance the initial cause of the flat anterior chamber was also deficient resistance to outflow. This was even more marked than in the first example, as indicated by the lower intraocular pressure. Prolonged hypotony led to the development of a choroidal detachment and eventual diminution of aqueous inflow. With absence of

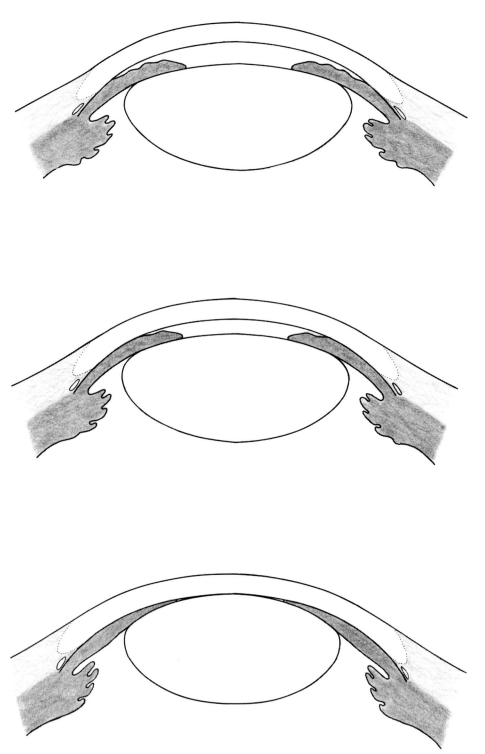

FIGURE 11–130. Not all "flat anterior chambers" are the same. In type 1 *(top)* there is contact between the peripheral iris and the corneal endothelium, but the chamber is formed centrally over the iris. In type 2 *(middle)* the iris touches the posterior surface of the cornea in all areas, even centrally. In a type 3 flat anterior chamber *(bottom)* no chamber is present anywhere.

TABLE 11–42. Causes for Shallow or Flat Anterior Chamber

CAUSE	IMPORTANT ASSOCIATED FINDINGS
1. Inadequate resistance to aqueous outflow	High bleb or positive Seidel test
2. Fluid in the suprachoroidal space	Ophthalmoscopic or ultrasound evidence of choroidal or ciliary body detachment
3. Inadequate aqueous formation	Low bleb, low intraocular pressure, and inflamed eye
4. Interference with flow of aqueous from the posterior to the anterior chamber	Adherence of the iris to lens or vitreous; positive fluorescein appearance test
5. Anterior displacement of the lens-iris diaphragm	
a. Misdirection of aqueous flow into the vitreous	High intraocular pressure; positive intravenous fluorescein appearance test
b. Ciliary body swelling	Inflamed eye; tight scleral band
c. Constriction of the ciliary body sphincter	Use of strong miotic
d. Increase in size of lens	Slit lamp evidence of increasing cataract
e. Partial or complete dislocation of lens	Phakodonesis
f. Swelling of vitreous contents	Intravitreal blood or gas (SF_6)

inflow the hypotony persisted and the bleb collapsed, allowing adhesions to develop between Tenon's capsule and the sclera. When the choroidal detachment spontaneously absorbed, aqueous production resumed, but there was no sclerostomy and, consequently, the pressure rose rapidly.

In a third variation on this case, the same patient has gone through the same clinical course up until the last point; that is, hypotony is persisting rather than disappearing spontaneously. Additional complications that can be expected to develop in the face of prolonged hypotony include continuing marked inflammation, posterior synechias that may lead to occlusion of the pupil and of the iridectomy,

decompensation of the cornea, progression to a type 3 flat chamber with contact between the lens and corneal endothelium, decompensation of the cornea, and premature development of cataract. Clearly this is an unfortunate sequence of events.

Diagnostic Features Related to Flat Anterior Chamber

Diagnostic features that help to determine the cause of the flat chamber include *the level of intraocular pressure, the nature of the filtering bleb, the patency of the pupil and iridotomy*, the nature of aqueous flow as determined by intravenous fluorescein, and the findings on diagnostic ultrasound. The change with time in

TABLE 11–43. Diagnosis of Postoperative Complications of Glaucoma Filtering Surgery

CONDITION	INTRAOCULAR PRESSURE	BLEB	ANTERIOR CHAMBER	OTHER FINDINGS
No filtration	High	None	Deep	—
Malignant glaucoma	Often high	None	Flat—II–III	Fluorescein pools behind vitreous face
Excessive filtration	Less than 10 mm Hg	High	Normal to flat	—
Inadequate aqueous production	Less than 5 mm Hg	Low and getting lower	Flat (I–III) until sclerostomy closes, then deep	Inflamed eye
Excessive filtration with developing inadequate aqueous production	Less than 5 mm Hg and falling	Low or none	Flattening	Increasingly inflamed eye
Pupillary block				
Early in association with excess filtration	5–15 mm Hg	Moderate	Flat with iris bombé	Posterior synechias
In association with inadequate aqueous production	0–10 mm Hg	None	Flat	Posterior synechias
After closure of sclerostomy	High	None	Flat	Posterior synechias
Suprachoroidal hemorrhage	5–50 mm Hg	High	Flat	Severe pain
Ciliary body detachment	0–10 mm Hg	None–high	Flat	Detachment visible

Modified from Spaeth, G. L.: Glaucoma Surgery, in Duane, T. D. (ed.): Clinical Ophthalmology, Philadelphia, J. B. Lippincott Co., 1988.

the nature of these findings is most revealing (Table 11–42).

Intraocular Pressure. If the pressure is below 5 mm Hg, there must be excessive outflow of aqueous humor or decreased formation of aqueous humor, or both. In such patients the area of the bleb should be examined. Proper surgical technique will have assured the absence of leakage in the form of buttonholes or improperly closed Tenon's-conjunctival flap. However, it is possible that an error was unrecognized, and therefore such leaks must be sought out. The conjunctival incision is inspected for wicks of extruding Tenon's capsule. A Seidel test is performed with pressure being placed on the eye at the time one is watching for leakage.

Persistent leaks almost invariably lead to the sequence of prolonged hypotony, hyposecretion, formation of adhesions, and failure of the surgery. Therefore, in cases in which such leaks are identified, serious consideration must be given to their surgical repair. If the leak is due to a dehiscence of the incision of the conjunctival flap, it is usually relatively easy to repair surgically. When it is due to a tear in the conjunctiva, repair is more difficult, especially when the tear occurs at the limbus. In patients with healthy conjunctiva a purse-string suture of 10–0 nylon with a noncutting, "vascular" needle can usually be placed without too much difficulty, and if pulled up gently and firmly often cures the problem. However, when the conjunctiva is tissue paper–thin, such an attempt may only make matters worse. This is also true when the leak is at the limbus, where it is difficult to pull the tissue together because of the unyielding cornea.

When clinical judgment suggests that the repair of the tear will be difficult, it is usually best to instill timolol and administer acetazolamide and patch the eye for 24 to 48 hours in hope that the tear will close off. Because other medications that play a role in the healing of the eye cannot be instilled in the eye during the period of time that the patch is in place, it is often appropriate to administer these subconjuctivally before applying the patch. Betamethasone, 3 mg, is given through the inferior cul-de-sac so that the conjunctiva is not ballooned up. Atropine ointment is placed in the eye, and the eye is then firmly patched with a pressure patch. The other eye can also be patched in order to immobilize the eyes more fully.

At the next dressing a Seidel test is again performed to determine the state of the leak. If the leak has stopped, the prognosis will have vastly improved. The eye is again pressure-patched for one more day, and if no leak is seen on the next day, it is probable that no conjunctival repair will be necessary.

If, on the other hand, the leak is still patent, it is probably best to try light patching for several more days, depending on the other clinical findings in the eye. Usually somewhere around the 3rd to 7th day one has to make a decision to choose one of three major options: (1) continue to watch the eye in hope that the tear will close off before the conjunctiva scars down to the sclera or the hypotony has resulted in a shut-down of aqueous flow; (2) conclude that healing is not going to take place and that salvage of a successful glaucoma procedure is a first priority and therefore repair must be attempted; or (3) give up hope of achieving a successful glaucoma operation and try to salvage the eye with minimal permanent complications, planning to perform a further glaucoma procedure in the future.

The frequency with which a choroidal detachment develops appears to be closely related to the level of intraocular pressure; the lower the pressure, the more frequent the choroidal detachment. Intraocular pressure is not the only causal factor; a choroidal detachment can occasionally develop spontaneously in an eye in which hypotony has not been documented, but it is my clinical impression that this is unusual. The success of glaucoma filtering procedures is closely related to the continuing production of aqueous humor. The aqueous appears to play three essential roles. First, it has a direct mechanical role, elevating the Tenon's-conjunctival flap from the underlying sclera and preventing adhesions between these two tissues. Second, aqueous humor flowing through the sclera appears to prevent the sclera from healing.[134] The greater the flow of aqueous, the greater the likelihood that sclerostomies will remain patent. Finally, the aqueous appears to have a flushing effect on the anterior chamber, carrying the debris of inflammation with it as it leaves the anterior chamber; the capacity of absorption of a hyphema is more rapid when aqueous secretion is not decreased. Aqueous suppressants, therefore, such as the carbonic anhydrase inhibitors and timolol, are generally contraindicated in cases in which the surgeon is attempting to achieve a development of filtration, either gross or microscopic. Because intraocular pressure is an indicator of rate of aqueous humor production, the intraocular pressure is itself a valuable prognostic indicator, especially when one considers the other indicators of aqueous inflow and outflow. If the bleb is high and the pressure around 10 mm Hg, then clearly the inflow is also high. If there is no apparent external filtration and the intraocular pressure is around 10 mm Hg, then presumably aqueous secretion must be poor or else aqueous is escaping in some way that is not immediately apparent (such as through a cyclodialysis cleft). If the intraocular pressure is 35 mm Hg and there is an iris bombé, the prognosis is probably better than in cases in which an iris bombé is found in association with an intraocular pressure of 10 mm Hg; in the former situation treatment need be directed only toward curing the pupillary block, whereas in the hypotonous eye the complication of pupillary block is compounded by that of hyposecretion.

It is not unusual for the intraocular pressure to be relatively unstable during the first 3 or 4 days after filtration surgery. An intraocular pressure that is lower on the 2nd or 3rd day than it was on the 1st postoperative day is not necessarily an unfavorable sign. The decrease in pressure may be a reflection of a lower outflow resistance in the trabecular meshwork or in the surgically created outflow channels owing to a flushing of inflammatory debris. However, when the intraocular pressure shows a progressive downward trend continuing after the 3rd or 4th postoperative day, the likelihood of hyposecretion becomes greater.

When the surgeon believes that low intraocular pressure is due to absence of aqueous production, and the bleb is seen to flatten and the chamber to remain shallow, the likelihood that reformation of the anterior chamber will need to be performed becomes great. As long as a type 1 chamber is present, reformation is usually unnecessary. However, if it progresses to a type 2, drainage of the choroidal detachment with reformation of the anterior chamber is usually required. In almost every situation in which a type 3 flat anterior chamber develops, surgical reformation is required. Type 3 flat anterior chambers rapidly predispose to corneal damage and to cataract. They constitute surgical emergencies and should be repaired as rapidly as can be reasonably achieved.

There are three major situations in which a shallow or flat anterior chamber occurs in association with high intraocular pressure. These include failure to filter in an eye with an extremely shallow anterior chamber, pupillary block glaucoma, and "malignant" glaucoma.

The intraocular pressure can be elevated after a filtering procedure simply because the resistance to outflow is not adequately eliminated by the surgical procedure. The sclerostomy may not have been made completely, or it may be so small that adjacent edges are forced together, preventing outflow. The sclerostomy can be blocked by iris or by ciliary processes. Blockage of the sclerostomy is especially likely to occur in patients in whom the anterior chamber is shallow preoperatively and the anterior segment small, as occurs with chronic angle-closure glaucoma. In an eye that has an extremely shallow chamber, the sclerostomy must be placed sufficiently anterior that the likelihood of its being blocked by iris or ciliary processes is minimized. The procedure of choice in these cases is trabeculectomy with a fairly thickly fashioned scleral flap that is sutured well in place so that the chamber is well formed at the end of the procedure. In the patient who has a high pressure postoperatively because of failure to filter, the anterior chamber should not be more shallow than it was preoperatively. Gonioscopy should reveal the cause of the problem.

Obstruction to the anterior movement of aqueous must also be considered as a possible cause for a high pressure in association with a shallow anterior chamber after glaucoma surgery. In these cases an iris bombé is usually present. However, in some patients who appear to have a rigid iris, or in whom the anterior chamber is almost totally collapsed, iris bombé is not always easy to spot. Surprisingly, the anterior chamber in most cases of pupillary block glaucoma is not completely flat, but is rather a type 1 or type 2 flat anterior chamber. Intravenous fluorescein, as described,[137] can be of considerable help in establishing an obstruction to aqueous flow. The examiner should try to determine whether the margin of the pupil is adherent 360 degrees to the anterior surface of the lens (or anterior vitreous face, or other retropupillary membrane). Furthermore, the iridectomy must be carefully inspected to see whether it is patent.

If pupillary block is present, the appropriate treatment is almost always nd:YAG laser iridotomy, unless the chamber is totally flat or the cornea hazy, in which case a surgical iridotomy is usually needed. The laser is an excellent means of performing this type of iridotomy. (The technique of laser iridotomy is discussed on p. 325.) The hole in the iris need not be large. If a laser is not available and the degree of iris bombé is marked, iris transfixation is probably the easiest way to relieve the pupillary block. This procedure eliminates the need to open the anterior chamber. The lens must be avoided in the phakic patient. Should the an terior chamber not deepen immediately after penetration of the iris, it must be assumed that the aqueous block is not at the level of the iris itself; there must be some type of retropupillary membrane blocking the passage of the aqueous humor into the anterior chamber.

Elimination of the pupillary block will not necessarily eliminate the glaucoma that has developed because of obstruction to aqueous. If there has been a significant iris bombé, or if the chamber has collapsed so that there is actual iris-cornea contact, it is extremely difficult to predict the rate at which peripheral anterior synechias will form in conjunction with an iris bombé. Pressure gonioscopy may not be successful, as the anterior chamber contains too little aqueous humor to permit displacement of the iris posteriorly and the eye is too firm to allow indentation of the cornea. Even when the chamber has been flat for as long as several weeks, cure of the pupillary block may be followed by complete deepening of the anterior chamber; the surgeon will be surprised to find no synechias present in such situations. In other cases adhesions will form within a period of hours.

The third major cause for a flat anterior chamber in association with elevated intraocular pressure after glaucoma surgery is the most uncommon and the most serious—"malignant glaucoma." Here aqueous humor is misdirected posteriorly into the vitreous cavity. Some authors have suggested that this type of glaucoma be called "ciliary block glaucoma."[135] However, a more precise diagnostic phrase would be glaucoma caused by posterior misdirection of aqueous.

The treatment for flat anterior chamber associated with high intraocular pressure owing to posterior misdirection of aqueous is combined use of topically applied atropine 1%, phenylephrine 10%, an osmotic agent in full dose, and a carbonic anhydrase inhibitor in full dose (such as acetazolamide 500 mg intravenously in an adult).[136] The atropine and phenylephrine help to pull the lens-iris diaphragm posteriorly and to break the pupillary block, the osmotic agents lower the intraocular pressure and shrink the vitreous, helping the lens-iris diaphragm return to its proper position, and the carbonic anhydrase inhibitors reduce the flow of aqueous humor that is causing the problem to start with. Many patients respond to this medical treatment, in which case the therapy can be gradually tapered, but it may be necessary to continue atropine for the remainder of the patient's life. If medical treatment is not effective, vitreous should be removed with a vitreous cutting instrument introduced through the pars plana, and the anterior chamber reformed. In rare cases the lens needs to be removed in conjunction with a vitrectomy.

Nature of the Filtering Bleb. The character of the filtering bleb provides valuable information regarding the mechanism of flat chamber. This has already been discussed (see Table 11–42) and need not be detailed further here.

Patency of the Pupil and Iridotomy. Interference with aqueous flow as a cause for flat anterior chamber has already been mentioned. The presence of an anterior convexity of the iris—the classic "iris bombé"—is an indication that pupillary block is present. However, the absence of an iris bombé does not prove that pupillary block is not present. When aqueous inflow is low, there may be pupillary block with low intraocular pressure and without iris bombé. The possibility of aqueous block must come to mind regardless of the level of intraocular pressure.

Nature of Aqueous Flow as Determined by Intravenous Fluorescein. A highly useful test to help determine the mechanism of flat anterior chamber is the fluorescein appearance test.[137]

Ultrasound. The important role that choroidal detachment assumes among postoperative complications has been stressed. Ultrasound is highly useful in evaluating the presence, extent, location, and natural history of such choroidal detachments. It also helps to distinguish between effusions and hemorrhages.

However, a large ciliary body detachment may be present and yet not be detected by ultrasound. Thus a negative ultrasound examination does not mean the absence of a choroidal detachment.

In summary, careful attention to a few attributes will usually allow correct diagnosis of the cause for a flat anterior chamber, leading to effective treatment.

The techniques for reforming the anterior chamber, performing a posterior sclerostomy, and draining a choroidal detachment are described in detail in the following section on surgical treatment.

Surgical Treatment

Reformation of the anterior chamber may be accomplished by a variety of means. The two primary methods are direct reformation with a viscoelastic substance and drainage of the choroidal detachment with reformation of the anterior chamber secondary to this.

Reformation of the Anterior Chamber with a Viscoelastic Substance. A paracentesis track (keratostomy) should have been placed at the time of the initial filtering surgery. The patient's eye is well anesthetized. The patient is seated at a slit lamp or, preferably, placed on a stretcher under an operating microscope.

A 30-gauge blunt needle (cannula) is placed on a 2-ml syringe that contains balanced salt solution. The anesthetized eye is well irrigated to lessen the number of surface contaminants. The cannula on the saline-containing syringe is cautiously introduced into the anterior chamber through the previously placed paracentesis, and saline is slowly injected. Once the surgeon is sure that the keratostomy is patent, the injection with balanced salt solution is usually stopped. Rarely the chamber deepens adequately with the saline solution alone, and no further treatment is needed. The intraocular pressure should come up to a firm level (at least 5 mm Hg, and preferably around 20 mm Hg). If this cannot be achieved with balanced salt solution, a 30-gauge blunt cannula is placed on a syringe containing a viscoelastic substance (I prefer Healon [sodium hyaluronate]). The Healon is then slowly introduced into the anterior chamber through the previously placed keratostomy. The surgeon must watch closely to be sure that the Healon does not force the iris out of the sclerostomy or cause an excessive rise of intraocular pressure. At the conclusion a small (2–5 mm) bubble of air is injected into the anterior chamber through the keratostomy. The effect of the injection of balanced salt solution and viscoelastic material into the anterior chamber on the appearance of the bleb is carefully monitored, as this gives important clues regarding the presence or absence, as well as deficiency or excess, of filtration.

In those cases in which a paracentesis was not previously made at the time of surgery, this needs to be done in order to permit reformation of the anterior chamber. This must be managed in a way that does not tear the conjunctiva, damage the bleb, or injure the internal contents of the eye, most notably the lens. As fixation of the globe may be difficult, it may be necessary to place a small, partial-thickness incision into the cornea near the limbus. An incision approximately 2 mm long and one-third thickness is usually adequate. A very sharp blade needs to be used. This groove is then used for fixation, permitting development of a keratostomy using a short, sharp 27-gauge disposable needle. This needle is placed on a small syringe, such as a tuberculin syringe, and cautiously introduced through the cornea into the anterior chamber.

The technique is similar to that described earlier for paracentesis (Figs. 11–93 to 11–95) in which the fixating hand pulls the globe back over the needle, and the plane of the needle is kept parallel to the iris. This is far more difficult in a soft eye, but it still can be accomplished. If the surgeon is having difficulty introducing the needle through the cornea, it is helpful to twist the syringe in the fingers, using a "coring" type of motion.

When balanced salt solution is injected through the paracentesis track slowly, the chamber should become deeper before the intraocular pressure rises. If the intraocular pressure rises before the chamber deepens, the balanced salt solution must be going through the plane of the iris into the vitreous, causing a "malignant glaucoma." In such circumstances the mechanism of the flat anterior chamber is probably not excessive filtration or hyposecretion, but aqueous misdirection, and efforts to correct it must be directed at that mechanism.

It is important to monitor both the depth of the anterior chamber and the pressure of the globe (with a finger) as balanced salt solution or other fluid is injected into the anterior chamber. If the chamber remains shallow and the pressure does not rise, then probably there is excessive filtration. This will be noted by a high bleb developing, unless there is a tear in the conjunctiva, permitting the injected fluid to go into the chamber and out through the sclerostomy and then out the conjunctiva. If the anterior chamber remains shallow and the pressure rises, then the most likely mechanism is aqueous misdirection, as just described. If the chamber remains shallow and the pressure rises somewhat, it may also be that the fluid is passing into the suprachoroidal space through a cyclodialysis cleft. If the anterior chamber becomes deep and the pressure becomes firm, then it is probable that the cause of the anterior chamber was hyposecretion and that there is no patent fistula; in such cases it is to be expected that as soon as the eye starts secreting aqueous once again, the pressure will rise markedly because the filtration procedure has failed. In such circumstances it may be necessary to release a suture in the trabeculectomy flap or undertake another maneuver to assure that aqueous injected into the anterior chamber will pass out through an opening in the sclera. If the anterior chamber deepens but the pressure remains soft, then one is describing what is usually the ideal situation, in which the chamber has become reformed but filtration is still present. If the chamber collapses over the next few minutes after injection of balanced salt solution has been stopped, then the surgeon knows that flattening of the anterior chamber will most likely recur owing to excessive filtration through the sclerostomy. In such situations the surgeon must decide whether to close down the sclerostomy further or inject a viscoelastic substance as mentioned earlier.

After the chamber has been adequately deepened and before the intraocular pressure is restored to normal, air may be injected into the anterior chamber. This air bubble may be pushed around inside the anterior chamber using a blunt instrument such as a muscle hook, to remove remaining anterior synechias. Air should not be placed in the anterior chamber until after the chamber has been partially deepened with saline. When air is placed into the anterior chamber it will form a bubble that causes deepening of the central chamber, but may not open the periphery. In fact, as the iris is pushed peripherally by the air and a partial pupillary block develops, the peripheral chamber may actually become more shallow. Thus air alone should not be used as the primary means of deepening the anterior chamber (Fig. 11–131).

Air should not be placed into the anterior chamber if there is a reasonable chance that it will become displaced into the posterior chamber or into the vitreous postoperatively. Should this happen, the air may actually produce exactly the opposite effect of what the surgeon desires; specifically, the air may push the iris anteriorly, helping to occlude the angle recess. The ideal intraocular pressure after reformation of the anterior chamber is usually around 15 to 20 mm Hg.

Posterior Sclerostomy. A variety of procedures involve the performance of a posterior sclerostomy. These include cyclodialysis, reformation of the flat anterior chamber, drainage of a choroidal detachment, and a posterior vitrectomy. A similar technique can be used regardless of the purpose.

The surgeon first decides how far posteriorly the sclerostomy is to be placed. Preferably the position is determined with a measuring caliper. The conjunctiva is opened by an appropriate technique to expose the area in which the scleral incision is to be made. The point on the sclera is located precisely. A ring of cautery is placed, the diameter being approximately 2 mm wider than the intended incision. The purpose of the cautery is merely to cauterize the surface vessels supplying the area to be incised; it should not be so hot that it chars or shrinks the sclera.

The sclera is well fixated and the scleral incision started. If the eye is firm, a sharply pointed knife such as a razor blade fragment should not be used; it is too likely to cut the underlying uvea as it is pushed up against the sclera by the firm intraocular pressure. A #67 Beaver blade is, in many ways, ideal. If the eye is mushy-soft, as may be the case if there is a choroidal detachment, then it may be necessary to use a sharper blade.

After the sclera has been incised through one-half to two-thirds of its thickness, a traction suture may be placed. This facilitates (1) incising through the depth of the sclera while minimizing the risk of damaging underlying tissue, (2) holding open the lips of the sclerostomy in order to aid drainage of fluid, and (3) closing rapidly should that be necessary. Any of a

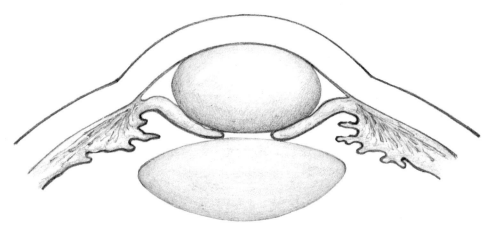

FIGURE 11–131. The anterior chamber should be deepened with saline and not with air alone. If air alone is used, the iris will be pushed peripherally and posteriorly, predisposing to pupillary block and narrowing of the peripheral angle. Some surgeons prefer a viscoelastic material such as sodium hyaluronate.

variety of suture materials can be used, but it should be recalled that it may take months for a sclera to heal. If insertion of an instrument through the sclerostomy is planned, it may be advisable to use a horizontal mattress suture with bites separated the correct distance to permit insertion of the instruments between the sutures.

The incision should not be closed so tightly with the permanent suture that it deforms the globe.

Drainage of a Choroidal Detachment. A posterior sclerostomy is performed approximately 6 mm posterior to the limbus. Choroidal detachments usually can be drained from any point on the globe, although there may be some advantage in selecting the position at which the choroidal detachment appears to be highest.

Preoperative evaluation may include ultrasound examination, which is often helpful in identifying the presence of a choroidal detachment even when it cannot be visualized ophthalmoscopically. Fluid between the uvea and the sclera may be localized to the area anterior to the equator, even as far as the ciliary body. In such cases the fluid may be difficult to visualize.

A choroidal detachment is present in virtually any eye with persistent hypotony. Even in cases in which the ultrasound examination does not reveal a choroidal detachment there is almost always enough fluid sequestered between the sclera and the choroid that it can be drained. If one is planning to reform an anterior chamber, one should almost invariably attempt to drain subchoroidal fluid. This removes space from the inside of the globe, permitting the chamber to be deepened without causing excessive rise of intraocular pressure. If the fluid is not drained, sometimes there is not enough volume in the globe to accept the amount of saline and air that is often necessary to deepen an anterior chamber adequately.

If the choroidal detachment is not localized, it may be easiest to drain the fluid inferotemporally.

After posterior sclerostomy the incision can be held apart by the traction sutures. It may take many minutes for the subchoroidal fluid to drain fairly completely. One way in which this can be helped is by injecting balanced salt solution through a paracentesis opening into the anterior chamber. If injected sufficiently slowly, this will trickle back into the posterior chamber and the vitreous cavity, flattening out the choroidal detachment and forcing the sub-

choroidal fluid out the sclerostomy opening. It is often helpful to alternate draining and injecting until the pressure within the globe is returned to a normal level—about 10 to 20 mm Hg.

After drainage of the choroidal detachment is relatively complete the anterior chamber is then reformed as described earlier.

Postoperative care after posterior sclerostomy usually consists of administration of cycloplegics and corticosteroids.

The conjunctiva is closed with a minimally irritating, fine absorbable suture, such as 8–0 chromic collagen.

Failure to Filter

If the intraocular pressure is elevated after a glaucoma filtering procedure, one must conclude that the resistance to outflow is still excessively high. Such a high intraocular pressure does not necessarily imply a surgical failure. Indeed, I much prefer to see mildly elevated intraocular pressure rather than hypotony in the immediate postoperative period. In the former case one or more sutures in the scleral flap may be released, using an argon laser. When the surgeon's goal is a relatively small lowering of intraocular pressure it is not unusual to see moderate elevation of pressure for a few days postoperatively. This is not infrequent after a trabeculectomy in which the scleral flap was sutured securely, as would be done in a patient with moderate disc damage and chronic angle-closure glaucoma. The explanation for this transient pressure rise is presumably decompensation of the trabecular meshwork owing to the trauma of the surgery; as the trabecular meshwork regains its normal function, the additional filtration effect of the trabeculectomy comes into play and the final intraocular pressure is lower than the pressure before surgery.

In other circumstances there appears to be a more frankly mechanical blockade, perhaps caused by a fibrinous clot. In some of these cases a mechanical method of increasing the flow is helpful.

Treatment

A component in aqueous humor appears to inhibit wound healing. This is probably true, but unproven assumption lies at the base of the belief that the expression of aqueous humor through a fistula will help to keep the fistula patent.

Compression. There are no studies that document the long-term value of mechanical expression of aqueous. In contrast, one study suggests that there is no long-term benefit. Furthermore, "massage" can certainly cause damage. The intraocular pressure rises to a level of around 120 mm Hg during standard massage. Incisions have been ruptured, significant hyphema has been caused, and it is likely that other damage has also been produced by compression of the globe in an attempt to encourage filtration. Therefore, I question the value of routine massage postoperatively, and I believe that, except for the third method described below, massage is probably inadvisable. I do not use massage in the postoperative period, except for the Carlo Traverso maneuver, in highly selected cases during the first 2 weeks postoperatively (see p. 345).

The usefulness of massage in the immediate postoperative period appears to be valuable in certain instances. Here the goal is quite simple. In the immediate postoperative period a sclerostomy may be blocked by fibrin or a clot or other inflammatory debris. Pressure on the globe may mechanically expel the cause of the blockade and permit the flow of aqueous through an otherwise patent sclerostomy. Were pressure not placed on the globe, the inflammatory debris might form a scar that would permanently block the exodus of aqueous. Thus this type of massage has not only a clinical impression of value but a logical explanation as well.

Massage is the term that has traditionally been used to describe the application of pressure on the globe to force aqueous out of a fistula. It is a poor term for several reasons, and probably should be discarded. Massage implies motion rather than pressure, and it is the pressure rather than the motion that is probably responsible for any effect. For this reason I greatly prefer the term compression to massage.

In patients in whom the surgeon hopes to develop a fistula, examination of the eye approximately 4 to 8 hours after the surgery is most useful. If at that time the chamber is deep, the intraocular pressure is too high as indicated by a firm globe, and there is little or no bleb, it may appear that the surgeon has failed to develop a sclerostomy. But pressure applied at that moment may often be effective in opening a plugged fistula and establishing transscleral flow of aqueous humor. Often such compression does not need to be repeated. When the patient is examined 8 to 12 hours later it may be that again the fistula is noticeably

nonfunctional, and again compression may reestablish it. This type of postoperative compression may be effective in helping to establish a fistula and assist in the long-term success of the procedure.

There are three quite different ways of applying pressure for the purpose of enhancing aqueous outflow through a glaucoma fistula. Two are used after full-thickness procedures and the third after trabeculectomy or other guarded procedures.

Should the intraocular pressure after a procedure designed to produce a full-thickness fistula be elevated in the immediate postoperative period, the surgeon can press on the eye through the closed lid, trying to place the pressure directly in the area where the fistula was made, or slightly to the side of that area. This results in an indentation of the sclerostomy, which forces apart the edges of the incision and thus allows the exodus of aqueous humor. The surgeon may often note an immediate softening of the globe with an elevation of the bleb and a shallowing of the anterior chamber. For this type of pressure to be effective, the sclerostomy must be able to be opened mechanically. Consequently this maneuver is usually not successful if first used later than a week after the glaucoma surgery. If the sclerostomy has been closed for that length of time, it is usually sufficiently scarred down that pressure will not reestablish a gross fistula.

The compressive force applied should be adequate to indent the globe. In procedures without scleral sutures, such as a peripheral iridectomy with thermal sclerostomy or trephination, there is good likelihood that this method of compression in the first 2 weeks after surgery may clear the sclerostomy and assist in the development of a functioning fistula. Clearly the pressure must not be applied so vigorously that it ruptures the sutures. The duration of pressure should be 10 seconds or less.

A second and quite different type of compression is that used for long-term maintenance of a fistula or improvement of a partially functioning fistula. This technique entails having the patient himself administer the pressure. There may be some circumstances in which this method is effective, but I believe that the risks are greater than the benefits. I do *not* recommend this type of long-term compression. In fact, I do *not* recommend *any* type of long-term compression by the surgeon or by the patient. Because I am almost alone in this belief, I provide here a description of the method.

The patient is instructed to squeeze the eyeball between the thumb and the index finger as if he were squeezing a grape. The fingers must be pushed quite vigorously back into the orbit in order to "hold" the globe between the two fingers. When the globe is thus held the patient squeezes firmly 10 times. The physician can demonstrate the proper degree of firmness to the patient by squeezing a knuckle of the patient's hand and then having the patient squeeze the physician's knuckle, and finally by applying pressure to the patient's eye so that the patient feels exactly how much pressure should be exerted. A variation of this technique is the first type of compression described above. The patient applies pressure to the eye for approximately 1 second at a time for 10 consecutive squeezes once or twice daily.

The third type of compression is the Carlo Traverso maneuver. This I recommend highly. It is applicable in all cases of filtration surgery, but especially in those such as trabeculectomy (Fig. 11–132). The eye is well anesthetized with topical proparacaine. A cotton-tipped applicator is moistened with anesthetic agent. With the patient at the slit lamp, focal pressure is discreetly applied with the applicator on the conjunctiva directly over or slightly to the side of one of the radial grooves in the scleral flap (Fig. 11–132). There should be an immediate gush of aqueous through the edge of the flap and the immediate development of a higher bleb. This is accompanied by fall of intraocular pressure and, in some cases, a shallowing of the anterior chamber. This very controlled compression ap-

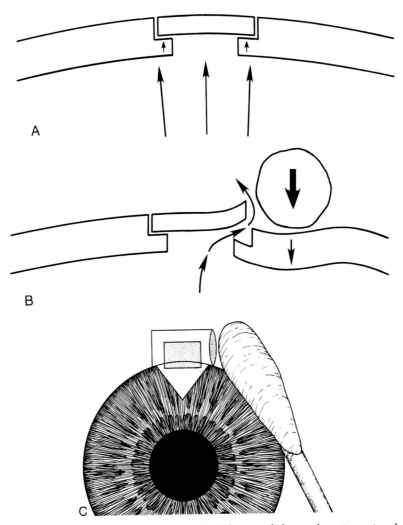

FIGURE 11–132. The Carlo Traverso maneuver. *A*, With a guarded procedure, increasing the pressure inside the eye is not a good way to cause increasing filtration. *B*, Deforming the sclera adjacent to the radial groove allows exodus of aqueous humor. *C*, Schematic depiction of method of performing a Carlo Traverso maneuver.

pears to be without complication, can be repeated several times a day for the first few days, and appears to be extremely helpful. It is of no value after the sclera heals, around 4 weeks postoperatively.

Suprachoroidal Hemorrhage

Suprachoroidal hemorrhage is one of the most dreaded complications of ophthalmic surgery. However, much has been learned about the cause and the management of this previously devastating complication.

The prevalence of suprachoroidal hemorrhage in patients with glaucoma is approximately 10 times greater than in those who do not have glaucoma. Therefore, it is obvious that appropriate precautions must be taken to limit the development of suprachoroidal hemorrhage during or after surgery.

Factors that predispose to suprachoroidal hemorrhage include the presence of glaucoma, systemic hypertension, sudden increase in venous pressure, many years of greatly elevated intraocular pressure, increasing age of the patient, myopia, and hypotony. It is no surprise, then, that suprachoroidal hemorrhage is not infrequent during cataract extraction performed with local anesthesia in the inadequately sedated, elderly, hypertensive patient who has had severe, uncontrolled glaucoma for many years.

It is prudent to lower intraocular pressure before surgery for as long as possible and to as great a degree as possible. However, this goal is not always achievable.

It is usually possible to make sure that the patient's blood pressure is well controlled during surgery and that sedation is satisfactory. General anesthesia is probably preferable to local anesthesia in such cases.

Hypotony should be minimized, and this can be partially achieved by performing guarded filtering procedures such as trabeculectomy, and by suturing the scleral flap tightly. Should the intraocular pressure be too high postoperatively, the scleral sutures can be released with an argon laser. Should hypotony develop, the patient should be cautioned not to strain or perform other maneuvers that will suddenly increase blood pressure or venous pressure. Patients should be routinely given stool softeners or laxatives to prevent them from becoming constipated during the period that their globe is hypotonous. Patients should be cautioned vigorously against any type of activity that puts

them at greater risk until the intraocular pressure rises to a range of 6 to 8 mm Hg. I am opposed to restricting activity of patients postoperatively unless there is a real anticipated benefit, which is rarely the case with restriction of activity. However, for the patient predisposed to suprachoroidal hemorrhage I am vigorous in recommending that the patient avoid those activities that will predispose to this serious complication.

The hallmark of suprachoroidal hemorrhage is the sudden development of excruciating pain. This sign is usually absent during surgery, or at any rate severely blunted by the anesthetic. But the patient who narrates a history of coughing or straining at stool, after which there is sudden excruciating pain, has provided the surgeon with a diagnosis of an acute suprachoroidal hemorrhage. When the hemorrhage occurs intraoperatively and the globe is open, there is an immediate expression of the intraocular contents unless it is possible to promptly close the incision.

Safety sutures or other means of closing the incision should be used in patients at high risk for developing suprachoroidal hemorrhage. The moment a hemorrhage is suspected intraoperatively, the sutures are closed and the immediate disastrous consequences of the hemorrhage prevented. There is usually a marked immediate rise of intraocular pressure, and this is treated with intravenous acetazolamide and mannitol. Once the pressure has fallen and the active bleeding stopped, the eye can be returned to the best condition possible. If after 10 or 15 minutes the intraocular pressure is still around 80 mm Hg and the globe does not appear to be softening, drainage of the suprachoroidal hemorrhage through the sclera is usually appropriate. Intraoperative drainage of a suprachoroidal hemorrhage is usually not necessary.

When a suprachoroidal hemorrhage that occurs intraoperatively does not clear spontaneously postoperatively, or when a suprachoroidal hemorrhage develops postoperatively or spontaneously at a later date, the preferred management is observation. When the pain is intolerable, or the hemorrhage is so extensive that the retina comes in contact with itself ("kissing choroidals"), or the retina is pushed up against the lens or an intraocular lens, drainage is usually necessary and appropriate. If the vitreous is markedly inflamed, drainage in association with a vitrectomy is usually the procedure of choice. Medical management of suprachoroidal hemorrhage is largely aimed at control of pain and control of the intraocular pressure. The timing of drainage of the suprachoroidal hemorrhage is dictated by the urgency posed by the signs and symptoms. As mentioned, this may need to be done in some cases at the time of the initial surgery. The pain often appears to be completely out of proportion to the size of the suprachoroidal hemorrhage or the extent of ocular inflammation. There is an understandable tendency to attribute the intensity of the discomfort to emotional factors. The patient is to be believed.

Although theoretically there is an advantage in waiting 4 or 5 days after the hemorrhage for the clot to lyse, when surgical management is required it is usually required urgently.

Drainage of the hemorrhage is usually best performed with general anesthesia.

A paracentesis is performed into the anterior chamber so that the globe can be reformed and kept "pressurized" during the drainage of the suprachoroidal hemorrhage, and the anterior chamber can be reformed at the conclusion of the procedure.

The suprachoroidal hemorrhage should be located precisely by direct visualization and with B-scan ultrasound. This is important because the incision must be placed directly over the suprachoroidal hemorrhage. Unlike a choroidal effusion, which can be drained virtually anywhere, suprachoroidal hemorrhage remains localized and will not be successfully drained unless the incision is placed over the hemorrhage. The incision into the sclera may be radial or circumferential, but should be so designed that it can be enlarged without involving the vortex veins.

Once the scleral incision has been completed, if the incision is properly located, there will be an immediate seepage of dark viscous blood that resembles motor oil. Immediately adjacent to the hemorrhage there is often a choroidal effusion. If xanthochromic or frankly bloody, watery fluid is obtained, the incision is probably not properly placed. If the hemorrhage is liquid and direct visualization reveals that most of it has been drained, the sclera should be closed tightly enough to permit the restoration of intraocular pressure by infusion of balanced salt solution through the paracentesis. It may be helpful to inject such a solution during drainage of the hemorrhage in order to facilitate the drainage and to maintain the intraocular pressure. If fundus examination shows that indeed the hemorrhage has been largely or totally drained, the sclera can then be closed with a suture such as 7–0 Mersilene.

In many instances the hemorrhage will be clotted. The surgeon must resist any temptation to try to reach through the scleral incision and pull out the clot. In the first place, this will not work. In the second, the clot is difficult to distinguish from choroid and the surgeon may inadvertently break through the choroid. This is an extremely serious complication because blood then enters the vitreous. If blood is retained in the suprachoroidal space and does not enter into vitreous, the prognosis for recovery is totally different. When blood enters the vitreous the likelihood of retinal detachment and poor final result is great; when the blood is retained in the suprachoroidal space the likelihood of an excellent result is high.

When a clot is present the incision almost invariably needs to be enlarged to permit the clot to expel itself spontaneously from the suprachoroidal space. In some cases the incision must involve almost 180 degrees of the globe. Although this seems alarming, in actuality the globe tolerates this well, and the sclera can be well closed with a strong, "permanent" suture such as Mersilene.

It should be stressed that the prognosis for an eye with a suprachoroidal hemorrhage is good, so long as extrusion of essential intraocular contents can be prevented, bleeding into the vitreous does not occur, and excessive inflammation of the vitreous can be avoided.

Repair of Leaking or Excessive Conjunctival Blebs

One should try to avoid repairing a functioning conjunctival bleb. The technique is moderately difficult, although by no means impossible. However, repairing a conjunctival bleb is usually associated with a rise in pressure. The surgeon must consider the ultimate purpose of the surgery, specifically to preserve the quality of life of the patient by means of maintaining the health of the optic nerve. If the optic nerve is severely damaged, it may be preferable to have the patient bear with the side effects of the leaking conjunctival bleb. When the optic nerve is fairly healthy, however, a prompt repair of the deficient bleb is usually advisable. Other factors that indicate a need to repair a filtering bleb are recurrent bleb infections, and hypotony that is sufficiently severe that it is associated with a choroidal detachment or macular edema. Hypotony by itself is not an indication for repair. Some patients may tolerate intraocular pressures as low as 4 mm Hg without symptoms and without apparent problems.

Other patients will develop macular edema with intraocular pressures in the range of 10 mm Hg.

The first approach to the problematic, excessively filtering bleb, then, in most instances, is medical, treating the patient with an antibiotic ointment and watchfully waiting. When the bleb does not recover by itself or the conditions mentioned above indicate the need for repair, the surgeon may try "gluing" the bleb by placing a tiny drop of "super glue" directly on the leaking area of the bleb. In some cases this is effective, but in most it is not. When bleb repair is required the following technique is suggested.

A peritomy is done. The faulty conjunctiva is excised. If possible, Tenon's capsule is freed by extensive dissection from the globe, and also is meticulously separated from the overlying conjunctiva, care being taken to avoid making buttonholes in the conjunctiva. If the surgeon does not believe that this can be accomplished, it is best not to separate Tenon's from the conjunctiva. The corneal epithelium is removed where the fornix-based flap is to be pulled down over the filtering area.

Tenon's capsule is then pulled inferiorly to cover the area of the filtration and sutured into the sclera just anterior to the sclerostomy, using a 10–0 nylon running suture. The conjunctiva is then pulled inferiorly anterior to Tenon's capsule and is sutured into the denuded cornea anterior to the Tenon's capsule–scleral juncture, using a 10–0 nylon running suture. An antibiotic ointment is instilled and the eye pressure-patched for at least 24 hours.

In some cases the sclerostomy will be so excessively large that it needs to be repaired itself before being covered with Tenon's capsule. A one-third–thickness flap of sclera is developed immediately adjacent to the sclerostomy, the hinged end of the flap being adjacent to the sclerostomy. The flap is then rotated on itself to cover the sclerostomy and sutured into the sclera firmly. This patched area is then covered with Tenon's capsule and conjunctiva as previously described.

Endophthalmitis

Endophthalmitis poses a special problem in patients with glaucoma. With full-thickness procedures around 1 per cent of eyes eventually develop an endophthalmitis. Infections of the bleb spread from the conjunctiva through the anterior chamber and eventually into the more posterior portions of the globe. When such infections are caught early the prognosis is excellent, and treatment should not include vitrectomy and intravitreal injection of antibiotics. Such procedures are excessively traumatic and do not increase the success rate in these cases. On the other hand, some types of late bacterial endophthalmitis after glaucoma filtering surgery are more similar to the typical postoperative endophthalmitis, rapidly causing serious and permanent damage. Distinction between these types of infections should be made so that the appropriate therapy can be given. When the reaction is slight, the vitreous clear, and vision not affected, usually the problem can be treated as a "bleb infection" without vitrectomy. However, when the vitreous is involved, or there is a direct connection between an infected bleb and the vitreous cavity, then the general principles for endophthalmitis are more likely to apply.

When endophthalmitis develops immediately after glaucoma surgery it, too, should be treated as operative endophthalmitis, and the principles and management techniques described elsewhere in this text on the diagnosis and management of endophthalmitis apply.

REFERENCES

1. Chandler, P. A., Grant, W. M.: Lectures on Glaucoma. Philadelphia, Lea & Febiger, 1965.
2. McLean, J. M.: Atlas of Glaucoma Surgery. St. Louis, C. V. Mosby Co., 1967, p. 17.
3. Swan, K. C.: Iridectomy for closed- (narrow) angle glaucoma. Am. J. Ophthalmol., 61:601, 1966.
4. Duke-Elder, W. S., Wybar, K. C. (eds.): System of Ophthalmology, Vol. II: The Anatomy of the Visual System. St. Louis, C. V. Mosby Co., 1961, pp. 186–215; 420.
5. Last, R. J. (ed.): Eugene Wolff's Anatomy of the Eye and Orbit. 6th ed. Philadelphia, W. B. Saunders Co., 1968, p. 59.
6. Hollows, F. C., Graham, P. A.: The Ferndale Glaucoma Survey. In Hunt, L. B. (ed.): Glaucoma: Epidemiology, Early Diagnosis and Some Aspects of Treatment. London, Williams & Wilkins, 1966.
7. Armaly, M.: Ocular pressure and visual fields. A ten-year follow-up study. Arch. Ophthalmol., 81:25, 1969.
8. Schappert-Kimmijser, J.: A five-year follow-up of subjects with intra-ocular pressure of 22-30 mm Hg without anomalies of optic nerve and visual field typical for glaucoma at first investigation. Ophthalmologica, 162:289, 1971.
9. Davanger, M.: Intraocular pressure in normal eyes and in eyes with glaucoma simplex. Acta Ophthalmol., 43:299, 1965.
10. Spaeth, G. L.: Low tension glaucoma: Its diagnosis and management. In Documenta Ophthalmologica Proceedings, Series 22, Glaucoma Symposium, Di-

agnosis and Therapy, Amsterdam, 1979. Greve, E. L. (ed.). The Hague, Dr. W. Junk Publishers, 1980, pp. 263–288.

11. Becker, B.: Diabetes mellitus and primary open-angle glaucoma. Trans. Am. Acad. Ophthalmol. Otolaryngol., 75:239, 1971.

12. Becker, B., Kolker, A., Roth, D.: Glaucoma family study. Am. J. Ophthalmol., 50:557, 1960.

13. Bertelsen, T. I.: The relationship between thrombosis in the retinal veins and primary glaucoma. Acta Ophthalmol., 39:603, 1961.

14. Drance, S. M.: Some factors involved in the production of low-tension glaucoma. Br. J. Ophthalmol., 56:229, 1972.

15. Werner, E. B., Drance, S. M.: The interrelationship of intraocular pressure and other risk factors in the development of optic nerve excavation and nerve fiber bundle field defects. Perspect. Ophthalmol., 1:153, 1977.

16. Francois, J., Heintz-DeBree, C.: Personal research on the heredity of chronic simple glaucoma. Am. J. Ophthalmol., 62:1067, 1966.

17. Hansen, E., Sellevold, O. J.: Pseudoexfoliation of the lens capsule. III. Ocular tension in eyes with pseudoexfoliation. Acta Ophthalmol., 48:446, 1970.

18. Harrington, D. O.: The pathogenesis of the glaucoma field; clinical evidence that circulatory insufficiency in the optic nerve is the primary cause of visual field loss in glaucoma. Am. J. Ophthalmol., 47:177, 1959.

19. Hitchings, R. A., Spaeth, G. L.: Chronic retinal vein occlusion in glaucoma. Br. J. Ophthalmol., 60:694, 1976.

20. Kass, M. A., Kolker, A. E., Becker, B.: Prognostic factors in glaucomatous visual field loss. Arch. Ophthalmol., 94:1274, 1976.

21. Kellerman, L., Posner, A.: The value of heredity in the detection and study of glaucoma. Am. J. Ophthalmol., 40:681, 1955.

22. Knapp, A.: Glaucoma in myopic eyes. Trans. Am. Ophthalmol. Soc., 23:61, 1925.

23. Layden, W. E., Shaffer, R. N.: The exfoliation syndrome. Am. Acad. Ophthalmol. Otolaryngol., 78:326, 1974.

24. Lichter, P. R.: Pigmentary glaucoma—current concepts. Trans. Am. Acad. Ophthalmol. Otolaryngol., 78:309, 1974.

25. Lowe, R. F.: Primary angle-closure glaucoma: Family histories and anterior chamber depths. Br. J. Ophthalmol., 48:191, 1967.

26. Moller, H. V.: Excessive myopia and glaucoma. Arch. Ophthalmol., 26:185, 1948.

27. Podos, S. M., Becker, B., Morton, W. R.: High myopia and primary open-angle glaucoma. Am. J. Ophthalmol., 62:1308, 1966.

28. Phojanpelto, P. E., Hurskainen, L.: Studies on relatives of patients with pseudo-exfoliation of the lens capsules. Acta Ophthalmol., 50:255, 1972.

29. Reese, A. B., McGavic, J. S.: Relation of field contraction to blood pressure in chronic primary glaucoma. Arch. Ophthalmol., 27:845, 1942.

30. Safir, A., Paulsen, E. P., Klaymen, J., et al. (eds.): Ocular abnormalities in juvenile diabetics: Frequent occurrence of abnormally high tensions. Arch. Ophthalmol., 76:557, 1966.

31. Spaeth, G. L.: Visual loss in glaucoma clinic. I. Sociological considerations. Invest. Ophthalmol., 9:73, 1970.

32. Spaeth, G. L.: The normal development of the human anterior chamber angle. A new system of descriptive grading. Trans. Ophthalmol. Soc. UK, 91:709, 1971.

33. Sugar, H. S.: Pigmentary glaucoma: A 25 year review. Am. J. Ophthalmol., 62:499, 1966.

34. Wilensky, J. T., Podos, S. M., Becker, B.: Prognostic indicators in ocular hypertension. Arch. Ophthalmol., 91:200, 1974.

35. Levene, R. Z.: Review: Low-tension glaucoma: A critical review and new material. Surv. Ophthalmol., 24:621, 1980.

36. Bankes, J. L. K., Perkins, E. S., Tsolakis, S., et al: Bedford Glaucoma Survey. Br. Med. J., 1:791, 1968.

37. Linnér, E., Strömberg, U.: Ocular hypertension: A five year study of the total population in a Swedish town, and subsequent discussions. In Leydhecker, W. (ed.): Glaucoma: Tutzing Symposium. Basel, S. Karger, 1967, p. 187.

38. Norskøv, K.: Routine tonometry in ophthalmic practice. I. Primary screening and further examinations for diagnostic purposes. Acta Ophthalmol., 48:838, 1970.

39. Perkins, E. S.: Recent advances in the treatment of glaucoma. Trans. Ophthalmol. Soc. UK, 86:199, 1966.

40. Spaeth, G. L.: Ocular hypertension: Reasons for abandonment of the term. In Spaeth, G. L. (ed.): Early Primary Open-Angle Glaucoma: Diagnosis and Management. Boston, Little, Brown & Co., 1979, pp. 37–49.

41. Spaeth, G. L.: Appearances of the optic disc in glaucoma: A pathogenetic classification. In New Orleans Academy of Ophthalmology: Symposium on Glaucoma. St. Louis, C. V. Mosby Co., 1981, pp. 114–153.

42. Chandler, P. A., Grant, W. M.: Lectures on Glaucoma. Philadelphia, Lea & Febiger, 1965, p. 11.

43. Hetherington, J., Jr., Shaffer, R. N., Hoskins, H. D.: The disc in congenital glaucoma. In Etienne, R., Paterson, G. D. (eds.): International Glaucoma Symposium, Albi. Marseille, Diffusion Générale de Librairie, 1975, pp. 127–143.

44. Quigley, H. A.: The pathogenesis of reversible cupping in congenital glaucoma. Am. J. Ophthalmol., 84:358, 1977.

45. Read, R. M., Spaeth, G. L.: The practical clinical appraisal of the optic disc in glaucoma: The natural history of cup progression and some specific disc-field correlations. Trans. Am. Acad. Ophthalmol. Otolaryngol., 78:255, 1974.

46. Hitchings, R. A., Spaeth, G. L.: The optic disc in glaucoma: Classification. Br. J. Ophthalmol., 60:778, 1976.

47. Kolker, A. E., Hetherington, J., Jr.: Becker and Shaffer's Diagnosis and Therapy of the Glaucomas. 3rd ed. St. Louis, C. V. Mosby Co., 1970, pp. 131, 161.

48. Spaeth, G. L.: Morphological damage of the optic nerve. In Heilmann, K., Richardson, K. T. (eds.): Glaucoma: Conceptions of a Disease. Pathogenesis, Diagnosis, Therapy. Philadelphia, W. B. Saunders Co., 1978, pp. 138–156.

49. Spaeth, G. L., Fernandes, E., Hitchings, R. A.: The pathogenesis of transient or permanent improvement in the appearance of the optic disc following glaucoma surgery. In Documenta Ophthalmologica Proceedings, Series 22, Glaucoma Symposium, Diagnosis and Therapy. Amsterdam, 1979. Greve, E. L. (ed.): The Hague, Dr. W. Junk Publishers, 1980, pp. 111–126.

49a. Pederson, J. E., Herschler, J.: Reversal of glaucomatous cupping in adults. Arch. Ophthalmol., 100:426, 1982.

49b. Greenidge, K. C., Spaeth, G. L., Traverso, C. E.: Change in appearance of the optic disc associated with lowering of intraocular pressure. Ophthalmology, 92:897, 1985.

50. Drance, S. M.: The early field defects in glaucoma. Invest. Ophthalmol., 8:84, 1969.

51. Werner, E. B., Drance, S. M.: Early visual field disturbances in glaucoma. Arch. Ophthalmol., 95:1173, 1977.

52. Aulhorn, E., Harms, H.: Early visual field defects in glaucoma. *In* Leydhecker, W. (ed.): Glaucoma: Tutzing Symposium. Basel, S. Karger, 1967, p. 151.

53. Peter, L. C.: Principles and Practice of Perimetry. Philadelphia, Lea & Febiger, 1938, pp. 14, 186.

54. Drance, S. M., Anderson, D.: Automatic Perimetry in Glaucoma: A Practical Guide. Orlando, Fla., Grune & Stratton, 1985.

55. Caprioli, J., Sears, M., Miller, J. M.: Patterns of early visual field loss in open-angle glaucoma. Am. J. Ophthalmol., 103:512, 1987.

56. Whalen, W. R., Spaeth, G. L.: Computerized Visual Fields: What They Are and How to Use Them. Thorofare, N.J., Slack, 1985.

57. Gloor, B., Stürmer, J., Vökt, B.: Was hat die automatisierte Perimetrie mit den Octopus für neue Kenntnisse über glaukomatöse Gesichtsfeldveränderungen gebracht? Klin. Mbl. Augenheilk, 184:249, 1984.

58. Kolker, A. E.: Visual prognosis in advanced glaucoma: A comparison of medical and surgical therapy for retention of vision in 101 eyes with advanced glaucoma. Trans. Am. Ophthalmol. Soc., 75:539, 1977.

59. Spaeth, G. L.: Primary angle-closure glaucoma: Methodology of diagnosis and management of patients with glaucomatous disease. *In* New Orleans Academy of Ophthalmology: Symposium on Glaucoma. St. Louis, C. V. Mosby Co., 1981, pp. 203–220.

60. Spaeth, G. L.: Gonioscopy: Uses old and new. The inheritance of occludable angles. Ophthalmology, 85:222, 1978.

61. Benedikt, O.: Prophylaktische Iridektomie nach Winkelblockglaukom am Partnerauge. Klin. Mbl. Augenheilk., 156:80, 1970.

62. Snow, J. T.: Value of prophylactic peripheral iridectomy on the second eye in angle-closure glaucoma. Trans. Ophthalmol. Soc. UK, 97:189, 1977.

63. Murphy, M., Spaeth, G. L.: I. Iridectomy as treatment for angle-closure glaucoma. II. Differential diagnosis of glaucoma associated with narrow angles. Arch. Ophthalmol., 91:114, 1974.

64. Shaffer, R. N., Weiss, D. I.: Congenital and Pediatric Glaucomas. St. Louis, C. V. Mosby Co., 1970.

65. Shaffer, R. N., Hoskins, H. D.: Goniotomy in the treatment of isolated trabeculodysgenesis (primary congenital (infantile) developmental glaucoma). Trans. Ophthalmol. Soc. UK, 103:581, 1983.

66. Jerndal, T.: Goniodysgenesis and hereditary juvenile glaucoma. Acta Ophthalmol., Suppl. 107. Copenhagen, Munksgaard, 1970.

67. Barkan, O.: Goniotomy. Trans. Am. Acad. Ophthalmol. Otolaryngol., 59:322, 1955.

68. Richardson, K. T.: Optic cup asymmetry in normal newborn infants. Invest. Ophthalmol., 7:138, 1968.

69. Bigger, J. F., Becker, B.: Cataracts and primary open-angle glaucoma: The effect of uncomplicated cataract extraction on glaucoma control. Trans. Am. Acad. Ophthalmol. Otolaryngol., 75:260, 1971.

70. Linn, J. G.: Cataract extraction in management of glaucoma. Trans. Am. Acad. Ophthalmol. Otolaryngol., 75:273, 1971.

71. Rich, W. J., Radtke, N. D., Cohan, B. E.: Early ocular hypertension after cataract extraction. Br. J. Ophthalmol., 58:725, 1974.

72. Spaeth, G. L.: The management of patients with cataract and glaucoma. Ophthalmic Surg., 11:780, 1980.

73. Dannheim, R., Hetzinger, A.: Trabekulotomie und Kataraktextraktion—simultan oder sukzessiv? Klin. Mbl. Augenheilk., 173:542, 1978.

74. Brown, S. V. L., Thomas, J. V. Budenz, D. L., et al.: Effect of cataract surgery on intraocular pressure reduction obtained with laser trabeculoplasty. Am. J. Ophthalmol., 100:373, 1985.

75. Shields, M. B.: Combined cataract extraction and guarded sclerectomy: Reevaluation in the extracapsular era. Ophthalmology, 93:366, 1986.

76. Oyakawa, R. T., Maumenee, A. E.: Clear-cornea cataract extraction in eyes with functioning filtering blebs. Am. J. Ophthalmol., 93:294, 1982.

77. Shuster, J. N., Krupin, T., Kolker, A. E., et al.: Limbus- v. fornix-based conjunctival flap in trabeculectomy: A long-term randomized study. Arch. Ophthalmol., 102:361, 1984.

78. Douglas, W. H. G., Ramsell, T. G.: Results of preoperative antiglaucomatous treatment and of Scheie's operation. Br. J. Ophthalmol., 53:472, 1969.

79. Jerndal, T., Lundström, M.: 330 Trabeculectomies: A long time study (3–5½ years). Acta Ophthalmol., 58:947, 1980.

80. Moro, F.: Antiglaukomatose Trabekulektomie. Klin. Mbl. Augenheilk., 172:670, 1978.

81. Wilson, P.: Trabeculectomy: Long-term follow-up. Br. J. Ophthalmol., 61:535, 1977.

82. Spaeth, G. L., Joseph, N. H., Fernandes, E.: Trabeculectomy: A reevaluation after three years and a comparison with Scheie's procedure. Trans. Am. Acad. Ophthalmol. Otolaryngol., 79:349, 1975.

83. Mackool, R. J., Buxton, J. N.: Anterior chamber depth after intrascleral filtering surgery. Ophthalmic Surg., 8:40, 1977.

84. Watson, P.: Trabeculectomy: A modified ab externo technique. Ann. Ophthalmol., 2:199, 1970.

85. Cairns, J. E.: Trabeculectomy. Trans. Am. Acad. Ophthalmol. Otolaryngol., 2:384, 1972.

85a. Watson, P. G., Grierson, I.: The place of trabeculectomy in the treatment of glaucoma. Ophthalmology, 88:175, 1981.

86. Spaeth, G. L.: A prospective, controlled study to compare the Scheie procedure with Watson's trabeculectomy. Ophthalmic Surg., 11:688, 1980.

86a. Starita, R. J., Fellman, R. L., Spaeth, G. L., et al.: Effect of varying size of scleral flap and corneal block on trabeculectomy. Ophthalmol. Surg., 15:484, 1984.

86b. Starita, R. J., Fellman, R. L., Spaeth, G. L., et al.: Short- and long-term effects of postoperative corticosteroids on trabeculectomy. Ophthalmology, 92:938, 1985.

86c. Kapetansky, F. M.: Trabeculectomy or trabeculectomy plus tenectomy: A comparative study. Glaucoma, 2:451, 1980.

86d. Draeger, J., Winter, R., Wirt, H.: Visco elastic

glaucoma surgery. Trans. Ophthalmol. Soc. UK, 103:270, 1983.

87. Galin, M. A., Obstbaum, S. A., Asano, Y., et al.: Trabeculectomy, cataract extraction and intra-ocular lens implantation. Trans. Ophthalmol. Soc. UK, 104:570, 1985.

88. Coleiro, J. A.: Combined intracapsulary cataract extraction and trabeculectomy with Severin five-loop posterior chamber intraocular lens. Br. J. Ophthalmol., 70:638, 1986.

89. Johns, G. E., Layden, W. E.: Combined trabeculectomy and cataract extraction. Am. J. Ophthalmol., 88:973, 1979.

90. McAllister, J. A., Spaeth, G. L.: Intrakapsuläre kataraktextraktion mit zyklodialyse eine nützliche methode. Klin. Mbl. Augenheilk, 184:283, 1984.

91. Galin, M. A., Baras, I., Sambursky, J.: Glaucoma and cataract. A study of cyclodialysis lens extraction. Am. J. Ophthalmol., 67:522, 1969.

92. Shields, M. B., Simmons, R. J.: Combined cyclodialysis and cataract extraction. Trans. Am. Acad. Ophthalmol. Otolaryngol., 81:286, 1976.

93. Spaeth, G. L., Sivalingam, E.: The partial-punch: A new combined cataract-glaucoma operation. Ophthalmic Surg., 7:53, 1976.

94. Stewart, R. H., Loftis, M. D.: Combined cataract extraction and thermal sclerostomy versus combined cataract extraction and trabeculectomy. Ophthalmic Surg., 7:93, 1976.

95. McGuigan, L. J. B., Gottsch, J.: Extracapsular cataract extraction and posterior chamber lens implantation in eyes with preexisting glaucoma. Arch. Ophthalmol., 104:1301, 1986.

96. Simmons, S. T., Litoff, D., Nichols, D. A., et al.: Extracapsular cataract extraction with posterior chamber intraocular lens implantation combined with trabeculectomy in patients with glaucoma. Am. J. Ophthalmol., 104:465, 1987.

97. Papst, W.: Zur kombinierten Trepanation mit Skleradeckel (Elliot-Fronimopoulos) und intrakapsulären Kataraktextraktion. Klin. Mbl. Augenheilk., 171:343, 1977.

98. Ostbaum, S., Galin, M.: The effects of timolol on cataract extraction and intraocular pressure. Am. J. Ophthalmol., 88:1017, 1979.

99. Balogou, P., Matta, C., Asdourian, K.: Cataract extraction after filtering operations. Arch. Ophthalmol., 88:12, 1972.

100. Regan, E. F., Day, R. M.: Cataract extraction after filtering procedures. Am. J. Ophthalmol., 71:331, 1971.

101. Fanta, H.: Die Kataraktextraktion nach fistelbildender Operation. Klin. Mbl. Augenheilk., 171:331, 1977.

102. de Roetth, A.: Ciliary body temperatures in cryosurgery. Arch. Ophthalmol., 85:204, 1971.

103. Lohse, K., Fuhrmeister, H.: Examinations on experimental animals after cryocyclotherapy. Klin. Mbl. Augenheilk., 162:505, 1973.

104. Green, K., Hull, D. S., Bowman, K.: Cyclocryotherapy and ocular blood flow. Glaucoma, 1:141, 1979.

105. Quigley, H. A.: Histological and physiological studies of cyclocryotherapy in primate and human eyes. Am. J. Ophthalmol., 82:722, 1976.

106. Paton, D., Butner, R. W.: Cyclocryotherapy. Ophthalmic Surg., 5:24, 1974.

107. Bellows, A. R., Grant, W. M.: Cyclocryotherapy of chronic open-angle glaucoma in aphakic eyes. Am. J. Ophthalmol., 85:615, 1978.

108. Krupin, T., Mitchell, K. B., Becker, B.: Cyclocryotherapy in neovascular glaucoma. Am. J. Ophthalmol., 86:24, 1978.

109. Caprioli, J., Strang, S. L., Spaeth, G. L.: Cyclocryotherapy in the treatment of advanced glaucoma. Ophthalmology, 92:947, 1985.

110. Faulborn, J., Birnbaum, F.: Zyklokryotherapie hämorrhagischer Glaukome: Langzeitbeobachtungen und histologische Befunde. Klin. Mbl. Augenheilk., 170:651, 1977.

111. Kaiden, J. S., Serniuk, R. A., Bader, B. F.: Choroidal detachment with flat anterior chamber after cyclocryotherapy. Ann. Ophthalmol., 11:1111, 1979.

112. Krupin, T., Johnson, M. F., Becker, B.: Anterior segment ischemia after cyclocryotherapy. Am. J. Ophthalmol., 84:426, 1977.

113. Caprioli, J., Sears, M.: Regulation of intraocular pressure during cyclocryotherapy for advanced glaucoma. Am. J. Ophthalmol., 101:542, 1986.

114. Beckman, H., Sugar, H. S.: Laser iridectomy therapy of glaucoma. Arch. Ophthalmol., 90:453, 455, 1973.

115. Abraham, R. K., Miller, G. L.: Outpatient argon laser iridectomy for angle closure glaucoma: A two-year study. Trans. Am. Acad. Ophthalmol. Otolaryngol., 79:529, 1975.

116. Anderson, D. R.: Laser iridotomy for aphakic pupillary block. Arch. Ophthalmol., 93:343, 1975.

117. Pollack, I. P., Patz, A.: Argon laser iridotomy: An experimental and clinical study. Ophthalmic. Surg., 7:22, 1976.

118. Theodossiadis, G.: A new argon-laser approach for the management of aphakic pupillary block. Klin. Mbl. Augenheilk., 169:153, 1976.

119. Rodrigues, M. M., Streeten, B., Spaeth, G. L., et al.: Argon laser iridotomy on primary angle closure or pupillary block glaucoma. Arch. Ophthalmol., 96:2222, 1978.

120. Podos, S. M., Kels, B. D., Moss, A. P., et al.: Continuous wave argon laser iridectomy in angle-closure glaucoma. Am. J. Ophthalmol., 88:836, 1979.

120a. Maltzman, B. A., Agin, M.: Árgon peripheral iridotomy and cataract formation. Ann. Ophthalmol., 20:28, 1988.

121. Bass, M. S., Cleary, C. V., Perkins, E. S., et al.: Single treatment laser iridotomy. Br. J. Ophthalmol., 63:29, 1979.

121a. Klapper, R. M.: Q-switched neodymium:YAG laser iridotomy. Ophthalmology, 91:1017, 1984.

121b. Robin, A. L., Pollack, I. P.: Q-switched neodymium-YAG laser angle surgery in open-angle glaucoma. Arch. Ophthalmol., 103:793, 1985.

121c. Wishart, P. K., Hitchings, R. A.: Neodymium YAG and dye laser iridotomy—a comparative study. Trans. Ophthalmol. Soc. UK, 105:521, 1986.

121d. Schwartz, L. W., Moster, M. R., Spaeth, G. L., et al.: Neodymium-YAG laser iridectomies in glaucoma associated with closed or occludable angles. Am. J. Ophthalmol., 102:41, 1986.

121e. Moster, M. R., Schwartz, L. W., Spaeth, G. L., et al.: A controlled study comparing argon and neodymium:YAG laser iridectomies. Ophthalmology, 93:20, 1986.

121f. Karjalanien, K., Lastikainen, L., Raitta, C.: Bilateral nonrhegmatogenous retinal detachment following neodymium-YAG laser iridotomies. Arch. Ophthalmol., 103:1134, 1986.

121g. Goldberg, M. F., Tso, M. O. M., Mirolovich, M.:

Histopathological characteristics of neodymium-YAG laser iridotomy in the human eye. Br. J. Ophthalmol., 71:623, 1987.

121h. Del Priore, L. V., Robin, A. L., Pollack, I. P.: Long-term follow-up of neodymium:YAG laser angle surgery for open-angle glaucoma. Ophthalmology, 95:277, 1988.

122. Beckman, H., Fuller, T. A.: Carbon dioxide laser scleral dissection and filtering procedure for glaucoma. Am. J. Ophthalmol., 88:73, 1979.

123. van der Zypen, E., Fankhauser, F.: Effekte eines neuartigen Lasertyps auf fixiertes Gewebe der Kammerwinkelregion des Affenauges. Klin. Mbl. Augenheilk., 172:436, 1978.

124. Wise, J. B., Witter, S. L.: Argon laser therapy for open-angle glaucoma. Arch. Ophthalmol., 97:319, 1979.

125. Fechner, P. U., Teichmann, I., Teichmann, K. D.: Long-term results of laser-trabecular puncture. Klin. Mbl. Augenheilk., 167:102, 1975.

126. Worthen, D. M., Wickham, M. G.: Laser trabeculotomy in monkeys. Invest. Ophthalmol., 12:707, 1973.

127. Hager, H., Hauck, W., Heppke, G., et al.: Experimentelle Grundlagen zur Trabekulo-Elektropunktur (TEP). Albrecht von Graefes Arch. Klin. Ophthalmol., 185:95, 1972.

128. Krasnov, M. M.: Laseropuncture of anterior chamber angle in glaucoma. Am. J. Ophthalmol., 75:674, 1973.

129. Ticho, U., Cadet, J. C., Mahler, J., et al.: Argon laser trabeculotomies in primates: evaluation by histological and perfusion studies. Invest. Ophthalmol., 17:667, 1978.

129a. Schwartz, L. W., Spaeth, G. L., Traverso, C., et al.: Variation of techniques on the results of argon laser trabeculoplasty. Ophthalmology, 90:781, 1983.

129b. Traverso, C. E., Greenidge, K. C., Spaeth, G. L.: Formation of peripheral anterior synechiae following argon laser trabeculoplasty. Arch. Ophthalmol., 102:861, 1984.

129c. Hotchkiss, M. L., Robin, A. L., Pollack, I. P., et al.: Nonsteroidal anti-inflammatory agents after argon laser trabeculoplasty: A trial with flurbiprofen and indomethacin. Ophthalmology, 91:969, 1984.

129d. Starita, R. J., Fellman, R. L., Spaeth, G. L., et al.: The effect of repeating full-circumference argon laser trabeculoplasty. Ophthalmol. Surg., 15:41, 1984.

129e. Sherwood, M. B., Svedbergh, B.: Argon laser trabeculoplasty in exfoliation syndrome. Br. J. Ophthalmol., 69:886, 1985.

129f. Sharpe, E. D., Simmons, R. J.: Argon laser trabeculoplasty as a means of decreasing intraocular pressure from "normal" levels in glaucomatous eyes. Am. J. Ophthalmol., 99:704, 1985.

129g. Schwartz, A. L., Love, D. C., Schwartz, M. A.: Long-term follow-up of argon laser trabeculoplasty for uncontrolled open-angle glaucoma. Arch. Ophthalmol., 103:1482, 1985.

129h. Brown, S. V. L., Thomas, J. V., Simmons, R. J.: Laser trabeculoplasty re-treatment. Am. J. Ophthalmol., 99:8, 1985.

129i. Gelfand, Y. A., Wolpert, M.: Effects of topical indomethacin pretreatment on argon laser trabeculoplasty: A randomized, double-masked study on black Africans. Br. J. Ophthalmol., 69:668, 1985.

129j. Yablonski, M. E., Cook, D. J., Gray, J.: A fluorophotometric study of the effect of argon laser trabeculoplasty on aqueous humor dynamics. Am. J. Ophthalmol., 99:579, 1985.

129k. Gilbert, C. M., Brown, R. H., Lynch, M. G.: The effect of argon laser trabeculoplasty on the rate of filtering surgery. Ophthalmology, 93:362, 1986.

129l. Krupin, T., Patkin, R., Kurata, F. K., et al.: Argon laser trabeculoplasty in black and white patients with primary open-angle glaucoma. Ophthalmology, 93:811, 1986.

129m. Migdal, C., Hitchings, R.: Control of chronic simple glaucoma with primary medical, surgical and laser treatment. Trans. Ophthalmol. Soc. UK, 105:653, 1986.

129n. Perkins, T. W., Hoskins, H. D., Hetherington, J., et al.: Effect of argon laser trabeculoplasty on subsequent trabeculectomy. ARVO, 27:252, 1986.

129o. Schultz, J. S., Werner, E. B., Krupin, T., et al.: Intraocular pressure and visual field defects after argon laser trabeculoplasty in chronic open-angle glaucoma. Ophthalmology, 94:553, 1987.

129p. Blondeau, P., Roberge, J. F., Asselin, Y.: Long-term results of low power, long duration laser trabeculoplasty. Am. J. Ophthalmol., 104:339, 1987.

129q. Bergeå, B.: Repeated argon laser trabeculoplasty. Acta Ophthalmol. (Copenh), 64:246, 1986.

129r. Grinich, N. P., Van Buskirk, E. M., Samples, J. R.: Three-year efficacy of argon laser trabeculoplasty. Ophthalmology, 94:858, 1987.

129s. Melamed, S., Epstein, D. L.: Alterations of aqueous humor outflow following argon laser trabeculoplasty in monkeys. Br. J. Ophthalmol., 71:776, 1987.

129t. Messner, D., Siegel, L. I., Kass, M. A., et al.: Repeat argon laser trabeculoplasty. Am. J. Ophthalmol., 103:113, 1987.

130. James, W. A., Jr., de Roetth, A., Jr., Forbes, M., et al.: Argon laser photomydriasis. Am. J. Ophthalmol., 81:62, 1976.

130a. Beckman, H., Sugar, H. S.: Neodymium laser cyclocoagulation. Arch. Ophthalmol., 90:27, 1973.

130b. Fankhauser, F., van der Zyphen, E., Kwasniewska, S., et al.: Transscleral cyclophotocoagulation using a neodymium:YAG laser. Ophthalmol. Surg., 17:94, 1986.

130c. Shields, M. B.: Intraocular cyclophotocoagulation. Trans. Ophthalmol. Soc. UK, 105:237, 1986.

130d. Shields, S. M., Stevens, J. L., Kass, M. A., Smith, M. E.: Histopathologic findings after Nd:YAG transscleral cyclophotocoagulation. Am. J. Ophthalmol., 106:100, 1988.

130f. Fankhauser, F., van der Zyphen, E., Kwasniewska, S., et al.: Transscleral cyclophotocoagulation using a neodymium:YAG laser. Ophthalmol. Surg., 17:94, 1986.

130g. Molteno, A. C. B.: New implant for drainage in glaucoma. Clinical trial. Br. J. Ophthalmol., 53:606, 1969.

130h. Freedman, J.: The use of the single stage Molteno long tube seton in treating cases of glaucoma. Ophthalmol. Surg., 16:480, 1985.

130i. Ritch, R., Liebmann, J. M., Krupin, T.: Reoperations using setons. In Spaeth, G. L., Katz, L. J. (eds.): Current Therapy in Ophthalmic Surgery. Philadelphia, B. C. Decker, 1989, pp. 208–211.

130j. Sherwood, M. B., Hitchings, R. A.: The Schoket procedure. In Spaeth, G. L., Katz, L. J. (eds.): Current Therapy in Ophthalmic Surgery. Philadelphia, B. C. Decker, 1989, pp. 211–218.

130k. Minckler, D. S., Baerveldt, G., Heuer, D. K.,

Hasty, B.: The Molteno implant. *In* Spaeth, G. L., Katz, L. J. (eds.): Current Therapy in Ophthalmic Surgery. Philadelphia, B. C. Decker, 1989, pp. 218–221.

130l. Gressel, M. G., Parrish, R. K., II, Folberg, R.: 5-Fluorouracil and glaucoma filtering surgery. I. An animal model. Ophthalmology, 91:378, 1984.

130m. Herschler, J.: What makes filtering procedures filter? Ophthalmol. Surg., 15:471, 1984.

130n. Parrish, R. K.: Filtering procedures in patients predisposed to failure. *In* Spaeth, G. L., Katz, L. J. (eds.): Current Therapy in Ophthalmic Surgery. Philadelphia, B. C. Decker, 1989, pp. 182–186.

130o. Weinreb, R.: Adjusting the dose of 5-fluorouracil after filtration surgery to minimize side effects. Ophthalmology, 94:564, 1987.

131. Allen, J. C.: Delayed anterior chamber formation after filtering operations. Am. J. Ophthalmol., 62:640, 1966.

131a. Hoskins, H. D., Jr., Migliazzo, C.: Management of failing filtering blebs with the argon laser. Ophthalmol. Surg., 15:731, 1984.

131b. Traverso, C. E., Greenidge, K. C., Spaeth, G. L., et al.: Focal pressure: A new method to encourage filtration after trabeculectomy. Ophthalmol. Surg., 15:62, 1984.

132. Chandler, P. A., Grant, W. M.: Lectures on Glaucoma. Philadelphia, Lea & Febiger, 1965, pp. 393–407.

133. Sampaolesi, R.: Postoperative flat anterior chamber after glaucoma surgery. La Atalamia Postoperatoria en el Glaucoma-An. Inst. Barraquer, 10:124, 1972.

134. Herschler, J., Clafin, A. J., Florentino, G.: The effect of aqueous humor on the growth of subconjunctival fibroblasts in tissue culture and its implications for glaucoma surgery. Am. J. Ophthalmol., 89:245, 1980.

135. Shaffer, R. N., Hoskins, H. D.: Ciliary block (malignant) glaucoma. Ophthalmology, 85:215, 1978.

136. Simmons, R. J.: Malignant glaucoma. Br. J. Ophthalmol., 56:263, 1972.

137. Ray, R. R., Binkhorst, R. D.: The diagnosis of pupillary block by intravenous injection of fluorescein. Am. J. Ophthalmol., 61:481, 1966.

138. Christensen, R. E., Rundle, H. L.: Repair of filtering blebs following cataract surgery. Arch. Ophthalmol., 84:8, 1970.

139. Cohen, J. S., Shaffer, R. N., Hetherington, J., Jr., et al.: Revision of filtration surgery. Arch. Ophthalmol., 95:1612, 1977.

140. Galin, M. A., Hung, P. T.: Surgical repair of leaking blebs. Am. J. Ophthalmol., 83:328, 1977.

141. Gehring, J. R., Ciccarelli, E. C.: Trichloracetic acid treatment of filtering blebs following cataract extraction. Am. J. Ophthalmol., 74:622, 1972.

142. Giebmann, H. G., Pambor, R.: Covering of fistulae after operations of glaucoma. Klin. Mbl. Augenheilk., 166:205, 1975.

143. Grady, F. J., Forbes, M.: Tissue adhesive for repair of conjunctival buttonhole in glaucoma surgery. Am. J. Ophthalmol., 68:656, 1969.

144. Mackensen, G., Atkinson, A.: Zur Technik des Verschlusses äusserer Fisteln an Sickerkissen nach Glaukomoperationen. Klin. Mbl. Augeheilk., 169:557, 1976.

145. Scheie, H. G., Guehl, J. J., III.: Surgical management of overhanging blebs after filtering procedures. Arch. Ophthalmol., 97:325, 1979.

146. Sugar, H. S.: Complications, repair and reoperation of antiglaucoma filtering blebs. Am. J. Ophthalmol., 63:825, 1967.

147. Romanchuk, K. G.: Seidel's test using 10% fluorescein. Can. J. Ophthalmol., 14:253, 1979.

148. Kanski, J. J.: Treatment of late endophthalmitis associated with filtering blebs. Arch. Ophthalmol., 91:339, 1974.

149. Katz, L. J., Cantor, L. B., Spaeth, G. L.: Complications of surgery in glaucoma. II. Early and late bacterial endophthalmitis following glaucoma filtering surgery. Ophthalmology, 92:959, 1985.

150. Kanski, J. J., McAllister, J. A.: Trabeculodialysis for inflammatory glaucoma in children and young adults. Ophthalmology, 92:927, 1985.

12

RETINAL DETACHMENT

by William E. Benson

To repair a retinal detachment the surgeon must (a) find the retinal breaks and (b) seal them adequately. First established by Jules Gonin in the 1920's,[26, 27] these basic principles are still valid. Surgical techniques, on the other hand, have undergone and are undergoing constant change. Current management of retinal detachment is discussed in this chapter.

PREOPERATIVE EVALUATION

Initial Diagnosis

The possibility of a retinal detachment should be considered in any patient who complains of light flashes or "floaters," the symptoms of posterior vitreous detachment (PVD).[68] When the vitreous liquefies, collapses, and moves forward (PVD), traction on the retina causes the sensation of brief flashes of light in the periphery of the visual field. Glial tissue torn free from the epipapillary area as the vitreous

advances is the source of a single centrally located opacity ("floater"), which the patient often likens to a cobweb or a fly. More ominous, however, are the symptoms of vitreous hemorrhage: myriad small floaters and blurred vision. Retinal tears or detachments are seldom found in patients who have PVD without vitreous hemorrhage, but detachments do occur in 60 to 70 per cent of such patients with vitreous hemorrhage.[42, 57, 98, 101] Although nearly all retinal detachments are preceded by PVD, 50 per cent of patients with retinal detachments have no symptoms before the visual field loss or decreased visual acuity caused by the detachment itself.[16, 68, 69]

Initial Diagnostic Examination

Findings That Suggest Retinal Detachment

The intraocular pressure is usually lower in the eye with retinal detachment than in the fellow eye.[19, 46, 70] In patients with glaucoma, an

354

unexpected drop in intraocular pressure may signify that a retinal detachment is present. On the other hand, occasional detachment patients have increased intraocular pressure (with or without cells in the anterior chamber), and are mistakenly treated for uveitis or glaucoma.[59, 88] When the retinal detachment is found and repaired, the intraocular pressure often returns to normal.

Clumps of pigment ("tobacco dust") in the vitreous of patients without previous ocular surgery are virtually pathognomonic of a retinal tear or detachment.[34, 93, 96]

Confirmation

Although the findings above suggest retinal detachment, confirmation usually requires a fundus examination by indirect ophthalmoscopy.

The most common entities that can be confused with rhegmatogenous retinal detachment are intraocular neoplasms with or without secondary retinal detachment, inflammatory diseases such as Harada's disease and posterior scleritis, idiopathic central serous chorioretinopathy with bullous retinal detachment, retinal detachment caused by an optic pit, traction retinal detachment caused by diabetic retinopathy, juvenile and senile retinoschisis, and choroidal detachment. The differential diagnosis of retinal detachment is beyond the scope of this chapter and has been covered elsewhere.[4, 37, 67]

Further Eye Examination

Blepharoconjunctivitis, when present, should be treated before retinal surgery. If the pupil will not dilate enough to allow peripheral retinal examination, it must be enlarged, either by photocoagulation of the iris or by iridectomy. Iridectomy is also indicated in patients with angle-closure glaucoma. If a dense cataract prevents complete examination, it must be removed. The retinal surgery can immediately follow the extraction at the same operative session; otherwise, it should be delayed for 1 month.

Indirect Ophthalmoscopy

Why Indirect Ophthalmoscopy?

The first principle of retinal detachment surgery is to find all of the breaks. The binocular indirect ophthalmoscope is invaluable for this

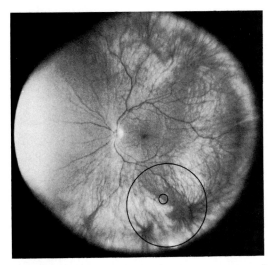

FIGURE 12–1. The area that can be seen at one time with the indirect ophthalmoscope and the large 20-diopter lens is indicated by the large circle. The area that can be seen with the direct ophthalmoscope is indicated by the small circle.

purpose, offering several advantages over the direct ophthalmoscope.[35, 40, 80] First, it allows simultaneous viewing of wide areas of the retina, thereby helping to ensure that no abnormalities will be missed (Fig. 12–1). Second, the hand lens can be used to neutralize refractive error, thus providing a clear image of the retinal periphery. Third, the good illumination supplied by the headlamp, coupled with the light-gathering capability of the hand lens, allows the examiner to see through hazy media. Fourth, it provides stereopsis. Fifth, indirect ophthalmoscopy, combined with scleral depression, provides the best view of the far periphery. In addition, the indirect ophthalmoscope is invaluable during surgery. (The hand lens can be sterilized so that the operative field is not contaminated.)

The Examination

The large, aspheric lenses provide a sharper image and a wider field of view than do the smaller spheric lenses. As for power, the 14-diopter lens magnifies the most ($3.6\times$) of the commonly used lenses,[81] but is difficult to use because of its long focal length (7 cm). The 30-diopter lens (f = 33 cm) is easy to use, but gives inadequate magnification ($1.5\times$) for finding small breaks. We prefer the 20-diopter lens (f = 5 cm), which is easy to use and provides adequate magnification ($2.3\times$). Any lens should be held with the more convex surface toward the observer. It should be tilted to move the

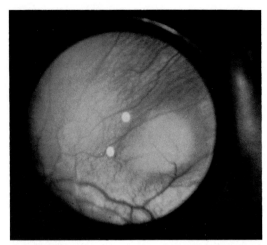

FIGURE 12–2. The lens is slightly tilted to separate the light reflections on its surface. (Courtesy of Dr. Jerry Shields.)

light reflexes away from the center of the lens (Fig. 12–2).

The patient should be reclining comfortably for the examination. Bilateral cycloplegia combined with topical anesthesia reduces photopsia and enhances cooperation. Bell's phenomenon is avoided if the patient keeps both eyes open. A fixation target, such as the patient's own thumb or a mark on the ceiling, is helpful (Fig. 12–3).

The superior periphery should be examined first because photopsia is minimized in upgaze

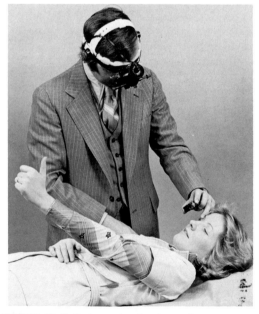

FIGURE 12–3. Patient using thumb as a fixation target to facilitate examination of the inferior retina.

and because the periphery is less sensitive to light than is the posterior pole. Initially the transformer rheostat should be set at a low voltage. Higher light intensities can be used later as the patient becomes less light-sensitive. Sensitivity to light is inversely proportional to the size of the area of detached retina. A patient with a total retinal detachment will usually tolerate the full voltage.

The examiner should hold his head so that he looks directly into the quadrant being examined. To examine the temporal periphery, he should stand on the side opposite the eye being examined (Fig. 12–4); for the nasal periphery, on the same side (Fig. 12–5). The hand lens is shifted from his right to his left hand as necessary to avoid awkward maneuvering, especially during scleral depression. The nose becomes less of an obstacle to viewing the temporal periphery when the patient rolls his head toward the observer while looking temporally.

Beginners frequently make the error of standing too close to the patient (Fig. 12–6). It is much easier for the examiner to obtain a clear fundus image if his arm is extended. This is especially important if the pupil is small.

A detailed drawing of the fundus should be made. The drawing may help to locate the tears during surgery if the media become opaque or if the pupil constricts. Retinal hemorrhages, pigment, blood vessels, and folds should be represented.

There are two ways to correct for the inverted image of the indirect ophthalmoscope. The first is to observe the retina and then mentally correct for the inverted image, drawing the findings as they are, not as they are seen. The second method is to invert the drawing pad and then draw the findings as they are seen. When the drawing is finished, the findings will be correctly positioned.

After the limits of the detachment have been sketched, all retinal breaks must be found.[51, 61] To this end, one may start at the optic nerve and follow each of the retinal vessels to the periphery. A scanning technique should also be used. Keeping his eyes and the hand lens aligned, the observer swings his gaze along the periphery, examining 90 degrees of retina in one swing.

Scleral Depression

After the retina has been thoroughly scanned, the sclera should be depressed for 360 degrees to detect small holes, especially those near the ora serrata. In some patients this region cannot

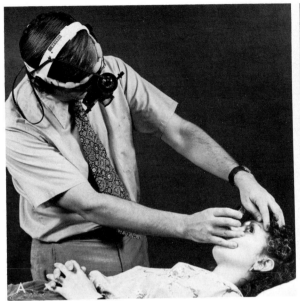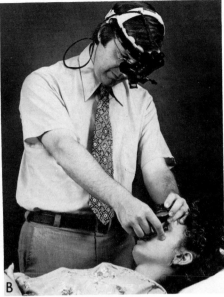

FIGURE 12–4. *A*, Examination of the left eye, superotemporal periphery. The lens is held in the right hand. The patient looks up and to the left. *B*, Examination of the left eye, inferotemporal periphery. The lens is held in the left hand. The patient looks down and to the left.

be seen without indentation. Scleral depression should not be attempted by beginners until they can routinely examine the retina anterior to the equator without difficulty. Otherwise, scleral depression will cause the patient unnecessary pain, and the examiner will probably learn little from the procedure.

Scleral depression helps in three ways to detect small breaks. First, it increases the contrast between the intact retina and the break; the indented choroid/retinal epithelium is darker than the unindented choroid/retinal pigment epithelium and darker still than the intact retina. The break then appears as a dark spot

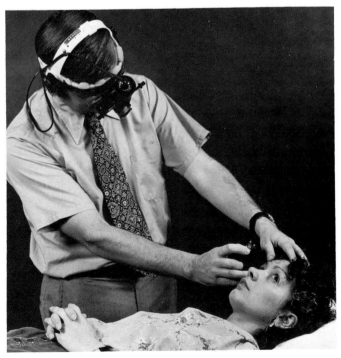

FIGURE 12–5. Examination of the right eye, superonasal periphery. The lens is held in the right hand. The patient looks up and to the left.

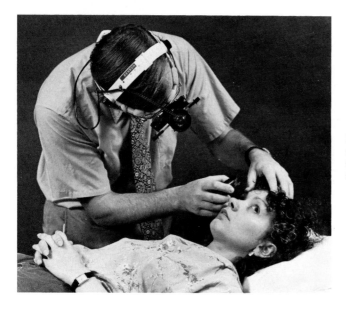

FIGURE 12–6. Examiner standing too close to the patient. Focusing is difficult, and it is difficult to get sufficient light into the eye while viewing the fundus.

(Fig. 12–7). Second, as the depressor tilts the retina downward, retinal translucency is decreased because the retina is seen at a more acute angle. This increases the contrast between the hole and the retina and allows the hole to be seen. Also, as the examiner looks at a more acute angle, he can sometimes see the posterior edge of a break (Fig. 12–7). Third, sometimes the flaps of tiny breaks at the posterior vitreous base can be seen as the eye is indented. In all cases, constant movement of the scleral depressor maximizes the chances of finding a small break.

There are few contraindications to scleral depression. Originally it was thought that it would enlarge retinal holes, but even after examination of thousands of patients this has not been found to be the case. Scleral depression should be avoided, however, in patients who have recently had intraocular surgery.

Scleral depression may cause pain. It raises the intraocular pressure and is, therefore, especially painful in eyes with a high initial pressure because adequate scleral depression raises the pressure still higher. Oral acetazolamide and topical timolol may lower the pressure enough for adequate scleral depression. Stretching and compressing the eyelids can also cause pain. Therefore, scleral depression should be started superiorly because the upper lid is looser and more flexible than the lower. We ask the patient to look down, place the depres-

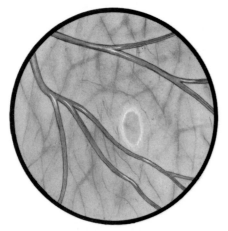
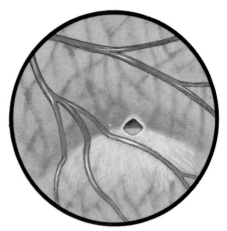

FIGURE 12–7. *Left,* A retinal break that can barely be seen because of little contrast between the retina and the underlying choroid. *Right,* Scleral depression darkens the underlying choroid. The break is more easily seen as a dark spot. Also, the posterior edge of the break is more easily seen because it is viewed at a more acute angle.

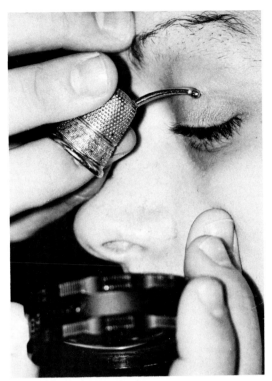

FIGURE 12–8. Scleral depression of the superior retina. The patient looks down and the depressor is placed on the lid fold.

sor near the lid margin (Fig. 12–8) and then follow the eyelid up as the patient is asked to look up (Fig. 12–9). Again, if the depressor is held vertically, it should be easy to locate the indentation on the inside of the eye. If the indentation is not readily seen, the beginner should make a scanning movement from side to

side. If the indentation is still not seen, he should begin all over again. If the ora serrata is to be viewed, the patient should look as far superiorly as possible (Fig. 12–9). Beginners will see the ora serrata most easily in highly myopic eyes and in aphakic eyes that have had a sector iridectomy. If areas posterior to the equator are to be examined, the patient must look slightly inferiorly (Fig. 12–10).

Scleral depression is most difficult at the 9 o'clock and 3 o'clock positions because the canthal ligaments resist the posterior movement of the depressor. Direct scleral depression at the canthus is painful. Moreover, the depressor may slip off the eyelid and strike the patient's eye. The following techniques help to avoid these problems. First, the depressor is placed on the superior eyelid and pushes the eyelid down to the horizontal meridian (Fig. 12–11). The lid becomes more slack when the patient, his head rolled away from the examiner, is not looking into an extreme position of gaze.[12] Second, a cotton-tipped applicator, being blunter and softer, may be better tolerated. Finally, after topical anesthesia, one can easily depress directly on the conjunctiva (Fig. 12–12).

After a thorough examination by indirect ophthalmoscopy and scleral depression, we use the slit lamp and the Goldmann three-mirror lens to search for small breaks and to evaluate vitreous traction. It is essential that the fellow eye be carefully examined for retinal breaks or other abnormalities that might require prophylactic treatment.[3]

The bilateral incidence of retinal detachment in phakic eyes is approximately 10 per cent. If there is a flap tear in the fellow eye, the

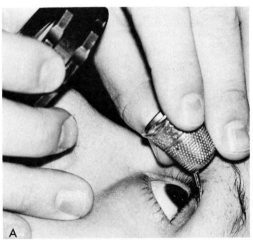

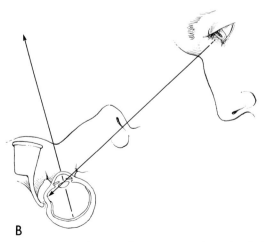

FIGURE 12–9. *A*, Scleral depression of the ora serrata of the superior retina. *B*, Viewing the ora serrata—the patient looks up as far as possible.

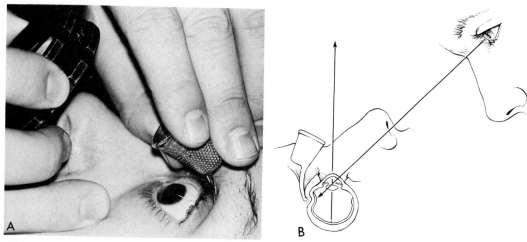

FIGURE 12–10. *A,* Examination of the midperiphery. The patient looks downward. *B,* Viewing the midperiphery.

incidence rises to about 20 per cent, and if there is lattice degeneration, to about 25 per cent. The bilateral incidence of retinal detachment has been reported to be between 21 and 36 per cent.[3]

PREOPERATIVE MANAGEMENT

After admission, the patient receives scopolamine 0.25% in both eyes twice per day. This avoids the need for repeat dilation each time another member of the operating team exam-

ines the patient. In addition, maximal cycloplegia is obtained. Rarely does the pupil constrict during surgery.

On the day of surgery, in addition to scopolamine, the patient is given cyclopentolate 1% and phenylephrine 2.5% every 15 minutes for three applications.

Binocular patching will, in almost all cases, prevent the spread of the retinal detachment. Moreover, significant quantities of subretinal fluid may be absorbed, especially in recent retinal detachments with small retinal breaks and superior detachments with a mobile retina. The fluid is not as readily absorbed in aphakic

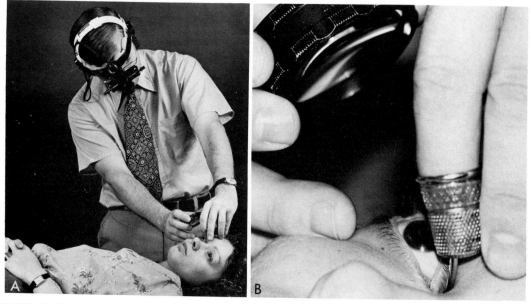

FIGURE 12–11. *A,* Scleral depression of the horizontal meridian. The patient rolls her head away from the examiner and looks straight ahead. *B,* The eyelid is pushed down so the horizontal periphery can be examined.

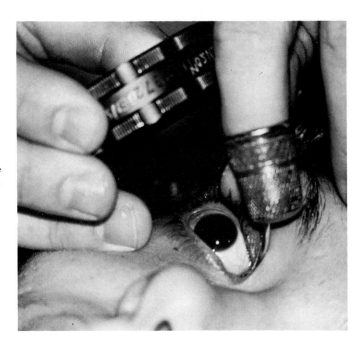

FIGURE 12–12. After topical anesthesia, one can easily depress directly on the conjunctiva.

and inferior retinal detachments.[39, 49] The decreased elevation of the detachment facilitates the localization of breaks and sometimes allows a nondrainage procedure to be performed.

A careful medical examination is important, since many retinal detachment procedures last for 2 or more hours and are done under general anesthesia. Allergic reactions must also be avoided.

OPERATIVE TECHNIQUE

Anesthesia

Local anesthesia has three advantages: total operating room time is decreased, there is less bleeding, and operative mortality may be slightly decreased. Disadvantages include possible retrobulbar hemorrhage, central retinal artery occlusion, respiratory arrest, and more difficult exposure during surgery. In addition, the patient may experience pain during the procedure, may become disoriented and restless if he is oversedated, and may have discomfort from having to lie still during a long procedure. One cannot always predict that an operation will be "easy" or short. Occasionally unexpected findings or operative complications necessitate a longer procedure than originally planned. For these reasons we prefer general anesthesia.

Opening

In primary operations the peritomy can be made either at the limbus[45] or 3 to 5 mm from it. Between two rectus muscles and near the limbus the conjunctiva and Tenon's capsule are tented up with toothed forceps and are incised with blunt scissors down to the sclera (Fig. 12–13). Blunt dissection separates Tenon's capsule from the sclera so that a 360-degree incision can be made (Fig. 12–14). (When a single radial sponge is to be placed, a 180-degree incision suffices.) Two relaxing incisions, 180 degrees apart, serve to avoid tearing the conjunctiva (Fig. 12–15). Additional blunt dissection is used posteriorly to further separate Tenon's capsule from the sclera so that the muscles can be hooked and bridled. A 4-0 black silk suture is passed under the muscle and tied. Before proceeding further the surgeon must search the sclera for staphylomas. In the rare cases in which adequate exposure cannot be obtained, a lateral canthotomy is performed, and one or more muscles are disinserted. A traction suture is placed into the stump of the tendon.

Localization of the Break(s)

In order to place the scleral buckle correctly, the surgeon must localize all breaks within the detachment (i.e., the sclera underlying them

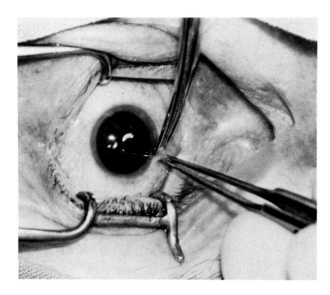

FIGURE 12–13. Opening for a scleral buckling procedure. The conjunctiva and Tenon's capsule are grasped with toothed forceps and incised down to the sclera.

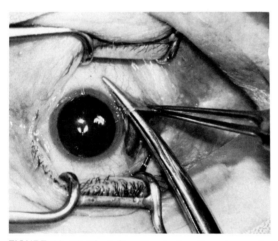

FIGURE 12–14. Blunt dissection to free Tenon's capsule from the episclera.

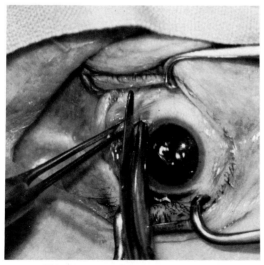

FIGURE 12–15. Radial relaxing incision.

must be marked). We localize with a blunt-tipped diathermy electrode. The intensity of the diathermy should be tested on anterior sclera. The assistant then steadies the eye by holding two bridle sutures while the surgeon, using a cotton-tipped applicator for scleral depression, locates the meridian of the break. The diathermy electrode is introduced into this meridian and is used to localize the breaks precisely under indirect ophthalmoscopic control (Fig. 12–16A and B). The surgeon cocks his wrist to ensure that only the tip of the instrument indents the sclera. A few gentle applications of diathermy are made on the sclera underlying the retinal break. The eye is then rolled forward and additional diathermy is applied to make a permanent mark.

For small breaks the posterior edge alone is localized; for large flap tears, the posterior edge and both anterior horns (Fig. 12–16C); for lattice degeneration with holes, both ends of the degeneration; for dialyses, the ends of the dialysis as well as the point in the center of the dialysis where the surgeon estimates that the retina will fall when the subretinal fluid is drained or is absorbed. Anterior and posterior localization of long tears is important, since many are not radial in direction.

If either a staphyloma or very thin sclera is present in the area of the hole, the diathermy technique is dangerous because the electrode may penetrate the globe. Instead, the surgeon can use the blunt end of a cotton-tipped applicator or can make a mark in thicker adjacent sclera.

Once the apparent holes have been localized, the retina should be examined once again for

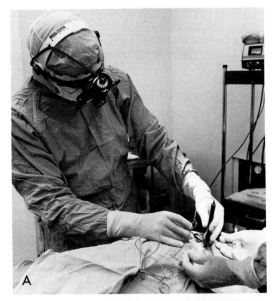

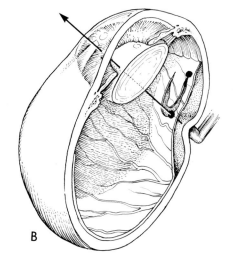

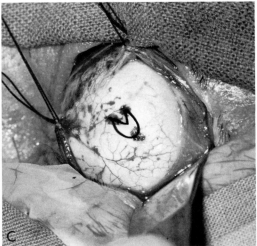

FIGURE 12–16. *A*, The surgeon indents *and marks* the sclera under the retinal break with the blunt diathermy probe. *B*, The localizing instrument, functioning as a scleral depressor, is slid posteriorly under indirect ophthalmoscopic control until the surgeon determines that the apex has been reached. He marks the sclera at this point. Then the anterior horns are marked. *C*, Localizing marks on the sclera overlying both anterior horns and the apex of a flap tear. (Methylene blue has been dabbed on the marks for purposes of illustration.)

any overlooked break. A cotton-tipped applicator serves as a scleral depressor for this final check, which is especially important if the preoperative examination has been difficult.

Cryotherapy

Most retinal surgeons currently use cryotherapy[54, 73] to make a firm adhesion between the retina and the retinal pigment epithelium, or Bruch's membrane. Some believe that an adequate adhesion results from cryotherapy of the pigment epithelium surrounding a break, even if the overlying detached retina is not frozen.[35] Experimental evidence indicates, however, that such treatment results in a relation between the sensory retina and the pigment epithelium similar to the relatively weak adhesion found in eyes without detachment.[47] A histologically strong adhesion results when the pigment epithelium and the sensory retina are both frozen during treatment, for tight junctions are later seen between Müller cells and the pigment epithelium, or Bruch's membrane.[21, 47, 55]

The pressure of the cryoprobe on the sclera forces fluid from the eye. As the eye softens, high indentation by the probe is possible. Therefore, breaks in nondetached retina should be frozen first; breaks in highly detached retina, last. As the assistant steadies the eye with the rectus muscle bridle sutures, the surgeon, viewing with the indirect ophthalmoscope (Fig. 12–17), surrounds the tears with 2 to 3 mm of retinal freezing to ensure adequate adhesion. It

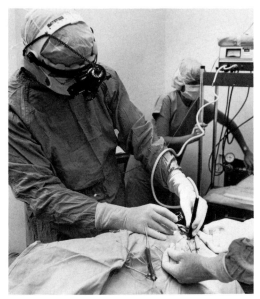

FIGURE 12–17. Cryotherapy of a retinal tear under direct visualization.

is important that the surgeon keep his wrist cocked outward so that only the tip of the cryoprobe indents the eye. Beginners tend to indent the eye with the shaft of the probe, which may cause severe posterior freezing to occur beyond the area of visualization. Most cryoprobes have a small knob 180 degrees away from the freezing tip to aid the surgeon in orienting the probe. The freezing portion of the tip must be pressed squarely against the globe. After the first application the surgeon waits for the iceball to thaw, and then, watching retinal landmarks, he gently slides the probe sufficiently to place the next contiguous lesion. Obviously, freezing the pigment epithelium within the hole does not increase the strength of the adhesion. Such freezing only releases more pigment into the vitreous, increasing postoperative glare.

The firmer the indentation, the faster the rate of freezing because choroidal blood flow (an insulator) is stopped.[8] Excessive indentation can close the central retinal artery. After a few consecutive applications, the surgeon must relax the pressure on the eye, to permit ocular circulation. If a break is highly elevated, the surgeon should not indent excessively, especially in patients who have recently undergone intraocular surgery or in those with staphylomatous sclera. Instead, he should drain the subretinal fluid before applying the cryotherapy.

When the sensory retina has been frozen, it becomes slightly opaque, helping the surgeon

to verify that his treatment applications have been contiguous. Scleral depression makes this opacity easier to see. The opaqueness also aids in differentiating small retinal breaks from small patches of thin retina. Normal and thin retina both turn white where frozen. Full-thickness retinal breaks appear dark in contrast to the adjacent frozen retina.

Scleral Buckling Procedures

Ernst Custodis made a great contribution to retinal detachment surgery when he introduced the scleral buckling procedure.[14, 15] He sutured a synthetic material, polyviol, onto the sclera to "buckle" (indent) it toward the retinal breaks. This explant procedure offered two major advantages over previous treatment: it made nondrainage operations possible and it permanently reduced vitreous traction on retinal breaks.

Before Custodis it was considered essential to drain all of the subretinal fluid in order to bring the sensory retina into contact with the pigment epithelium. His procedure effected successful reattachment of the retina without drainage. Sometimes the two tissues are brought into contact in the operating room; once the break is so closed, whatever subretinal fluid remains will subsequently be absorbed. In other cases the break closes postoperatively. If the sutures are tightly tied, fluid is forced from the eye and the height of the buckle increases. In addition, a certain amount of spontaneous absorption of subretinal fluid goes on postoperatively, even before the break is closed, decreasing the height of the detachment. Bilateral patching facilitates this postoperative settling of the detached retina.

Strong vitreous traction impedes the development of a firm chorioretinal scar. Even after thorough drainage of subretinal fluid plus proper treatment with cryotherapy or diathermy, unrelieved vitreous traction can reopen a retinal break before the sealing scar has developed. Custodis' scleral buckle, by relieving the traction, allows the scar to form.

Explants

An explant is a foreign material attached by sutures to the sclera. Explants may be radial (perpendicular to the ora serrata) or circumferential (parallel to the ora serrata). All explant material currently used is made of silicone. There are two varieties, silicone sponge and solid silicone. Available sponges are 80 mm

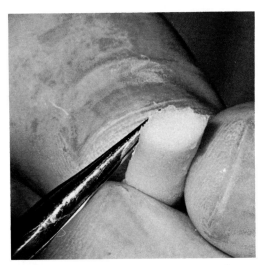

FIGURE 12–18. The sponge is cut in half lengthwise to reduce its bulk.

long and are either round (3, 4, or 5 mm in diameter) or elliptical (7.5 × 5.5 mm). Solid silicone is available in a variety of sizes and shapes. Explants are held in place by mattress sutures of 5-0 monofilament nylon, 4-0 or 5-0 Dacron, or 4-0 or 5-0 Supramyd. Thinner sutures tend to erode out of the sclera. Colored sutures are easier to locate in reoperations than white ones. The sponge is bisected lengthwise to reduce its bulk (Fig. 12–18).

The assistant provides exposure and steadies the globe by using the bridle sutures adjacent to the break. He also holds back Tenon's capsule with a blade or a Schepens retractor. The surgeon further prevents movements of the globe by grasping the tendon of a rectus muscle. It is difficult to place deep scleral sutures in a hypotonic eye without accidental penetration of the choroid. If the eye is soft, the assistant must increase the pressure to a nearly normal level by gentle indentation.

If the break is located under a rectus muscle, the assistant can aid in the placement of sutures by retracting the muscle with a muscle hook. Alternatively, the muscle can be temporarily tenotomized. Finally, a circumferential explant can be used instead of a radial one.

It is easier to stabilize the globe if the suture needle moves away from rather than toward the muscle grasped. Therefore, if a double-armed suture is used, both bites are made from anterior to posterior. An added benefit of tying the suture posteriorly is that Tenon's capsule is thicker there, and late erosion of the suture is therefore unlikely. Scleral bites should be both deep and long, so that the suture will not erode out of the sclera postoperatively. A spatula

needle must be used. Its tip is introduced slowly into the sclera. When the proper depth has been reached, the needle is carefully pushed along between scleral lamellae. Proper depth can be verified by gently lifting the needle while keeping it parallel to the sclera. The needle must not be allowed to lose its depth because it is difficult and dangerous to regain depth once it has been lost. When the bite has been completed, the surgeon should push the suture through to its hub and remove it following the curve of the needle. If the spatula needle is twisted while still in the sclera, the sharp edge may cut through the choroid and cause bleeding. If it cuts through the overlying sclera, it will weaken it.

Radial Explants. The indentation of the scleral buckle should extend 1 to 2 mm beyond the margins of the break. A 5-mm sponge will adequately close a break 3 mm wide; a 7.5 × 5.5-mm sponge, a break 5 mm wide. Larger breaks require two sponges placed side by side. The height of the indentation is determined not only by the diameter of the explant, but also by the distance between the arms of the mattress suture. How tightly the mattress suture is tied is also important. We place the arms of the suture 2 to 3 mm farther apart than the width of the sponge (Fig. 12–19). For small holes one suture is adequate. For larger breaks two are needed. To prevent the fishmouth phenomenon, we begin the posterior bite at the level of the apex of the tear and carry it 3 mm posteriorly. The anterior suture starts 2 mm anterior to the horns of the tear.

Radial explants are preferred over circumferential explants for closing wide horseshoe tears because they cause much less fishmouthing of the posterior edge.[53] In addition, for very posterior breaks it is easier to place the sutures necessary for a radial explant than those required for a circumferential explant.

Circumferential Explants. A circumferential explant is indicated for wide retinal breaks (80 to 90 degrees), for multiple breaks at different distances from the ora serrata (Fig. 12–20), and for detachments in which no break is found. The width of the explant depends on the anterior-posterior *length*, not width, of the break. The sutures are asymmetrically placed so that the hole will lie on the crest or anterior slope of the buckle. The posterior bite of the mattress suture usually must be made 3 to 4 mm posterior to the localizing mark of the apex of the tear.

Using similar principles, solid silicone can be used as an explant.

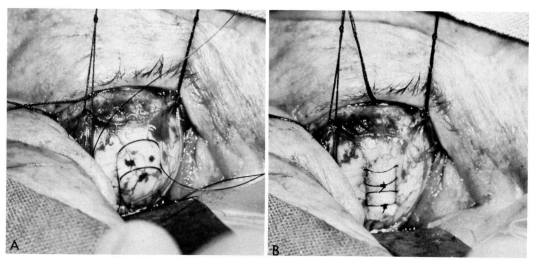

FIGURE 12–19. *A*, Suture placement for a flap tear. *B*, Sutures tied over the sponge.

Implants

An implant is a foreign material placed within the sclera to obtain a buckling effect. Its insertion necessitates a lamellar scleral dissection procedure. To ensure proper closure of retinal breaks, the scleral bed of the lamellar dissection should extend 3 to 4 mm beyond each edge of the break or breaks. A circumferential incision is made through the most posterior localization

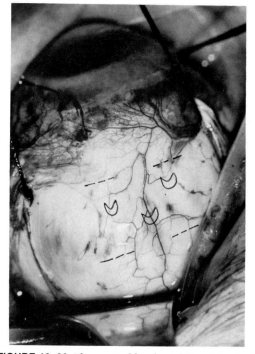

FIGURE 12–20. Three retinal breaks at different levels. A circumferential explant is required. Dashed lines indicate location of mattress sutures.

mark on the sclera. Gentle cutting strokes are used. To avoid cutting too deeply, the wound is spread frequently by a lateral movement of the blade. The proper level has been reached when the blue color that denotes the choroid is seen. A scraping motion is used to begin the dissection of the posterior flap. After a small flap has been made, it is grasped with a forceps and pulled; traction on the flap facilitates the dissection (Fig. 12–21*A*).

Sometimes vortex veins are encountered when the retinal breaks are posteriorly located. Although the vortices should be preserved if at all possible, the surgeon should not compromise posterior dissection if it is necessary to seal a break. One or two vortices can be sacrificed if necessary, especially in younger people. Elderly patients and those with a high degree of myopia are more prone to complications such as choroidal bleeding and anterior segment necrosis. First, the extrabulbar portion of the vein to be sacrificed is carefully cauterized. We then cauterize the intrascleral branches. Repeated diathermy as the dissection continues usually prevents bleeding.

After the anterior flap has been dissected, the blunt conical electrode is used to apply staggered rows of diathermy lesions in the scleral bed (Fig. 12–21*B*).[85, 86] The power of the diathermy machine should be set so that a short application of the electrode results in slight scleral shrinkage and desiccation. Too high a setting unnecessarily destroys tissues. If the surgeon prefers cryotherapy, he must apply it before the bed is dissected or he may penetrate the thin sclera with the probe. If a permanent indentation by an implant is desired, an encir-

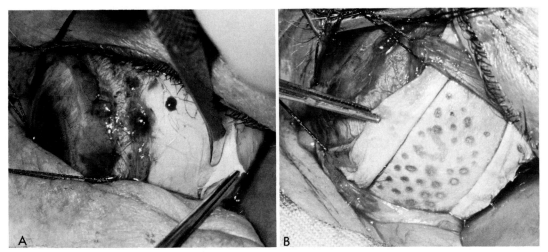

FIGURE 12–21. *A,* Traction on the posterior flap facilitates the dissection. *B,* Anterior and posterior flaps of the lamellar dissection have been completed. Diathermy has been applied in staggered rows.

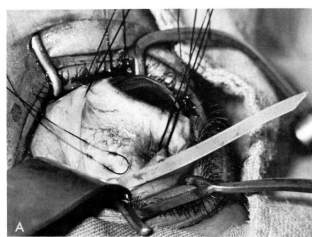

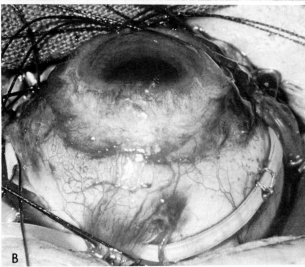

FIGURE 12–22. *A,* Mattress suture placed in the sclera to anchor an encircling band. *B,* Encircling band anchored by a mattress suture.

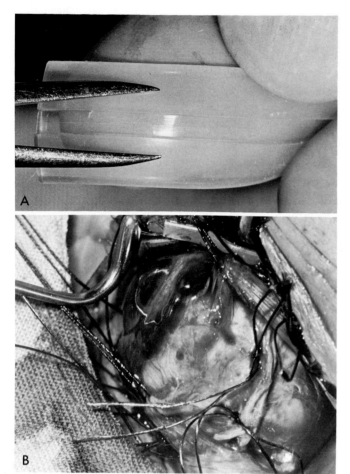

FIGURE 12–23. *A,* A solid silicone piece about to be trimmed to fit the bed. A #40 band will fit in the groove on the piece. *B,* The scleral flaps are closed with mattress sutures over the silicone piece and encircling band.

cling procedure is necessary (Fig. 12–22). After drainage, the scleral flaps are closed over the implant (Fig. 12–23).

Drainage of Subretinal Fluid

Complications

Since Custodis,[14, 15] the drainage of subretinal fluid has not been considered essential in all retinal detachment surgery. We believe that drainage should be avoided whenever possible because its complications result in postoperative loss of vision in 1 to 2 per cent of the cases in which it is performed. The four major complications are choroidal bleeding, retinal incarceration (Fig. 12–24), loss of formed vitreous, and retinal perforation. When vessels are lacerated by the drainage perforation, choroidal bleeding may result, especially in high myopes, in elderly patients, and in patients with Ehlers-Danlos syndrome. If the blood accumulates under the fovea, the eye almost never regains central visual acuity. Retinal incarceration and loss of formed vitreous can both cause macular pucker. Moreover, vitreous loss is followed by a high incidence of massive periretinal proliferation (MPP).[41] Retinal perforation by the drainage instrument usually does not cause postoperative visual loss, but does require treatment and buckling of the iatrogenic hole.

Indications for Use

Despite its complications, drainage of subretinal fluid must be performed in some cases. Eyes with poor retinal circulation, staphylomatous sclerae, or recent intraocular surgery require a drainage procedure because the indentation of the scleral buckle causes a rise in intraocular pressure that could close the central retinal artery or rupture the globe. Drainage of the fluid softens the eye and allows it to accommodate the indentation without a precipitous rise in pressure. Because of their poor outflow facility, glaucomatous eyes also require a drain-

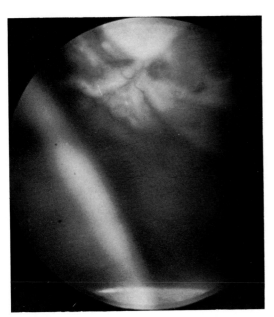

FIGURE 12–24. Retinal incarceration at drainage site.

age procedure; without it they may sustain damage before their pressure has returned to normal. When the retinal break cannot be closed at surgery and it is apparent that vitreous traction (as in massive periretinal proliferation or diabetic traction detachment) will prevent postoperative settling of the retina, the subretinal fluid should be drained. Finally, drainage of the subretinal fluid is indicated in cases of retinal detachment with giant tears because such detachments usually do not settle with bedrest and because space must be created for the intraocular gas or air often used in their therapy.

Although Lincoff[50, 52] and others[10, 38, 75, 90] believe that most other cases can be managed without drainage of subretinal fluid, we and the majority of retinal surgeons choose to drain in a high percentage of cases.[76, 104] The reason for this is that nondrainage procedures have a lower initial rate of reoperation.[11] Common causes of failure in nondrainage procedures are inadequate indentation, inaccurate placement of the scleral buckle, vitreous traction, and meridional folds (fishmouthing). Although the reoperation is usually successful, it has its own complications. First of all, if drainage is required, the inflammation caused by the initial operation increases the likelihood of choroidal bleeding. Second, postoperative infection and explant extrusion are more common after reoperations. In addition, the patient again faces the danger of anesthesia and the psychic trauma of surgery,

as well as having his hospital stay lengthened. Finally, some patients refuse the reoperation.

Technique of Drainage of Subretinal Fluid

Because there are few large choroidal blood vessels just above or below the medial or lateral rectus muscles and under the superior or inferior rectus muscles, these are prime drainage sites. The chances of hemorrhage are further minimized if the choroid is perforated anteriorly. It is best to drain through a sclera that will be buckled by the intended implant or explant; then, if the retina should be perforated or incarcerated at the drainage site, the repair will not entail placing additional sutures in a soft eye. Drainage under a large bulla of subretinal fluid allows a good quantity of fluid to drain before the retina settles over the drainage site and closes it. It also helps to avoid retinal perforation by the drainage needle. One final consideration in selecting a drainage site is that the stiff retina of a fixed fold will seldom incarcerate.

Once the drainage site has been selected, transillumination can be used to reveal the presence of large choroidal blood vessels. This is especially helpful if the drainage site is located posteriorly. The surgeon must be especially careful with the occasional rhegmatogenous retinal detachment with shifting fluid. The fluid may move away from the selected drainage site and the retina may be perforated accidentally.

It is important that the eye be normotensive for drainage. If the intraocular pressure is too high, it must be lowered by administration of acetazolamide or mannitol, or by an anterior chamber paracentesis. Otherwise, when the choroid is perforated, sudden decompression can cause choroidal hemorrhage or rapid evacuation of the subretinal fluid followed by retinal or vitreous incarceration. If the intraocular pressure is too low, the assistant indents the eye with a cotton-tipped applicator to restore the pressure nearly to normal, thus facilitating scleral dissection and choroidal perforation.

Best drainage is obtained if no scleral fibers overlie the choroid at the drainage site. In a lamellar dissection procedure a radial cutdown to the choroid is made through the prepared lamellar bed. If fluid must be drained outside of the bed, or if an explant is to be used, we expose the choroid in the bed of a small triangular scleral flap (Fig. 12–25) or simply through a radial cutdown. A longer cutdown provides better exposure, allowing safe removal of the deep scleral fibers. The thicker the sclera, the

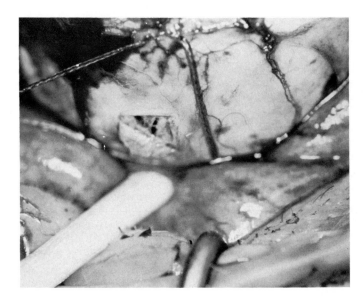

FIGURE 12–25. Drainage in an explant procedure. The choroid is exposed in the base of a triangular scleral flap.

longer the cutdown necessary. If the drainage site is made in a lamellar bed, no suture is needed to close it. If it will be under an explant, the scleral flap or cutdown is closed with an absorbable suture (Fig. 12–26). If the drainage site will not be covered by an implant or an explant, it should be closed with a nonabsorbable suture. Before perforation, a 20-diopter lens is used to examine the choroid for large choroidal blood vessels. In order to further reduce the possibility of hemorrhage, the exposed choroid is next treated with applications of low-intensity diathermy, using the blunt conical electrode (Fig. 12–27).[23]

The choroid is then perforated with the diathermy needle electrode, a 27-gauge hypodermic needle, a tapered suture needle, or a Ziegler knife. Before the perforation the surgeon must verify that the pressure in the eye is not elevated. A gentle thrust penetrating 1 mm is sufficient to perforate. Alternatively, the argon laser can be used for the choroidotomy.[6]

When the subretinal fluid begins to drain, gentle indentation of the globe opposite the drainage site helps to shift subretinal fluid toward it. Excessive pressure on the eye to force out subretinal fluid may cause retinal incarceration and must be avoided. Traction on the edge of the scleral flap with a small forceps helps to hold the sclera and choroid away from the retina, reducing the chances of incarceration.

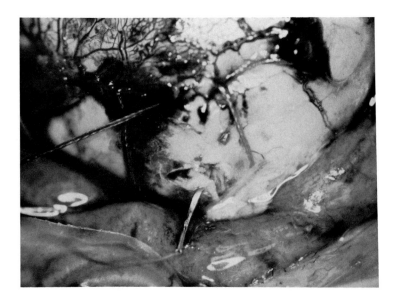

FIGURE 12–26. After drainage, the scleral flap, which will lie under the explant, is closed with an absorbable suture.

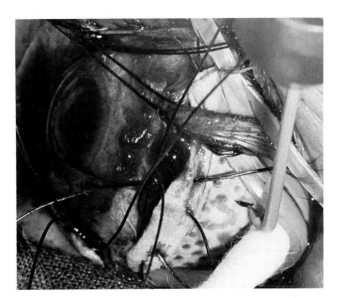

FIGURE 12–27. Drainage in a lamellar dissection bed. The exposed choroid is coagulated with diathermy before perforation.

When little or no subretinal fluid remains, a small hemorrhage or pigment granules may appear at the drainage site. When the drainage stops, the fundus must be inspected to see if there is subretinal fluid over the drainage site. If there is, gentle lateral traction on the scleral flap may allow further drainage. Occasionally another choroidal perforation is required. It is almost never necessary to drain until all of the subretinal fluid is gone or even until the break is flat on the buckle, so long as the buckle is properly placed and of adequate height. When adequate fluid has been drained, the suture over the drainage site is immediately tied. This prevents the retinal incarceration that might otherwise result from a sudden elevation in intraocular pressure caused by manipulation of the globe. If the perforation site is in a lamellar dissection bed, the scleral flap suture closest to it is immediately closed to prevent retinal incarceration.

Encircling Procedures

Vitreous traction can be permanently reduced by a silicone band or sponge that encircles and constricts the eye. The introduction of encircling procedures is one of Schepens' invaluable contributions to retinal surgery.[28, 87] Encircling is indicated if there is evidence of early massive periretinal proliferation, such as fixed folds or strong vitreous traction. If additional indentation is needed (e.g., to close large breaks), solid silicone or sponge explants are placed under the encircling band. Aphakic retinal detachments usually receive encircling procedures both because of their higher incidence of massive periretinal proliferation and because they characteristically have small breaks, some of which may be missed.

Encircling can also be used when no break can be found. In these cases the posterior vitreous base is treated with cryotherapy for the whole length of the detached retina. An encircling silicone band or sponge is then placed so as to buckle the posterior vitreous base.

The encircling element (usually a 2-mm wide silicone band) is placed at the posterior vitreous base (2 to 3 mm posterior to the ora serrata). The band is anchored to the sclera by mattress sutures (Fig. 12–22B) and is tied with a suture. The surgeon should try to obtain an indentation of from 1 to 2 mm. Excessive indentation may cause severe postoperative pain or anterior segment necrosis.

Intraoperative Problems

Central Retinal Artery Occlusion

If, after retrobulbar anesthesia, the eye becomes rock hard owing to an expanding hemorrhage in the closed orbital space, the surgeon must act immediately to avoid retinal artery occlusion. He decompresses the orbit by a lateral canthotomy and by a rapid 360-degree peritomy. This is a rare complication of retrobulbar anesthesia.

Small Pupil

If the pupil will not dilate preoperatively, a sector iridectomy can be performed just before the retinal detachment surgery. Xenon or argon photocoagulation can also be used to widen the pupil. Several small burns 2 mm from the pupil will shrink the iris, pulling the pupil open.

Hazy Cornea

Corneal transparency may be decreased by contact with the solutions used for sterile preparation of the operative field. Excessive scleral depression during localization or treatment may cause epithelial edema. A clearer view of the fundus can be obtained if the corneal epithelium is then removed with a rounded blade. The epithelium usually heals postoperatively in 1 to 2 days, though healing may take longer in diabetics.

Posteriorly Located Breaks

Sometimes it is difficult to place sutures for posteriorly located breaks. Adequate exposure is usually provided by a lateral canthotomy. If this does not suffice, disinsertion of a rectus muscle may be necessary. A traction suture placed through the stump of the muscle enables the surgeon to manipulate the eye in order to obtain the desired exposure. Breaks in the posterior pole itself are best managed by vitrectomy techniques.

Oblique Muscles

In order to place an explant correctly, it may be necessary to put a scleral suture where the superior or inferior oblique muscle inserts into the globe. If the muscle cannot be adequately retracted, it should be partially disinserted to give the surgeon an unobstructed view of the sclera.

Staphyloma

Placing sutures into very thin sclera is dangerous because the choroid may accidentally be perforated. Moreover, the sutures may pull out postoperatively. The scleral sutures should be placed in adjacent thicker sclera. Because the mattress suture is then wider than actually required, one must use a larger explant than is needed to close the break. Silicone sponges should be used over staphylomatous sclera because they are less likely to intrude into the eye than is solid silicone. When a true staphyloma exists, the surgeon must be careful not to raise the intraocular pressure too high during the procedure, or the globe may rupture.

Premature Drainage

If the needle accidentally penetrates the choroid while sutures are being placed, subretinal fluid may drain, causing the eye to become markedly hypotonic. The suture should be removed and its replacement suture positioned so that the accidental drainage site will later fall under the buckle. Pressure with a cotton-tipped applicator over the accidental drainage site can be used to make the eye firm enough for correct placement of the remaining sutures. If too much fluid has drained, even this will not suffice, and an intraocular injection of saline solution will be necessary to restore the intraocular pressure. If a deep suture perforates attached retina, the area should be treated with cryotherapy and scleral buckling.

Increased Intraocular Pressure Owing to Indentation from the Scleral Buckle

If a nondrainage procedure is anticipated, intravenous acetazolamide and topical timolol can be given before surgery, to lower the intraocular pressure. Even with these precautions, as the surgeon ties the scleral sutures he must constantly monitor the intraocular pressure. An estimate can be obtained by palpation ("finger tension") or by indentation with a muscle hook. More accurate readings can be taken with the Schiøtz or Perkins tonometer. If the pressure is high, the surgeon must inspect the optic disc to see whether the central retinal artery is pulsating or occluded. If the media are hazy, arterial patency can be confirmed by observing the artery while pressing gently on the eye. If pulsations can be produced, it is apparent that the artery is patent.

If all of the scleral sutures cannot be tied because of increased intraocular pressure, several maneuvers are possible. First, if the eyelids have been pushed behind the globe, decreasing the available orbital space, they should be pulled forward and the globe reposited. Second, with nonglaucomatous eyes the surgeon must be patient enough to wait for the excess fluid to drain through the trabecular meshwork. In phakic patients an anterior chamber paracentesis is helpful. This is not advised for aphakic eyes because vitreous may become incarcerated in the wound. If these measures are insufficient, the surgeon can loosen some of the sutures or decrease the constriction of the encircling band. A last resort is vitreous aspiration.

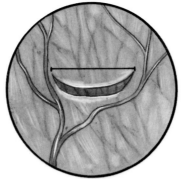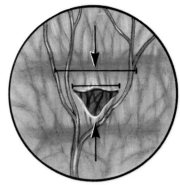

FIGURE 12–28. The fishmouth phenomenon. *Left*, Flap tear in detached retina. Solid line indicates width of the tear. *Right*, A circumferential buckle (between arrows) compresses the tear (large line indicates original width), keeping its posterior edge open.

The Fishmouth Phenomenon

The scleral buckling may result in a meridional fold formed by redundant retina on the posterior slope of the buckle. The buckle, in this case, actually prevents reattachment (Fig. 12–28). It keeps the break open and allows a free passage of subretinal fluid posteriorly. This phenomenon, called "fishmouthing," is more likely to occur with circumferential than with radial buckling.[53] If the break is superiorly located, an intravitreal injection of air will close the break. If not, the meridional folding can be reduced by decreasing the height of the buckle (by loosening the sutures). Another approach is to place a radial element under the circumferential buckle.

Intraocular Air or Gas

Indications for Use

Tamponade of a retinal break with air or gas temporarily closes a break as effectively as a scleral buckle.[74] The choroid/pigment epithelium then absorbs the subretinal fluid, effecting contact between the treated retinal pigment epithelium and the sensory retina. Intraocular air or gas is also useful in closing giant tears or, as mentioned earlier, tears showing the fishmouthing phenomenon and posterior pole tears.

In some cases in which drainage of subretinal fluid is attempted near large tears, liquid vitreous can pass through the tear and out of the eye. The eye becomes very soft, but the amount of fluid under the retina remains the same. In these cases we close the drainage site, place the scleral buckle, and inject air to tamponade the retinal hole. Once the hole has been so closed, the subretinal fluid is absorbed.

When the tamponading effect is needed to last longer than 2 days, gas should be used rather than air. Sulfur hexafluoride is an inert gas that remains in the vitreous for 7 to 10 days.[22, 44] Perfluoropropane (C_3F_8) lasts for approximately 5 weeks.[56]

Technique

Sterile air can be obtained by drawing room air through a Millipore filter. After the filter is removed, the air is injected into the vitreous cavity through a 30-gauge needle. The injection of intraocular air or gas is made 4 to 5 mm from the surgical limbus, through the pars plana. It is important that a sharp needle be used and that the needle have passed through the nonpigmented epithelium of the pars plana before the injection. This must be confirmed by indirect ophthalmoscopy. As the air is injected, the assistant monitors intraocular pressure to prevent excessive injection.

Complications

Hemorrhage from such injections is rare but can occur. The surgeon must be careful not to strike the lens with the needle as it enters the eye. If the needle does not pass cleanly through the pars plana epithelium before the air is injected, a dialysis may occur. If too much air or gas is injected, the excessive rise in intraocular pressure may occlude the central retinal artery, rupture the globe through a weakened area, or tear out scleral sutures. Although fibrous ingrowth through the site of penetration is rare, it may occur. Finally, before injection of the air or gas, the surgeon must make certain that nitrous oxide is not being used for anesthesia.[24] The nitrous oxide would quickly diffuse into the injected air or gas bubble, and would cause a marked elevation in the intraocular pressure.

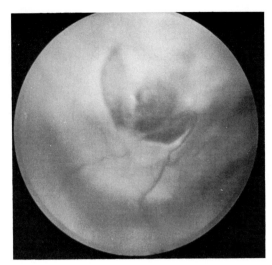

FIGURE 12–29. Flap tear correctly placed on a radial scleral buckle.

Final Inspection and Adjustments

If all of the subretinal fluid has been drained, it is easy to determine whether the scleral buckle has been correctly placed (Fig. 12–29). If subretinal fluid remains under the hole, the surgeon can push gently on the scleral buckle. The increased indentation helps him to assess the buckle's relation to the break.

When an implant is being used and the buckle has not been placed far enough posteriorly, it is necessary to dissect farther back and use a larger implant than previously intended. If an explant is not properly placed anteriorly or posteriorly, the surgeon can place a new scleral suture and remove the old one. Finally, if the posterior edge of an encircling explant is near to but not fully buckling the hole, a trimmed piece of sponge can be slipped under the explant. This technique is particularly helpful in cases in which there is fishmouthing of the posterior edge of the break.

It is important not to trim a radial explant until adequate closure of the retinal break has been confirmed. If it has not been correctly placed posteriorly or anteriorly, an additional suture can be easily placed. If a radial sponge has not been placed in the correct radial meridian, it is necessary to replace the original mattress suture. Usually it is best to place the new scleral suture before removing the old. This will maintain the intraocular pressure so that the new sutures can be safely placed.

When it has been ascertained that the scleral buckle has been correctly placed and that the intraocular pressure is not too elevated, a culture sample is taken and the orbit is irrigated with an antibiotic solution. Separate closure of Tenon's capsule is important, to prevent late extrusions (Fig. 12–30). We attach Tenon's capsule to the tendon of a rectus muscle in each quadrant. The conjunctiva is closed with plain catgut suture (Fig. 12–31). Atropine and antibiotic ointment are then applied, and the eye is patched with a semipressure dressing to reduce postoperative eyelid edema.

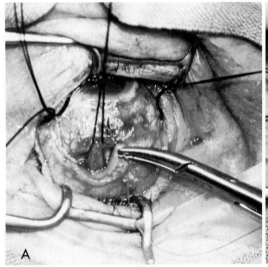
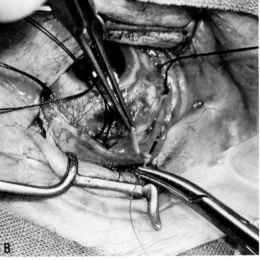

FIGURE 12–30. *A,* Closure of the peritomy. The posterior flap is stretched forward by a suture needle so that Tenon's capsule can be firmly grasped. *B,* Tenon's capsule is anchored to the rectus muscle tendon in all four quadrants.

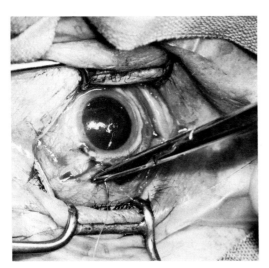

FIGURE 12–31. The relaxing incision is closed with an absorbable suture.

POSTOPERATIVE MANAGEMENT

Postoperatively, the patient is mobilized as quickly as possible.[7] If there is air or sulfur hexafluoride in the vitreous cavity, the patient is positioned so that the air rises against the break to tamponade it. Bilateral patches are occasionally used after nondrainage procedures if the retina has not settled. Atropine 1% is given twice daily, and an antibiotic-corticosteroid mixture is given three times daily. Most patients require only mild analgesics.

The patients are discharged on the third or fourth postoperative day and are told to return in 1 week for follow-up examination.

COMPLICATIONS

Early Complications

Acute Angle-Closure Glaucoma

Choroidal congestion resulting from the surgery can cause a forward rotation of the ciliary body and closure of the filtration angle.[78] The consequent increased intraocular pressure causes pain and corneal edema. This condition may be misdiagnosed because the central portion of the anterior chamber may remain deep. The diagnosis is made by applanation tonometry. Schiøtz tonometry may give a falsely low reading because of decreased scleral rigidity. Because pupillary block is not a contributing factor, treatment with pilocarpine or with iri-

dectomy is not effective. Proper management includes the use of acetazolamide, timolol, topical or systemic corticosteroids, and, if necessary, mannitol. Sometimes it is necessary to loosen the encircling band.

Symblepharon

The eye must be carefully inspected for adhesions between the bulbar and palpebral conjunctiva, especially after a lateral canthotomy has been performed. Early adhesions can be broken with a glass rod.

Anterior Segment Necrosis

Anterior segment necrosis is common after operations in which three muscles have been disinserted,[25] three vortex veins have been occluded,[36] diathermy has been applied over the long ciliary arteries, or a tight posteriorly located encircling band has been used.[17, 18, 108] Patients with sickle cell disease are especially prone to this condition.[83] The earliest finding is striate keratopathy. Later there is corneal edema without elevated intraocular pressure. Many patients have marked chemosis. A diagnostic finding is white flakes floating in the anterior chamber or deposited on the lens. Large keratic precipitates may be present. Late findings are hypotony owing to atrophy of the ciliary processes, an irregularly dilated pupil, iris atrophy, posterior synechiae, and cataract.[5, 94] If anterior segment necrosis is suspected, the patient should be treated with high doses of topical and systemic corticosteroids. The encircling band should be loosened.

Infection

The risk of infection can be decreased by soaking the sponges in an antibiotic solution before suturing them to the globe.[1, 20] If infection occurs, the best indicator is unusually severe pain. In addition, there is marked chemosis and injection of the conjunctiva, mucopurulent discharge, and progressive swelling of the lid. Some patients have numerous inflammatory cells in the vitreous. A localized exudate over a scleral buckle is a particularly ominous sign, for it may indicate early scleral necrosis and endophthalmitis.

If these signs of intraocular infection are present, pending culture results, we treat with systemic methacillin and gentamicin and topical broad-spectrum antibiotics. If there are no signs of intraocular involvement, we use topical antibiotics alone. The most common bacteria involved are *Staphylococcus aureus, Pseudo-*

monas, and *Proteus.* The infection cannot be cured with antibiotics alone; the implant or explant must be removed.[33, 50, 82, 89, 97, 103]

Choroidal Detachments

Choroidal detachments are common after retinal detachment surgery, especially in elderly or aphakic patients. They are also seen in patients with broad or posteriorly located buckles and in patients who have undergone reoperations.

The choroidal fluid characteristically accumulates during the first 3 to 4 days and then remains stable for 1 to 2 weeks. Because of decreased aqueous secretion, the intraocular pressure remains low despite apparent occlusion of the filtration angle. Treatment is seldom indicated, as the fluid nearly always reabsorbs spontaneously.

Failure to Reattach the Retina

The most common cause of failure of retinal detachment surgery is massive periretinal proliferation. Metaplastic pigment epithelial and glial cells proliferate on the retina and on vitreous strands and then contract, preventing settling of the retina or causing its redetachment.[48, 62–64, 71, 84] The goal of the reoperation is to relieve vitreous traction. If a higher scleral buckle is unsuccessful, vitrectomy is indicated.[62, 66, 95]

If any break in the detached retina has been missed, the surgery cannot be successful. If the subretinal fluid has been drained, new fluid will accumulate; if it has not, the retina will not settle. The only remedy is a reoperation to close the missed break.

Reoperation is also necessary if the cause of the failure is an inaccurately placed buckle. On the other hand, if the break remains elevated over a correctly placed scleral buckle, reoperation may be avoided. If the hole is nearly closed, argon laser or xenon arc photocoagulation may seal the break, repairing the detachment.[13] If the break is superiorly located, an intravitreal air injection may tamponade it so that the subretinal fluid is absorbed. If these remedies fail, drainage of the subretinal fluid is indicated.

If a reoperation is performed within 2 weeks, opening the conjunctiva and Tenon's capsule is swiftly accomplished because these tissues have not yet scarred down to the sclera. The surgeon must take great care not to inadvertently penetrate the eye through a drainage site or through sclera thinned by a lamellar scleral dissection and diathermy.

It is difficult to assess, in cases of failure,

when and where reapplication of cryotherapy or diathermy is necessary. If the sensory retina has been thoroughly frozen in the first operation, tight junctions will probably form between the pigment epithelium and Müller's cells without retreatment (see above). However, if only the pigment epithelium was frozen in the original operation, retreatment probably is indicated after 4 to 5 days. By this time the treated pigment epithelium will have been replaced by pigment epithelial cells sliding over from untreated areas, and a firm adhesion will not result.

Late Complications

Refractive Error

Encircling procedures usually cause a slight increase in myopia. Segmental buckling procedures may cause astigmatism.[29] Sometimes an irregular astigmatism that cannot be corrected by spectacles is seen after radial explants have been used.[9]

Muscle Imbalance

Disturbances in ocular motility are especially common when a vertical muscle has been disinserted,[43] when a large implant or explant has been placed under a rectus muscle,[79, 92, 102] or when Tenon's capsule has been broken.[107] This most commonly occurs in the muscle sheath 10 mm posterior to the limbus. Scarring then causes loss of elasticity in the extraconal septae.[77] Excessive scarring after reoperations is another important contributing factor. Because many patients have temporary diplopia after a scleral buckling procedure, it is advisable to wait at least 6 months before considering corrective muscle surgery.[65] It is then important to determine whether the diplopia is due to scar tissue preventing rotation of the eye, or to the underaction of a muscle that is adherent to the globe. Forced ductions aid greatly in this determination.[79]

Extrusion of Implants or Explants

Pain, mucopurulent discharge, and subconjunctival hemorrhage are all signs of an extruding explant. In some cases mechanical erosion of the sponge through the conjunctiva probably precedes the infection. In others the reverse occurs. If a sponge explant has been used in addition to an encircling band, we generally do not remove the band or the sutures when removing the explant. Fifteen to 30 per cent of retinas will redetach after removal of the scleral buckle.[33, 50, 58, 82, 89, 97, 103, 106]

Macular Pucker

Macular pucker, which usually occurs 6 to 8 weeks after surgery, can ruin an otherwise good visual result.[32, 60, 99] In many cases the macular pucker probably results from the same vitreous traction that caused the retinal detachment. Other contributing factors are loss of formed vitreous at surgery, retinal incarceration, subretinal hemorrhage, or vitreous hemorrhage.[99] Some authors believe that macular pucker is more common after diathermy procedures than after cryotherapy.[32]

Late Redetachment of the Retina

In patients observed at the Wills Eye Hospital the most common cause of late redetachment of the retina has been found to be a new break posterior to an encircling band. New breaks can also be seen overlying an encircling band or in quadrants without a buckle.[91]

We have found that late redetachments caused by new breaks have an excellent prognosis for successful repair. Extensive operations are not necessary; all that is required is to close the new breaks with a local explant. Careful surgery is required to expose the sclera, especially if the original operation involved a lamellar scleral dissection and diathermy.

A less common cause of late redetachment is reopening of the original break by increased vitreous traction. This may be caused by incomplete diathermy or cryotherapy, by extrusion of the scleral sutures, or by removal of the implant or explant. A higher scleral buckle is usually successful; rarely, vitrectomy is necessary.

PROGNOSIS

Anatomical Reattachment

With current techniques, 95 per cent of detached retinas can be repaired. Success rates for different types of retinal detachment vary as follows:

1. *Excellent prognosis* (nearly 100 per cent): detachments caused by dialysis, or by small or round holes; detachments with demarcation lines; detachments with minimal subretinal fluid

2. *Slightly poorer prognosis* (90 per cent): aphakic detachments,[2, 72] total detachments, detachments with associated detachment of nonpigmented epithelium of pars plana

3. *Poor prognosis* (50 to 75 per cent): detachments with associated choroidal detachment, detachments with breaks larger than 180 degrees

Postoperative Visual Acuity

Overall, approximately 50 per cent of patients will regain a visual acuity of 20/50 (6/15) or better; 25 per cent, 20/60 to 20/100; and 25 per cent, 20/200 or worse.[72] Postoperative visual acuity chiefly depends on whether or not and how long the macula was detached before surgery.[29–31] When the macula has detached, necrosis of photoreceptors may prevent good postoperative visual acuity. Seventy-five per cent of patients with a macular detachment of less than 1 week's duration will obtain a final visual acuity of 20/70 (6/21) or better, as opposed to 50 per cent with a macular detachment of 1 to 8 weeks' duration.[30]

The prognosis for vision is far better in cases in which the macula has not detached, though up to 15 per cent of these patients lose vision from macular pucker or cystoid macular edema.[30, 100, 105] Obviously, intraoperative complications (see above) also affect the final visual acuity.

REFERENCES

1. Arribas, N. P., Olk, R. J., Schertzer, M., et al.: Preoperative antibiotic soaking of silicone sponges: Does it make a difference? Ophthalmology, 91:1684, 1984.
2. Ashrafzadeh, M. T., Schepens, C. L., Elzeneiny, I. I., et al.: Aphakic and phakic retinal detachment. Arch. Ophthalmol., 89:476, 1973.
3. Benson, W. E.: Prophylactic therapy of retinal breaks. Surv. Ophthalmol., 22:41, 1977.
4. Benson, W. E.: Differential diagnosis of retinal detachment. *In* Retinal Detachment, Diagnosis and Management. Hagerstown, Md., Harper & Row, 1979, Chapter 5.
5. Boniuk, M., Zimmerman, L. E.: Pathological anatomy of complications of retinal surgery. *In* Schepens, C. L., Regan, C. D. J. (eds.): Controversial Aspects of the Management of Retinal Detachment. Boston, Little, Brown & Co., 1965, pp. 263–311.
6. Bovino, J. A., Marcus, D. F., Nelsen, P. T.: Argon laser choroidotomy for drainage of subretinal fluid. Arch. Ophthalmol., 103:443, 1985.
7. Bovino, J. A., Marcus, D. F.: Physical activity after retinal detachment surgery. Am. J. Ophthalmol., 98:171, 1984.
8. Brihaye, M., Oosterhuis, J. A.: Experimental cryoapplication with variations in the pressure exerted on the sclera. Ophthalmol. Res., 3:129, 1972.

9. Burton, T. C.: Irregular astigmatism following episcleral buckling procedures. Arch. Ophthalmol., 90:447, 1973.

10. Chignell, A. H.: Retinal detachment surgery without drainage of subretinal fluid. Am. J. Ophthalmol., 77:1, 1974.

11. Chignell, A. H., Fison, L. G., Davies, E. W. G., et al.: Failure in retinal detachment surgery. Br. J. Ophthalmol., 57:525, 1973.

12. Curtin, V. T.: Management of retinal detachment. In Duane, T. D. (ed.): Clinical Ophthalmology, Vol. 5, Chapter 16, p. 2. Hagerstown, Md., Harper & Row, 1978.

13. Curtin, V. T., Norton, E. W. D., Gass, J. D. M.: Photocoagulation: its use in the prevention of reoperations after scleral buckling. Trans. Am. Acad. Ophthalmol. Otolaryngol., 71:432, 1967.

14. Custodis, E.: Bedeutet die Plombenaufnähung auf die Sklera einen Fortschritt im der operativen Behandlung der Netzhautablösung? Ber. Dtsch. Ophthalmol. Ges., 58:102, 1953.

15. Custodis, E.: Scleral buckling without excision and with polyviol implant. In Schepens, C. L. (ed.): Importance of the Vitreous Body in Retina Surgery with Special Emphasis on Reoperations. St. Louis, C. V. Mosby Co., 1960, p. 175.

16. Delany, W. V., Jr., Oates, R. P: Retinal detachment in the second eye. Arch. Ophthalmol., 96:629, 1978.

17. Diddle, K. R., Ernest, J. T.: Uveal blood flow after 360 degrees constriction in rabbit. Arch. Ophthalmol., 98:719, 1980.

18. Dobbie, J. G.: Circulatory changes in the eye associated with retinal detachment and its repair. Trans. Am. Ophthalmol. Soc., 78:503, 1980.

19. Dobbie, J. G.: A study of the intraocular fluid dynamics in retinal detachment. Arch. Ophthalmol., 69:159, 1963.

20. Doft, B. H., Lipkowitz, J., Kowalski, R., et al.: An experimental model to assess factors associated with scleral buckle infection. Retina, 3:212, 1983.

21. Fernan, S. S.: Electron microscopy study of cryogenic chorioretinal adhesions. Am. J. Ophthalmol., 81:823, 1976.

22. Fineberg, E., Machemer, R., Sullivan, P., et al.: Sulfur hexafluoride in the owl monkey vitreous cavity. Am. J. Ophthalmol., 79:67, 1975.

23. Freeman, H. M., Schepens, C. L.: Innovations in the technique of drainage of subretinal fluid: Transillumination and choroidal diathermy. Trans. Am. Acad. Ophthalmol. Otolaryngol., 78:829, 1974.

24. Fuller, D., Lewis, M. L.: Nitrous oxide anesthesia with gas in the vitreous cavity. Am. J. Ophthalmol., 80:778, 1975.

25. Girard, L. J., Beltranena, F.: Early and late complications of extensive muscle surgery. Arch. Ophthalmol., 64:576, 1960.

26. Gonin, J.: Guérison opératoires des décollements rétiniens. Rev. Gén. Ophthalmol., 37:295, 1923.

27. Gonin, J.: Le Décollement de la Rétine. Lausanne, Librairie Payot, 1934.

28. Griffith, R. D., Ryan, E. A., Hilton, G. F.: Primary retinal detachment without apparent breaks. Am. J. Ophthalmol., 81:420, 1976.

29. Grupposo, S.: Visual results after scleral buckling with silicone implant. In Schepens, C. L., Regan, C. D. J. (eds.): Controversial Aspects of the Management of Retinal Detachment. Boston, Little, Brown, & Co., 1965, pp. 254–363.

30. Grupposo, S. S.: Visual acuity following surgery for retinal detachment. Arch. Ophthalmol., 93:327, 1975.

31. Gundry, M. F., Davies, E.W.G.: Recovery of visual acuity after retinal detachment surgery. Am. J. Ophthalmol., 77:310, 1974.

32. Hagler, W. S., Aturaliya, U.: Macular pucker after retinal detachment surgery. Br. J. Ophthalmol., 55:451, 1971.

33. Hahn, Y. S., Lincoff, A., Lincoff, H., Kreissig, I.: Infection after sponge implantation for scleral buckling. Am. J. Ophthalmol., 87:180, 1979.

34. Hamilton, A. M., Taylor, W.: Significance of pigment granules in the vitreous. Br. J. Ophthalmol., 56:700, 1972.

35. Havener, W. H., Gloeckner, S.: Atlas of Diagnostic Techniques and Treatment of Retinal Detachment. St. Louis, C. V. Mosby Co., 1967.

36. Hayreh, S. S., Baines, J.A.B.: Occlusion of the vortex veins: An experimental study. Br. J. Ophthalmol., 57:217, 1973.

37. Hilton, G. F., McLean, E. B., Norton, E.W.D.: Retinal Detachment. A Manual. Rochester, Minn., American Academy of Ophthalmology, 1979.

38. Hilton, G. F.: The drainage of subretinal fluid. A randomized controlled clinical trial. Trans. Am. Ophthalmol. Soc., 79:517, 1981.

39. Hofmann, H., Hanselmayer, H.: Frequency and extent of spontaneous flattening of retinal detachments by patient immobilization. Klin. Monatsbl. Augenheilkd., 162:178, 1973.

40. Hovland, K. R., Elzeneiny, I. H., Schepens, C. L.: Clinical evaluation of small pupil indirect ophthalmoscope. Arch. Ophthalmol., 82:466, 1969.

41. Humphrey, W. T., Schepens, C. L., et al.: The release of subretinal fluid and its complications. In Pruett, R. C., Regan, C. D. J. (eds.): Retina Congress. New York, Appleton-Century Crofts, 1974, pp. 383, 390.

42. Jaffe, N. S.: Complications of acute posterior vitreous detachment. Arch. Ophthalmol., 79:568, 1968.

43. Kanski, J. J., Elkington, A. R., Davies, M. S.: Diplopia after retinal detachment surgery. Am. J. Ophthalmol., 76:38, 1973.

44. Kelley, F. P., Edelhauser, H. F., Aaberg, T. M.: Intraocular sulfur hexafluoride and octofluorocyclobutane. Arch. Ophthalmol., 96:511, 1978.

45. King, L. M., Schepens, C. L.: Limbal peritomy in retinal detachment surgery. Arch. Ophthalmol., 91:295, 1974.

46. Langham, M. E., Regan, C.D.J.: Circulatory changes associated with the onset of primary retinal detachment. Arch. Ophthalmol., 81:820, 1969.

47. Laqua, H., Machemer, R.: Repair and adhesion mechanisms of the cryotherapy lesion in experimental retinal detachment. Am. J. Ophthalmol., 81:833, 1977.

48. Laqua, H., Machemer, R.: Glial cell proliferation in retinal detachment (massive periretinal proliferation). Am. J. Ophthalmol., 80:602, 1975.

49. Lean, J. S., Mahmood, M., Manna, R., et al.: Effect of preoperative posture and binocular occlusion on retinal detachment. Br. J. Ophthalmol., 64:94, 1980.

50. Lincoff, H.: Should retinal breaks be closed at the time of surgery? In Brockhurst, R. J., et al. (eds.): Controversy in Ophthalmology. Philadelphia, W. B. Saunders Co., 1977, pp. 582–598.

51. Lincoff, H., Geiser, R.: Finding the retinal hole. Arch. Ophthalmol., 85:565, 1971.

52. Lincoff, H., Kreissig, I.: The treatment of retinal detachment without drainage of subretinal fluid. Trans. Am. Acad. Ophthalmol. Otolaryngol., 76:1221, 1972.

53. Lincoff, H., Kreissig, I.: Advantages of radial buckling. Am. J. Ophthalmol., 79:955, 1975.

54. Lincoff, H. A., McLean, J. M., Nano, H.: Cryosurgical treatment of retinal detachment. Trans. Am. Acad. Ophthalmol. Otolaryngol., 68:412, 1964.

55. Lincoff, H., Kreissig, I., Jakobiec, F., et al.: Remodeling of cryosurgical adhesion. Arch. Ophthalmol., 99:1845, 1981.

56. Lincoff, H., Coleman, J., Kreissig, I., et al.: The perfluorocarbon gases in the treatment of retinal detachment. Ophthalmology, 90:546, 1983.

57. Lindner, B.: Acute posterior vitreous detachment and its retinal complications. Acta Ophthalmol., Suppl. 87:1, 1966.

58. Lindsey, P. A., Pierce, L. H., Welch, R. B.: Removal of scleral buckling elements. Arch. Ophthalmol., 101:570, 1983.

59. Linner, E.: Intraocular pressure in retinal detachment. Acta Ophthalmol., 84:101, 1966.

60. Lobes, L. A., Burton, T. C.: The incidence of macular pucker after retinal detachment surgery. Am. J. Ophthalmol., 85:72, 1978.

61. Lyall, M.: Correspondence. Arch. Ophthalmol., 88:228, 1972.

62. Machemer, R., Laqua, H.: A logical approach to the treatment of massive periretinal proliferation. Ophthalmology, 85:584, 1978.

63. Machemer, R., Laqua, H.: Pigment epithelial proliferation in retinal detachment (massive periretinal proliferation). Am. J. Ophthalmol., 80:1, 1975.

64. Machemer, R., Van Horn, D., Aaberg, T. M.: Pigment epithelial proliferation in human retinal detachment with massive periretinal proliferation. Am. J. Ophthalmol., 85:181, 1978.

65. Mets, M. B., Wendell, M. E., Gieser, R. G.: Ocular deviation after retinal detachment surgery. Am. J. Ophthalmol., 99:667, 1985.

66. Michels, R. G.: Surgery of retinal detachment with proliferative vitreoretinopathy. Retina, 4:63, 1984.

67. Morse, P. H.: Vitreoretinal Disease. A Manual for Diagnosis and Treatment. Chicago, Year Book Medical Publishers, 1979.

68. Morse, P. H., Scheie, H. G., Aminlari, A.: Light flashes as a clue to retinal disease. Arch. Ophthalmol., 91:179, 1974.

69. Morse, P. H., Scheie, H. G.: Prophylactic cryotherapy of retinal breaks. Arch. Ophthalmol., 92:204, 1974.

70. Moses, R. A., Becker, B.: Clinical tonography: the scleral rigidity factor. Am. J. Ophthalmol., 45:196, 1958.

71. Newsome, D. A., Rodrigues, M. M., Machemer, R.: Human massive periretinal proliferation. Arch. Ophthalmol., 99:873, 1981.

72. Norton, E.W.D.: Retinal detachment in aphakia. Trans. Am. Ophthalmol. Soc., 61:770, 1963.

73. Norton, E.W.D.: Present status of cryotherapy in retinal detachment surgery. Trans. Am. Acad. Ophthalmol. Otolaryngol., 73:102, 1969.

74. Norton, E.W.D.: Intraocular gas in the management of selected retinal detachments. Trans. Am. Acad. Ophthalmol. Otolaryngol., 77:85, 1973.

75. O'Connor, P. R.: Absorption of subretinal fluid after external scleral buckling. Am. J. Ophthalmol., 76:30, 1973.

76. Okun, E.: Discussion of Lincoff, H., Kreissig, I.: The treatment of retinal detachment without drainage of subretinal fluid. Trans. Am. Acad. Ophthalmol. Otolaryngol., 76:1232, 1972.

77. Parks, M. M.: Discussion of Wright, K. W.: The fat adherence syndrome and strabismus after retina surgery. Ophthalmology, 93:411, 1986.

78. Perez, R. N., Phelps, C. D., Burton, T. C.: Angle-closure glaucoma following scleral buckling operations. Trans. Am. Acad. Ophthalmol. Otolaryngol., 81:247, 1976.

79. Portney, G. L., Campbell, L. H., Casebeer, J. C.: Acquired heterophoria after surgery for retinal detachment. Am. J. Ophthalmol., 73:985, 1972.

80. Rosenthal, M. L., Fradin, S.: The technique of binocular indirect ophthalmoscopy. Highlights Ophthalmol., 9:179, 1967.

81. Rubin, M. L.: The optics of indirect ophthalmoscopy. Surv. Ophthalmol., 9:449, 1964.

82. Russo, C. E., Ruiz, R. S.: Silicone sponge rejection. Arch. Ophthalmol., 85:647, 1971.

83. Ryan, S. J., Goldberg, M. F.: Anterior segment ischemia following scleral buckling in sickle cell hemoglobinopathy. Am. J. Ophthalmol., 72:35, 1971.

84. Ryan, S. J.: The pathophysiology of proliferative vitreoretinopathy and its management. Am. J. Ophthalmol., 100:188, 1985.

85. Schepens, C. L.: Current management of retinal detachment: Progress or chaos? Ann. Ophthalmol., 3:21, 1971.

86. Schepens, C. L., Okamura, I. D., Brockhurst, R. J.: The scleral buckling procedures. I. Surgical techniques and management. Arch. Ophthalmol., 58:797, 1957.

87. Schepens, C. L.: Scleral buckling with circling element. Trans. Am. Acad. Ophthalmol. Otolaryngol., 68:959, 1964.

88. Schwartz, A.: Chronic open-angle glaucoma secondary to rhegmatogenous retinal detachment. Am. J. Ophthalmol., 75:205, 1973.

89. Schwartz, P. L., Pruett, R. C.: Factors influencing retinal detachment following removal of buckling elements. Arch. Ophthalmol., 95:804, 1977.

90. Scott, J. D.: Retinal detachment surgery without drainage. Trans. Ophthalmol. Soc. U.K., 90:57, 1970.

91. Seelenfreund, M. H., Silverstone, B-Z., Hirsch, I., et al.: Recurrent tears following successful retinal detachment surgery. Ann. Ophthalmol., 18:319, 1986.

92. Sewell, J. J., Knobloch, W. H., Eifrig, D. E.: Extraocular muscle imbalance after surgical treatment for retinal detachment. Am. J. Ophthalmol., 78:321, 1974.

93. Shafer, D. M.: Comment in Schepens, C. L., Regan, C.D.J. (eds.): Controversial Aspects of the Management of Retinal Detachment. Boston, Little, Brown & Co., 1965, p. 51.

94. Shea, M.: Complications common to all surgical procedures. In Schepens, C. L., Regan, C.D.J. (eds.): Controversial Aspects of the Management of Retinal Detachment. Boston, Little, Brown & Co., 1965, pp. 207–221.

95. Sternberg, P., Machemer, R.: Results of conventional vitreous surgery for proliferative vitreoretinopathy. Am. J. Ophthalmol., 100:141, 1985.

96. Stratford, T. P.: Comment in Schepens, C. L., Regan, C.D.J. (eds.): Controversial Aspects of the Manage-

ment of Retinal Detachment. Boston, Little, Brown & Co., 1965, p. 51.

97. Stratford, T. P.: Fate of the re-attached retina following removal of silicone elements. *In* Pruett, R. C., Regan, C.D.J. (eds.): Retina Congress. New York, Appleton-Century-Crofts, 1974, p. 623.

98. Tabotabo, M. M., Karp, L. A., Benson, W. E.: Posterior vitreous detachment. Ann. Ophthalmol., 12:59, 1980.

99. Tanenbaum, H. L., Schepens, C. L., Elzeneiny, I., Freeman, H. M.: Macular pucker following retinal detachment surgery. Arch. Ophthalmol., 83:286, 1970.

100. Tani, P., Robertson, D. M., Langworthy, A.: Rhegmatogenous retinal detachment without macular involvement treated with scleral buckling. Am. J. Ophthalmol., 90:503, 1980.

101. Tasman, W.: Posterior vitreous detachment and peripheral retinal breaks. Trans. Am. Acad. Ophthalmol. Otolaryngol., 72:271, 1968.

102. Theodossiadis, G.: Diplopia after retinal detachment surgery with cryotherapy and episcleral Silastic sponges. Klin. Monatsbl. Augenheilkd., 166:423, 1975.

103. Ulrich, R. A., Burton, T. C.: Infections following scleral buckling procedures. Arch. Ophthalmol., 92:213, 1974.

104. Wilkinson, C. P., Bradford, R. H.: The drainage of subretinal fluid. Trans. Am. Ophthalmol. Soc., 81:162, 1983.

105. Wilkinson, C. P.: Visual results following scleral buckling for retinal detachments sparing the macula. Retina, 1:113, 1981.

106. Wiznia, R. A.: Removal of solid silicone rubber exoplants after retinal detachment surgery. Am. J. Ophthalmol., 95:495, 1983.

107. Wright, K. W.: The fat adherence syndrome and strabismus after retina surgery. Ophthalmology, 93:411, 1986.

108. Yoshida, A., Feke, G. T., Green, G. J., et al.: Retinal circulatory changes after scleral buckling procedures. Am. J. Ophthalmol., 95:182, 1983.

13

RETINAL PHOTOCOAGULATION

by William Tasman

HISTORY OF PHOTOCOAGULATION

The effect of solar light on the retina has been known for centuries.[29] Indeed, Socrates mentioned the danger of viewing the sun during an eclipse and suggested instead viewing its reflection in water. The first description of a central scotoma after a solar burn of the retina dates back to Theophilus Bonetus, who practiced in Geneva during the 17th century.[6] Even the artist Degas may have sustained a solar retinal burn, since he dates his visual impairment from a sunny day when he painted near a moat surrounding a chateau. In 1853, two years after Helmholtz invented the ophthalmoscope, Coccius described an exudative burn that gradually developed into a pigmented scar,[9] and in 1912 an eclipse of the sun on a cloudless day caused many macular burns in Europe.

Experimental research on the effect of light damage on the retina was first carried out by Czerny in 1867.[17] In 1882 Deutschmann duplicated Czerny's experiments.[19] Both of these investigators used a concave mirror and a convex lens to focus sunlight on the retinas of rabbits whose pupils had been dilated. After a few seconds of exposure, grayish burns of varying sizes developed, which gradually turned into pigmented scars. Widmark in 1893 produced the same effect using a carbon arc lamp.[48] The first experimental photocoagulation of the human retina was performed by Maggiore in 1927.[37] He focused sunlight for 10 minutes into an eye that was to be enucleated because of a malignant tumor. Hess' hammer light was focused into the eye of a second patient. Histologic sections of these eyes showed hyperemia and edema of the retina.

Meyer-Schwickerath made one of the major contributions to ophthalmology when he developed an instrument for light coagulation of retinal disorders. His experiments began in the spring of 1946 after he had observed a number of patients with macular damage that followed an eclipse of the sun on July 10, 1945.

Initial experiments with a carbon arc showed that the intensity of radiation required to treat the human retina was greater than that required for the rabbit retina. This led Meyer-Schwickerath to develop an instrument that used the sun as its light source.[39] The instrument, developed in 1949, consisted of a Galillean telescope with a mirror that had a central aperture suspended on a universal joint in front of the ocular. In order to get significant coagulation burns one had to produce a fivefold magnification of the retinal image of the sun. However, the overriding dependence on weather conditions, time of day and year, and rotation of the earth made the instrument unreliable for clinical use. Therefore, in 1949 Meyer-Schwickerath tried using the Beck high-intensity carbon arc, which proved to be a suitable light source.[40] However, because the filaments of all carbon arcs become used up in the process of burning, there were, once again, built-in limitations to this prototype light source. Another disadvantage was the liberation of gases saturated with soot and carbon particles.

The next stage in development utilized a xenon high-pressure lamp. When xenon is made to glow by high-intensity currents, the spectrum of the light emitted is similar to that of ordinary daylight. The xenon lamp burns steadily, and no adjustments are necessary during coagulation. Over the years xenon has proved an extremely useful light source, and has permitted the clinical application of light coagulation as an accepted therapeutic tool.

However, it has been superseded by additional instruments such as the argon blue-green laser, the argon green laser, the krypton red laser, and dye lasers with variable wavelengths, including yellow. Each of these instruments possesses certain features that produce a specific tissue reaction in a photocoagulated retina and choroid. The intensity of the lesion produced by any mode of photocoagulation is largely dose related. The major source of heat is the retinal pigment epithelium, which absorbs the light energy and converts it to heat. In addition, the blue-green light of the argon laser is absorbed and converted to heat by hemoglobin.

The histopathologic characteristics of xenon arc photocoagulation have been extensively studied. Curtin and Norton described the histologic changes produced by low intensities of light energy on the human retina with the xenon photocoagulator.[16] They confirmed the findings of Geeraets and associates that high-intensity light energy involves all layers of choroid, pigment epithelium, and sensory retina, whereas very low energy light intensity primarily involves the pigment epithelium and photoreceptor elements with sparing of the inner retinal layers.[25]

Zweng and co-workers noted that ruby laser photocoagulation burns cause an early adhesion of the sensory retina to the pigment epithelium and choroid.[23, 49, 50] In addition, after mild burns they detected marked destruction and clumping of retinal pigment epithelium and marked disruption of the outer half of the sensory retina. Blair and Gass noted one lesion produced with the ruby laser that had destroyed all retinal layers.[1] They observed that the retina in this particular area was thinner than the papillomacular bundle, in which no fiber layer damage had occurred, and concluded that only a small range existed between the energy density of

light that produces partial-thickness destruction and that that produces full-thickness destruction.

Laser light is characterized by waves that are all in the same phase. This contrasts with the white light of the original xenon photocoagulator, in which the waves were completely out of phase. Thus the beam of laser energy remains collimated along its path, with only minimal loss of power caused by divergence.

Originally, as indicated earlier, the laser was primarily developed for its thermal effect. Now, however, Q-switched neodymium-YAG lasers have been developed that operate on a different principal and produce molecular disruption. This technique has been tried experimentally on the retina,[3–5] but as yet it is not widely accepted for treatment of retinal conditions.

All current types of lasers (i.e., argon, krypton, neodymium-YAG, excimer, and carbon dioxide) operate through a noncontact system. However, a new method of delivering laser energy to tissue, the contact laser probe, has recently been developed. The goal of the contact laser probe has been to cut, vaporize, coagulate, and deliver interstitial radiation.[22] This is an evolving area of treatment, and one in which more will be forthcoming in the near future.

Table 13–1 provides a list of indications for fundus photocoagulation for various ophthalmic conditions.

RETINAL DISEASES

Neovascularization

Proliferative Diabetic Retinopathy

Proliferative diabetic retinopathy has become one of the leading causes of blindness, especially among patients under 40 year of age. In a population-based study in southern Wisconsin 1370 patients diagnosed as being diabetic at age 30 years or older were noted to have a prevalence of diabetic retinopathy, varying from 28.8 per cent of people who had diabetes for less than 5 years to 77.8 per cent of people who had diabetes for 15 or more years.[31] The rate of proliferative diabetic retinopathy varied from 2 per cent of people who were diabetic for less than 5 years to 15.5 per cent of people who had diabetes for 15 or more years. The severity of retinopathy was related to a longer duration of diabetes, younger age of diagnosis, higher glycosylated hemoglobin levels, higher systolic

TABLE 13–1. Indications for Fundus Photocoagulation

CONDITION	ALTERNATIVE TREATMENT METHODS	PREFERRED METHOD	COMMENT
Angioid streaks Paget's disease Pseudoxanthoma elasticum Sickle-cell disease	—	—	Value not documented
Arterial macroaneurysm	—	Photocoagulation	Only if exudation threatens fovea
Background diabetic retinopathy	Aspirin, dipyridamole	Photocoagulation	Clinically significant macular edema (ETDRS)
Capillary retinal hemangioma	Cryotherapy	Cryotherapy	Cryotherapy effective
Central serous chorioretinopathy	—	Photocoagulation	Generally resolves without treatment
Choroidal hemangioma	Radioactive plaque, diathermy, cryotherapy	Treatment modality depends on tumor size	Treat tumor surface
Choroidal melanoma	Radioactive plaques, resection, enucleation	Treatment depends on tumor size and location	—
Congenital pit of optic nerve	Vitrectomy	Photocoagulation	Effectiveness controversial
Degenerative retinoshisis (outer layer breaks)	—	Observation	Do not treat schisis unless symptomatic retinal detachment
Eales' disease	—	Photocoagulation	Treat avascular retina
Iris neovascularization	Cyclocryotherapy	Depends on degree of rubeosis and angle involvement	Panretinal photocoagulation if media clear
Lattice degeneration	Photocoagulation	Cryotherapy	—
Proliferative diabetic retinopathy	—	Photocoagulation	DRS showed PRP to be effective
Retinal breaks	Cryotherapy, scleral buckle	Cryotherapy	Break should be flat without bridging vessels
Retinal telangiectasia (Coats' disease)	Cryotherapy	Cryotherapy and photocoagulation	Modality depends on location of lesions and degree of exudation
Retinal vascular occlusion Branch vein	—	Photocoagulation if edema present	(BVO study)
Branch vein	—	Photocoagulation if NVE present	Lessens chance of hemorrhage (BVO study)
Central vein	Cryotherapy	Photocoagulation (cryotherapy if vitreous)	Treat if NVE, NVD, or retinal ischemia present
Retinoblastoma	Cryotherapy, radiation, enucleation	Depends on size and location of tumor(s)	—
Sarcoid	—	Photocoagulation	—
Sickle cell (SC)	—	Photocoagulation	Treat avascular retina
Subretinal neovascular membranes Macular degeneration (drusen)	—	Photocoagulation of SRNVM	Membrane preferably outside capillary-free zone
Optic nervehead drusen	—	Photocoagulation of SRNVM	Membrane preferably outside capillary-free zone
Presumed ocular histoplasmosis syndrome	—	Photocoagulation of SRNVM	Membrane preferably outside capillary-free zone
Traumatic choroidal rupture	—	Photocoagulation of SRNVM	Membrane preferably outside capillary-free zone

NVE, neovascularization of retina; DRS, diabetic retinopathy study; PRP, panretinal photocoagulation; NVD, neovascularization of disc; SRNVM, subretinal neovascular membranes. ETDRS, early treatment diabetic retinopathy study; BVO, branch vein occlusion study.

blood pressure and use of insulin, presence of protein urea, and small body mass.

The relation of vitreous traction to new vessel formation on the disc and retina has been well described by Davis.[18] In 1976 the National Eye Institute completed a collaborative study to evaluate the effectiveness of peripheral retinal photocoagulation for this disorder.[44] More than 1500 patients were enrolled in the study. One eye was arbitrarily assigned to treatment either by xenon arc or argon laser photocoagulation, and those patients with neovascularization of the disc who were assigned to argon laser therapy had focal treatment to the vessels on the disc as well as the panretinal photocoagulation. However, those who were allotted to the xenon group had only the peripheral retinal photocoagulation. The results of this study showed that treated eyes had a much lower incidence of severe visual loss (5/200 or less) than untreated eyes. There was no significant difference between the xenon-treated group and the argon-treated group, except for the fact that xenon photocoagulation caused a greater decrease in visual acuity, visual field, and night vision. For this reason the second eyes of patients in this study were treated with argon laser therapy.

Because the xenon group and argon group showed no difference with respect to the disc

TABLE 13–2. Results of PRP in Preventing Visual Loss

	PERCENT-AGE OF TREATED EYES	PERCENT-AGE OF CONTROL EYES
NVE greater than 0.5 DD and vitreous hemorrhage	7	30
NVD less than 0.5 DD and vitreous hemorrhage	4	26
NVD greater than 0.5 DD and no hemorrhage	9	26
NVD greater than 0.5 DD and vitreous hemorrhage	20	37

neovascularization, it was not thought mandatory to treat directly on the disc if neovascularization was present when the second eye was treated.

Subsequent follow-up reports from the Diabetic Retinopathy Study showed that photocoagulation reduced the risk of severe visual loss by 50 per cent or more.[45] Eyes with new vessels on or within 1-disc diameter of the optic disc equaling or exceeding one-fourth to one-third of the disc area in extent (Fig. 13–1A and B), and eyes with new vessels and preretinal vitreous hemorrhage were at particular risk without treatment[46] (Table 13–2).

New vessel formation is thought to be a response to a possible angiogenic factor that may be secreted from zones of ischemic retina. Such areas are characteristic of preproliferative diabetic retinopathy and can be detected by fluorescein angiography (Figs. 13–2 and 13–3A

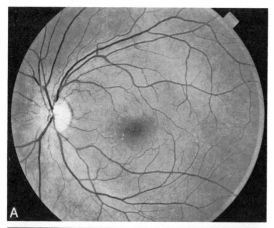
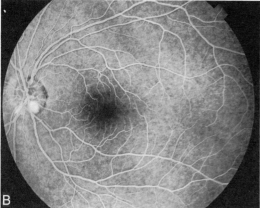

FIGURE 13–1. *A,* Red-free picture of a diabetic fundus with little or no apparent change. *B,* Fluorescein angiography confirms the presence of neovascularization occupying less than one-quarter of a disc diameter.

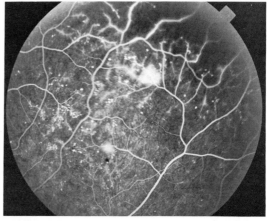

FIGURE 13–2. Diabetic fundus showing proliferative changes just posterior to an area of retinal ischemia.

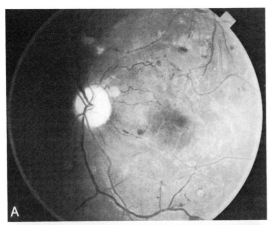

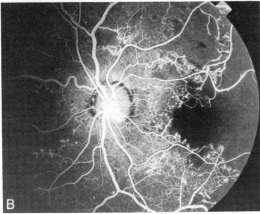

FIGURE 13–3. *A*, Red-free picture of the posterior pole of a patient with diabetes. Scattered hemorrhages can be seen. *B*, Fluorescein angiography reveals marked loss of capillary function in the retina in this patient with diabetic retinopathy.

and *B*). This is common to other proliferative retinopathies as well. Examples include central retinal vein occlusion, branch vein occlusion, SC sickle disease, sickle thalassemia, retinopathy of prematurity, Eales' disease, dominant familial exudative retinopathy, and X-linked dominant incontinentia pigmenti.

Despite the importance of these findings and widespread publicity about them, the photocoagulation technique was slow in becoming widely known to a population of physicians, whose practice included an appreciable number of diabetic patients.[20]

Technique of Panretinal Photocoagulation

The immediate goal of laser photocoagulation, when applied specifically to areas of flat

neovascularization of the retina (NVE) while performing panretinal photocoagulation, is fragmentation of the blood column in all new vessels, insofar as this can be done without damaging central vision, and the application of burns to cover a major portion of the retina in all quadrants. All new vessels elsewhere (NVE), with the exception of new vessels within one-half the disc diameter of the center of the macula and over the papillomacular bundle, can be treated. New vessels greater or equal to 125 μm (the size of major veins) should be treated at the discretion of the individual ophthalmologist. In addition, discretion should also be used when evaluating vessels accompanied by fibrous proliferations or neovascular patches equal to or greater than four disc areas in size. Treatment should not be used for preretinal sheets of blood (subhyaloid hemorrhages) or for walling off of localized retinal detachments.

If hemorrhage occurs from neovascularization of the disc (NVD) or elevated NVE during the application of treatment, the bleeding site should be treated as follows: (a) The spot size should be 200 or 500 μm. (b) Duration of application should be from 0.2 to 0.5 second, and pressure should be applied to the eye with the contact lens to slow blood flow. (c) Next, the power should gradually be increased until the bleeding stops. Sometimes it is necessary to produce charring of blood to stop the hemorrhage.

If the bleeding site is over the papillomacular bundle, the risk of damage to the nerve fiber layer with treatment must be balanced against the additional bleeding that may occur if the bleeding site is not treated. In this situation the ophthalmologist must use his best judgment, and treatment of the hemorrhage is optional.

Secondary glaucoma owing to choroidal detachment is another complication of panretinal photocoagulation and can usually be treated medically with antiglaucoma agents. Even though this complication has become rare with multiple-session treatments, it is advisable to check each patient gonioscopically before laser therapy. If the angle is narrow and later becomes occluded, it may be necessary to do an iridectomy. On the other hand, if the angle is known to be deep, the patient can be treated with carbonic anhydrase inhibitors and topical steroids until the choroidal detachment subsides and the pressure once again returns to normotensive levels.

A 500-μm-spot size is used unless the media makes it difficult to get a reaction in the retina, or a panfunduscopic lens is used to treat the posterior pole. In the latter case a 200-μm-spot is used. When vitreous hemorrhage is present, it is again often necessary to reduce the size of the spot to 200 μm, or to use a krypton, rather than an argon, laser, since the longer wavelengths of light penetrate through lens opacities and vitreous hemorrhage better than argon. Krypton is generally more uncomfortable for the patient, however.

Care should be taken to avoid hitting any visible retinal vessels. The power setting should be such that a moderate white retinal coagulation is apparent. The power setting required to achieve this endpoint is recorded for future reference, and is defined as the baseline power setting for the treatment session. Frequently it needs to be higher for a panfunduscopic lens than for a three-mirror contact lens.

To complete scatter treatment, burns should be applied to the retina beginning at points on an oval defined as two disc diameters above, below, and temporal to the center of the macula and one disc diameter nasal to the disc, and should extend peripherally to the equator at least past the vortex veins. In general, application should be scattered uniformly throughout this area, the distance between burns being one burn diameter. In order to minimize impairment of the temporal visual field, burns within four to five disc diameters of the disc on the nasal side should be arranged in rows parallel to the nerve fibers. Treatment should not be directed over large retinal vessels or over small vessels supplying the macula. In carrying out this treatment the ophthalmologist should deviate from the uniform spacing of burns described above in order to treat intraretinal microvascular abnormalities, hemorrhages, and/or microaneurysms, so long as this does not lead to more than five or ten confluent burns. The 500-μm-spot size is generally used for the treatment described in this section, except for the area posterior to the major temporal vascular arcades, where 200-μm-spot sizes should be used. Exposure time should be set at 0.1 or 0.05 second. In general, at least 1200 to 1600 burns of 500-μm-spot size should be applied.

Microaneurysms and intraretinal microvascular abnormalities are treated by applying discrete spots of coagulation to each lesion with 0.05 to 0.2 second exposure times, and with 50-μm- to 100-μm-spot sizes, using the smaller-spot size near the macula. The described endpoint is moderately intense whitening of the microaneurysm or the adjacent retina.

Most ophthalmologists usually attempt to complete peripheral retinal photocoagulation treatment over three sessions; some, however, prefer to do it all at one sitting.

Another major complication of laser photocoagulation is rupture of Bruch's membrane, leading to neovascularization originating in the choroid. Such neovascularization is under a high head of pressure and can be difficult to eliminate with laser therapy. Other complications include puckering of the macula and persistent macular edema. Visual field loss can also occur with argon laser photocoagulation, and there can be a marked reduction in dark adaptation. These findings are less pronounced with argon laser than with xenon photocoagulation. Finally, although traction retinal detachment is a devastating complication, it can frequently be avoided by careful selection of patients to eliminate those who have evidence of marked vitreoretinal traction before treatment.[38]

Occasionally the panretinal photocoagulation fails, and vision decreases. This can be due to increased macular edema, focal bleeding from NVE, increasing neovascularization or persistent NVD (this usually regresses in 3 to 4 weeks after treatment), retinal detachment, or neovascularization of the iris. If macular edema does not regress in 2 to 3 months, focal treatment in the posterior pole may help. In the case of focal bleeding from NVE, confluent laser treatment using a 200- to 500-μm-spot size can be applied heavily if the NVE is less than two disc diopters in size. Scanning fluorescein angiography may be helpful in identifying additional areas of NVE, since 90 per cent of NVE occurs within six disc diopters of the optic nervehead.

In the case of increasing NVD or persistent NVD with bleeding, supplemental treatment may be helpful. Many patients receive up to 8000 (500-μm) burns with the Goldmann lens or 5000 (200-μm) burns with the panfunduscopic lens. Peripheral retinal cryoablation, if the fundus can be visualized, may also be effective in causing regression of NVD or NVE. Approximately six applications are applied to each quadrant.

If vitreous hemorrhage has occurred, the supplemental treatment can only be applied as the blood clears. In some cases, however, vitrectomy becomes necessary. Generally this is recommended if vision is 5/200 or less for at least 1 month, since the diabetic vitrectomy study has shown that after two years' follow-up, 25 per cent of vitrectomized eyes had 20/40 or better vision if vitrectomized early (3 months), whereas only 15 per cent of eyes achieved this result when vitrectomy was deferred for 1 year.[47]

Technique of Focal Photocoagulation

Diabetic Macular Edema

Because of the success of the Diabetic Retinopathy Study, the Early Treatment Diabetic Retinopathy Study was initiated to see whether or not aspirin and/or focal photocoagulation might be beneficial before the development of proliferative changes. Data from the Early Treatment Diabetic Retinopathy Study published in 1985 showed that focal photocoagulation of "clinically significant" diabetic macular edema substantially reduced the risk of visual loss.[21] It was noted that focal treatment also increased the chance of visual improvement, decreased the frequency of persistent macular edema, and caused only minor visual field loss. In this randomized clinical trial 1154 eyes that had macular edema and mild to moderate diabetic retinopathy were randomly assigned to focal argon laser photocoagulation, while 1490 such eyes were randomly assigned to deferral of photocoagulation.[42] The beneficial effects of treatment demonstrated in the trial suggested that all eyes with clinically significant diabetic macular edema should be considered for focal photocoagulation. Clinically significant macular edema was defined as retinal thickening that involved or threatened the center of the macula (even if visual acuity was not yet reduced), and was assessed by stereo contact lens biomicroscopy or stereo photography.

A pretreatment fluorescein angiogram was used during photocoagulation to identify treatable lesions, and was prescribed for all such lesions located within two disc diameters of the center of the macula, but at least 500 μ from the center (Figs. 13–4A and B and 13–5A, B, and C). Microaneurysms and other focal leakage sites received about 50- to 100-μ argon blue-green or green-only burns of 0.1 second or less duration, with adequate power to obtain definite whitening around the microaneurysm or leakage site. For all microaneurysms greater than 40 μ in diameter, an attempt was made to obtain actual whitening or darkening of the microaneurysm itself, which was generally accomplished using a 50-μ-spot size. Sometimes repeated burns were needed.

Treatment of lesions closer than 500 μ to the macula was not required initially. However, if vision was less than 20/40, and the retinal edema and leakage persisted, treatment of lesions up to 300 μ from the center was recommended, unless there was perifoveal capillary

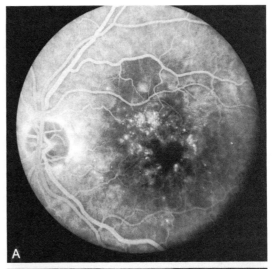

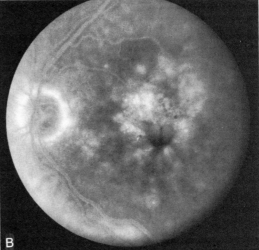

FIGURE 13–4. A, Posterior pole of a patient with macular edema secondary to diabetic retinopathy. B, Late stages of the angiogram show macular edema in the foveal area.

dropout, which might be worsened by this treatment.

Areas of diffuse leakage or nonperfusion within two disc diameters of the center of the macula were treated with a grid pattern. The goal of treatment in such cases was to produce a burn of light to moderate intensity, not more than 200 μ in diameter. Toward this end a 50- to 200-μ-spot size was used, and a space one burn wide was left between each lesion. Burns were placed in the papillomacular bundle, but no closer than 500 μ from the center of the macula. In the study it was also noted that aspirin did not modify the effect of focal photocoagulation. The indications for treatment of macular edema as outlined by the ETDRS are listed in Table 13–3.

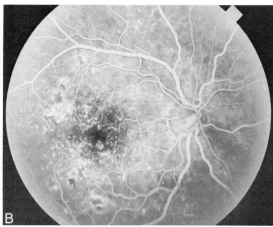

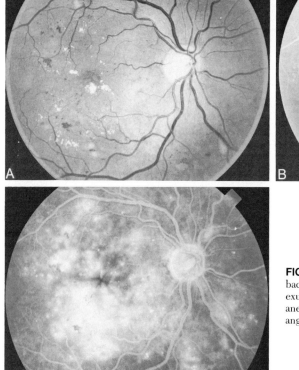

FIGURE 13–5. *A*, Red-free picture of a patient with background diabetic retinopathy showing hemorrhages and exudates. *B*, Fluorescein angiogram begins to reveal microaneurysmal changes and macular edema. *C*, Late stages of angiogram show marked macular edema.

OTHER RETINAL VASCULAR DISORDERS

Proliferative Sickle Cell Retinopathy and Sickle Thalassemia

Proliferative sickle cell retinopathy is most common in the SC form of this disorder. The initial event is peripheral arteriolar occlusions,

---

TABLE 13–3. ETDRS Indications for Laser Treatment of Diabetic Macular Edema

1. Thickening of the retina at or within 500 microns of the center of the macula if associated with retinal thickening.

2. Hard exudates at or within 500 microns of the center of the macula if associated with retinal thickening.

3. A zone or zones of retinal thickening one disc area or larger in size, any part of which is within one disc diameter of the center of the macula.

---

which cause retinal ischemia.[10–14] Arteriovenous connections develop in the temporal periphery and lead to the typical sea fan formation and, ultimately, to vitreous hemorrhage (Fig. 13–6). In the past it has been recommended that these arteriovenous communications be treated focally in an attempt to eliminate the feeder vessel entering the frond.[26] This form of treatment has some degree of risk, since it is not uncommon for high-intensity burns to occlude feeder vessels to rupture Bruch's membrane, resulting in neovascularization from the choroid. As a result, peripheral photocoagulation to eliminate the ischemic zone from the equator anteriorly is suggested as an initial alternative to eliminate the fronds.

Retinal Vein Occlusion

Branch retinal vein occlusion is another common cause of retinal neovascularization. Most frequently this is seen along the superior temporal vein, with the inferior temporal vein the next most commonly affected. It should be

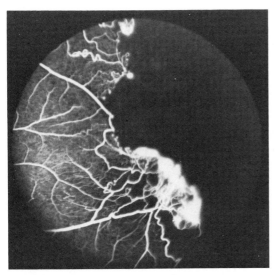

FIGURE 13–6. Fronds of neovascularization in a patient with SC sickle disease. The fronds have occurred at the junction between vascularized and avascular retina.

remembered that a large number of branch vein occlusions spontaneously improve without treatment, and it is only when persistent macular edema and intraretinal microvascular abnormalities develop that one should begin to consider laser therapy (Figs. 13–7A, B, and C and 13–8A, B, and C).

This is in contrast with central retinal vein occlusion, in which the incidence of rubeosis after demonstrated retinal ischemia on fluorescein angiography may be as high as 60 per cent. Patients with hemispheric or central retinal vein occlusion and good capillary perfusion have a much lower incidence of rubeosis, on the order of only 1 per cent (Fig. 13–9). Thus panretinal photocoagulation is usually indicated in patients after central retinal vein occlusion, when marked retinal ischemia can be demonstrated (Fig. 13–10A, B, and C).

Just as with diabetic retinopathy, any form of therapy for retinal vein occlusion should be

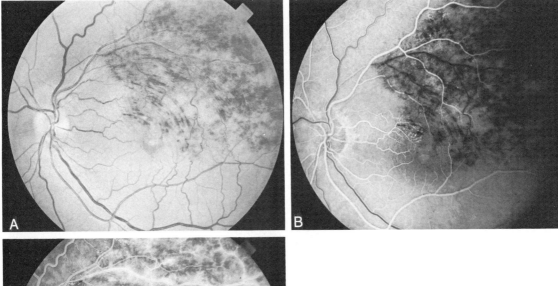

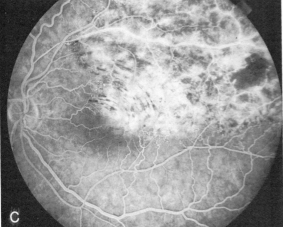

FIGURE 13–7. A, Red-free picture of a patient with a superotemporal branch vein occlusion. B, Early fluorescein angiogram of the fundus shown in A. C, In the late stages of the angiogram there is marked edema in this patient with branch vein retinal occlusion.

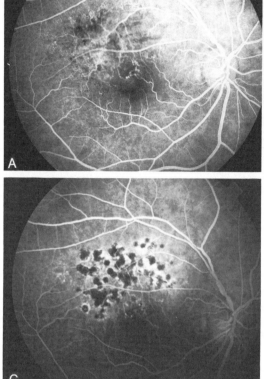

FIGURE 13–8. *A,* Early fluorescein angiogram in a patient with superotemporal branch vein occlusion showing some leakage of fluorescein dye. *B,* Marked edema is present in the late stage of the angiogram in this patient with superotemporal branch vein occlusion. *C,* After photocoagulation, edema has been eliminated.

preceded by a medical work-up to detect any underlying disease, such as hypertension, diabetes, or carotid artery narrowing, predisposing to the vein occlusion.

The natural course of vein occlusion is extremely variable, particularly when only a branch is involved, and because visual acuity is often better than 20/40 when branch vein occlusion occurs, results of photocoagulation or other forms of therapy have been difficult to evaluate until recently.[27] The Branch Vein Occlusion Study, however, has provided new information about the effectiveness of treatment.[42]

This study was designed to learn whether argon laser photocoagulation was useful in improving visual acuity in eyes with branch vein occlusion and macular edema that reduced vision to 20/40 or worse. One hundred thirty-nine eligible eyes were randomly assigned to either a treated or an untreated control group. After 3.1 years follow-up the gain of at least two lines of visual acuity from baseline maintained for two consecutive visits was significantly greater in treated eyes. As a result, laser photocoagulation is now recommended for patients with macular edema from branch vein occlusion.

The Branch Vein Occlusion Study also accumulated data suggesting that peripheral scatter treatment should be applied after the develop-

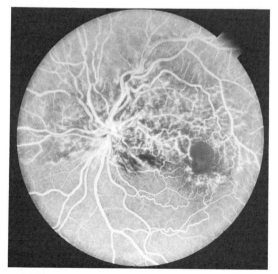

FIGURE 13–9. Good retinal perfusion is seen in a patient with a superior hemispheric branch vein occlusion.

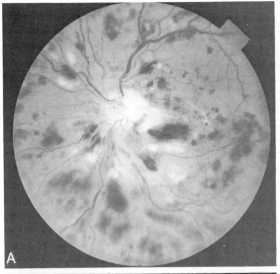

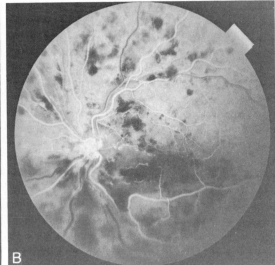

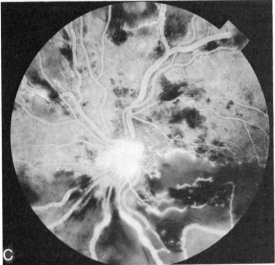

FIGURE 13–10. *A*, Red-free picture of a patient with central retinal vein occlusion. *B*, Early fluorescein angiogram already revealing nonperfusion of the retina inferiorly. *C*, Marked nonperfusion can be diagnosed inferiorly despite the fact that there is marked retinal hemorrhage secondary to the central retinal vein occlusion.

ment of neovascularization rather than before the development of neovascularization.[43] It was noted that scatter argon laser photocoagulation to the affected segments, as determined by color photography and fluorescein angiography, and extending no closer than two disc diameters from the center of the fovea, lessened the occurrence of vitreous hemorrhage.

The Branch Vein Occlusion Study, which was a collaborative one, demonstrated that an average visual acuity increase of 1.33 lines was present in eyes that were treated compared with those not receiving photocoagulation.[42] Many eyes, however, experienced a far more substantial visual improvement. In addition, the study demonstrated that laser treatment applied in a grid pattern can be effective for treating macular edema. It also documented that scatter treatment can reduce the risk of vitreous hemorrhage in nondiabetic patients with retinal neovascularization, and that vitreous hemorrhage is a complication of neovascularization in patients with branch vein occlusion (Fig. 13–11),[2] although it is not nearly as frequent or as devastating visually as when vitreous hemorrhage occurs as a complication of neovascularization in patients with diabetes. Furthermore, the Branch Vein Occlusion Study demonstrated that retinal neovascularization can occur outside an area of retinal ischemia.

Eales' Disease

Diagnosis of Eales' disease is difficult to establish. Characteristically the condition is thought to occur predominantly in males under the age of 40 who otherwise appear healthy. It

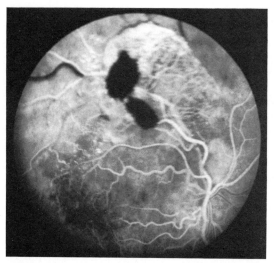

FIGURE 13–11. Neovascularization of the retina has developed along the superotemporal branch vein occlusion. Preretinal hemorrhage is present overlying the neovascularization.

starts often as a periphlebitis in the retinal periphery and may lead to central retinal vein occlusion. Sometimes periphlebitis resolves spontaneously, but extensive vascular occlusions may lead to the proliferation of new vessels. Areas of neovascular formation can lead to massive vitreous hemorrhage, and for this reason they are usually treated by applying laser therapy to areas of avascular retina with argon laser photocoagulation in the manner described for neovascularization after branch vein occlusion.

Sarcoidosis

In addition to causing a granulomatous uveitis, a sarcoidosis can produce inflammatory changes along the vessels, often characterized as "candle wax drippings." Less common is the occurrence of peripheral arteriovenous connections, which lead to neovascular formation and leakage on fluorescein angiography. These neovascular changes can precede vitreous hemorrhage and act in many ways like the proliferative retinopathies of diabetes and sickle-cell disease. In severe cases traction retinal detachment may result. Treatment of the peripheral lesion is usually satisfactorily carried out with focal 500-μ burns.

Retinal Telangiectasia (Coats' Disease)

In 1908 Coats published the first of two articles in which he described a condition char-

acterized by retinal vascular changes and exudation.[8] Through the years this has frequently been confused with Leber's multiple miliary aneurysms, and in truth the two conditions are probably similar, or even the same. Clinically, retinal telangiectasia (Coats' disease) occurs in juvenile males, although occasionally females are affected. Ninety per cent of the cases are unilateral. The superior temporal quadrant is most commonly involved. The hallmark of Coats' disease is development of "light bulb" telangiectasis in the retinal periphery, which leads to subretinal exudation that has an affinity for the posterior pole (Fig. 13–12A and B).

When subretinal exudation is increasing, treatment is directed at obliterating the abnormal telangiectatic vascular changes by photocoagulation or cryotherapy. Because many of

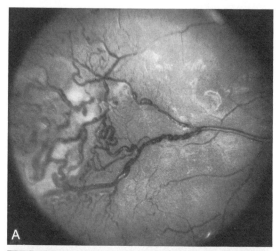

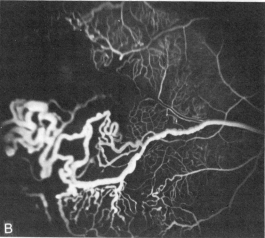

FIGURE 13–12. A, Red-free picture showing retinal telangiectasia in a 4-year-old boy with Coats' disease. B, Fluorescein angiogram delineates the retinal telangiectasia and areas of nonperfusion in the temporal fundus periphery.

the affected patients are children, treatment usually has to be done under general anesthesia; cryotherapy is preferred. This is particularly so if large areas of exudate are present beneath the telangiectatic areas because it is difficult to get adequate photocoagulation reaction when an underlying exudate is present. Using cryotherapy, the ophthalmologist freezes the "light bulbs" until the retina adjacent to them is white and the vessels are narrowed or engulfed in the iceball.

The prognosis with treatment is best when only one or two quadrants are affected and diminishes significantly when the disease involves more than 180 degrees of the retinal periphery.

Retinal telangiectasia can ultimately lead to exudative retinal detachment, in which case it may be necessary to perform a scleral buckling procedure. The vascular abnormality is eliminated by either diathermy or cryotherapy, and subretinal fluid is drained. Despite the fact that these are, for the most part, nonrhegmatogenous retinal detachments, drainage of subretinal fluid is surprisingly easy, and the retina may become reattached. Subsequent argon laser or xenon arc photocoagulation on the buckle may be necessary if all of the vascular abnormalities have not been eliminated.

With the successful obliteration of the abnormal vasculature, exudate will begin to absorb in about 6 to 8 weeks. It may take as long as 10 to 12 months, however, before it is entirely gone. Even after complete obliteration of all abnormal vessels and resorption of all exudate, follow-up examinations are mandatory for several years. If new exudate begins to appear later, it can be assumed that new vascular abnormalities have developed. We have seen recurrences of the disease as long as 5 years after an apparent cure.[41]

Arterial Macroaneurysm

Arterial macroaneurysms may occur without apparent antecedent cause. Often they are associated with surrounding exudation and in some cases present because of hemorrhage either into the retina or into the vitreous cavity. Fluorescein angiography is helpful in establishing the diagnosis, since the macroaneurysm usually retains the fluorescein and appears as a discrete light bulb (Fig. 13–13).

Treatment of these lesions is controversial. Many resolve spontaneously after bleeding, and

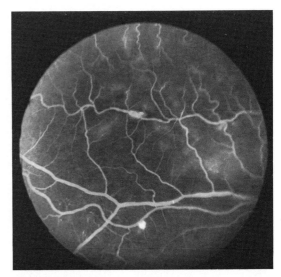

FIGURE 13–13. Fluorescein angiogram showing a macroaneurysm without hemorrhage or exudation.

treatment is generally reserved for those that have an exudative component threatening the macula.

Capillary Retinal Hemangioma

Capillary retinal hemangioma was first seen clinically in 1882 by Fuchs, who mistakenly called it a traumatic arteriovenous aneurysm.[24] In 1894 Collins described its pathology.[15] He called it a capillary nevus. Von Hippel earned the academic credit after his presentation, and in 1904 accurately described its natural history.

Approximately 20 per cent of patients with angiomas of the retina develop central nervous system involvement, characteristically cerebellar hemangioblastoma, although hemangioblastomas of the medulla, pons, spinal cord, and, rarely, cerebrum have been reported. The classic fundus lesion is an angiomatous tumor that resembles a red balloon lodged temporally in the equatorial or pre-equatorial region (Fig. 13–14A, B, and C). It is a round or oval globular red nodule that may be so small that it cannot be seen ophthalmoscopically, or it may be several disc diameters in size and project into the vitreous. The exudation from the lesion may reach the posterior pole. The hallmarks of the disease are the large tortuous afferent and efferent retinal vessels that accompany the tumor. They are enormously dilated, and show focal swellings, numerous kinkings, and sausage-like constriction.

Early attempts to eradicate these lesions by

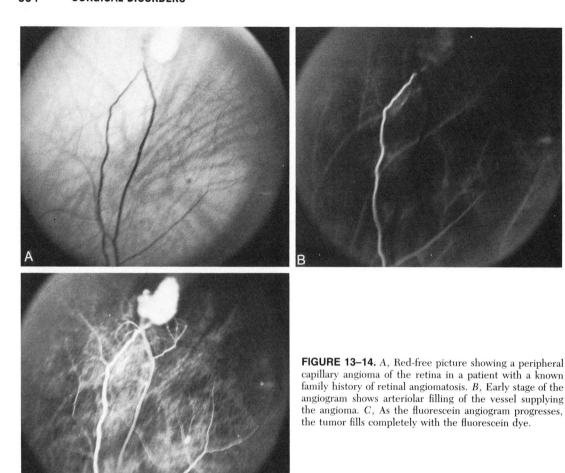

FIGURE 13–14. *A*, Red-free picture showing a peripheral capillary angioma of the retina in a patient with a known family history of retinal angiomatosis. *B*, Early stage of the angiogram shows arteriolar filling of the vessel supplying the angioma. *C*, As the fluorescein angiogram progresses, the tumor fills completely with the fluorescein dye.

applying radium directly to the orbit, as well as subconjunctivally, led to some fibrosis of the angioma and a decrease in size of the feeder vessels, but the use of radon seed sutured directly to the sclera over the angioma had a more pronounced effect. Roentgen radiation was found to be unsuccessful when applied after the lesion had advanced to scarring and retinal detachment or when applied indiscriminately to the whole head. Before photocoagulation penetrating diathermy proved to be effective, and it was noted that if the tumor could be destroyed, the exudate also disappeared.

Photocoagulation has provided another means for successfully treating angiomatosis retinae. It offers significant advantages over the other modes of treatment. It requires no conjunctival incision and causes no scleral necrosis. The technique involves mild photocoagulation burns to the surface of the angioma. These are just intense enough to cause blanching on the surface of the tumor. The feeder vessels are avoided. The treatments are frequently spread out over several sessions and have as their major complications hemorrhage and secondary retinal detachment.

More recently cryotherapy has been used to treat angiomas, and seems to be an effective way of eliminating the tumors. Frequently even large tumors can be eradicated with only one treatment when the individual lesion is frozen and then thawed.

RETINAL BREAKS AND DEGENERATION

Retinal Breaks

Before discussing the treatment of retinal breaks with photocoagulation, some discussion of the types of retinal breaks that may occur is warranted. Common usage has led to the classification of some breaks as horseshoe or flap tears, and of others as operculated tears, in which a plug of retina has been pulled into the vitreous cavity on the posterior surface of the detached vitreous gel. Retinal breaks may also be round or oval atrophic areas, whereas others, such as lattice breaks, are associated with degenerative conditions of the retina.

It is important to know which breaks need treatment and which merely need to be followed. Byer has followed 240 untreated patients with lattice degeneration and noted only a 0.3 per cent incidence of detachment in the eyes he followed.[6] Similarly, round or oval atrophic areas infrequently lead to retinal detachment. Those most ominous in significance are symptomatic horseshoe tears because these have a high incidence of subsequent retinal detachment. It has been our policy to treat such breaks, as well as operculated breaks, when they occur and produce symptoms.

Breaks that may be treated with laser therapy or cryotherapy are horseshoe tears that are totally flat and have no subretinal fluid under the edges. In addition, there should not be a bridging retinal vessel if either photocoagulation or cryotherapy is contemplated. Breaks with patent vessels have a tendency to bleed later and, in our opinion, are better treated by localized scleral buckling techniques.

Many breaks today are treated with cryotherapy rather than photocoagulation. We have reserved photocoagulation for breaks that are located posterior to the equator, where they are inaccessible to cryotherapy unless a conjunctival incision is made. Adequate treatment of the break necessitates encircling it with two or three rows of laser application. Usually a 200-μm-spot size with a time exposure of 200 mW is adequate to produce a reaction. One should be cautious about the use of laser photocoagulation if the retinal break has produced a vitreous hemorrhge. In such cases, if at all possible, we prefer to use cryotherapy.

Breaks in lattice degeneration primarily occur as round holes within the lattice or as horseshoe tears at the edge of the lattice. The latter are more serious and generally require treatment. Here, again, we prefer cryotherapy if the break can be reached with the cryoprobe. When laser therapy is used for such areas of lattice with break formation, we prefer to encircle the lattice by placing two or three rows of laser burns in sound retina around the area (Fig. 13–15A and B). The settings are generally the same as described for treatment of retinal breaks.

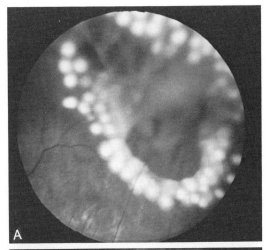
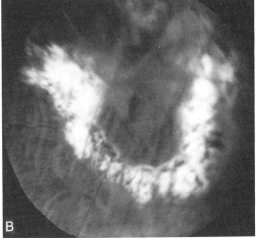

FIGURE 13–15. A, Laser photocoagulation surrounding a horseshoe tear at the edge of lattice degeneration. B, Three months later the tear is well sealed by the photocoagulation.

Degenerative Retinoschisis

In the early 1960's photocoagulation was used to treat bullous degenerative retinoschisis. Xenon photocoagulation was applied through the diaphanous inner layer of the senile schisis in an attempt to flatten the cavity. This, of course, did nothing to restore visual field to the patient, since bullous retinoschisis creates an absolute field defect as a result of the separation at the outer plexiform layer, which interrupts the neuronal pathway. In our experience this treatment seldom succeeded in flattening the schisis. Because the inner layer was so transparent, one often looked right through it after photocoagulation had been performed. In addition, retinoschisis only infrequently leads to detached retina and seldom progresses to the macula, so a more conservative approach of careful follow-up, rather than treatment, is advocated.

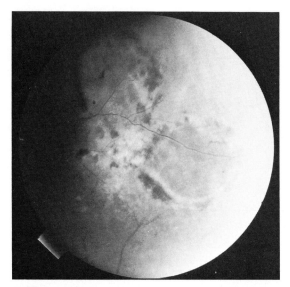

FIGURE 13–16. Localized schisis detachment with pigmentary changes around outer layer breaks. This patient was followed and not treated.

Occasionally patients develop outer-layer retinal breaks, but these seldom become associated with symptomatic retinal detachment secondary to the schisis (Fig. 13–16). As a result of Byer's report, when outer-layer retinal breaks are present we do not recommend treatment.[7] If clinically symptomatic retinal detachment occurs, then scleral buckling is indicated.

Subclinical Retinal Detachment

A subclinical retinal detachment is one that occurs in the periphery and has not yet caused visual symptoms. These should be treated surgically, and usually have a good prognosis with scleral buckling. Attempting to wall off the detachment with photocoagulation is not recommended, since it has been shown that traumatic retinal detachments that frequently have a delayed onset between the time of injury and the time of diagnosis often demonstrate successive demarcation lines tht have failed to stem the tide of subretinal fluid.

CHORIORETINAL DISEASES

Subretinal Neovascular Membranes

Many ocular diseases are known to cause subretinal neovascular membranes. Probably the one most frequently encountered is age-related macular degeneration. This disorder has a higher incidence in people with drusen in the posterior pole, and unfortunately it is only infrequently that the subretinal neovascular membrane develops at a distance remote enough from the foveal area to be amenable to treatment. When present extrafoveally it can rapidly extend into the fovea, so prompt treatment is imperative (Fig. 13–17*A* and *B*).

Choroidal rupture is another condition that leads to subretinal neovascular membrane formation, and is also amenable to photocoagulation if the membrane is remote enough from the capillary-free zone (Fig. 13–18).

Other conditions associated with subretinal neovascular membrane include histoplasmosis, myopic degeneration, angioid streaks, rubella retinopathy, serpiginous choroiditis, vitelliform degeneration, choroidal nevus, choroidal osteoma, idiopathic subretinal neovascularization, and iatrogenic formation of a subretinal neovascular membrane after laser therapy, to mention a few.

Studies related to the effectiveness of argon laser photocoagulation for age-related macular

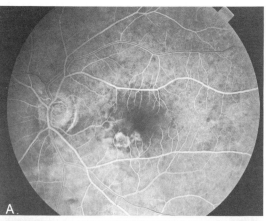

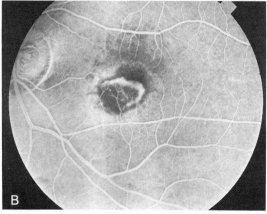

FIGURE 13–17. *A*, Subretinal neovascular membrane inferior to the foveola. *B*, Within 4 weeks the membrane has extended.

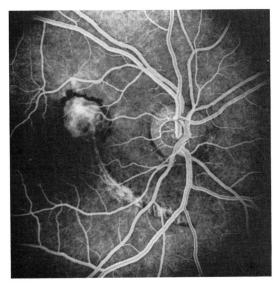

FIGURE 13–18. Subretinal neovascular membrane associated with a choroidal rupture that occurred secondary to a tennis ball injury.

degeneration have been carried out in a randomized manner.[28, 32–36] In the first report by the macular photocoagulation study group[32] it was noted that after 15 months of follow-up, 60 per cent of untreated eyes versus only 25 per cent of treated eyes had experienced severe visual loss (Fig. 13–19A and B). By August 1985 three more years of scheduled follow-up examination had been completed for 208 (88 per cent) of 236 eyes in the age-related macular degeneration study, 203 (77 per cent) of 262 eyes in the ocular histoplasmosis study, and 51 (76 per cent) of 67 eyes in the idiopathic neovascularization study. The relative risk of experiencing severe visual loss after three years in eyes initially assigned to the no-treatment group, in comparison with the eyes assigned to the argon laser photocoagulation group, was 1.4 in the age-related macular degeneration study, 5.5 in the ocular histoplasmosis study, and 2.3 in the idiopathic neovascularization study. This gave a 95 per cent confidence level for each of these groups. The beneficial effects of argon laser treatment have persisted in all three studies despite the fact that some eyes in the no-treatment groups were treated later in their clinical course as a result of the evidence of early benefit.[33–36]

Subfoveal neovascular membranes were not treated, but their prognosis in eyes with relatively good initial visual acuity has been shown to be poor.[28]

Unfortunately, however, laser treatment has not been entirely successful in permanently eradicating active neovascularization from these eyes. Recurrent neovascularization in the form of either neovascularization contiguous with the treatment scar or independent neovascular membranes have been observed in 70 (59 per cent) of 119 age-related macular degeneration eyes originally assigned to treatment, 40 (30 per cent) of 132 ocular histoplasmosis eyes, and 11 (33 per cent) of 33 idiopathic neovascularization study eyes. Recurrence was accompanied by an increased frequency of severe visual loss. Characteristics of the patients and their original lesion and treatment were examined to see if there was any clue to predict recurrence. In the age-related macular degeneration group, as well as in the idiopathic neovascularization study patients, cigarette smoking appeared to be related to the rate of recurrence. Younger age and female gender were associated with an increased frequency of recurrence in the ocular histoplasmosis study. The study points out,

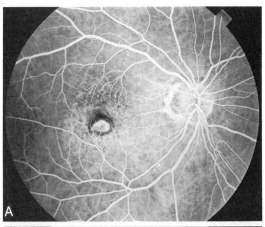

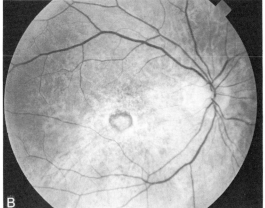

FIGURE 13–19. A, Subretinal neovascular membrane in a patient with age-related macular degeneration. B, After krypton laser photocoagulation the membrane has been eradicated.

however, that predictions of which eyes will suffer recurrence cannot be made totally accurately.[36]

Central Serous Chorioretinopathy

Central serous chorioretinopathy has been thought to be a fairly benign condition. Various reports in the literatue have pointed out that there is almost a 100 per cent spontaneous cure rate if one waits long enough. As our experience with this condition has grown over the years, we have come to recognize that some of the patients with recurrent episodes do indeed develop retinal pigment epithelial changes and reduction of central vision. We do not treat central serous chorioretinopathy unless the foveola has been detached for 6 months or the patient has lost vision from this condition in his other eye.

When performed, laser treatment is applied to a pigment epithelial detachment, which is identified by fluorescein angiography. In contrast to the treatment of subretinal neovascular membranes, in which a long burn is used, the treatment of a pigment epithelial detachment should be light. A 100- to 200-μ-spot size is used, and the duration of exposure should not exceed 0.1 second. An exposure of 100 to 200 mW is satisfactory to accomplish the treatment.

One should remember that in treating patients over the age of 45 years, there is an increased incidence of subretinal neovascular membrane formation, and what appears as a pigment epithelial detachment may actually be an early subretinal neovascular membrane viewed on end. If there is any doubt as to whether the lesion in question is a pigment epithelial detachment of a subretinal neovascular membrane, conservatism is indicated, since a rip in the pigment epithelium may occur.[30] This is a devastating complication of laser therapy, and may occur in the treatment of subretinal neovascular membranes as well.

CONTRAINDICATIONS TO LASER THERAPY

The contraindications to laser therapy include the presence of opaque media or small pupil. In order to adequately visualize the fundus and perform satisfactorily laser photocoagulation the pupil must be well dilated. Mid-dilation fre-

quently compromises photocoagulation of the retinal periphery, and as a result, the surgeon is more apt to hit the edge of the iris. Interestingly enough, however, intraocular lenses are not necessarily a contraindication to laser photocoagulation. If the lens implant permits dilation, treatment can be applied.

When photocoagulation was first devised, many macular holes were treated with the xenon photocoagulator. We have now come to recognize that it is not necessary to treat the majority of macular holes. Only a small percentage of retinal detachments are due to macular holes, and these most often occur in patients who are highly myopic.

In our opinion there is also no justification for treatment of cystoid macular edema after cataract surgery with laser photocoagulation.

REFERENCES

1. Blair, C. J., Gass, J.D.M.: Photocoagulation of the macula and papillomacular bundle in the human. Arch. Ophthalmol., 88:167, 1972.
2. Branch Vein Occlusion Study Group: Argon laser scatter photocoagulation for prevention of neovascularization and vitreous hemorrhage in branch vein occlusion. Arch. Ophthalmol., 104:34, 1986.
3. Brown, G. C., Benson, W. E.: Treatment of diabetic traction retinal detachment with the pulsed neodymium-YAG laser. Am. J. Ophthalmol., 99:258, 1985.
4. Brown, G. D., Green, W. R., Shah, H. G., et al.: Effects of the ND-YAG laser on the primate retina and choroid. Ophthalmology, 91:1397, 1984.
5. Brown, G. C., Scimeca G., Shields, J.: Effects of the pulsed neodymium:YAG laser on the posterior segment. Ophthalmic Surg., 17:470, 1986.
6. Byer, N.: Changes in and prognosis of lattice degeneration of the retina. Trans. Am. Acad. Ophthalmol. Otolaryngol., 78:114, 1974.
7. Byer, N.: Long-term natural history study of senile retinoschisis with implications for management. Ophthalmology, 93:1127, 1986.
8. Coats, G.: Forms of retinal diseases with massive exudation. R. London Ophthalmol. Hosp. Rep., 17:440, 1908.
9. Coccius: Anwendung des Augenspiegels, 1853, p. 111.
10. Cohen, S., Fletcher, M. E., Goldberg, M. F., Jednock, N.: Diagnosis-management of ocular complications of sickle hemoglobinopathies. Part I. Ophthalmic Surg., 17:57, 1986.
11. Cohen, S., Fletcher, M. E., Goldberg, M. F., Jednock, N.: Diagnosis-management of ocular complications of sickle hemoglobinopathies. Part II. Ophthalmic Surg., 17:110, 1986.
12. Cohen, S., Fletcher, M. E., Goldberg, M. F., Jednock, N.: Diagnosis-management of ocular complications of sickle hemoglobinopathies. Part III. Ophthalmic Surg., 17:184, 1986.
13. Cohen, S., Fletcher, M. E., Goldberg, M. F., Jednock, N.: Diganosis-management of ocular complications of sickle hemoglobinopathies. Part IV. Ophthalmic Surg., 17:312, 1986.
14. Cohen, S., Fletcher, M. E., Goldberg, M. F., Jednock,

N.: Diagnosis-management of ocular complications of sickle hemoglobinopathies. Part V. Ophthalmic Surg., 17:369, 1986.

15. Collins, E. T.: Two cases, brother and sister, with peculiar vascular new growth, probably primarily retinal, affecting both eyes. Trans. Ophthalmol. Soc. U.K., 14:141, 1894.

16. Curtin, V. T., Norton, E.W.D.: Early pathological changes of photocoagulation in the human retina. Arch. Ophthalmol., 69:744, 1963.

17. Czerny: Ber. Wien. Acad. Wiss., 56:II, 1912.

18. Davis, M. D.: Clinical observations concerning the pathogenesis of diabetic retinopathy. In Goldberg, M. D., Fine, S. L. (eds.): Symposium on the Treatment of Diabetic Retinopathy. Washington, D.C., USPHS Publication No. 1890, 1969.

19. Deutschmann, R.: Ueber die Blendung der Netzhaut durch directes Sonnenlicht von Graefe's. Arch. Ophthalmol., 28:241, 1882.

20. Dunn, D.R.F.: Dissemination of the published results of an important clinical trial: An analysis of the citing literature. Bull. Med. Libr. Assoc., 69:301, 1981.

21. Early Treatment Diabetic Retinopathy Study Research Group: Photocoagulation for diabetic macular edema. Arch. Ophthalmol., 103:1796, 1985.

22. Federman, J. L.: Contact laser surgery with potential applications in ophthalmology. Cont. Ophthalmic Forum, 4:97, 1986.

23. Flocks, M., Zweng, H. C.: Laser coagulation of ocular tissues. Arch. Ophthalmol., 72:604, 1964.

24. Fuchs, E.: Aneurysma arterio-venosum. Arch. F. Ophthalmol., 11:440, 1882.

25. Geeraets, W. J., Williams, R. C., Chan, G., et al.: The relative absorption of thermal energy in retinal and choroid. Invest. Ophthalmol., 1:340, 1962.

26. Goldbaum, M., Goldberg, M., Nappal, K., et al: Proliferative sickle retinopathy. In L'Esperance, F. (ed.): Current Diagnosis and Management of Chorioretinal Diseases. St. Louis, C. V. Mosby Co., 1977.

27. Gutman, F. A., Zegarra, H.: The natural course of temporal retinal branch vein occlusion. Trans. Am. Acad. Ophthalmol. Otolaryngol., 78:178, 1974.

28. Guyer, D. R., Fine, S. L., Maguire, M. G., et al.: Subfoveal choroidal neovascular membranes in age-related macular degeneration: Visual prognosis in eyes with relatively good initial visual acuity. Arch. Ophthalmol., 104:702, 1986.

29. Hamm, H.: Zentralskotom nach Sonnenblendung. Dissertation, Hamburg, 1947.

30. Hoskin, A., Bird, A. C., Schmi, K.: Tears of detached retinal pigment epithelium. Br. J. Ophthalmol., 65:417, 1981.

31. Klein, R., Klein, B.E.K., Moss, S. E., et al.: The Wisconsin Epidemiologic Study of Diabetic Retinopathy. III. Prevalence and risk of diabetic retinopathy when age at diagnosis is 30 or more years. Arch. Ophthalmol., 102:527, 1984.

32. Macular Photocoagulation Study Group: Argon laser photocoagulation for senile macular degeneration: Results of a randomized clinical trial. Arch. Ophthalmol., 100:912, 1982.

33. Macular Photocoagulation Study Group: Argon laser photocoagulation for ocular histoplasmosis: Results of a randomized clinical trial. Arch. Ophthalmol., 101:1347, 1983.

34. Macular Photocoagulation Study Group: Argon laser photocoagulation for neovascular maculopathy: Three-year results from randomized clinical trials. Arch. Ophthalmol., 104:694, 1986.

35. Macular Photocoagulation Study Group: Argon laser photocoagulation for idiopathic neovascularization: Results of a randomized clinical trial. Arch. Ophthalmol., 101:1358, 1983.

36. Macular Photocoagulation Study Group: Recurrent choroidal neovascularization after argon laser photocoagulation for neovascular maculopathy. Arch. Ophthalmol., 104:503, 1986.

37. Maggiore, L.: Soc. Ital. Oftal. Rome, 1927.

38. McMeel, J. W.: Photocoagulation approach with various diabetic vitreoretinal problems. In L'Esperance, F. (ed.): Current Diagnosis and Management of Chorioretinal Diseases. St. Louis, C. V. Mosby Co., 1977, pp. 269–275.

39. Meyer-Schwickerath, G.: Ber. Vers. Deutsch. Ophth. Ges. Heidelberg, 55:256, 1949.

40. Meyer-Schwickerath, G.: Ber. Vers. Deutsch. Ophth. Ges. Heidelberg, 57:144, 1951.

41. Ridley, M. E., Shields, J. A., Brown, G. C., Tasman, W.: Coats' disease: Evaluation of management. Ophthalmology, 89:1381, 1982.

42. The Branch Vein Occlusion Study Group: Argon laser photocoagulation for macular edema in branch vein occlusion. Am. J. Ophthalmol., 98:271, 1984.

43. The Branch Vein Occlusion Study Group: Argon laser scatter photocoagulation for prevention of neovascularization and vitreous hemorrhage in branch vein occlusion. Arch. Ophthalmol., 104:34, 1986.

44. The Diabetic Retinopathy Study Research Group: Preliminary reports on effects of photocoagulation therapy. Am. J. Ophthalmol., 81:383, 1976.

45. The Diabetic Retinopathy Study Research Group: Photocoagulation treatment of proliferative diabetic retinopathy: The second report of diabetic retinopathy study findings. Trans. Am. Acad. Ophthalmol. Otolaryngol., 85:82, 1978.

46. The Diabetic Retinopathy Study Research Group: Photocoagulation treatment of proliferative diabetic retinopathy: Clinical application of diabetic retinopathy study (DRS) findings, DRS Report Number 8. Ophthalmology, 88:583, 1981.

47. The Diabetic Retinopathy Vitrectomy Study Research Group: Early vitrectomy for severe vitreous hemorrhage in diabetic retinopathy: Two-year results of a randomized trial: Diabetic retinopathy vitrectomy study Report 2. Arch. Ophthalmol., 103:1644, 1985.

48. Widmark: Skand. Arch., 4:281, 1893 (cited from Birch-Hirschfeld).

49. Zweng, H. C., Flocks, M., Peabody, R. R.: Histology of human ocular laser coagulation. Arch. Ophthalmol., 76:11, 1966.

50. Zweng, H. C., Little, H. L., Peabody, R. R.: Laser Photocoagulation and Retinal Angiography. St. Louis, C. V. Mosby Co., 1969.

14

VITRECTOMY

by J. Arch McNamara and William E. Benson

INTRODUCTION

Pars plana vitrectomy, introduced by Machemer,[1, 2] has revolutionized the management of numerous ocular conditions. It has restored the vision of countless diabetics. Previously "inoperable" retinal detachments can now be repaired. It facilitates the sterilization of eyes with endophthalmitis. The management of these and other conditions is discussed below.

EVALUATION OF THE PATIENT

A complete eye examination is performed. Vitrectomy is nearly always contraindicated in eyes that do not perceive light. In eyes with opaque media it is critical to evaluate the status of the retina and the optic nerve before proceeding with surgery. Tests normally considered useful in the evaluation of visual function are often unreliable in these cases.[3] For example, when a patient with opaque media in an otherwise normal eye is tested for light projection, color perception, two-point discrimination, or the entoptic (Purkinje) phenomenon, his inability to perceive the stimulus may be because inadequate light is reaching the retina. On the other hand, some patients with detached

retina may be able to respond normally to these stimuli. In addition, a patient with a dense vitreous hemorrhage in an otherwise normal eye may even have a Marcus Gunn pupil (afferent pupillary defect). Because subjective tests are frequently misleading, we have come to rely heavily on ultrasonography,[4, 5] electroretinography,[6] and the visual evoked response. Ultrasound, especially with recent refinements, can accurately diagnose vitreous membranes, retinal detachments (Fig. 14–1A), intraocular foreign bodies (Fig. 14–1B), double perforation of the globe by a foreign body (Fig. 14–1C), choroidal detachment (Fig. 14–1D), intraocular tumors, and other conditions. It is important to recognize the distinctive funnel-shaped pattern (Fig. 14–1E) that identifies retinal detachment with severe proliferative vitreoretinopathy[7, 8;] such detachments are often inoperable. Computerized tomography (CT) scans have been helpful in localizing foreign bodies in or near the sclera (Fig. 14–1F).

Electroretinography (ERG) helps to evaluate the functional status of the retina. In cases of extremely dense vitreous hemorrhage, however, the light provided by the standard Grass photosimulator may not be bright enough to stimulate even a normal retina. The resultant flat tracing falsely indicates a nonfunctioning or detached retina. In order to solve this problem, Fuller and co-workers developed the bright-

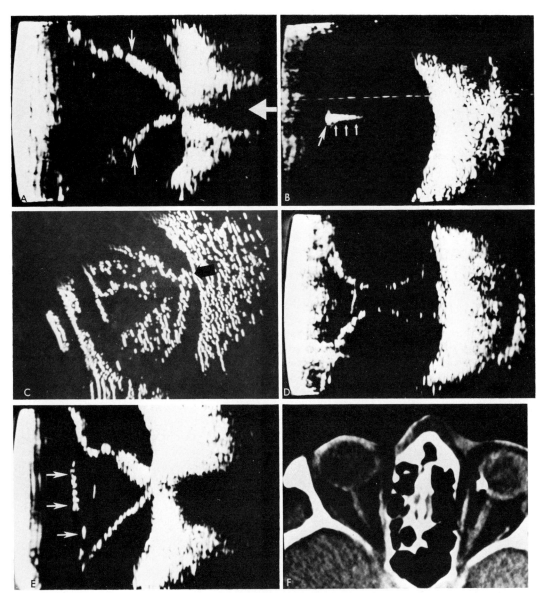

FIGURE 14–1. *A,* B-scan ultrasonography of retinal detachment. Notice that the retina (small arrows) is attached to the optic nerve (large arrow). *B,* Metallic foreign body in the anterior vitreous (large arrow). The "tail" (small arrows) is caused by reverberation echoes. *C,* B-scan ultrasonography of a double perforating injury. The intravitreal echoes represent vitreous hemorrhage. The vitreous is adherent to the retina, choroid, and sclera at the site of the posterior perforation (arrow). *D,* Choroidal detachment. Notice that the choroid inserts much further anteriorly than does the retina in a retinal detachment. *E,* B-scan ultrasonography of retinal detachment with proliferative vitreoretinopathy. The anterior line (arrows) indicates an equatorial transvitreal membrane. *F,* CAT scan localizing a foreign body embedded in the nasal sclera. (*C* courtesy of Dr. Dwain G. Fuller; *F* courtesy of Dr. Louis A. Lobes.)

flash ERG, which uses a much brighter light source, able to penetrate any vitreous hemorrhage.[6] A positive bright-flash ERG tracing indicates that at least some retina is functioning. A flat bright-flash tracing may indicate either a total retinal detachment or a severely damaged retina. Therefore, if no retinal detachment is found on ultrasonography, and if the bright-flash ERG tracing is flat, the retina may be nonfunctioning. Occasionally, however, eyes with a flat bright-flash ERG and an attached retina may regain some useful vision after vitrectomy.[9] The ERG may even become recordable.

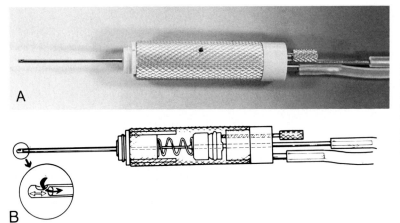

FIGURE 14–2. *A*, Ocutome vitrectomy probe. *B*, Schematic diagram of Ocutome probe; pneumatically activated piston drives cutting tip, which moves up and down (open arrows). Material is aspirated through the hollow inner tube (closed arrow).

INSTRUMENTATION

Numerous instruments for pars plana vitrectomy have been designed.[2, 10–17] All instruments feature a probe that is capable of simultaneous suction and cutting (Fig. 14–2). In nearly all cases we use a three-port approach with separate sites for the vitrectomy probe, an endoillumination fiberoptic probe, and an infusion cannula. Other intraocular instruments, such as motorized scissors, picks, foreign body or membrane forceps, extrusion needles, and magnets, can be exchanged for the vitrectomy probe. The fiberoptic diathermy tissue manipulator,[18] which combines mild suction and diathermy with the fiberoptic probe, may be used instead of the standard fiberoptic probe.

An operating microscope and a corneal contact lens are used for visualization of the vitreous cavity. Illumination can be provided by the microscope's coaxial light source when surgery is being performed anteriorly.

GENERAL TECHNIQUE OF VITRECTOMY

A hand support is essential for intravitreal surgery (Fig. 14–3). The surgeon rests both hands throughout the operation, avoiding fatigue and permitting fine control of the intravitreal manipulations. A plastic drape is pushed down into the space between the patient's head and the hand support, forming a trough to collect fluid that would otherwise spill onto the floor.

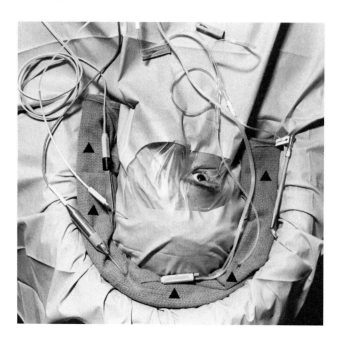

FIGURE 14–3. Patient draped for vitrectomy. The hand support is indicated by triangles.

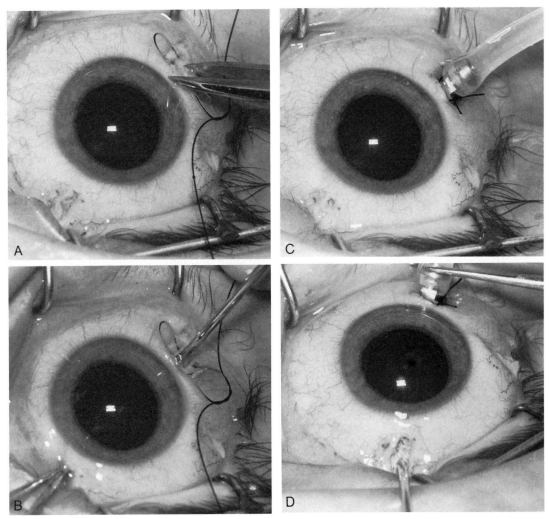

FIGURE 14–4. *A,* The sclera is marked 4 mm from the corneoscleral limbus. *B,* A microvitreoretinal knife is used to incise the sclera, choroid, and pars plana epithelium (a 5-0 nylon suture has been preplaced to secure the infusion cannula). *C,* The infusion cannula is secured. *D,* Sclerostomies are prepared superotemporally and superonasally.

Radial incisions are made superotemporally, superonasally, and inferotemporally through the conjunctive and Tenon's capsule. Entry incisions through the sclera and pars plana are made parallel to the corneoscleral limbus and are 3.5 to 4 mm from it (Fig. 14–4). All knives used for incisions must be sharp so that when introduced into the eye, the instruments do not push pars plana epithelium or vitreous base ahead of them, causing a retinal dialysis. It is important that these sclerotomies (through the sclera, uvea, and pars plana) be just large enough to permit entry of the desired instrument(s). If the incisions are too long, irrigation fluid leaks out of the eye. This leads to three potential problems. First, the intraocular pressure cannot be raised high enough to tampon-

ade small intraocular bleeding vessels. Second, currently available irrigation solutions are slightly toxic to the cornea.[19-21] If the incision is not watertight, more irrigating fluid must be used, theoretically increasing the chances of corneal endothelial damage. Third, if silicone oil is to be used, it escapes from the eye, greasing all sutures, making them difficult to tie, and mixing with the infusion from the infusing contact lens, interfering with visibility.

An infusion cannula is inserted inferotemporally and secured into place with a 5-0 nylon suture. The fiberoptic light probe and the cutting instrument (or forceps and the like) are inserted through the superior incisions.

Before entering the eye the surgeon must be certain that all parts of the instrument are functioning correctly. Immediately after entering the eye he should verify that the tip is cutting well by removing vitreous well away from the vitreous base.

When the vitrectomy has been completed, the scleral incisions are closed with 8-0 nylon sutures and the conjunctival incisions, with 6-0 plain catgut. We routinely inject subconjunctival antibiotic and steroid at the end of the case. Antibiotic ointment is then instilled into the conjunctival cul-de-sac.

MAJOR INDICATIONS

A. Opaque Vitreous
   1. Hemorrhage
      a. Proliferative diabetic retinopathy
      b. Retinal vein occlusion
      c. Proliferative sickle cell retinopathy
      d. Trauma
      e. Eales' disease
   2. Amyloidosis
   3. Inflammatory cells
   4. Asteroid hyalosis
B. Lens Removal
   1. Lensectomy preliminary to vitrectomy
   2. Dislocated lens or lens fragments
C. Retinal Detachment
   1. Proliferative vitreoretinopathy
   2. Diabetic traction retinal detachment
   3. Giant tear with rolled-over retina
   4. Aphakic retinal detachment made "inoperable" by vitreous incarceration
   5. Retinal detachment following penetrating injury
D. Intraocular Foreign Bodies
E. Macular Pucker
F. Glaucoma
G. Cystoid Macular Edema
H. Endophthalmitis

SPECIFIC INDICATIONS AND TECHNIQUES

Opaque Vitreous

Vitrectomy is successful in removing vitreous that is opaque as a result of hemorrhage, amyloidosis, or inflammatory cells. Vitreous hemorrhage caused by proliferative diabetic retinopathy is the most common indication for vitrectomy. Other common causes of vitreous hemorrhage are branch and central retinal vein occlusion, retinal vessel avulsion owing to posterior vitreous detachment, sickle cell retinopathy, trauma, and Eales' disease. Because vitreous hemorrhage is often reabsorbed spontaneously, and because of the many possible complications mentioned below, most surgeons wait 6 months or longer before recommending vitrectomy, especially if the patient's other eye has good visual function. Occasionally, however, during the waiting period, an undetected traction retinal detachment develops and spreads; early removal of the vitreous might prevent this.[22] In other cases the original hemorrhage clears only to be followed by another, denser hemorrhage. Finally, removal of the formed vitreous commonly arrests the progression of proliferative retinopathy, and often effects complete regression.[23, 24] For these reasons some surgeons believe that the eye fares better if vitrectomy is undertaken soon after the vitreous hemorrhage occurs.

The National Eye Institute is sponsoring the ongoing Diabetic Retinopathy Vitrectomy Study (DRVS).[25, 26] The second report of the DRVS studied 1616 eyes with severe vitreous hemorrhage that had reduced visual acuity to 5/200 or less for at least 1 month. These eyes were randomized to either early vitrectomy or deferral of vitrectomy for 1 year. After 2 years of follow-up 25 per cent of the early vitrectomy group had visual acuity of 20/40 or better compared with 15 per cent in the deferral group. There was no significant difference between the early and deferral groups in the percentage of eyes with visual acuity of no light perception (NLP) at 2 years. The information indicated that early vitrectomy provides an advantage for obtaining visual acuity of 20/40 or better at 2 years.

In cases of simple vitreous hemorrhage with complete posterior detachment (Fig. 14–5A), only clearing of the central vitreous is required (Fig. 14–5B). Complete removal of the vitreous near its base is not indicated because opaque peripheral vitreous does not significantly diminish the visual field. In addition, there is the risk that traction on the vitreous base may cause a retinal dialysis.

If the vitreous has pulled a stalk of neovascular tissue forward into the vitreous cavity (Fig. 14–6A), it is necessary to release all of the vitreous traction in order to prevent future bleeding and also to prevent a later traction retinal detachment (Fig. 14–6B). When new vessels are cut, the bleeding usually stops spontaneously. If it does not, increasing the intra-

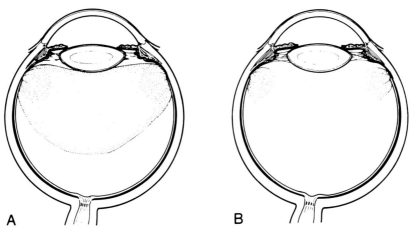

FIGURE 14–5. *A*, Simple vitreous hemorrhage with complete posterior vitreous detachment. *B*, Central vitreous removed by vitrectomy.

ocular pressure by raising the height of the infusion bottles may suffice, provided there is no loss of irrigation fluid through a sclerotomy that is too long. If the bleeding should continue, endodiathermy of the vessel is indicated.[27] Intravitreal thrombin is useful to control hemorrhage during vitrectomy in patients at high risk of intraoperative bleeding.[28]

Approximately three-fourths of the patients who undergo vitrectomy for simple vitreous hemorrhage have a significant improvement in vision.[3, 28–34] Those with a successful result 6 months after surgery almost always retain functional vision.[23] Patients with severe renal dysfunction have a relatively poor prognosis.[3, 35] Many vitreous surgeons believe that young patients with florid proliferative retinopathy also do poorly because of late rebleeding and because of anterior segment complications.

Lens Removal

Lensectomy Preliminary to Vitrectomy

Because neovascular glaucoma, postoperative iritis, and corneal complications are more common in aphakic eyes,[36–40] clear lenses are almost never removed. However, if a cataract is dense enough to prevent visualization of the posterior pole, it must be removed. There is considerable evidence that eyes are much less likely to progress to neovascular glaucoma after extracapsular cataract extraction (ECCE) than after intracapsular cataract extraction. We prefer to have a cataract surgeon perform an ECCE with a posterior chamber intraocular lens implantation. In many cases the vitrectomy can be done at the same sitting. If not, it is delayed a few weeks. When retinal detachment is present the

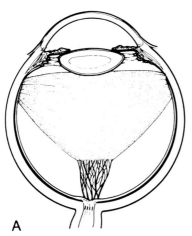
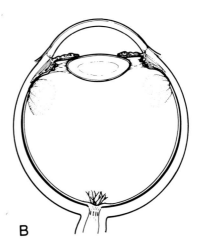

FIGURE 14–6. *A*, Stalk of neovascular tissue pulled forward by contracting vitreous body. *B*, Vitrectomy relieves traction on the stalk, which then retracts toward the optic nerve.

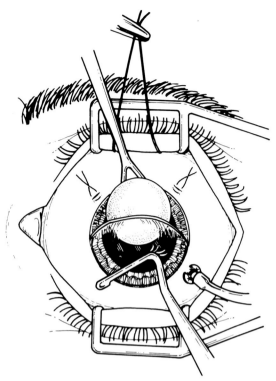

FIGURE 14–7. Extracapsular cataract extraction. The scler-otomies are made and the infusion cannula is preplaced before lens removal.

cataract operation and vitrectomy must be performed at the same time. An ECCE can be performed if the nucleus is too dense for fragmentation[41] (Fig. 14–7), or else the lensectomy can be done through the pars plana[42] (Fig. 14–8).

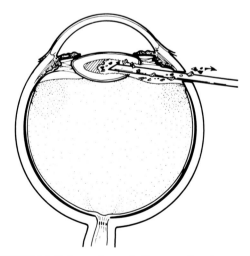

FIGURE 14–8. Lensectomy via the pars plana by use of the Shock phacofragmentation technique. The nucleus is removed before the cortex.

Dislocated Lens or Lens Fragments

Vitrectomy instruments have been helpful in the removal of spontaneously dislocated lenses and in the removal of nuclei and cortex dislocated during cataract surgery.[43–45] The technique of choice depends on the degree of nuclear sclerosis. If the nucleus is 1+ or 2+ sclerotic, a vitrectomy instrument, introduced through the pars plana, will easily remove the lens. Sometimes a second instrument, such as a bent needle, is helpful; firm pieces of nucleus can be crushed between it and the vitrectomy instrument (Fig. 14–9A and B).

An open-sky approach is preferred for dislocated lenses with 3+ and 4+ nuclear sclerosis because most vitrectomy instruments are incapable of sucking the nucleus into the cutting port and because crushing such nuclei can be difficult. A Flieringa ring is first placed to support the sclera. Then a 180- to 210-degree limbal corneal incision is made. After a sector iridectomy the formed vitreous is removed with a vitrectomy instrument. Finally, the nucleus is removed with a thin cryoprobe (Fig. 14–9C).

Vitrectomy techniques are also useful in the management of a posteriorly dislocated intraocular lens (IOL).[46] Occasionally at the time of cataract surgery or postoperatively an IOL may fall into the vitreous cavity. At the time of surgery an open-sky vitrectomy is done, and the IOL can then be retrieved with foreign body forceps. If the dislocation occurs postoperatively, a pars plana vitrectomy can be done and foreign body forceps used to manipulate the IOL back into position (Fig. 14–10). Once in position, a McCannel-type iris-fixation suture[47] should be used to maintain the IOL in place.

Retinal Detachment

Retinal Detachment with Proliferative Vitreoretinopathy

In some retinal detachments retinal pigment epithelial and/or glial cells proliferate on both surfaces of the retina and on the posterior vitreous face, pulling the retina into fixed folds (Fig. 14–11). This process, now called proliferative vitreoretinopathy, is the most common cause of failure to reattach (or keep attached) the retina. In advanced cases, when standard scleral buckling procedures have failed, vitrectomy may be indicated. The central vitreous is first removed with the vitrectomy instrument, after which the contracted posterior face of the vitreous, which often causes circumferential

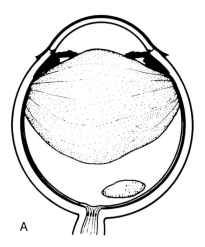

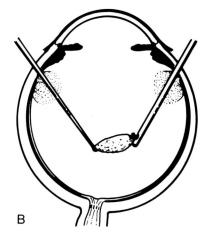

FIGURE 14–9. *A*, Lens nucleus dislocated during cataract extraction. *B*, Nucleus crushed between bent needle and vitrectomy instrument to facilitate its removal. *C*, Alternate technique. After placement of a Flieringa ring (arrows), the cataract wound is reopened, the vitreous is removed, and the nucleus is removed with a cryoprobe.

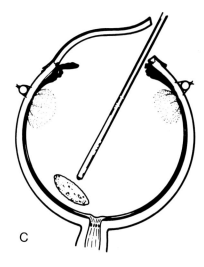

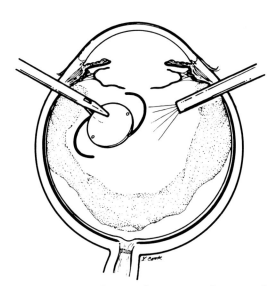

FIGURE 14–10. After partial vitrectomy, the intraocular lens is grasped with intraocular forceps so that repositioning can be performed.

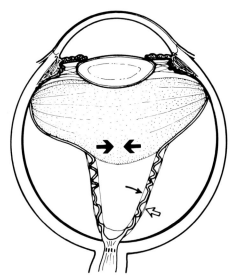

FIGURE 14–11. Retinal detachment with proliferative vitreoretinopathy. Preretinal (thin arrow), subretinal (open arrow), and vitreous proliferations (heavy arrows) pull the retina into a funnel shape with fixed folds.

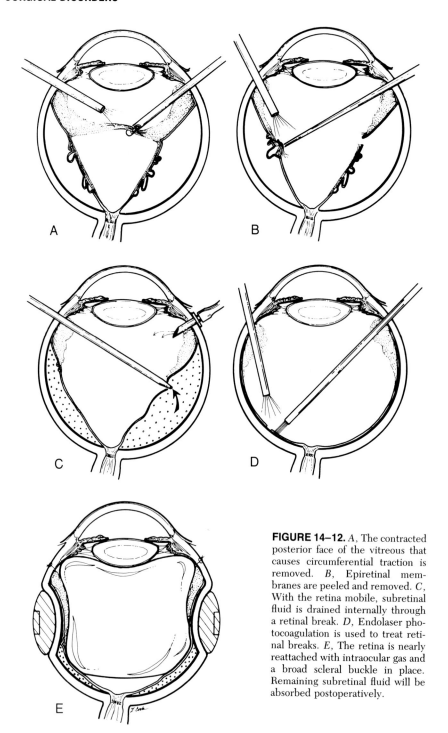

FIGURE 14–12. *A*, The contracted posterior face of the vitreous that causes circumferential traction is removed. *B*, Epiretinal membranes are peeled and removed. *C*, With the retina mobile, subretinal fluid is drained internally through a retinal break. *D*, Endolaser photocoagulation is used to treat retinal breaks. *E*, The retina is nearly reattached with intraocular gas and a broad scleral buckle in place. Remaining subretinal fluid will be absorbed postoperatively.

traction on the retina, is also removed (Fig. 14–12*A*). Epiretinal membranes are cut and/or peeled by a bent needle or membrane peeler-cutter[48] (Fig. 14–12*B*). Once the retina is again freely mobile, subretinal fluid is drained either internally through a retinal break (Fig. 14–12*C*) or externally through the sclera. Occasionally

relaxing retinotomies are required if the membranes cannot be removed sufficiently.[49] The retinal breaks are then treated to prevent reopening with either endolaser photocoagulation[50] (Fig. 14–12*D*) or transvitreal or external cryoretinopexy. Intraocular gas (air or a long-acting gas such as sulfur hexafluoride[51] or perfluoropropane[52–54]) is then infused into the globe to maintain the retina in approximation with the retinal pigment epithelium while the chorioretinal adhesion around the retinal break(s) is taking place. Most patients already have an encircling scleral buckle in place from previous surgery. If not, and if persistent peripheral circumferential retinal traction exists, then a broad encircling element should be placed (Fig. 14–12E). This technique can repair about one-half of the retinal detachments judged inoperable without vitrectomy.[54–62]

In some cases proliferation of periretinal membranes recurs and the retina redetaches. It may be judged at that stage that the aforementioned techniques will not be sufficient to repair the retinal detachment. Silicone oil injection into the vitreous cavity can be used in these cases. Liquid silicone oil is an inert, clear liquid with a specific gravity of 0.97 and a surface tension of approximately 50 with respect to water. Clinically useful viscosities have ranged between 1,000 and 12,500 centistokes, with 1,000 being the most commonly used. The refractive index of silicone oil is 1.4, and therefore, relatively mild refractive shifts occur when silicone fills the posterior segment. It is the high surface tension of silicone oil that allows for it to close retinal breaks and to permit internal drainage of subretinal fluid during fluid/silicone exchange.[63, 64]

Cibis[65] was the first to use this treatment in the management of complicated retinal detachments. More recently, with the realization that extensive removal of retinal membranes is necessary and with the refinements in vitrectomy techniques, silicone oil has regained a place in the treatment of these complex cases.[64–72]

Most patients will already have had a scleral buckling procedure and a vitrectomy. A repeat vitrectomy is performed to divide and/or remove as much epiretinal proliferation as possible. There is often severe "anterior loop traction" involving the vitreous base, ciliary body, and iris, which may cause foreshortening of the retina (Fig. 14–13). Careful dissection of this area must be performed, and this often necessitates lensectomy (Fig. 14–14). A high, broad 360-degree scleral buckle should be in place to treat residual anterior loop traction and anterior retinal breaks. Once all membranes have been removed or divided, a fluid/air exchange is performed. Subretinal fluid is drained through a posterior retinal break or through a retinotomy made superior nasal to the optic disc. Once the retina is flattened by this technique, silicone oil is injected into the eye (Fig. 14–

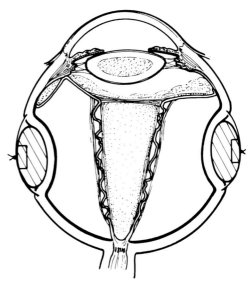

FIGURE 14–13. Anterior loop traction. In this example the peripheral retina is pulled forward and is adherent to the ciliary body, causing foreshortening of the retina.

15). The silicone is occasionally exchanged for fluid without a preceding air exchange. All retinal breaks are treated with either endolaser photocoagulation or transvitreal cryoretinopexy. Confluent endolaser photocoagulation lesions are applied to the encircling buckle for 360 degrees to try and close any nonvisualized, small retinal breaks as well as to try to isolate the posterior retina from any anterior retinal redetachment that may occur postoperatively (Fig. 14–16).

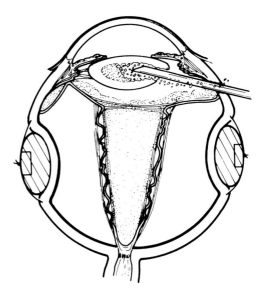

FIGURE 14–14. Pars plana lensectomy is performed to allow complete removal of anterior membranes.

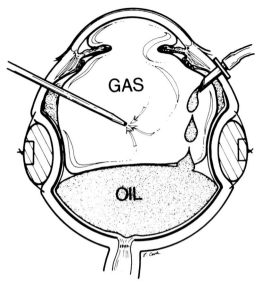

FIGURE 14–15. Silicone oil is exchanged for air once the retina has been flattened.

Many complications can occur in eyes treated with silicone oil.[69, 70, 72–74] These include persistent or recurrent retinal detachment, corneal decompensation, cataract, glaucoma, hypotony, and fibrous proliferation on the surface of the silicone.[75] Removal of the silicone oil after the proliferative phase is over (approximately 3 months) may diminish some of these complications, but approximately one-third of successfully reattached retinas redetach after its removal.

The National Eye Institute is currently spon-soring a multicenter, prospective, controlled clinical trial to evaluate the place of silicone oil in the management of proliferative vitreoretinopathy.[76] It is hoped that many of the controversies regarding silicone oil will be resolved by this study.

Diabetic Traction Retinal Detachment

Because diabetic retinal detachments often remain stationary for long periods,[77] vitrectomy should be undertaken only if there is demonstrated progression of the detachment into the macula. Recent detachments caused by a small focus of vitreous traction (Fig. 14–17) have the best prognosis among detachments of this kind, for the vitrectomy instrument easily releases the traction. Detachments with broader areas of traction involving the macula (Fig. 14–18) and longstanding diabetic traction retinal detachments have a poor prognosis.[3] Vitrectomy is not indicated for longstanding nonprogressive detachments because the eye usually does not regain useful visual function even after anatomical reattachment of the retina.

When surgery is undertaken, vitreous traction must be markedly reduced or the procedure may fail (Fig. 14–19).[48, 78–80] Peeling of fibrovascular membranes from the retina is hazardous, as the retina may be torn. It is much better to segment membranes by cutting bridges with motorized scissors or delaminating them from the retina. Broad membranes adherent to the retinal surface pose specific problems. They may strongly resist removal, and an inadvertent retinal tear may result. Moreover,

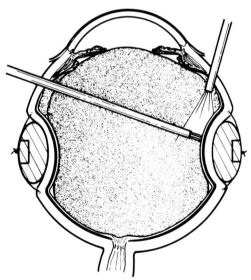

FIGURE 14–16. Confluent endolaser photocoagulation is applied to the encircling buckle for 360 degrees.

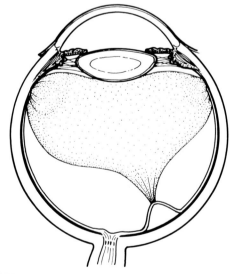

FIGURE 14–17. Traction retinal detachment with small area of vitreoretinal adhesion. Good prognosis.

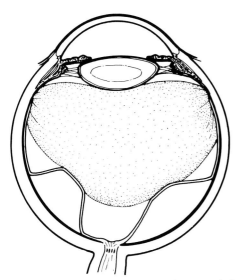

FIGURE 14–18. Traction retinal detachment with broad areas of vitreoretinal contact. Poor prognosis.

because these membranes shorten the retina, the release of vitreous traction alone will not result in reattachment. Therefore, when these broad membranes are present, a combined vitrectomy/scleral buckling procedure may be indicated. Eyes with dense premacular hemorrhage but without traction retinal detachment may benefit from prompt vitrectomy, since these eyes are at risk for developing macular traction detachment.[81, 82]

Giant Tear with Rolled-Over Retina

There are two major problems in the treatment of giant tears (circumferential tears 90 degrees or larger) with rolled-over retina (Fig. 14–20): first, initially unrolling the retina and, second, keeping it unrolled while cryosurgical, laser, or diathermy scarring takes place. Vitrectomy aids in solving both of these problems.[83] The patient is placed on a Stryker frame to

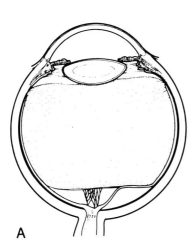

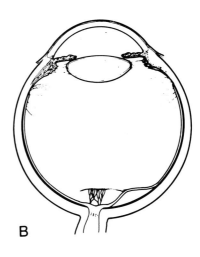

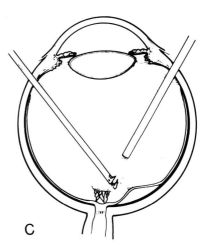

FIGURE 14–19. *A*, Contracting vitreous body pulling on neovascular stalk and retina. *B*, Vitreous traction relieved, but retina remains detached because of a bridge between the stalk and the retina (arrow). *C*, The stalk is pulled away from the retina by a bent needle so that it can be safely cut.

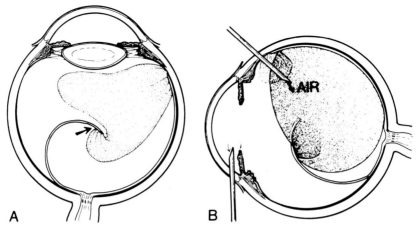

FIGURE 14–20. *A,* Giant tear with rolled-over retina. The vitreous remains attached to the anterior retina (arrow). *B,* After lensectomy and vitrectomy, the patient is positioned so that as air (or SF_6) is injected (arrow), it unrolls the retina. As the air is injected, fluid leaves the eye through a needle passed into the anterior chamber.

permit later repositioning. Cryoretinopexy is applied to the retinal pigment epithelium in the region of the retinal break, as well as to the attached retina in the remainder of the circumference of the globe. Michels believes that to minimize subsequent proliferative vitreoretinopathy, the cryotherapy should be done before the vitrectomy so that retinal pigment epithelium debris and viable retinal pigment epithelium cells can be washed out of the eye. An encircling scleral buckle that will provide a broad, low buckling effect is then placed. The vitrectomy is then performed. Generally, lensectomy is required to permit removal of all the anterior vitreous. Once the formed vitreous has been removed, the retina is unrolled by a bent needle. If the posterior retinal flap is completely inverted, then these techniques may not be sufficient to unroll the retina. The patient may then be turned into a prone position on the Stryker frame to allow the retina to unroll by gravity.[84] As air is slowly injected from below, the retina is flattened against the retinal pigment epithelium from posterior to anterior. The inert gas remains in the eye long enough to keep the retina in contact with the treated pigment epithelium until a firm surgical adhesion develops (Fig. 14–21). When the entire vitreous volume must be replaced by a gas, a mixture of 20 per cent SF_6 and 80 per cent room air should be used to prevent the severe elevation of the intraocular pressure that would otherwise result from postoperative expansion of pure SF_6.[85] Once the retina is completely flattened, five or six rows of endolaser photocoagulation are placed under the control of the operating microscope or the indirect ophthal-

moscope. Other techniques useful in the treatment of giant retinal tears have been described.[86–88] These include an intraocular balloon to help unfold the retina[89] and silicone oil,[90] sodium hyaluronate,[91] transscleral retinal sutures,[92] and retinal tacks[93, 94] to maintain the unrolled retina in place.

Aphakic Retinal Detachment Made "Inoperable" by Vitreous Incarceration

Sometimes traction on the retina caused by vitreous incarceration in a cataract wound prevents reattachment of an aphakic retinal detachment by a scleral buckling procedure (Fig. 14–

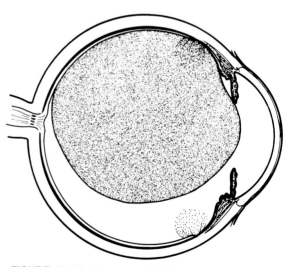

FIGURE 14–21. Postoperatively the patient is positioned so that the previously detached retina is superiorly located. The air (or gas) keeps the retina in contact with the pigment epithelium.

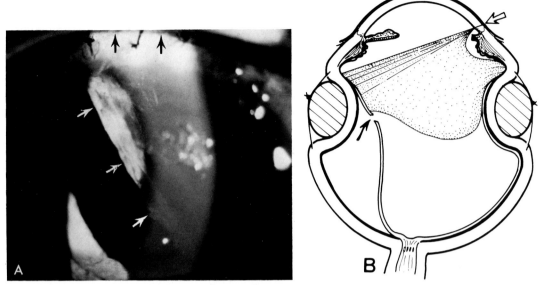

FIGURE 14–22. *A*, Vitreous base (white arrows), avulsed during anterior vitrectomy, is caught in the cataract wound (black arrows). *B*, Aphakic retinal detachment with vitreous caught in the cataract wound (open arrow), preventing closure of the retinal break (thin arrow) by the scleral buckle.

22).[95] This condition usually results from inadequate removal of vitreous lost during a complicated cataract extraction. A pars plana approach is used to completely remove the anterior vitreous. No longer pulled forward, the retina can fall back onto the scleral buckle.

Retinal Detachment After Penetrating Injury

A late complication of penetrating injury is the proliferation of episcleral fibrovascular tissue into the eye along the path of the foreign body (Fig. 14–23). The vitreous fibers act as a scaffold on which the tissue grows. When the fibrovascular membrane contracts, it can cause a retinal tear 90 to 180 degrees from the site of penetration. The resultant retinal detachment often can be repaired by a scleral buckling procedure, but vitrectomy is indicated when traction prevents the retina from settling.[96–102] Scissors must be used if the vitrectomy instrument cannot cut the dense membrane from the eye, and a scleral buckling procedure is then performed (Fig. 14–24). Even with the aid of vitreous surgery, the prognosis for these cases remains poor.

A new multicenter, randomized, controlled clinical trial, the Vitrectomy for Trauma Study, is currently under way, and this will, it is hoped, provide insight into the many unanswered questions regarding the management of severe ocular trauma.

Intraocular Foreign Bodies

Most magnetic intraocular foreign bodies can be removed easily and safely by a giant magnet. If the foreign body is encapsulated by fibrin, however, the magnet may fail. In such cases,

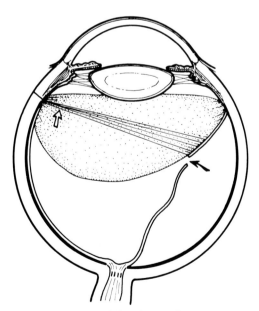

FIGURE 14–23. Retinal detachment after penetrating injury. The break (thin arrow) is caused by contraction of fibrovascular tissue that has proliferated from the entry wound (open arrow).

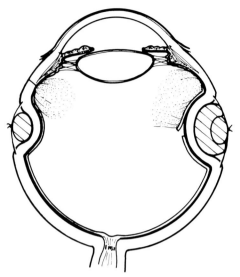

FIGURE 14–24. After vitrectomy has cut the proliferative tissue, the detachment is repaired by a scleral buckle.

and in cases in which the intraocular foreign body is nonmagnetic, vitrectomy is indicated.[96-98, 103-105] Vitrectomy is also indicated in cases in which the retina cannot be examined because of a dense vitreous hemorrhage or a cataract. A retinal tear may be present, and a retinal detachment may develop as the hemorrhage clears.

After the vitreous has been removed, a foreign body forceps, under direct visualization, safely removes the object (Fig. 14–25). All retinal tears are then treated with cryotherapy and scleral buckling.

Macular Pucker

Epiretinal membrane growth can lead to significant visual loss by causing distortion or "puckering" of the central macula. Epiretinal membranes can occur in a variety of situations. The most common is idiopathic or spontaneous. Macular pucker can also occur after retinal reattachment surgery and treatment for retinal breaks, intraocular inflammation, and retinal vascular disease; blunt or penetrating trauma; and vitreous hemorrhage.

The surgical technique for removal of an epiretinal membrane requires a core vitrectomy to be performed first. The membrane is then removed by stripping with a bent 23-gauge needle (Fig. 14–26) or vitreoretinal pick. Occasionally intraocular forceps are used to peel the membrane.[106, 107] Improvement in vision postoperatively is more likely if the duration of blurred vision preoperatively is short. Additionally, eyes with poorer vision preoperatively are more likely to have a greater amount of visual improvement postoperatively.[108] We generally do not operate on eyes with a visual acuity of 20/60 or better.

Glaucoma

Conventional therapies for malignant glaucoma after cataract surgery include maximal mydriasis, iridectomy, disruption of the hyaloid

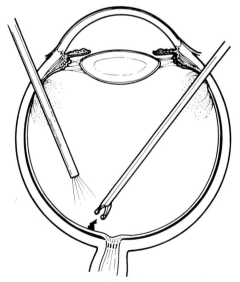

FIGURE 14–25. Foreign-body forceps are used to remove a nonmagnetic intraocular foreign body.

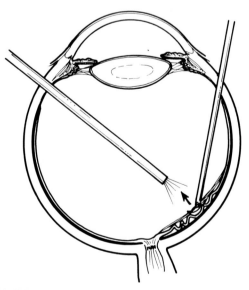

FIGURE 14–26. A bent 23-gauge hypodermic needle is used to peel the epiretinal membrane.

faces, aspiration of liquid vitreous, and injection of air into the anterior chamber. If these methods fail, removal of the formed vitreous by vitrectomy provides a definitive cure.

Erythrocyte debris that diffuses into the anterior chamber from a vitreous hemorrhage may cause hemolytic glaucoma because the trabecular meshwork becomes blocked by macrophages that phagocytize the debris. Temporary relief can be obtained by an anterior chamber washout. A permanent cure, however, requires removal of the vitreous hemorrhage by pars plana vitrectomy. When the hemorrhage has been removed, there is no longer any debris to come forward into the anterior chamber.

Cystoid Macular Edema

Cystoid macular edema (CME) frequently occurs after cataract surgery if vitreous becomes adherent to the wound. Many cases of CME resolve spontaneously; however, if CME and associated poor vision (less than 20/80) persist beyond several months, then pars plana vitrectomy to remove the adherent vitreous should be performed.[109, 110]

Endophthalmitis

Vitrectomy has been advanced as an adjunct to the antibiotic treatment of endophthalmitis (see Chapter 6), for several reasons.[111–117] First, it helps to control the infection by removing live bacteria from the eye. Second, it washes out bacterial enzymes, preventing further ocular damage. Third, it removes bacterial debris and necrotic inflammatory cells, both of which attract additional inflammatory cells. Fourth, it may allow better diffusion of antibiotics throughout the vitreous cavity.

Laboratory studies have shown that vitrectomy and intravitreal antibiotics combined were more effective than either treatment modality alone.[111] In addition, the combined treatment has cured endophthalmitis in humans.[112–117]

The role of vitrectomy, and even intravitreal antibiotics, in the treatment of endophthalmitis remains controversial. Cases have been successfully treated by systemic and periocular antibiotics alone.[118–120] Intravitreal antibiotics alone have also been effective.[112, 121–123] Our current approach is as follows. If the clinical diagnosis is "possible endophthalmitis," we do an anterior chamber and vitreous tap for smears and cultures and inject antibiotics periocularly.

If the clinical diagnosis is "probable endophthalmitis," or if smears and cultures from a tap are positive, we perform a vitrectomy and inject intravitreal antibiotics.

POSTOPERATIVE CARE AND COMPLICATIONS

Routine Care

The patients are mobilized as quickly as possible. Acetaminophen or other mild analgesics usually control the mild postoperative pain. Topically, we use a cycloplegic such as atropine 1% or scopolamine 0.25% two times per day and a combination corticosteroid-antibiotic four times per day. We do not use systemic antibiotics. The patients are discharged on the 1st or 2nd postoperative day. To prevent a fresh hemorrhage, the patients are advised to avoid heavy lifting or athletics, but, vision permitting, they are allowed to return to work 2 to 3 weeks after surgery.

Complications

Opaque Cornea in Diabetics

Predisposition. Vitreous surgery has many complications that can lead to permanent loss of vision. A permanently opaque cornea may result from persistent postoperative corneal edema and/or epithelial erosions. Diabetics are particularly prone to these complications, probably because of preexistent corneal abnormalities. First, the somewhat increased thickness of a diabetic's cornea indicates endothelial dysfunction. Second, diabetic corneas have slightly decreased sensation. Therefore, a neurotrophic component may contribute to their postoperative complications. Finally, the adhesion between the epithelium and the stroma is abnormally weak in diabetics. Indeed, the epithelium in diabetic patients can be easily brushed off with cotton-tipped applicator, whereas that of nondiabetics must be removed with a scalpel.

Management. In the immediate preoperative period corneal contact such as by tonometry, contact lens examination, and electroretinography should be minimized. The surgeon must avoid touching the cornea with solutions used for sterile preparation of the operative field. During surgery the cornea must be kept moist. Removal of the epithelium predisposes to late corneal complications,[37, 124] and should be performed only if the epithelium becomes hazy and prevents posterior visualization.

There are conflicting reports in the literature as to whether aphakia is a factor in corneal complications.[3, 36, 37, 123] Certainly if the toxicity of the intraocular irrigation solutions contributes to the corneal complications of vitrectomy, aphakic eyes should fare worse than phakic ones. In some series this is indeed the case.[37, 124] In other series the incidence of corneal complications is the same for both phakic and aphakic eyes.[3, 36] Because lensectomy may increase these complications, the lens should not be routinely removed during vitrectomy.

Postoperatively, the eye should be pressure-patched until any epithelial defects have healed. Phenylephrine drops are toxic to the corneal endothelium, especially if there are any epithelial defects;[125] they should be avoided. Finally, the intraocular pressure should be controlled because the epithelial edema caused by a high pressure predisposes to epithelial erosions.

Although early vitrectomy series reported a high incidence of corneal complications, by using the precautions above, we seldom see them unless the patient develops neovascular glaucoma.

Cataract

A cataract may develop as a result of toxicity of the intraocular irrigating solutions,[19, 126, 127] an inadvertent touch by the vitrectomy instrument,[128] or prolonged touch of the posterior lens surface by intravitreal gas.[129] Newer intraocular irrigating solutions such as BSS Plus are much less toxic to the lens.[19] In diabetic patients the addition of supplemental glucose to BSS Plus greatly reduces lens opacification during vitrectomy.[127]

Retinal Detachment

In vitreous surgery the surgeon can cause retinal tears that may lead to detachment. Therefore, when cutting a vitreous membrane close to the retina, he should lessen the suction of the instrument. The two-instrument technique offers an added safety feature: the membrane is elevated by a bent needle so that it can be cut by the vitrectomy instrument without involving the retina.[48] Excessive pulling on the membrane while it is being stripped can also tear the retina. Such tears must be repaired by a scleral buckling procedure or fluid-gas exchange with endolaser photocoagulation or endocryotherapy. Only by experience can a surgeon know when he has removed enough membrane and when he is taking an unnecessary risk in removing more. In some cases removal of all preretinal membranes is requisite to success; in others, such as diabetic traction retinal detachments, good visual function can be restored with some of the membranes still in place.

If ultrasonography has indicated the presence of a retinal detachment before surgery, special care should be taken to avoid contact between the retina and the vitrectomy instrument. The surgeon should then use the "land-to-sea" technique advocated by Machemer, which is as follows. When trying to enlarge a hole that he has cut in an opaque posterior vitreous membrane, the surgeon turns the cutting tip tangential to the membrane so that the suction pulls the membrane, and not the retina, into the tip.[83] Only when he can clearly see the retina should the surgeon direct the cutting tip toward it. A rare late complication of vitrectomy is retinal detachment owing to the contraction of a fibrovascular ingrowth from the entry site.[130–132]

Neovascular Glaucoma

Neovascular glaucoma is a frequent complication of vitrectomy in diabetic patients, occurring in 11 to 26 per cent of cases.[3, 29, 133–138] The risk of neovascular glaucoma is much greater if lensectomy is performed at the time of vitrectomy.[40] Once neovascular glaucoma is well established, the intraocular pressure can seldom be controlled without attendant loss of vision. Rubeosis iridis, present either before or after vitrectomy, may progress to postoperative neovascular glaucoma in diabetic eyes. Early rubeosis is not, however, an absolute contraindication to vitrectomy because it may not advance to neovascular glaucoma; moreover, if the vitrectomy is required, the risk of neovascular glaucoma must be taken.

Retinal detachment and severe iritis predispose diabetic eyes to rubeosis. After vitrectomy nearly all diabetic eyes with unrepaired retinal detachment develop rubeosis. Postoperative iritis must be vigorously controlled by cycloplegics and corticosteroids.

In our recent series of vitrectomies for nonclearing vitreous hemorrhage only 4 per cent of the patients who did not develop an inoperable retinal detachment developed neovascular glaucoma. We attribute this to the use of endolaser panretinal photocoagulation in cases not previously photocoagulated. Also, any patient who develops rubeosis iridis receives supplemental photocoagulation[139] or peripheral retinal cryotherapy. Fortunately neovascular glaucoma seldom develops later than 6 months after vitrectomy.[23] (For other comments regarding treatment of neovascular glaucoma, see Chapter 12.)

Hemolytic and Erythroclastic Glaucoma

If all of the red blood cells and red blood cell debris are not removed during vitrectomy, hemolytic glaucoma may ensue. Erythroclastic glaucoma is another possible complication of vitrectomy.[131, 132, 138] It is due to blockage of the trabecular meshwork by erythrocyte ghost cells (erythroclasts), which, unlike living erythrocytes, are inflexible and cannot pass through the meshwork. Occasionally the anterior chamber must be irrigated to decrease the intraocular pressure.

Recurrent Hemorrhage

Sometimes recurrent vitreous hemorrhage is seen after vitrectomy, especially in diabetics who have florid retinitis proliferans.[140, 141] These recurrent hemorrhages can be treated by simple irrigation of the vitreous cavity using two 23-gauge needles—one to infuse clear fluid and the other to aspirate the hemorrhage. Unfortunately many of these eyes will later rebleed.

SUMMARY

Vitrectomy is a high-risk procedure and must be undertaken only after careful evaluation. In cases for which a less dangerous remedy is not available, vitrectomy may preserve or restore vision that would otherwise be lost.

REFERENCES

1. Machemer, R., Buettner, H., Norton, E. W. D., Parel, J. M.: Vitrectomy: A pars plana approach. Trans. Am. Acad. Ophthalmol. Otolaryngol., 75:813, 1971.
2. Machemer, R., Buettner, H., Parel, N. J.: A new concept for vitreous surgery. I. Instrumentation. Am. J. Ophthalmol., 73:17, 1972.
3. Mandelcorn, M. S., Blankenship, B., Machemer, R.: Pars plana vitrectomy for the management of severe diabetic retinopathy. Am. J. Ophthalmol., 81:561, 1976.
4. Coleman, D. J., Abramson, D. H.: Ocular ultrasonography. In Duane, T. D. (ed.): Clinical Ophthalmology, Vol. 2, Ch. 26. Hagerstown, Md., Harper & Row, 1976.
5. Jack, R. L., Hutton, W. L., Machemer, R.: Ultrasonography and vitrectomy. Am. J. Ophthalmol., 78:2651, 1974.
6. Fuller, D. G., Knighton, R. W., Machemer, R.: Bright-flash electroretinography for the evaluation

of eyes with opaque vitreous. Am. J. Ophthalmol., 80:214, 1976.
7. Coleman, D. J., Jack, R. L.: B-scan ultrasonography in diagnosis and management of retinal detachment. Arch. Ophthalmol., 90:29, 1973.
8. Fuller, D. B., Laqua, H. Machemer, R.: Ultrasonographic diagnosis of massive periretinal proliferation in eyes with opaque media (triangular retinal detachment). Am. J. Ophthalmol., 83:460, 1977.
9. Abrams, G. W., Knighton, R. W.: Falsely extinguished bright flash electroretinogram. Arch. Ophthalmol., 100:1427, 1982.
10. Brightbill, F. S., Kaufman, H. E., Levenson, J. E. L.: A vitreous suction cutter for aphakic keratoplasty. Am. J. Ophthalmol., 76:331, 1973.
11. Douvas, N. G.: The cataract roto-extractor. Trans. Am. Acad. Ophthalmol. Otolaryngol., 77:792, 1973.
12. Federman, J. L.: The "S.I.T.E." instrument (suction infusion tissue extractor). In McPherson, A. (ed.): New and Controversial Aspects of Vitreoretinal Surgery. St. Louis, C. V. Mosby Co., 1977, pp. 184–190.
13. Kloti, R.: Vitrektomie. I. Ein neues instrument fur die hintere Vitrektomie. Abrecht von Graefes Arch. Klin. Exp. Ophthalmol., 187:161, 1973.
14. Krieger, A. E., Straatsma, B. R., Griffin, J. R., et al.: A vitrectomy instrument in stereotaxic intraocular surgery. Am. J. Ophthalmol., 76:527, 1973.
15. O'Malley, C., Heintz, R. M.: Vitrectomy with an alternative instrument system. Ann. Ophthalmol., 7:585, 1972.
16. Peyman, G. A., Dodich, N. A.: Experimental vitrectomy. Arch. Ophthalmol., 86:548, 1971.
17. Schepens, C. L.: Vitreous surgery: Tissue removal. In Pruett, R. C., Regan, C. D. J. (eds.): Retina Congress, New York. New York, Appleton-Century-Crofts, 1972, pp. 677–701.
18. McCuen, B. W. II, Hickingbotham, D.: A fiberoptic diathermy tissue manipulator for use in vitreous surgery. Am. J. Ophthalmol., 98:803, 1984.
19. Haimann, M. H., Abrams, G. W., Edelhauser, H. F., Hatchell, D. L.: The effect of intraocular irrigating solutions on lens clarity in normal and diabetic rabbits. Am. J. Ophthalmol., 94:594, 1982.
20. Edelhauser, H. F., Van Horn, D. C., Shultz, R. O., Hyndiuk, R. A.: Comparative toxicity of intraocular irrigation solutions on the corneal endothelium. Am. J. Ophthalmol., 81:483, 1976.
21. Edelhauser, H. F., Van Horn, D. C., Hyndiuk, R. A., Shultz, R. O.: Intraocular irrigation solutions. Their effect on the corneal endothelium. Arch. Ophthalmol., 93:648, 1975.
22. Diabetic Retinopathy Vitrectomy Study Group: Early vitrectomy for severe vitreous hemorrhage in diabetic retinopathy (two-year results of a randomized trial. Diabetic Retinopathy Vitrectomy Study Report #2). Arch. Ophthalmol., 103:1644, 1985.
23. Blankenship G. W., Machemer, R.: Pars plana vitrectomy for the management of severe diabetic retinopathy. An analysis of results five years after surgery. Ophthalmology, 85:553, 1978.
24. Federman, J. L., Boyer, D., Lanning, R., Breit, P.: An objective analysis of proliferative retinopathy before and after pars plana vitrectomy. Ophthalmology, 86:276, 1979.
25. Diabetic Retinopathy Vitrectomy Study Group: Two-year course of visual acuity in severe proliferative diabetic retinopathy with conventional management (Diabetic Retinopathy Vitrectomy Study Group Report #1). Ophthalmology, 92:492, 1985.

26. Charles, S., White, J., Dennison, C., Eichenbaum, D.: Bimanual, bipolar intraocular diathermy. Am. J. Ophthalmol., 81:101, 1976.

27. Thompson, J. T., Glaser, B. M., Michels, R. G., deBustros, S.: The use of intravitreal thrombin to control hemorrhage during vitrectomy. Ophthalmology, 93:279, 1986.

28. Michels, R. G.: Vitrectomy for complications of diabetic retinopathy. Arch. Ophthalmol., 96:237, 1978.

29. Michels, R. G., Ryan, S. J.: Results and complications of 100 consecutive cases of pars plana vitrectomy. Am. J. Ophthalmol., 80:24, 1975.

30. Peyman, G. A., Huamonte, F. U., Goldberg, M. F.: One hundred consecutive pars plana vitrectomies using the vitreophage, Am. J. Ophthalmol., 81:263, 1976.

31. Peyman, G. A., Huamonte, F. U., Goldberg, M. F.: Four hundred consecutive pars plana vitrectomies with the vitreophage. Arch. Ophthalmol., 96:45, 1978.

32. Machemer, R., Blankenship, G.: Vitrectomy for proliferative diabetic retinopathy associated with vitreous hemorrhage. Ophthalmology, 88:643, 1981.

33. Michels, R. G., Rice, T. A., Rice, E. F.: Vitrectomy for diabetic vitreous hemorrhage. Am. J. Ophthalmol., 95:12, 1983.

34. Blankenship, G. W., Machemer, R.: Long-term diabetic vitrectomy results. Report of 10 year follow-up. Ophthalmology, 92:503, 1985.

35. Aaberg, T. M.: Pars plana vitrectomy. In Brockhurst, R. J., Boruchoff, S. A., Hutchinson, B. T., Lessell, S. (eds.): Controversy in Ophthalmology. Philadelphia, W. B. Saunders Co., 1977, pp. 478–487.

36. Blankenship, G., Cortez, R., Machemer, R.: The lens and pars plana vitrectomy for diabetic retinopathy complications. Arch. Ophthalmol., 97:1263, 1979.

37. Foulks, G. N., Thoft, R. A., Perry, H. D., Tolentino, F. I.: Factors related to corneal epithelial complications after closed vitrectomy in diabetics. Arch. Ophthalmol., 97:1076, 1979.

38. Irvine, A. R., Shorb, S.: Removal of the lens at vitrectomy: Its advantages and disadvantages. In McPherson, A. (ed.): New and Controversial Aspects of Vitreoretinal Surgery. St. Louis, C. V. Mosby Co., 1977, pp. 295–300.

39. L'Esperance, F. A.: Influence of cataract extraction on the outcome of pars plana vitrectomy in eyes with proliferative diabetic retinopathy. In McPherson, A. (ed.): New and Controversial Aspects of Vitreoretinal Surgery. St. Louis, C. V. Mosby Co., 1977, pp. 301–311.

40. Rice, T. A., Michels, R. G., Maguire, M. G., Rice, E. F.: The effect of lensectomy on the incidence of iris neovascularization and neovascular glaucoma after vitrectomy for diabetic retinopathy. Am. J. Ophthalmol., 95:1, 1983.

41. Tasman, W.: Intracapsular cataract extraction and sector iridectomy combined with pars plana vitrectomy. In McPherson, A. (ed.): New and Controversial Aspects of Vitreoretinal Surgery. St. Louis, C. V. Mosby Co., 1977, pp. 281–285.

42. Coleman, D. J.: Phacoemulsification with vitrectomy through the pars plana. Ophthalmic Surg., 6:95, 1975.

43. Hutton, W. L., Snyder, W. B., Vaiser, A.: Management of intravitreal lens fragments by pars plana vitrectomy. Ophthalmology, 85:176, 1978.

44. Machemer, R.: Vitrectomy: A Pars Plana Approach. New York, Grune & Stratton, 1975, pp. 11–113.

45. Michels, R. G., Shacklett, D. R.: Vitrectomy technique for removal of retained lens material. Arch. Ophthalmol., 95:1767, 1977.

46. Stark, W. J., Michels, R. G., Bruner, W. E.: Management of posteriorly dislocated intraocular lenses. Ophthalmic Surg., 11:495, 1980.

47. McCannel, M. A.: A retrievable suture idea for anterior uveal problems. Ophthalmic Surg., 7:98, 1976.

48. Machemer, R.: Removal of pre-retinal membranes. Ophthalmology, 81:420, 1976.

49. Machemer, R., McCuen, B. W., de Juan, E.: Relaxing retinotomies and retinectomies. Am. J. Ophthalmol., 102:7, 1986.

50. Parks, D. W. II, Aaberg, T. M.: Intraocular argon laser photocoagulation in the management of severe proliferative vitreoretinopathy. Am. J. Ophthalmol., 97:434, 1984.

51. Abrams, G. W., Swanson, D. E., Sabates, W. J., Goldman, A. I.: The results of sulfur hexafluoride gas in vitreous surgery. Am. J. Ophthalmol., 94:165, 1982.

52. Lincoff, H., Coleman, J., Kreissig, I., et al.: The perfluorocarbon gases in the treatment of retinal detachment. Ophthalmology, 90:546, 1983.

53. Chang, S., Coleman, D. J., Lincoff, H., et al.: Perfluorocarbon gas in the management of proliferative vitreoretinopathy. Am. J. Ophthalmol., 98:180, 1984.

54. Chang, S., Lincoff, H. A., Coleman, D. J., et al.: Perfluorocarbon gases in vitreous surgery. Ophthalmology, 92:651, 1985.

55. Brown, G. C., Tasman, W. S.: Vitrectomy and Wagner's vitreoretinal degeneration. Am. J. Ophthalmol., 86:485, 1978.

56. Machemer, R., Laqua, H.: A logical approach to the treatment of massive periretinal proliferation. Ophthalmology, 85:584, 1978.

57. Michels, R. G.: Surgery of retinal detachment with proliferative vitreoretinopathy. Retina, 4:63, 1984.

58. Ratner, C. M., Michels, R. M., Auer, C., Rice, T. A.: Pars plana vitrectomy for complicated retinal detachments. Ophthalmology, 90:1323, 1983.

59. de Bustros, S., Michels, R. G.: Surgical treatment of retinal detachments complicated by proliferative vitreoretinopathy. Am. J. Ophthalmol., 98:694, 1984.

60. Jalkh, A. E., Avila, M. P., Schepens, C. L., et al.: Surgical treatments of proliferative vitreoretinopathy. Arch. Ophthalmol., 102:1135, 1984.

61. Sternberg, P., Jr., Machemer, R.: Results of vitreous surgery for proliferative vitreoretinopathy. Am. J. Ophthalmol., 100:141, 1985.

62. de Bustros, S., Michels, R. G.: Surgical treatment of retinal detachments complicated by proliferative vitreoretinopathy. Am. J. Ophthalmol., 102:20, 1986.

63. Haut, J., Larricart, J. P., Van Effenterre, G., Pinon-Pignero, Fl.: Some of the most important properties of silicone oil to explain its action. Ophthalmologica (Basel), 191:150, 1985.

64. McCuen, B. W., II, de Juan, E., Machemer, R.: Silicone oil in vitreoretinal surgery. I. Surgical techniques. Retina, 5:189, 1985.

65. Cibis, P. A., Becker, B., Okun, E., Canaan, S.: The use of liquid silicone in retinal detachment surgery. Arch. Ophthalmol., 68:590, 1962.

66. Scott, J. D.: A rational for the use of liquid silicone. Trans. Ophthalmol. Soc. U. K., 97:235, 1977.

67. Lean, J. S., Leaver, P. K., Cooling, R. J., McLeod, D.: Management of complex retinal detachments by vitrectomy and fluid/silicone exchange. Trans. Ophthal. Soc. U.K., 102:203, 1982.

68. Gonvers, M.: Temporary use of silicone oil in the treatment of special cases of retinal detachment. Ophthalmologica (Basel), 187:202, 1983.

69. McCuen, B. W., II, de Juan, E., Landers, M. B., III, Machemer, R.: Silicone oil in vitreoretinal surgery. II. Retina, 5:198, 1985.

70. McCuen, B. W., II, Landers, M. B., III, Machemer, R.: The use of silicone oil following failed vitrectomy for retinal detachment with advanced proliferative vitreoretinopathy. Ophthalmology, 92:1029, 1985.

71. Gonvers, M.: Temporary use of silicone oil in the management of retinal detachment with proliferative vitreoretinopathy. Am. J. Ophthalmol., 100:239, 1985.

72. Cox, M. S., Trese, M. T., Murphy, P. L.: silicone oil for advanced proliferative vitreoretinopathy. Ophthalmology, 93:646, 1986.

73. Chan, C., Okun, E.: The question of ocular tolerance to intravitreal liquid silicone; a long-term analysis. Ophthalmology, 93:651, 1986.

74. Watzke, R. C.: Use of silicone oil. Arch. Ophthalmol., 100:1354, 1985.

75. Laroche, L., Paviakis, C., Saraux, H., et al.: Ocular findings following intravitreal silicone injection. Arch. Ophthalmol., 101:1422, 1983.

76. The Silicone Study Group: Proliferative vitreoretinopathy. Am. J. Ophthalmol., 99:593, 1985.

77. Cohen, H. B., McMeel, J. W., Franks, E. P.: Diabetic traction detachment. Arch. Ophthalmol., 97:1268, 1979.

78. Machemer, R.: Results of vitreous surgery. In Symposium on Retinal Disease. Transactions of the New Orleans Academy of Ophthalmology. St. Louis, C. V. Mosby Co., 1977, pp. 81–88.

79. Aaberg, T.: Pars plana vitrectomy for diabetic traction retinal detachment. Ophthalmology, 88:639, 1981.

80. Rice, T. A., Michels, R. G., Rice, E. F.: Vitrectomy for diabetic traction retinal detachment involving the macula. Am. J. Ophthalmol., 95:22, 1983.

81. O'Hanley, G. P., Canny, C. L. B.: Diabetic dense premacular hemorrhage. A possible indication for prompt vitrectomy. Ophthalmology, 92:507, 1985.

82. Ramsay, R. C., Knobloch, W. H., Cantrill, H. L.: Timing of vitrectomy for active proliferative diabetic retinopathy. Ophthalmology, 93:283, 1986.

83. Machemer, R., Allen, A. W.: Retinal tears 180° and greater. Management with vitrectomy and intravitreous gas. Arch. Ophthalmol., 94:1340, 1976.

84. Schepens, C. L., Freeman, H. M.: Current management of giant retinal breaks. Trans. Am. Acad. Ophthalmol. Otolaryngol., 71:474, 1967.

85. Norton, E. W. D.: Intraocular gas in the management of selected retinal detachments. Trans. Am. Acad. Ophthalmol. Otolaryngol., 77:85, 1973.

86. Freeman, H. M., Castillejos, M. E.: Current management of giant retinal breaks: Results with vitrectomy and total air fluid exchange in 95 cases. Trans. Am. Ophthalmol. Soc., 79:89, 1981.

87. Michels, R. G., Rice, T. A., Blankenship, G.: Surgical techniques for selected giant retinal tears. Retina, 3:139, 1983.

88. Vidaurri-Leal, J., de Bustros, S., Michels, R. G.: Surgical treatment of giant retinal tears with inverted posterior retinal flaps. Am. J. Ophthalmol., 98:463, 1984.

89. Freeman, H. M.: Vitreous Surgery, 10. Current status of vitreous surgery in cases of rhegmatogenous retinal detachment. Trans. Am. Acad. Ophthalmol. Otolaryngol., 77:202, 1973.

90. Leaver, P. K., Lean, J. S.: Management of giant retinal tears using vitrectomy and silicone oil/fluid exchange. A preliminary report. Trans. Ophthalmol. Soc. U.K., 101:189, 1981.

91. Brown, G. C., Benson, W. E.: Use of sodium hyaluronate for the repair of giant retinal tears. Arch. Ophthalmol., 107:1246, 1989.

92. Federman, J. L., Shakin, J. L., Lanning, R. C.: The microsurgical management of giant retinal tears with trans-scleral retinal sutures. Ophthalmology, 89:832, 1982.

93. de Juan, E., Jr., Hickingbotham, D., Machemer, R.: Retinal tacks. Am. J. Ophthalmol., 99:272, 1985.

94. Ando, F., Kondo, J.: Surgical techniques for giant retinal tears with retinal tacks. Ophthalmic Surg., 17:408, 1986.

95. Norton, E. W. D., Machemer, R.: New approaches to the treatment of selected retinal detachments secondary to vitreous loss at cataract surgery. Am. J. Ophthalmol., 72:705, 1971.

96. Benson, W. E., Machemer, R.: Severe perforating injuries treated with pars plana vitrectomy. Am. J. Ophthalmol., 81:729, 1976.

97. Conway, B. P., Michels, R. G.: Vitrectomy techniques in the management of selected penetrating ocular injuries. Ophthalmology, 85:560, 1978.

98. Hutton, W. L., Snyder, W. B., Vaiser, A.: Vitrectomy in the treatment of ocular perforating injuries. Am. J. Ophthalmol., 81:733, 1976.

99. Michels, R. G.: Vitrectomy methods in penetrating ocular trauma. Ophthalmology, 87:629, 1980.

100. Ramsey, R. C., Cantrill, H. L., Knobloch, W. H.: Vitrectomy for double penetrating injuries. Am. J. Ophthalmol., 100:586, 1985.

101. Coleman, D. J.: Early vitrectomy in the management of the severely traumatized eye. Am. J. Ophthalmol., 93:543, 1982.

102. De Juan, E., Sternberg, P. Jr., Michels, R. G., Auer, C.: Evaluation of vitrectomy in penetrating ocular trauma: A case-control study. Arch. Ophthalmol., 102:1160, 1984.

103. Shock, J. P., Adams, D.: Long-term visual acuity results after penetrating and perforating ocular injuries. Am. J. Ophthalmol., 100:714, 1985.

104. Howcroft, M. J., Shea, M.: Management of posterior-segment foreign bodies. Can. J. Ophthalmol., 17:265, 1982.

105. Peyman, G. A., Raichand, M., Goldberg, M. F., Brown, S.: Vitrectomy in the management of intraocular foreign bodies and their complications. Br. J. Ophthalmol., 64:476, 1980.

106. Michels, R. G.: Vitrectomy for macular pucker. Ophthalmology, 91:1384, 1984.

107. Margherio, R. R., Cox, M. S., Trese, M. T., et al.: Removal of epimacular membranes. Ophthalmology, 92:1075, 1985.

108. Rice, T. A., de Bustros, S., Michels, R. G., et al.: Prognostic factors in vitrectomy for epiretinal membranes of the macula. Ophthalmology, 93:602, 1986.

109. Fung, W., Vitrectomy-ACME Study Group: Vitrectomy for chronic aphakic cystoid macular edema. Results of a national, collaborative, prospective, randomized investigation. Ophthalmology, 92:1102, 1985.

110. Federman, J. L., Annesley, W. H., Sarin, L. K.,

Remer, P.: Vitrectomy and cystoid macular edema. Ophthalmology, 87:622, 1980.

111. Cottingham, A. J., Forster, R. K.: Vitrectomy in endophthalmitis. Results of study using vitrectomy, intraocular antibiotics, or a combination of both. Arch. Ophthalmol., 94:2078, 1976.

112. Peyman, G. A.: Antibiotic administration in the treatment of bacterial endophthalmitis. Intravitreal injections. Surv. Ophthalmol., 21:332, 1977.

113. Peyman, G. A., Vastine, D. W., Diamond, J. G.: Vitrectomy and intraocular gentamycin management of Herellea endophthalmitis after incomplete phacoemulsification. Am. J. Ophthalmol., 80:764, 1975.

114. Peyman, G. A., Vastine, D. W., Diamond, J. G.: Vitrectomy in exogenous *Candida* endophthalmitis. Albrecht von Graefes Arch. klin. exp. Ophthalmol., 197:55, 1975.

115. Snip, R. C., Michels, R. G.: Pars plana vitrectomy in the management of endogenous *Candida* endophthalmitis. Am. J. Ophthalmol., 82:699, 1976.

116. Peyman, G. A., Raichand, M., Bennett, T. O.: Management of endophthalmitis with pars plana vitrectomy. Br. J. Ophthalmol., 64:472, 1980.

117. Driebe, W. T., Mandelbaum, S., Forster, R. K., et al.: Pseudophakic endophthalmitis. Diagnosis and management. Ophthalmology, 93:442, 1986.

118. Baum, J. L.: Antibiotic administration in the treatment of bacterial endophthalmitis. Periocular injections. Surv. Ophthalmol., 21:332, 1977.

119. Griffin, J. R., Pettit, T. H., Fishman, L. S., Foos, R. Y.: Blood-borne *Candida* endophthalmitis. Arch. Ophthalmol., 9:450, 1973.

120. Robertson, D. M., Riley, F. C., Herman, P. E.: Endogenous *Candida* oculomycosis. Report of two patients treated with flucytosine. Arch. Ophthalmol., 91:33, 1974.

121. Forster, R. K., Zachary, I. G., Cottingham, A. J., Norton, E. W. D.: Further observations on the diagnosis, cause and treatment of endophthalmitis. Am. J. Ophthalmol., 81:52, 1976.

122. Peyman, G. A., Herbst, R.: Bacterial endophthalmitis treatment with intraocular injections of gentamycin and dexamethasone. Arch. Ophthalmol., 91:416, 1974.

123. Stern, G. A., Fetkenhour, C. L., O'Grady, R. B.: Intravitreal amphotericin-B treatment of *Candida* endophthalmitis. Arch. Ophthalmol., 95:89, 1977.

124. Brightbill, F. S., Myers, F. L., Bresnick, G. H.: Postvitrectomy keratopathy. Am. J. Ophthalmol., 85:651, 1978.

125. Edelhauser, H. F., Hine, J. E., Pederson, H., et al.: The effect of phenylephrine on the cornea. Arch. Ophthalmol., 97:937, 1979.

126. Christiansen, J. M., Kollarits, C. R., Fukui, H., et al.: Intraocular irrigating solutions and lens clarity. Am. J. Ophthalmol., 82:594, 1976.

127. Haimann, M. H., Abrams, G. W.: Prevention of lens opacification during diabetic vitrectomy. Ophthalmology, 91:116, 1984.

128. Faulborn, J., Conway, B. P., Machemer, R.: Surgical complications of pars plana vitreous surgery. Ophthalmology, 85:116, 1978.

129. Novak, M. A., Rice, T. A., Michels, R. G., Auer, C.: The crystalline lens after vitrectomy for diabetic retinopathy. Ophthalmology, 91:1480, 1984.

130. Buettner, H., Machemer, R.: Histopathologic findings in human eye after pars plana vitrectomy and lensectomy. Arch. Ophthalmol., 95:2029, 1977.

131. Pulhorn, G., Teichmann, K. D., Teichmann, I.: Intraocular fibrous proliferation as an incisional complication in pars plana vitrectomy. Am. J. Ophthalmol., 83:810, 1977.

132. Tardif, Y. M., Schepens, C. L.: Closed vitreous surgery. II. Surgical technique and complications. Am. J. Ophthalmol., 74:1022, 1972.

133. Aaberg, T. M., Van Horn, D. L.: Late complications of pars plana vitreous surgery. Ophthalmology, 85:125, 1978.

134. Campbell, D. G., Simmons, R. J., Tolentino, F. I., McMeel, J. W.: Glaucoma occurring after closed vitrectomy. Am. J. Ophthalmol., 83:63, 1977.

135. Gitter, K. A., Cohen, G.: Complications of vitrectomy. *In* Gitter, K. A. (ed.): Current Concepts of the Vitreous Including Vitrectomy. St. Louis, C. V. Mosby Co., 1976, pp. 253–262.

136. Machemer, R.: Special problems of the diabetic eye after vitrectomy. *In* Symposium on Retinal Diseases. Transactions of the New Orleans Academy of Ophthalmology. St. Louis, C. V. Mosby Co., 1977, pp. 165–169.

137. Weinberg, R. S., Peyman, G. A., Huamonte, F. U.: Elevation of intraocular pressure after pars plana vitrectomy. Albrecht von Graefe Arch. kin. exp. Ophthalmol., 200:157, 1976.

138. Wilensky, J., Goldberg, M. F., Alward P.: Glaucoma after pars plana vitrectomy. Trans. Am. Acad. Ophthalmol. Otolaryngol., 83:114, 1977.

139. Little, H. L., Rosenthal, R., Dellaporta, A., Jacobson, D. R.: The effect of panretinal photocoagulation on rubeosis iridis. Am. J. Ophthalmol., 81:804, 1976.

140. Blankenship, G. W.: Management of vitreous cavity hemorrhage following pars plana vitrectomy for diabetic retinopathy. Ophthalmology, 93:39, 1986.

141. Schachat, A. P., Oyakawa, R. T., Michels, R. G., Rice, T. A.: Complications of vitreous surgery for diabetic retinopathy. II. Postoperative complications. Ophthalmology, 90:522, 1983.

15

SURGERY OF THE ORBIT

by Arthur S. Grove, Jr.

The management of orbital disorders requires knowledge of the pathogenesis of orbital disease and familiarity with appropriate diagnostic studies as well as skill in surgical techniques. Before treatment is begun, a patient with an orbital disorder should be carefully evaluated. The abnormality should be localized, and a preliminary diagnosis should be established if possible. In many cases a diagnosis can be reached without surgical intervention because some lesions can be recognized by their characteristic clinical features. Sometimes orbital surgery can be avoided when a lesion is thought to be benign or when resolution of the abnormality is possible. It is important to avoid unnecessary surgery when injury to normal adjacent structures is likely to result from an operation. However, even in patients with benign lesions it may be necessary to obtain tissue to establish a definite diagnosis or to correct secondary abnormalities such as eyelid malposition or strabismus.

Patients with nontraumatic orbital disorders, including unexplained exophthalmos, are usually evaluated and treated differently from those who have sustained recent orbital trauma. However, blood cysts, sinus mucoceles, and carotid-cavernous sinus (CCS) fistulas may result from trauma and cause exophthalmos long after the original injury.

ORBITAL DISORDERS AND EXOPHTHALMOS

Evaluation

An orderly sequence of diagnostic steps should be used for the evaluation of a patient who is suspected of having an orbital disorder (Table 15–1).

Maintain Index of Suspicion

In the absence of recent trauma, a high index of suspicion should be maintained for the occurrence of the most common orbital disorders.[1-6] The incidence of orbital disorders differs in adults (Table 15–2) from that in children (Table 15–3). It is also necessary to consider whether these abnormalities may be mimicked by conditions that cause pseudoexophthalmos, such as an enlarged globe, eyelid retraction, contralateral ptosis, extraocular muscle weakness, and asymmetrical orbital sizes.

History and Physical Examination

A careful history and physical examination should precede laboratory and radiographic studies. In most cases a preliminary diagnosis can be made with a high degree of accuracy based on a knowledge of the behavior of com-

421

TABLE 15–1. Diagnostic Steps in the Evaluation of Orbital Disorders and Exophthalmos

1. *Maintain index of suspicion.*
   a. Consider common orbital disorders (see Tables 15–2 and 15–3)
   b. Consider causes of pseudoexophthalmos
2. *Take history and perform physical examination.*
   a. History
   b. Ocular examination
   c. Neurological examination
   d. Orbital examination
3. *Perform systemic examinations.*
   a. Hematologic and urine examinations
   b. Chest x-rays
   c. Breast examination (women)
   d. Blood tumor factors
   e. Neuroblastoma tests (children)
   f. Evaluation of ophthalmic Graves' disease (see Table 15–4)
4. *Perform orbital imaging studies.*
   a. X-rays
   b. Ultrasonography
   c. Computed tomography
   d. Magnetic resonance imaging
   e. Radionuclide scans
   f. Venography
   g. Arteriography
5. *Use tissue processing techniques as needed.*
   a. Light microscopy
   b. Electron microscopy
   c. Immunohistochemistry
   d. Hormone receptor assay

TABLE 15–3. Common Orbital Disorders in Children*

Cellulitis
Idiopathic inflammations (pseudotumors)
Dermoids
Vascular tumors (especially capillary hemangiomas)
Sarcomas (especially rhabdomyosarcomas)
Neurogenic tumors (especially neurofibromas and optic gliomas)
Bone tumors
Metastatic tumors (especially neuroblastomas)
Histiocytic and eosinophilic tumors
Leukemias

*These disorders are listed in approximate order of frequency and do not include trauma.

mon orbital abnormalities together with a meticulous history and physical examination.

The *history* should focus attention on important features, such as the duration of symptoms; the occurrence of tumors elsewhere in the body, including lung cancer, breast cancer, and melanoma; the presence of thyroid disease in the patient or other members of his family; evidence of head trauma; the presence of sinus disease; and the awareness of pulsations or bruits. Among the most common symptoms of orbital disease are decreased vision, pain, and diplopia.

TABLE 15–2. Common Orbital Disorders in Adults*

Graves' disease
Idiopathic inflammations (pseudotumors)
Lymphomas
Vascular tumors (especially cavernous hemangiomas)
Neurogenic tumors (especially meningiomas)
Metastatic tumors (especially from breast or lung)
Lacrimal gland tumors
Sinus mucoceles and tumors
Dermoids
Vascular communications and malformations

*These disorders are listed in approximate order of frequency and do not include trauma.

Rapidly evolving symptoms, especially if pain is a prominent feature, are usually the result of acute inflammations, such as infections or pseudotumors, or of malignant tumors. Symptoms that have been present for many months or years are probably caused by chronic inflammations or benign tumors. Breast cancer and melanoma may metastasize to the orbit years after the primary lesions have been treated. Almost any systemic malignancy should be considered a possible origin for an orbital metastasis. Ophthalmic Graves' disease is the most common cause of both unilateral and bilateral exophthalmos in adults. Most patients with Graves' disease have thyroid abnormalities, and many have a family history of thyroid disorders. Head trauma may cause CCS fistulas or blood cysts and may imbed foreign bodies within the orbital tissues. Fractures of the orbital floor may cause enophthalmos, and thus mimic prominence of the contralateral eye. Sinus disease commonly causes orbital abnormalities as a result of spread of infection, extension of tumors, or expansion of sinus mucoceles. Dynamic abnormalities such as pulsations or bruits may result from vascular disorders or from bony defects between the orbit and the intracranial space.

The *ocular examination* should precede evaluation of the orbits. Visual acuities, refractive errors, and intraocular pressures should be measured. Anterior segments must be carefully examined to locate abnormalities such as tortuous conjunctival vessels, which may indicate the presence of an arteriovenous (AV) communication. Fundus examination may reveal an intraocular tumor, papilledema, or chorioretinal folds.

The *neurological examination* of a patient with an orbital disorder should include documentation of visual fields and eye movements. Pupil reactions and sizes should be measured.

Corneal and cutaneous sensation should be recorded. Color vision testing may be useful if an optic nerve lesion is suspected.

The *orbital examination* may reveal abnormalities such as displacement of the eye, a palpable mass, distortion of the eyelids, or dynamic changes that fluctuate with time. A real or apparent prominence of the eye is one of the most frequent and dramatic consequences of an orbital disorder. Photographs and sketches in the patient's chart are useful for documenting clinical features with which the patient's future appearance may be compared.

Exophthalmos is an abnormal prominence of one or both eyes, and usually results from an orbital tumor, an inflammation, or a vascular disorder. Reference measurements may conveniently be made from the lateral orbital rim to the corneal apex with use of a Hertel exophthalmometer. The usual distance from the orbital rim to the cornea is approximately 16 mm in adults. It is uncommon for an eye to normally protrude more than 21 mm beyond the orbital rim. An asymmetry of more than 2 mm between the prominence of the two eyes is suggestive of unilateral exophthalmos.

In adults (Table 15–2) unilateral exophthalmos is most often caused by ophthalmic Graves' disease. Cavernous hemangiomas are the most common benign tumors found in the orbits of adults. The most common orbital malignancies among adults are secondary tumors extending from the paranasal sinuses and metastatic tumors from the breast or lung.

In children (Table 15–3) prominence of one eye is most frequently caused by orbital cellulitis as a complication of either ethmoidal sinus disease or a respiratory tract infection. Dermoids and capillary hemangiomas are the most common benign orbital tumors of childhood, whereas rhabdomyosarcomas are the most common primary orbital malignancies in this age group.

Bilateral exophthalmos in adults is most often caused by ophthalmic Graves' disease, and less often by lymphoma or inflammations such as pseudotumor or Wegener's granulomatosis. In children bilateral exophthalmos is most frequently caused by leukemia or metastatic neuroblastoma.

Pseudoexophthalmos is usually defined as the simulation of abnormal prominence of the eye, as occurs in patients with asymmetrical eyelid positions caused by eyelid retraction or contralateral ptosis. In addition, pseudoexophthalmos may be used to describe a truly abnormal prominence of the eye that is not due to a mass, an inflammation, or a vascular disorder. Causes of such pseudoexophthalmos include an enlarged globe in patients with myopia, relaxation of the extraocular muscles resulting from nerve or muscle damage, a shallow orbit, and contralateral enophthalmos resulting from fractures or cicatricial tumors. Metastatic breast carcinoma is the most common tumor causing cicatricial enophthalmos. Even if a patient is found to have pseudoexophthalmos, it is appropriate to carefully examine the orbits clinically and to obtain orbital x-rays as a reference for future examinations.

Palpation around the globe may disclose the presence of a mass in the anterior orbit, particularly if the lacrimal gland is enlarged or if a sinus mucocele is present. Increased resistance to retrodisplacement of the globe (decreased orbital resilience) suggests the presence of a retrobulbar mass. This is a nonspecific abnormality that may occur with tumors and with inflammatory disorders.

Eyelid distortion is characteristic of certain orbital disorders. Among the most common ophthalmic signs of Graves' disease are retraction of the lower or upper eyelids (Dalrymple's sign), lag of the upper eyelid on downgaze, and restriction of downward traction on the upper eyelid (Grove's sign). Dermoid cysts often present as firm, subcutaneous nodules beneath the brow and upper lip. Capillary hemangiomas may involve the skin of the lids during infancy and produce "strawberry birthmarks" that usually regress spontaneously within several years. Plexiform neurofibromas usually occur in patients with von Recklinghausen's disease. These tumors often cause ptosis and grow within the lateral upper eyelids as a mass that resembles a "bag of worms."

Dynamic orbital abnormalities are those that pulsate, that are associated with bruits, or that rapidly change in size, shape, or position. Pulsating exophthalmos may result from vascular abnormalities such as CCS fistulas, dural shunts, and other AV communications, or from bony defects between the orbit and the intracranial space. Large mucoceles can allow the transfer of intracranial pulsations to the globe or to the orbit, as can developmental abnormalities of the orbital bones in patients with von Recklinghausen's disease. Highly vascularized tumors can cause orbital pulsations on occasion. A tonometer may detect minimal pulsations that are not otherwise evident. Bruits may be objectively detected with a stethoscope or may be subjectively described by patients with AV communications. Rapid changes in the amount of exophthalmos or in the size of an orbital mass may be associated with crying, raised intrathoracic pressure, or dependence of the head. Such fluctuations in prominence or size may be caused by a varix, an AV communication, or a meningoencephalocele. Rarely, this phenomenon occurs with hemangiomas or lymphangiomas.

Systemic Examinations

Hematological examination with a complete blood count can help to determine whether a blood dyscrasia such as leukemia is present. Some patients with lymphocytic abnormalities may have abnormal circulating white blood cells. An abnormal sedimentation rate may be found in patients with inflammatory disorders such as vasculitis. Forms of vasculitis that may involve the orbit include giant cell arteritis, polyarteritis nodosa, and Wegener's granulomatosis.[7]

Urine examination may occasionally reveal abnormalities associated with orbital disease. Patients with amyloidosis and plasma cell proliferations such as Waldenström's macroglobulinemia may have immunoglobulin fragments in the urine as Bence Jones proteins. If a patient is suspected of having such a disorder, a 24-hour urine collection should be analyzed for protein abnormalities.[7] Children with possible neuroblastoma should be studied by a 24-hour urine collection that is analyzed for vanillylmandelic acid (VMA), a norepinephrine metabolite that is often elevated in patients with this tumor.[1] Although renal and other urological tumors rarely metastasize to the orbit, sometimes they may be detected by the presence of blood in the urine.

Chest x-rays should be performed on almost all patients, since lung cancer is one of the most frequent tumors that metastasize to the orbit in adults. Sometimes tumors originating in other locations may metastasize to both the orbit and the lungs, and may therefore be detected by chest examination.

Breast examination in women should be performed as part of the complete physical examination that all patients suspected of having orbital tumors should undergo. In women breast carcinoma is the most frequent tumor that metastasizes to the orbit. Mammography might be considered if a breast tumor is thought to be present.

Blood tumor factors may be elevated in some patients with malignant tumors. Plasma levels of carcinoembryonic antigen (CEA) are abnormal in many patients with gastrointestinal malignancies as well as in some patients with other tumors, such as neuroblastoma and breast carcinoma.[8] Serum levels of human chorionic gonadotropin (HCG) are elevated during pregnancy and in a significant number of women with metastatic breast cancer and trophoblastic tumors.[9] A number of other blood factors have been found to be elevated in the presence of certain tumors, and their use as screening tests may be indicated in patients with orbital abnormalities.

Neuroblastoma tests are commonly used to study children who are suspected of having a malignant orbital tumor. Neuroblastoma is the most frequent solid tumor found in children, usually occurring before 2 years of age. This neoplasm may metastasize to the orbits and may produce ecchymosis of the eyelids and bilateral exophthalmos. Neuroblastomas usually arise from sympathetic neuroblasts within the abdomen, and computed tomographic (CT) scans may reveal a retroperitoneal mass. As previously mentioned, neuroblastomas may cause elevated levels of plasma CEA and urinary VMA.

Evaluation of ophthalmic Graves' disease should be a basic part of the study of most patients with orbital disease (Table 15–4). Graves' disease is the most common cause of both unilateral and bilateral exophthalmos among adults. Graves' disease is an inflammatory disorder of unknown cause that is often,

---

TABLE 15–4. Evaluation of Ophthalmic Graves' Disease

Ophthalmic Signs of Graves' Disease
 1. Extraocular muscle enlargement
 2. Eye movement limitation
 3. Lid retraction (Dalrymple's sign), lid lag, and restriction of downward traction on lid (Grove's sign)
 4. Lid and orbital edema
 5. Unilateral and bilateral exophthalmos
 6. Optic neuropathy (defects in acuity, color sense, visual fields, and pupil reactions)

Serum Thyroid Tests
 1. Thyroxine (T_4) levels
 2. Triiodothyronine (T_3) levels
 3. Thyrotropin (thyroid-stimulating hormone or TSH) levels
 4. Thyrotropin releasing hormone (TRH) test*

Anatomical Studies
 1. Ultrasonography
 2. Computed tomography (especially with both axial and coronal or sagittal scans)

---

*The TRH test is usually reserved for evaluation of patients whose T_4, T_3, and TSH levels are normal or equivocal, but in whom Graves' disease is still suspected because of clinical signs or other test results.

but not always, related to thyroid abnormalities such as hyperthyroidism. Thyroid function tests are valuable both in guiding the management of endocrine dysfunction and in establishing the diagnosis of Graves' disease. The diagnosis of this disorder is usually made chiefly on the basis of typical clinical signs and the results of anatomical studies such as ultrasonography and computed tomography.[10] These signs and studies are discussed under Ophthalmic Graves' Disease.

Although some patients with ophthalmic Graves' disease have no thyroid abnormality, most will have elevated serum thyroxine (T_4) or serum triiodothyronine (T_3) levels. Serum thyrotropin (thyroid-stimulating hormone [TSH]) levels may also be used to detect thyroid dysfunction. If these tests are normal or equivocal but Graves' disease is still suspected because of clinical signs or anatomical study results, then a thyrotropin releasing hormone (TRH) test may be ordered. Sometimes TRH tests disclose a thyroid abnormality in patients whose other blood tests are normal.[11–13]

Orbital Imaging Studies

After the history and physical examination have been completed and systemic examinations with tests for Graves' disease have been initiated, the orbits can be evaluated by a variety of imaging studies. The most important of these are x-rays, ultrasonography, computed tomography, and magnetic resonance imaging. Examples of some of these studies are given under discussion of specific orbital disorders.

X-rays are a fundamental part of the evaluation of nearly all orbital abnormalities. Although tomographic x-rays can be used to visualize thin sections of the body, these studies have been almost superseded by computed tomography and magnetic resonance imaging.

Optic canal enlargement may be an important diagnostic feature of certain tumors such as optic gliomas and meningiomas. Therefore, the anatomy of this structure must be thoroughly understood. The optic canal is 5 to 10 mm long and is located within the lesser wing of the sphenoid. The optic nerve, ophthalmic artery, and sympathetic nerves pass through this canal. The orbital end of the canal is the optic foramen, which normally is less than 6.5 mm in diameter. An optic foramen that is 7 mm in diameter is usually abnormal. In young children whose optic canals have not yet reached adult dimensions, the sizes of both foramens should be compared. In such patients a foramen that is 6.5 mm in diameter and at least 1 mm larger

than the contralateral foramen is usually considered to be abnormal.[14]

Ultrasonography uses high-frequency sound waves to produce echoes as the waves strike interfaces between acoustically different structures. These sound waves are electrically generated by a transducer crystal, which also serves as the sound wave receiver.

A-scan ultrasonography produces single-dimensional images composed of vertical spikes that represent interfaces from which sound waves are reflected. A-scan equipment is relatively compact and can be used to measure the dimensions of the eye with great accuracy. The usefulness of A-scan ultrasonography is somewhat limited for orbital examinations because of the single-dimensional images and the difficulty in maintaining orientation during the study.[10]

B-scan ultrasonography produces two-dimensional images of ocular and orbital structures while the transducer is mechanically or manually moved in front of the eye. Because B-scan images resemble anatomical cross sections of the orbit, they are more easily interpreted by clinicians than A-scans. The orbit can be most effectively studied when B-scan ultrasonography is used with a water bath and low-frequency (5 to 10 MHz) transducers.

Because ultrasonography does not use x-rays or ionizing radiation, it is of value as a screening technique. It can be considered part of an initial office examination and may be repeated without risk to the patient. The usefulness of any ultrasonography is limited because sound waves cannot penetrate the bony orbital walls and because tissues at the orbital apex and along the orbital roof are often poorly visualized.[1, 15]

Computed tomography is performed by using thin (collimated) x-ray beams to obtain tissue density values, from which detailed cross section images of the body are formed by computers. CT scans of the orbits visualize details of the eyes, the extraocular muscles, the optic nerves, and the lacrimal glands. In addition, orbital CT scans usually visualize the orbital bones, the sinuses, and intracranial structures. These studies have been used for the evaluation of orbital tumors and inflammations, both for diagnosis and for planning therapy.[15–18] CT scans are valuable for the study of orbital trauma, since soft tissue injuries and fractures can be visualized, as well as foreign bodies that are not radiographically opaque.[19, 20] The information obtained from CT scanning can be maximized by using several special techniques: (a) contrast enhancement, (b) narrow density window measurement, (c) three-dimensional computed tomography, and (d) image reversal.

Contrast enhancement is performed by administering iodine-containing materials intravenously. These materials increase the radiographic density within vascular structures. Therefore, blood vessels and vascularized abnormalities can be seen more distinctly than is possible without enhancement.

Density windows are electronically controlled ranges of radiographic densities that can be selected to appear on the imaging device of a CT scanner. By using a narrow density window, structures and tissues that have relatively similar densities can be separated from one another. This technique is particularly useful in evaluating and localizing foreign bodies.

Three-dimensional computed tomography can be achieved by using a combination of axial, coronal, and sagittal or oblique scans. Sometimes extraocular muscle enlargement can be distinguished from tumors when both axial and coronal views are used to study orbital detail. This is particularly valuable in studying patients with ophthalmic Graves' disease. Three-dimensional computed tomography can also aid in distinguishing solid tumors from cystic lesions and in evaluating traumatic abnormalities such as fractures and foreign bodies.

Image reversal is a technique of displaying bone and dense objects as black images against a white or light gray background. On normal CT scans bone appears white against a black background. When these images are reversed, bone defects resulting from tumors, fractures, or other causes may be more clearly visualized.

Magnetic resonance imaging (MRI) is a tech-nique of visualizing thin anatomical sections by exposing patients to a magnetic field and then recording the radiofrequency emissions from protons. Protons are the nuclei of hydrogen atoms, which are distributed throughout biological tissues. After protons have been stimulated by a strong magnet they emit faint signals that can be received and translated by a computer into an anatomical image.

Magnetic resonance characteristics differ according to tissue water content and cellularity. Two types of images can be produced, which are described as T1 and T2, and which can be used to help recognize different tissues.[21, 22]

Advantages of MRI include the lack of ionizing radiation and the ability to distinguish among certain vascular and neurological abnormalities. The optic nerve can readily be distinguished from adjacent structures and from most tumors by MRI (Fig. 15–1). A disadvantage is that bone does not give magnetic resonance signals; therefore, some lesions may be better evaluated by x-rays or CT scans. In addition, the patient must be confined to a small space during the examination and the equipment is bulky, since the magnets must be carefully shielded.

The localization of an orbital abnormality and a presumptive diagnosis can usually be reached after completion of the systemic examinations and other diagnostic studies that have been described. In unusual circumstances, especially if a vascular abnormality is suspected, additional studies may be performed. These additional diagnostic studies include radionuclide scans, venography, and arteriography.

Radionuclide scans visualize anatomical de-

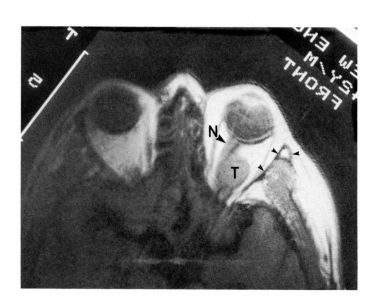

FIGURE 15–1. *Schwannoma.* Scan by magnetic resonance imaging (MRI) shows neurogenic tumor (T) at apex of right orbit. Optic nerve (N) is distinguished from adjacent tumor. Bones of lateral orbital wall and rim (small arrows) are not as well visualized by magnetic resonance as by x-rays or computed tomography.

tails by the localization of various gamma ray–emitting radionuclides, usually after their intravenous injection. Gallium-labeled compounds frequently localize in lymphoid foci within the orbit and elsewhere in the body.[1]

Radionuclide cisternography is a technique of localizing radioactive compounds that are injected into the cerebrospinal fluid (CSF) by lumbar puncture. Sometimes CSF leaks that may result from skull fractures can be detected by this method.[23]

Venography is usually performed by injecting radiopaque iodine-containing dye into the angular, frontal, or facial veins in order to visualize veins within the orbit. Displacement or obstruction of the superior ophthalmic and other orbital veins may give a clue about the location of a mass, but such information can usually be obtained more easily with ultrasonography or CT scans. Venography is most useful for the evaluation of varices, lymphangiomas, or lesions involving the cavernous sinus.[1]

Arteriography of the orbit requires the injection of radiopaque dye into carotid arteries. Although both orbital and intracranial arteries can be visualized, these examinations carry the low, but significant, risk of serious neurological complications. Vascular abnormalities that involve the arterial circulation, such as AV communications and aneurysms, are best evaluated by arteriography. Maximum information can be obtained from these studies by use of selective internal and external carotid injections, magnification, and radiographic subtraction.[1, 24]

Tissue Processing Techniques

Except in some patients with inflammations, vascular abnormalities, and clinically distinctive tumors, it is usually necessary to either biopsy or excise an orbital lesion to establish a definite diagnosis.

Light microscopy should be used for the basic examination of all tissues removed at surgery. Special stains should be requested if specific tumors are suspected, such as fat stains in the case of sebaceous cell carcinomas. Frozen-section examination of most orbital tumors should be performed while the patient is in the operating room. However, in most cases radical or mutilative surgery should not be carried out solely on the basis of a frozen-section diagnosis. Before the excised tissue is placed into formalin, consideration should be given to reserving some of the specimen for study by other techniques.[25–27]

Electron microscopy is useful to study poorly differentiated tumors, particularly metastatic lesions and childhood sarcomas. Tissues fixed in glutaraldehyde usually provide more satisfactory specimens for electron microscopy than those fixed in formalin.

Immunohistochemistry can be used to detect component cellular antigens that can aid in the diagnosis of orbital lesions. Among the substances that can be differentiated are myoglobins, glial proteins, and immunoglobulins. By using such techniques it may be possible to help distinguish benign from malignant lymphoid tumors, which may be difficult to identify solely on the basis of histological morphology. Lymphocytes can be divided into B (bone marrow–derived) cells and T (thymus-derived) cells. Immunoglobulins are located on the cell surfaces of B lymphocytes, which are primarily responsible for antibody production. Most malignant lymphomas are composed of B cells on which a single class of immunoglobulin predominates (monoclonal origin). Benign lymphocytic tumors are usually composed of T cells, or B cells with multiple classes of cell surface immunoglobulins (polyclonal origin). Fresh tissues must be used for immunoglobulin typing, and surgical specimens should be sent directly from the operating room for these studies.[24–26, 28, 29]

Hormone receptor assay can be performed on metastatic breast cancer tissue found at the time of orbital surgery. Breast cancer is the distant malignancy that most commonly metastasizes to the orbit. A certain percentage of patients with breast cancer respond favorably to endocrine therapy. This response usually correlates with the presence of estrogen and other hormone receptors in the tumor tissue. When such a malignancy is found, fresh tissue may be submitted for assay of estrogen and progesterone receptor activity.[8]

FEATURES OF COMMON ORBITAL DISORDERS

The examinations and studies that have been described should be used to localize and characterize orbital disorders. In order to select the appropriate treatment for the most common of these abnormalities (Tables 15–2 and 15–3), it is necessary to understand their histological and clinical features.

Ophthalmic Graves' Disease

As previously stated, Graves' disease is an inflammatory disorder of unknown cause that is usually associated with thyroid abnormalities. It is a multisystem disorder characterized by one or more of three pathognomonic clinical entities: (1) infiltrative ophthalmopathy; (2) infiltrative dermopathy; and (3) hyperthyroidism associated with diffuse hyperplasia of the thyroid gland.[1, 30] Although many patients with Graves' disease have hyperthyroidism, it has not been established that the thyroid disorder is a direct cause of the ophthalmic changes. Indeed, some patients with the ophthalmic changes of Graves' disease have no thyroid abnormality.

Ophthalmic Graves' disease is the term used to describe the orbital, eyelid, and ocular changes that may occur with this disorder. These abnormalities include exophthalmos, eyelid retraction and edema, limited eye movements, and optic neuropathy. Secondary cor-

neal changes may be caused by exposure of the eye, and optic neuropathy may result from nerve compression or vascular insufficiency.

Exophthalmos caused by Graves' disease may be unilateral or bilateral. Pseudoexophthalmos is a common finding, in which the eye is in a normal position but appears to be prominent because of a wide palpebral fissure. A great many eyelid changes have been described in patients with Graves' disease. Among the most common of these are upper eyelid retraction (Dalrymple's sign), eyelid lag on downgaze, and restriction of downward traction (Grove's sign) (Fig. 15–2). The downward traction test is useful to distinguish ophthalmic Graves' disease from other causes of a wide palpebral fissure. When the lashes of the upper eyelid are grasped and pulled downward, restriction of downward traction is often met in patients with Graves'

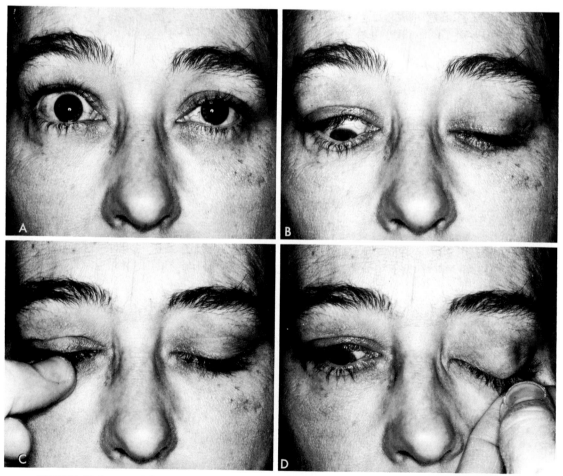

FIGURE 15–2. *Graves' disease.* Common eyelid signs (see Table 15–4). *A,* Retraction of right upper eyelid (Dalrymple's sign). *B,* Lag of right upper eyelid in downgaze. *C,* Downward traction test. Restriction when lashes of involved right upper eyelid are grasped and pulled downward (Grove's sign). Upper lid crease is accentuated by subcutaneous adhesions near the levator. *D,* No restriction when uninvolved left upper eyelid is pulled downward.

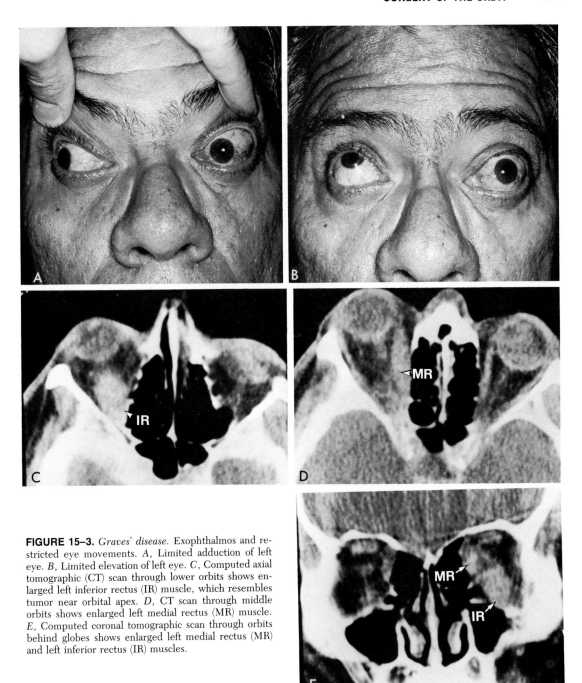

FIGURE 15–3. *Graves' disease.* Exophthalmos and restricted eye movements. *A,* Limited adduction of left eye. *B,* Limited elevation of left eye. *C,* Computed axial tomographic (CT) scan through lower orbits shows enlarged left inferior rectus (IR) muscle, which resembles tumor near orbital apex. *D,* CT scan through middle orbits shows enlarged left medial rectus (MR) muscle. *E,* Computed coronal tomographic scan through orbits behind globes shows enlarged left medial rectus (MR) and left inferior rectus (IR) muscles.

disease because of changes involving the levator muscle and levator aponeurosis. The most frequent ocular motility disorder associated with Graves' disease is restriction of vertical eye movement, caused by contracture and fibrosis of the inferior rectus muscle. The medial rectus muscle may also be involved by similar changes, and less commonly other extraocular muscles may be involved (Fig. 15–3). Although eyelid

edema is a common feature of Graves' disease, this is a nonspecific abnormality that accompanies many orbital disorders.

Histologically, the orbital tissues become swollen by edema, which may involve the extraocular muscles, the retrobulbar fat, the lacrimal gland, and the eyelids. This edema fluid contains increased mucopolysaccharides, especially hyaluronic acid. The edema is usually accompanied by infiltration of plasma cells, lymphocytes, mast cells, and macrophages. These inflammatory cells usually group near blood vessels (perivascular cuffing) in the early stages of the disorder. As the inflammation becomes chronic, fibrosis may develop within the extraocular muscles and produce restrictive myopathy.[12] Upper eyelid retraction in Graves' disease may be due to overaction of Müller's muscle (which is sympathetically innervated); overaction of the levator muscle in association with superior rectus action against a contracted inferior rectus muscle; atrophy and/or fibrosis of the levator; or abnormal subcutaneous adhesions near the levator.[31]

As previously mentioned, ophthalmic Graves' disease is usually diagnosed on the basis of clinical findings and changes in the orbital anatomy that are characteristic of this disorder. The diagnostic studies that give the most useful information about characteristic anatomical changes caused by Graves' disease are ultrasonography and computed tomography. Ultrasonography often demonstrates enlargement of one or more extraocular muscles together with inflammatory changes in the muscles, fat, and optic nerve sheath.[15] CT scans similarly demonstrate enlargement of multiple extraocular muscles. Because enlarged muscles near the orbital apex sometimes resemble neoplasms on CT scans, abnormalities in this area must be carefully studied and correlated with clinical findings. Three-dimensional computed tomography, using both axial and coronal scans, is a useful technique to study details of the extraocular muscles and optic nerve (Fig. 15–3).[2, 3, 16, 18]

Most patients with Graves' disease have abnormal serum thyroid tests, including elevated T_4 or T_3 levels, and often decreased TSH levels. If these tests are normal or equivocal, and if Graves' disease is still suspected on the basis of clinical signs or the anatomical studies just described, then a TRH test may demonstrate thyroid nonsuppressibility.[11–13] An outline of important clinical features and diagnostic steps that are useful in the evaluation of ophthalmic Graves' disease is provided in Table 15–4.

Treatment of ophthalmic Graves' disease should usually be as conservative as possible because of the unpredictable development of eyelid malpositions, motility disorders, and orbital congestion. Some of these abnormalities improve after treatment of thyroid dysfunction, but occasionally they become more severe after control of hyperthyroidism (Fig. 15–4). In many instances the orbital disease is self-limited, with resolution of the acute inflammatory changes after a period of months or years.

Early ophthalmic Graves' disease is usually treated by topical lubricants to prevent corneal drying. When possible, thyroid abnormalities should be stabilized for several months before corrective eyelid or muscle surgery is performed. If corneal damage becomes severe because of lid retraction or exophthalmos, the palpebral fissure may be narrowed by raising the inferior lid or lowering the retracted upper lid (Fig. 15–5).[31–33]

If orbital congestion becomes severe, and particularly if optic neuropathy occurs, the use of high-dose systemic steroids should be considered. Radiation therapy may be used in the treatment of severe inflammation, especially in debilitated patients.[34] Surgical decompression of the orbit can provide dramatic reduction of exophthalmos and congestion, especially if portions of the medial wall and orbital floor are removed to allow prolapse of the congested tissues into the maxillary and ethmoidal sinuses (Fig. 15–4).[12, 35, 36]

Pseudotumors

Orbital pseudotumors are idiopathic inflammations with no identified cause.[7, 37–39] Consequently pseudotumors are unrelated to a specific local or systemic disease. When an orbital inflammation is associated with a well-defined disorder such as sarcoidosis or polyarteritis nodosa, it is usually excluded from the category of pseudotumor. Similarly, when an orbital inflammation is part of an identifiable syndrome, such as ophthalmic Graves' disease, it is not considered a pseudotumor.

Although some pseudotumors are chronic and indolent, the most common clinical findings include orbital pain, restricted eye movements, exophthalmos, and evidence of acute inflammation. Pseudotumors are common in both adults and children (Tables 15–2 and 15–3), and may be either unilateral or bilateral. Bilateral orbital inflammation in adults is frequently associated with a systemic disorder such as vasculitis or Graves' disease, even though that disease may not be apparent at the time of the initial orbital presentation. However, most children with bilateral orbital inflammation never develop any signs of a systemic disorder.[38, 39]

Specific categories of orbital pseudotumors have been proposed, based on criteria such as their histological character and the anatomical

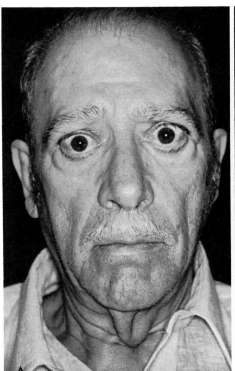

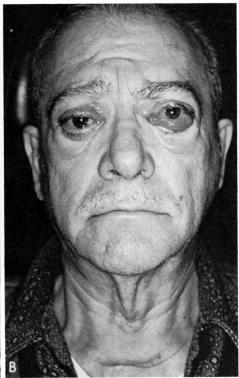

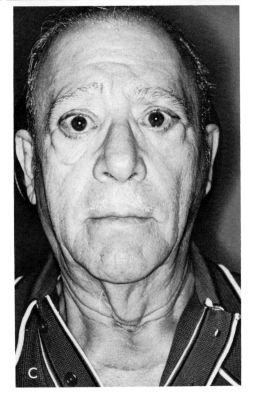

FIGURE 15–4. *Graves' disease.* Bilateral exophthalmos and optic neuropathy treated by orbital decompression. *A*, Moderate orbital congestion and exophthalmos in patient with hyperthyroidism before treatment. *B*, After treatment of hyperthyroidism by thyroidectomy (note horizontal scar in lower neck), patient developed severe orbital congestion and optic neuropathy. Visual acuity in left eye was reduced to ability to count fingers and did not improve with systemic steroid therapy. *C*, After bilateral orbital decompressions by partial removal of medial walls and floors of both orbits, optic neuropathy resolved and visual acuity improved to 20/40 in left eye.

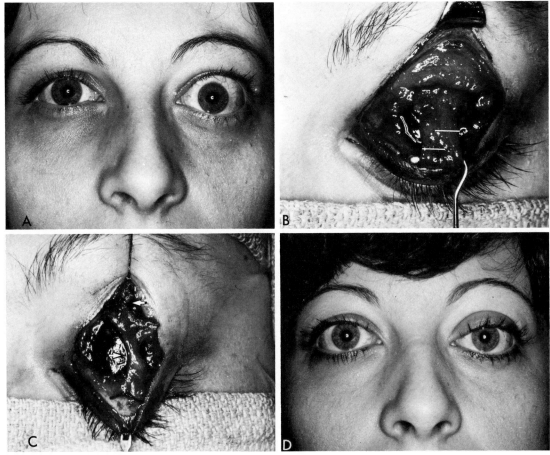

FIGURE 15–5. *Graves' disease.* Upper eyelid retraction treated by levator marginal myotomy. *A*, Left upper lid retracted 5 mm above normal position. *B*, Marginal myotomy incisions (parallel lines) are made through levator and Müller's muscles. Incisions are made in opposite margins, and each extends more than half the width of the muscles. *C*, Lid is pulled downward after myotomy incisions (arrows) have been made. Incisions should be long enough to lengthen levator by 1.25 to 1.50 times the desired amount of eyelid lowering. In this patient the levator was lengthened 7 mm to lower the lid 5 mm. *D*, One year after myotomy left upper lid remains in satisfactory position.

structures involved as demonstrated by ultrasonography and computed tomography.

Histologically, most pseudotumors are composed of a mixture of lymphocytes, plasma cells, and eosinophils. When lymphocytes predominate, the process is usually described as benign lymphoid hyperplasia. These lesions and related abnormalities are discussed under the topic of lymphocytic tumors. Because it may be difficult to histologically distinguish such benign lymphoid pseudotumors from malignant lymphomas, cell surface immunology studies may help to identify pseudotumors or lymphomas. Some pseudotumors are granulomas, composed of epithelioid cells that usually accumulate in noncaseating foci or nodules. Sarcoidosis may produce conjunctival or lacrimal gland granulomas that may be confused with idiopathic pseudotumors. Fibrosclerosis, in which dense collagenous tissue is formed, may involve the orbital periosteum (periorbita) and produce a thick membrane on the orbital walls. Less common histological forms of pseudotumors include vascular inflammations and lipogranulomas, in which orbital fat may become necrotic and degenerate, with infiltration of macrophages and giant cells. Lesions that contain both lymphocytes and plasma cells may represent Waldenström's macroglobulinemia, which is discussed under the topic of plasmacytic tumors. In Sjögren's syndrome lymphocytes and plasma cells may infiltrate the lacrimal gland and lead to enlargement of the gland, with decreased tear formation.

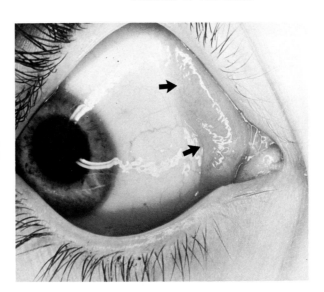

FIGURE 15–6. *Pseudotumor.* Conjunctival benign lymphoid hyperplasia (arrows) located near superior fornix and caruncle.

Anatomically, orbital pseudotumors may be categorized by the structures that they involve and by their focal or diffuse growth pattern. Most focal pseudotumors involve the extraocular muscles (myositis), the lacrimal gland (dacryoadenitis), tissues adjacent to the globe (episcleritis), or the conjunctiva. Conjunctival pseudotumors are relatively common, and usually present as an elevated "salmon pink" lesion on the surface of the globe or near the fornices (Fig. 15–6). These conjunctival lesions are usually composed primarily of lymphocytes, and may be difficult to distinguish from lymphomas. When the lacrimal gland is involved in a chronic inflammation, the disorder may represent a specific disease process such as sarcoidosis or Sjögren's syndrome. Less commonly, focal pseudotumors may involve the periosteum (periosteitis), blood vessels (vasculitis), or tissues adjacent to nerves (perineuritis). Diffuse pseudotumors are those in which the inflammatory process involves multiple tissues throughout the orbit.

The Tolosa-Hunt syndrome, or idiopathic painful ophthalmoplegia, is a form of pseudotumor in which the inflammatory process probably involves the cavernous sinus, or the superior orbital fissure and optic canal. Orbital pain and restriction of all eye movements are the most common features of this disorder, and visual acuity may be reduced as well.

Ultrasonography and CT scans may show involvement of specific tissues, such as thickened extraocular muscles (Figs. 15–7 and 15–8), enlargement of the lacrimal gland (Fig. 15–9), or increased density of tissues surrounding the globe ("ring sign"; see Fig. 15–10).[19] Some-

times other focal masses may be seen around the optic nerve, within the orbital fat, or near the periorbita.

Treatment of orbital pseudotumors usually involves the use of high-dose systemic steroids (Fig. 15–10).[7, 37, 38] Oral prednisone may be given to adults in doses of 60 to 80 mg each day unless medically contraindicated. Sometimes this therapy can be initiated after establishing a presumptive diagnosis based on clinical findings and diagnostic studies. Often it is necessary to perform a surgical exploration and obtain tissue for histological examination.

Some neoplasms may produce a secondary inflammation that subsides as a result of steroid therapy. Therefore, patients should continue to be followed even after a response to steroids is apparent. In the case of lacrimal gland lesions it may be necessary to remove the entire lacrimal gland because of the possibility that the lesion is a mixed tumor. When a pseudotumor fails to respond to these measures, radiation therapy may be effective, especially when the lesion is composed primarily of lymphocytes.[40]

Secondary Tumors

The most common malignant tumors involving the orbit in adults are those that extend directly by secondary growth from adjacent structures such as the paranasal sinuses, the nose, the eyelids, the globe, and the intracranial area.[41] The paranasal sinuses and nose are the most common areas from which tumors extend secondarily into the orbit.

Sinus and nasal tumors that invade the orbit

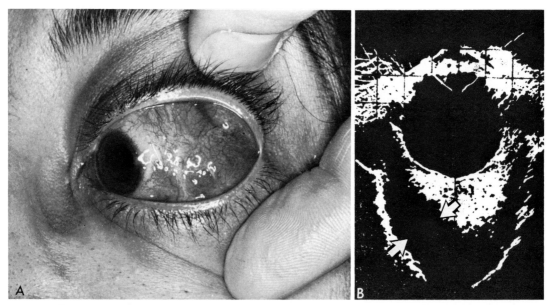

FIGURE 15–7. *Pseudotumor.* Myositis involving lateral rectus muscle. *A,* Left lateral rectus muscle enlarged with conjunctival vascular congestion. *B,* Horizontal ultrasound B scan shows enlarged left lateral rectus muscle (arrows).

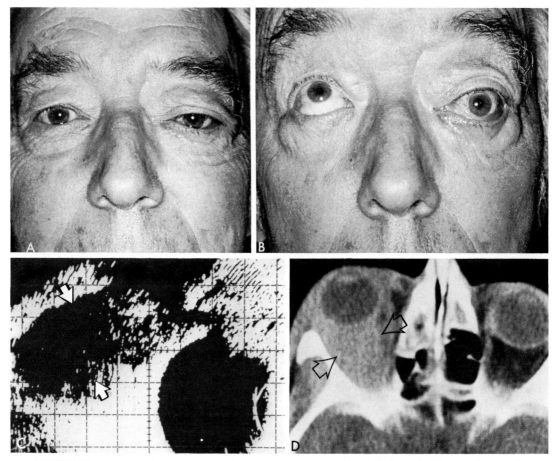

FIGURE 15–8. *Pseudotumor.* Myositis involving superior rectus muscle. *A,* Left exophthalmos and ptosis of left upper eyelid. *B,* Limited elevation of left eye. *C,* Vertical ultrasound B scan shows enlarged left superior rectus muscle (arrows). *D,* CT scan through upper orbits shows enlarged left superior rectus muscle (arrows).

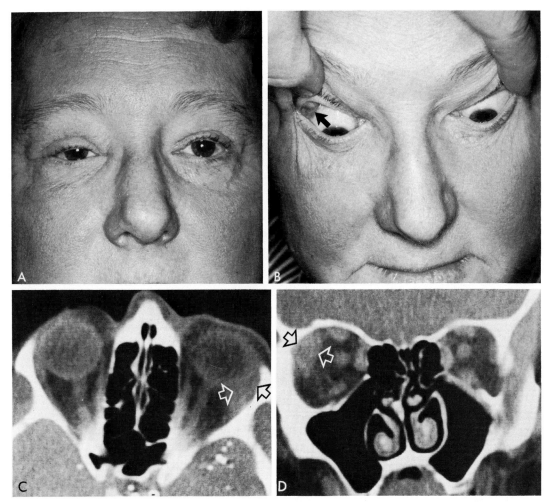

FIGURE 15–9. *Pseudotumor.* Benign lymphoid hyperplasia (lymphoid dacryoadenitis) of lacrimal gland. *A,* Right exophthalmos and ptosis of right upper eyelid. *B,* Right lacrimal gland (arrow) protrudes when upper lids are pulled back. *C,* CT scan shows enlarged right lacrimal gland (arrows). *D,* CT scan shows enlarged right lacrimal gland (arrows).

are most frequently squamous cell carcinomas. Most of these carcinomas arise from the maxillary sinus, in which they are the most common epithelial malignant tumor.[41, 42] Other, more unusual sinus malignancies such as adenocarcinomas and chondrosarcomas may also extend into the orbit. Inverted papillomas are benign tumors that usually arise in the lateral nasal wall and may secondarily invade the orbit. Although inverted papillomas are histologically benign, they have a tendency to persist and recur as diffuse, infiltrative lesions if excision is incomplete.[42] These tumors may also undergo malignant transformation to squamous cell carcinoma.[43]

Orbital x-rays are almost always abnormal in patients with sinus and nasal tumors involving the orbit. CT scans are useful for the study of secondary tumors because they demonstrate details of both soft tissues and bones (Fig. 15–11).

Treatment of sinus and nasal tumors should be planned after examining tissue removed by biopsy, which can often be obtained from the nasal fossa. Many sinus malignancies are treated by orbital exenteration in addition to resection of the involved sinuses (Fig. 15–12). Radiation is frequently used as adjunctive therapy before or after surgical resection. Some nonepithelial malignancies such as lymphomas and rhabdomyosarcomas are treated by radiation and systemic chemotherapy alone.

Eyelid tumors can invade the orbit from the skin, the subcutaneous tissues, or the conjunctiva. Basal cell carcinomas are the most common malignant tumors of the eyelids. Less com-

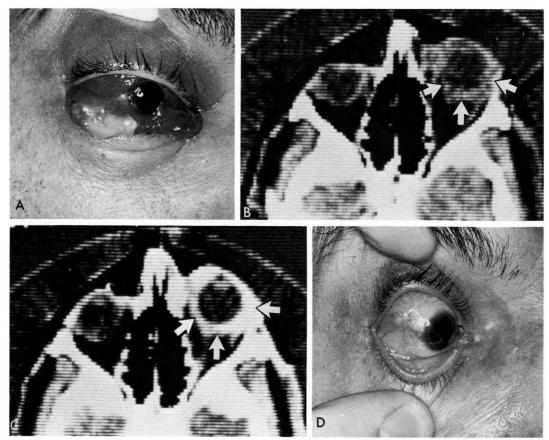

FIGURE 15–10. *Pseudotumor.* Episcleral inflammation and computed tomographic "ring sign." *A,* Right exophthalmos with severe conjunctival congestion and edema. *B,* CT scan shows increased density (arrows) of tissues surrounding right eye ("ring sign"). *C,* CT scan after intravenous administration of iodine-containing materials (contrast enhancement) shows additional increase in density (arrows) around right eye. *D,* After treatment with oral prednisone, exophthalmos and congestion resolved completely.

monly, squamous cell carcinomas, sebaceous cell carcinomas, and malignant melanomas arise within the eyelids.[41, 45] Any of these tumors can secondarily extend into the orbit. Deep orbital extension is usually more frequent when a tumor recurs or persists after treatment, especially if the lesion was initially treated by radiation or surgery with extensive reconstruction.

Orbital x-rays and CT scans are useful to evaluate the integrity of the orbital walls in patients with invasive eyelid tumors. However, these studies may appear normal in some patients even when the tumors involve the periosteum and bones. Therefore, if the clinical findings suggest that bones are involved, normal x-rays or scans should not deter removal of the clinically abnormal tissues.

Treatment of eyelid tumors that secondarily invade the orbit depends on the biological behavior of the tumor and the depth of invasion. Because basal cell carcinomas almost never me-

tastasize, wide local excision with histological evaluation of all margins is usually the most effective means of control. Such histological control of the margins around basal cell carcinomas is particularly important in the case of morpheaform tumors, which have a leather-like surface and irregular edges. These morpheaform tumors often extend histologically beyond their clinical margins and may invade deep tissue planes (Fig. 15–13).

Some basal cell carcinomas can be described as "extensive facial-orbital tumors" because of having the following features: tumor involvement of more than 1 square inch of the skin surface near the eyelids; tumor fixation to orbital periosteum or bone; and tumor extension onto the inner eyelid surface or through the orbital septum. Such tumors, as well as tumors that recur after initial treatment, are often effectively treated by Mohs' technique (chemosurgery) or a variation of this technique known

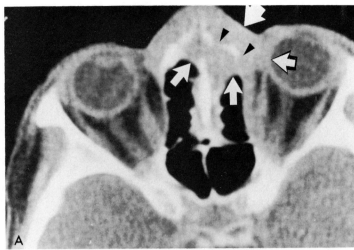

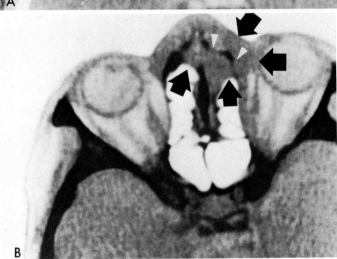

FIGURE 15–11. *Nasal carcinoma.* Adenoid cystic carcinoma extending from nasal fossa into anterior orbit. *A,* CT scan shows tumor (large arrows) extending through destroyed nasal bones (small arrowheads). *B,* Same CT scan displayed by image reversal, which clearly visualizes bone defects (small arrowheads) caused by tumor (large arrows).

as lamellar resection.[46, 47] In both Mohs' technique and lamellar resection the tumor is excised in small lamellar tissue blocks, each of which is 5 to 10 mm square and 2 to 4 mm thick. The undersurface of each lamellar block is then histologically examined, and if tumor is present, additional lamellar blocks are excised from the adjacent tissues until all of the malignancy is removed (Fig. 15–13).

Although both radiation therapy and cryotherapy can be used to destroy some eyelid tumors, neither of these techniques provides histological confirmation that the margins surrounding the treated area are free of tumor. In most cases surgical resection of both primary and recurrent (persistent) eyelid tumors is the preferred treatment. Unfortunately some eyelid tumors that invade the deep orbit or extend over a wide area of the skin or conjunctiva cannot be completely removed unless the eye

is also excised. In such cases exenteration may be necessary in order to provide the best opportunity for complete tumor eradication (Fig. 15–14).

Intraocular tumors are usually detected before they extend into the orbit. The most common intraocular malignancies in children are retinoblastomas and in adults are choroidal malignant melanomas. If these tumors secondarily invade the optic nerve or extend through the sclera, and if they have not metastasized to other areas of the body, orbital exenteration is frequently performed in an attempt at local control (Fig. 15–15). Sometimes systemic chemotherapy is used to suppress the growth of residual cells or metastases.[41]

Intracranial tumors that invade the orbit are most often meningiomas arising adjacent to the spheroid wings, the base of the skull, or the frontal area.[41, 48] Meningiomas and other fibro-

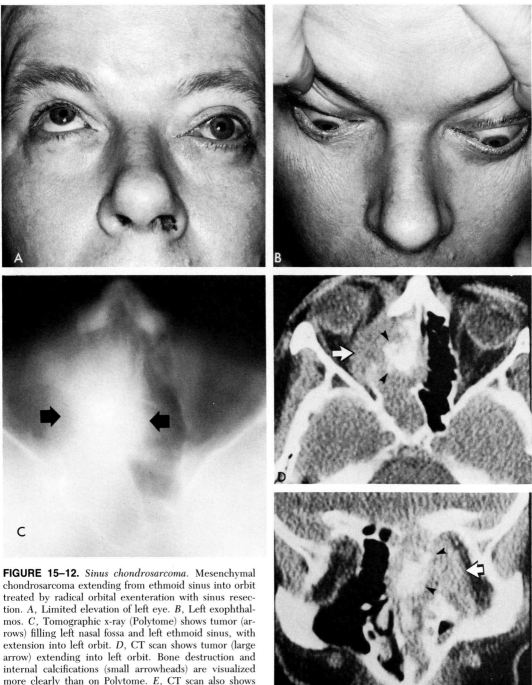

FIGURE 15–12. *Sinus chondrosarcoma.* Mesenchymal chondrosarcoma extending from ethmoid sinus into orbit treated by radical orbital exenteration with sinus resection. *A,* Limited elevation of left eye. *B,* Left exophthalmos. *C,* Tomographic x-ray (Polytome) shows tumor (arrows) filling left nasal fossa and left ethmoid sinus, with extension into left orbit. *D,* CT scan shows tumor (large arrow) extending into left orbit. Bone destruction and internal calcifications (small arrowheads) are visualized more clearly than on Polytome. *E,* CT scan also shows tumor (large arrow) and internal calcifications (small arrowheads).

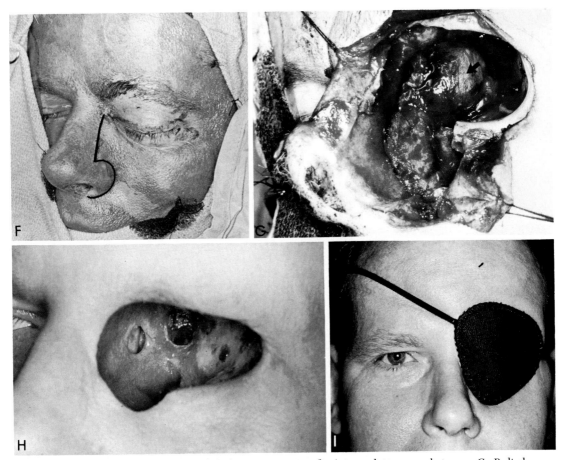

FIGURE 15–12 *Continued F,* Lateral rhinotomy incision (line) is used to approach tumor. *G,* Radical exenteration of left orbit has been performed with removal of left eye, medial orbital rim, and segment of inferior orbital rim, exposing tumor (arrow) extending from ethmoid sinus. *H,* Orbital cavity 2 years after tumor removal, orbital exenteration, and radiation therapy. Openings into sphenoid sinus are visible in posterior surface of cavity. *I,* Black patch is used to cover exenteration defect.

osseous tumors that may involve the skull and orbit are discussed separately. Less frequently intracranial tumors such as gliomas may extend into the orbit.

Metastatic Tumors

Metastatic spread of malignancies to the orbit occurs much less frequently than metastases to the eye. In adults the most common distant tumors that metastasize to the orbit arise in the breast or the lung. In children neuroblastoma and Ewing's sarcoma are the most common tumors to cause orbital metastases.[41, 49, 50]

Breast carcinoma is the most frequent primary source of orbital metastasis in women. Metastases may occur and cause inflammation many years after the primary lesion has been removed.[51] The findings of exophthalmos, ophthalmoplegia, and bone destruction should raise the suspicion of a metastatic tumor. Metastatic breast carcinoma may elicit a fibrous response that produces cicatrization and enophthalmos (Fig. 15–16). Breast examination, and sometimes mammography, should be performed on women who are suspected of having an orbital tumor. In some patients with metastatic breast carcinoma certain blood tumor factors such as CEA or HCG may be elevated. Lung cancer frequently metastasizes to the orbit, and therefore a chest x-ray should be performed on almost all patients with an unexplained orbital abnormality. Less commonly tumors such as carcinoids and malignant melanomas may metastasize to the orbit.

Text continued on page 446

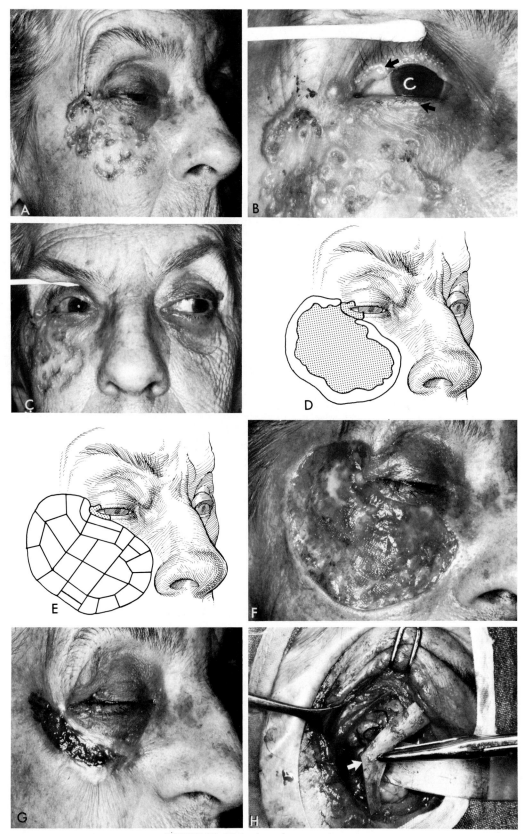

FIGURE 15–13 *See legend on opposite page*

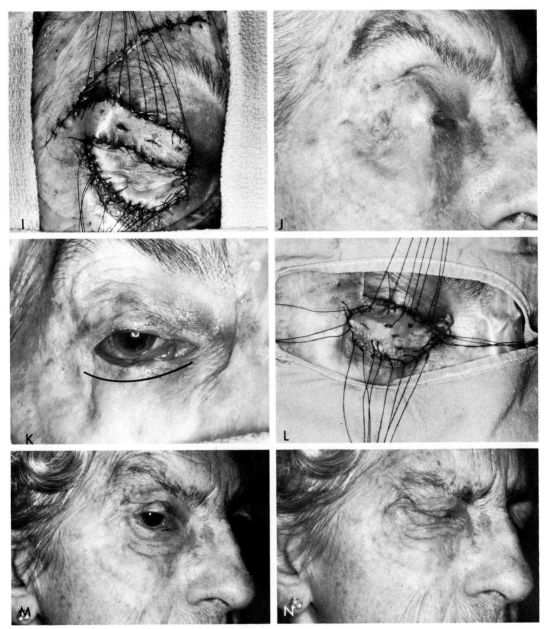

FIGURE 15–13. *A*, Morpheaform basal cell carcinoma has leather-like surface and irregular edges. Extensive tumor involves right cheek, lateral canthus, and lateral eyelids. *B*, Tumor extending from lateral canthus along margins of upper and lower eyelids (arrows). *C*, Limited adduction of right eye caused by growth of tumor onto conjunctiva near lateral rectus muscle. *D*, Lamellar resection, first excision. Effort is made to remove all clinically evident tumor (dotted area) except the portion at lateral canthus and along lid margins. Outer solid line shows extent of peripheral skin incision placed beyond clinical margins of tumor. Tissue is removed to a depth that includes full-thickness skin in most areas. *E*, Lamellar resection, second excision. After removal of the tissue shown previously, the surface and all margins surrounding the original surgical defect are then removed in a group of lamellar blocks. These tissue blocks are each 2 to 4 mm thick and 5 to 15 mm wide. Each lamellar block is identified by a letter and is drawn as illustrated on a "map" of the face. Each specimen is histologically examined so that if tumor is present, additional tissue can be removed from the appropriate location. *F*, Surgical defect several days after completion of lamellar resection, with all tissue blocks free of tumor except those at lateral canthus and lid margins. *G*, One month after lamellar resection, surgical defect has grown much smaller as a result of spontaneous granulation. *H*, Residual tumor at lateral canthus, lid margins, and conjunctiva is excised, with frozen-section control used to assure complete tumor removal. Lateral orbital rim (arrow) is also removed because overlying periosteum was invaded by tumor. *I*, Defect over eye is covered by inner mucosal graft from nasal septum and outer full-thickness skin grafts. *J*, Several months later grafts have completely healed. *K*, New palpebral fissure is created by horizontal incision through grafts. Skin incision (line) is made in lower eyelid so that skin graft can be placed. *L*, Full-thickness skin graft is used to maintain elevation of lower eyelid. *M*, Four months after completion of eyelid reconstruction. *N*, Complete eyelid closure is possible and no evidence of residual tumor is apparent.

441

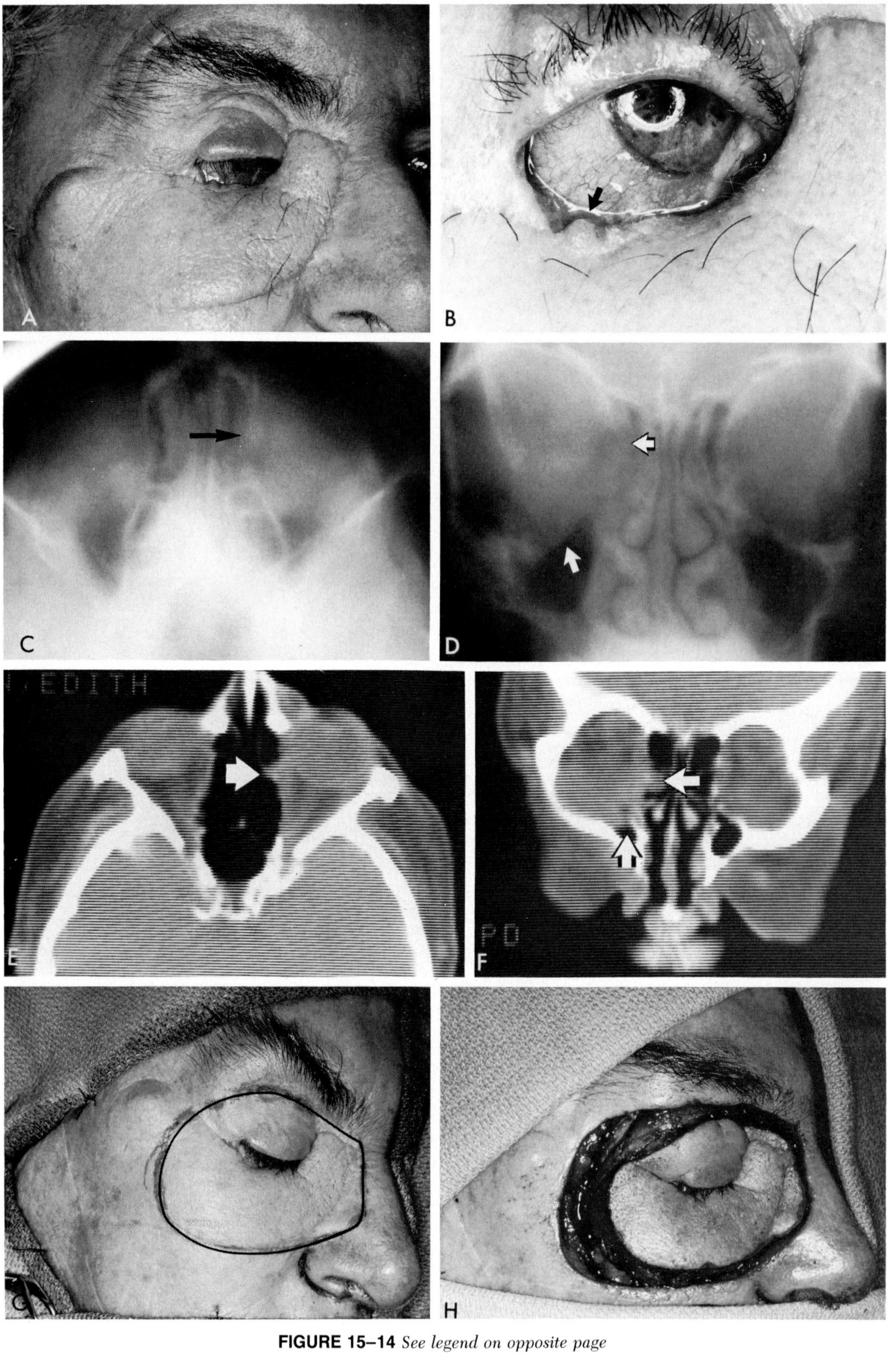

FIGURE 15–14 *See legend on opposite page*

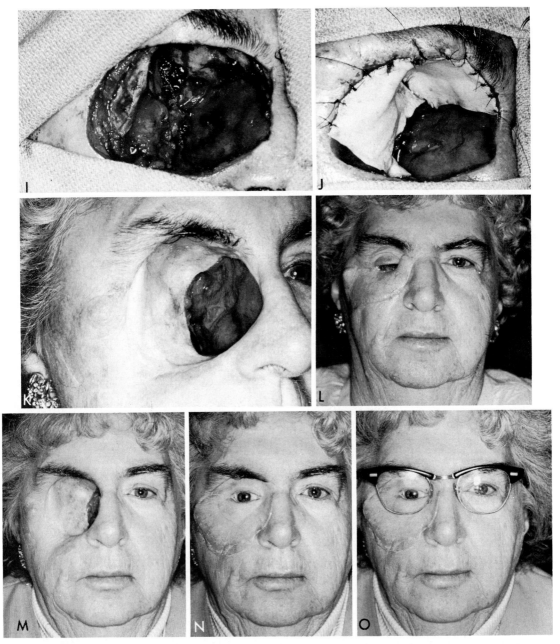

FIGURE 15–14. *Basal cell carcinoma.* Recurrent (persistent) eyelid tumor extending beneath skin grafts and into orbital bones treated by radical orbital exenteration with sinus resection. *A,* Right eye is unable to move normally because of basal cell carcinoma that has invaded orbit after multiple operations. *B,* Lower eyelid destroyed by tumor (arrow) adjacent to conjunctiva. *C,* Axial Polytome shows tumor (arrow) extending into right ethmoid sinus. *D,* Coronal Polytome shows tumor (arrows) extending through orbital walls into adjacent sinuses. *E,* Axial CT scan shows tumor (arrow) within right ethmoid sinus. *F,* Coronal CT scan shows tumor (arrows) within right ethmoid and maxillary sinuses. *G,* Skin incision (line) placed to include eyelids, lateral surface of nose, and previous skin grafts. *H,* Incision is continued through deeper tissues beyond the areas of bone involvement seen on x-rays and CT scans. Margins around exenteration site are histologically examined to determine whether tumor is totally removed. *I,* After removal of lids and orbital exenteration, the right ethmoid sinus and medial maxillary sinus are excised. *J,* Several weeks after exenteration and completion of histological examination of margins, split-thickness skin grafts are used to cover granulating surfaces of orbit. *K,* Orbital cavity 1 year after orbital exenteration. Opening into nasal fossa is visible medially. *L,* Recurrent (persistent) tumor before orbital exenteration. *M,* One year after orbital exenteration. *N,* Plastic prosthesis is used to cover exenteration defect. *O,* Eyeglasses partially disguise prosthesis and protect left eye.

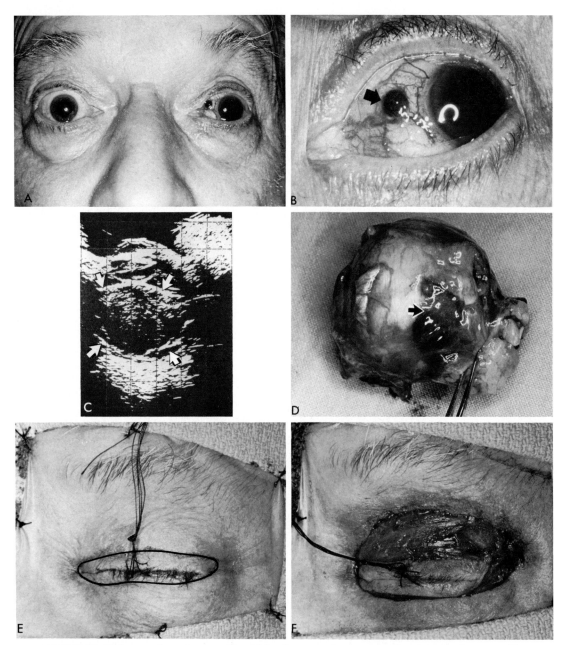

FIGURE 15–15. *Intraocular melanoma.* Choroidal malignant melanoma extending through sclera treated by orbital exenteration. *A,* Blind left eye with black nodule beneath conjunctiva. *B,* Subconjunctival black nodule (arrow) in eye with opaque media and no view of fundus. *C,* Horizontal ultrasound B scan shows solid tumor (arrows) filling most of left eye. *D,* Left eye enucleated and black nodule found emerging from posterior sclera. Frozen-section examination revealed malignant melanoma. *E,* Skin incision (line) is placed several millimeters from eyelashes and canthi. *F,* Skin is dissected from underlying orbicularis muscle.

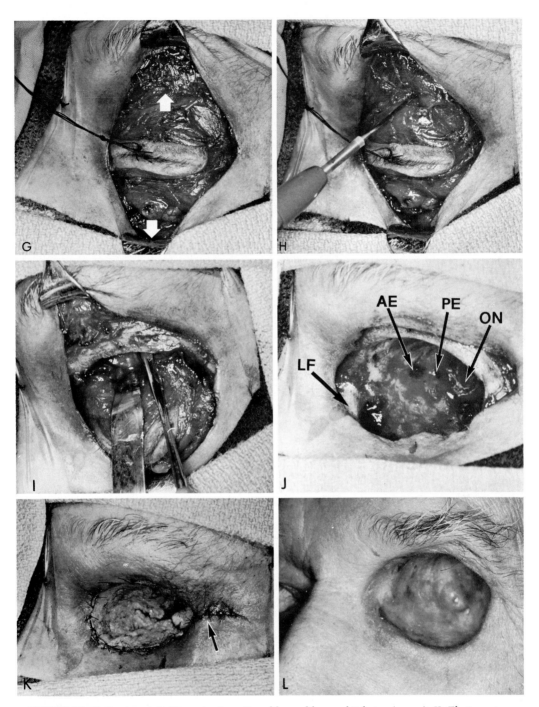

FIGURE 15–15 *Continued G,* Dissection is continued beyond bony orbital rims (arrows). *H,* Electrocautery is used to cut muscles and subcutaneous tissues near orbital rims. *I,* Periosteal elevator used to dissect periosteum (periorbital) from orbital walls. *J,* Orbital walls exposed after completion of exenteration and removal of orbital contents. Lacrimal sac fossa (LF), anterior ethmoid foramen (AE), posterior ethmoid foramen (PE), and transected optic nerve (ON) can be seen along medial wall of orbit. *K,* Skin is undermined and directly closed (arrow) to cover lateral orbital rim, after which a split-thickness skin graft is used to line orbital cavity. *L,* Orbital cavity with healed skin graft.

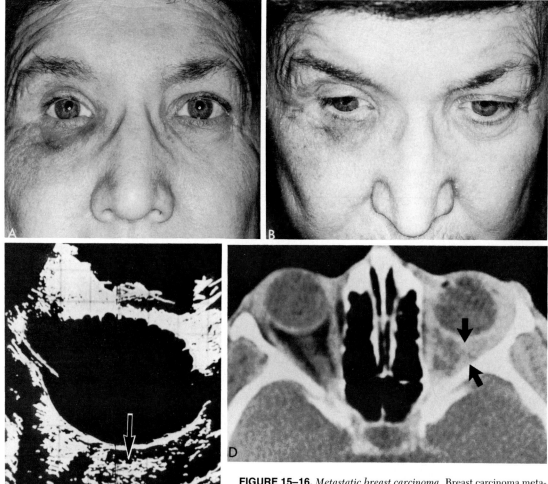

FIGURE 15–16. *Metastatic breast carcinoma.* Breast carcinoma metastatic to orbit, producing cicatrization and enophthalmos. *A*, Right eye pulled inward by fibrous response to infiltrative tumor. *B*, Right enophthalmos. *C*, Horizontal ultrasound B scan shows tumor infiltration (arrows) within retrobulbar fat. *D*, CT scan shows right enophthalmos and diffuse tumor infiltration (arrows) within retrobulbar fat.

Neuroblastoma usually arises in the retroperitoneal area and almost always occurs in patients younger than 2 years of age. Metastatic orbital neuroblastoma typically produces abrupt exophthalmos and eyelid ecchymosis that may be bilateral. Histologically, these tumors are composed of primitive neuroectodermal cells (neuroblasts) originating in the adrenal medulla, in sympathetic ganglia, or in the peripheral nervous system. Scans may demonstrate adrenal abnormalities, and bone defects may be found on x-rays. Increased urinary excretion of VMA is common, and sometimes plasma levels of CEA are elevated. Bone marrow aspiration may show tumor cells in some patients with neuro-

blastoma. These studies have been described earlier under the topic of systemic examinations.

A metastatic tumor may appear as a focal mass or as a diffuse infiltrative lesion on ultrasonography and CT scans (Fig. 15–16). Although bone destruction is common in patients with metastatic tumors, the lesion may be confined to the soft tissues, and x-rays may appear normal.

Treatment of metastatic tumors is usually palliative, consisting of local radiation therapy. Because hormone therapy may be useful in the treatment of some patients with metastatic breast carcinoma, tissue removed at the time of orbital exploration can be submitted for assay of estrogen and progesterone receptor activity. Occasionally metastatic tumors should be treated by wide local excision, since patients with some primary lesions such as carcinoids may survive for many years after their metastasis is removed.

Vascular Abnormalities

Cavernous hemangiomas, capillary hemangiomas, lymphangiomas, and venous malformations are the most common vascular abnormalities that involve the orbit.[52, 53] Many of these lesions are not considered to be neoplasms, but are thought to be benign developmental hamartomas. Hamartomas are growths arising from tissue elements that are usually found at the position in which the tumor is located.

Venous malformations include a number of abnormalities, including varices, varicoceles, and venous angiomas.[52] The most common of these lesions are orbital varices, which are enlarged venous channels and which may be either primary or secondary. Primary varices are usually congenital, whereas secondary varices are often caused by intracranial abnormalities or by tumors near the orbital apex. Because some varices share features in common with lymphangiomas, sometimes these two lesions are considered the same.

Hemangiopericytomas are among the most frequent true vascular neoplasms found in the orbit. Fibrous histiocytomas have many features in common with hemangiopericytomas, but have fewer vascular elements. Both of these neoplasms occur in benign and malignant forms.

Arteriovenous (AV) communications that involve the orbit may be classified as malformations, fistulas, or shunts.[24] AV malformations usually present as pulsatile tumors within the orbit. Fistulas and shunts are commonly communications between the cavernous sinus and the carotid arteries or their branches. Orbital changes are usually secondary to vascular congestion and resulting inflammation.

Cavernous hemangiomas are the most common benign tumors of the orbit in adults. Although a rudimentary lesion may be present at birth, symptoms do not usually occur until the hemangioma enlarges during the second to fourth decade of life. These tumors are usually located within the muscle cone behind the eye, but they may also lie against an orbital wall and cause bone displacement. Exophthalmos, optic nerve compression, and chorioretinal striae (Fig. 15–17) are common sequelae of cavernous hemangiomas. Histologically, these tumors are composed of large vascular spaces lined by endothelial cells. These vascular channels are often separated by fibrous septa. Cavernous hemangiomas have few significant feeding arteries or draining veins. They are usually well circumscribed and are surrounded by a firm capsule.

Orbital x-rays may show fossa formation caused by chronic pressure against the orbital walls. Ultrasonography commonly demonstrates a well-circumscribed lesion with multiple high-amplitude internal echoes. CT and magnetic resonance scans usually show smooth surfaces around a discrete solid tumor (Fig. 15–17). Enhancement is usually seen on CT scans after contrast material is administered.

The treatment of cavernous hemangiomas is surgical excision, most often by a lateral approach because of the usual position within the muscle cone (Fig. 15–17). Some lesions can be removed through anterior approaches, especially if the eye has been greatly displaced. Complete removal of cavernous hemangiomas is usually possible because of the presence of a firm capsule and the relative lack of significant feeding or draining vessels. Sometimes tumors that lie in less accessible areas, such as the medial orbit, may be cut into pieces before removal by means of electrocautery (Fig. 15–18). Cavernous hemangiomas rarely undergo spontaneous involution.

Capillary hemangiomas are among the most common benign tumors of the orbit in children. These lesions typically appear during the first month after birth as elevated red nodules within or near the eyelids. The surface of the lesion may be dimpled, giving rise to the name strawberry birthmark. A mass is often found within the deep lids and the anterior orbit (Fig. 15–19). In addition, lesions may arise elsewhere in the head and neck, or in other locations on the body. Displacement of the eye, astigmatism, and ptosis may be caused by eyelid involvement. Histologically, these tumors are typified by a proliferation of capillaries and endothelial cells with rare mitoses. Large feeding vessels are common, and the margins of the tumors are relatively indistinct.[52–54]

Because capillary hemangiomas have such a typical clinical appearance, the diagnosis can usually be made without resorting to elaborate tests. Sometimes orbital x-rays show enlargement of the bony orbit. Ultrasonography and

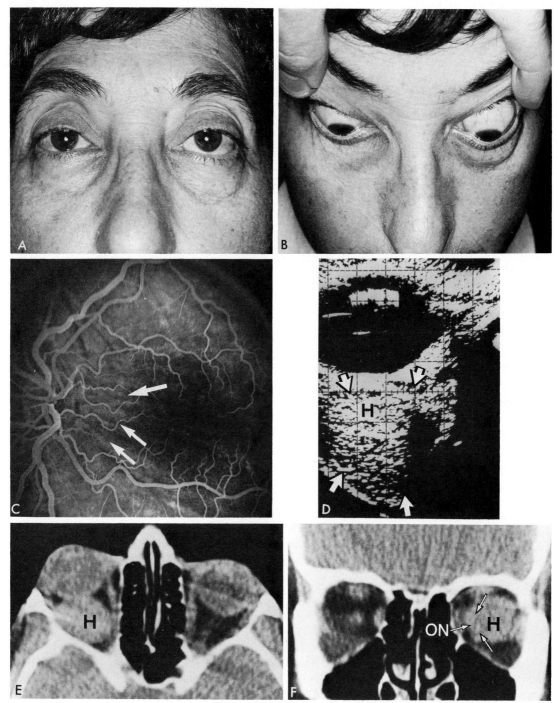

FIGURE 15–17. *Cavernous hemangioma.* Retrobulbar cavernous hemangioma treated by lateral orbital exploration. *A,* Left eye pushed forward with widened left palpebral fissure. *B,* Left exophthalmos. *C,* Fluorescein angiogram shows chorioretinal striae (arrows) temporal to optic disc. *D,* Horizontal ultrasound B scan shows well-circumscribed cavernous hemangioma (H, arrows) with multiple internal echoes behind left eye. *E,* CT scan shows cavernous hemangioma (H) within muscle cone behind left eye. *F,* CT scan shows cavernous hemangioma (H) displacing optic nerve (ON, arrows) medially.

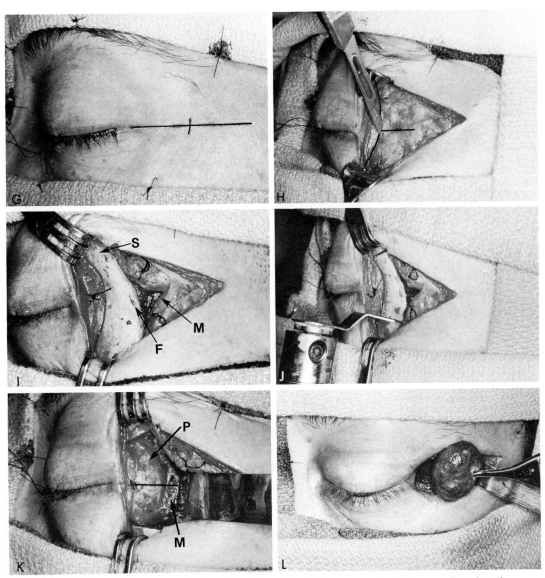

FIGURE 15–17 *Continued G,* Skin incision (line) extends parallel to zygomatic arch from near lateral canthus toward base of helix. Incision is approximately 30 mm long and is bisected by perpendicular scratch incision to aid reapproximation of skin margins. Suture is placed beneath insertion of lateral rectus muscle to aid in identification during orbital exploration. *H,* Periosteum covering lateral orbital rim is exposed by retracting skin and subcutaneous tissues. Incisions (lines) are made through periosteum on temporal surface of lateral orbital rim (position of knife blade) and through fascia over temporalis muscle. *I,* Lateral orbital rim is exposed by elevating periosteum and retracting temporalis muscle (M). Zygomaticofrontal suture (S) and zygomatico-facial foramen (F) can be seen on outer surface of rim. *J,* Oscillating saw is used to cut lateral orbital rim above zygomaticofrontal suture and near zygomatic arch. *K,* Periosteum covering orbital walls (periorbita, P) is exposed after segment of lateral orbital rim is removed from between bone cuts. Temporalis muscle (M) is retracted toward ear. Incision (line) is made in periorbital parallel to lateral rectus muscle. If necessary, a relaxing incision can be made perpendicular to the first incision. *L,* Cavernous hemangioma is removed from within muscle cone in position seen on ultrasound and CT scans. Firm capsule can usually be grasped with toothed forceps and dissected from surrounding tissues with blunt instruments.

Illustration continued on following page

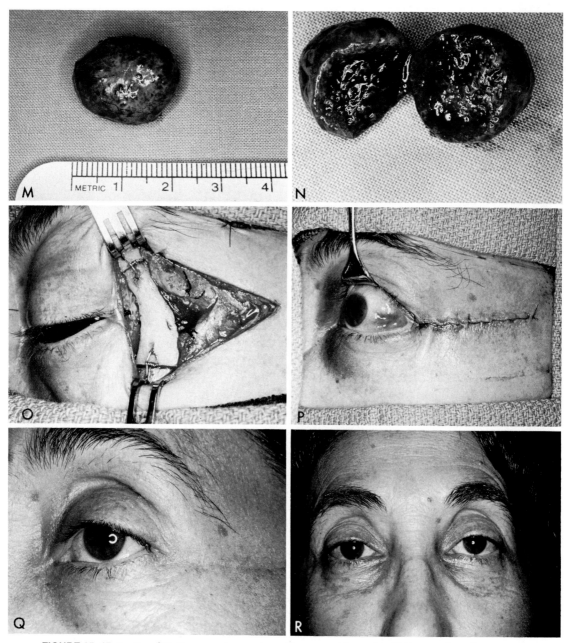

FIGURE 15–17 *Continued M,* Cavernous hemangioma after removal from orbit. *N,* Incision through cavernous hemangioma reveals outer capsule and inner complex of vascular channels. *O,* Periorbita is approximated and lateral orbital rim is wired back into original position. *P,* Periosteum is closed over lateral orbital rim, after which subcutaneous tissues and skin are carefully approximated. *Q,* Several months after operation, skin incision is well healed. *R,* Postoperatively eyes are in symmetrical positions.

scans may be performed if a deep lesion cannot be distinguished from other orbital lesions of childhood, such as dermoids, rhabdomyosarcomas, or meningoceles.

Most capillary hemangiomas undergo partial or complete involution by the time the child is 5 years of age. Because of this, treatment should be delayed if possible. Amblyopia should be combated by correction of significant refractive errors. If some treatment must be initiated, intralesional injection with steroids may hasten resolution of the tumor.[55, 56] Systemic steroids have also been used to decrease the size of capillary hemangiomas in some patients. Steroid responsiveness is often greatest in young children. Low-dose radiation therapy may cause reduction in tumor size, and sometimes surgical excision can be used to remove portions of particularly large lesions. After capillary hemangiomas have regressed or been treated, the patient may be left with crepe-like skin and ptosis that may require surgical correction.

Lymphangiomas are benign vascular tumors that most often appear during childhood. These tumors may be found in the conjunctiva, the eyelids, the orbit, or elsewhere in the head and neck.[52, 57]

One of the most common manifestations of orbital lymphangiomas is spontaneous hemorrhage that may cause sudden exophthalmos and limited eye movement. The hemorrhage usually subsides without treatment, but a chronic blood cyst may form and require surgical drainage or removal. Lymphangiomas may rapidly enlarge during acute respiratory tract infections, probably because of lymphoid hyperplasia. Histologically, these tumors consist of cystic spaces filled with clear fluid and lined by flattened endothelial cells. Smooth muscle cells are usually absent in the vascular walls of lymphangiomas. However, true arteries and veins may also be found in these tumors. This may explain why some abnormalities that clinically resemble lymphangiomas have dilated veins thought to represent congenital orbital varices.[57] Lymphoid follicles may be found within the interstitial stroma. Chronic lymphangiomas may contain phleboliths and calcified nodules.

Orbital x-rays are usually normal, although a blood cyst may produce enlargement of the orbit, and calcifications are occasionally seen in chronic lesions. Ultrasonography and CT scans usually show irregular internal densities and may demonstrate cystic spaces that can contain blood. Lymphangiomas are commonly infiltrative, with irregular outlines.

Treatment of lymphangiomas may involve surgical excision of disfiguring portions of the tumors, or drainage of blood cysts that fail to resolve spontaneously (Fig. 15–20). Because these benign tumors often infiltrate deeply into the orbit, complete excision is often difficult or impossible. Therefore, extensive surgery should be avoided if possible. Systemic steroids may reduce the size of lymphoid nodules and the amount of inflammation. Sometimes radiation therapy by external sources or implantation has been recommended, but this has not been found to be of significant value in the control of most lymphangiomas.

Varices of the orbit are usually primary, in which case they are believed to be of congenital origin and may even be classed as hamartomas. Other varices are secondary, and are acquired as a result of other abnormalities, such as intracranial AV communications or lesions near the orbital apex. One of the hallmarks of congenital varices is intermittent exophthalmos that may be caused by placing the head in a dependent position or by crying. Histologically, smooth muscle fibers are usually found in the walls of varices. In some varices the smooth muscle may atrophy as the vascular lumen enlarges. The resulting absence or paucity of muscle fibers together with the presence of lymphoid infiltration may produce a lesion that resembles a lymphangioma.[52, 53, 57]

Orbital x-rays may demonstrate calcifications if phleboliths have formed in a chronic varix. Orbital venography will often visualize these tortuous vascular structures, although blood flow may be reversed in secondary varices and the vessel may not fill by conventional injection of contrast material into superficial veins. Ultrasonography may show the outline of a dilated vessel. CT scans may demonstrate the enlarged vessels by contrast enhancement.

Treatment of orbital varices should be conservative, and surgery should usually be performed only in progressive cases when vision is threatened or deformity is severe. If the abnormality is primary and involves the posterior orbit, a neurosurgical approach may be necessary. If the varix is secondary, the deformity may resolve if the cause of the venous dilation is treated.

Hemangiopericytomas are uncommon, but they are among the most frequent true neoplasms of vascular origin found in the orbit. These tumors usually appear after the second decade of life and cause slowly progressive exophthalmos. Sometimes they cause intermittent orbital edema. Histologically, endothelial cells proliferate with reticulin formation and

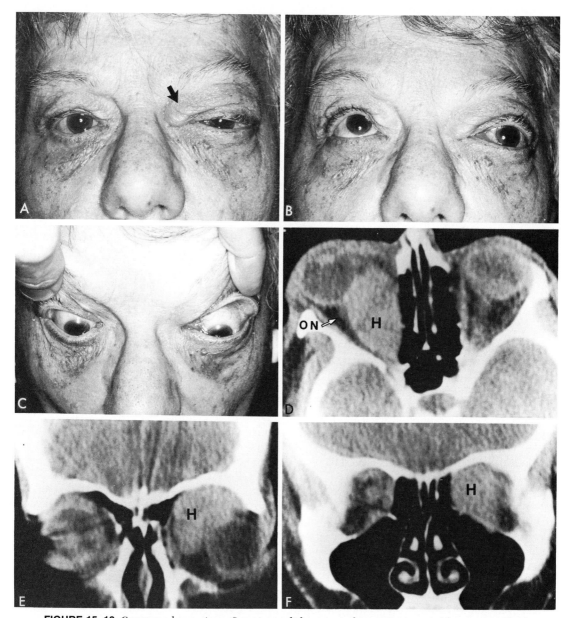

FIGURE 15–18. *Cavernous hemangioma.* Superior-medial cavernous hemangioma treated by anterior orbital exploration with division of eyelid margin. *A,* Ptosis of left upper eyelid and palpable mass (arrow) in superior-medial left orbit. *B,* Limited elevation of left eye. *C,* Left exophthalmos. *D,* CT scan shows cavernous hemangioma (H) displacing optic nerve (ON) laterally. *E,* CT scan through anterior orbits shows cavernous hemangioma (H) in superior-medial orbit displacing left eye down and laterally. *F,* CT scan through orbits behind globes shows cavernous hemangioma (H) filling most of medial orbit.

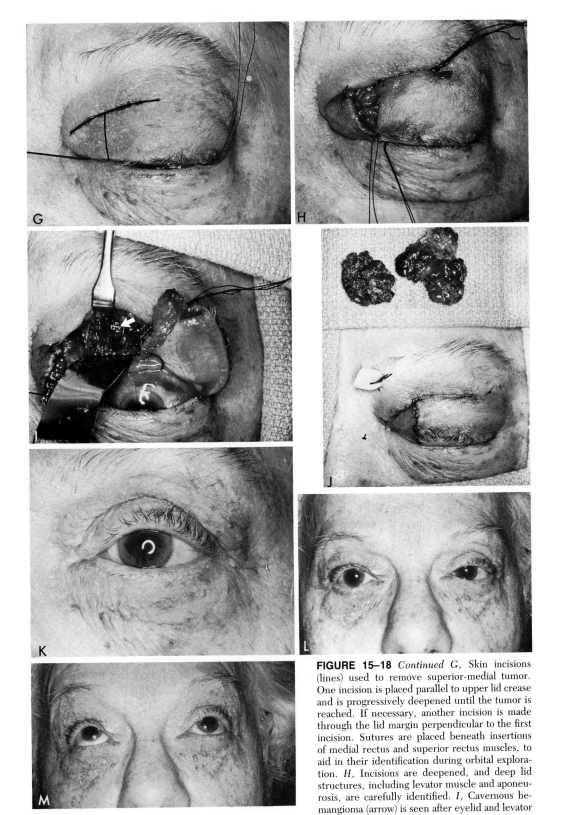

FIGURE 15–18 *Continued G*, Skin incisions (lines) used to remove superior-medial tumor. One incision is placed parallel to upper lid crease and is progressively deepened until the tumor is reached. If necessary, another incision is made through the lid margin perpendicular to the first incision. Sutures are placed beneath insertions of medial rectus and superior rectus muscles, to aid in their identification during orbital exploration. *H*, Incisions are deepened, and deep lid structures, including levator muscle and aponeurosis, are carefully identified. *I*, Cavernous hemangioma (arrow) is seen after eyelid and levator aponeurosis are divided. *J*, Electrocautery was used to cut cavernous hemangioma into pieces, since tumor extending behind eye could not be removed intact. Tumor fragments are seen above eyebrow. Eyelid tissues are anatomically reapproximated, and rubber drain is placed through stab incision near medial brow. *K*, Several months after operation eyelid incisions are well healed. *L*, Postoperatively left upper eyelid is less ptotic. *M*, Eye movements are almost symmetrical.

453

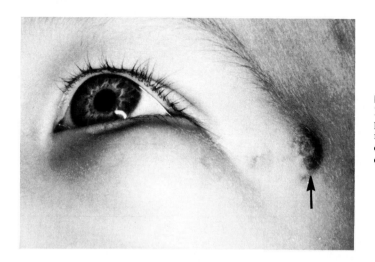

FIGURE 15–19. *Capillary hemangioma.* Elevated capillary hemangioma with dimpled surface (strawberry birthmark, arrow) is located near lateral eyebrow. Separate capillary hemangioma is located in anterior orbit beneath lower eyelid.

irregularly scattered small vascular spaces. A fibrous stroma may predominate, and indeed these tumors closely resemble fibrous histiocytomas.[52, 58] Hemangiopericytomas can be benign or malignant, and they may become infiltrative and metastasize. Although a capsule is often present, these neoplasms may be multinodular. Complete excision of hemangiopericytomas is usually more difficult than removal of cavernous hemangiomas.

Orbital x-rays seldom show any abnormality in patients with hemangiopericytomas unless the tumors are present for many years. Ultrasonography usually shows internal echoes similar to those seen in cavernous hemangiomas. CT scans usually visualize a relatively circumscribed mass that enhances significantly after contrast is administered.

AV communications may be divided into three main groups: (1) arteriovenous malformations (AVMs); (2) carotid-cavernous sinus (CCS) fistulas; and (3) dural shunts. In all of these abnormalities blood flows from the arterial circulation directly into the venous circulation without passage through intervening capillaries. However, the cause and vascular dynamics are different in each of the conditions.[24, 52, 53]

AVMs are usually supplied by branches of both the internal and external carotid arteries. An AVM frequently presents as a pulsatile mass within the orbit or eyelids. Such malformations may occur spontaneously or may result from trauma. Although they are seldom found in young children, some spontaneous lesions may be congenital. Histologically, these tumors are composed of mature arteries and veins. These vessels are usually hypertrophied, and the arteries lead directly into the draining veins. AVMs often enlarge progressively and are dif-

ficult to completely excise because they may recur after apparent obliteration of the feeding vessels.

CCS fistulas are direct communications between an internal carotid artery and the cavernous sinus. The abnormalities are frequently the result of a basal skull fracture, of rupture of an intracavernous carotid aneurysm, or of rupture of an atherosclerotic internal carotid artery in a hypertensive person. The common clinical features of CCS fistulas include severe exophthalmos and orbital congestion, tortuous episcleral vessels (Fig. 15–21), limited ocular motility, and loud bruits. Treatment may involve vascular embolization or surgical occlusion of feeding arteries.

Dural shunts are indirect communications between meningeal branches of the internal or external carotid arteries and intracranial venous channels such as the cavernous sinus. In contrast to CCS fistulas, in which high blood flow and high blood pressure directly enter the venous circulation, dural shunts have relatively low blood flow and low blood pressure. Therefore, dural shunts may go unrecognized for long periods of time because most of the arterial blood is drained off slowly into systemic veins rather than abruptly into orbital veins.

The common clinical features of dural shunts include mild exophthalmos, moderate elevation of intraocular pressure, and conjunctival vascular congestion. Bruits are infrequent, and because of the relatively mild signs and symptoms, sometimes the misdiagnosis of pseudotumor may be made. Most dural shunts are found in postmenopausal women and may be associated with intracranial venous occlusions. The clinical manifestations, such as exophthalmos and glaucoma, may resolve spontaneously without treatment. Conservative treatment and observation are usually warranted in patients with dural shunts.[24]

Orbital x-rays may reveal fractures in patients with traumatic AVMs and CCS fistulas; otherwise, they seldom reveal any evidence of AV communications. Detailed study of AV communications and their blood supply requires the use of positive contrast arteriography with selective injection of the internal and external carotid arteries followed by radiographic subtraction. Ultrasonography and CT scans with contrast enhancement may reveal enlarged vessels as well as secondary inflammatory changes in the orbit.

Lacrimal Gland Tumors

Although most mass lesions in the superior temporal quadrant of the orbit arise within the lacrimal gland, other tumors, such as dermoids, may also be found in this location. Of the tumors that involve the lacrimal gland, approximately half are nonepithelial and half are epithelial in origin.[59]

Nonepithelial lacrimal gland lesions include idiopathic inflammatory pseudotumors (Fig. 15–9) that may present in a variety of histologic forms, but especially as lymphocytic proliferations (benign lymphoid hyperplasias) and granulomas. Sarcoidosis and Sjögren's syndrome may cause lacrimal gland enlargement that sometimes is bilateral. Malignant lymphomas may involve the lacrimal gland, and as previously mentioned, these tumors may be difficult to distinguish from benign lymphocytic pseudotumors.

Epithelial lacrimal gland lesions are approximately half benign and half malignant.[59, 60] Almost all of the benign epithelial lesions, totaling nearly one quarter of all lacrimal gland tumors, are mixed tumors. These benign mixed tumors usually produce a slowly enlarging mass beneath the lateral upper lid with no significant pain or inflammation. These lesions are usually discovered during the third through sixth decade of life. Although the presence of a mass and symptoms are usually present for at least 12 months, the duration often cannot be accurately determined by history alone. Histologically, mixed tumors are composed primarily of epithelial tissue. In addition, they contain mesenchymal elements, some of which appear to be formed by metaplastic transformation of myoepithelium. Malignant epithelial tumors include adenoid cystic carcinomas, malignant forms of mixed tumors, and uncommon lesions such as squamous carcinomas.

Orbital x-rays are usually normal in patients with nonepithelial lacrimal gland lesions such as pseudotumors or lymphomas. Because benign mixed tumors are usually painless and slow growing, they may produce localized pressure erosion of the bone overlying the lacrimal gland. These findings are variable, however, and some benign mixed tumors may have a relatively short duration of symptoms and no bony changes. Irregular bone destruction is frequently due to a malignant lesion, although some benign mixed tumors, dermoids, and inflammatory lesions such as foreign body granulomas may occasionally produce similar changes. Ultrasonography and CT scans can usually demonstrate the extent of lacrimal gland tumors and may help to determine the kind of lesion that is present.[61]

Treatment of lacrimal gland tumors involves some of the most important decisions in orbital surgery. Benign mixed tumors should be completely removed without preliminary biopsy whenever possible, since if their contents are spilled or seeded within the orbit, they can recur as widely infiltrative and even truly malignant lesions.

When a benign mixed tumor is thought to be present, surgical excision is usually best accomplished by using a superior-lateral approach with removal of the upper portion of the lateral orbital rim (Fig. 15–22). The adjacent lacrimal gland, the periosteum, and the capsule that is adherent to the tumor should be removed en bloc in order to prevent residual tumor from being left within the orbit. Sometimes a very small tumor can be completely excised through an anterior incision without bone removal.

When a lacrimal gland mass is believed to be inflammatory but a biopsy is planned to confirm that suspicion, the possibility of a benign mixed tumor should be kept in mind. For this reason the biopsy incision should be placed so that it can be extended to a superior-lateral incision if a benign mixed tumor is found on frozen-section examination.

Malignant epithelial tumors of the lacrimal gland are among the most lethal tumors of the orbit. Adenoid cystic carcinomas are the most malignant of these neoplasms, with a common growth pattern along vessels, nerves, and the orbital periosteum. Even if a complete exenteration is performed, local recurrence within the orbital bones or metastatic spread is common. For this reason radical exenteration with re-

Text continued on page 460

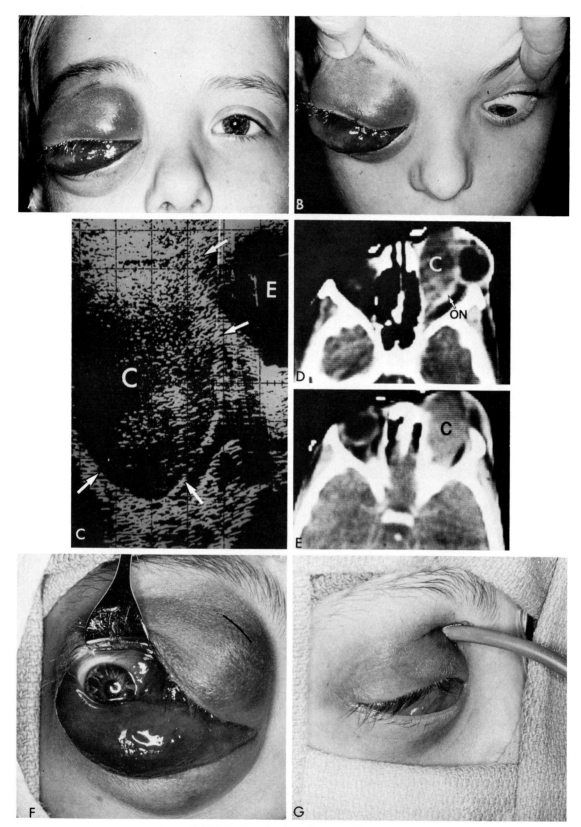

FIGURE 15–20 *See legend on opposite page*

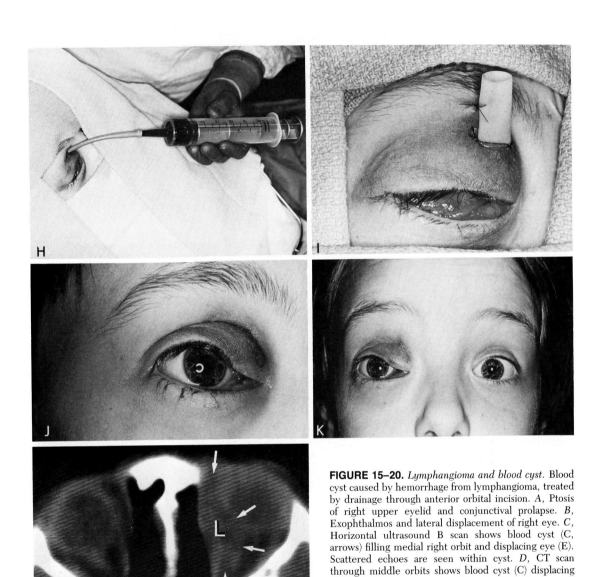

FIGURE 15–20. *Lymphangioma and blood cyst.* Blood cyst caused by hemorrhage from lymphangioma, treated by drainage through anterior orbital incision. *A,* Ptosis of right upper eyelid and conjunctival prolapse. *B,* Exophthalmos and lateral displacement of right eye. *C,* Horizontal ultrasound B scan shows blood cyst (C, arrows) filling medial right orbit and displacing eye (E). Scattered echoes are seen within cyst. *D,* CT scan through middle orbits shows blood cyst (C) displacing right eye and optic nerve (ON). *E,* CT scan through upper orbits shows large blood cyst (C) above right eye. *F,* Eyelid ecchymosis and edema with conjunctival prolapse. Upper eyelid incision (line) is used to reach blood cyst. *G,* Catheter is placed through incision into blood cyst. *H,* Blood is aspirated from cyst into syringe. *I,* Rubber drain is placed into cyst cavity through upper eyelid incision. *J,* Postoperatively right upper eyelid is less ptotic. *K,* Eyes are in almost symmetrical positions. *L,* CT scan after drainage of blood cyst shows infiltrative lymphangioma (L, arrows) in medial right orbit.

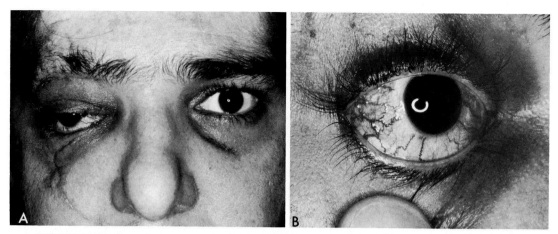

FIGURE 15–21. *Carotid–cavernous sinus fistula.* A, Right CCS fistula caused by trauma to orbit and basal skull fracture. B, Dilated, tortuous episcleral vessels caused by CCS fistula.

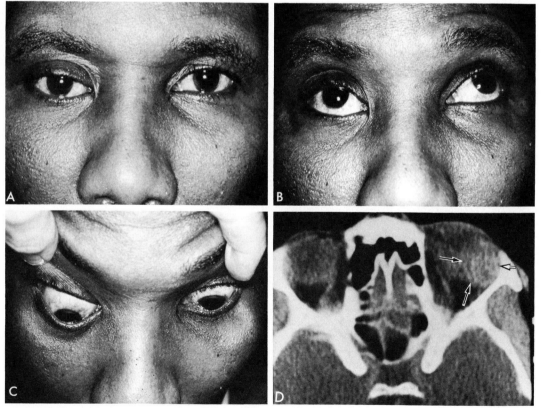

FIGURE 15–22. *Lacrimal gland benign mixed tumor.* Benign mixed tumor of lacrimal gland treated by superior-lateral orbital exploration. A, Ptosis of right upper eyelid and downward displacement of right eye. B, Limited elevation of right eye. C, Right exophthalmos. D, CT scan shows lacrimal gland tumor (arrows) in anterior orbit above right eye.

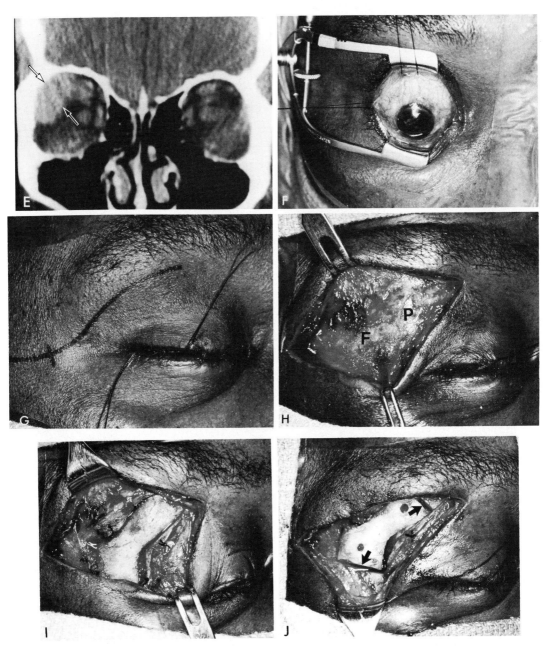

FIGURE 15–22 *Continued E*, CT scan shows lacrimal gland tumor (arrows) in superior-lateral right orbit. *F*, Sutures are placed beneath insertions of superior rectus and lateral rectus muscles, to aid in identification during orbital exploration. *G*, Skin incision (line) extends from below the unshaved eyebrow in an arc approximately 1 cm temporal to the lateral canthus and then toward the ear parallel to the zygomatic arch. A short perpendicular scratch incision is made to aid reapproximation of skin margins. *H*, Skin and subcutaneous tissues are retracted to expose periosteum (P) covering lateral orbital rim and fascia (F) covering temporalis muscle. *I*, Lateral orbital rim is exposed by elevating periosteum and retracting temporalis muscle. *J*, Lateral orbital rim is cut (arrows) with oscillating saw, and holes are drilled to allow passage of wires for bone fixation after removal of tumor.

Illustration continued on following page

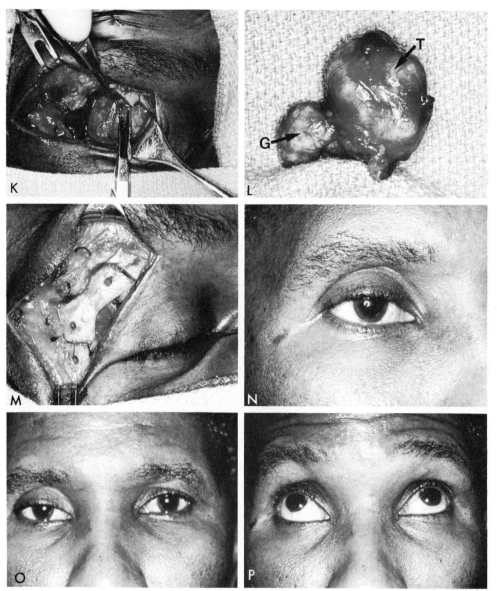

FIGURE 15–22 *Continued K,* Lacrimal gland tumor is removed together with adherent periosteum (grasped by forceps). *L,* Lacrimal gland tumor (T) and attached lacrimal gland (G) after removal from orbit. *M,* Lateral orbital rim is replaced and wired into original position. *N,* Six months after operation, skin incision is well healed. *O,* Postoperatively, eyes are in symmetrical positions, but right upper eyelid ptosis persists. *P,* Postoperatively, both eyes move without restriction.

moval of major portions of the superior and lateral bony walls of the orbit seems to offer the best chance of survival in such patients (Fig. 15–23).

If the clinical or radiographic appearance of a lacrimal gland tumor is such that an epithelial malignancy seems likely, a biopsy through an anterior incision is usually preferable to a lateral approach. If the lateral orbital rim is not removed at the time of biopsy, there is less chance of spreading tumor cells, and a more circumscribed exenteration can be performed. Because of the mutilative nature of exenteration, the diagnosis of a malignant lacrimal gland tumor should be based on permanent-section histological evaluation rather than frozen-section examination. In some patients radiation therapy may be used in addition to exenteration, especially if the orbital bones are involved by tumor at the time of initial surgery (Fig. 15–24).

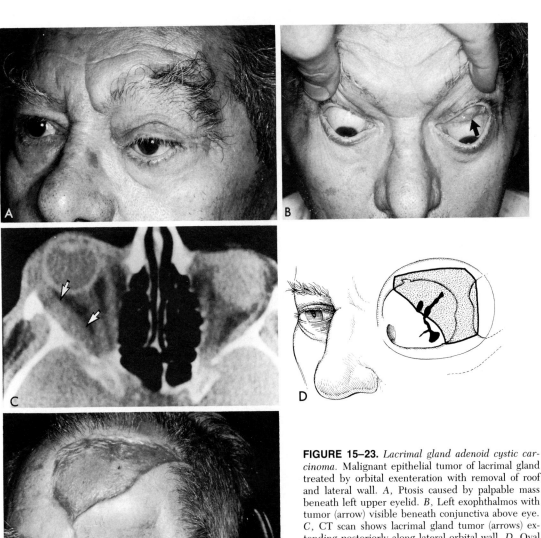

FIGURE 15–23. *Lacrimal gland adenoid cystic carcinoma.* Malignant epithelial tumor of lacrimal gland treated by orbital exenteration with removal of roof and lateral wall. *A,* Ptosis caused by palpable mass beneath left upper eyelid. *B,* Left exophthalmos with tumor (arrow) visible beneath conjunctiva above eye. *C,* CT scan shows lacrimal gland tumor (arrows) extending posteriorly along lateral orbital wall. *D,* Oval line shows skin incision used for orbital exenteration. Shaded area shows extent of bone removed from roof and lateral wall of orbit. *E,* Exenteration defect is covered by rotation flap from forehead.

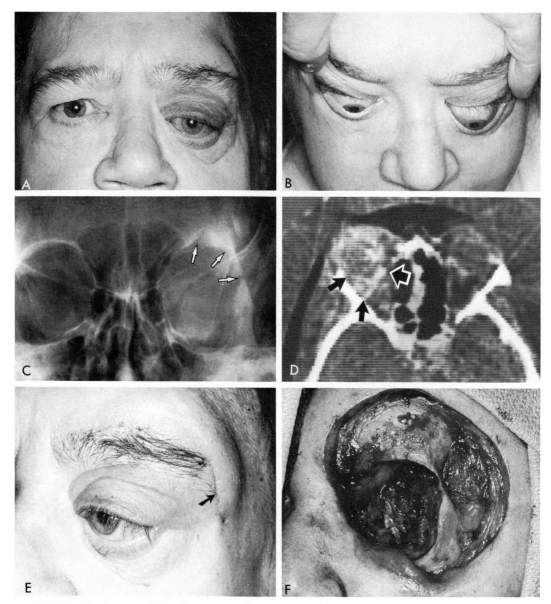

FIGURE 15–24. *Lacrimal gland squamous cell carcinoma.* Malignant epithelial tumor of lacrimal gland treated by orbital exenteration, bone removal, and radiation. *A,* Downward displacement of left eye caused by palpable mass beneath left brow. *B,* Left exophthalmos. *C,* X-ray shows destruction of orbital rim (arrows) caused by lacrimal gland tumor. *D,* CT scan shows lacrimal gland tumor (arrows) above and behind left eye. *E,* Biopsy of tumor was taken through brow incision (arrow). *F,* Exenteration of left orbit has been performed with removal of skin above brow and over anterior temporalis muscle.

Lymphocytic and Related Tumors

The white blood cell–macrophage system gives rise to a diverse group of lesions that can be classified into lymphocytic, plasmacytic, leukemic, and histiocytic tumors. This rather amorphous group of abnormalities includes malignancies such as lymphomas and leukemias, as well as benign lesions such as lymphoid hyperplasias and plasma cell pseudotumors.[7, 28]

Lymphocytic tumors of the orbit occur predominantly in adults and are rare in children. On the basis of features such as lymphocyte maturity and growth pattern, lymphocytic tumors can be classified into three groups: (1) benign lymphoid hyperplasia (idiopathic lym-

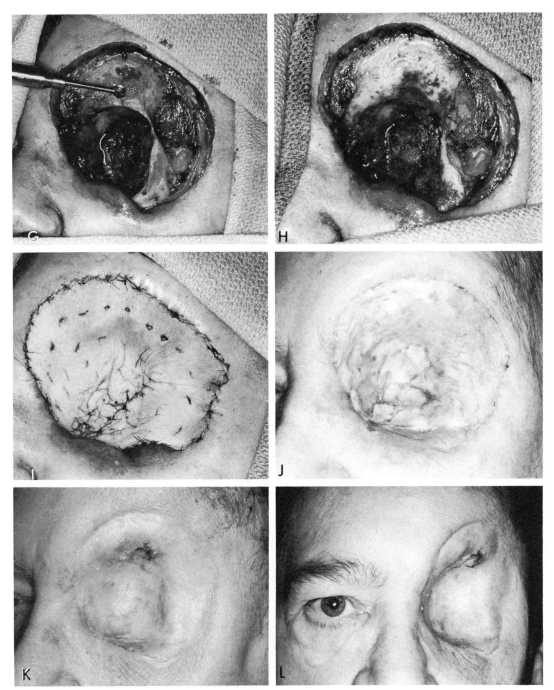

FIGURE 15–24 *Continued G*, Drill is used to remove bone in area from which tumor was removed. *H*, Exenteration defect after removal of bone and anterior temporalis muscle. *I*, Exenteration defect covered by split-thickness skin graft from anterior thigh. *J*, Skin graft, 1 month after operation. *K*, Two years after exenteration and postoperative radiation therapy, wound is well healed, and there is no recurrence of tumor. Small scab is present near brow. *L*, Exenteration defect can be covered by a patch or prothesis.

phocytic pseudotumor), (2) atypical lymphoid hyperplasia, and (3) malignant lymphoma.

Benign lymphoid hyperplasia or idiopathic lymphocytic pseudotumor is typified by a combination of mature lymphocytes and plasma cells with occasional eosinophils. These lesions may appear reactive, and frequently contain germinal centers and areas of fibroblastic proliferation. Mitoses are rare, and lymphoid follicle formation is common. Atypical lymphoid hyperplasia is an intermediate category of tumor in which atypical mononuclear cells are found among more mature cells. Some histological features of lymphoma are present, but the lesion is not clearly malignant. Lymphomas make up the malignant group of these lymphocytic tumors. Malignant lymphoma may either take the form of a systemic disease or may arise as a lesion confined to the orbit with the potential for dissemination. Histologically, lymphomas are usually composed of immature large lymphocytes with frequent mitoses and a random distribution of cells in diffuse sheets.

Because it is not always possible to distinguish benign lymphoid hyperplasia from malignant lymphoma on the basis of histological criteria alone, immunological features have been used to help classify lymphocytic tumors. Most human lymphocytes can be categorized as B or T cells.[29] B lymphocytes chiefly originate in the bone marrow. These cells are primarily responsible for antibody production, as a consequence of which immunoglobulins are located on their surface membranes. These B lymphocytes tend to localize in lymph nodes and the spleen, and can transform into plasma cells. T lymphocytes are predominantly derived from the thymus and are primarily responsible for cell-mediated immunity. These cells make up most of the circulating lymphocytes in the blood.

The origin of groups of B lymphocytes can be determined by analysis of the classes of immunoglobulins found on their cell surfaces. A monoclonal proliferation is one in which a single immunoglobulin class predominates in a tumor. Polyclonal proliferations are those in which multiple classes of immunoglobulins are found.

Malignant lymphomas are commonly composed of B cells with a monoclonal origin. Benign lymphoid hyperplasia is usually composed either of B cells of polyclonal origin or of T cells. Some lymphomas of T cell origin do exist, as in Hodgkin's disease, but these are less common than B cell lymphomas and rarely involve the orbit. If a lymphoid tumor is found at the time of surgery, consideration should be given to submitting some fresh tissue for cell surface immunology analysis to aid in diagnosis and classification.[25–27]

Histiocytic lymphoma (reticulum cell sarcoma) and poorly differentiated lymphocytic lymphoma are among the most common forms of malignant lymphoma involving the orbit. Histiocytic lymphoma is more likely to be widely disseminated and is more rapidly lethal than lymphocytic lymphoma.[28]

Burkitt's lymphoma is a distinctive tumor that usually occurs among children in tropical Africa. Many patients with this tumor have maxillary involvement with orbital extension. Rare cases of Burkitt's lymphoma have been found in the United States, and it has been suspected that a virus may be the cause. Histologically, these tumors contain poorly differentiated lymphoblasts and clear phagocytic histiocytes that produce a characteristic "starry sky" appearance. Although this tumor may be lethal, sometimes it is cured by a combination of chemotherapy, radiation therapy, and local surgical excision.[28]

Lymphocytic tumors near the eye may be superficial beneath the skin or conjunctiva, or may be located deep within the orbit. Superficial tumors frequently appear as salmon-colored or pale nodules under the conjunctiva (Fig. 15–25). Such subconjunctival lesions may be either malignant or benign, and unless an acute viral illness occurs coincident with the appearance of the nodule, a large conjunctival biopsy is usually necessary to establish a diagnosis. Lymphoid tumors must be distinguished from other common subconjunctival lesions such as prolapsed orbital fat and epibulbar dermoids or lipodermoids. The lacrimal gland is a common location for lymphocytic tumors in the deep orbit. It is often difficult to clinically distinguish these lymphocytic lesions from epithelial neoplasms such as lacrimal gland mixed tumors, which should be completely excised rather than examined by biopsy.

Although orbital x-rays are usually normal in patients with lymphoma, bone destruction may be present. Ultrasonography and CT scans frequently demonstrate an orbital mass with irregular margins and infiltration near the extraocular muscles (Fig. 15–26). Sometimes radionuclide body scans with gallium-labeled compounds demonstrate foci of lymphoma outside the orbit (Fig. 15–25).

Patients with benign or malignant lymphocytic tumors of the orbit should be given a systemic evaluation that includes a general physical examination, chest x-ray, and serum

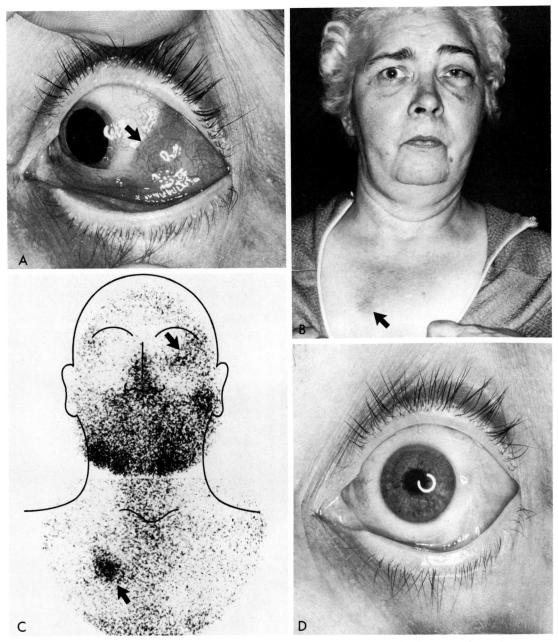

FIGURE 15–25. *Malignant lymphoma.* Multifocal lymphoma presenting as orbital tumor. *A,* Lymphoma (arrow) infiltrating beneath temporal conjunctiva of left eye. *B,* Subcutaneous tumor (arrow) was palpated near sternum. *C,* Gallium radionuclide scan shows localization of tumor (arrows) in left orbit and chest. *D,* Resolution of subconjunctival lymphoma after systemic chemotherapy.

immunoprotein electrophoresis for the detection of abnormal immunoglobulins. When a malignant lesion is suspected, bone marrow aspiration, abdominal computed tomography, and lymphangiography for the detection of involved retroperitoneal lymph nodes should be considered. Periodic follow-up examinations of

patients with lymphocytic tumors is appropriate because systemic lymphoma can appear years after the presentation of an orbital lesion.

The treatment of choice for malignant lymphoma that is localized to the orbit is usually radiation therapy. Sometimes even benign lymphoid hyperplasia is treated with low-dose ra-

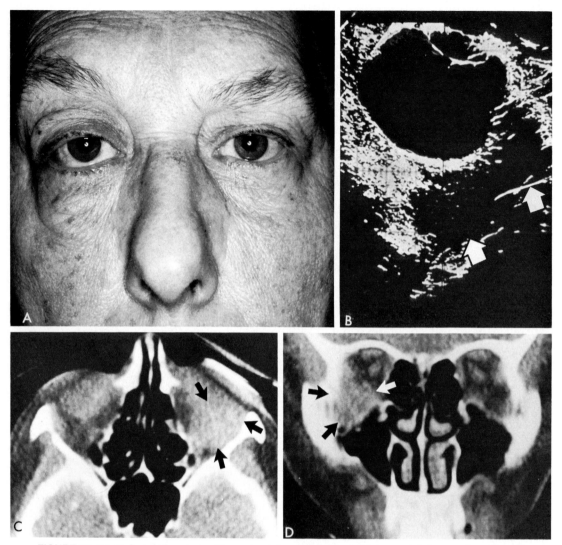

FIGURE 15–26. *Malignant lymphoma.* Tumor involving right orbit. *A,* Right exophthalmos and swelling of right lower eyelid. *B,* Horizontal ultrasound B scan shows tumor (arrows) adjacent to right eye, extending along lateral orbital wall. *C,* CT scan through lower orbits shows infiltrative tumor (arrows) beneath right eye. *D,* CT scan shows tumor (arrows) filling the inferior right orbit.

diation.[40] Systemic chemotherapy is usually given if orbital lymphoma is part of a systemic disease process (Fig. 15–25).

Plasmacytic tumors are closely related to lymphocytic tumors, and indeed, plasma cells may originate from B lymphocyte stem cells. The most common plasma cell tumor involving the orbit is the plasmacytoma, which may be either unifocal or part of disseminated multiple myeloma (plasma cell myeloma). In multiple myeloma, tumor cells involve the bone marrow to produce anemia, bleeding disorders, and frequent bone pain. Benign plasma cell pseudo-

tumors are uncommon; if found, the patient must be carefully evaluated to determine whether multiple myeloma is present.

Plasmacytic tumors often produce elevated levels of serum immunoglobulins. In some diseases characterized by plasma cell proliferation—such as Waldenström's macroglobulinemia—immunoglobulin fragments may appear in the urine as Bence Jones proteins.

Histologically, plasma cells can assume a variety of forms. Plasma cell pseudotumors are chiefly composed of relatively small plasma cells with eccentric nuclei in which chromatin is dispersed in a cartwheel pattern. Plasmacytomas and the tumors associated with multiple myeloma contain larger plasma cells that have multiple nuclei with widely dispersed chromatin. In Waldenström's macroglobulinemia, lymphocytoid plasma cells may be found. These cells have characteristics of both lymphocytes and plasma cells, and may contain eosinophilic intranuclear immunoglobulin inclusions known as Dutcher bodies. Dutcher bodies may be found in other disorders as well, including systemic lymphoma with immunoglobulin production.[28]

Although orbital x-rays seldom show abnormalities in patients with plasma cell tumors, multiple myeloma may involve the skull and produce the appearance of punched-out lesions in the calvarium. Ultrasonography and CT scans may show a highly cellular solid tumor within the orbit. Treatment of orbital plasmacytoma usually consists of local excision or biopsy followed by radiation therapy.

Leukemic tumors may be classed as hematopoietic tumors because they involve malignant white blood cells that proliferate within blood-forming tissues and the circulating blood. The leukemic tumors most frequently involving the orbit are acute lymphocytic leukemia and acute myelogenous leukemia (granulocytic sarcoma). These malignancies occur more often in children than in adults. Leukemias are diffuse disorders that usually involve multiple internal organs and may cause sudden hemorrhage. In some patients exophthalmos may be caused by orbital hemorrhage rather than by cellular proliferation and tumor growth. Spontaneous eyelid ecchymosis in a child should raise the possibility that either leukemia or metastatic neuroblastoma is present. On some occasions an orbital mass may appear before systemic signs of leukemia such as blood changes are apparent. Careful ophthalmic examination may reveal leukemic infiltration of the fundus or the anterior segment of the eye.

Histologically, the cells of both lymphocytic and myelogenous leukemia may resemble the reticulum cells of histiocytic lymphoma (reticulum cell sarcoma). Sometimes myelogenous leukemia is termed chloroma because of the green color that may be given to the tumor by the enzyme myeloperoxidase.[28]

The findings on orbital x-rays, ultrasonography, and CT scans are similar to those seen in patients with lymphoma. Orbital leukemia usually responds to treatment of the systemic disease.

Histiocytic tumors are primarily composed of histiocytes (macrophages), which are phagocytes and do not play a significant role in antibody or immunoglobulin production. These abnormalities usually occur in children who are younger than 16 years of age. The most common of such tumors that involve the orbit are grouped together as histiocytosis X, which includes eosinophilic granuloma, Hand-Schüller-Christian disease, and Letterer-Siwe disease. Another histiocytic condition that is not part of the histiocytosis X complex is benign juvenile xanthogranuloma (nevoxanthoendothelioma). This latter disorder rarely involves the orbit, and is usually a self-limited cutaneous disease that may occur in the skin and within the eye.

Histologically, the tumors of the histiocytosis X group contain mixtures of histiocytes and chronic inflammatory cells. Eosinophilic granuloma contains a predominant number of eosinophils and usually occurs as a solitary lesion within bone rather than as a systemic disorder. Hand-Schüller-Christian disease and Letterer-Siwe disease are believed to be two forms of a panoramic disorder that is usually disseminated throughout the body. Hand-Schüller-Christian disease is a chronic condition in which bone destruction is very common, especially in the sphenoid and near the sella. Letterer-Siwe disease is an acute condition that occurs in infants and very young children in which the liver and spleen are usually enlarged, with frequent involvement of bones and bone marrow. The histiocytes in all of these disorders appear relatively benign, giving rise to the term differentiated histiocytoses. Giant cells are relatively common. In the chronic (Hand-Schüller-Christian) form of the disease lipid phagocytosis within the histiocytes is more prominent than in the acute (Letterer-Siwe) form.[28]

Orbital x-rays may show lytic defects in the skull or orbital walls, or may demonstrate a bony sclerosis that resembles fibrous dysplasia. Ultrasonography will detect only soft tissue lesions, while CT scans may also confirm the presence and extent of abnormalities in the bone. Hand-Schüller-Christian disease may involve the orbit, skull, and pituitary gland to produce a characteristic triad of exophthalmos, bone destruction in the calvarium, and diabetes insipidus.

The most lethal of these conditions is Letterer-Siwe disease, while eosinophilic granuloma is almost never fatal. Localized eosinophilic granuloma may be adequately treated by surgical excision, sometimes accompanied by radiation therapy. In some cases these tumors may spontaneously resolve after biopsy alone.

Disseminated histiocytoses usually require combined treatment with radiation and chemotherapy.

Meningiomas and Other Fibro-osseous Tumors

Mesenchymal tissues give rise to fibro-osseous tumors, including meningiomas, osteomas, fibrous histiocytomas, and a group of lesions related to fibrous dysplasia.[48, 62–65] Most of these tumors are locally invasive and are either slow growing or benign. Many of these abnormalities extend into the orbit from the adjacent skull or sinuses.

Less frequently highly malignant tumors such as osteogenic sarcomas and chondrosarcomas may arise from the orbital bones or sinuses. The treatment of these malignancies often requires radical exenteration, which has been mentioned under the topic of secondary tumors (Fig. 15–12).

Meningiomas are tumors that arise from arachnoidal tissues that cover the central nervous system. Although meningiomas are invasive and locally destructive, they grow slowly and rarely metastasize. Most orbital meningiomas are secondary tumors that originate intracranially near the sphenoid wing. These tumors usually cause painless exophthalmos and may produce a soft tissue swelling beneath the temporalis muscle

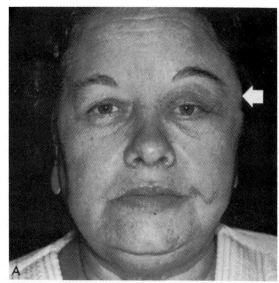

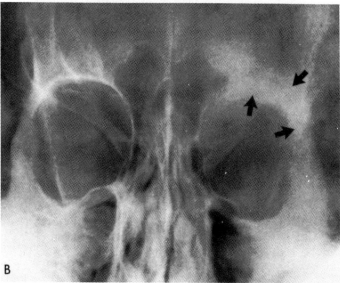

FIGURE 15–27. *Meningioma.* Sphenoid wing meningioma invading left orbit. *A,* Left exophthalmos and swelling (arrow) beneath temporalis muscle. *B,* X-ray shows both thickening and destruction (arrows) of orbital bones.

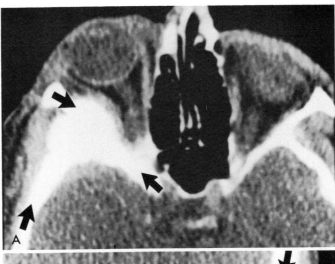

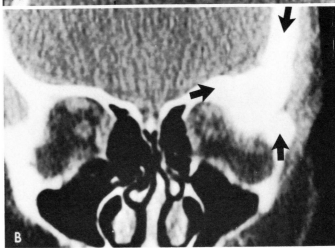

FIGURE 15–28. *Meningioma.* Sphenoid wing meningioma invading left orbit. *A,* CT scan shows hyperostosis (arrows) of skull and orbital walls invaded by tumor. *B,* CT scan shows similar hyperostosis (arrows).

(Fig. 15–27). Primary intraorbital meningiomas are much less common than intracranial tumors. These primary tumors usually arise from the optic nerve sheath, but rarely they may be ectopic and unassociated with the optic nerve.[48] Meningiomas involving the optic nerve usually cause decreased vision, as well as exophthalmos. Secondary tumors may displace the eye without visual loss. An intraocular feature of some orbital meningiomas is the presence of opticociliary shunt vessels that direct retinal venous blood into the choroidal circulation near the optic nerve head.[48, 66]

Orbital x-rays usually show characteristic changes in the sphenoid bone when intracranial tumors invade the orbit. The involved bones are usually thickened with abnormal calcifications (Fig. 15–27). Occasionally bone absorption and destruction are apparent. Primary optic nerve sheath meningiomas generally enlarge and demineralize the optic canal. Arteriography usually demonstrates an abnormal blood supply, which most often originates from enlarged branches of the external carotid artery. Ultrasonography can be used to demonstrate some intraorbital meningiomas, but may fail to outline tumors growing *en plaque* against the orbital walls. CT scans are useful for outlining both the soft tissue components and bony changes of many meningiomas (Fig. 15–28).[67] The visualization of most meningiomas is enhanced after contrast administration (Fig. 15–29).

Surgical excision of those meningiomas that have an intracranial component is best accomplished through a neurosurgical approach. After removal of the involved orbital walls the orbital tumor can often be excised through the same transcranial incision. Because intracranial meningiomas have usually undergone considerable growth by the time they are recognized, it is common that only partial tumor removal is

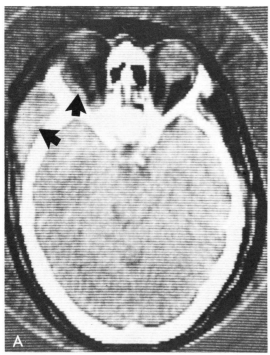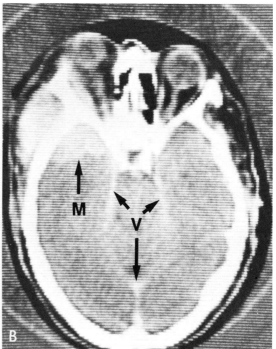

FIGURE 15–29. *Meningioma.* Sphenoid wing meningioma invading left orbit. *A*, CT scan without contrast shows tumor within left orbit and beneath temporalis muscle (arrows). *B*, CT scan with contrast shows normal intracranial vessels (V) and intracranial meningioma (M).

possible. The slow growth of a meningioma may allow a normal life span, despite tumor persistence or recurrence after surgery.

The treatment of primary intraorbital meningiomas of the optic nerve sheath is somewhat controversial. If the vision in the involved eye remains good, and if the optic canal is radiographically normal, some surgeons would recommend that a biopsy be done and the patient observed until the vision deteriorates severely. In some cases meningiomas adjacent to the optic nerve have been surgically removed with preservation of useful vision.[68] Most surgeons recommend excision of the involved optic nerve and the tumor by a craniotomy approach, in order to try to prevent posterior extension into the orbital chiasm. This approach is usually recommended when the optic canal is radiographically abnormal. Although radiation therapy seldom destroys meningiomas, it may be useful as adjunctive therapy when tumors extend to the optic chiasm and brain stem, or when patients refuse surgery.[69]

Osteomas are benign tumors that arise in membranous bones of the skull and face, with frequent extension into the orbit and sinuses. These tumors are composed of osteoblastic connective tissue that forms abundant osteoid and

new bone. Although this bone is usually exceptionally dense, it is otherwise normal. Osteomas can be categorized as ivory, mature, or fibrous, depending on their cellular features. Despite such histological differences, osteomas are similar in their clinical behavior and seldom recur after excision.[62, 64]

Extension of osteomas into the orbit may cause ptosis or exophthalmos. Other signs and symptoms may be the result of intracranial involvement or of secondary sinus disease. Osteomas are most commonly found within the frontal sinuses, and less frequently occur within the ethmoid, maxillary, and sphenoid sinuses.

Orbital x-rays usually show a dense radiopaque tumor with characteristically smooth margins. Occasionally the tumor contour may be irregular or pedunculated (Fig. 15–30). Although ultrasonography may show some distortion of the contour of the orbital wall, sound waves will not penetrate an osteoma and cannot distinguish such tumors from normal bone. CT scans clearly outline osteomas and may also show soft tissue abnormalities within the adjacent sinus cavities (Fig. 15–31).

If an osteoma is radiographically diagnosed but does not produce significant symptoms, it is appropriate to follow its growth by periodic

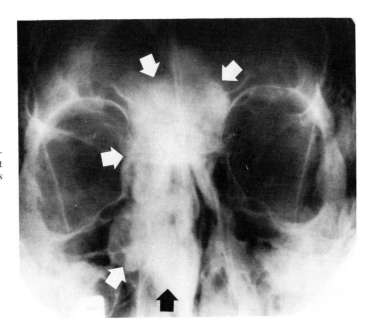

FIGURE 15–30. *Osteoma.* X-ray shows extensive osteoma (arrows) involving right maxillary and ethmoid sinuses, as well as both frontal sinuses.

x-rays or computed tomographic scans. If the tumor has grown rapidly and, especially, if calcifications are mottled rather than uniform, the diagnosis of another tumor such as chondrosarcoma should be considered (Fig. 15–12). Such malignant tumors usually produce significant bone destruction, and a biopsy through the nose, sinus, or skin will reveal the nature of the lesion.

Surgical excision of small osteomas that project primarily into the orbit can usually be performed through incisions near the brow or medial canthus. Excision of large frontal osteomas is most effectively performed through an osteoplastic approach similar to that used for treatment of frontal sinus mucoceles. In most patients the frontal sinus can best be reached through a coronal skin incision, with obliteration of the sinus cavity by insertion of an adipose implant.[61] On rare occasions a neurosurgical approach may be used to remove extensive osteomas that have an intracranial component.

Fibrous histiocytomas are tumors that contain a fibrous stroma, histiocytes (macrophages), and varying amounts of vascular tissue. Vascular channels lined with proliferating endothelial cells may predominate, and the lesions may appear similar to hemangiopericytomas.[65, 70] Fibrous histiocytomas, like hemangiopericytomas, may be benign or malignant. Although these tumors may appear circumscribed, they are usually found to be infiltrative at the time of surgical exploration and histological examina-

tion. Metastasis is uncommon, and despite the presence of histiocytes, these tumors do not appear to be related to the disseminated lesions that are found as part of histiocytosis X.

Orbital x-rays may reveal smooth displacement of the orbital walls but seldom show bone destruction. Ultrasonography shows a solid tumor that may or may not appear encapsulated. Internal echoes are usually present because of a heterogeneous structure. CT scans may demonstrate an apparently circumscribed mass that sometimes enhances after contrast is administered if the tumor contains a significant vascular component.

Treatment of fibrous histiocytomas usually consists of wide local excision. Complete removal may be difficult because of infiltration near normal tissues such as the extraocular muscles and optic nerve. The presence of malignant tumors and benign tumors that have recurred may necessitate orbital exenteration.[71] Radiation therapy is usually not very effective in the management of fibrous histiocytoma.

Fibrous dysplasia is a benign condition that most often involves the skull, facial bones, ribs, and long bones such as the femur and tibia. The involved bones are thickened by fibrous tissue that contains trabeculae of immature nonlamellar bone.[62, 65] The process may be localized to one bone (monostotic) or may involve multiple bones (polyostotic). Skull asymmetry and exophthalmos may result from frontal bone involvement and extension of the thickened tis-

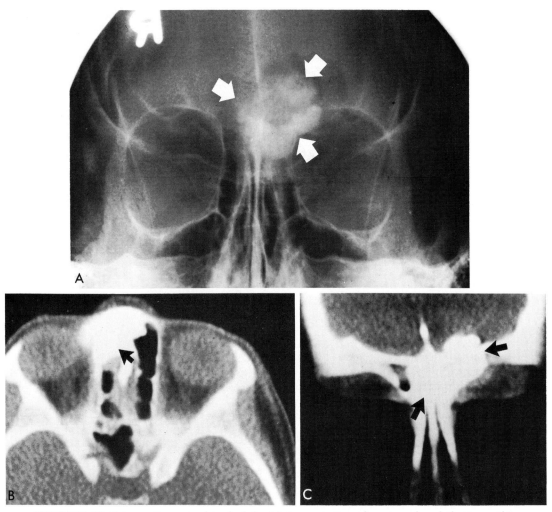

FIGURE 15–31. *Osteoma.* Tumor involving both frontal sinuses. *A,* X-ray shows irregular calcifications within osteoma (arrows). *B,* CT scan shows dense tumor (arrow) involving upper nasal cavity and left orbit. *C,* CT scan shows tumor (arrows) within frontal sinuses and extending into left orbit.

sues into the orbit. Diplopia, decreased vision, and hearing defects are common. The clinical abnormalities usually present during childhood or adolescence. Albright's syndrome consists of polyostotic fibrous dysplasia, irregular cutaneous pigmentation (with irregular margins shaped like the coast of Maine), and early puberty in the female.

Orbital x-rays of fibrous dysplasia often show thickened bones with a ground-glass appearance. Although the bones are usually densely sclerotic, radiolucent areas may be caused by fibrous tissue. Ultrasonography usually shows only a distorted contour of the orbital wall. CT scans show bony thickening with scattered areas of lesser density. These changes may be indistinguishable from those caused by meningiomas or other fibro-osseous tumors.

If the diagnosis of fibrous dysplasia is established on the basis of clinical findings and diagnostic studies, some patients may be followed without surgery when cosmetic and functional impairment is minimal. Orbital lesions are usually removed in part, often with the use of curettes, rongeurs, and drills. Complete excision is often impossible because of the extensive involvement of the lesion. A neurosurgical approach may be required to approach the sphenoid bones or to decompress the optic nerve.

Ossifying fibroma (fibrous osteoma) and *cementifying fibroma* (an odontogenic tumor) are lesions that may be confused with fibrous dysplasia.[62, 65, 72] Ossifying fibroma is a benign growth that usually arises as a solitary lesion within the jaw. Cementifying fibroma arises from tissues that normally form teeth; it usually involves the mandible, although it may occur in other facial bones as well. Even histological examination may not reveal a specific diagnosis, since a single lesion may contain areas that resemble more than one fibro-osseous tumor.

Radiographically, these tumors are usually more localized than fibrous dysplasia. If a tumor is circumscribed, complete excision may be attempted. Often the lesion is diffuse, and only portions can be removed without damage to adjacent structures.

Sinus Mucoceles

Mucoceles of the paranasal sinuses are benign cystic structures that may slowly expand to displace the orbital bones and secondarily invade the orbit. Most mucoceles are caused by obstruction of the sinus ducts and ostia through which fluid normally drains out of the air-filled sinus cavities. Trauma or tumors that involve the sinuses may lead to mucocele formation. Mucoceles usually contain mucoid fluid, which may appear brown if hemorrhage has occurred. These cysts are usually lined by pseudostratified ciliated columnar respiratory epithelium. Sometimes the epithelial lining may become attenuated and disappear.[7] A mucocele that becomes infected and fills with pus is termed a pyocele. Mucoceles most commonly arise in the frontal or ethmoid sinuses.

Frontal sinus mucoceles characteristically produce a palpable mass in the superior nasal quadrant of the orbit (Fig. 15–32). Ptosis and limited elevation of the eye may be caused by these lesions. Ethmoid sinus mucoceles may produce a mass in the medial portion of the orbit (Fig. 15–33). Maxillary sinus and sphenoid sinus mucoceles are uncommon and seldom extend into the orbit. Infected ethmoid mucoceles may cause pain and swelling, mimicking dacryocystitis, which is an infection of the lacrimal sac.

Orbital x-rays characteristically show the thinning and smooth expansion of the bony walls of the sinus. The sinus cavity is usually dense and may have an air-fluid level. Ultrasonography and CT scans commonly visualize a cystic lesion with smooth contours (Figs. 15–32 and 15–33). Occasionally cholesterol crystals or debris within the mucocele may show densities or echoes that distort the otherwise homogeneous pattern of the cyst contents.

Treatment of sinus mucoceles usually involves aspiration of the contents with removal of the mucosal lining, together with establishment of an ostium into the nasal cavity. Infections should be treated with appropriate antibiotics. Recurrence of frontal mucoceles is common if they are simply treated by intranasal drainage through an external frontal-ethmoid incision. Frontal mucoceles are most effectively treated by an osteoplastic approach, with removal of all the sinus mucosa followed by obliteration of the sinus cavity by use of abdominal fat.[73] A coronal incision may be placed in the scalp behind the hairline to hide the surgical scar in most patients (Fig. 15–32). Ethmoid mucoceles are usually approached through a medial incision with wide drainage of the sinus cavity into the nose (Fig. 15–33).

Developmental Cysts

Dermoids, epidermoids, teratomas, and meningoceles are among the most common cystic lesions that involve the orbit. Some lesions have noncystic components and may be completely solid. Most of these abnormalities are not neoplastic, but rather benign developmental lesions that are present in some form at the time of birth.[74, 75]

Most dermoids, epidermoids, and teratomas are thought to be developmental choristomas. Choristomas are growths that arise from tissue elements not usually found at the position in which the tumor is located. Meningoceles are cysts that consist of herniated meninges and cerebrospinal fluid. These intracranial tissues can project into the orbit through congenital dehiscences in the skull. If brain tissue is also found within the herniated meninges, the defect is termed an encephalocele.

Dermoids are benign and usually cystic. Most of these tumors are caused by developmental sequestrations of surface epidermis, often adjacent to bony suture lines. Some dermoids are solid subconjunctival tumors that often have a significant fatty component, in which case they are described as dermolipomas or lipodermoids.

Dermoids can be anatomically classified into three groups: (1) superficial subcutaneous dermoids, (2) subconjunctival dermoids, and (3) deep orbital dermoids. Superficial dermoids are usually discovered during childhood, when they appear as painless subcutaneous nodules most often found beneath the lateral brow. Subconjunctival dermoids or dermolipomas are usually located on the temporal surface of the globe

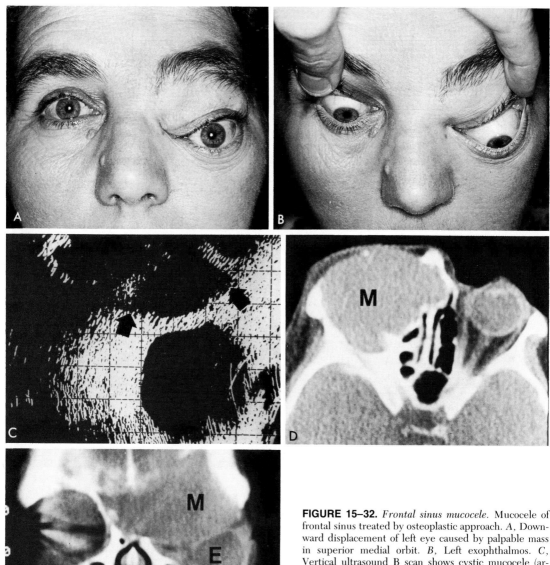

FIGURE 15–32. *Frontal sinus mucocele.* Mucocele of frontal sinus treated by osteoplastic approach. *A,* Downward displacement of left eye caused by palpable mass in superior medial orbit. *B,* Left exophthalmos. *C,* Vertical ultrasound B scan shows cystic mucocele (arrows) in superior orbit indenting left eye. *D,* CT scan shows mucocele (M) filling entire orbit above left eye. *E,* CT scan shows mucocele (M) displacing left eye (E) downward.

and may extend into the posterior orbit. In adults deep orbital dermoids are often found after a long period of slow growth. These tumors frequently displace the eye and cause exophthalmos.

Histologically, dermoids are composed of epidermal tissue together with one or more dermal adnexal structures and skin appendages such as hair follicles, sebaceous glands, and sweat glands. The cystic component is lined by keratinizing epidermis and may be filled with keratin, hairs, and fatty material. If these contents are released into the orbit either spontaneously or during surgery, an inflammatory reaction may result.

Orbital x-rays are usually normal in patients with superficial subcutaneous dermoids and subconjunctival dermoids or dermolipomas. However, deep orbital dermoids often displace the orbital walls or cause sharply marginated

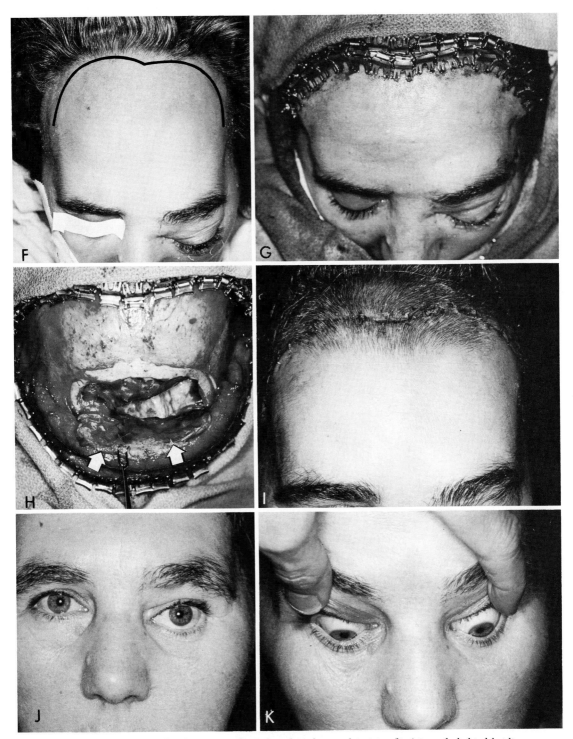

FIGURE 15–32 *Continued F,* Anterior scalp is shaved, and coronal incision (line) is made behind hairline. *G,* Hemostatic clips are used to control bleeding. *H,* Osteoplastic flap (arrows) is turned inferiorly to expose mucocele. Sinus mucosa is then removed, and mucocele cavity is obliterated with abdominal fat. *I,* Postoperatively, incision is hidden by scalp hair. *J,* Six months after operation left eye has almost returned to normal position. *K,* No exophthalmos is present.

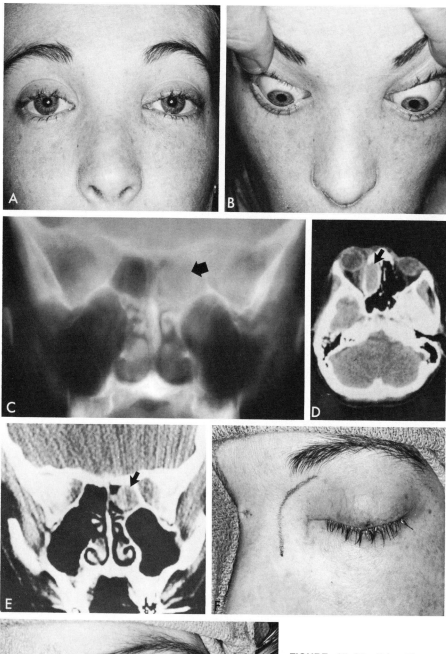

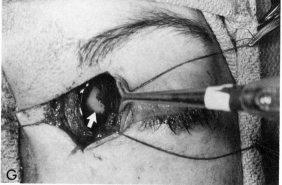

FIGURE 15–33. *Ethmoid sinus mucocele.* Mucocele of ethmoid sinus treated by medial orbital approach. *A,* Swelling and tenderness near left medial canthus. *B,* Minimal left exophthalmos. *C,* Polytome shows opacification of left ethmoid sinus (arrow). *D,* CT scan shows density in left ethmoid sinus (arrow). Medial wall of orbit is displaced toward left eye, but bone is not destroyed. *E,* CT scan shows similar sinus density (arrow). *F,* Curved incision (line) is made along lateral surface of nose. *G,* Pus and mucus (arrow) are visible within left ethmoid sinus.

defects in the orbital bones adjacent to the lesion. Ultrasonography and CT scans usually demonstrate a cyst, and sometimes an adjacent solid component can be seen as well (Fig. 15–34).

Superficial subcutaneous dermoids can usually be removed through a skin incision directly over the lesion. The deep surface of the tumor is nearly always adherent to periosteum, from which it must be sharply divided. The diagnosis

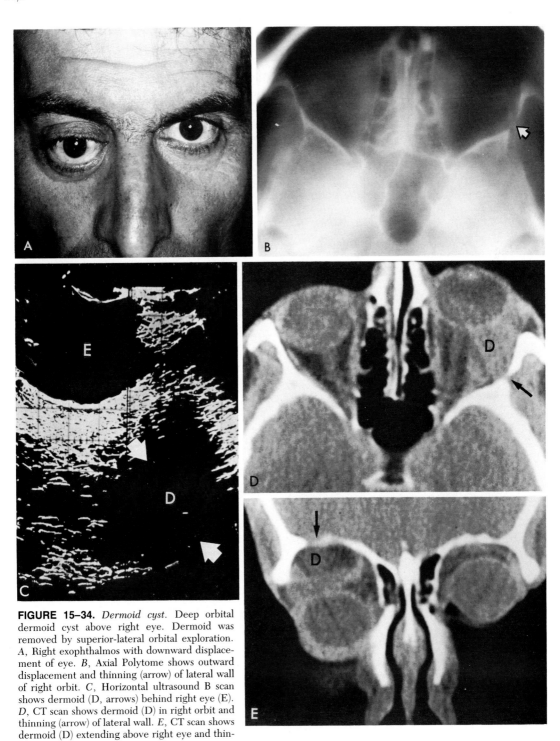

FIGURE 15–34. *Dermoid cyst.* Deep orbital dermoid cyst above right eye. Dermoid was removed by superior-lateral orbital exploration. *A,* Right exophthalmos with downward displacement of eye. *B,* Axial Polytome shows outward displacement and thinning (arrow) of lateral wall of right orbit. *C,* Horizontal ultrasound B scan shows dermoid (D, arrows) behind right eye (E). *D,* CT scan shows dermoid (D) in right orbit and thinning (arrow) of lateral wall. *E,* CT scan shows dermoid (D) extending above right eye and thinning (arrow) of orbital roof.

of these lesions can commonly be made from their clinical appearance, and excision may be delayed when the abnormality is discovered in young children (Fig. 15–35).

Subconjunctival dermoids or dermolipomas can also be recognized by their location and appearance in most instances. These lesions are usually located on the temporal surface of the globe and are commonly yellow or white (Fig. 15–36). Hairs may project from the surface of the tumor and irritate the eye. Solid epibulbar dermoids may occur in Goldenhar's syndrome, in association with eyelid colobomas and auricular appendages (Fig. 15–37).[76] Subconjunctival dermoids may have deep orbital extensions that lie near the levator and extraocular muscles. Excision of these tumors may be complicated by damage to the eye, by restricted eye movement, and by ptosis.[77] Because of the potential for complications, excision of subconjunctival dermoids or dermolipomas should usually be avoided if possible. If excision is necessary because of enlargement, cosmetic deformity, or irritation, then surgery should be performed with great care.

Removal of deep orbital dermoids usually requires a lateral orbital incision with removal of the lateral orbital rim. If the lesion is located in the upper orbit, a superior-lateral approach similar to that described for removal of lacrimal gland tumors may be used. Deep dermoid cysts located in the lower orbit may be removed by using an inferior-lateral approach (Fig. 15–38). Excision is made easier if the cyst is preliminarily decompressed by careful removal of the contents before dissection of the cyst wall.[75] Some deep orbital dermoids extend through the orbital bones and involve the intracranial space, in which case they should usually be removed through a neurosurgical approach.

Epidermoids are benign cystic choristomas that differ from dermoids in that they are composed only of epidermal tissues without adnexal structures or skin appendages. The cyst may be filled with cholesterol crystals and epithelial debris such as keratin. X-rays frequently show bony defects with sharp margins similar to those produced by deep dermoid cysts. Treatment consists of incision and aspiration of the cyst contents followed by removal of the cyst wall.

Teratomas are rare tumors that arise from multiple germinal layers and usually include tissues of ectodermal, endodermal, and mesodermal origin. Although orbital teratomas have

Text continued on page 483

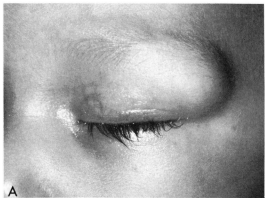

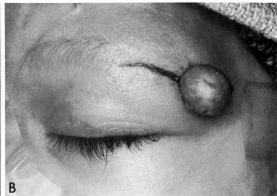

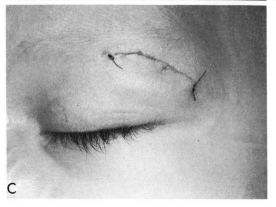

FIGURE 15–35. *Dermoid cyst.* Subcutaneous dermoid cyst beneath left brow. *A,* Palpable mass attached to lateral rim of left orbit. *B,* Dermoid is removed through skin incision, which is beveled parallel to brow hairs. *C,* Incision is closed with subcuticular suture.

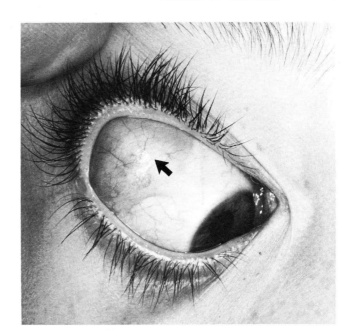

FIGURE 15–36. *Dermolipoma.* Subconjunctival dermolipoma (arrow) presents as white nodule on temporal surface of right eye.

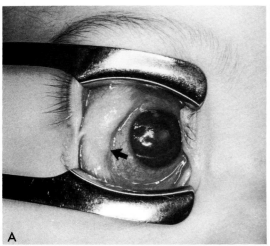

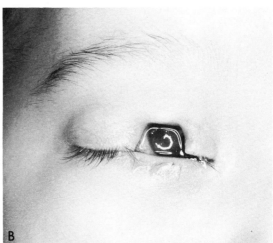

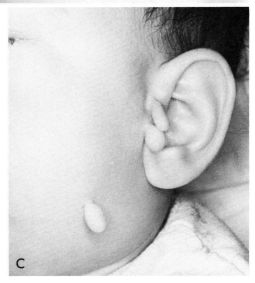

FIGURE 15–37. *Goldenhar's syndrome.* Multiple congenital deformities in young child. *A*, Epibulbar dermoid (arrow) on lateral surface of right eye. *B*, Coloboma of right upper eyelid. *C*, Preauricular skin appendages.

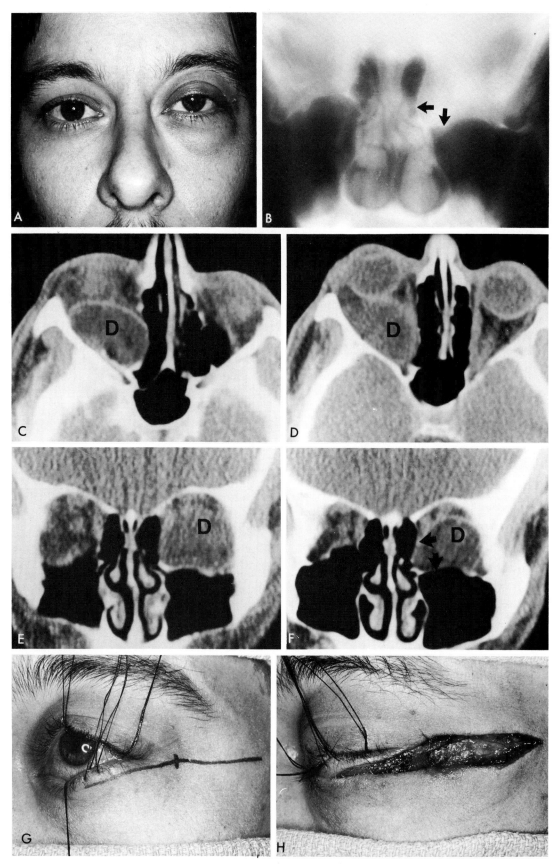

FIGURE 15–38 *See legend on opposite page*

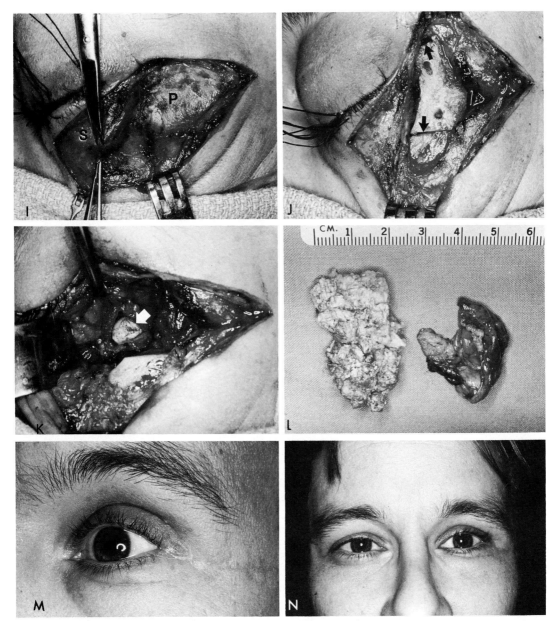

FIGURE 15–38. *Dermoid cyst.* Deep orbital dermoid cyst below left eye, treated by inferior-lateral orbital exploration. *A,* Left exophthalmos with swelling of lower eyelid and upward displacement of eye. *B,* Coronal Polytome shows smooth displacement (arrows) of medial wall and floor of left orbit. *C,* CT scan through lower orbits shows dermoid (D) with smooth surface. *D,* CT scan through middle orbits shows dermoid (D) behind left eye. *E,* CT scan through orbits behind globes shows dermoid (D) filling most of lower left orbit. *F,* CT scan near apex of orbits shows dermoid (D) displacing left orbital floor and medial wall (arrows). *G,* Skin incision (line) is made several millimeters below the eyelashes of lower lid and extends temporally to the lateral canthus and parallel to the zygomatic arch. A short perpendicular scratch incision is made to aid reapproximation of skin margins. Sutures are placed beneath insertions of inferior rectus, lateral rectus, and superior rectus muscles and through the lower eyelid, to aid in identification and retraction during orbital exploration. *H,* Skin and subcutaneous tissues are incised. *I,* Skin is retracted downward, and orbicularis muscle is grasped by forceps and dissected from underlying orbital septum (S). Periosteum (P) covering lateral orbital rim is exposed. *J,* Lateral orbital rim is cut (arrows) with oscillating saw, and holes are drilled to allow passage of wires for bone fixation after removal of dermoid. *K,* Dermoid cyst is opened with great care to avoid spilling irritating contents (arrow) into orbit. *L,* Dermoid contents (left) and cyst wall (right) after removal from orbit. *M,* Four months after operation skin incision is well healed. *N,* Postoperatively, eyes are in almost symmetrical positions.

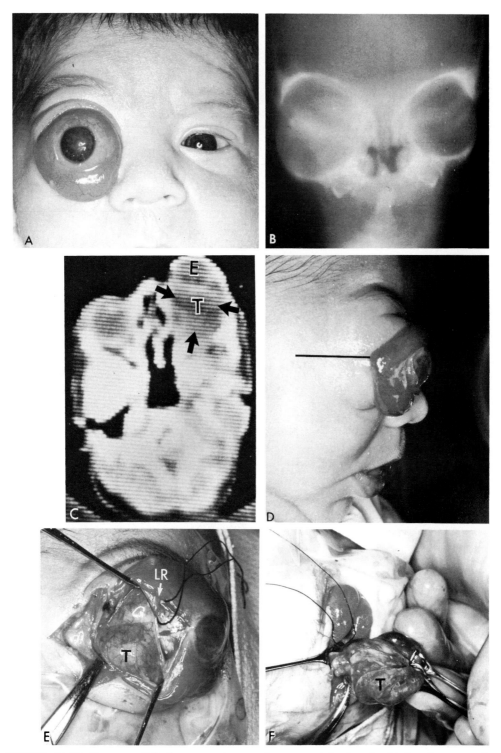

FIGURE 15–39. *Teratoma.* Orbital teratoma in a newborn treated by lateral orbital exploration with preservation of eye. *A,* Right exophthalmos present at birth. *B,* Coronal Polytome shows enlarged right orbit and calcifications within teratoma. *C,* CT scan shows large cystic teratoma (T, arrows) behind right eye (E). *D,* Skin incision (line) extends from lateral canthus toward ear, parallel to zygomatic arch. *E,* Skin, subcutaneous tissues, conjunctiva, and lateral rectus muscle (LR) are retracted to expose teratoma (T). *F,* Cyst is decompressed by aspirating contents. Teratoma (T) is then dissected from behind eye and removed from orbit.

been found in adults, most of these tumors are present at the time of birth and are the most common cause of dramatic exophthalmos in newborn infants. These tumors may be primarily solid, but a cystic component is almost always present.

Histologically, teratomas may contain diverse tissues such as enteric mucosa, respiratory epithelium, central nervous system elements, cartilage, and bone. The presence of relatively immature tissues does not necessarily indicate malignancy, especially if the teratoma occurs in a young infant.

Orbital x-rays often visualize an enlarged orbit and may demonstrate calcifications if cartilage or bone is present in the tumor. Ultrasonography and CT scans demonstrate multiple internal densities and commonly show cystic areas (Fig. 15–39).

Treatment of teratomas should be directed

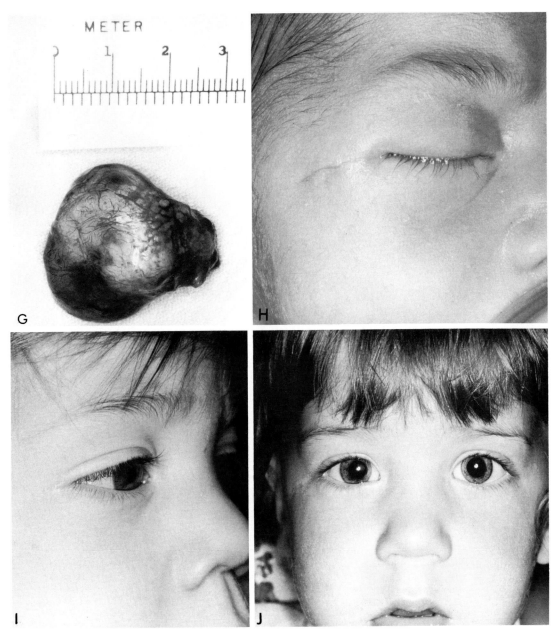

FIGURE 15–39 *Continued G,* Teratoma after removal from orbit. *H,* One month after operation. *I,* Two years after operation. *J,* Two years after operation eyes are in symmetrical positions.

toward removal of the tumor for careful histological examination. Although exenteration is sometimes performed because of fear of malignancy, many teratomas are benign, and in some instances these tumors can be carefully removed with preservation of the eye (Fig. 15–39).

Meningoceles are cysts that extend into the orbit from the adjacent intracranial space. These cysts are lined by meningeal tissues and may contain only cerebrospinal fluid or they may contain brain as well, in which case they are encephaloceles. The most common orbital me-

ningoceles are associated with neurofibromatosis (von Recklinghausen's disease), which is discussed under Neurogenic Tumors. In neurofibromatosis the posterior sphenoid and other orbital bones may become dysplastic and produce pulsating exophthalmos (Fig. 15–40). Less commonly meningoceles and encephaloceles may cause a swollen mass in the superior-medial quadrant of the anterior orbit. Although such anterior meningoceles usually produce a mass that lies on one side of the nose, the swollen area may cross the bridge of the nose and involve the glabella. Intracranial vascular pul-

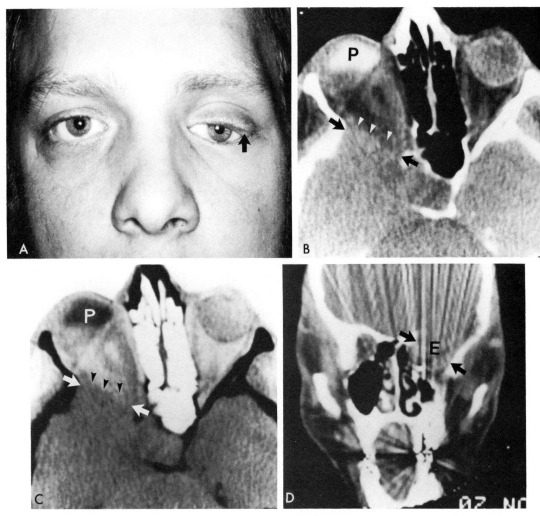

FIGURE 15–40. *Neurofibromatosis* (von Recklinghausen's disease). Eyelid neurofibroma and sphenoid dysplasia. Left eye was enucleated because of retinal detachment and glaucoma. *A,* Left upper eyelid is thickened (arrow) and ptotic because of neurofibroma. *B,* CT scan shows prosthesis (P) replacing enucleated left eye. Greater wing of left sphenoid is dysplastic and partially absent (large arrows). Encephalocele (small arrowheads) results from anterior herniation of left temporal lobe and causes orbital pulsations. *C,* Same CT scan displayed by image reversal, which shows sphenoid dysplasia (large arrows) and encephalocele (small arrowheads). *D,* CT scan shows sphenoid dysplasia (arrows) and encephalocele (E). Radiating lines are scan artifacts caused by dental fillings.

sations may be transmitted to the cyst, and crying may cause intermittent enlargement.

Orbital x-rays usually demonstrate a dehiscence in the orbital walls, but such defects may not be apparent unless tomographic x-ray techniques are used. CT scans usually demonstrate both the cyst and the bony abnormalities. Because meningoceles are often located at the orbital apex, ultrasonography is somewhat less useful for the evaluation of these lesions than for many other orbital cysts. The possibility that a meningocele may be present should always be considered in the evaluation of any child with an orbital cyst, particularly if the lesion pulsates or intermittently changes in size.

Treatment of posterior orbital meningoceles is usually not necessary unless they produce severe disfiguring exophthalmos. Anterior meningoceles should be treated with a neurosurgical approach, so that the base of the cyst and the bony defect can be covered with a graft of fascia or other suitable material.

Infections

Bacterial infection that leads to orbital cellulitis is the most common cause of exophthalmos in young children, but is somewhat less frequent in adults. Cellulitis is usually the result of an infection that spreads from the nasopharynx or the paranasal sinuses. In children most orbital infections extend through the lamina papyracea from the ethmoid sinus. Cellulitis may occasionally result from a hordeolum, from dacryocystitis, or from hematogenous dissemination. Clinical features of orbital cellulitis include fever, pain, exophthalmos, lid edema, and restricted eye movements.

Cavernous sinus thrombosis may result from orbital cellulitis. This life-threatening complication often produces rapidly progressive exophthalmos, ophthalmoplegia with pupillary abnormalities, and diffuse neurological disorders. Meningitis may develop, in which case the cerebrospinal fluid obtained by lumbar puncture often contains acute inflammatory cells and organisms that may grow in culture.

Most orbital cellulitis in adults is caused by *Staphylococcus aureus* or *Streptococcus*. When cellulitis is suspected, cultures should be obtained from the nasopharynx and conjunctiva, after which initial treatment usually involves the systemic administration of a penicillinase-resistant drug such as methicillin. In young children *Haemophilus influenzae* is a common

cause of orbital cellulitis, and initial treatment with ampicillin should be considered.[78–80]

Orbital x-rays often show sinus opacification if the cellulitis is caused by sinus disease. Ultrasonography and CT scans may visualize either diffuse inflammatory changes or a focal abscess cavity if the infection is localized (Fig. 15–41).

Most patients with orbital cellulitis respond to medical therapy alone. Sometimes an infected sinus must be drained if a pyocele is present. It is rarely necessary to surgically explore an infected orbit unless an abscess cavity is present.[81]

Fungal infection of the orbit is usually caused by fungi of the genera *Rhyzopus* or *Mucor*, in which case the infection is termed mucormycosis. These fungi belong to the class Phycomycetes, which gives rise to the more general diagnosis of phycomycosis. Phycomycosis usually results from extension of the organisms from the nasal cavity or the sinuses. The fungi often invade blood vessels, with resultant thrombosis and intracranial extension. Almost all patients with phycomycosis are systemically debilitated, and many have metabolic acidosis. The majority of such patients have diabetes or have been treated with antimetabolites and steroids.

Orbital x-rays often show sinus opacification, while ultrasonography and CT scans may visualize inflammatory changes in the orbit. The diagnosis of phycomycosis is made by biopsy of the involved tissues and demonstration of nonseptate branching hyphae.

Treatment usually involves control of the underlying metabolic disorder, the administration of amphotericin B, and local surgical excision of the infected tissues, which are frequently necrotic.[82] Exenteration may be necessary if the infection involves tissues near the orbital apex, especially if vision has been destroyed.[7, 82, 83]

Rhabdomyosarcomas

Rhabdomyosarcomas are the most common malignant tumors of the orbit in children. More than three-quarters of these tumors are found in patients under 15 years of age. On rare occasions rhabdomyosarcomas have been found in newborn infants, and sometimes they arise in adults. The most common clinical manifestation of these tumors is exophthalmos that becomes rapidly progressive over several days or weeks. Although any portion of the orbit can be involved, many of these tumors arise above

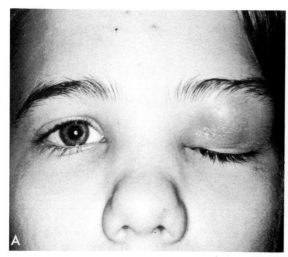

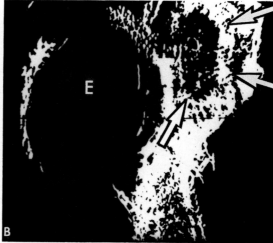

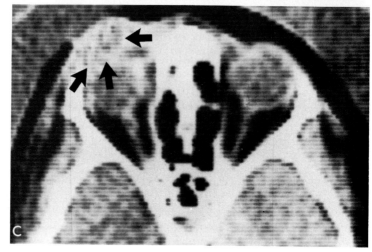

FIGURE 15–41. *Abscess.* Bacterial infection causing abscess of anterior orbit and eyelid. Abscess was treated by drainage and systemic antibiotics. *A,* Ptosis and swelling caused by mass beneath left upper eyelid. *B,* Vertical ultrasound B scan shows abscess (arrows) beneath left upper eyelid in front of eye (E). *C,* CT scan shows abscess (arrows) within left anterior orbit and upper eyelid.

or medial to the globe. Sometimes a palpable nodule appears beneath the eyelids or conjunctiva. Pain is usually not an early symptom, and bone involvement is variable.

Histologically, rhabdomyosarcomas are composed of malignant mesenchymal cells that frequently resemble immature striated muscle. They have been traditionally classified according to the degree of cellular differentiation and histologic pattern into three types: (1) embryonal, (2) pleomorphic, and (3) alveolar. Embryonal rhabdomyosarcoma is the most common type in children. Poorly differentiated cells called rhabdomyoblasts are arranged in a loose syncytial pattern. Mitoses are frequent, and intracytoplasmic cross striations may be found in some of the cells. A variety of the embryonal type of tumor is called botyroid rhabdomyosarcoma, which grows in grapelike clusters beneath the conjunctival mucosa. Pleomorphic rhabdomyosarcoma is a relatively well differ-

entiated type of tumor frequently found in older patients. Cells are arranged in a disorganized pattern, but may contain multiple nuclei in the form of straps. Cross striations are found easily in most of these tumors. Alveolar rhabdomyosarcoma is found in both children and adults. Cells are poorly differentiated and are arranged in a distinctive alveolar pattern, with connective tissue trabeculae. Tumor cells line the surfaces of the alveolar spaces and float freely with the cavities. Among these three types of tumors, alveolar rhabdomyosarcomas have the worst prognosis, and pleomorphic rhabdomyosarcomas seem to have the best prognosis.[84]

Orbital x-rays may be normal when rhabdomyosarcomas are confined to the soft tissues. When bone destruction is present in a child with rapidly evolving exophthalmos, a rhabdomyosarcoma is frequently present. Sometimes tomographic x-rays detect focal areas of bone destruction that are not seen in other diagnostic studies. Ultrasonography and CT scans may demonstrate either a solid tumor with well-circumscribed margins, or an infiltrative lesion that extends irregularly into adjacent tissues (Fig. 15–42).

The preauricular and cervical lymph nodes should be palpated to locate regional metastases. Chest x-rays may demonstrate more distant metastases. The diagnosis of rhabdomyosarcoma is established by biopsy, which should

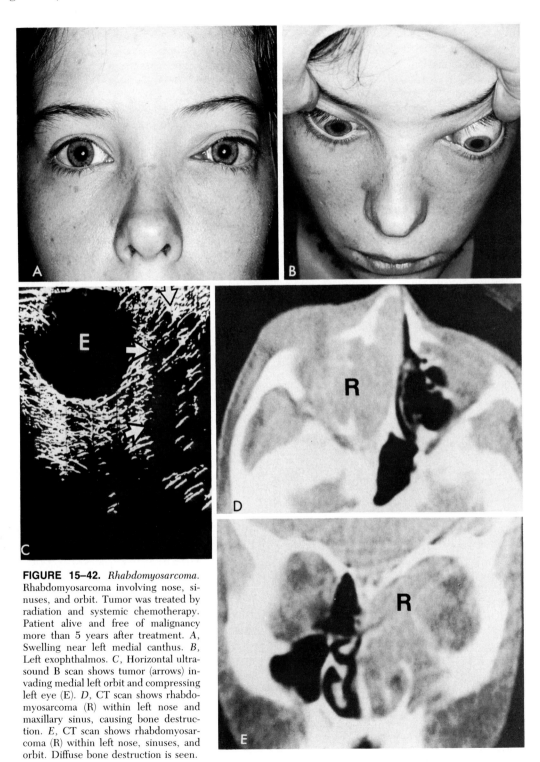

FIGURE 15–42. *Rhabdomyosarcoma.* Rhabdomyosarcoma involving nose, sinuses, and orbit. Tumor was treated by radiation and systemic chemotherapy. Patient alive and free of malignancy more than 5 years after treatment. *A,* Swelling near left medial canthus. *B,* Left exophthalmos. *C,* Horizontal ultrasound B scan shows tumor (arrows) invading medial left orbit and compressing left eye (E). *D,* CT scan shows rhabdomyosarcoma (R) within left nose and maxillary sinus, causing bone destruction. *E,* CT scan shows rhabdomyosarcoma (R) within left nose, sinuses, and orbit. Diffuse bone destruction is seen.

be performed expeditiously when this tumor is clinically suspected. If the lesion is located in the anterior orbit, an anterior approach through the conjunctiva or eyelid is appropriate. When a retrobulbar tumor is present, it is usually necessary to utilize a lateral orbital approach. Surgery should be performed with minimal trauma, and the tumor should not be excessively manipulated, in order to minimize the chance of dissemination.

In addition to routine histological examination of the tumor, a specimen should be submitted for electron microscopy, preferably after fixation in glutaraldehyde. Some poorly differentiated rhabdomyosarcomas may not be diagnosed by light microscopy, and characteristic cross striations may be found only by electron microscopy. In children, rhabdomyosarcomas may be confused with a number of rare, poorly differentiated neoplasms such as neuroblastomas, lymphomas, and soft tissue sarcomas. Electron microscopy and selective histological staining may help to distinguish among these tumors.[25-27]

The treatment of orbital rhabdomyosarcomas usually consists of local radiation therapy, with the total dose reaching 5000 to 6000 rad. If the tumor extends beyond the orbit, the sinuses and neck may also be treated with radiation. Systemic chemotherapy with a combination of cyclophosphamide, vincristine, and dactinomycin is usually given as an adjunct to radiation treatment.[75] Orbital exenteration, which in the past was the preferred treatment of these tu-

mors, is rarely indicated. The survival rate when radiation therapy is combined with systemic chemotherapy is greater than 70 per cent, as compared with less than 50 per cent with exenteration. Some patients can be cured of rhabdomyosarcoma even when the bones and sinuses are involved, and when cervical metastases are present. High-dose local radiation therapy may cause ocular damage, including keratopathy and cataract formation, as well as atrophy and hypoplasia of the orbital tissues (Fig. 15–43).

Neurogenic Tumors

A variety of orbital tumors arise from tissues that are intimately associated with the central and peripheral nervous systems. Most of these tumors originate from the meninges, from Schwann cells, or from glial astrocytes.

Meningiomas grow from arachnoidal cells, which usually form tissues covering the central nervous system. Although most meningiomas arise intracranially, some originate as primary tumors within the orbit. Features and management of these fibro-osseous tumors have been discussed separately.

Schwannomas, granular cell tumors, and neurofibromas are among the lesions that arise from Schwann cells.[48, 86, 87] Plexiform neurofibromas, which are usually associated with the neurofibromatosis syndrome (von Recklinghausen's

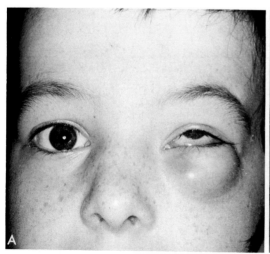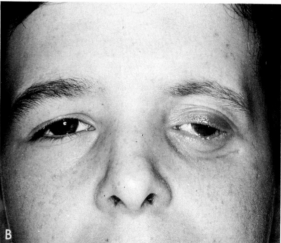

FIGURE 15–43. *Rhabdomyosarcoma.* Rhabdomyosarcoma within left orbit treated by radiation and systemic chemotherapy. *A,* Upward displacement of left eye caused by rhabdomyosarcoma within anterior orbit. *B,* Six years after treatment by radiation and systemic chemotherapy, left eye is still present, but lids and orbital tissues are atrophic. Patient shows no evidence of malignancy.

disease), are the most common of these tumors found in the orbit. Schwann cells help to insulate and support peripheral nerves. These cells originate from neuroectoderm and envelope peripheral nerve axons. The myelin sheath of peripheral nerves is a lipid product of Schwann cells. Schwann cells are in turn surrounded by extracellular basement membranes.

Optic nerve gliomas arise from glial astrocytes that normally help to support tissues within the optic nerves. The most common form of optic nerve glioma usually occurs in children. These juvenile gliomas are often found in patients with the neurofibromatosis syndrome, in whom plexiform neurofibromas may also occur.[14, 86]

Schwannomas are usually benign and encapsulated, originating as solitary lesions within the orbit. In these tumors, sometimes described as neurilemmomas, the Schwann cells often proliferate in an orderly palisading arrangement known as the Antoni A pattern. Alternatively, the Schwann cells may lie in a haphazard distribution within a myxomatous matrix, described as the Antoni B pattern. Although the Antoni B pattern is more commonly found in neurofibromas, schwannomas may contain either or both of these arrangements of Schwann cells.[48]

Ultrasonography and CT scans usually reveal a solid, well-circumscribed tumor. Although encapsulated schwannomas can usually be completely removed, they may recur if excision is incomplete. Truly malignant schwannomas may extend intracranially and may metastasize, but fortunately such tumors are quite uncommon.

Granular cell tumors have been described as myoblastomas because they were originally believed to arise from striated muscle. Histologically, granular cell tumors are composed of large cells with prominent nuclei and a granular cytoplasm. The granules within the cytoplasm stain with periodic acid–Schiff (PAS), a reaction that is unaffected by diastase. Electron microscopy has demonstrated morphological similarities between granular cells and Schwann cells, including cytoplasmic features and basement membrane configurations. Granular cell tumors are uncommon in the orbit, and may be either malignant or benign. The malignant lesions may be lethal and may metastasize, whereas benign tumors can usually be completely excised and will not recur.[48, 87]

Neurofibromas are benign, slow-growing tumors that are not encapsulated. Although neurofibromas are sometimes circumscribed, they often infiltrate diffusely within normal tissues of the orbit and eyelids. Some neurofibromas occur as solitary lesions, especially within the skin. However, the majority of neurofibromas within the orbit are diffuse lesions known as plexiform neurofibromas.

Plexiform neurofibromas seem to occur only as part of the neurofibromatosis syndrome. They typically grow within the superior-temporal orbit, where they often thicken the lateral portion of the upper lid and cause ptosis (Figs. 15–40 and 15–44). Plexiform neurofibromas are more extensive than solitary tumors, and usually are heavily vascularized. Sometimes the subcutaneous cordlike growth of these lesions feels like a bag of worms.

Histologically, neurofibromas contain proliferating nerve axons as well as Schwann cells and have a myxomatous matrix with abundant mucopolysaccharides that stain with alcian blue. The Schwann cells are commonly distributed in a haphazard arrangement (Antoni B pattern).[48]

Neurofibromatosis (von Recklinghausen's disease) is a syndrome that is usually inherited as an autosomal dominant trait with irregular penetrance. Neurofibromatosis is considered to be a phakomatosis or neurocutaneous syndrome. A phakomatosis is a syndrome in which hamartomas involve the central nervous system and skin, as well as the viscera and eye on occasion. In addition to the presence of plexiform neurofibromas, von Recklinghausen's disease is commonly typified by flat brown pigmented skin lesions known as café au lait spots (with smooth margins shaped like the coast of California). Other variable features of the syndrome include fibromata molluscum (pedunculated skin nodules), congenital glaucoma, pigmented iris nodules, bone abnormalities, including dysplasia of the sphenoid, and central nervous system tumors such as optic nerve gliomas.

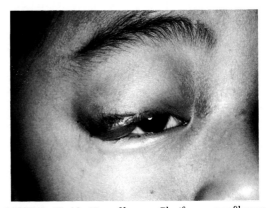

FIGURE 15–44. *Neurofibroma.* Plexiform neurofibroma causes ptosis and thickening of lateral upper eyelid with conjunctival prolapse.

Developmental defects in the orbital bones can allow dynamic exophthalmos to be caused by transfer of intracranial vascular pulsations.[48, 86] When a patient has a mild form of the syndrome with only one classic abnormality, such as a plexiform neurofibroma or sphenoid dysplasia, the condition is known as a *forme fruste.*

Orbital x-rays of patients with plexiform neurofibromas often show bony abnormalities of the orbital walls. The optic canal may be abnormal in size or shape as a result of sphenoid dysplasia or from growth of an associated optic nerve glioma. Ultrasonography may show distortion of the posterior orbital contour, while CT scans can reveal bone defects together with herniated meninges or brain tissue within the orbit (meningocele or encephalocele) (see Fig. 15–40).

Surgical treatment of patients with orbital neurofibromas is usually limited to correction of eyelid abnormalities. When the upper eyelid is elongated, a full-thickness horizontal resection of the most involved lid segment may produce cosmetic improvement. Ptosis repair is often difficult, since the levator may be infiltrated by the neurofibroma. It may be necessary to perform a frontalis suspension in order to elevate the lid. In most patients it is not possible, by any surgical procedure, to produce lids that appear completely normal. A neurosurgical approach is seldom required, since it is rarely necessary to cover defects in the posterior orbital walls.

Optic nerve gliomas are tumors that originate from astrocytes within the optic nerve. Three-quarters of these lesions are present during the first decade of life, and most are found between 2 and 6 years of age. Approximately one-quarter to one-half of all patients with optic nerve gliomas have neurofibromatosis. Therefore, the findings of multiple café au lait spots or other stigmata of von Recklinghausen's disease in a child with exophthalmos and optic nerve abnormalities suggest that an optic nerve glioma is present.[14, 86]

Decreased vision is the most common initial sign of an optic nerve glioma, and an afferent pupillary defect (Marcus Gunn sign) is often present. Exophthalmos and optic disc abnormalities such as edema and atrophy are frequently seen as early findings (Fig. 15–45).

The great majority of optic nerve gliomas, which occur primarily in children and young adults, are described as juvenile gliomas. The enlargement of these tumors occurs at irregular intervals, and in some cases growth may cease or become clinically inapparent. This unusual pattern of limited growth has led to a dispute over whether juvenile gliomas should be considered hamartomas or true neoplasms. Even though some juvenile gliomas do cease growing, others have enlarged and have extended intracranially to the optic chiasm.

A small minority of optic nerve gliomas, most of which occur in adults, are highly invasive tumors known as malignant gliomas. These lesions grow rapidly and may be multicentric. They are usually lethal and are considered malignant neoplasms.[88]

Histologically, a juvenile glioma is usually composed of well-differentiated fibrillary astrocytes, which leads to its classification as a grade I astrocytoma. Because the astrocytes are often hair-shaped, they are sometimes referred to as juvenile pilocytic astrocytomas. In addition to proliferating astrocytes, the enlarged optic nerve may contain cystic, myxomatous areas. Gliomas that arise in patients who have neurofibromatosis usually grow on the outer surface of the optic nerve in a circumferential-perineural pattern.[89] The meninges over an optic nerve glioma often thicken as a result of a reactive arachnoid hyperplasia. This hyperplasia may resemble a meningioma of the optic nerve sheath both clinically and histologically.[14] Therefore, a biopsy of an optic nerve tumor should usually include both meninges and tissue from the nerve itself. A malignant glioma is usually composed of pleomorphic astrocytes with hyperchromatic nuclei and frequent mitotic figures. Such a poorly differentiated, rapidly growing neoplasm may be classified as a glioblastoma multiforme or grade IV astrocytoma.

Orbital x-rays frequently show enlargement of the involved optic foramen or optic canal. Although optic canal projections on plain films may reveal abnormalities, axial Polytomography is useful for detailed examination of the two canals simultaneously. Details of radiographic anatomy of the optic canals have been separately discussed. Ultrasonography and CT scans show the contours and sizes of the optic nerves, so that tumors can usually be easily localized (Fig. 15–45). On occasion enlarged extraocular muscles may mimic optic nerve enlargement. Three-dimensional computed tomography usually allows the muscles and nerve to be separately identified. Although CT scans usually provide adequate information about the intracranial anatomy of the optic nerves, pneumoencephalography is sometimes necessary to evaluate the area near the optic chiasm.

Treatment of juvenile optic nerve gliomas is

controversial, since these tumors are characterized sometimes as hamartomas and sometimes as invasive neoplasms. In nearly all patients with an optic nerve tumor, tissue should be obtained to establish a histological diagnosis.[90] Some young children with neurofibromatosis who have optic nerve enlargement, apparently good vision, and no evidence of intracranial tumor extension might be followed closely without surgery. In such patients repeated CT scans can be used to document any growth, and surgical exploration should be performed if vision is severely depressed or if tumor enlargement is significant.

Biopsy of optic nerve tumors frequently can be performed along the medial side of the globe after disinsertion of the medial rectus muscle. A lateral approach may be required to reach tumors near the orbital apex or to excise a significant segment of the optic nerve. As previously mentioned, optic nerve gliomas may stimulate a reactive arachnoid hyperplasia that can resemble a meningioma. For this reason a biopsy should usually include tissue that is clearly from the optic nerve as well as from the meninges.

When the tumor is confined to the orbit and vision is severely decreased, excision of the tumor is justified. If the glioma has invaded the globe, enucleation may be performed and sometimes the involved optic nerve can be excised anteriorly without bone removal (Fig. 15–45). If the glioma is retrobulbar, the eye may be left in place and the tumor may be excised by a lateral approach.

When the optic canal is enlarged and the tumor extends intracranially, many surgeons recommend a neurosurgical approach with excision of the intracranial tumor if the optic chiasm is not involved (Fig. 15–45). In some cases such a resection can be performed with preservation of the eye. Care should be taken to minimize trauma to the innervations of the levator and superior rectus muscles, so that upper lid function and eye movements can be preserved.[91]

Some authors have recommended that no surgery be performed on juvenile optic nerve gliomas, unless the eye is blind and exophthalmos is disfiguring, or unless intracranial pressure is elevated.[92] However, because many of these tumors grow progressively, it seems appropriate to remove most or all of the lesion if vision is severely decreased, or if intracranial extension is suspected. Radiation therapy may be considered if the tumor cannot be completely resected and if severe neurological symptoms progress because of intracranial growth.

ORBITAL TRAUMA

Evaluation

Orbital trauma can damage soft tissues, embed foreign bodies, and cause fractures. Soft tissue injuries may involve the eye as well as any other structures within the orbit. Foreign bodies may be extremely difficult to detect and localize, particularly if they are not radiopaque. Fractures of the orbit may be extensive and may involve the midfacial skeleton and the skull. Orbital injuries may be associated with damage to the brain, the paranasal sinuses, or the nasolacrimal pathways. CCS fistulas and cerebrospinal fluid (CSF) leaks may be associated with orbital trauma and with fractures that involve the base of the skull.[23]

An orderly sequence of diagnostic steps, including a careful history and physical examination, should be used to evaluate a patient who has sustained orbital trauma. Most of the basic principles of orbital examination and the diagnostic techniques available to study patients who suffer orbital trauma have been described under Orbital Disorders and Exophthalmos.

History and Physical Examination

In most cases ocular or orbital abnormalities occur shortly after the trauma that caused them. However, some traumatic abnormalities first appear long after the injury has occurred and been forgotten. Therefore, even in the absence of recent trauma, a patient with an orbital disorder should be questioned about past injuries that may have produced chronic abnormalities such as CCS fistulas and blood cysts. Foreign bodies may lie dormant for years before they cause an abscess or bony erosion. Fractures may produce an enophthalmos that mimics contralateral exophthalmos, and is known as pseudoexophthalmos.

A detailed ocular examination should include measurement of visual acuities and intraocular pressures. Anterior segment and fundus details should be evaluated. Neurological and orbital examinations should be performed to determine eye movements, pupil reactions, sensory abnormalities, and positions of the eyes. Photographs and sketches are useful to document clinical features for future reference.

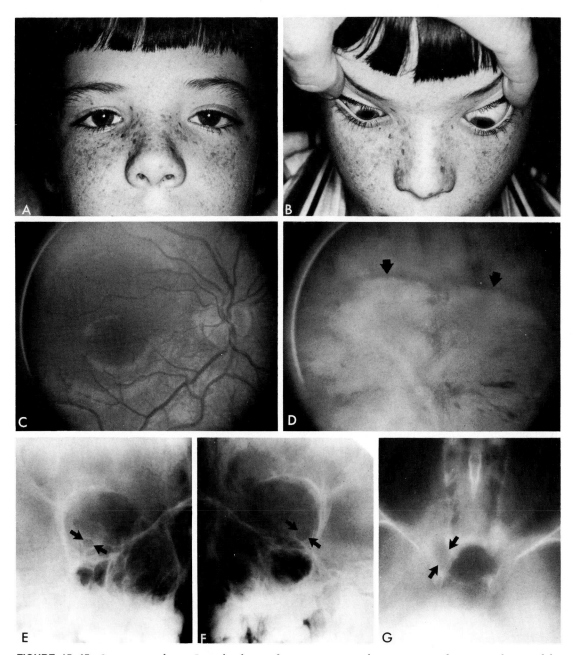

FIGURE 15–45. *Optic nerve glioma.* Juvenile glioma of optic nerve extending into eye and optic canal, treated by enucleation and intracranial resection. *A*, No vision in left eye, but eyes appear almost symmetrical. *B*, Left exophthalmos. *C*, Right optic disc and fundus are normal. *D*, Left optic disc is obliterated by elevated tumor (arrows). *E*, X-ray shows right optic foramen (arrows) is normal, 5.5 mm in diameter. *F*, X-ray shows left optic foramen (arrows) is enlarged, 8 mm in diameter. *G*, Axial Polytome shows enlarged left optic canal (arrows).

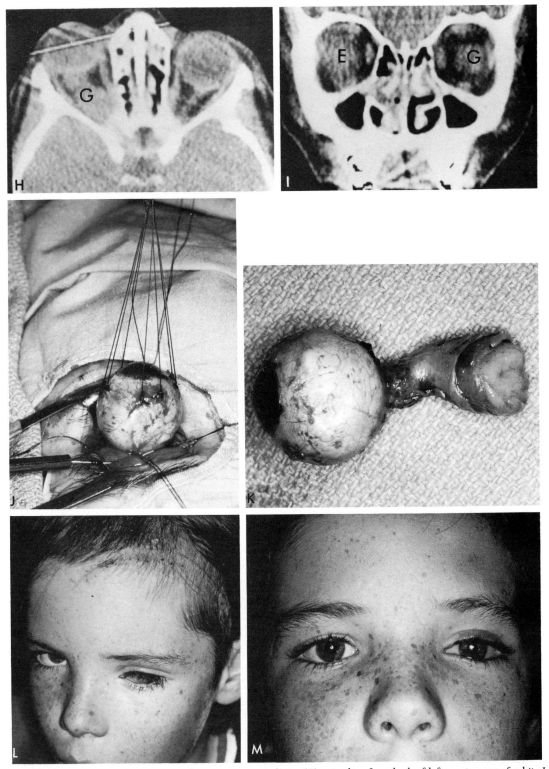

FIGURE 15–45 *Continued H,* CT scan shows optic nerve glioma (G) extending from back of left eye to apex of orbit. *I,* CT scan through anterior orbits shows normal right eye (E) and glioma (G) in left orbit. Scan does not show left eye, which has been pushed forward by tumor. *J,* Left eye is enucleated because of intraocular extension of tumor. *K,* Enucleated left eye and orbital segment of optic nerve glioma. *L,* Scalp incision is healing satisfactorily after resection of intracranial segment of optic nerve glioma. *M,* Three months after operation patient wears left ocular prosthesis.

Diagnostic Studies

The most valuable diagnostic studies for the evaluation of patients who have sustained orbital trauma are x-rays and computed tomography. Ultrasonography is useful for the evaluation of intraocular injuries, especially when direct visualization of the fundus is prevented by hemorrhage or lens opacity. However, ultrasonography is not as useful as radiographic studies or CT scans for the evaluation of extraocular trauma.[19, 20, 23] On occasion radionuclide scanning may provide useful information about the location of CSF leaks.[23]

Consequences of Orbital Trauma

Soft Tissue Injuries

Hemorrhage into the orbital soft tissues may cause exophthalmos and limited movements of the eyes and eyelids. In adults the posterior surface of the globe is usually less than 20 mm from the optic foramen, while the orbital segment of the optic nerve is approximately 25 mm long. Therefore, some exophthalmos may occur without damaging the optic nerve by stretching. Drainage or aspiration of an orbital hemorrhage is seldom necessary, unless visual function is compromised by compression of the optic nerve or the globe. Extravasated blood usually resorbs, although a chronic blood cyst may form and require surgical removal.

Optic neuropathy may result from direct injury (contusion of the nerve), from secondary vascular ischemia, or from damage caused by foreign bodies or bone fragments. Although spontaneous improvement of visual function may occur, treatment with systemic steroids, surgical decompression, or removal of impinging foreign bodies or bone might be considered in some cases.

Limited movement of the extraocular muscles or levator can be caused by either soft tissue injury to nerves or muscles alone, or by mechanical restriction associated with orbital fractures. It is important to distinguish between neuromuscular injury, which often improves spontaneously, and mechanical restriction associated with fractures, which may require surgical exploration. Fortunately many orbital fractures do not mechanically restrict eye movement or cause significant cosmetic facial deformity, and therefore do not require surgical intervention.

Many patients whose eye movements are limited in both horizontal and vertical gaze will have spontaneous improvement to at least some movement. Limitation of eye movements chiefly in upgaze and downgaze is more likely to be the result of mechanical restriction of movement of the inferior rectus muscle and possibly of the inferior oblique muscle. The forced traction test is useful to determine whether eye movements are mechanically restricted. Cocaine (4%) on a cotton pledget may be applied to the inferior surface of the globe and allowed to remain in place for several minutes. The insertion of the inferior rectus muscle is then firmly grasped, and the globe is

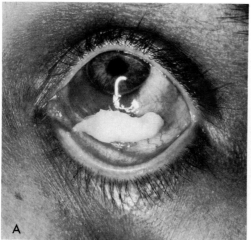 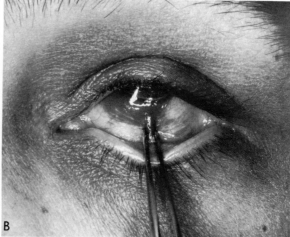

FIGURE 15–46. *Forced traction test.* Test is used to help determine whether vertical eye movements are mechanically restricted. *A,* Topical anesthesia is administered by application of a cotton pledget containing 4% cocaine. *B,* Insertion of inferior rectus muscle is grasped with heavy forceps, and eye is moved up and down.

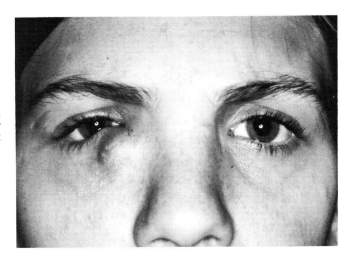

FIGURE 15–47. *Lacrimal sac mucocele.* Right lacrimal sac mucocele and dacryocystitis after medial orbital fracture with nasolacrimal duct obstruction.

passively moved up and down (Fig. 15–46). Restriction of such movements suggests that the muscle is mechanically bound by direct entrapment within a fracture, by connective tissue septa between a muscle and the fracture, or by secondary adhesions.

Decreased sensation in the distribution of the infraorbital nerve is common in patients who suffer fractures of the orbital floor. This numbness may involve the lower eyelid, the cheek, the palate, and the upper lip, but it usually improves spontaneously.

Nasolacrimal obstructions may result from fractures of the medial orbit or nose. Lacrimal sac mucoceles (Fig. 15–47), dacryocystitis, and epiphora can result from such obstructions and may require dacryocystorhinostomy to reestablish tear drainage into the nose. Medial orbital trauma may also disrupt attachments of the medial canthal tendon and cause displacement of the medial canthus and eyelids (Fig. 15–48).

Orbital emphysema and epistaxis are frequent sequelae of medial orbital fractures because of injury to the ethmoid sinus.

Frontal sinus mucoceles may result from fractures that involve the frontal bones, the orbital walls, and the nose. The frontal sinuses normally drain into the nasal cavities by the nasofrontal duct. If this duct is lacerated or obstructed so that it cannot be repaired, it may be necessary to obliterate the sinus with adipose tissue. Such an obliteration may be performed by an osteoplastic approach as recommended for the treatment of frontal sinus mucoceles.[73]

Sometimes CCS fistulas result from tears in the wall of the segment of the internal carotid artery, which lies within the cavernous sinus. These injuries are usually associated with basal skull fractures. A bruit is usually heard when such a fistula is present. Dilated, tortuous vessels are usually seen on the surface of the eye (Fig. 15–21). CT scans with contrast enhance-

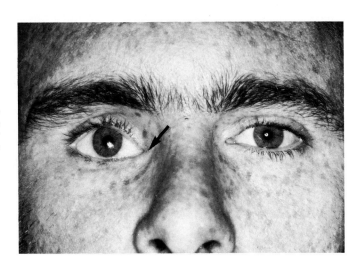

FIGURE 15–48. *Medial canthal displacement.* Right medial canthus and eyelids are displaced laterally and inferiorly (arrow) after medial orbital fracture with disruption of medial canthal tendon.

ment may visualize these vascular communications with minimal risk to the patient. Fine anatomical details of these vessels can be seen by using positive contrast arteriography with selective injections and radiographic subtraction.

Sometimes CSF leaks into the nose (rhinorrhea) occur after severe midfacial trauma. Such leaks should be suspected if the patient notes the drainage of clear fluid from the nose or frequently swallows when recumbent. Fluorescein dye may be injected by lumbar puncture to determine whether CSF is leaking into the nose. Radionuclides have also been injected by lumbar puncture so that radioactivity can be detected by nasal pledgets or followed by cisternography with use of photographic imaging.[23]

Orbital Foreign Bodies

The detection, localization, and removal of foreign bodies from the orbit is often extremely difficult. Although bone details are usually ad-

equately seen with conventional x-rays, these studies are of little value in the detailed study of soft tissues and low-density foreign bodies such as plastic, glass, or wood. Sometimes even radiopaque foreign bodies are difficult to accurately localize with x-rays unless mathematical computations or devices such as contact lenses are used.[23] By using x-rays alone it may be impossible to determine the position of foreign bodies with reference to the globe, the optic nerve, or the extraocular muscles.

CT scans visualize most soft tissue, bone details, and foreign bodies regardless of their density. Accurate foreign body localization by CT scanning can be most effectively achieved by use of narrow density windows and three-dimensional tomography with both axial and coronal scans (Figs. 15–49 and 15–50).

Clinically, it is important to maintain a high index of suspicion that a foreign body may be embedded within the orbit after a penetrating wound has occurred. Wooden objects may lac-

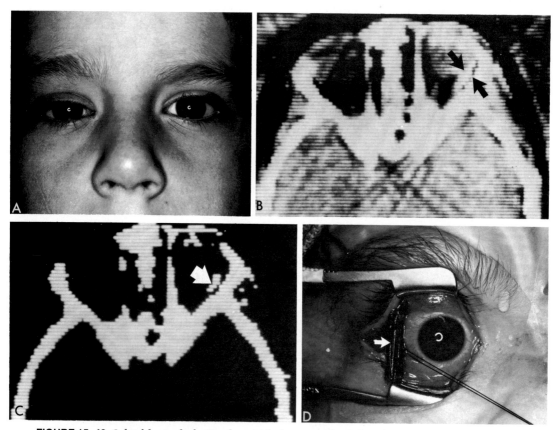

FIGURE 15–49. *Orbital foreign body.* Wooden stick had penetrated right lateral conjunctiva 1 year previously. *A,* Ptosis of right upper eyelid, x-rays normal. *B,* CT scan shows wooden foreign body (arrows) between right eye and lateral orbital wall. *C,* Same CT scan using narrow density window shows wooden foreign body (arrow) more clearly in same location. Soft tissues are eliminated by this technique. *D,* Wooden foreign body (arrow) removed from lateral right orbit in location shown by CT scans.

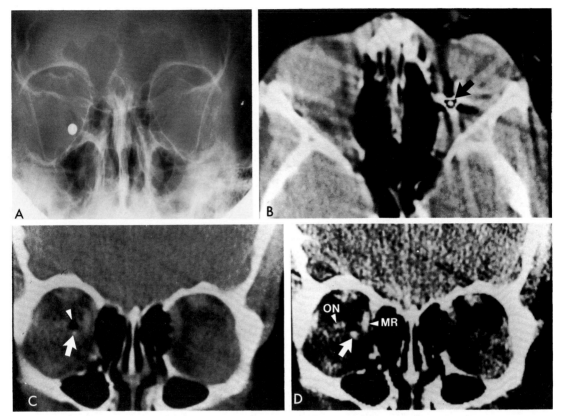

FIGURE 15–50. *Orbital foreign body.* Metallic pellet from air gun penetrated right medial conjunctiva without damage to eye. *A,* X-ray shows metallic foreign body in right orbit. Specific localization of foreign body in relation to eye and other soft tissues cannot be made by x-rays. *B,* CT scan shows metallic foreign body (arrow) behind right eye. Radiating lines are scan artifacts produced by metallic objects. *C,* CT scan through orbits behind globes shows metallic foreign body (large arrow) and air shadow (small arrowhead) that was not seen on x-rays. *D,* Same CT scan using narrow density window shows metallic foreign body (arrow) more clearly by eliminating many soft tissue details and air shadow. Foreign body lies between optic nerve (ON) and medial rectus muscle (MR).

erate the eyelid or the conjunctiva and appear to be completely withdrawn from the point of entry. However, portions of these objects may remain buried within the orbit and may be initially asymptomatic. Vegetable matter foreign bodies such as wood fragments may cause chronic abscesses that drain to the skin surface through a fistula. By surgically following such a fistula tract, these fragments may usually be reached and removed even from remote areas of the orbit (Fig. 15–51). The most likely position of an embedded foreign body may be predicted by reconstructing the direction of entry into the orbit and then approaching the orbital wall that lies opposite the original wound.

General principles of management when a foreign body has entered the orbit include culturing the wound or culturing the foreign body if it is removed, and administering systemic antibiotics. Foreign objects should usu-

ally be removed if they are composed of vegetable matter, if they are anterior in the orbit, or if they have sharp edges. Objects may sometimes be safely left in place if they are inert, if they are in the posterior orbit, or if they have relatively smooth surfaces.

Orbital Fractures

Most fractures of the middle segment of the face involve at least a portion of the orbit. These midfacial fractures may be classified into several categories: (1) LeFort fractures, (2) zygomatic fractures, (3) orbital apex fractures, (4) orbital roof fractures, (5) medial orbital fractures, and (6) orbital floor fractures. Some of the soft tissue injuries that may be associated with these fractures have already been discussed.

LeFort fractures involve the maxilla to varying degrees and are divided into three types. These fractures are frequently complex and

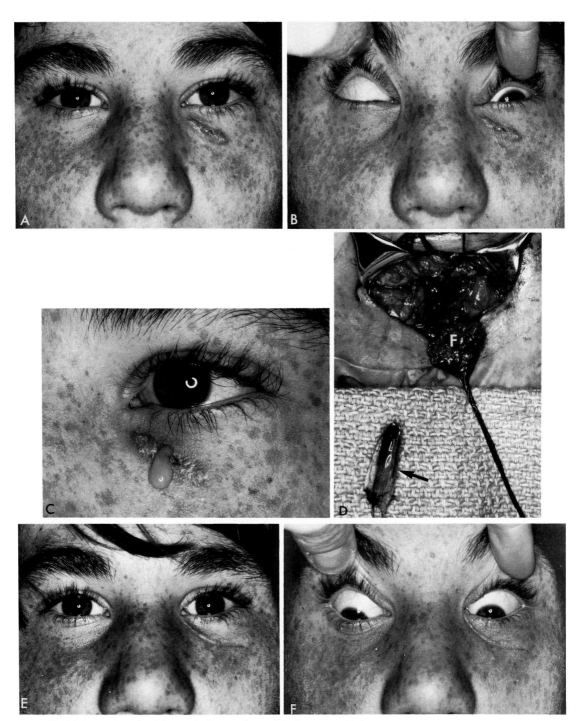

FIGURE 15–51. *Orbital foreign body.* Wooden stick had penetrated left lower eyelid several years previously. *A*, Left exophthalmos and elevated scar on lower eyelid. *B*, Limited downgaze of left eye. *C*, Pus flows from scar when pressure is applied to eye or eyelid. *D*, Large wooden foreign body (arrow) was removed from beneath optic nerve by surgically following fistula (F) posteriorly from scar. *E*, Postoperatively eyes are in symmetrical positions and eyelid scar is flattened. *F*, Eye movements have improved.

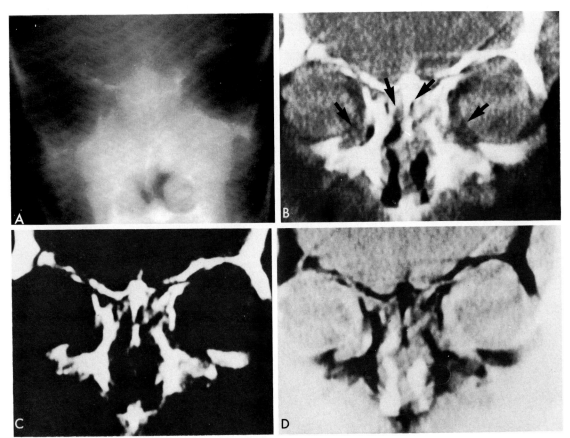

FIGURE 15–52. *Complex orbital fractures.* Fractures of skull and orbits caused by automobile accident. *A,* Polytome shows multiple fractures of skull and orbits, but many bone details are obscured. *B,* CT scan shows details of bilateral orbital roof fractures and of LeFort II fractures (arrows). *C,* Same CT scan using narrow density window shows bones and fractures more clearly by eliminating soft tissues. *D,* Same CT scan displayed by image reversal shows increased detail of fractures.

asymmetrical, with more damage on one side of the face than on the other. *LeFort I (Guerin)* fractures are low transverse maxillary fractures that do not involve the orbit. *LeFort II* fractures are pyramidal fractures that involve the maxilla, the nasal bones, and the medial orbital floors (Fig. 15–52). *LeFort III* fractures are complex fractures that extensively involve both orbits to produce separation of the maxilla from the skull (craniofacial dysjunction or free-floating maxilla). Treatment of these maxillary fractures may require reduction of displaced bone fragments with fixation and dental stabilization. Severe LeFort fractures are frequently associated with skull fractures and intracranial injuries that necessitate neurosurgical treatment.[93]

Zygomatic fractures involve the cheek bone (zygoma or malar bone), which forms a significant portion of the floor and lateral wall of the orbit. The zygoma is composed of an arch, which extends laterally over the temporalis muscle to articulate with the temporal bone, and a body, which forms the prominence of the cheek. Zygomatic fractures may involve the arch alone, without extension into the orbit. If a zygomatic fracture involves the body, sometimes it is termed a tripod fracture, since breaks almost always occur in three locations: the zygomatic arch, the lateral orbital rim, and the inferior orbital rim (Fig. 15–53). If the bones are not significantly depressed or rotated, no reduction or fixation may be required. Simple fractures that produce a cosmetic deformity or limit jaw motion may be treated by reduction without fixation. Some fractures require both reduction and open fixation by wires, suspension, or packing.[93] In some cases it may be appropriate to repair the orbital floor if the bones are severely comminuted. It is uncommon for extraocular muscle entrapment to occur with zygomatic fractures.

Orbital apex fractures usually occur in asso-

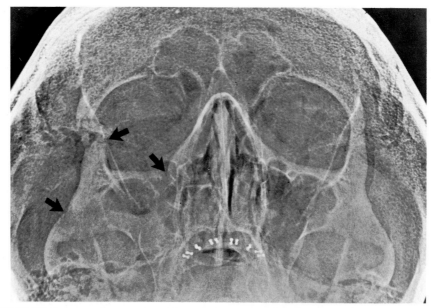

FIGURE 15–53. *Zygomatic fracture.* Xeroradiograph shows tripod fracture of right zygoma with bone defects (arrows) involving lateral orbital rim, inferior orbital rim, and zygomatic arch.

ciation with other fractures of the face, orbit, or skull. LeFort fractures may extend posteriorly to the orbital apex, and complex zygomatic fractures may extend medially through the sphenoid wings. Orbital apex fractures may encroach on the optic canal and the base of the skull, with damage to the optic nerves or production of CCS fistulas or CSF leaks. When visual acuity is decreased in patients with orbital fractures and with no significant intraocular injury, involvement of the orbital apex and optic canal should be suspected.

Orbital roof fractures may involve the frontal sinuses or the brain. Because frontal sinus mucoceles sometimes occur after severe injuries involving the nasofrontal duct, sinus obliteration may be recommended at the time of initial surgical repair.[73] Intracranial injuries and CSF leaks should be suspected when an orbital roof fracture is found. Limited eye movements and ptosis may result from injuries that involve the orbital roof, but surgical reduction of fractures over the posterior orbit is seldom required.

Medial orbital fractures are usually the result of direct trauma to the nose or the medial orbital rim. Such direct fractures may involve the frontal process of the maxilla, the ethmoid labyrinth (including the "paper plate" or lamina papyracea), and the lacrimal bone. Medial orbital direct fractures may damage the lacrimal sac or nasolacrimal duct, to cause epiphora or a lacrimal sac mucocele (Fig. 15–47). Cosmetic

deformity may be produced by damage to the nose or displacement of the medial canthus and eyelids (Fig. 15–48).

Indirect or blow-out fractures are those in which the orbital rims are intact and only the bony wall is fractured. The mechanism of most blow-out fractures is believed to be the hydraulic transmission of forces produced by a blow to the globe or eyelids.[94] Because the lamina papyracea is one of the thinnest surfaces of the orbit, this portion of the medial wall is frequently fractured by such injuries. In many patients medial orbital blow-out fractures produce few consequences and may be overlooked. Epistaxis and orbital emphysema may occur but are usually self-limited and do not require treatment except to caution the patient to avoid blowing the nose. Movement of the medial rectus muscle may be mechanically restricted by a medial orbital fracture and may require surgical exploration. Prolapse of orbital fat and other tissues into the ethmoid sinus may play a role in the production of enophthalmos in some patients.

Orbital floor fractures may also be either direct or indirect, depending on whether or not the orbital rims are fractured. Direct fractures of the floor are those that involve the inferior orbital rim. Because much of the inferior orbital rim is part of the zygoma, these injuries are usually classified as zygomatic fractures. Although the floor may have to be repaired in some severe zygomatic fractures, it is unusual for true entrapment of the extraocular muscles to occur with such injuries.

Indirect or blow-out fractures, as previously explained, are those in which the inferior orbital rim is intact and the bony injury usually results from hydraulically transmitted forces. In most instances the injury is due to a sudden increase of intraorbital pressure applied by a nonpenetrating object such as a fist or a ball.[93, 94]

Orbital x-rays usually demonstrate defects in the orbital bones, and tomographic x-rays may provide increased details of bone distortion (Fig. 15–54). Computed tomography is valuable because it demonstrates both orbital bones and soft tissues, including the extraocular muscles (Fig. 15–55).[19, 20]

Decreased sensation in the distribution of the infraorbital nerve is common in patients with blow-out fractures of the orbital floor, since the bones covering the infraorbital canal are very thin and subject to fragmentation. Orbital floor fractures may lead to displacement of the eye or mechanical restriction of eye movement. These two features are the most common indications for surgical repair of blow-out fractures of the orbital floor.

Displacement of the eye may take the form of enophthalmos (decreased prominence) or ptosis of the globe (drop of the eye toward the maxillary sinus). The mere presence of measurable enophthalmos is not always an indication for surgical repair. Significant enophthalmos or ptosis of the globe usually occurs only in patients with relatively large bony defects. It is common for blow-out fractures to involve both the floor and the medial wall of the orbit. The medial wall defect may be the cause of persistent enophthalmos even after the floor defect has been repaired. In some cases the presence of enophthalmos may be responsible for abnormal eye movements because of a shift of the plane of action through which the vertical rectus muscles move. Although it may be possible to arrest the progress of enophthalmos by covering the fracture defect with a plate such as a plastic prosthesis, it is often difficult to correct enophthalmos that has already occurred.[94] Surgical repair of an orbital floor fracture may be indicated when a significant cosmetic defect seems to be evolving because of progressive enophthalmos or ptosis of the globe.

Restriction of eye movements in patients with orbital floor fractures may be due to generalized orbital edema or hemorrhage, to neuromuscular injury, or to mechanical restriction of the vertical rectus muscles. In most cases any surgical repair should be delayed until significant orbital edema and hemorrhage have resolved. If eye movements are chiefly restricted in vertical fields of gaze, a forced traction test (Fig. 15–46) may confirm that the eye either is or is not mechanically restricted. Surgical repair may be indicated when the forced traction test is positive (when passive movements are restricted), when double vision is present in a functionally

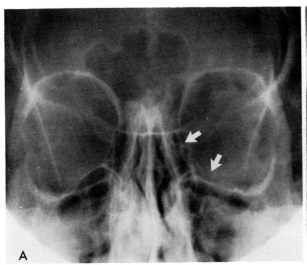
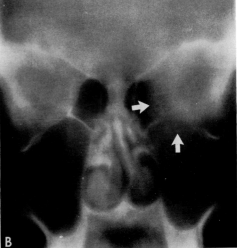

FIGURE 15–54. *Orbital floor fracture.* Indirect (blow-out) fracture of left orbital floor and medial wall. *A,* X-ray shows discontinuity (arrows) of floor and medial wall of left orbit. *B,* Polytome shows orbital soft tissues (arrows) herniating through bone defects into maxillary and ethmoid sinuses.

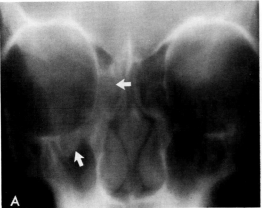
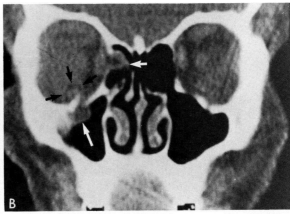
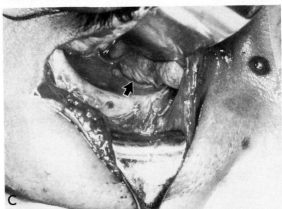

FIGURE 15–55. *Orbital floor fracture.* Indirect (blow-out) fracture of right orbital floor and medial wall. *A,* Polytome shows soft tissue densities (arrows) in right maxillary and ethmoid sinuses. *B,* CT scan through middle orbits shows densities (white arrows) in maxillary and ethmoid sinuses. A soft tissue density (black arrows) adjacent to angulated floor fracture is entrapped inferior rectus muscle. *C,* Exploration of right orbital floor shows soft tissues, including inferior rectus muscle, entrapped within linear fracture (arrow).

important position of gaze (usually in primary gaze or downgaze), and when the diplopia fails to abate after several days of observation.

In general, the best time for surgical exploration of an orbital floor fracture is within the first 2 weeks after injury. However, if the eye or the optic nerve has been damaged, a longer delay is usually appropriate. If eye movements are restricted but seem to be improving, surgery may be delayed for weeks or months. Except when a linear fracture is actually compressing the inferior rectus muscle and causing fibrosis, a delay of several weeks probably has little effect on the ultimate results of surgical repair. In many patients with mechanical limitation of eye movement, the restriction may be due to connective tissue septa extending between the fracture and the extraocular muscles.[95] However, in some patients the muscles themselves may actually be entrapped within the fracture, necessitating surgical release.

The usual surgical approach to blow-out fractures of the orbital floor is through a skin incision (blepharoplasty incision) placed several millimeters beneath the lashes of the lower lid (Fig. 15–56). A skin and muscle flap is dissected free from the underlying orbital septum until the inferior orbital rim is reached. The periosteum is elevated from the orbital floor until the area of the fracture is located. Entrapped or prolapsed tissues are removed from the defect, and if necessary, the continuity of the orbital floor is restored. The bony defect is usually covered by a plastic prosthesis such as a Silastic or Supramid implant. It is important to avoid using an unnecessarily large prosthesis so that the risk of optic nerve damage and implant extrusion is minimized. Sometimes no implant is needed, especially when the fracture is small. Small defects may be covered with Gelfilm, which is rapidly absorbed, but which may prevent secondary adhesions from forming during the postoperative period. Some surgeons prefer to cover the defect with autogenous cartilage or bone.

Complications of blow-out fracture surgery include diplopia, lower eyelid retraction, infraorbital nerve damage, implant extrusion, and blindness.[94] Loss of vision has occurred several days after orbital fractures, even when surgery was not performed.

ORBITAL SURGERY

If a diagnosis can be established on the basis of the clinical features and diagnostic studies that have been described, and if the abnormality is apparently benign and not progressive, then it may be advisable to avoid surgical intervention. However, even benign lesions can produce such severe cosmetic defects or functional disturbances that surgical correction is appropriate.

When surgery is necessary in order to establish a diagnosis, to correct a deformity, or to remove a tumor, then the procedure selected should be the one that is the least extreme that will still accomplish the goal of the operation. It is important that biopsy specimens be adequately large and not deformed or crushed, so that an accurate diagnosis can be made. It is also important not to perform a radical, mutilative operation when a diagnosis has not been clearly established by preliminary tissue examination.

Most orbital lesions can be effectively reached through an anterior or lateral approach.[96–101] The risk of complications and the morbidity associated with these approaches are relatively low, compared with a neurosurgical (transcranial) approach. However, some lesions at the orbital apex, tumors extending into the optic canal, and lesions associated with defects of the sphenoid or orbital roof are usually best reached by a transcranial approach (Fig. 15–45).[91] Sinus and nasal lesions that extend into the orbit are usually reached through a sinus or nasal approach (Figs. 15–12, 15–32, and 15–33).

General Principles

By means of a careful physical examination, the taking of a complete history, and the use of appropriate diagnostic studies, most orbital tumors can be anatomically localized. Localization and a preliminary diagnosis are the most important factors in selecting a surgical approach to the orbit. It is necessary to have a thorough knowledge of orbital anatomy in order to interpret diagnostic studies and to perform orbital surgery. In addition, potential complications should be considered, appropriate instruments chosen, and satisfactory anesthesia selected.

Localization and Diagnosis

The techniques of evaluating patients with orbital disorders and orbital trauma were described earlier in this chapter. In general, if a malignant tumor is thought to be present, it is best to perform a biopsy of the lesion, using an anterior approach so that the integrity of the lateral wall is not compromised. However, it may not be possible to reach some retrobulbar tumors through an anterior incision, and a lateral approach may be required. Some benign tumors with a high potential for recurrence, such as benign mixed tumors of the lacrimal gland, should usually be completely removed through a lateral approach (Fig. 15–22), in order to avoid incomplete excision, which may leave residual tumor cells within the orbit.

Orbital Anatomy

Surgical exploration of the orbit demands a thorough understanding of the anatomical features of the orbital bones and soft tissues. The anterior entrance to the orbit is composed of portions of the zygomatic, maxillary, and frontal bones (Figs. 15–57 and 15–58).

The lateral orbital rim, which can be palpated beneath the skin adjacent to the lateral canthus, is composed of the frontal process of the zygomatic bone and the zygomatic process of the frontal bone. These two bones join at the zygomaticofrontal suture (Fig. 15–58). Inferior to this suture the orbital tubercle serves as a bony attachment of the lateral canthal tendon. On the posterior edge of the rim the zygomatic (marginal) tubercle is a projection that serves as an attachment of the temporalis muscle. The lateral orbital rim terminates inferiorly at the zygomatic arch, which is formed by horizontal processes of the zygomatic and temporal bones.

The orbital bones are covered by periosteum, which is perforated by vessels and nerves that enter and leave the orbit. The periosteum lining the inner surfaces of the orbital bones is termed the periorbita. The lacrimal gland lies adjacent to the periorbita in a shallow fossa within the superior-temporal orbit (Fig. 15–57).

Many orbital lesions can be reached without bone removal by anterior approaches through the conjunctiva or the eyelids. Much of the orbital cavity is filled with fat that lies between the globe and the orbital walls (Fig. 15–59). Structures such as the lacrimal gland, fascia, nerves, vessels, and the extraocular muscles are surrounded by this fat, which must be retracted

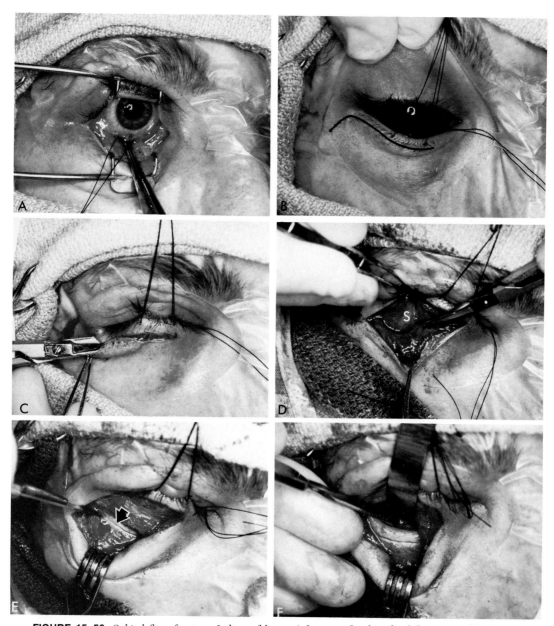

FIGURE 15–56. *Orbital floor fracture.* Indirect (blow-out) fracture of right orbital floor treated by lower eyelid (blepharoplasty) approach. *A,* Suture is placed beneath insertion of inferior rectus muscle to aid in identification and retraction during surgery. Muscle is grasped with forceps, and forced traction test is performed. *B,* Skin incision (line) is made several millimeters below eyelashes of lower lid. *C,* Scissors are used to dissect skin flap from orbicularis muscle for a short distance inferior to skin incision. *D,* Skin and orbicularis muscle are retracted downward and dissected from underlying orbital septum (S). *E,* Incision (arrow) is made through periosteum below inferior orbital rim. *F,* Periosteum and orbital soft tissues are elevated from orbital floor behind rim.

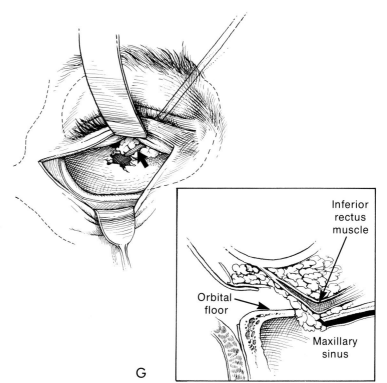

FIGURE 15–56 *Continued G,* Fracture is exposed, and prolapsed soft tissues are carefully elevated from defect in orbit floor. Inferior rectus muscle (arrow) may be identified by pulling on traction suture. Insert shows sagittal view of inferior rectus muscle restricted by adhesions to fracture.

Inferior rectus muscle

Orbital floor

Maxillary sinus

G

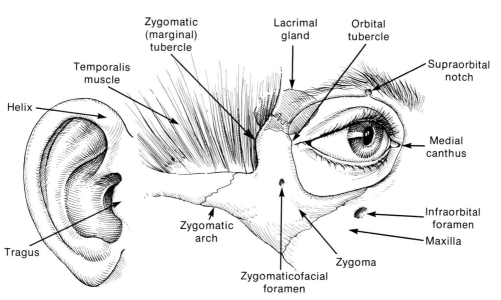

Zygomatic (marginal) tubercle

Lacrimal gland

Orbital tubercle

Supraorbital notch

Temporalis muscle

Helix

Medial canthus

Infraorbital foramen

Maxilla

Zygomatic arch

Tragus

Zygoma

Zygomaticofacial foramen

FIGURE 15–57. *Right orbit and face.* Skin and superficial muscles have been removed to show anterior entrance to orbit and zygomatic arch. Temporalis muscle lies within fossa beneath the zygomatic arch and is most firmly attached to lateral orbital rim at zygomatic (marginal) tubercle. The lateral canthal tendon is attached to lateral orbital rim at orbital tubercle. Lacrimal gland lies in shallow fossa within superior-temporal orbit. External auditory canal opens behind tragus near posterior end of zygomatic arch.

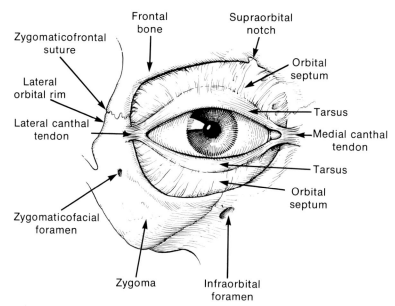

FIGURE 15–58. *Right orbit viewed from front.* Skin and orbicularis muscle have been moved, exposing orbital septum, tarsal plates, and canthal tendons. Orbital septum is fused to periosteum near anterior orbital rim and helps to retain fat within orbital cavity. Sensory nerves emerge through supraorbital notch or foramen, infraorbital foramen, and zygomaticofacial foramen.

during surgery to provide adequate visualization.

Potential Complications

Bleeding is usually moderate during orbital operations, and it is rarely necessary to provide blood replacement. However, severe hemorrhage is a possibility, especially during exenterations, sinus operations, and excisions of vascular lesions. If significant blood loss is believed to be likely, it is appropriate to prepare for possible blood replacement by typing and crossmatching the patient's blood. Hypotensive anesthesia may be of value both to control blood

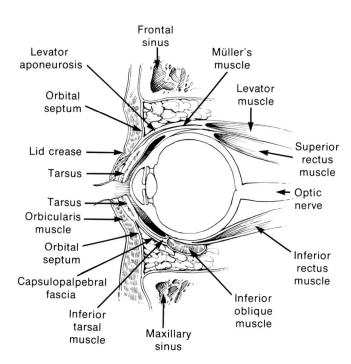

FIGURE 15–59. *Sagittal view of orbit.* The upper eyelid is elevated by the levator muscle and Müller's muscle, and the lower eyelid is retracted by the capsulopalpebral fascia and the inferior tarsal muscle. Abundant fat surrounds the muscles and lies between globe and orbital walls. Upper lid crease is partly formed by subcutaneous attachments of the levator aponeurosis.

loss and to improve visualization of structures during surgery. Cauterization of vessels should be performed under direct visualization and with great care to avoid unnecessary damage to nerves and the eye. Bipolar electrocoagulation forceps will cauterize tissue between the instrument tips, thus minimizing injury to surrounding structures. It is not necessary to routinely place drains beneath incisions used for orbital exploration. If postoperative bleeding is considered likely, a drain may be inserted through the skin or the incision, to allow blood to drain externally.

Blindness may be a necessary result of orbital surgery if a tumor involves the optic nerve, or if the eye is removed by enucleation or exenteration. However, unplanned blindness may result from almost any retrobulbar operation because of damage to blood vessels or the optic nerve. Even anterior orbital operations and orbital fracture repairs have been followed by loss of vision. Careful tissue dissection, adequate exposure, and minimal application of pressure to the eye should help to reduce the risk of blindness.

Ocular damage can usually be minimized by shielding the eye as much as possible during surgery. The cornea can be protected by a curved plastic shell, by a moistened Gelfoam patch, or by temporary approximation of the lids with sutures. When bone is being cut or drilled, especially along the lateral orbital rim, the eye may be protected by a malleable band retractor.

Extraocular muscle damage often follows orbital surgery, and may be reversible or permanent. The edema and hemorrhage that accompany almost any surgical procedure can cause transient upper eyelid ptosis and some limitation of eye movement. The removal or biopsy of lesions that involve the extraocular muscles often causes restricted eye movement. Muscle injury may be avoided if traction sutures are placed beneath the muscle insertions before operation. These muscles may then be identified during surgery by pulling on the sutures. Muscle damage can usually be minimized during orbital exploration if the muscles are simply identified and gently pushed aside by smooth retractors, rather than being dissected and pulled away from surrounding tissues.

Decreased sensation may occur as a result of injury to the branches of the trigeminal nerve that supply the brow, the cheek, and the temple. Incisions near the superior orbital rim may damage the supraorbital or supratrochlear nerves that supply the scalp, forehead, brow,

and upper eyelid. Incisions near the inferior orbital rim and orbital floor may damage the infraorbital nerve, which runs through the inferior orbital fissure, along the infraorbital canal, and out of the infraorbital foramen. This nerve supplies part of the mouth, upper lip, lateral nose, cheek, and lower eyelid. Incisions near the lateral orbital rim may damage the zygomaticofacial or zygomaticotemporal nerves that supply the skin over the temple and zygomatic bone. Sensory abnormalities may be transient or permanent after orbital exploration in any of these areas.

Infection is an unusual complication of orbital surgery, and routine use of systemic antibiotics is not necessary in conjunction with orbital exploration. If an infected lesion such as an abscess or a sinus pyocele is suspected, appropriate cultures and stains should be performed and antibiotics administered.

Instruments

The instruments used for orbital exploration can be divided into those necessary for bone manipulation and those used for soft tissue dissection. Air-driven oscillating saws and drills are extremely useful for cutting or removing bone (Figs. 15–17J and 15–24G). Rongeurs can be used to grasp bone flaps and to bite off small bone fragments. Osteotomes, chisels, and a mallet are useful to remove lamellar pieces of bone, to complete incisions into bone, and to help remove fibro-osseous tumors. Periosteal elevators are primarily used to dissect the adherent periosteum free from underlying bone. In addition, periosteal elevators that have a slightly curved, flat blade are often useful in dissecting soft tissues within the orbit, especially near the optic nerve. If necessary, bone that has been removed can be replaced and fixed in position by passing a stainless steel wire of small diameter (approximately 28-gauge) through drilled holes (Figs. 15–17O and 15–22M).

Soft tissues must be retracted to provide exposure of subcutaneous and deep orbital structures. Rake or hook retractors are useful for retracting skin margins. Deeper tissues are usually retracted by smooth ribbon or blade retractors. Adequate retraction is especially important to provide good visualization when orbital fat is pushed aside and when the optic nerve is approached. Self-retaining retractors have been designed for use with the operating microscope.[102]

Scissors, forceps, and scalpels used for most orbital surgery are generally the same as the

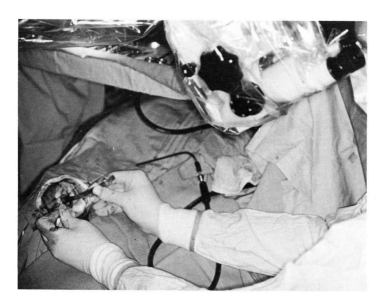

FIGURE 15–60. *Lateral orbital exploration using binocular operating microscope.* Coaxial illumination and 250-mm objective lens allow space for instrument manipulation.

instruments used for eyelid and facial plastic surgery. Microsurgical instruments with long arms are useful in deep orbital dissection and tumor removal.

A binocular operating microscope with coaxial illumination is of great value when surgery is performed near the optic nerve (Fig. 15–60). By using a 150- to 250-mm objective lens, depending on the location of the tumor and the length of the surgeon's arms, adequate space is provided between the patient and the microscope for instrument manipulation. In most cases the microscope itself should be covered by a sterile drape to prevent contamination of the operative field. Side arms on the microscope allow assistants to view the same operative field as the surgeon.

Both unipolar and bipolar electrocautery devices are useful for providing hemostasis during orbital surgery. Any electrocoagulation instrument should be used with care in patients who have a cardiac pacemaker. The unipolar cautery (Bovie) can be used to cut tissues with minimal blood loss, and is therefore of value in procedures such as exenteration (Fig. 15–15*H*). The bipolar cautery (Codman-Wetfield) minimizes tissue damage by cauterizing structures between the tips of the instrument forceps.

Anesthesia

Orbital surgery is most often performed using general inhalation anesthesia, although some procedures can be carried out with local infiltration or nerve block anesthesia. General anesthesia is usually selected when the retrobulbar area is explored, when bone is to be removed,

and when the operation may exceed several hours in length. By using controlled vascular hypotension in a healthy patient, bleeding can often be minimized and visualization improved during orbital dissection.

Regional anesthesia can be provided by injecting medications near the supraorbital, supratrochlear, infratrochlear, infraorbital, zygomaticofacial, or lacrimal nerves. Anterior or superficial surgery of the orbit, such as biopsy of lesions beneath the conjunctiva, can sometimes be performed using local infiltration of anesthetics. Although the choice of anesthetic agents for nerve block or local infiltration varies among surgeons, a mixture of lidocaine hydrochloride and bupivacaine hydrochloride offers rapid onset of anesthetic with a prolonged effect and little discomfort after surgery.

Wound Closure and Dressings

In order to create a wound that is both cosmetically and functionally optimal, it is important to accurately reapproximate deep and subcutaneous tissues. When lateral orbital approaches are used, the lateral canthus should be firmly approximated to bone or periosteum in its normal location, to prevent canthal sag and eyelid displacement. If the canthi are divided, they should be accurately reapproximated.

It is seldom necessary to completely close periosteum that has been cut. In fact, periosteum can often be completely excised without apparent complication. A running subcuticular monofilament suture is useful to firmly close linear incisions. Firm wound closure should be provided chiefly by deep and subcutaneous absorbable sutures.

In order to assure accurate closure of skin edges, small scratch incisions can be made perpendicular to the principal incision (Figs. 15–17G, 15–22G, and 15–38G). Skin sutures should usually be relatively small and should not exert tension on the wound, which should be initially closed by adequate subcutaneous sutures.

As previously mentioned, drains are seldom necessary if bleeding vessels have been satisfactorily closed during surgery. Sometimes drains are inserted through the skin or through the incision itself (Fig. 15–20I) if a severe hemorrhage has occurred, or if postoperative bleeding is considered likely.

In most cases relatively light wound dressings should be used after orbital surgery. Postoperative hemorrhage beneath a tight bandage may cause loss of vision as a result of occlusion of intraocular vessels or optic nerve ischemia.

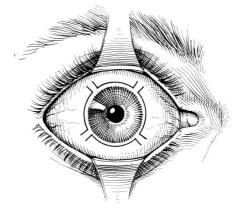

FIGURE 15–61. *Conjunctival incisions.* Anterior orbit can be explored through conjunctival incision near corneal limbus. Incision is made near lesion and extended radially to expose deep tissues.

Surgical Approaches

Most orbital abnormalities can be reached through anterior or lateral approaches by use of a variety of techniques and incisions. Many of these techniques have already been illustrated earlier in this chapter. The principal types of anterior and lateral approaches to the orbit will be described in the following diagrams.

Anterior Approaches to the Orbit

Lesions that lie in front of the equator of the globe, or that can be visualized or palpated beneath the conjunctiva or eyelids, can usually be reached by an anterior approach through the conjunctiva or skin. Some lesions near the optic nerve may be approached through a medial conjunctival incision. Lesions adjacent to the lamina papyracea of the ethmoid sinus may be approached through a nasal skin incision.

Conjunctival Approaches. Conjunctival approaches are usually appropriate when tumors lie adjacent to the surface of the globe. Incisions through the conjunctiva may be made at the corneal limbus and extended radially to provide adequate exposure (Fig. 15–61). If a conjunctival lesion is visible, the incision may be made directly over the abnormality.

Incisions into the upper fornix should usually be avoided unless a tumor appears to be located near the levator or superior rectus muscles. Most lesions in the upper orbit and most lacri-

mal gland masses are best approached through a skin incision.

Among the most common lesions that may appear as subconjunctival masses are prolapsed orbital fat, lymphoid tumors (Figs. 15–6 and 15–25A), dermolipomas (Fig. 15–36), and epibulbar dermoids (Fig. 15–37A). Prolapsed fat may be excised for cosmetic purposes. Lymphoid tumors may be studied by biopsy to establish a diagnosis but seldom require wide excision. Excision of dermolipomas and epibulbar dermoids may cause restricted eye movements and ptosis.[77] Therefore, excision of these benign tumors should be avoided or performed very cautiously.

Tumors that lie near the anterior portion of a rectus muscle can be approached through a conjunctival incision (Fig. 15–62). Lesions within or adjacent to the optic nerve can be reached by a medial conjunctival incision with detachment of the medial rectus muscle (Fig. 15–63). Removal of the lateral orbital rim and displacement of the eye can give even greater access to the posterior portion of the medial orbit and the optic nerve (Fig. 15–64).

Skin Approaches. Most lesions in the anterior orbit that are not directly adjacent to the globe can be approached through skin incisions. These anterior skin approaches are usually grouped into three anatomical regions: superior, medial, and inferior (Fig. 15–65).

Superior incisions may be made near the brow or near the upper lid crease (Fig. 15–66A). An incision above, within, or below the brow allows dissection along the orbital roof. Incisions in the brow should be beveled parallel to the direction of the hair shafts, to prevent

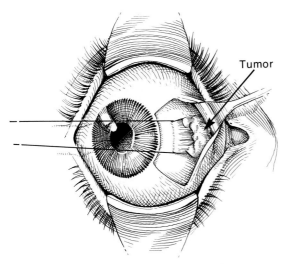

FIGURE 15–62. *Medial conjunctival approach to anterior orbit.* Conjunctiva is retracted toward nose by smooth retractor. Eye is retracted in opposite direction by suture passed beneath insertion of medial rectus muscle, exposing tumor adjacent to muscle.

loss of hair. Incisions near the central portion of the brow may damage the supraorbital nerves and vessels. If this area cannot be avoided, the patient should be alerted to the possibility of decreased or absent sensation over a portion of the forehead after surgery.

An incision used to reach the lacrimal gland when a nonepithelial lesion is believed to be present should be placed near the brow so that it can be extended if a benign mixed tumor is found (Fig. 15–66B). When a benign mixed tumor is found it should be completely removed together with adjacent tissues, which may require removal of the lateral orbital rim.

Incisions made within or near the lid crease are suitable for approaching lesions behind the orbital septum. The levator aponeurosis, which lies immediately behind the lid crease (Fig. 15–59), should be identified during exploration in the superior orbit, to prevent unnecessary damage.

Medial incisions may be made near the brow, along the nose, or through the eyelid (Fig. 15–67). Lesions along the medial orbital wall, near the lacrimal sac, and within the frontal sinus or ethmoid sinus may be approached through these incisions.

A curved incision extending downward and medially from the brow toward the lateral surface of the nose (Lynch approach) may be used to reach the superior-medial orbit, the floor of the frontal sinus, and the ethmoid sinus (Fig. 15–33F). Some frontal sinus tumors such as osteomas can be removed through a brow or superior-medial incision.[64] When performing surgery in this area care must be taken to avoid unnecessary damage to the superior oblique muscle and the trochlea. The trochlea may be elevated from its bony fossa with the attached periosteum and reflected toward the orbit (Fig. 15–68). After the exploration is completed the trochlea can be replaced by suturing the periosteum. The Lynch approach was at one time preferred for treatment of frontal sinus muco-

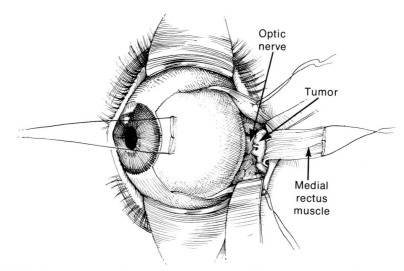

FIGURE 15–63. *Medial conjunctival approach to optic nerve.* Medial rectus muscle is detached and gently pulled toward nose. Orbital fat is held aside by smooth retractors, exposing optic nerve and retrobulbar tumor.

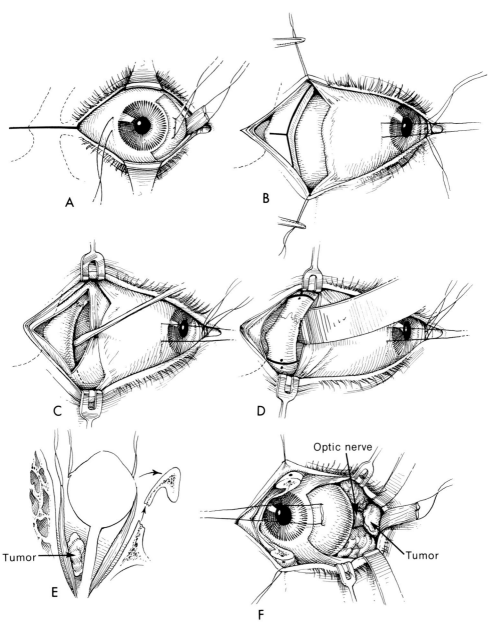

FIGURE 15–64. *Medial conjunctival approach with removal of lateral orbital rim.* A, Medial rectus muscle is detached from insertion to globe through conjunctival incision. Suture is placed beneath insertion of lateral rectus muscle. Lateral canthal incision (line) is made parallel to zygomatic arch. B, Eye is retracted toward nose, and lids are retracted by sutures placed through superior and inferior portions of lateral canthus. Lateral orbital rim is exposed, and incisions (lines) are made in periosteum. C, Periosteum is dissected from lateral orbital rim. D, Smooth retractor is used to protect the eye and displace soft tissues from lateral orbital wall. Lateral orbital rim is cut (lines) with oscillating saw, and holes are drilled to allow fixation of bone with wires. E, Lateral orbital rim is removed (arrows) with rongeur. F, Eye is retracted laterally into space provided by removal of orbital rim. Medial rectus muscle and fat are retracted to expose posterior optic nerve and tumor.

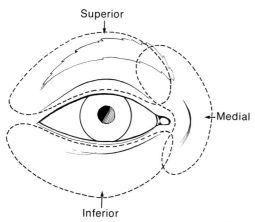

FIGURE 15–65. *Skin approaches to anterior orbit.*

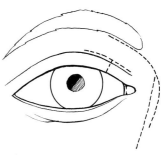

FIGURE 15–67. *Medial skin incisions.* Incisions (broken lines) can be placed near the brow (Lynch incision), along the nose, or through the eyelid.

celes. However, mucoceles treated in this way frequently recur, an osteoplastic operation with removal of the sinus mucosa and obliteration of the sinus cavity is the operation of choice for treating most frontal sinus mucoceles (Fig. 15–32).[73]

A nasal incision placed from 8 to 12 mm from the inner canthus provides an approach to the medial orbit, the ethmoid sinus, and the lacrimal sac. Lacrimal drainage operations such as dacryocystorhinostomies can be performed

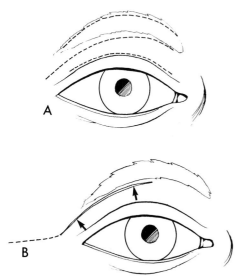

FIGURE 15–66. *Superior skin incisions.* A, Incisions (broken lines) can be placed near upper brow margin, lower brow margin, or lid crease. B, Incision near brow (arrows) used in taking a biopsy of lacrimal gland is curved to allow extension (broken line) for removal of lateral orbital rim if benign mixed tumor is found.

using this approach. Because some tumors in this area involve the lacrimal drainage structures, tearing may be an unavoidable consequence of surgery. Posterior dissection along the medial orbital wall (lamina papyracea of the ethmoid) exposes the ethmoid vessels, which should be identified and occluded to prevent significant bleeding.

A full-thickness incision through the upper lid margin provides good visualization of the superior-medial orbit.[100] A separate skin incision that approximately parallels the upper lid crease can be placed to intersect the marginal incision and give even greater exposure (Figs. 15–18 and 15–69). Because these incisions involve transsection of both the tarsus and portions of the levator aponeurosis, it is important for the surgeon to have a detailed knowledge of eyelid anatomy and of plastic surgical techniques for tissue reapproximation.

Inferior incisions may be made several millimeters below the eyelashes (blepharoplasty incision) or near the inferior orbital rim (Fig. 15–70). A less noticeable scar usually results from a blepharoplasty incision, which is partly hidden by the eyelashes (Figs. 15–56, 15–71, and 15–72). At the lateral canthus the incision is usually continued downward at a slight angle, in the direction of natural skin creases ("crow's feet"). If greater exposure is necessary, the lateral end of the incision can be continued temporally in a line parallel to the zygomatic arch, and part of the lateral orbital rim may be removed.

A skin and muscle flap is dissected downward toward the inferior orbital rim (Fig. 15–72A). Most inferior orbital tumors can be reached through the orbital septum. The same approach can be used to elevate the periosteum and repair fractures of the orbital floor (Fig. 15–72B).

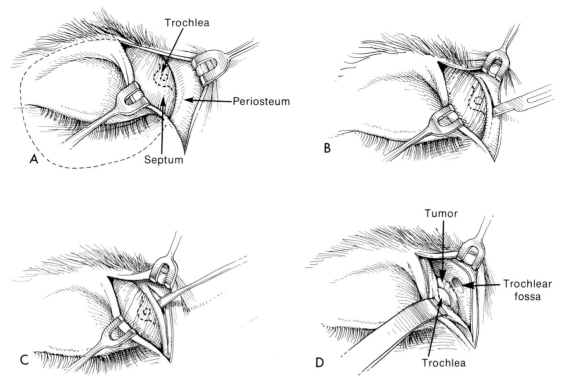

FIGURE 15–68. *Superior-medial (Lynch) approach with elevation of trochlea. A,* Skin and subcutaneous tissues are retracted to expose periosteum and orbital septum anterior to trochlea, which is not actually visualized. *B,* Incision is made in periosteum medial to trochlea along orbit rim. *C,* Periosteum is elevated from superior-medial orbital rim together with attached trochlea. *D,* Periosteum and trochlea are reflected toward orbit, exposing tumor and trochlear fossa in frontal bone. After tumor is removed, the periosteum along with attached trochlea is replaced in normal position.

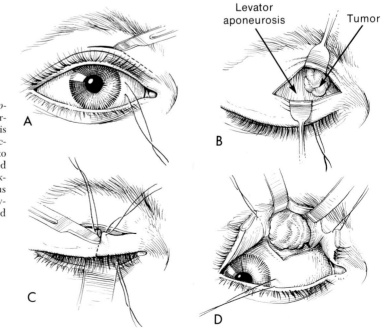

FIGURE 15–69. *Medial eyelid approach. A,* Skin incision is made parallel to upper lid crease. Suture is placed beneath insertion of medial rectus muscle. *B,* Tissues are retracted to expose tumor, which is partly covered by levator aponeurosis. *C,* Full-thickness incision is made through tarsus and upper lid margin. *D,* Eyelid, levator, and orbital tissues are retracted to expose entire tumor.

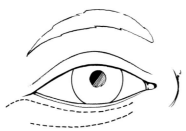

FIGURE 15–70. *Inferior skin incisions.* Incisions (broken lines) can be placed near the eyelashes (blepharoplasty incision) or near the inferior orbital rim.

Lateral Approaches to the Orbit

Lesions lying within the muscle cone, lacrimal gland tumors, and lesions that are posterior to the equator of the globe can usually be reached by a lateral orbital approach. As previously discussed, some optic nerve and other posterior orbital lesions can be reached through a medial anterior approach (Figs. 15–63 and 15–64). Some lesions near the orbital apex should be approached through the orbital roof by a craniotomy. When the orbit is approached from above, care should be taken to avoid unnecessary damage to the levator and superior rectus muscles.[91]

Lateral Canthotomy. Incisions made directly into the lateral canthus (lateral canthotomy) are frequently used to explore the orbit in infants or children (Figs. 15–39 and 15–73). A large canthotomy alone may provide sufficient exposure to remove some tumors from within the muscle cone in children.

Lateral canthotomy in adults is used primarily as an approach for taking biopsies of infiltrative tumors that lie near the lateral rectus muscle. Most posterior tumors are approached by removing the lateral orbital rim through orbitotomy incisions that do not divide the lateral canthus (Fig. 15–74).

Lateral Orbitotomy. A lateral orbitotomy can be used to reach lesions behind the eye that cannot be reached through an anterior approach. A lateral orbitotomy approach provides good visualization and access to the retrobulbar area with minimal deformity (Figs. 15–16 and 15–75). The eponym Krönlein operation has often been used to describe a lateral orbitotomy; however, Krönlein's original operation involved an unsightly crescent-shaped incision that is no longer used.

The skin incision used for a lateral orbitotomy is approximately 30 mm long and extends from near the lateral canthus toward the helix of the ear, parallel to the zygomatic arch (Fig. 15–75A). Although Berke[96] described a lateral orbitotomy incision that divides the canthus, adequate retrobulbar exposure is provided with-

Text continued on page 520

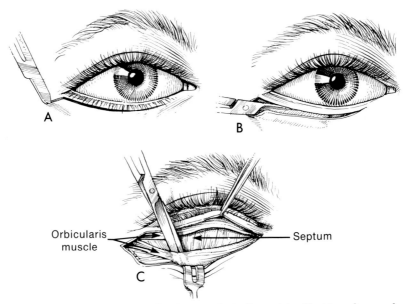

Orbicularis muscle — Septum

FIGURE 15–71. *Inferior eyelid (blepharoplasty) approach. A,* Skin incision (line) is made several millimeters below eyelashes of lower lid. At lateral canthus, incision is extended in natural skin crease. *B,* Scissors are used to dissect skin flap from orbicularis muscle for a short distance inferior to skin incision. *C,* Scissors are used to incise orbicularis muscle and to dissect muscle from underlying orbital septum.

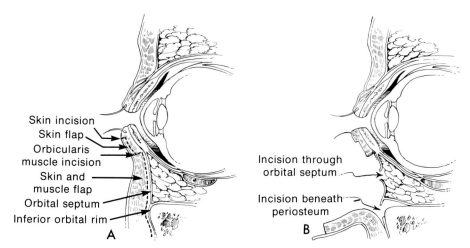

FIGURE 15–72. *Sagittal views of inferior eyelid (blepharoplasty) approach.* A, Incision (broken line) is carried in steps through skin and orbicularis muscle. Skin and muscle flap is dissected from orbital septum. B, Skin and muscle flap is reflected downward. An incision can be made through orbital septum to reach tissues beneath eye, or periosteum can be elevated to reach orbital floor.

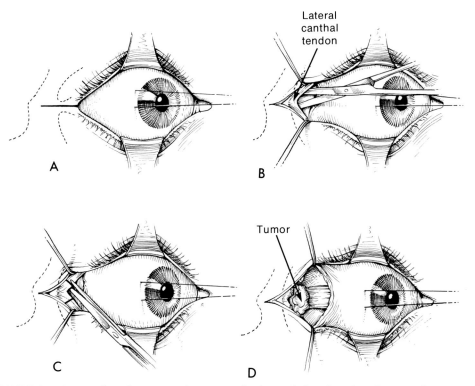

FIGURE 15–73. *Lateral canthotomy.* A, Skin incision (line) extends from lateral canthus toward ear parallel to zygomatic arch. Suture is placed beneath insertion of lateral rectus muscle. B, Skin and orbicularis muscle are dissected and retracted from anterior surface of lateral canthal tendon. Scissors are used to dissect conjunctiva from behind tendon. C, The superior and inferior limbs of lateral canthal tendon are cut (lines) to free the eyelids. D, Canthal margins and lids are retracted to expose tumor near lateral rectus muscle.

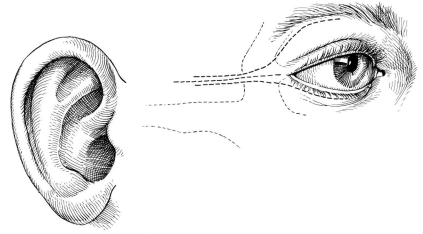

FIGURE 15–74. *Orbitotomy incisions.* Incisions (broken lines) are used for superior-lateral orbitotomy, lateral orbitotomy, and inferior-lateral orbitotomy.

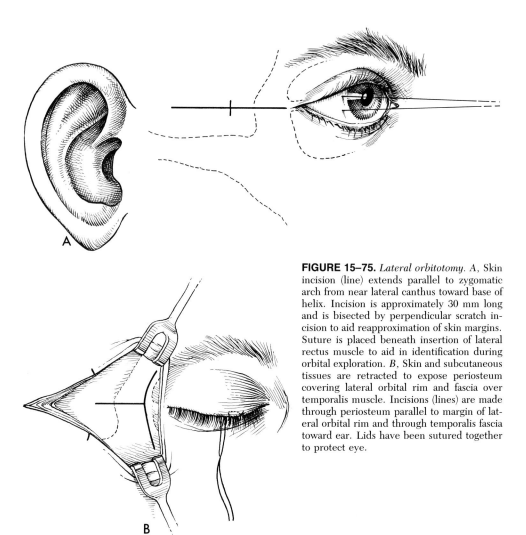

FIGURE 15–75. *Lateral orbitotomy. A,* Skin incision (line) extends parallel to zygomatic arch from near lateral canthus toward base of helix. Incision is approximately 30 mm long and is bisected by perpendicular scratch incision to aid reapproximation of skin margins. Suture is placed beneath insertion of lateral rectus muscle to aid in identification during orbital exploration. *B,* Skin and subcutaneous tissues are retracted to expose periosteum covering lateral orbital rim and fascia over temporalis muscle. Incisions (lines) are made through periosteum parallel to margin of lateral orbital rim and through temporalis fascia toward ear. Lids have been sutured together to protect eye.

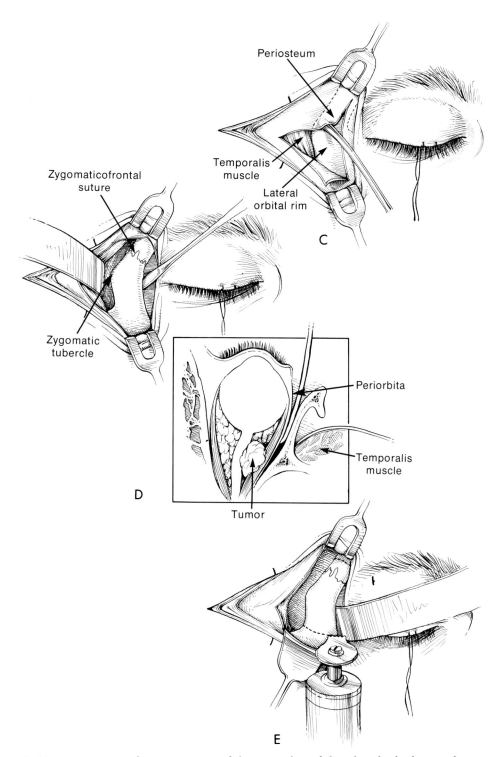

FIGURE 15–75 *Continued C,* Periosteum and fascia are elevated from lateral orbital rim and anterior temporalis muscle. *D,* Temporalis muscle is retracted from outer lateral orbital rim. Orbital periosteum (periorbita) is dissected from lateral wall of orbit. Inset shows tumor within muscle cone displacing optic nerve. *E,* Oscillating saw is used to cut lateral orbital rim (broken lines) above zygomaticofrontal suture and near zygomatic arch. Eye is protected by smooth retractor.

Illustration continued on following page

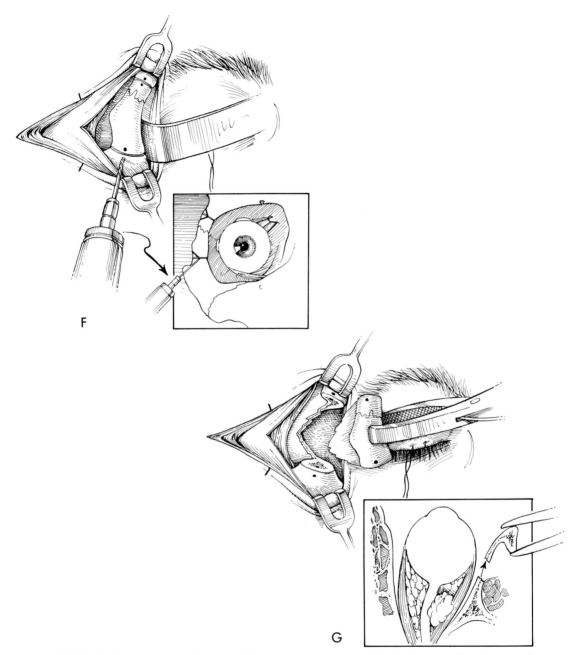

FIGURE 15–75 *Continued F,* Holes are drilled adjacent to cuts in lateral orbital rim to allow fixation with wires when bone is replaced. *G,* Heavy forceps or rongeur is used to remove lateral orbital rim together with attached segment of orbital wall. *H,* Rongeur is used to remove additional bone from lateral orbital wall. *I,* Incisions are made in periorbita (inset). Periorbita is retracted to expose lateral rectus muscle and tumor. *J,* Lateral rectus muscle is gently retracted downward, and tumor is removed from muscle cone. *K,* Insets show: (I) closure of periorbita; (II) replacement of lateral orbital rim and fixation with stainless steel wire; and (III) closure of periosteum and temporalis fascia. Subcutaneous tissues are firmly approximated with absorbable sutures, and skin incision is closed with running subcuticular monofilament suture such as nylon.

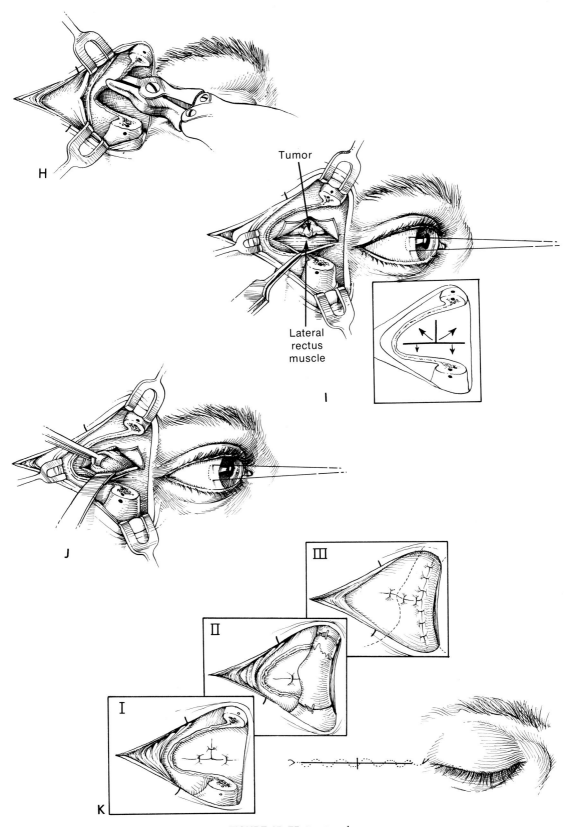

Tumor

Lateral
rectus
muscle

FIGURE 15–75 *Continued*

out cutting the lateral canthus. After the skin and subcutaneous tissues are retracted, the periosteum and temporalis muscle are elevated from the lateral orbital rim (Fig. 15–75C). The temporalis muscle is firmly attached to the lateral orbital rim at the zygomatic (marginal) tubercle, and the muscle must usually be cut free with a scalpel at that point (Fig. 15–75D).

To remove the lateral orbital rim an oscillating saw is used to cut the bone near the zygomatic arch and above the zygomaticofrontal suture (Fig. 15–75E). A hammer and osteotome or chisel can be used to complete cuts begun by the saw and to cut bone in awkward positions. Before the rim is removed, an air-driven drill is used to make holes in the bone adjacent to the saw cuts so that the rim can later be wired in place (Fig. 15–75F). The eye should be protected by a retractor when instruments such as mechanical saws or drills are used in the orbit.

By completely removing the lateral orbital rim, rather than simply pushing it aside, the size of the operative field is increased (Fig. 15–75G). If necessary, additional bone can be removed with a rongeur from the thin sphenoid bone of the temporalis muscle fossa (Fig. 15–75H).

The periorbita should be incised with great care to avoid unnecessary damage to the underlying lateral rectus muscle (Fig. 15–75I). Identification of this muscle is simplified if a suture is passed beneath its insertion at the beginning of the operation. If exploration of the upper or lower orbit is planned, the superior rectus or inferior rectus muscles should be tagged with sutures as well. After the lateral rectus muscle is identified it should be gently retracted to the side so that the muscle cone can be explored (Fig. 15–75J).

When deep intraorbital dissection is performed, an operating microscope provides valuable illumination and magnification (Fig. 15–60). Sharp dissection should be avoided unless good visualization is available. Orbital tissues should usually be retracted with smooth tools and instruments so as to avoid unnecessary trauma.

A good cosmetic result after an orbital exploration is largely dependent on the care taken to accurately reapproximate tissues. Normal facial contour is maintained by replacing the lateral orbital rim. The subcutaneous tissues must be firmly closed in multiple layers (Fig. 15–75K).

Superior-Lateral Orbitotomy. A superior-lateral orbitotomy, popularized by Stallard,[91] provides a wider operative field than a lateral orbitotomy (Figs. 15–22 and 15–76). This approach is used to reach lesions in or near the lacrimal gland and along the orbital roof. It may also be used to remove large tumors from within the muscle cone.

The skin incision extends in an arc from beneath the brow toward the helix of the ear (Fig. 15–76A). A portion of the superior orbital rim that covers the lacrimal gland is removed together with the lateral rim (Fig. 15–76C). Lesions suspected of being benign mixed tumors of the lacrimal gland should be removed together with adherent periosteum.

Inferior-Lateral Orbitotomy. An inferior-lateral orbitotomy combines an inferior eyelid (modified blepharoplasty) incision with a lateral incision and removal of the lateral orbital rim (Figs. 15–38 and 15–77). This approach can be used to reach lesions near the orbital floor and within the muscle cone, which are not accessible through an anterior approach.

A skin and muscle flap is dissected downward below the eyelid margin to expose the orbital septum, the lateral orbital rim, and part of the inferior orbital rim (Fig. 15–77B). After the lateral orbital rim is removed an incision is made through the periorbita and the septum (Fig. 15–77E). This approach provides access to the retrobulbar area as well as to the area beneath the eye.

Exenteration

Exenteration is removal of the eye together with a significant portion of the orbital tissues (Figs. 15–11, 15–13, 15–14, 15–23, 15–24, 15–78, and 15–79). The amount of tissues removed depends on the origin and extent of the abnormality to be removed. Although exenterations are usually performed for malignant lesions, some benign diseases, such as phycomycosis, may require exenteration.

On the basis of the amount of tissue removed, exenterations may be classified as (a) subtotal exenteration, (b) total exenteration (with or without preservation of the eyelid skin), and (c) radical exenteration.

Subtotal or limited exenteration is an extended enucleation. The eye and epibulbar tissues are removed, but the periosteum and some orbital soft tissues are left. Sometimes the eyelids may be spared, leaving a cavity that can retain a cosmetic prosthesis. More often the conjunctiva must be removed, and the skin of the eyelids, frequently with orbicularis muscle, is sewn together over the retrobulbar tissues. This operation is most often used to remove tumors that involve the anterior portion of the

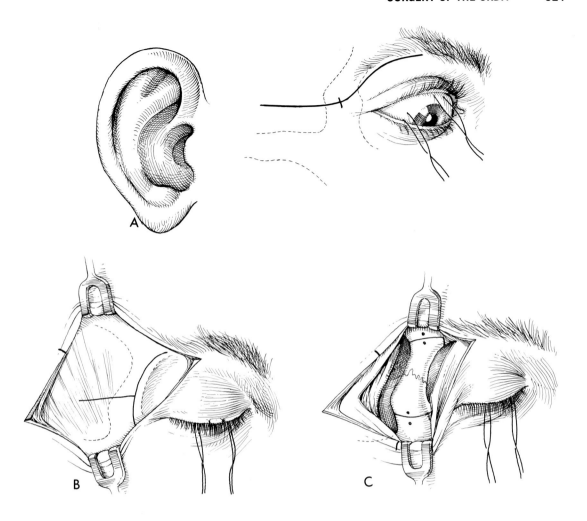

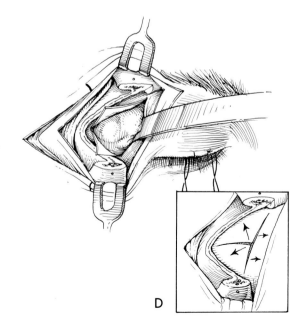

FIGURE 15–76. *Superior-lateral orbitotomy. A,* Skin incision (line) extends from below the unshaved eyebrow in an arc approximately 1 cm temporal to the lateral canthus and then toward the ear parallel to the zygomatic arch. A short perpendicular scratch incision is made to aid reapproximation of skin margins. Sutures are placed beneath insertions of superior rectus and lateral rectus muscles to aid in identification during orbital exploration. *B,* Skin and subcutaneous tissues are retracted to expose periosteum covering lateral orbital rim and fascia covering temporalis muscle as high as its anterior origin at the frontal bone. Incisions (lines) are made through periosteum behind margin of lateral orbital rim, extending onto superior orbital rim and through temporalis fascia. Lids have been sutured together to protect eye. *C,* Cuts in orbital rim are made higher than those for lateral orbitotomy. Upper cut is angled across frontal bone and through superior orbital rim; lower cut is made below orbital tubercle. Holes are drilled to allow fixation with wires when bone is replaced. *D,* Incisions are made in periorbita (inset) after orbital rim is removed. Periorbita, levator, and rectus muscles are retracted to expose tumor.

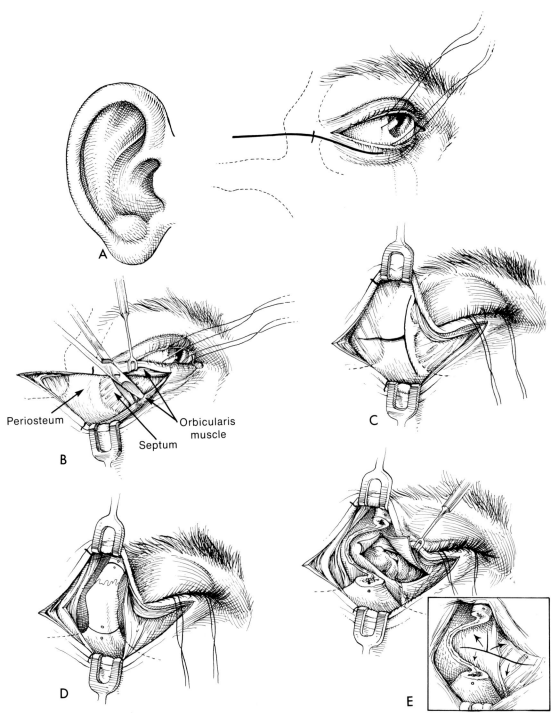

FIGURE 15–77. *Inferior-lateral orbitotomy. A,* Skin incision (line) is made several millimeters below eyelashes of lower lid and is extended temporal to the lateral canthus and parallel to the zygomatic arch. A short perpendicular scratch incision is made to aid reapproximation of skin margins. Sutures are placed beneath insertions of inferior rectus and lateral rectus muscles to aid in identification during orbital exploration. *B,* Skin and subcutaneous tissues are retracted downward, and orbicularis muscle is dissected from underlying orbital septum and periosteum. *C,* Additional tissues are dissected and retracted to expose periosteum covering lateral orbital rim and fascia covering temporalis muscle. Incisions (lines) are made through periosteum behind margin of lateral orbital rim extending onto inferior orbital rim and through temporalis fascia. Lids have been sutured together to protect eye. *D,* Cuts in orbital rim are made above zygomaticofrontal suture and near zygomatic arch. Holes are drilled to allow fixation with wires when bone is replaced. *E,* Incisions are made in periorbita and lateral orbital septum (inset). Periorbita and other tissues are retracted to expose tumor.

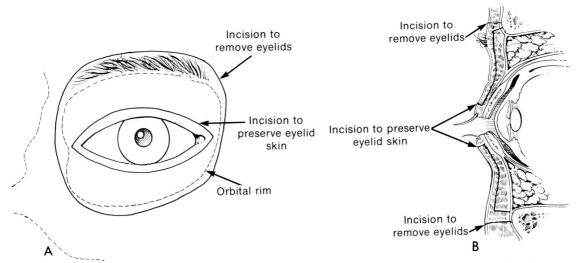

FIGURE 15–78. *Exenteration incisions.* A, Incisions (lines) can be placed near lashes to preserve skin of eyelids, or near orbital rim (broken line). B, Sagittal view shows incisions (lines).

eye and the conjunctiva, without significant posterior extension.

Total or complete exenteration involves removal of all tissues within the bony orbit, including the periorbita. The eyelids may be totally removed, or the eyelid skin may be preserved and folded into the orbital cavity to help line the walls (Figs. 15–15, 15–78, and 15–79). Total exenteration is indicated when an intraocular tumor such as a melanoma extends through the sclera into the orbit. A malignant tumor that does not involve bone and that does not respond well to radiation may be treated by total exenteration.

Bleeding can be minimized by visualization and cauterization of the ethmoid vessels and the vessels in the superior and inferior orbital fissures. During elevation of the periosteum care should be taken to avoid perforation of the bony walls, especially the ethmoid lamina papyracea (Fig. 15–79D). Perforation into the sinuses or nasal cavity can cause mucus or fluid to drain into the orbit. This drainage is usually minimal, however, and can be absorbed with a dressing if necessary.

The lateral skin margins should be undermined and sutured over the lateral orbital rim, to reduce the size of the cutaneous defect. The bony orbital walls can be covered by a split-thickness (0.012- to 0.015-inch thick) skin graft, usually taken from a donor site on hairless portions of the upper leg or abdomen (Fig. 15–79E). The skin graft should be held against the bone with a firm dressing for 7 to 10 days. The orbital cavity can be packed with gauze impregnated with an antibiotic ointment. Dressing changes usually cause little discomfort if care is used in removing the packing.

The bone surfaces may also be allowed to heal and epithelialize spontaneously without grafting. Spontaneous healing requires months for complete coverage of the bone surfaces, and dressings must be changed at intervals of approximately 1 week. However, orbital cavities that epithelialize spontaneously are usually more shallow and are less sensitive to extremes of heat and cold than are those that are covered with skin grafts.

Radical exenteration involves removal of one or more of the bony orbital walls in addition to soft tissues and periosteum. Such an operation may be required when a malignant sinus tumor has invaded the orbit (Fig. 15–12), or when a malignant skin tumor has involved the orbital bones (Fig. 15–14). Malignant epithelial tumors of the lacrimal gland often involve the periosteum and bone along the lateral orbital roof. Therefore, parts of the roof and lateral orbital wall should be removed when such tumors are present (Figs. 15–23 and 15–24).

After exenteration wounds have healed, the resulting cavity may be covered by a black patch (Fig. 15–12). Some patients prefer a cosmetic plastic prosthesis, which is held in place with adhesive (Fig. 15–14N). A prosthesis gives the appearance of a normal eye and lids. Even though the lids do not blink, eyeglasses help to reduce the cosmetic asymmetry.

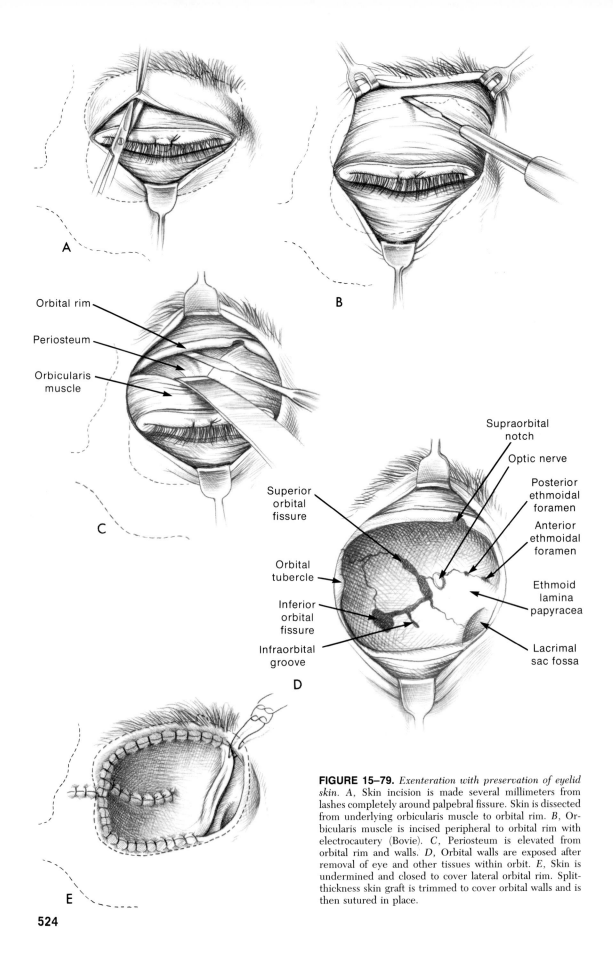

Orbital rim

Periosteum

Orbicularis
muscle

Supraorbital
notch

Optic nerve

Posterior
ethmoidal
foramen

Superior
orbital
fissure

Anterior
ethmoidal
foramen

Orbital
tubercle

Ethmoid
lamina
papyracea

Inferior
orbital
fissure

Infraorbital
groove

Lacrimal
sac fossa

FIGURE 15–79. *Exenteration with preservation of eyelid skin. A,* Skin incision is made several millimeters from lashes completely around palpebral fissure. Skin is dissected from underlying orbicularis muscle to orbital rim. *B,* Orbicularis muscle is incised peripheral to orbital rim with electrocautery (Bovie). *C,* Periosteum is elevated from orbital rim and walls. *D,* Orbital walls are exposed after removal of eye and other tissues within orbit. *E,* Skin is undermined and closed to cover lateral orbital rim. Split-thickness skin graft is trimmed to cover orbital walls and is then sutured in place.

REFERENCES

1. Grove, A. S., Jr.: Evaluation of exophthalmos. N. Engl. J. Med., 292:1005, 1975.
2. Grove, A. S., Jr.: Orbital disease: Examination and diagnostic evaluation. Ophthalmology, 86:854, 1979.
3. Grove, A. S., Jr.: Orbital diagnosis. Head Neck Surg., 2:12, 1979.
4. Jones, I. S., Jakobiec, F. A., Nolan, B. T.: Patient examination and introduction to orbital disease. In Duane, T. D. (ed.): Clinical Ophthalmology, Vol. 2: The Orbit. Hagerstown, Md., Harper & Row, 1979, Ch. 21.
5. Shields, J. A., Bakewell, B., Augsburger, J. J., Flanagan, J. C.: Classifications and incidence of space-occupying lesions of the orbit. A survey of 645 biopsies. Arch. Ophthalmol., 102:1606, 1984.
6. Shields, J. A., Bakewell, B., Augsburger, J. J., et al.: Space-occupying orbital masses in children. A review of 250 consecutive biopsies. Ophthalmology, 93:379, 1986.
7. Jakobiec, F. A., Jones, I. S.: Orbital inflammations. In Duane, T. D. (ed.): Clinical Ophthalmology, Vol. 2: The Orbit. Hagerstown, Md., Harper & Row, 1979, Ch. 35.
8. Bullock, J. D., Yanes, B.: Ophthalmic manifestations of metastatic breast cancer. Ophthalmology, 87:961, 1980.
9. Tormey, D. C., Waalkes, T. P., Simon, R. M.: Biological markers in breast carcinoma. II. Clinical correlations with human chorionic gonadotropin. Cancer, 39:2391, 1977.
10. Byrne, S. F., Glaser, J. S.: Orbital tissue differentiation with standardized echography. Ophthalmology, 90:1071, 1983.
11. Surks, M. I.: Assessment of thyroid function. Ophthalmology, 88:476, 1981.
12. Gorman, C. A., Waller, R. R., Dyer, J. A. (eds.): The Eye and Orbit in Thyroid Disease. New York, Raven Press, 1984.
13. Klee, G. G., Hay, I. D.: Assessment of sensitive thyrotropin assays for an expanded role in thyroid function testing: Proposed criteria for analytic performance and clinical utility. J. Clin. Endocrinol. Metab., 64:461, 1987.
14. Eggers, H., Jakobiec, F. A., Jones, I. S.: Optic nerve gliomas. In Duane, T. D. (ed.): Clinical Ophthalmology, Vol. 2: The Orbit. Hagerstown, Md., Harper & Row, 1979, Ch. 42.
15. Coleman, D. J., Lizzi, F. L., Jack, R. L.: Ultrasonography of the Eye and Orbit. Philadelphia, Lea & Febiger, 1977.
16. Trokel, S. L., Hilal, S. K.: Recognition and differential diagnosis of enlarged extraocular muscles in computed tomography. Am. J. Ophthalmol., 87:418, 1979.
17. Alper, M. G.: Computed tomography in planning and evaluating orbital surgery. Ophthalmology, 87:418, 1980.
18. Trokel, S. L., Jakobiec, F. A.: Correlation of CT scanning and pathologic features of ophthalmic Graves' disease. Ophthalmology, 88:553, 1981.
19. Grove, A. S., Jr., Tadmor, R., New, P. F. J., Momose, J. K.: Orbital fracture evaluation by coronal computed tomography, Am. J. Ophthalmol., 85:679, 1978.
20. Grove, A. S., Jr.: Orbital trauma and computed tomography. Ophthalmology, 87:403, 1980.
21. Moseley, I., Brant-Zawadski, M., Mills, C.: Nuclear magnetic resonance imaging of the orbit. Br. J. Ophthalmol., 67:333, 1983.
22. Zimmerman, R. A., Bilaniuk, L. T., Yanoff, M., et al.: Orbital magnetic resonance imaging. Am. J. Ophthalmol., 100:312, 1985.
23. Grove, A. S., Jr.: New diagnostic techniques for the evaluation of orbital trauma. Trans. Am. Acad. Ophthalmol. Otolaryngol., 83:626, 1977.
24. Grove, A. S.: The dural shunt syndrome. Pathophysiology and clinical course. Ophthalmology, 91:31, 1984.
25. Messmer, E. P., Font, R. L.: Applications of immunohistochemistry to ophthalmic pathology. Ophthalmology, 91:701, 1984.
26. Rootman, J., Quenville, N., Owen, D.: Recent advances in pathology as applied to orbital biopsy. Ophthalmology, 91:708, 1984.
27. Kincaid, M. D., Green, W. R.: Diagnostic methods in orbital diseases. Ophthalmology, 91:719, 1984.
28. Jakobiec, F. A., Jones, I. A.: Lymphomatous, plasmacytic, histiocytic, and hematopoietic tumors. In Duane, T. D. (ed.): Clinical Ophthalmology, Vol. 2: The Orbit. Hagerstown, Md., Harper & Row, 1979, Ch. 39.
29. Knowles, D. M., II, Jakobiec, F. A., Halper, J. P.: Immunologic characterization of ocular adnexal lymphoid neoplasms. Am. J. Ophthalmol., 87:603, 1979.
30. Solomon, D. H., Chopra, I. J.: Graves' disease—1972. Mayo Clin. Proc., 47:803, 1972.
31. Grove, A. S.: Upper eyelid retraction and Graves' disease. Ophthalmology, 88:499, 1981.
32. Putterman, A. M.: Surgical treatment of thyroid-related upper eyelid retraction. Graded Müller's muscle excision and levator recession. Ophthalmology, 88:507, 1981.
33. Harvey, J. T., Anderson, R. S.: The aponeurotic approach to eyelid retraction. Ophthalmology, 88:513, 1981.
34. Ravin, J. G., Sisson, J. C., Knapp, W. T.: Orbital radiation for the ocular changes of Graves' disease. Am. J. Ophthalmol., 79:285, 1975.
35. Leone, C. R., Bajandas, F. J.: Inferior orbital decompression for thyroid ophthalmopathy. Arch. Ophthalmol., 98:890, 1980.
36. McCord, C. D.: Current trends in orbital decompression. Ophthalmology, 92:21, 1985.
37. Chavis, R. M., Garner, A., Wright, J. E.: Inflammatory orbital pseudotumor. Arch. Ophthalmol., 96:1817, 1978.
38. Mottow, L. S., Jakobiec, F. A.: Idiopathic inflammatory orbital pseudotumor in children. I. Clinical characteristics. Arch. Ophthalmol., 96:1410, 1978.
39. Mottow-Lippa, L., Jakobiec, F. A., Smith, M.: Idiopathic inflammatory orbital pseudotumor in childhood. II. Results of diagnostic tests and biopsies. Ophthalmology, 88:565, 1981.
40. Kennerdell, J. S., Johnson, B. L., Deutsch, M.: Radiation treatment of orbital lymphoid hyperplasia. Ophthalmology, 86:942, 1979.
41. Jakobiec, F. A., Rootman, J., Jones, I. S.: Secondary and metastatic tumors of the orbit. In Duane, T. D. (ed.): Clinical Ophthalmology, Vol. 2: The Orbit. Hagerstown, Md., Harper & Row, 1979, Ch. 46.
42. Batsakis, J.: Tumors of the Head and Neck. Baltimore, Williams & Wilkins, 1979.
43. Lawton, A. W., Karesh, J. W., Gray, W. C.: Proptosis from maxillary sinus inverted papilloma with malig-

nant transformation. Arch. Ophthalmol., 104:874, 1986.

44. Cheng, V. S. T., Wang, C. C.: Carcinomas of the paranasal sinuses. Cancer, 40:3038, 1977.

45. Grove, A. S., Jr.: Melanomas of the conjunctiva. Int. Ophthalmol. Clin., 20(2):161, 1980.

46. Groves, A. S., Jr.: Staged excision and reconstruction of extensive facial-orbital tumors. Ophthalmic Surg., 8:91, 1977.

47. Mohs, F. E.: Micrographic surgery for microscopically controlled excision of eyelid cancers. Arch. Ophthalmol., 104:901, 1986.

48. Jakobiec, F. A., Jones, I. S.: Neurogenic tumors. In Duane, T. D. (ed.): Clinical Ophthalmology, Vol. 2: The Orbit. Hagerstown, Md., Harper & Row, 1979, Ch. 41.

49. Ferry, A. P., Fort, R. L.: Carcinoma metastatic to the eye and orbit. I. A clinicopathologic study of 227 cases. Arch. Ophthalmol., 92:276, 1974.

50. Fort, R. L., Ferry, A. P.: Carcinoma metastatic to the eye and orbit. III. A clinicopathologic study of 28 cases metastatic to the orbit. Cancer, 38:1326, 1976.

51. Mottow-Lippa, L., Jakobiec, F. A., Iwamoto, T.: Pseudoinflammatory metastatic breast carcinoma of the orbit and lids. Ophthalmology, 88:575, 1981.

52. Jakobiec, F. A., Jones, I. S.: Vascular tumors, malformations and degenerations. In Duane, T. D. (ed.): Clinical Ophthalmology, Vol. 2: The Orbit. Hagerstown, Md., Harper & Row, 1979, Ch. 37.

53. Flanagan, J. C.: Vascular problems of the orbit. Ophthalmology, 86:896, 1979.

54. Haik, B. G., Jakobiec, F. A., Ellsworth, R. M., Jones, I. S.: Capillary hemangioma of the lids and orbit: An analysis of the clinical features and therapeutic results in 101 cases. Ophthalmology, 86:760, 1979.

55. Kushner, B. J.: Intralesional corticosteroid injection for infantile hemangioma. Am. J. Ophthalmol., 93:496, 1982.

56. Bonavolonta, G., Vassallo, P., Uccello, G., Tranfa, F.: Our experience with intralesional corticosteroid injection therapy for infantile adnexal hemangioma. Orbit, 4:177, 1985.

57. Iliff, W. J., Green, W. R.: Orbital lymphangiomas. Ophthalmology, 86:914, 1979.

58. Jakobiec, F. A., Howard, G. M., Jones, I. S., Wolf, M.: Hemangiopericytoma of the orbit. Am. J. Ophthalmol., 78:816, 1974.

59. Fort, R. L., Gamel, J. W.: Epithelial tumors of the lacrimal gland: An analysis of 265 cases. In Jakobiec, F. A. (ed.): Ocular and Adnexal Tumors. Birmingham, Ala., Aesculapius Publishing Co., 1978, pp. 787–805.

60. Stewart, W. B., Krohel, G. B., Wright, J. E.: Lacrimal gland and fossa lesions: An approach to diagnosis and management. Ophthalmology, 86:886, 1979.

61. Jakobiec, F. A., Yeo, J. H., Trokel, S. L., et al.: Combined clinical and computed tomographic diagnosis of primary lacrimal fossa lesions. Am. J. Ophthalmol., 94:785, 1982.

62. Fu, Y. S., Perzin, K. H.: Non-epithelial tumors of the nasal cavity, paranasal sinuses, and nasopharynx: A clinicopathologic study. II. Osseous and fibroosseous lesions, including osteoma, fibrous dysplasia, ossifying fibroma, osteoblastoma, giant cell tumor, and osteosarcoma. Cancer, 33:1289, 1974.

63. Blodi, F. C.: Pathology of orbital bones. Am. J. Ophthalmol., 81:1, 1976.

64. Grove, A. S., Jr.: Osteomas of the orbit. Ophthalmic Surg., 9:23, 1978.

65. Jakobiec, F. A., Jones, I. S.: Mesenchymal and fibroosseous tumors. In Duane, T. D. (ed.): Clinical Ophthalmology, Vol. 2: The Orbit. Hagerstown, Md., Harper & Row, 1979, Ch. 44.

66. Zakka, K. A., Summerer, R. W., Yee, R. D., et al.: Opticociliary veins in a primary optic nerve sheath meningioma. Am. J. Ophthalmol., 87:91, 1979.

67. Jakobiec, F. A., Depot, M. J., Kennerdell, J. S., et al.: Combined clinical and computed tomographic diagnosis of orbital glioma and meningioma. Ophthalmology, 91:137, 1984.

68. Mark, L. E., Kennerdell, J. S., Maroon, J. C., et al.: Microsurgical removal of a primary intraorbital meningioma. Am. J. Ophthalmol., 86:704, 1978.

69. Smith, J. L., Vuksanovik, M. M., Yates, B. M., Bienfang, D. C.: Radiation therapy for primary optic nerve meningiomas. J. Clin. Neuroophthalmol., 1:85, 1981.

70. Jakobiec, F. A., Howard, G. M., Jones, I. S., Tannenbaum, M.: Fibrous histiocytoma of the orbit. Am. J. Ophthalmol., 77:333, 1974.

71. Rodrigues, M. M., Furgiuele, F. P., Weinreb, S.: Malignant fibrous histiocytoma of the orbit. Arch. Ophthalmol., 95:2025, 1977.

72. Becker, S. P., Sisson, G. A.: Unilateral proptosis secondary to fibrous cementoma. Trans. Am. Acad. Ophthalmol. Otolaryngol., 84:159, 1977.

73. Montgomery, W. W.: Surgery of the frontal sinuses. Otolaryngol. Clin. North Am., 4(1):97, 1971.

74. Howard, G. M.: Cystic tumors. In Duane, T. D. (ed.): Clinical Ophthalmology, Vol. 2: The Orbit. Hagerstown, Md., Harper & Row, 1979, Ch. 31.

75. Grove, A. S., Jr.: Giant dermoid cysts of the orbit. Ophthalmology, 86:1513, 1979.

76. Mandelcorn, M. S., Merin, S., Cardarelli, J.: Goldenhar's syndrome and phocomelia. Am. J. Ophthalmol., 72:618, 1971.

77. Paris, G. L., Beard, C.: Blepharoptosis following dermolipoma surgery. Ann. Ophthalmol., 5:697, 1973.

78. Watters, E. C., Wallar, P. H., Hiles, D. A., Michaels, R. H.: Acute orbital cellulitis. Arch. Ophthalmol., 94:785, 1976.

79. Weiss, A., Friendly, D., Eglin, K., et al.: Bacterial periorbital and orbital cellulitis in childhood. Ophthalmology, 90:195, 1983.

80. Bergin, D. J., Wright, J. E.: Orbital cellulitis. Br. J. Ophthalmol., 70:174, 1986.

81. Krohel, G., Krauss, H. R., Winnick, J.: Orbital abscess. Presentation, diagnosis, therapy, and sequelae. Ophthalmology, 89:492, 1982.

82. Bullock, J. D., Jampol, L. M., Fezza, A. J.: Two cases of orbital phycomycosis with recovery. Am. J. Ophthalmol., 78:811, 1974.

83. Ferry, A. P., Abedi, S.: Diagnosis and management of rhinoorbitocerebral mucormycosis (phycomycosis). A report of 16 personally observed cases. Ophthalmology, 90:1096, 1983.

84. Knowles, D. M., II, Jakobiec, F. A., Jones, I. S.: Rhabdomyosarcoma. In Duane, T. D. (ed.): Clinical Ophthalmology, Vol. 2: The Orbit. Hagerstown, Md., Harper & Row, 1979, Ch. 43.

85. Abramson, D. H., Ellsworth, R. M., Tretter, P., et al.: The treatment of orbital rhabdomyosarcoma with irradiation and chemotherapy. Ophthalmology, 86:1330, 1979.

86. Fort, R. L., Ferry, A. P.: The phakomatoses. Int. Ophthalmol. Clin., 12(1):1, 1972.

87. Drummond, J. W., Hall, D. L., Steen, W. H., Jr., Maxey, S. A.: Granular cell tumor (myoblastoma) or the orbit. Arch. Ophthalmol., 97:1492, 1979.

88. Spoor, T. C., Kennerdell, J. S., Martinez, A. J., Zorub, D.: Malignant gliomas of the optic nerve pathways. Am. J. Ophthalmol., 89:284, 1980.

89. Stern, J., Jakobiec, F. A., Housepian, E. M.: The architecture of optic nerve gliomas with and without neurofibromatosis. Arch. Ophthalmol., 98:505, 1980.

90. Miller, N. R., Iliff, W. J., Green, W. R.: Evaluation and management of gliomas of the anterior visual pathways. Brain, 97:743, 1974.

91. Housepian, E. M.: Surgical treatment of unilateral optic nerve gliomas. J. Neurosurg., 31:604, 1969.

92. Hoyt, W. F., Baghdassarian, S. A.: Optic glioma of childhood: Natural history and rationale for conservative management. Br. J. Ophthalmol., 53:793, 1969.

93. Converse, J. M.: Surgical Treatment of Facial Injuries, Vol. 1, 3rd ed. Baltimore, Williams & Wilkins, 1974.

94. Converse, J. M., Smith, B.: On the treatment of blow-out fractures of the orbit. Plastic Reconstr. Surg., 62:100, 1978.

95. Koornneff, L.: Orbital septa: Anatomy and function. Ophthalmology, 86:876, 1979.

96. Berke, R. N.: A modified Krönlein operation. Arch. Ophthalmol., 51:609, 1954.

97. Leone, C. R., Jr.: Surgical approaches to the orbit. Ophthalmology, 86:930, 1979.

98. McCord, C. D., Jr.: A combined lateral and medial orbitotomy for exposure of the optic nerve and orbital apex. Ophthalmic Surg., 9:58, 1978.

99. Sevel, D.: Lateral orbitotomy. Ophthalmic Surg., 10:29, 1979.

100. Smith, B.: The anterior surgical approach to orbital tumors. Trans. Am. Acad. Ophthalmol. Otolaryngol., 70:607, 1966.

101. Stallard, H. B.: A plea for lateral orbitotomy with certain modifications. Br. J. Ophthalmol., 44:718, 1960.

102. Kennerdell, J. R., Maroon, J. C.: Microsurgical approach to intraorbital tumors. Arch. Ophthalmol., 94:133, 1976.

16

PLASTIC SURGERY

by Charles R. Leone, Jr.

INTRODUCTION

General Principles

Ophthalmic plastic surgery involves the repair and reconstruction of the structures surrounding the eye, specifically the eyelids and orbit. A pleasing cosmetic appearance is a desired goal. More important, however, is restoration of function. Little is gained, for example, from surgery that results in an eyelid that looks pleasing but does not adequately protect the eye or assist in lacrimal function. Knowledge of basic plastic surgery principles is necessary to utilize optimally the techniques necessary to achieve the most satisfactory function.[1, 2]

In the region of the eyelids and orbit the tissues are thin and delicate. One must therefore keep in mind that gentle surgical technique tends to minimize postoperative reaction and thus helps to ensure a good result. Instruments should be applied as infrequently as possible and care taken to avoid crushing of tissue. Cautery should be used judiciously, particularly near the skin edges, since necrosis can occur. The bipolar cautery is a useful hemostatic instrument, since it functions in a wet field and the patient need not be grounded. On the other hand, the electrocautery applied to microforceps can effectively achieve hemostasis with a minimum of secondary tissue reaction. The electrocautery can also be used as an effective cutting instrument in the thicker skin of the periorbital area with the appropriate blending of the cutting and coagulation modes.

During surgery in the orbital area the eye should be protected, to prevent corneal abrasions or the even more serious trauma that can be caused by heavy instruments, such as the drills used for lacrimal and orbital surgery, which can inadvertently brush the eye. This protection is accomplished with thin, opaque methyl methacrylate scleral shells. If unilateral surgery is being done, it is wise to tape the opposite eye closed, to prevent its slipping open with movement of the overlying drapes. After mucous membrane grafting to reconstruct cul-de-sacs, scleral lenses with the central corneal portion removed help to maintain the fornices during the postoperative period.

Skin grafts are commonly used in ophthalmic plastic surgery. Both free grafts and those that carry their own circulation are used. A free graft may be either full thickness (including epidermis and dermis) or split thickness (mainly epidermis). Split-thickness grafts do not require surgical closure of the donor site. Grafts devoid of epidermis are termed dermal grafts. When attached to the underlying fat these are known as dermal-fat grafts. Fat, when transplanted by itself, tends to absorb and, consequently, is seldom used. The various types of flaps are sliding, advancement, rotational, transpositional, and pedicle. A *sliding flap* is created by simple undermining of the tissue adjacent to the defect. An *advancement flap* is similar, with the exception that parallel incisions on either side of the flap are extended for the purpose of relaxation and elongation of the flap. *Rotational flaps* are constructed by extending the incision along one edge in the design of an arc of a circle. *Transpositional flaps* differ from advancement flaps in that the distal portion is released from the base and then transposed across normal tissue to a recipient bed. A pedicle graft is similar but does not cross normal tissue. These donor areas are closed directly or covered by free graft.

In the orbital area, skin graft necrosis is infrequent, since the circulation is plentiful. Free grafts fuse rapidly to the recipient bed and create less peripheral deformity than is seen with local flaps. However, free grafts tend to contract in an inverse proportion to their thickness. The same principle of contraction applies to mucous membrane grafts taken from the buccal area. Other tissues used in the orbital area are composite graft from the opposite eyelid, tarsus from the opposite lid, preserved sclera, and fascia lata. Grafts that carry their own circulation tend to contract less, and reduce the chance of a poor take.

When there is good subcutaneous support, surface sutures may be removed early. Buried absorbable sutures should be kept to a minimum, since they cause tissue reaction and may subsequently lead to a hypertrophic scar. Sutures left in place more than 7 days usually leave a suture mark and tend to produce suture tract epithelialization and suture line cysts; this is particularly true of silk. If such sutures are removed too early, an external support should be applied; otherwise, wound disruption could occur. Sterile tape strips are useful in this regard. Accurate apposition of skin is important, as invagination of skin edges can cause inclusion cysts because of the implanted surface epithelium. This is more common with continuous rather than interrupted suturing, since there is a tendency for rolling under of the skin edges.

In periorbital skin closure a minimum of buried suture should be used, augmented by subcuticular pullout Prolene or nylon sutures and interrupted surface sutures of the same material. The interrupted skin sutures can be removed within 5 days, and the subcuticular suture in 7 to 10 days. Silk is pleasant to use because of its ease of handling as compared with the wiry nature of Prolene; silk does, however, produce more tissue reaction than Prolene or nylon. Six-0 plain catgut suture is an ideal skin suture in children, since it does not need to be removed; it has also been satisfactory with adults.

Secondary surgery on scars and deformities should be delayed until the primary wound has softened and regained normal color. In some patients this takes 3 to 6 months; one would be wise to wait even longer. If surgery is attempted before the wound matures, a greater scar formation can result because of stimulation of further fibroblastic proliferation. Massage is not recommended for at least 6 weeks, as before that time the mechanical trauma can stimulate rather than lessen the scar. Steroid injection may be considered to reduce a hypertrophic scar, since it retards fibroblast accumulation. Triamcinolone, 40 mg/ml, mixed in an equal amount with lidocaine, is injected into the scar area. One must, however, be cautious about overtreating, since subcutaneous atrophy and depigmentation can occur, particularly in dark-skinned people.

Bandaging in the orbital area is done to protect against accidental manipulation of a fresh wound and to soak up ooze from the wound edges. Pressure dressings are avoided,

since the eye can be tamponaded between the tight dressing, and retrobulbar edema or hemorrhage with compromise of the ocular circulation (both venous and arterial) can occur. It is far better to tend carefully to bleeding points while the wound is open than to rely on postoperative pressure dressings to seal vessels.

In dressing the surgical area, wet saline eye pads may be placed over the orbit after an antibiotic ointment is spread over the incisions and globe. A dry eye pad is placed over the wet one, and plastic or paper tape is used to secure it to the check and forehead. Tincture of benzoin may be lightly applied to the skin to make the tape more adherent; this is especially helpful in cases of oily or moist skin. If the patient is monocular, or if bilateral surgery was done, eye pads with the centers removed are used.

Waking up from anesthesia into darkness is a frightening experience for the patient; thus bilateral dressings are avoided in young children. Adults should also be forewarned about the need for patches, so that they will be spared a period of frantic worry postoperatively.

The dressing is routinely removed the day after surgery, and can usually be left off after that. Wet saline pads can be applied during the day and at bedtime; in addition to providing a soothing effect, they help to prevent the patient's rubbing the operative area during sleep. This is particularly true in cases where exposure could be a problem and when manipulation of a newly grafted area is not desired. If protection only is desired, a malleable metal shield is worn during periods of sleep. In most situations the patient can, within a day or two, leave the dressing off and use sunglasses to cover the surgical area.

Choice of Anesthetic

Most adult oculoplastic procedures can be done under local anesthesia, and thus the hazards and complications of general anesthesia can be avoided. General anesthesia may be better from a practical standpoint for cases that require more than 1½ to 2 hours of surgery, since local anesthesia patients may become restless. Operations that involve the lacrimal system, fractures, decompression of the orbit, and the taking of mucous membrane grafts can usually be more easily done with general anesthesia, since deep local infiltration anesthesia would be necessary and the threat of aspiration in a sedated patient would be eliminated. However, our policy is to have an anesthesiologist monitor most local anesthesia patients, which allows for the titration of sedation to keep the patient comfortable, sleepy, and yet cooperative for even lengthy procedures or those that would generally call for general anesthesia. The exception is healthy people who are having cosmetic surgery.

The local anesthetic used is a mixture of 12 ml (60%) of 2% lidocaine with 1:100,000 epinephrine, 8 ml (40%) of bupivacaine 0.75% with 1:200,000 epinephrine, and 1500 units of hyaluronidase. In patients with hypertension or arrhythmias the epinephrine may be further diluted, injected slowly to determine response, or eliminated. The epinephrine aids in hemostasis if injected 10 to 15 minutes before incising the tissues; therefore, the patient is marked and injected before he is prepped. Hyaluronidase will help in dispersing the large bolus of local agent that could distort and thicken the tissues. Bupivacaine gives the added advantage of prolonging anesthetic effect for several hours. Even with general anesthesia, bupivacaine with epinephrine is usually injected in the operative area to reduce bleeding and prolong anesthesia.

Preparation of Patient

Because oculoplastic surgery almost always results in a change in the external appearance of the orbital area, it is mandatory to discuss in detail with the patient, and possibly a family member, what the problem is, how you plan to correct it, and the expected results. Many times the patient's expectations, particularly with cosmetic blepharoplasty, are not realistic, and it is incumbent on the surgeon to be frank about what the patient can anticipate, to avoid postoperative misunderstandings. Be sure the patient realizes that reconstructive surgery on, for instance, a congenitally ptotic lid will, if successful, result in a normal-appearing eyelid, but will not produce a normally functioning eyelid. Enumerating the possible complications and their approximate frequency is necessary so that the patient is fully informed before his making a decision on whether to undergo surgery. Make certain the patient clearly understands what you are saying, and always ask if he or she has any questions. Never assume that the patient understands what you are saying, despite your best efforts at an articulate, detailed explanation. All of this information can also be presented to the patient in written form, but it is still necessary to go over it verbally, to make certain the patient understands what he is reading.

Before admission or outpatient surgery it will allay patients' anxiety, particularly if it is their first admission, to explain the admission process and any preliminary procedures that they may undergo, such as the taking of blood, x-rays, and electrocardiogram. Inform patients of their time of surgery and when they may leave the room, and advise them of fluid and food restrictions. If they are outpatients, they must arrive at the center before the scheduled time of surgery. Let them know that the anesthesiologist will be monitoring their vital signs and tending to their sedation, and, if the operation is to be under local anesthesia, that they will feel the injection for a few seconds followed by complete numbness for the rest of the procedure. Mention that they may have some discomfort and nausea postoperatively, but that medication is ordered to keep them as comfortable as possible. Give them the feeling that you care about them and appreciate their anxiety, and that you will be available if they need you. On the day of admission review again with the patient the procedure you intend to do, the side or sides to be operated on, and the type of anesthesia. This is also the time to ask if there are any last-minute questions. Ideally, the patient and surgeon should feel that nothing has been left uncovered and that the patient, with the proper preparation, has developed confidence in his surgeon and is prepared for any eventuality.

ANATOMY

Complete familiarity with the anatomy of the orbit and eyelids is essential for proper performance of oculoplastic surgery.[3, 4] Having a thorough knowledge of the functional anatomy leads to an appreciation of how and why procedures work or do not work, and why complications occur or do not occur. Furthermore, this helps the surgeon to develop confidence in planning and executing surgical repairs.

In defining regions of the eyelid it is convenient to refer to the tarsal, septal, and orbital portions (Fig. 16–1). For example, the orbicularis over these areas is called the pretarsal, preseptal, and orbital orbicularis, respectively. The tarsal area is confined to the region overlying the tarsus, the septal area to the region overlying the orbital septum, and the orbital

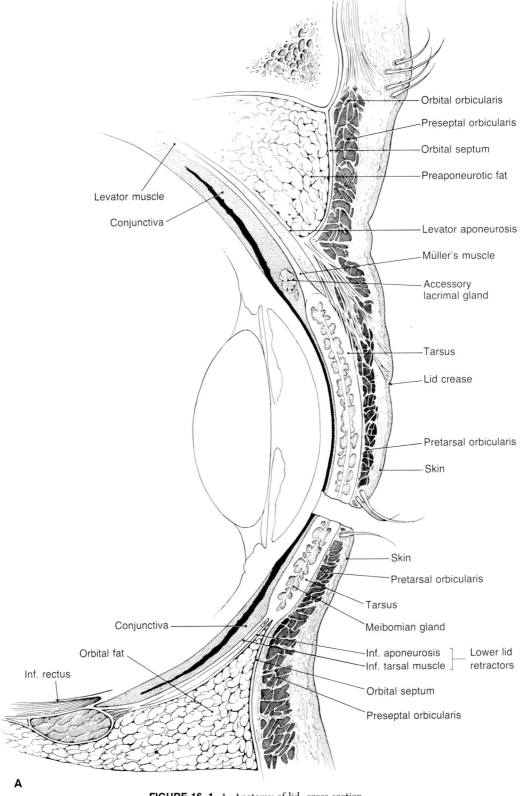

Orbital orbicularis

Preseptal orbicularis

Orbital septum

Preaponeurotic fat

Levator muscle

Conjunctiva

Levator aponeurosis

Müller's muscle

Accessory
lacrimal gland

Tarsus

Lid crease

Pretarsal orbicularis

Skin

Skin

Pretarsal orbicularis

Tarsus

Meibomian gland

Conjunctiva

Inf. aponeurosis ⎤ Lower lid
Inf. tarsal muscle ⎦ retractors

Orbital fat

Orbital septum

Inf. rectus

Preseptal orbicularis

A

FIGURE 16–1. *A*, Anatomy of lid, cross section.

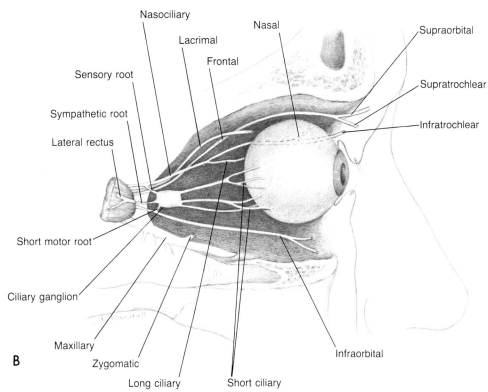

Nasociliary

Lacrimal

Frontal

Nasal

Supraorbital

Sensory root

Supratrochlear

Sympathetic root

Infratrochlear

Lateral rectus

Short motor root

Ciliary ganglion

Maxillary

Zygomatic

Long ciliary

Short ciliary

Infraorbital

B

FIGURE 16–1 *Continued B*, Nerves supplying orbital area.

area to the part that overlies the circumference of the bony rims. The meibomian glands are sebaceous glands within the tarsus, number approximately 25 in the upper and 20 in the lower, and empty through orifices at the posterior lid margin. There are more than 40 accessory lacrimal glands in the upper fornix and 10 in the lower fornix that account for the basic secretion of tears.

The tarsus in the lower lid is approximately 5 mm in vertical height, or roughly half that of the upper eyelid, which is 10 mm in the midline but curves to a somewhat smaller size on either side. The orbital septum is an extension of the periosteum of the inferior and superior orbital rims. It lies deep to the orbicularis, and fuses with the retractors of the eyelid near the tarsus. The orbital septum acts as a diaphragm, keeping the fat within the orbit. In the upper eyelid the preaponeurotic fat lies between the septum and the levator aponeurosis. Preseptal cellulitis refers to infection anterior to the septum, as opposed to the more serious orbital cellulitis that occurs deep to the septum.

In the upper eyelid the levator muscle originates from the annulus of Zinn and runs forward over the superior rectus muscle (Fig. 16–2). Before it emerges from under the rim the condensation of its sheath forms the superior transverse ligament (Whitnall's ligament). The muscle divides into the aponeurosis and superior tarsal muscle (Müller's muscle). The aponeurosis inserts into the tarsus and sends fibers to the skin, creating the lid crease. The superior tarsal muscle inserts at the superior border of the tarsus.

The medial and lateral horns are tendinous extensions from the aponeurosis and act as check ligaments. The medial horn passes above the sheath of the superior oblique tendon and fuses with the medial canthal tendon. The lateral horn divides the lacrimal gland into the orbital and palpebral lobes and attaches to the upper portion of the lateral canthal tendon.

The lower eyelid retractors emanate from the capsulopalpebral head of the inferior rectus muscle. The inferior aponeurosis and the inferior tarsal muscle beneath it make up the lower eyelid retractors, inserting into the lower tarsal border. These two structures are the counterparts of the levator aponeurosis and superior tarsal muscle in the upper eyelids.

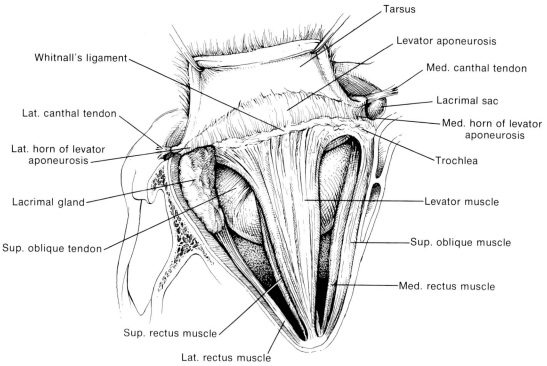

Tarsus

Levator aponeurosis

Med. canthal tendon

Lacrimal sac

Med. horn of levator aponeurosis

Trochlea

Levator muscle

Sup. oblique muscle

Med. rectus muscle

Whitnall's ligament

Lat. canthal tendon

Lat. horn of levator aponeurosis

Lacrimal gland

Sup. oblique tendon

Sup. rectus muscle

Lat. rectus muscle

FIGURE 16–2. Anatomy of lid, viewed from above.

BASIC TECHNIQUE OF EYELID MARGIN CLOSURE

Proper apposition of the tarsus, and to a lesser extent the orbicularis muscle, is an important element in allowing the margin of the lid to heal without notching. The following technique is designed to produce an optimal cosmetic and functional approach.

Standard Three-Layer Closure of Full-Thickness Eyelid

Technique (Fig. 16–3)

A. The three-suture technique is used in the lid margin. A 6-0 silk suture is placed through the gray line and just anterior and posterior to the lash line. Together, these untied sutures are placed on moderate traction to facilitate the placement of the tarsal sutures.

B. Conjunctiva and tarsus are approximated with 6-0 chromic catgut to the lid margin. The bites are taken through the tarsus, to avoid exposing the sutures to the cornea.

C. The orbicularis is approximated with interrupted 6-0 plain catgut where gaps exist.

D. The skin is closed with interrupted 6-0 silk.

E. The margin sutures are tied with the ends brought anteriorly and tied to one of the lower skin sutures, so that they are kept away from the globe.

Proper apposition of all layers in the eyelids is an important element in allowing the margin to heal without notching.

DERMATOCHALASIS, FAT HERNIATION

Dermatochalasis refers to a redundancy in the skin of the eyelid.[5] Usually associated with the aging process, it is occasionally found in younger people in whom there is a familial tendency. If a weakness or thinning develops in the orbital septum, the orbital fat protrudes, causing pouches or "bags" that are usually seen in the medial aspect of the upper lid and across the entire lower lid. In the lower lids the condition is more bothersome from a cosmetic standpoint; furthermore, it can cause difficulty with spectacle frames if the pouches abut against the inner part of the frame.

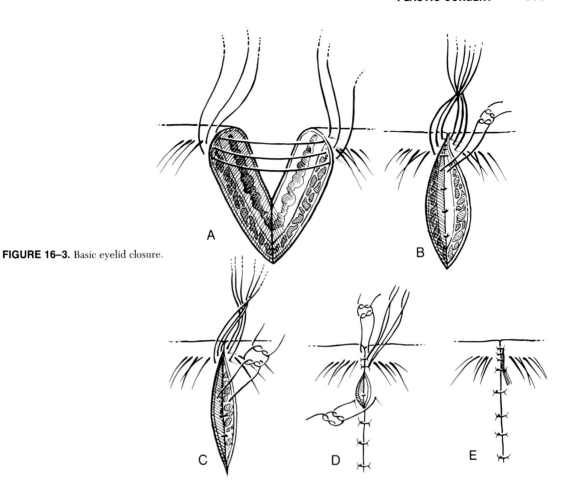

FIGURE 16–3. Basic eyelid closure.

True blepharochalasis is rare and refers to chronic lymphedema of the eyelids. It can be seen at any age, although it occurs more frequently in young females.

The excessive skin of dermatochalasis may hang in a fold over the anterior aspect of the upper lid or may even create a visor effect that reduces the upper and temporal visual field. It may be necessary for the patient to raise his eyebrows in order to have a full field of vsion. Common complaints include a feeling of pressure around the eyes, or a browache because of excessive frontalis and levator muscle action. In severe cases the lashes may be pushed into the visual axis and the patient may feel as if he is looking through a grid. Some women find that the extra skin fold prevents them from wearing eye shadow or using eye liner.

Every patient for a blepharoplasty should have a complete ophthalmologic examination, including visual field testing if necessary.[6] Estimation of tear function is advisable in older people; many have decreased lacrimal secretion and borderline keratitis sicca that may be ag-

gravated by removing the protective folds of skin. Lack of tonicity of the lower lids should alert the surgeon to the possibility of including a full-thickness horizontal shortening to avoid producing an ectropion. The position of the eyebrows may, in some cases, be excessively low, and may be largely responsible for creating a droopy lid appearance. If this is the case, the brows may need to be elevated. The upper eyelid crease must be noted; if a higher one is desired, and this is particularly true with women, supratarsal fixation will be required.[7] It is necessary to discuss with patients the anticipated result, to avoid their having expectations that are impossible to satisfy.

Preoperatively, if excessive skin is present in the medial canthal area, the surgery may need to be modified. A Z-plasty can be done in severe cases, or simply a triangular resection of skin in the upper medial canthal area in less severe situations. Ordinarily fixating the skin to the deeper tissues flattens out the area. Removing a large amount of skin may create an epicanthal fold that will require a Z-plasty postoperatively.

Relaxation of the brow area and frontalis muscle because of aging or 7th nerve palsy creates an overhang of the eyebrow. In evaluating a patient for blepharoplasty it is important to notice whether this has occurred, since, if it has, blepharoplasty alone may not provide a satisfactory result.[8] If the droop is severe, it can interfere with central vision because of brow hairs that appear in the visual axis; furthermore, it can significantly impair the visual field.

Blepharoplasty

Technique (Fig. 16–4)

A. A line is drawn in the upper eyelid crease, or where the crease across the eyelid is desired should a definite one not be present. Medially, the line is not carried beyond the level of the punctum. At the lateral canthus the line is gently curved upward for about 1 cm.

B. To estimate the amount of skin that can be removed, the lid skin is gently pinched with smooth forceps between the crease line and the brow. When the lashes begin turning upward, the amount of skin within the forceps can usually be safely removed; the upper limit of this folded skin is marked and the maneuver repeated across the eyelid. These marks are joined, forming the upper limit of the ellipse of skin to be removed.

C. After the upper lid is injected with the local anesthetic incisions are made in the marked area. The skin and orbicularis are removed, exposing the orbital septum, and bleeding points in the orbicularis are cauterized.

D. Pressure on the globe aids in identifying the septum, as the fat can be seen protruding forward.

E. The septum is cut completely across, exposing the preaponeurotic fat and the levator aponeurosis below.

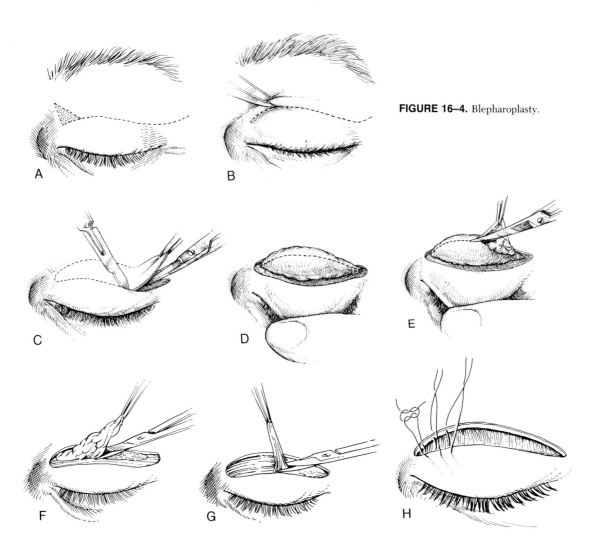

FIGURE 16–4. Blepharoplasty.

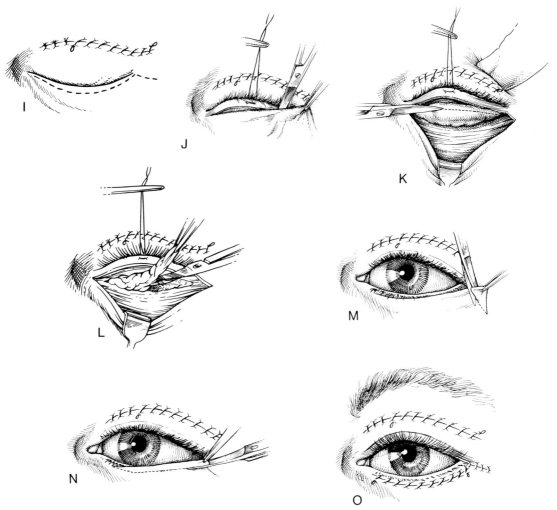

FIGURE 16–4 *Continued*

F. The intimate envelope surrounding the fat is cut, and the bare fat lobules are gently grasped and separated from the levator aponeurosis. The fat is gently lifted out of the wound and only that which protrudes beyond the superior rim is cut. This is followed by cauterization of the fat lobules with the bipolar cautery. The fat is spread on wet gauze to guide a similar fat removal on the other side.

G. (Optional) If a more definite crease is desired, a 3-mm wide horizontal strip of orbicularis is removed just above the tarsus, exposing the levator aponeurosis.

H. Medially, three interrupted sutures of 6-0 plain catgut are placed from the lower skin edge through the upper border of the tarsus or aponeurosis and then through the upper skin edge. This is done to flatten the skin and reduce the possibility of bulging.

I. Ordinarily, a continuous 6-0 Prolene suture is used to close the incision. A small suture loop is made medially instead of trying the suture to the skin to facilitate removal. Before closing, the same procedure is carried out on the other side. There should be an accurate assessment of hemostasis; all bleeding must have stopped completely before the skin is closed.

In the lower lid a line is drawn 2 mm below the lash line from the punctum to the lateral canthus, where it is angled 45 degrees downward for 0.5 to 1.0 cm.

J. The lower lids are treated consecutively as well, to match the amount done. A suture of 6-0 silk is placed through the lower lid margin to put the lid on stretch. An incision is made in the previously placed mark, and a thin skin-muscle flap is raised to the inferior orbital rim.

K. Posterior pressure on the globe will indicate the location of the herniated fat, and the orbital septum is cut completely across the lid.

L. The lobules are gently separated from

their fascial envelopes, lifted outward, and removed in the previously described manner. This maneuver is repeated across the lid until, with gentle pressure on the globe, no further fat protrudes. The same procedure is carried out on the other side, followed by inspection for any persistent bleeding.

M. The silk retraction suture is removed and the skin is smoothed over the lower lid and pulled laterally, allowing the redundancy to cover the lid margin in the lateral canthal area. With slight tension laterally, the redundant skin, which usually measures from 5 to 10 mm, is removed horizontally in line with the oblique incision.

N. The patient is asked to look up and open his mouth, to exaggerate the tension of the lower lids. The amount removed vertically is between 2 and 4 mm at the lateral canthal area, decreasing to zero as it approaches the medial aspect of the eyelid. Occasionally horizontal shortening of the skin is all that is necessary or safe to do.

O. The oblique incision is closed first with interrupted sutures, followed by the horizontal incision, using continuous 6-0 Prolene.

Antibiotic ointment is liberally placed over the globe and the incisions, and wet saline pads with the centers removed are lightly placed over each eye. The patient is kept in an elevated position and returned to the room. The eye pads are removed the next morning. The sutures are removed in 5 or 6 days.

Modifications of Blepharoplasty

1. *Excessive skin in the medial canthus.* If excessive skin is present in the medial canthal area, one of the following procedures may be done.

A. In Figure 16–4A a triangle of upper eyelid skin is removed in the medial aspect of the upper eyelid in order to tighten the loose skin in the medial canthal area. The base of the triangle, which is usually no more than 1 cm, is near the upper eyelid crease, and the other arms are 2 to 3 mm longer in the direction of the medial aspect of the eyebrow.

B. A Z-plasty (see Fig. 16–5) can be done by making an incision along the crest of the fold. Two incisions at either end are made in opposite directions 60 degrees from the original incision. The flaps are raised, transposed, and sutured with 6-0 silk or Prolene. It may be wise to use two small Z-plasties rather than one large one, to avoid a longer and more obvious scar line.

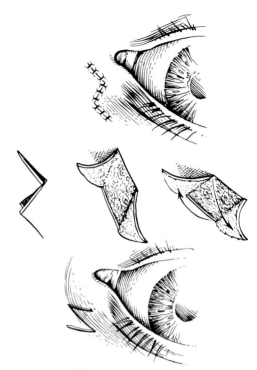

FIGURE 16–5. Z-plasty.

C. Fixating the skin to the deep tissues in the medial aspect of the incision will flatten the area (Fig. 16–4H).

2. *Formation of an upper eyelid crease.* Formation of an eyelid crease may be necessary in cases in which the upper eyelid crease has been lost as a result of surgery or trauma; this is due to lack of attachment of the skin to the levator aponeurosis. For the same reason the Oriental eyelid has a very low crease, or none at all. Supratarsal fixation with or without skin excision (Fig. 16–4H) is an effective method for forming an upper eyelid crease.

3. *Fornix approach to lower eyelid fat.* Approaching herniated fat through the inferior fornix has the advantage of avoiding a skin incision with its attendant potential problems.[9] However, this "back door" approach is more tedious because of the cramped space of the inferior cul-de-sac. Patients who are candidates for this procedure have fairly tight skin, such as younger patients whose primary problem is herniated fat.

Technique (Fig. 16–6)

A. A small canthotomy is made.

B. The skin is separated anteriorly, the conjunctiva posteriorly on either side of the lower arm of the canthal tendon, and the lower arm of the canthal tendon is cut.

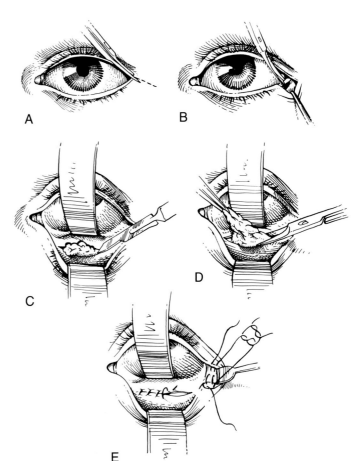

FIGURE 16–6. Fornix approach to lower eyelid fat.

C. The conjunctiva is stretched with two ribbon retractors over the inferior orbital rim, and an incision is made across the fornix through retractors of the lower eyelid.

D. The fat encountered between the lower lid retractors and septum is gently teased loose. It is then cut and cauterized. The procedure is done "simultaneously" on both sides to achieve symmetry.

E. The conjunctiva is closed with a continuous suture of 6-0 plain catgut, and the canthal tendon is reattached with 5-0 chromic catgut.

The inferior oblique muscle may be exposed at its origin at the posterior lacrimal crest; it is necessary to recognize this to avoid inadvertent injury. The canthus must be adequately re-established to re-form a sharp canthal angle. It is helpful to expose the fat on each side before cutting it in order to remove a proper amount to achieve the desired symmetry.

Complications of Blepharoplasty

The most common complication is undercorrection, which, although disappointing, can be remedied by another operation if the patient desires. Overcorrection can be a serious problem, jeopardizing the integrity of the eye and necessitating reparative surgery. In the upper eyelids overcorrection is a rare but troublesome problem, causing lagophthalmos and exposure keratopathy. Vertical shortening and ectropion of the lower lids is a not uncommon error that is sometimes caused by the surgeon's effort to achieve a perfect result. Vertical shortening can occur without removing skin and is due to a contraction of the orbital septum–lower lid retractor complex. This may occur from excessive cautery adjacent to the retractors. The proper and safe treatment of the lower lids demands accurate calculations and a conservative attitude; it is better to leave too much skin rather than too little. Immediate overcorrection of the lower eyelids should be treated conservatively, since many lids will loosen and return to a satisfactory position against the globe. If the condition persists for several months, it may be rectified, in mild cases, by releasing the vertical traction by horizontal shortening or lateral canthal sling. In severe cases skin grafting will be necessary.

Ptosis may occur postoperatively as a result

of injury to the levator aponeurosis. If supratarsal fixation is placed too far above the tarsus, it can compromise the lifting advantage of the levator. This is usually only a temporary problem.

Suture line cysts can occur. As mentioned in the introduction, these are usually the result of epithelialization of the suture tract caused by leaving the sutures in place for longer than 7 days. It can also occur as a result of invagination of the skin edges and implanted epithelium. This may be avoided by careful placement of interrupted sutures. Irregularity or bumpiness in a suture line is more common in the upper lid, but usually smoothes out within 2 to 3 months. If it remains and is a problem to the patient, local excision can be done.

In a poll of 3000 surgeons doing blepharoplasties, DeMere and associates found the incidence of blindness to be 0.04 per cent, or 1 in 2500.[10] Although this would be considered a rare complication, it is clearly a disastrous one. The surgeon must be aware of the possible pitfalls leading to this tragedy, the basic cause of which is a compromised ocular circulation, usually owing to raised intraorbital pressure after bleeding.[11] This is the reason for carefully cauterizing the fat that is returned to the orbit. Excessive pulling on the fat can also tear one of the deep vessels attached to the fat septae that would either bleed into the retrobulbar space or possibly affect nutritional supply to the optic nerve. Prolonged pressure on the globe should also be avoided, since this could retard circulation. Sometimes such pressure is inadvertently applied during the surgery, or it may result from excessively tight patching postoperatively.

If a patient complains of unusual pain or poor vision in the immediate postoperative period, prompt examination should be carried out.[12] If proptosis and an increase in intraocular pressure are present, immediate reduction of intraocular and intraorbital pressure is necessary. If a lateral canthotomy does not accomplish this virtually immediately, more extensive surgery may be required. While the patient is being readied for this, the intraocular pressure can be temporarily lowered by intravenous mannitol and acetazolamide, and topical timolol. Intravenous steroids (dexamethasone) will aid in reducing the edema. As a last resort, an anterior chamber tap could be done. If necessary, further decompression of the orbit should be carried out by widely opening the incision, evacuating the clots, and searching for and coagulating bleeding points.

DEEP UPPER EYELID SULCUS[13]

A deep upper eyelid sulcus associated with enophthalmos is often the result of fracture or an enucleation. Surgical attempts to fill the defect by bringing the globe or prosthesis forward are difficult. In the case of the seeing eye, the globe can be raised vertically, but medial or lateral implants are required to bring it forward. Further, the hazard of retrobulbar implants must be recalled. In the anophthalmic socket numerous attempts at secondary implants may still leave a recess in the upper eyelid.

A sulcus in a normal orbit can result from a higher crease of congenital, acquired, or iatrogenic origin. Most cases we have seen follow blepharoplasty with asymmetric supratarsal fixation or trauma.

Dermal-Fat Graft

A dermal-fat graft from the left lower abdominal quadrant and implanted into the preaponeurotic space of the upper lid can fill out the deep sulcus. It also serves as a barrier in those cases in which the crease is fixated at a higher level, allowing a lowering of the crease and filling out of the superior sulcus.

Technique (Fig. 16–7)

A. An incision is made in the proposed upper eyelid crease.

B. Dissection is carried superiorly, creating a plane between the skin-orbicularis layer and the orbital septum. The orbital septum is incised horizontally, superior to its attachment to the levator aponeurosis. The preaponeurotic fat is identified with the levator aponeurosis directly underneath.

C. The autogenous dermal-fat graft is excised from the region just superior to the iliac crest, preferably on the left side to avoid confusion with an appendectomy scar on the right side. An oblique elliptical incision is made 3 to 4 cm horizontally and 1 to 2 cm vertically and carried into the subcutaneous fatty tissue. The donor area is closed with deep interrupted 4-0 chromic catgut sutures, and the skin closed with 4-0 Prolene. A nonadherent absorbent dressing is placed over the incision followed by an elastic dressing.

D. The graft is stabilized with heavy forceps at either end; the epidermis is removed with a #15 Bard-Parker blade, using a sawing motion.

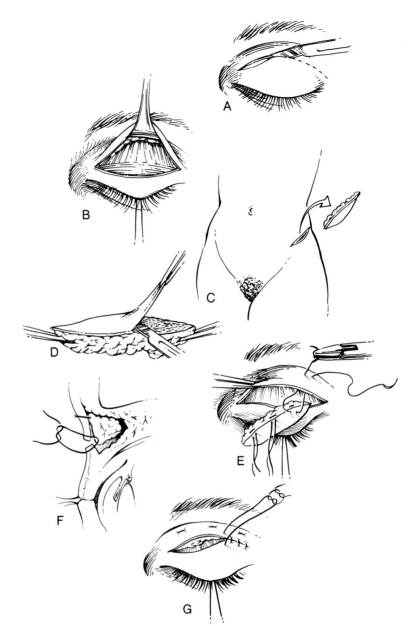

FIGURE 16–7. Dermal-fat graft.

E. The graft is then transported to the supra-tarsal area and trimmed to fit the defect, allowing for a slight over-correction. Three double-armed 6-0 Prolene sutures are placed first through the dermis on one side of the graft and then through the skin-orbicularis layer above the incision line and superior enough so that the lower edge of the graft meets the inferior edge of the incision.

F, G. The fat is tucked into the preaponeurotic space. Interrupted sutures of 6-0 Prolene are placed between the lower skin edges to incorporate the inferior edge of the dermis-fat

graft. The lid sutures are removed in 5 to 7 days, and the sutures from the donor site in 10 days.

BROW PTOSIS

Browplasty

If ptosis of the eyebrows is present, a browplasty is done. This procedure is usually performed in older people whose aging face shows a drop in the forehead, especially in the outer area of the brows. Younger people have probably had low-set brows all their lives and lifting their brows would change their normal appearance; a conservative blepharoplasty would probably be all that was needed to restore their more youthful appearance.

The direct brow lift leaves a scar above the brow that can usually be concealed with makeup if it is prominent. If a scar line would be undesirable and the patient wants the whole forehead to be lifted, a coronal lift would be more appropriate.[14]

Technique (Fig. 16–8)

A. An ellipse of skin and subcutaneous tissue to the deep fascia is removed just above the brow. The lower incision is placed adjacent to the hairs. The ellipse may be made larger laterally to create a more pleasing cosmetic effect. If one side is ptotic owing to a seventh nerve palsy, a desired level against the normal side should be determined with the patient in the upright position. When both brows are being elevated, a 7- to 10-mm excision is usually made.

B. In cases of seventh nerve paralysis sutures

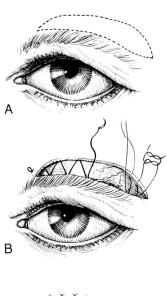

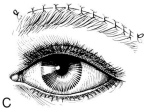

FIGURE 16–8. Browplasty.

of 5-0 Prolene are placed from the deep brow tissue to a deep frontalis fascia in order to fixate and suspend the tissue. To evaluate the position of the brow, they are tied with slip knots before being tied permanently. In a purely cosmetic brow lift it is not necessary to deeply fixate the tissues.

C. The subcutaneous tissue is approximated with a pull-out 4-0 Prolene suture and the skin with interrupted 6-0 Prolene.

ESSENTIAL BLEPHAROSPASM

Essential blepharospasm is characterized by involuntary spasms of the orbicularis muscle. These are usually bilateral, and range in intensity from mild twitches to forceful contractions. Afflicted patients are frequently quite miserable and may even be rendered virtually blind. Other muscles of the face are often involved as well. The cause is obscure.

Essential blepharospasm should be differentiated from hemifacial spasm, which is characteristically unilateral. Though hemifacial spasm occasionally becomes bilateral, it differs from essential blepharospasm by unsynchronous twitching of both sides. Thought to be due to vascular compression of the 7th nerve near the brain stem, hemifacial spasm responds to neurosurgical intervention.[15]

Essential blepharospasm should not be confused with the periodic blinking that is a rather common ocular complaint. Repeated blinking of the eyelids may be a manifestation of external ocular disease, but most frequently it is a reflection of an emotional problem. Recognition of the purely functional nature of the condition and proper counseling are often highly effective in correcting the difficulty.

In mild cases muscle relaxants or neurotropic drugs may provide temporary relief; however, when blepharospasm is so persistent and severe that it interferes with the affected person's life, the initial form of therapy is the periocular injection of botulinum A toxin.[16] This drug selectively binds motor-nerve terminals (end plates) and blocks the release of acetylcholine. The toxin is mixed to a concentration of 2.5 to 5.0 units per 0.1 ml in a tuberculin syringe. The injection sites are the medial and lateral aspects of both upper and lower eyelids in the pretarsal space, as well as the medial brow, to weaken the procerus and corrugator muscles. Initially 2.5 units are injected at each site. The onset of orbicularis weakness generally occurs within 2 to 5 days and reaches a maximum at 10 to 12 days. A beneficial effect may last for 8 to 12 weeks with a range between 2 weeks and 5 months.

No instances of systemic botulism have been reported. The local side effects are related to exposure keratopathy, making it necessary for patients to use ocular lubricants as needed. Repeated injections are given when the spasms return, and there has been no evidence of the development of immunity.

If the injections of botulinum A toxin are not totally successful, or if the patient is unhappy about the frequency of the injections needed to control the condition, surgery can be considered. Whereas differential section of the seventh nerve was a surgical procedure of choice in the past, myectomy of the orbicularis muscle, as well as the corrugator and procerus muscles of the brow, is preferred.[17]

Myectomy

Myectomy has the advantage of treating only the locally offending muscles; therefore, side effects are restricted to the orbital area. A combination of botulinum A toxin injections and orbicularis myectomy has given us the best results. The effect of the toxin is prolonged, since the number of myoneural end plates has been reduced.

Technique (Fig. 16–9)

The procedure is similar to a blepharoplasty except for the removal of the orbicularis muscle.

A. The initial marking line is placed in the upper eyelid crease, and the amount of excess skin is estimated. The incisions are made, and orbicularis muscle is included with the skin excision.

B. The skin is separated from the orbicularis

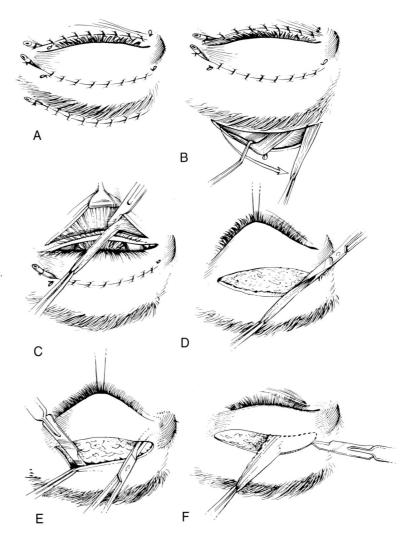

FIGURE 16–9. Myectomy.

above to the superior rim, and below to the lash line. Sometimes it is helpful to split the muscle from the skin with a #15 Bard-Parker blade.

C. The muscle is then excised from the medial to the lateral canthal area.

D. It is optional to do the lower lids; only the pretarsal orbicularis is removed to obviate any potential eyelid malposition.

E. It is optional to do the brow area. An incision is made across the brow just above the hairs followed by a parallel incision removing up to a 1-cm segment. The orbital portion of the orbicularis muscle is excised as well as the corrugator, which arises from the supraciliary ridge and passes laterally to the midbrow. The procerus is more difficult to expose because of its midline position, arising from the nasal bone and running upward into the forehead. Care must be taken to avoid injuring the supraorbital nerve.

F. The incisions are closed as described under blepharoplasty and browplasty. Bleeding is brisk because of the vascularity of the muscle; therefore, assiduous attention must be given to

hemostasis. Rubber-band drains or small silicone tubes, placed along the extent of the lid and exiting the most lateral incision, may be used and removed in 24 hours.

Differential Section of the Seventh Nerve

Because of the efficacy of botulinum A toxin with or without myectomy, differential section of the seventh nerve has limited usage. If it is to be considered, a facial nerve block will simulate the surgical result and aid the patient in making a decision regarding the surgery.

Technique (Fig. 16–10)

A. The procedure must be done under general anesthesia, since local anesthesia would preclude use of the nerve stimulator. An incision is made 2 cm in front of the area down to the parotid gland, through which the seventh nerve traverses. The tissue is gently separated with blunt dissection, permitting careful isolation of the distal branches of the nerve.

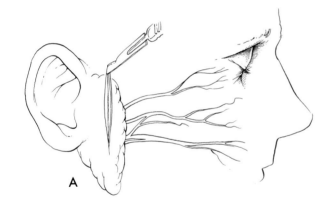

FIGURE 16–10. Blepharospasm repair.

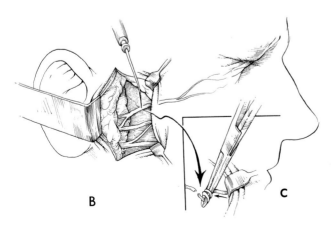

B. A nerve stimulator is used to identify the nerve branches and the muscle groups they supply. The plan is to section the branches that innervate the orbicularis oculi, and to avoid those that predominantly supply the other facial muscles.

C. The nerve branches are isolated as far distally as possible, transected, and wound around the tips of a hemostat. They are carefully avulsed. Care must be taken to avoid excessive trauma to the parotid gland or injury to Stenson's duct.

Unfortunately even this procedure does not promise permanent relief to all patients with essential blepharospasms; there is a 50 per cent recurrence rate of the blepharospasm within 2 years.[18]

After this operation all the problems related to seventh nerve palsy may occur: brow droop, ectropion, lagophthalmos, exposure keratopathy, and sagging of the mouth. These complications may not be permanent; if they are bothersome, secondary surgical repair can be carried out.

ENTROPION

Entropion is a turning in of the eyelid margin, which often causes the lashes to rub against the eye. Entropion should be differentiated from trichiasis, which refers to misdirected or aberrant lashes, and from distichiasis, which is a congenital accessory row of lashes emanating from the meibomian gland orifices. In both of these latter conditions the lid margin is in correct position.

Entropion has a variety of causes. In infants it can be caused by hypertrophy of the orbicularis muscle and, possibly, congenital malposition. The elderly can be affected as a result of involutional changes that alter the apposition of the eyelid to the globe. Cicatricial entropion is caused by shrinkage of the internal surface of the eyelid, forcing the lashes and margin against the eye; the underlying problem may be trauma, infection, or inflammation. Trichiasis may be an additional problem, especially in the cicatricial type of entropion. For cases in which the cornea is traumatized, prompt surgical correction is indicated.

Congenital Entropion, Epiblepharon

Congenital entropion is a rare condition associated with hypertrophy of the marginal and pretarsal orbicularis muscle and probable slippage of the lower eyelid retractors. A much more common condition is epiblepharon, which is due to a lack of skin fixation to the lower border of the tarsus where the lower lid retractors insert. A fold of skin based at the medial canthus is thus created, which is elevated against the lid and forces the lashes upward and against the globe, particularly in downward gaze. This situation is usually temporary and disappears as the facial structures enlarge. If it persists as the infant grows older, with irritation and staining of the cornea, surgical correction is indicated.[19]

Skin-Tarsal Fixation

Technique (Fig. 16–11)

A. A line is drawn 2 mm below the lash line, beginning lateral to the punctum and carried to the lateral canthus, or 5 mm beyond where the lashes are affected.

B. An incision is made below the lashes to

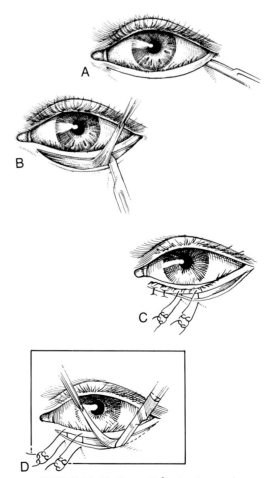

FIGURE 16–11. Congenital entropion repair.

the inferior border of the tarsus. The orbicularis over the tarsus is completely resected up to the margin.

C. Sutures of 6-0 plain catgut are placed first from the skin edge below the margin through the inferior border of the tarsus and then through the inferior skin edge, thus tacking the skin edges to the inferior border of the tarsus and rotating the eyelid margin outward. Several adjustments of the sutures may be necessary to obtain the correct eversion.

D. Rarely, it may be necessary to excise a 2-mm strip of skin in order to achieve a normal everted lash line.

Involutional Entropion

Internal Tarsal-Orbicularis Resection

When the canthal tendons retain their rigidity but the apposition of the lid to the globe is changed, the eyelid margin may turn inward. This is a frequent occurrence in the elderly, in whom atrophy of the orbital fat leads to enophthalmos. Moreover, there is often instability of the lower tarsus, which allows the orbicularis muscle to flip the lid inward. To unroll the eyelid and provide snug lid-globe apposition, we have found that tarsectomy with internal orbicularis resection,[20] combined with lid-bracing sutures, works well.

Technique (Fig. 16–12)

A. The eyelid is everted on a large chalazion clamp, and a triangle made in the tarsus, with the apex in the midline close to the lid margin and the base at the inferior aspect of the tarsus. The base is from 5 to 6 mm in length, depending on the severity of the entropion.

B. The section of tarsus is entirely removed, exposing the orbicularis muscle.

C. The orbicularis muscle is pulled up with forceps and completely incised.

D. A suture of 6-0 polyglactin 910 (Vicryl) is then placed through the cut ends of the pretarsal orbicularis, with both ends coming out inferiorly.

E. Sutures of 6-0 silk are then placed through

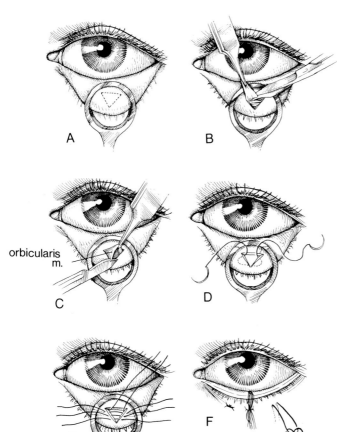

orbicularis m.

FIGURE 16–12. Internal tarsal-orbicularis resection.

the tarsal margins, and the chalazion clamp is removed.

F. The shortened orbicularis is approximated with the 6-0 Vicryl, stabilizing the tarsus against the globe. The silk sutures are then tied, with the ends left long and brought over the margin and tied to the skin. Lid-bracing sutures (see Fig. 17–11) of 5-0 chromic catgut can be added to augment the repair in severe entropion cases.

The overcorrected everted position lasts for several weeks and then gradually disappears. There is a small peak in the lid margin, which usually smooths out within 6 months.

Tucking of the Lower Eyelid Retractors

Jones and colleagues believe that involutional entropion is due to weakness of the retractors of the lower eyelid.[21] They have pointed out that when one is looking down, the lower lid should retract two-thirds the distance that the globe rotates. When this retraction fails to occur, because of the enophthalmos of old age as well as the attenuation of the retractor muscles, entropion develops. The tucking procedure is designed to restore the eyelid to a proper position.

Technique (Fig. 16–13)

A. A horizontal incision is made 5 mm below the lashes in the lateral two-thirds of the eyelid and taken down to the inferior tarsal border.

B. The lower eyelid retractors are exposed and are found overlying the conjunctiva of the inferior cul-de-sac. Sutures of 6-0 silk are placed first from the skin edge below the margin through the inferior tarsal border, catching the

retractors, then through the retractors again 5 to 8 mm inferiorly, and then through the inferior skin edge. Four or five of these sutures are so placed and then tied. If the eyelid margin is excessively pulled outward, the tuck should be reduced. When the patient is asked to look downward, the lid should move at least 4 mm.

One must be careful not to shorten the eyelid inadvertently; on the other hand, however, one should strive for a small overcorrection, which is usually apparent if the lid margin is no more than 1 mm away from the globe. In the immediate postoperative period a gross overcorrection can be remedied by removing a suture in the area of greatest traction.

Full-Thickness Horizontal Shortening at the Lateral Canthus

In situations in which there is extreme laxity in the entire lower lid associated with inversion of the eyelid margin, horizontal shortening is indicated. This occurs most often in elderly people who have a combination of sagging lids and entropion. Shortening the eyelid at the lateral canthus brings it up and against the globe and aids in restoring the eyelid margin to its proper position.

Technique (Fig. 16–14)

A. A 1.5-cm incision, angled toward the earlobe, is made at the lateral canthus.

B. The lid is pulled over the canthal angle to determine how much to resect to tighten the lid. Usually 4 to 7 mm is sufficient to bring the margin firmly against the globe.

C. Two sutures of 5-0 Vicryl are placed first in the tarsus and then through the remnant of

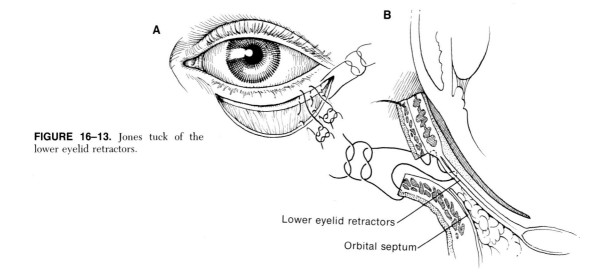

FIGURE 16–13. Jones tuck of the lower eyelid retractors.

Lower eyelid retractors

Orbital septum

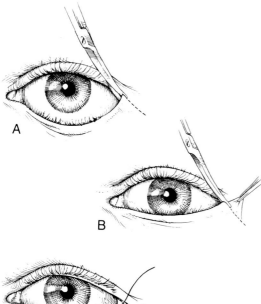

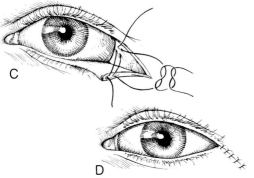

FIGURE 16–14. Full-thickness horizontal shortening at the lateral canthus for entropion.

the lateral canthal tendon near the rim and tied, resulting in a moderately overcorrected position.

D. The skin is closed with 6-0 silk.

Full-Thickness Horizontal Shortening Combined with Skin-Tarsal-Aponeurosis Approximation

In some cases of recurrent entropion a combination of procedures is necessary. A most effective combination is to shorten the eyelid horizontally at the lateral canthus and perform a skin-tarsal–inferior aponeurosis approximation. This brings the eyelid tightly against the globe with horizontal shortening, and braces the eyelid margin in an erect position with the skin-tarsal–inferior aponeurosis attachment.

Technique (Fig. 16–15)

A. A 1.5-cm incision, angled toward the earlobe, is made at the lateral canthus.

B. An incision is made 4 to 5 mm below the lash line across the lower lid, and the lower border of the tarsus is exposed as well as the anterior expansion of the inferior aponeurosis.

C. The lower lid is pulled across the canthus, and where it crosses the canthal angle the redundant portion is excised.

D. Sutures of 5-0 Vicryl are placed from the exposed tarsus to the remnant of the lateral canthal tendon and tied, achieving a firm position of the lid against the globe.

E. Absorbable 6-0 sutures are placed between the skin edges, catching the lower border of the tarsus and the anterior expansion of the inferior aponeurosis. This should result in a mildly overcorrected, everted position of the lid margin. The canthal incision is also closed with absorbable sutures.

Lid-Bracing Sutures

When transportation to the operating room is impractical, as with debilitated or nursing home patients, or for those who prefer not to have a surgical procedure, lid-bracing sutures can immediately correct an entropion and oftentimes produce a longlasting cure.[22] This procedure is also useful for those patients whose entropion has been activated by recent intraocular surgery. Here, a minimum of additional surgical trauma and irritation is advisable.

Technique (Fig. 16–16)

Double-armed sutures of 5-0 chromic catgut are brought from the inferior cul-de-sac through the pretarsal orbicularis and out below the lid margin. As a rule, three are placed and tied fairly tightly, causing an immediate eversion of the lid margin. The sutures produce enough inflammatory reaction to create a cicatrix that tends to keep the margin in position after absorption of the suture. However, with a severe degree of entropion, permanent correction should not be expected.

Cicatricial Entropion

This is caused by shrinkage of the tarsal conjunctival surface, which forces the lid margin and lashes against the globe. Its causes include trauma, chemical injuries (particularly lye burns), chronic infection, such as trachoma, and inflammations that include Stevens-Johnson syndrome and ocular pemphigoid. Correction of this deformity is aimed at mechanical rotation of the lid margin with and without mucous membrane–lined grafts.

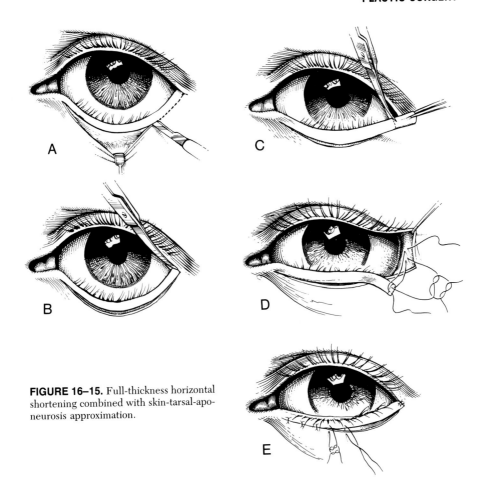

FIGURE 16–15. Full-thickness horizontal shortening combined with skin-tarsal-aponeurosis approximation.

Full-Thickness Transverse Tarsotomy with Marginal Rotation

This method fractures the tarsus and mechanically rotates the eyelid margin and lashes outward. It is similar to the one Wies described in 1955.[23]

Technique (Fig. 16–17)

A. A horizontal incision is made in the skin 3 mm from the lash line at least 5 mm on either side of the area involved, or, if the entire lid is affected, from the lateral canthus to a few millimeters lateral to the punctum. This is carried to the tarsus.

B. The eyelid is everted over a Desmarres retractor, and a separate incision made in the tarsus to prevent an irregular cut that may compromise the marginal artery.

C. The inner and outer incisions are then connected with scissors, and the lid margin is now virtually separated from the rest of the eyelid.

D. Three or four 6-0 double-armed sutures are placed from the cut border of the attracted tarsus through the pretarsal orbicularis of the detached portion to the lid margin, coming out near the cilia. The closer the sutures exit to the cilia, the greater the degree of eversion that will be obtained.

E. The sutures are tied over cotton pegs (rolled-up cotton measuring approximately 2 × 4 mm) to avoid excessive pressure on the margin. The cutaneous incision is closed with 6-0 silk. The marginal sutures are usually removed in 10 days; if a gross overcorrection is evident, the sutures are removed sooner.

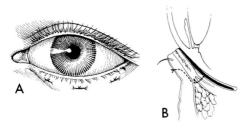

FIGURE 16–16. Lid-bracing sutures.

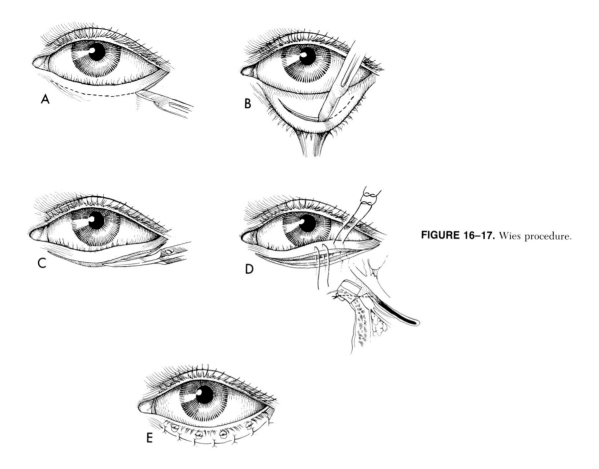

FIGURE 16–17. Wies procedure.

Partial-Thickness Transverse Tarsotomy with Marginal Rotation

This is preferable in cases in which the surgeon wants to minimize postoperative distortion in the contour of the lid margin. The procedure is especially suited for entropion of the upper lid.

Technique (Fig. 16–18)

A. With the eyelid everted over a Desmarres retractor, a horizontal incision 3 mm from the margin is made 5 mm beyond either side of the area involved.

B. Double-armed sutures of 5-0 chromic catgut are placed through the proximal tarsus away from the margin, to give a greater arc of rotation to the lid margin. The needle is then passed through the pretarsal orbicularis and then out near the anterior lid margin. Catching the pretarsal orbicularis with the needle augments the rolling-outward effect of the lid margin.

C. The sutures are tied over cotton pegs and removed in 7 to 10 days.

Free Tarsal-Conjunctival Graft

In cases of recurrent entropion after several surgical procedures, the tarsus has usually lost considerable substance. The placement of a tarsal graft in such cases will not only add support and stabilize the lid, but also give it vertical height and push the margin outward.[24] This is also suitable for frank cicatricial entropion that has produced shrinkage of the tarsus and rolling inward of the lid margin. The graft is usually taken from the ipsilateral upper lid; if an upper lid is involved, the graft can be taken from the opposite upper eyelid.

Technique (Fig. 16–19)

A. The eyelid is everted over a Desmarres retractor, and a horizontal incision made 2 mm below the margin across the length of the lid, separating the tissues from the orbicularis to create a bed. It is placed near the margin to force the margin up and outward.

B. The upper lid is then everted on a Desmarres retractor, and the graft taken from the

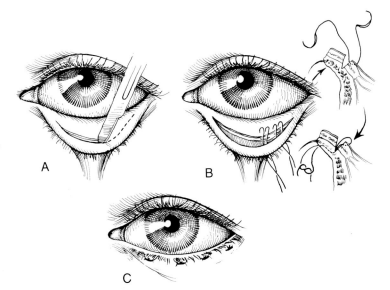

FIGURE 16–18. Partial Wies procedure.

midtarsal area; this is usually 2 to 3 mm wide. The tarsal defect is allowed to heal unsutured.

C. The graft is placed in the bed and sutured with continuous pull-out 6-0 Prolene sutures with the knots tied on the cutaneous surface.

D. Sutures of 6-0 double-armed silk are placed from the inferior cul-de-sac to below the lid margin and tied over silicone pegs (#40 silicone band). These keep the lid margin

braced in an everted position while the graft is healing. The Prolene pull-out sutures are removed in 1 week and the lid-bracing sutures in 2 weeks.

Recession of the Lid Margin with or without Mucous Membrane Graft

When there is marked scarring, as with trachoma or chronic tarsitis, or when there is

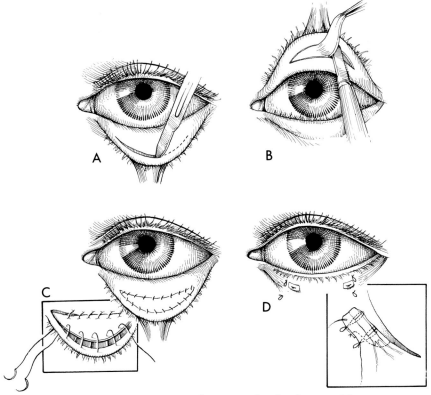

FIGURE 16–19. Free tarsal conjunctival graft to lower eyelid.

epidermalization of the conjunctiva near the lid margin, recessing the lid margin with or without mucous membrane grafting may be considered.[25] This procedure is used most often in treatment of the upper lid, but it can be used for the lower lid as well.

Technique (Fig. 16–20)

A. The eyelid is everted over a Desmarres retractor, and a horizontal incision is made the length of the eyelid just posterior to the lid margin.

B. The anterior aspect of the tarsus is exposed with the lid margin and skin recessed upward. It is stabilized in this position with through-and-through sutures of 4-0 silk tied over silicone pegs. The procedure can be terminated here, allowing the raw surfaces to epithelialize; it is preferable, however, to place a mucous membrane graft over the bare tarsal area.

C. To remove full-thickness mucous membrane, the lower lip is injected with lidocaine and epinephrine for hemostasis and with saline, if necessary, to give extra firmness, making it easier to cut. Towel clips can be placed at either end to evert the lip. The amount desired is outlined with a knife blade and then removed with sharp and blunt dissection. Full-thickness tissue is preferred to split-thickness, since the

shrinkage factor is less. An effort is made not to include the submucosal fat, since it must subsequently be removed before placing the graft in its bed. The raw donor bed is left open and covered with a wet saline sponge. The lip begins to heal in 3 to 4 days with a thin sheet of regenerating cells, and within several weeks it is completely healed.

D. The graft, one-third of which is left redundant to allow for shrinkage, is sutured to the tarsal edge with 6-0 silk and to the retracted lid marginal edge with interrupted 6-0 chromic catgut sutures. The silk sutures are removed in 7 days. Within 6 weeks the graft shrinks, pulling the retracted margin closer to the inferior edge. If it remains redundant after 3 months, the graft can be trimmed. It is necessary, however, to leave at least 2 mm of mucosa at the lid margin because of the ongoing nature of many of these cicatricial processes.

Distichiasis

Distichiasis is a rare anomaly consisting of an extra row of lashes along the posterior margin. The lash follicles emanate from the meibomian gland orifices. One or all four lids may be

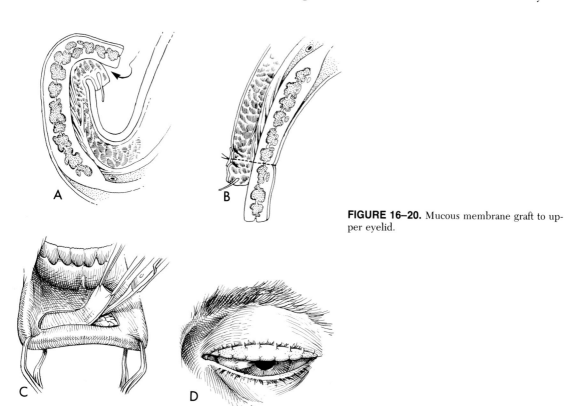

FIGURE 16–20. Mucous membrane graft to upper eyelid.

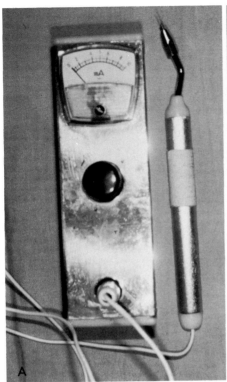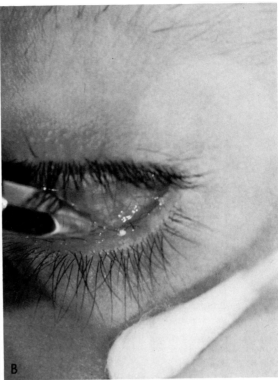

FIGURE 16–21. Electrolysis.

involved. Other members of the patient's family may be similarly affected. Many of these patients are photophobic and may even have corneal scarring.

Surgical remedies consist of electrolysis or resecting the posterior lid margin in association with mucous membrane grafting. This latter procedure may leave the margin irregular and beefy. Electrolysis, however, can destroy individual lash follicles and still leave the margin intact, and thus it is the preferred procedure.

Electrolysis

Technique (Fig. 16–21)

A. Electrolysis uses a galvanic current, requiring that the patient be grounded to the instrument to complete the circuit. We usually place the instrument against the patient's arm, with a thin coating of electrocardiographic conductive jelly against the back of the instrument. Any electrolysis unit is suitable, but it must have adjustable current that is just high enough to bring bubbles to the surface as the needle is positioned adjacent to the lash. The Prolectro instrument fulfills the above criterion.

B. The needle is directed along the lash into the root of the follicle. Power is turned on, and if bubbles come to the surface, the current is

sufficient. This is repeated with the needle brought out and then redirected a little differently along the lash until the lash can be wiped away or lifted out without resistance. All the lashes are removed similarly.

There are a few lashes that invariably grow back, and thus repeated procedures are necessary. However, there is little or no scarring on the lid margin.

Trichiasis

Trichiasis is an acquired condition in which aberrant lashes rub against the globe. In some cases the lashes emanate from the correct position on the lid margin but are misdirected posteriorly, whereas in others they may arise from anywhere on the lid margin, owing to distortion of the lash roots as a result of injury or chronic inflammation. Electrolysis (as described above) is one method used to eradicate a few individual lashes; however, in severe cases it is difficult to determine the direction of these distorted follicles to accurately guide the needle tip.

Cryotherapy[26] is a convenient and easily performed method for treating severe or recurrent trichiasis. Cryo instruments using nitrous oxide as a coolant, as used in retinal and cataract surgery, are suitable for this procedure.

Cryotherapy of Aberrant Lashes

Technique (Fig. 16–22)

A. The lash is marked every 5 mm within the area involved.

B. The retinal probe is placed on the lid margin and activated. The temperature on the instrument gauge must drop to its lowest reading ($-80°$ C) in order to deliver an effective freeze to the area. The probe is left in place for 2 minutes in regular-thickness lids (approximately 30 seconds less in thin lids and 30 seconds more in thick lids). The area is allowed to thaw while another freeze is delivered elsewhere, and then it is refrozen (freeze-thaw-refreeze technique).

The main complication from this procedure is recurrent lashes, which can be retreated in the same way. Because this procedure is not selective to single lashes, normal lashes can be destroyed as well. Depigmentation can also occur in dark-skinned patients. There can also be thinning of the lids from overfreezing. Most people are not concerned about these sequelae if they can obtain relief from this most annoying condition.

ECTROPION

Ectropion refers to an eversion of the eyelid margin. Aside from the rare entity of congenital ectropion, most ectropion conditions occur as a result of involutional changes that cause the canthal tendon to stretch and the lid tissue itself to become redundant. Paralytic ectropion, caused by seventh nerve paralysis, is due to a loss of orbicularis support and is aggravated by involutional changes already present. Cicatricial ectropion occurs at any age, and is due to a shortening of the external surface of the eyelid. The result of this poor eyelid apposition is tearing and exposure keratopathy. The basic surgical goal is to return the eyelid to its original position.

Patients for ectropion surgery should be reexamined before being put in a supine position on the operating table. The reason for this is that the lid may assume a more normal position when the patient is supine than when he is upright. Thus the surgeon may be misled at the time of the surgery unless he has rechecked the patient in the upright position.

Congenital Ectropion

Congenital ectropion is most often associated with Down's syndrome and consists of an elongation of the lid itself. Occasionally there is eversion of the upper eyelid with prolapse of the superior cul-de-sac; this may eventually right itself or it may require correction by temporary intermarginal sutures. Ectropion is also associated with a syndrome that includes blepharoptosis, blepharophimosis, epicanthus, and telecanthus. In these cases there frequently

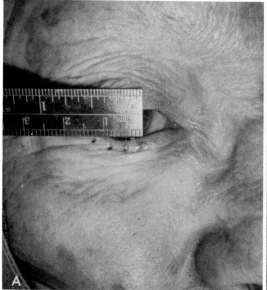
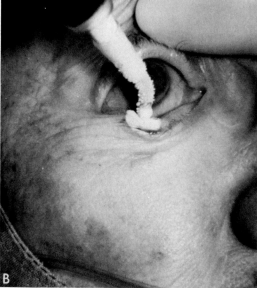

FIGURE 16–22. Cryotherapy.

is a deficit of skin in the lower lids and occasionally such a deficit in the upper lids. If closure is affected, or if keratopathy ensues, skin grafts are necessary.

Eversion of the Lacrimal Punctum

One of the most bothersome symptoms associated with ectropion is excessive tearing. This is caused by separation of the lacrimal punctum from the globe, owing to the external eversion of the lid. As ectropion progresses, the lid becomes more everted and the eye more chronically irritated because of conjunctival exposure. Though older people with eversion of the punctum are sometimes asymptomatic, owing to the diminution of tears that occurs with aging, if the patient is symptomatic and the punctum is out of the lacrimal lake, a tarsal-conjunctival resection may be indicated.

Tarsal-Conjunctival Resection Below the Lacrimal Punctum

Technique (Fig. 16–23)

A. The lid is everted, a probe is placed in the canaliculus as a precaution, and an ellipse of tarsus and conjunctiva is resected below the punctum. The resection usually measures 5 to 6 mm, divided into one-third on the medial and two-thirds on the lateral side of the punctum; the incision is 3 to 4 mm in a vertical direction.

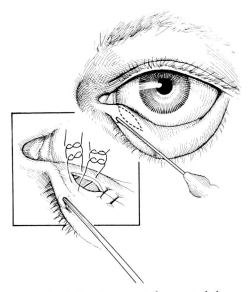

FIGURE 16–23. Tarsal-conjunctival resection below punctum.

B. The defect is closed with interrupted 6-0 plain catgut sutures, incorporating the anterior expansion of the lower lid retractors.

Medial Ectropion

If the lower arm of the medial canthal tendon has become stretched, the medial aspect of the eyelid everts. Moreover, involutional changes in the lid itself will cause it to lose its tone. When this occurs not only does the punctum need to be turned inward, but the redundant eyelid must be resected. The following procedure is modified from Byron Smith's description of the "lazy T" operation.[27]

"Lazy T" Procedure

Technique (Fig. 16–24)

A. A vertical incision is made into the inferior cul-de-sac in the eyelid, 5 mm lateral to the punctum.

B. A probe is placed in the canaliculus. On either side of the punctum, 2 mm below the margin, an incision is made in the tarsus extending to the edge of the vertical full-thickness incision.

C. The tarsal-conjunctival flap is undermined for 5 to 6 mm.

D. It is pulled upward and resected.

E. The tarsus and conjunctiva are approximated with 6-0 plain catgut. As a result of this vertical shortening, the punctum is pulled inward.

F. The two cut edges of the eyelid are overlapped with moderate tension; the redundant portion is excised with another vertical incision through the eyelid into the cul-de-sac.

G. The lid is approximated in the standard way (see basic eyelid repair, Fig. 16–3).

Involutional Ectropion

If the punctum is still everted despite the lid tightening, and the patient is middle aged or younger, a tarsal-conjunctival resection below the punctum may also be needed (see Fig. 16–18). In many older people, however, it is sufficient to merely approximate the lid to the globe, since it cures exposure and allows tears to make their way to the upper punctum.

Horizontal Shortening at the Lateral Canthus

For the usual type of involutional ectropion, in which the whole eyelid sags, horizontal short-

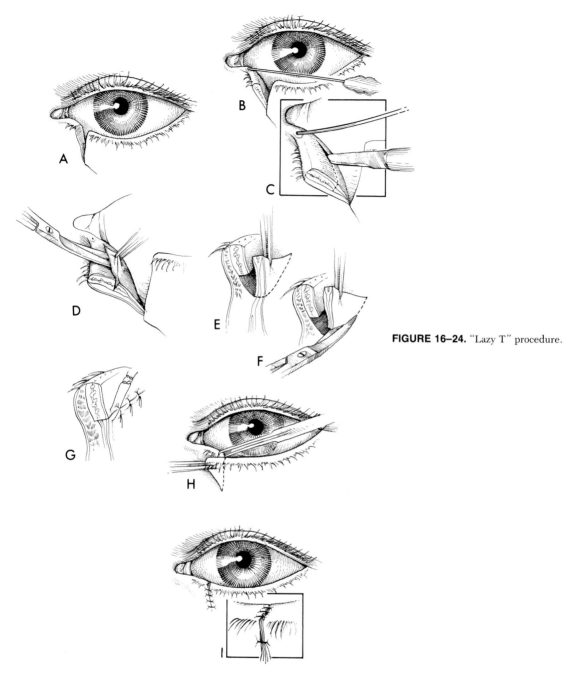

FIGURE 16–24. "Lazy T" procedure.

ening at the lateral canthus brings the lower lid into correct position.[28] The advantages of performing the surgery at the lateral canthus are that the incision is away from the globe, reducing any potential irritation, and lid margin irregularities are avoided. This procedure would work well in many cases of paralytic ectropion in which the lid has lost its tone and needs to be supported mechanically. It would also be appropriate in conjunction with lower lid bleph-

aroplasty when there is laxity in the lower lid. With the exception of the latter condition, it is necessary to achieve an overcorrected position in order to obtain the desired result.

Technique (Fig. 16–25)

A. An incision angled toward the earlobe is made from the lateral canthus for 1.5 cm; the lower lid is disinserted from the lateral canthal tendon.

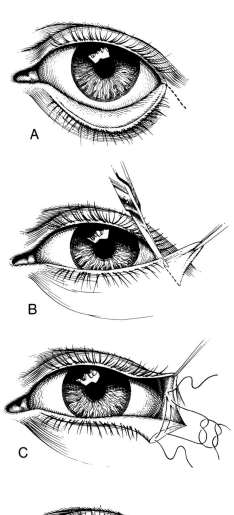

A

B

C

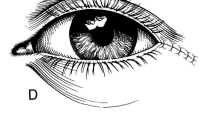

D

FIGURE 16–25. Horizontal shortening at lateral canthus for ectropion.

slight postoperative drop. It is also important to make certain that the sutures are along the inner aspect of the periosteum or tendon; this brings the eyelid snugly against the globe.

D. Sutures of 5-0 Vicryl through the epitarsal tissue and remnant of the lateral canthal tendon augment the suspension suture. The skin is closed with 6-0 silk or plain catgut.

Hypertrophic Conjunctiva

In cases of longstanding ectropion the conjunctiva may be hyperemic, dry, or hypertrophic. Usually this exposed conjunctiva will soften and normalize once it is repositioned and bathed with tears. In extreme cases it is impossible to achieve the correct apposition of the eyelid against the globe because of the extremely thick hypertrophic conjunctiva. In these cases it may be necessary to resect a portion of it in order to ensure a satisfactory result.

Technique (Fig. 16–26)

A. An ellipse of conjunctiva immediately below or adjacent to the lower border of the tarsus can be removed or shaved with a knife blade. Merely thinning the roll of conjunctiva may be enough to allow adequate apposition when the lid is pulled tight at the lateral canthus.

B. If there is still a rolling outward of the lid margin, a 6-0 Prolene suture is passed through

B. The lid is pulled upward and across the canthus until it is tight; where it crosses the canthus it is resected down to the inferior aspect of the original incision. Five to 7 mm is the usual amount removed.

C. Two 5-0 Vicryl sutures are placed from the cut edge of the tarsus into the remnant of the lateral canthal tendon or periosteum. An effort is made to place the superior suture a little above the lateral canthal angle to allow for

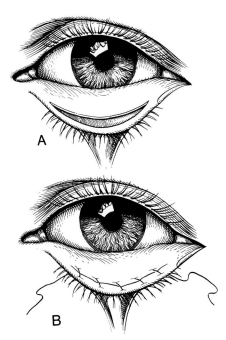

A

B

FIGURE 16–26. Hypertrophic conjunctiva.

the skin to the inner surface, closing the conjunctiva; the other end exits the skin at the opposite side of the eyelid.

Entropic Lid Margin Associated with Ectropion

In longstanding ectropion conditions, particularly when there are cicatricial changes, an irregularity of the lid margin may occur that creates a cicatricial entropion along with a frank involutional or cicatricial ectropion. In these situations approximating the eyelid to the globe results in an unhappy patient, since lashes are brought against the globe, although the cosmetic result may be satisfactory. In these situations it is necessary to do a combination ectropion-entropion repair.

Technique (Fig. 16–27)

A. After the eyelid is brought against the globe with horizontal shortening, an incision is made approximately 3 to 5 mm below the lash line, exposing the lower border of the tarsus.

B. Absorbable 6-0 sutures are placed between the skin edges, catching the lower border of the tarsus, which turns the lid margin and lash line outward.

This can also be done in cases of cicatricial ectropion in which a graft is placed in the lower lid. The sutures are brought from the skin below the lid margin first through the lower border of

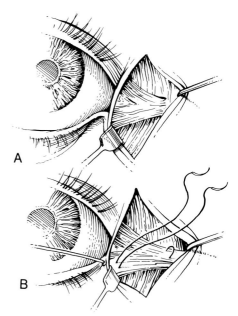

FIGURE 16–28. Tucking of the lower arm of the medial canthal tendon.

the tarsus and then through the graft edge, resulting in an eversion of the lash line.

Tucking the Lower Arm of the Medial Canthal Tendon

In some patients, in addition to ectropion, the inner aspect of the lower lid is laterally displaced. If the eyelid is pulled laterally to correct the ectropion, the punctum may end up in the middle of the eyelid or adjacent to the lower limbus. Therefore, in this unusual situation a combination of tucking the lower arm of the canthal tendon and a full-thickness excision of the eyelid at the lateral canthus would be more appropriate.

Technique (Fig. 16–28)

A. The medial canthal tendon is exposed through a vertical incision just medial to the canthal angle.

B. A probe is placed in the canaliculus as a precaution. A double-arm 5-0 Prolene suture is placed between the main canthal tendon and the stretched lower arm of the tendon and tied, thus tightening and stabilizing the lower lid medially. Because the canaliculus is directly under the medial canthal tendon, there could be kinking or collapse of the lumen, and this must be guarded against. The horizontal shortening of the lower lid is then carried out laterally as previously described.

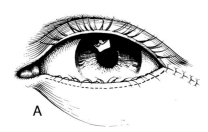

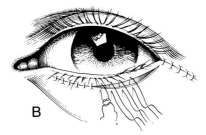

FIGURE 16–27. Entropic lid margin associated with ectropion.

Cicatricial Ectropion

Cicatricial ectropion is caused by abnormal vertical tension, which pulls the lid away from the globe. Anything that causes excessive scarring or shrinkage in the skin or subcutaneous tissue, such as injury with loss of tissue, poor tissue apposition, or third-degree burns, can cause ectropion.

Tearing, irritation, and exposure keratopathy may induce the surgeon to attempt repair as soon as possible. However, as a general rule, it is wise to wait at least 6 months from the time of injury, since there will be residual fibroblastic activity going on in and around the scar. Therefore, surgical interference, if carried out before the initial scars have reached a mature state, may result in a greatly increased scar tissue formation.

Horizontal Shortening with Transpositional Skin Graft for Mild Cicatricial Ectropion

Some people, especially those chronically exposed to the sun, develop shrinkage or tightening of the skin of their face, particularly on the lower lid and cheek. As they age, involutional changes allow the lids to be everted. Because of the downward pull of the skin, horizontal shortening alone would not be an adequate procedure. These cases, whatever the cause, are good candidates for a technique that combines horizontal shortening with a transpositional flap from the upper lid.[29]

Technique (Fig. 16–29)

A. An incision is made 2 mm below the lid margin across the lid, separating the right skin from the eyelid margin area.

B. The eyelid is separated from the lateral canthus by cutting through the lower arm of the lateral canthal tendon.

C. The separated lid is pulled tightly across the lateral canthus; usually 5 to 7 mm is resected.

D. The lid is reattached to the rim with a buried 5-0 Vicryl suture, joining the tarsus to the rim or remnant of the lateral canthal tendon. The transpositional graft from the upper lid, usually 5 to 7 mm in vertical height and hinged beyond the lateral canthus, is prepared. This includes both skin and orbicularis because a thicker flap is easier to handle and does not curl as much. Moreover, it will carry a greater blood supply and reduce the chances for necrosis.

E. In most cases the graft must reach beyond the midline; it is sutured in place with 6-0 silk with the ends left long.

F. Over the graft a cotton stent soaked in antibiotic drops is placed and the long suture ends are tied over the stent. This serves to keep the graft on stretch while it is healing, as well as to maintain its close adherence to the host bed, where vascular buds will grow into the graft. The upper lid defect is closed with a 6-0 silk suture, and in the hinge area the graft is arranged to conform to the defect.

The patient is instructed to wear a metal shield at bedtime to avoid inadvertently dislodging the cotton stent. The sutures are removed in 1 week.

Full-Thickness Skin Graft Repair of Cicatricial Ectropion

For cases of moderately severe cicatricial ectropion a full-thickness skin graft repair is indicated.[30] This would include cases after burns or trauma, or longstanding cases in older people that require a graft greater than 1 cm in vertical height. Even in mild cases it may be prudent to use a full-thickness skin graft rather than a transpositional graft from the upper lid, to prevent a disparity in the upper eyelid appearance. The preferred donor site is the postauricular area, since the skin there is thicker and has more supportive structures to reduce the amount of shrinkage. The color match is also very good.

Technique (Fig. 16–30)

A. An incision 3 mm below the lid margin is carried from one canthus to the other. In severe cases the incision must extend 3 to 5 mm beyond the canthi to allow for full upward mobilization of the lid.

B. Sutures of 6-0 silk through silicone pegs are placed on either side of the midline, and the lid is pulled up to exaggerate the skin defect. If all the cicatricial bands are released, the margin should easily pass over the cornea. Because the lid margin may be redundant after being released, it may be necessary to shorten it and reconnect it to the lateral canthus (see Fig. 16–25C and D).

C. In the lower lid, postauricular skin is preferred, since it is thicker, shrinks less, and gives better support. The color matchup after 3 months is more than acceptable. Alternate sites are the supraclavicular area and the inner surface of the arm. A pattern slightly larger than the defect is drawn over the postauricular area; this is followed by injection of local anesthesia. The area is removed with sharp dissec-

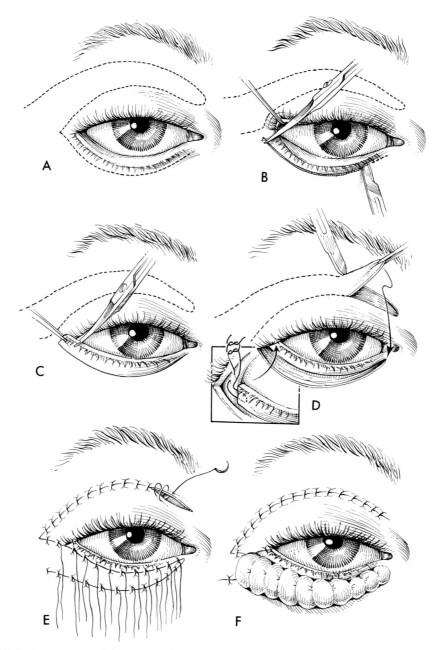

FIGURE 16–29. Horizontal shortening with transpositional flap from upper eyelid, for correction of cicatricial ectropion.

tion, with as much subcutaneous tissue left as possible, since it must be trimmed.

D. The defect is closed with a continuous 4-0 Prolene suture, with the ends left long and tied over a piece of rolled Telfa.

E. With the lid pulled up over the cornea, the graft is tailored to fit the defect and sutured with 6-0 silk sutures with the ends left long.

Stab incisions are made in the graft for drainage, as well as to give it more stretch to cover a greater area if necessary.

F. A cotton stent soaked in antibiotic drops is placed over the graft, and the sutures are tied over it. To facilitate removal of the stent a piece of Adaptic gauze is usually placed over the graft. The intermarginal sutures are contin-

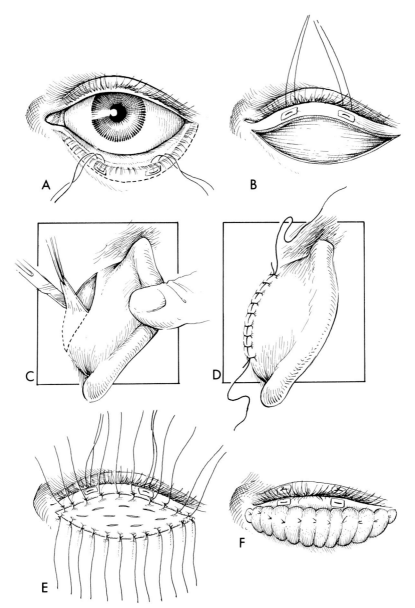

FIGURE 16–30. Full-thickness skin graft for cicatricial ectropion.

ued into the upper lid and tied over silicone pegs, to keep the lower lid splinted and on stretch. Immobilization of the grafted area is necessary in order to prevent early shrinkage.

The stent and sutures are removed in 7 days. The graft may look dusky and irregular, but as a rule, within several weeks it begins to assume the color of the surrounding skin and develops a smooth contour. The intermarginal sutures are removed in 2 or 3 weeks. The patient wears a metal shield at night during that time to protect the surgical area.

BLEPHAROPTOSIS

Classification

Congenital Blepharoptosis

Congenital ptosis of the lids is due to a congenital dystrophy of the levator muscle, which can be mild, moderate, or severe.[31] Many patients have a strong family history. The superior rectus muscle may be involved, owing to the fact that its embryological origin is similar to that of the levator muscle. An infrequent syndrome occurs in which blepharoptosis is one of the consistent findings; it may also include blepharophimosis, epicanthal folds, telecanthus, and, occasionally, ectropion.

Another and quite different type of congenital ptosis is that in which up and down movement of the lid occurs in association with motion of the jaw or tongue. This is the Marcus Gunn or "jaw-winking" ptosis. The phenomenon is almost always unilateral and occurs in 4 to 6 per cent of cases of congenital ptosis. At rest, there is a fairly constant ptosis of the involved eye. However, when the mouth is opened or the jaw is moved to the opposite side, the ptotic lid elevates, returning to its usually droopy condition with relaxation of the jaw. In most cases it is the side motion of the jaw rather than opening it that activates the lid elevation. Jaw-winking tends to be noticed early in life, when the infant is nursing or sucking on a bottle. In some cases the amount of winking decreases as the child grows older, but the degree of ptosis remains the same. In most cases the patient learns to control the winking as he grows older, giving the impression that it is less. The cause is obscure, but the condition appears to result from a misdirection of the fifth cranial nerve fibers into the third cranial nerve.

There is some controversy regarding the treatment of Marcus Gunn ptosis. Beard recommends excising the levator muscle on the affected side to obliterate the winking, followed by placement of a frontalis sling.[31] To make both sides similar with regard to elevation and lagophthalmos, he excised the levator and does a frontalis sling on the normal side as well. Many surgeons are reluctant to violate a normal eyelid; some prefer to treat the Marcus Gunn patient as a routine congenital ptosis case. Many of these patients on whom an external levator resection or frontalis sling is done have less winking because they are better able to control it as they grow older.

Acquired Ptosis

Neurogenic Ptosis. There are two quite different neurogenic causes for acquired ptosis: (1) paresis of the third cranial nerve, affecting the levator muscle of the lid; and (2) interference with the sympathetic nervous system innervation of Müller's muscle. The significance and treatment of the two types are quite different.

Paresis of the third cranial nerve often has ptosis of the lid as one of its most prominent symptoms. Frequently other extraocular muscles are also involved. Mydriasis is frequently

present with aneurysms and trauma but is seldom associated with diabetic neuropathy. If the superior division of the third nerve is selectively affected, ptosis and superior rectus weakness are the only apparent manifestations. Conditions involving the third cranial nerve are, in their order of frequency, diabetes, trauma, aneurysm, and tumor.

A lesion along the course of the sympathetic chain can affect the functioning of Müller's muscle. This type of ptosis is part of Horner's syndrome. The syndrome also includes miosis and a decrease in sweating on the affected side of the face. In a dimly lit room the relative difference in the size of the pupils becomes more apparent, thus making the diagnosis easier. Invariably pupillary involvement accompanies the ptosis, but the converse is not true.[32]

In a patient with Horner's syndrome phenylephrine 0.12% instilled in both eyes usually causes elevation of the affected side because of the hypersensitivity of the denervated sympathetic nerve endings in Müller's muscle. Phenylephrine 1% instilled in both eyes should cause dilatation of the affected pupil and raise the eyelid, but have little effect on the normal side.[33]

Myogenic Ptosis and Aponeurosis Defects. Myogenic causes of ptosis include myasthenia gravis, progressive external ophthalmoplegia, progressive levator muscle myopathy, and dehiscence of the levator aponeurosis.

MYASTHENIA GRAVIS. Myasthenia gravis is caused by a malfunction at the myoneural junction. The symptoms are more prominent toward the end of the day or after the eyes have been used for a prolonged period, especially when upward gaze is required. A highly valuable clinical sign is the inability to keep the lids elevated during prolonged upward gaze. In testing for this the patient is asked to fixate in upward gaze with the examiner carefully watching the lid margins; when myasthenia gravis is present the lid often quite suddenly droops.[32] Other muscles, including extraocular muscles, may also be involved, but in some cases the condition seems to be limited to the lids themselves. If myasthenia is suspected, confirmation of the diagnosis should be made using the Tensilon test.

Tensilon (edrophonium chloride) has a direct neuromuscular stimulating effect and, to a lesser extent, an anticholinesterase effect. It counteracts the effect of curare and improves the contraction of myasthenic muscles. The test is administered in the following way: A tuberculin syringe is used to draw up the contents of a 1-ml (10-mg) ampul; 2 mg is injected during a 15-second period and the patient is observed for a response. If there is no response after 1 minute, the remaining 8 mg is slowly injected. Atropine is the antidote and should be available in case excessive cholinergic effects occur.[33]

Should myasthenia be diagnosed, the treatment is medical, using a variety of agents, including cholinergics, parasympathomimetics, and corticosteroids. Frontalis sling procedures are indicated in cases that become refractory to medical treatment.

PROGRESSIVE EXTERNAL OPHTHALMOPLEGIA. This is a muscular dystrophy that affects all the extraocular muscles. Onset may be as early as middle age. The condition tends to progress until there is total paralysis of all of the external ocular muscles. In addition, there may be other associated neuromuscular problems in the face and neck, causing difficulty with speech and swallowing. Surgical correction of the ptosis that accompanies progressive external ophthalmoplegia is fraught with hazard because Bell's phenomenon is usually poor or totally absent. The Kearns-Sayre syndrome[34] is a pediatric form of this condition accompanied by pigmentary retinopathy, cardiac conduction defects, and a possible decrease in the ventilatory drive after general anesthesia.

PROGRESSIVE LEVATOR MUSCLE MYOPATHY. In elderly people myopathic changes may occur in the levator muscle, with the other extraocular muscles being spared. There may be a tendency for this to occur at around the same age in different members of a family.

DEHISCENCE OR STRETCHING OF THE LEVATOR APONEUROSIS. Defects in the levator aponeurosis may occur after trauma or severe upper eyelid swelling, or as a result of the aging process. In the two former conditions a definite line of separation is found at the time of surgery. In the gradually progressive cases in the older age groups a definite dehiscence may not be found; instead, a thinning in the aponeurosis may be apparent.

Blepharoptosis After Trauma and Ocular Surgery

Trauma. Horizontal lacerations across the upper eyelid may involve the levator muscle. A sign that this has occurred is the presence of orbital fat prolapsing through the wound; this idicates that the orbital septum has been cut, exposing the fat that overlies the levator. This sign is not proof of levator involvement, but it is strongly suggestive. An optimal functional result can be expected when correct repair is carried out at the time of injury. However, caution must be exercised in order to make certain that there has in fact been an actual dehiscence or laceration of the levator, since the trauma itself may cause a temporary paresis of the levator. Because these two conditions are sometimes impossible to differentiate, it is best to follow a conservative course in equivocal situations. If repair of a lacerated levator muscle is not accomplished within 24 hours of the time of trauma, it would be wise to delay definitive surgery until there is no change in the lid position for at least 6 months.

Ptosis After Ocular Surgical Procedures. Drooping of the upper lid after ocular surgery is not rare; it is most commonly seen after cataract extraction. The cause is unclear, but it is thought that the surgical trauma may accelerate a dehiscence of the levator aponeurosis or damage Müller's muscle. This permanent type of postsurgical ptosis should be differentiated from the temporary blepharoptosis that frequently follows surgical procedures, which is related to the external and internal ocular inflammation. Furthermore, after glaucoma procedures it is not unusual for the lid to assume a protective position covering the area of conjunctival filtration.

Mechanical Causes for Ptosis

1. Blepharochalasis may be severe enough to cause reduction in the width of the lid fissure by the overhanging folds of skin. In these situations blepharoplasty is curative.

2. After orbital fractures in which the globe becomes recessed back into the orbit, the mechanical function of the globe in elevating the upper lid is impaired. In this type of enophthalmos bringing the eye forward surgically is difficult; consequently surgical repair of the ptosis may be indicated to improve the cosmetic appearance. On the other hand, if the eye should be depressed (hypo-ophthalmic) as well as recessed, the preferred procedure is elevation of the globe with an implant. This improves the position of the eye and of the upper eyelid as well.

Evaluation of the Patient

The two major questions the examiner seeks to answer when evaluating a patient with ptosis are:

1. What is the cause of the ptosis?
2. How stable is the condition?

It is necessary to determine whether the ptosis has been present since birth and whether it is changing. Does the lid move with eating? If the ptosis was caused by trauma, is the lid position still improving? In cases of acquired ptosis ruling out a neurologic cause is essential.

The fissure size of both eyes must be measured in the primary position, and the position of the lid on the cornea noted. Normally the eyelid rests 1 to 2 mm from the limbus.

Levator function is determined by measuring the excursion of the eyelid; the change in position of the lid margin when the patient is looking down to that when he is looking up is measured. It is important to eliminate the action of the frontalis muscle by placing the thumb firmly on the brow; only by doing this can the examiner be sure that the lid elevation is really a function of the levator itself. Normally the lid should be elevated about 13 to 15 mm as a result of levator function. Elevation of 10 to 12 mm can be considered subnormal, 7 to 9 mm fair, 3 to 6 mm minimal, and 0 to 2 mm poor.[31] In congenital ptosis there is likely to be lagophthalmos because of a fibrotic condition of the levator.

It is important to observe whether a lid crease is present. In severe congenital ptosis the lid is usually flat. When some residual levator function is in fact present, a lid crease can usually be seen. The position of the lid crease on the normal side also serves as a guide for placing the incision on the lid to be operated on. The direction of the lashes on both the normal and the abnormal sides should also be noted.

It is extremely important to determine the function of the other extraocular muscles, most notably the superior rectus. Normally when the lids are closed the eye elevates, owing to activity of the superior rectus muscle. This is known as Bell's phenomenon. If the upper lid is firmly held by the examiner and the patient is asked to close his eyes firmly, it is possible to estimate the adequacy of Bell's phenomenon. In the normal state the cornea should almost completely disappear from view. The absence of Bell's phenomenon should alert the surgeon that postoperative problems may be likely. This consideration is especially important for adults, as children tend to adapt better to exposure.

It is important in adults to determine the adequacy of tear function by using the Schirmer test. A patient with low or borderline tear function would usually not be a candidate for a full ptosis correction.

As mentioned previously, neurological causes for acquired ptosis must be ruled out by appropriate testing. Specifically, the examiner must eliminate third cranial nerve palsies, myasthenia gravis, and Horner's syndrome. The nature of these conditions and appropriate tests were briefly described on pages 562 and 563.

Choosing the Operation

The following outline should serve as a guide for choosing the operation for a specific condition. The next section describes the procedures in detail.

I. CONGENITAL PTOSIS
  A. Mild ptosis (1.5 to 2.0 mm) with 10 mm or more function: Fasenella-Servat operation or aponeurosis tuck
  B. Mild ptosis with less than 10 mm function: small external levator resection (10 to 13 mm)
  C. Moderate ptosis (3 mm) with fair (7 to 9 mm) function: external levator resection (12 to 17 mm)
  D. Moderate ptosis (3 mm) with minimal (3 to 6 mm) function: external levator resection (18 to 25 mm)
  E. Moderate ptosis (3 mm) with poor (0 to 2 mm) function: external levator resection (20 to 25 mm) or frontalis sling
  F. Severe ptosis (4 mm or more): external levator resection (25 mm) or frontalis sling
II. ACQUIRED PTOSIS
  A. Neurogenic
    1. Third nerve palsy: frontalis sling (silicone rod)
    2. Horner's syndrome: Fasanella-Servat procedure
  B. Myogenic and aponeurosis defects
    1. Myasthenia gravis: frontalis sling (silicone rod)
    2. Chronic progressive external ophthalmoplegia: frontalis sling (silicone rod); aponeurosis tuck in mild cases
    3. Levator myopathy: aponeurosis tuck, external levator resection, or frontalis sling (silicone rod)
    4. Defects of the aponeurosis: aponeurosis repair or tuck
III. PTOSIS AFTER TRAUMA AND OCULAR SURGERY
  A. Traumatic ptosis: aponeurosis advancement or repair of aponeurosis dehiscence

B. Postocular surgery ptosis: Fasanella-Servat procedure or aponeurosis tuck

IV. MECHANICAL PTOSIS

   A. Blepharochalasis: blepharoplasty

   B. Enophthalmic ptosis: Fasanella-Servat procedure

Blepharoptosis Repair

External Levator Resection

External levator resection is indicated for cases of moderate to severe ptosis with fair to poor levator function. Most cases of congenital ptosis fall into this category. How much to resect is usually determined by the levator function and, to a lesser extent, by the amount of ptosis. Some surgeons use the position of the lid on the cornea at the time of surgery as a guide[18]; others calculate the amount beforehand; and still others use a combination of both methods.

Technique (Fig. 16–31)

A. A suture of 6-0 silk is placed in the lid margin to permit downward traction. The upper eyelid incision is placed where the crease is desired as measured on the normal side, or, if both eyes are to be done, 6 to 8 mm from the lash line. The incision is carried through the orbicularis to the superior border of the tarsus.

B. The upper one-half of the tarsus is exposed with sharp and blunt dissection.

C. The upper skin edge is grasped and the orbicularis separated from the orbital septum. It is wise to extend the dissection superiorly to avoid inadvertently injuring the levator aponeurosis. Pushing the globe into the orbit will further aid in identifying the orbital septum, as fat will be seen bulging. The orbital septum is cut completely across the lid, exposing the preaponeurotic fat.

D. The fat is retracted posteriorly under a Desmarres retractor, exposing the white tendinous aponeurosis. Filmy bands usually remain attached to the aponeurosis and can be severed or bluntly removed. The orbicularis overlying the leading edge of the levator aponeurosis is excised.

E. The eyelid is everted over a Desmarres retractor, and the conjunctiva is incised at the superior tarsal border and separated from Müller's muscle as far as the superior cul-de-sac.

F. The aponeurosis is buttonholed at its medial and lateral border, and a straight hemostat is placed across it and Müller's muscle at the superior tarsal border.

G. The muscles are transected from the tarsus and separated by blunt dissection from attachments to Tenon's capsule in the superior cul-de-sac.

H. The conjunctiva is reapproximated to the superior tarsal border with a continuous 6-0 plain catgut suture.

I. (Optional) An alternative way is to buttonhole the lateral aspect of the aponeurosis superior to the tarsus, opening the space between it and Müller's muscle. A hemostat is then placed in the space, clamping the aponeurosis.

J. (Optional) The aponeurosis is cut away from the superior tarsal border. This avoids the cutting and reattachment of the conjunctiva.

K. The medial and lateral horns are cut, releasing the muscle. Care must be exercised to avoid the superior oblique medially and the lacrimal gland laterally.

L. Three sutures are placed in the midtarsus: centrally, medially, and laterally. The central one is a white 5-0 Vicryl suture, and the others are purple 6-0 Vicryl; the color difference helps in identification. These sutures are placed in the levator at the predetermined level, or where the eyelid crosses the levator when it is lifted to the desired level on the cornea. Slip knots are tied to evaluate the position. Adjustments can be made, if necessary, to achieve the desired lid contour. The sutures are then finally tied.

M. The excess levator muscle is excised.

N. To reduce the bulk in the pretarsal area, the orbicularis is excised from the inferior skin edge.

O. The lid crease sutures of 6-0 silk or plain catgut are placed from the superior cul-de-sac through the levator, catching the upper and lower skin edges.

P. When tied, they invaginate the skin to form an attachment to the levator; the lashes should be everted at this point. A Frost suture of 6-0 silk through a silicone peg is placed through the lower lid margin, pulling it up over the globe. It is taped to the forehead and is removed the next day.

Q. When bilateral surgery is done in young children, the eyes are generally left open. Eye pads with the centers cut out are placed over the eyes with a great deal of lubricating ointment instead of Frost sutures.

Postoperatively, antibiotic ointment is placed over the eye and wound several times daily. At bedtime, an eye pad soaked with irrigating solution is placed over the eye for protection, since closure is usually poor for several weeks. Because ointment blurs vision, lubricating drops can be substituted during the day.

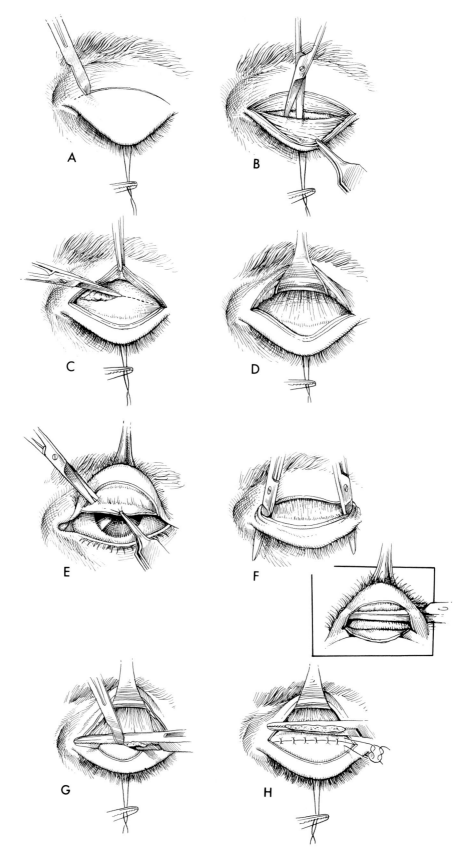

FIGURE 16–31. External levator resection.

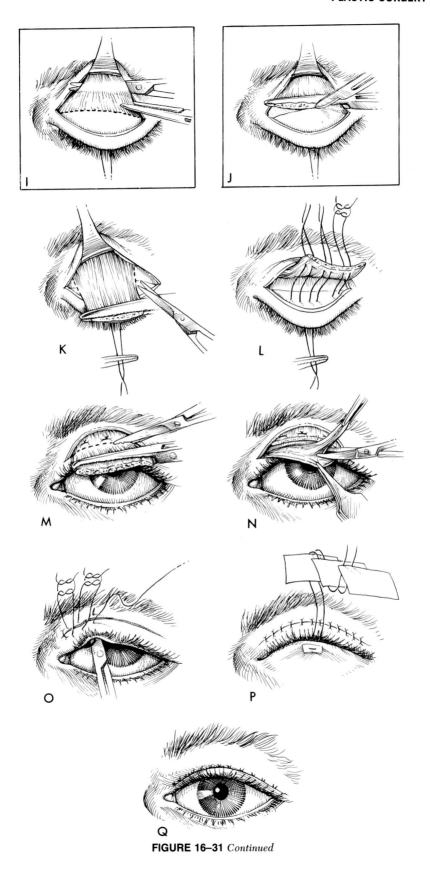

FIGURE 16–31 *Continued*

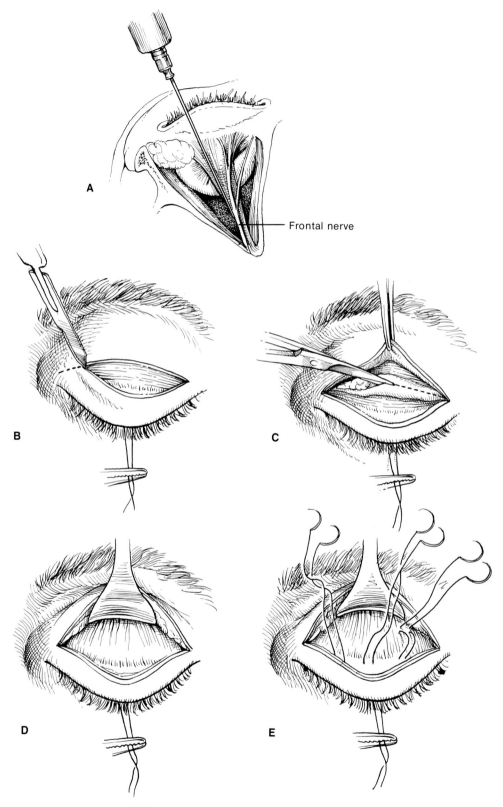

Frontal nerve

FIGURE 16–32. Aponeurosis tuck and advancement.

The severer the ptosis, the greater the levator resection must be to achieve a satisfactory result. Epstein and Putterman[36] described large levator resections of 30 mm or more for severe unilateral ptosis and compared them with a group who had bilateral brow suspensions with excision of the normal levator muscle.[25] Overall, cosmesis was judged better in those who had unilateral levator resection.

I have found that parents of children with severe unilateral ptosis were reluctant to accept the need for surgery on the normal eyelid, particularly if it is suggested that the normal levator muscle must be removed and lid function governed by brow movement. Therefore, when I make patients aware that lid lag will occur postoperatively in the maximal levator resection, I also inform them that a symmetrical lid lag could be created on the normal side, if they so desire, at any time in the future. In my experience, if the lid is satisfactory in the primary position, parents are generally pleased and seek no further surgery.

Advancement or Tucking of the Levator Aponeurosis

This procedure is usually indicated in cases of acquired ptosis. It can also be done in cases of mild congenital ptosis for which a Fasanella-Servat procedure (see below) is not quite enough, or when a lid crease is desired. This type of repair is particularly suited to traumatic ptosis, since this is often due to separations of the aponeurosis. The aponeurosis is often difficult to identify because of the scar tissue present; therefore, the procedure is best done under local anesthesia, so that the patient can move the levator while the surgeon attempts to identify it.[37]

Technique (Fig. 16–32)

A. Either local infiltration anesthesia or a frontal nerve block can be used. A frontal nerve block has the advantage of giving sensory anesthesia to the upper lid while preserving motor function. The midportion of the orbit is felt, and a 4-cm #24 needle is directed straight back along the roof of the orbit until the hub is reached. This should be at the superior orbital fissure, where the frontal and lacrimal nerves enter. To avoid infiltrating the annulus of Zinn, no more than 0.5 or 0.75 ml of 2% lidocaine or 0.75% bupivacaine with epinephrine should be injected. A disadvantage of the frontal nerve block technique is the rendering of the levator totally paretic if the anesthetic solution invades the levator–superior rectus complex.

B. An incision is made in the lid crease and the superior border of the tarsus exposed. A 6-0 silk suture is used for downward traction.

C. The upper part of the orbicularis is spread until the orbital septum is encountered. By going superiorly in the lid, inadvertent injury to the aponeurosis can be avoided. The septum is cut completely across the lid.

D. The preaponeurotic fat is retracted posteriorly with blunt dissection and the aponeurosis exposed. If there is a dehiscence, the leading edge will be separated from the tarsal attachment and the conjunctiva will be visible

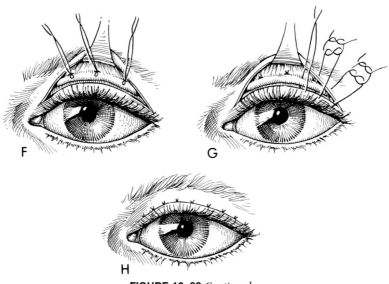

F

G

H

FIGURE 16–32 *Continued*

in the defect. Many times, however, the apo-neurosis appears normal, although subtle invo-lutional changes are present.

E. Three double-armed sutures of 6-0 Pro-lene or 5-0 Vicryl are placed in the tarsus near the superior border medially, centrally, and laterally; these are then carried through the aponeurosis anywhere from 5 to 15 mm above the tarsus, depending on the amount of ptosis.

F. The sutures are tied with slip knots and the patient is asked to look straight ahead. If the level is unsatisfactory, the amount tucked is either increased or decreased. In cases in which frontal nerve block is used, the lid should be placed at the desired level; with local infil-tration it should be overcorrected by at least 1 mm, since orbicularis function is paralyzed.

G. Lid crease sutures of 6-0 silk or plain catgut are placed, catching the aponeurosis at the superior tarsal border.

H. The operation is completed with lid crease sutures in place. A Frost suture is usually unnecessary.

Fasanella-Servat Procedure[38]

This operation is indicated when there is 10 mm of levator function and only mild ptosis (1 to 2 mm). If there is poor levator function, a satisfactory result cannot be expected. Ideal patients are those with Horner's syndrome and mild acquired ptosis, and some with very mild congenital ptosis.

Technique (Fig. 16–33)

A. A 2-mm incision is made in the lid crease medially and laterally.

B. The upper lid is everted and a mark is placed in the tarsus 3 mm from the superior border on either side of the midline. If there is normal levator function, as in patients with Horner's syndrome, the expected correction is about a millimeter for each millimeter resected. Patients with less than normal function may require 1.5 mm per millimeter of correction desired, up to a maximum of 4 mm tarsal resection. Straight hemostats are placed from either side along the 3-mm mark, meeting in

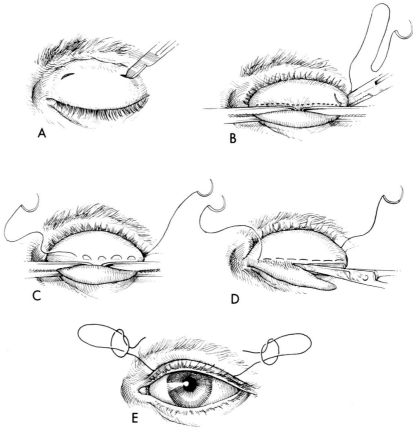

FIGURE 16–33. Fasanella-Servat procedure.

the midline. Before this maneuver, however, the superior tarsal border is grasped and pulled downward and outward to avoid including any of the levator aponeurosis. The tissue clamped in the hemostats will include tarsus, underlying Müller's muscle, and conjunctiva. A suture of 6-0 plain catgut is placed through the lateral cutaneous incision, coming out inferior to the lateral hemostat.

C. A continuous mattress placement is run across the lid, incorporating the tarsus, Müller's muscle, and conjunctiva.

D. The hemostats are removed and scissors used to cut across the crushed area.

E. The other end of the suture is brought from the internal surface through the lid and out the medial incision. Both free ends are individually tied to the orbicularis, and the skin incision is left open.

The 6-0 plain catgut does not usually produce corneal problems, although some people do complain of a foreign body sensation for several weeks. To avoid a medial droop postoperatively, it is necessary to place the hemostat across Müller's muscle even if the tarsus is not present there. A medial droop may occur because of a lateral shift in the tarsus, which makes it difficult to effectively carry out the resection in that area. This is usually due to involutional changes associated with levator aponeurosis dehiscence, in which case a levator advancement would be the procedure of choice.

Because this procedure consists of removing superior tarsus and conjunctiva, it has been accused of sacrificing some of the accessory lacrimal glands. However, we have had no cases of postoperatively acquired keratitis sicca; further, there is no difference in the preoperative and postoperative basic tear secretion test in a consecutive series of 50 patients. The operation is the most predictable of all the ptosis procedures, and does not require any intraoperative adjusting, thus relieving the surgeon of onerous decision making as to whether the lid level is too high or low.

Frontalis Suspension[39, 40]

Patients with severe ptosis and poor levator function may not have adequate elevating power for successful levator resection. In such patients frontalis suspension is required to correct the blepharoptotic eyelid. Frontalis suspension is also indicated in cases of synkinetic ptosis, such as third nerve paresis with aberrant regeneration and in ptosis associated with the Marcus Gunn jaw-winking phenomenon. The levator muscle should be excised to eliminate the synkinetic component before performing frontalis suspension. Frontalis suspension can be performed unilaterally, but to provide a symmetrical lagophthalmos in downward gaze, bilateral surgery is necessary.[31] A number of autogenous, homologous, and synthetic materials have been used, but we prefer preserved fascia lata, or the 1-mm solid silicone rod.

Frontalis Suspension, Silicone Rod. A silicone rod frontalis suspension is particularly indicated in those with severe acquired ptosis with ophthalmoplegia or third nerve paralysis.[41] The elastic quality of the silicone rod allows almost complete approximation of the lids with forced closure, which helps to minimize exposure keratopathy. Older patients usually have decreased tear secretion, which makes it desirable to achieve a slightly undercorrected lid position to avoid symptoms of exposure keratopathy. This is also important in patients with chronic progressive external ophthalmoplegia, since their extraocular muscle movements are impaired and Bell's phenomenon may be absent. A patient with a seventh nerve paralysis and ptosis would also fall into this category. Because silicone is nonbiodegradable and is usually surrounded with a connective tissue envelope, readjustment of the lid position can be accomplished months or years after the initial surgery. However, synthetic materials have the disadvantage of breaking or sliding through the tissues, which would cause a recurrence of the ptosis or promote infection if exposed through the skin.

Technique (Fig. 16–34)

A. The procedure can be performed under local or general anesthesia, but in either case the eyelid and brow are infiltrated with the usual anesthetic mixture. An incision is made in the area of the desired upper eyelid crease. The skin and orbicularis muscle are dissected to expose the anterior tarsal surface. The 1-mm silicone rod is sutured directly to the anterior tarsal surface in a semicircular manner with four or five 5-0 Mersilene sutures so that the inferior skin flap covers most of the sutures. A 2-cm horizontal incision is made just above the brow, centered over the pupil. The incision is undermined to expose the frontalis muscle, avoiding the supraorbital neurovascular bundle. A Wright fascia needle is threaded through the brow incision medially and laterally to the level of the superior rim, where it is directed first posterior to approximately the level of the levator aponeurosis and then forward to emerge at

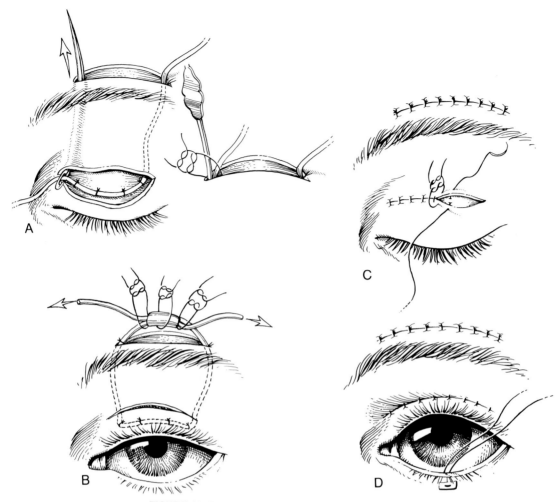

FIGURE 16–34. Frontalis suspension, silicone rod method.

the level of the tarsus. A large abdominal needle can be used to pass the silicone rod from the eyelid to the brow area. This produces a smaller tract for the rod and creates a path that is closer to the levator than when coming from the brow into the eyelid with the Wright fascia needle. To secure the rod medially and laterally, a 4-0 Ethibond suture is fixated to the deep frontalis fascia and then tied around the rod and a #1 Bowman probe, so that when the probe is removed there is a noose through which the rod can easily slide; this also prevents migration of the rod.

B. A silicone tube, 1.5 mm in diameter and 5 mm long, is used as a Watzke sleeve through which the two ends of the rod are passed. The rod is tightened and the eyelid is elevated to the desired position. For chronic progressive external ophthalmoplegia, a safe level is be-

tween the limbus and the pupil. The rods are secured on either side of the sleeve with several sutures of 5-0 Mersilene, and a dyed suture is placed around the sleeve itself to make identification easier if a reoperation is necessary. The ends of the silicone rod are cut, leaving 5 mm of excess rod on either side for later adjustment, if necessary. When dealing with a patient who has good extraocular muscle function without compromised corneal protective mechanisms, the level of the lid should be overcorrected by approximately 1 mm, or the lid level should be at least to the superior limbus.

C. The brow incision is closed with subcutaneous sutures of 6-0 plain catgut and the skin with the same material or, in the case of an adult, 6-0 Prolene. The lid crease sutures of 6-0 plain catgut are brought through the superior cul-de-sac, grasping the upper and lower skin edges, or they can be placed anteriorly between the skin edges, grasping the tarsal tissue.

D. In all cases it is necessary to evert the lash line. At the end of the procedure a Frost suture can be inserted, or eye pads with the centers cut out placed over the globe and ointment instilled.

In patients with chronic progressive external ophthalmoplegia a Frost suture should be placed to protect the globe, as these cases have poor or absent Bell's phenomenon and will be unable to close the eye until the effects of the anesthetic wear off. On the first postoperative day the suture can be let down to open the eye and then retaped to the forehead at night until it has been determined that the patient can tolerate the newly opened position of the eye. During this time lubricants are liberally used and wet eye pads applied at night until it has been determined what is necessary to keep the eye comfortable.

An overcorrection or undercorrection can be treated fairly easily by readjusting the rods within the silicone sleeve. Local anesthesia is infiltrated into the central brow area and the silicone sleeve is exposed. Usually the sleeve is within an envelope of connective tissue, and the dyed suture around the sleeve provides easy localization. The ends of the rod are either loosened or tightened, depending on the situation of the eyelid. Because the eyelid is not anesthetized, adjustment can be more accurately accomplished. It is rare for the rod to come loose from its tarsal attachment.

Frontalis Suspension, Fascia Lata. In children and young adults with good extraocular muscle movements we use fascia lata for cases of frontalis suspension. Our preferred material is preserved fascia lata, since there has not been a significant difference in our results when using a preserved or autogenous fascia lata. Using the preserved fascia lata eliminates the time necessary to obtain autogenous fascia as well as a secondary scar on the thigh.

TECHNIQUE (Fig. 16–35)

The procedure is carried out as described in the previous section for the silicone rod (Fig. 16–34), except for the tying of the fascia in the brow area. The fascia is tied with one loop and pulled tightly within the incision, until the eyelid reaches the superior limbus. With the knot secured, the lid is pulled downward to eliminate any kinks in the fascia. Sutures of 5-0 Mersilene are placed through the looped fascia in several places in order to secure it. The closure and formation of the upper eyelid crease is carried out as previously described (Fig. 16–34C and D).

We usually eliminate the Frost suture in children and use eye pads with the centers cut out and ointment placed over the globes. Systemic antibiotics are used in order to reduce the chance of infection.

The "open sky" frontalis suspension procedure has several advantages.

1. The suspensory material is fixated to the tarsus under direct visualization. This gives the

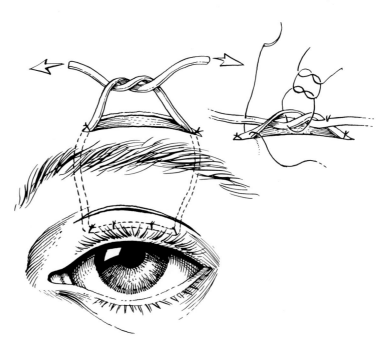

FIGURE 16–35. Frontalis suspension, fascia lata method.

surgeon better control over the eyelid contour and position when elevating the eyelid.

2. A better lid crease and fold can be achieved, since a complete incision is made in the eyelid. Thus lid crease sutures create an adhesion to the tarsus and aid in everting the lashes.

3. The eyelid has a less bulky appearance postoperatively, since only one strand of material is used.

Complications of Ptosis Surgery

The most common complication of ptosis surgery is undercorrection. This can be rectified after a period of 6 months by another procedure. The choice of a second procedure is based on the amount of remaining ptosis, the levator function, and what was done previously. For example, if a Fasanella-Servat procedure was done initially, a levator resection or aponeurosis tuck should be considered for the second operation, whereas a small undercorrection after a tuck or a resection can be corrected by a Fasanella-Servat operation.

Tarsectomy–Block Resection

In a case of an undercorrected ptosis procedure, particularly if it was an external levator resection, a tarsectomy–block resection could be considered.[41] The tarsectomy–block resection can improve an undercorrection after levator resection or advancement. This is particularly true when there is a tight band of cicatricial tissue caused by the fusion of the levator aponeurosis, tarsus, and orbital septum, producing a lid lag. A tarsectomy–block resection of this tissue can lift the lid almost millimeter for millimeter of desired correction.

Technique (Fig. 16–36)

A. An incision is made in the lid crease down to the tarsus, where the levator and orbital septum join the tarsus. Extensive dissection of tissue planes is avoided.

B. A rectangle is outlined in this area with the vertical height being 1 ml more than the number of millimeters of desired vertical correction. If the superior edge is not in tarsus but in levator, double-armed sutures of 6-0 Vicryl are placed through the superior cul-de-sac, coming out at the upper edge of the resection; the preplaced suture avoids the need to guess where the superior edge lies when the tissues retract after the full-thickness cut is made.

C. An initial scratch incision is made to outline the area to be removed, followed by careful incisions through all layers into the superior cul-de-sac. Scissors then excise the full-thickness block of tissue.

D. Sutures of 6-0 Vicryl are brought through partial-thickness tarsus, approximating the lid tissues and avoiding irritation of the cornea. If preplaced sutures are already present superiorly, they are left in place and brought through partial-thickness tarsus inferiorly.

E. Lid crease sutures are placed between the skin edges, grasping the epitarsal tissue to invaginate the skin edges.

Overcorrection is the most serious complication of surgery for blepharoptosis. Exposure keratopathy is not only uncomfortable, but it may also lead to ulceration, infection, and blindness. Overcorrection is unusual with congenital ptosis associated with fair to poor function but more common with acquired cases. In the early postoperative stages gross overcorrection is usually obvious and exposure keratopathy may develop rapidly. In this situation, if an external levator resection was done, the levator can be separated from the adjacent tissues and moved back to the superior tarsal border. It is, however, difficult to tell the first day postoperatively if a slight overcorrection is a true overcorrection because the operated side is usually a little stiff and there may be some splinting of the eyelid on the unoperated side. After a week of orbicularis movement the lid may be a little lower. If the overcorrection is mild, instructing the patient to forcibly squeeze his lid closed or to massage the lid downward may help loosen the levator attachment.

Overcorrection of the levator aponeuroris tuck, if recognized early, can be treated by removing one or all of the tucking sutures; this may allow the lid to drop several millimeters. Sometimes this can be done in the office by gently separating the wound edges to expose the Prolene tucking sutures. An overcorrected Fasanella-Servat operation or one with a high central arch can be corrected only by loosening the internal suture. Once it becomes permanent, a scleral graft is necessary. Frontalis suspensions that result in overcorrection must be released to allow the lid to drop downward; this is much easier with silicone, since it is inert and not incorporated into the tissues. If fascia lata was used, an early reversal would require loosening the fascia in the brow area while putting downward pressure on the lid. For late overcorrections it would be necessary to cut the cicatricial fascial bands in the lid and place the

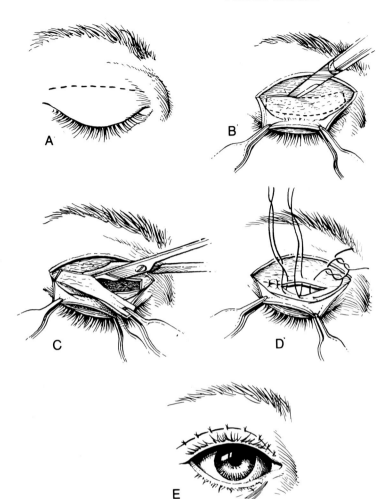

FIGURE 16–36. Tarsectomy-block resection.

lid on sustained stretch with a reverse Frost suture.

After 6 weeks, if overcorrection persists, it may become necessary to recess the levator from the superior tarsal border, using preserved sclera. Usually the size of the graft is equal to the amount of recession desired.

Levator Recession with Scleral Graft

Technique (Fig. 16–37)

The technique of standard external levator resection outlined in Figure 16–31 is used through step *K*. At this point the preserved sclera is cut as wide as the amount to be recessed and approximately 15 mm long horizontally; this is sutured to the anterior edge of the levator on one side and to tarsus on the other, using 5-0 Vicryl. The lid crease sutures are placed from the skin edges through the epitarsal tissue.

Entropion is caused by excessive shortening of the internal lamella of the lid (tarsus, conjunctiva, levator). It is usually associated with overcorrection and is remedied by levator recession. It may also be due to a lack of skin–levator attachment, which allows the skin to push the lashes downward. In this situation formation of the lid crease may correct the entropion by everting the lashes and lid margin.

Ectropion is usually due to excessive tension on the lower skin edge on placement of the lid crease sutures, resulting in an eversion of the lashes. Occasionally this occurs when the initial incision is placed low on the tarsus, with lid crease sutures to the superior tarsal border creating upward tension on the lower skin edge and lid margin. If this problem is recognized early, removing the sutures and massaging downward may correct the problem. Otherwise, it can be improved by making an incision in the superior tarsal area and then undermining and releasing the skin–tarsal attachment.

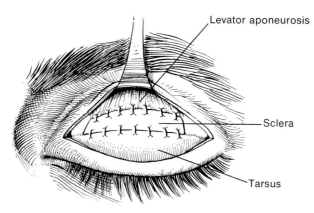

FIGURE 16–37. Levator recession with sclera.

SURGERY OF THE LACRIMAL SYSTEM

Anatomy

The lacrimal gland is located in the superior lateral quadrant of the orbit within the lacrimal gland fossa.[3] The levator aponeurosis indents the gland and divides it into an orbital and palpebral lobe (Fig. 16–2). The major lacrimal ducts empty into the superior cul-de-sac 5 mm above the lateral tarsal border. The ducts from the orbital portion run through the palpebral portion; therefore, removal or damage to the palpebral portion of the gland can seriously reduce reflex tear secretion. For reflex tearing, the afferent pathway is along the fifth cranial nerve, and the efferent pathway is along the seventh cranial nerve. Removal of the orbital portion of the lacrimal gland eliminates the efferent nerve supply, and, as a consequence, the palpebral portion, which depends on this innervation, cannot be activated. The glands of Krause and Wolfring, located mainly in the superior cul-de-sac, are the basic lacrimal secretors and have no efferent nerve supply.

The excretory system begins with the punctum (Fig. 16–38), which is the most distal portion and should be found slightly inverted against the globe.[42] It is vertically placed in the eyelid for 2 mm, and its location is usually identified by a slight pouting at the end of the cilia line. The canaliculus is approximately 8 to 10 mm long; in 90 per cent of people the upper and lower canaliculi join to form a single duct,

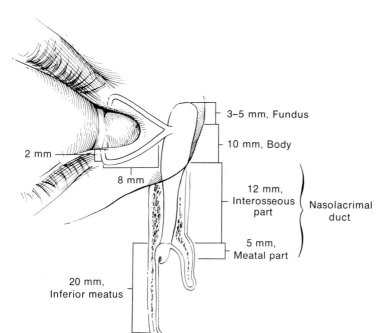

FIGURE 16–38. Lacrimal excretory anatomy.

the common canaliculus, which opens into the tear sac just posterior and superior to the center of its lateral wall. The lacrimal sac lies posterior to the medial canthal tendon and within the lacrimal sac fossa, which is adjacent to the middle meatus of the nose. The dome of the sac extends several millimeters superior to the tendon. The medial canthal tendon has two attachments: one—Horner's muscle—to the posterior lacrimal crest, and the other main portion to the frontal process of the maxillary bone. The nasal lacrimal duct is about 12 mm long and runs in the maxillary bone, slightly lateral and posterior, emptying into the inferior meatus of the nose. The angular vein lies approximately 8 mm from the canthal angle; sometimes this can be seen through the skin.

Lacrimal Pump

The concept of the lacrimal pump is basic to an understanding of tear excretion, as the lacrimal pump is the primary mechanism for excreting tears.[42] When the eyelids close during blinking, the superficial and deep heads of the pretarsal orbicularis muscles close the ampulla of the punctum and shorten the canaliculus. The punctum can be observed to move medially with lid closure. Simultaneously the deep heads of the preseptal orbicularis muscles pull the lacrimal periosteum—to which the lateral wall of the tear sac is firmly attached—laterally. This creates a negative pressure within the sac, and thus draws fluid from the ampulla and the canaliculus into the sac. On opening the eye the deep heads of the preseptal orbicularis muscle relax and the fibroelastic resilience of the lacrimal periosteum puts positive pressure on the tear sac, forcing tears into the nose. The punctum also moves laterally, and fluid enters it, filling the ampulla and the lengthened canaliculus.

Evaluation of Lacrimal Function

Tests of Secretory Function[42]

The Schirmer #1 test measures both reflex and basic secretion. A thin strip of filter paper is placed in the inferior cul-de-sac of the unanesthetized eye, where it remains for 5 minutes. The length of the strip that becomes moistened with tears is measured in millimeters of wetting. The tests may be expedited by reducing the wetting time to 1 minute and the result multi-

plied by 3. The normal range is between 10 and 30 mm.

The Basic Tear Secretion Test is the same test performed after topically anesthetizing the conjunctiva and blotting the inferior cul-de-sac dry. With reflex secretion eliminated, only basic secretion is measured. The patient must not feel the paper; otherwise, the test is invalid. The normal result is 10 mm of wetting within 5 minutes.

If the results of the Schirmer #1 test and the Basic Tear Secretion Test are low, the Schirmer #2 test can be done by irritating the middle turbinate of the unanesthetized nose. If this fails to wet the paper, there is a complete failure of the reflex secretors, not just a fatigue block. If there is more wetting, the reflex secretors are normal, but do not react because of a fatigue block of the efferent nerves of the conjunctiva.

Tests of Excretory Function[42]

The Primary Dye Test is the basic test to determine if there is a functioning excretory system. A drop of 2% fluorescein is instilled in the inferior cul-de-sac; after 5 minutes the meatus of the nose is swabbed with a cotton-tipped applicator. If fluorescein is found on the cotton, the test is positive, indicating an open and functioning excretory system. Because manipulations within the nose can be painful, this maneuver is facilitated by anesthetizing the nose with anesthetic spray or with a cotton pledget soaked in 5% cocaine or 4% lidocaine and placed under the inferior turbinate. An alternate way to perform this test is to place a drop of fluorescein in the side in question. After 5 minutes the patient is instructed to blow his nose into the tissue, while firmly holding the opposite nostril closed. If the dye cannot be recovered because of a dry nose, several drops of saline should be instilled into the nose; the dye then may be recovered either by blowing or by spitting out the fluid. Only one side can be tested in this manner, since it is sometimes difficult to tell from what side of the nose the dye has come. This test is especially helpful in children.

If there is epiphora with a normal Primary Dye Test, one must look for an ocular reason for the symptom.

When the Primary Dye Test is negative, all residual dye is wiped from the cul-de-sac, and lacrimal irrigation should be attempted; this is referred to as the Secondary Dye Test. If irrigation shows that the nasolacrimal duct is open and the fluid is tinged with fluorescein, it means not only that the ducts are at least partially patent but also that the lacrimal pump is normal, since dye made its way into the sac. It also indicates that there is an incomplete nasolacrimal block. If the fluid is clear, it means that dye did not reach the sac, indicating a punctal or canalicular stenosis, or, possibly, a lacrimal pump defect from a seventh nerve paresis.

Dacryocystography using radiopaque dye, or microscintigraphy using technetium 99, is indicated when the tests above are equivocal or when a mass is suspected within the sac. These tests reveal the site of many obstructions as well as the presence of diverticula and fistulas. In a normally functioning lacrimal system all radiopaque dye should disappear from the sac and the nasolacrimal duct within 30 minutes of injection. Failure to do so is evidence of a functional block.

To do a dacryocystogram, an angiocatheter #22 is stretched to narrow its lumen and then cut diagonally to form a more pointed catheter, which is threaded through the punctum. The catheter is taped to the cheek and face to allow injection of the dye. While the patient's head is against the x-ray machine, the physician can stand away while injecting the dye. A baseline Caldwell and lateral are taken first, followed by the same views immediately after injecting the dye. A final set is taken in 30 minutes.

If the patient is complaining of tearing, and pressure over the lacrimal sac produces regurgitation of tears and mucus, the diagnosis of obstruction of the nasolacrimal duct can be made with virtual certainty. However, when this helpful finding does not occur, instrument examination of the upper part of the lacrimal system is in order. Because the lower punctum is easier to expose, it is dilated with a sharp dilator and a #000 or #00 Bowman probe is passed along the canaliculus until it hits the bony fossa. As a rule, if the probe passes along the canaliculus for 12 to 15 mm, no block is present. If difficulty is encountered passing the probe into the sac, this could indicate a stenosis of the common canaliculus. This would be important to know preoperatively, since silicone intubation would be indicated to dilate the common canaliculus during the postoperative stage after a dacryocystorhinostomy.

The straight lacrimal cannula, attached to a syringe containing saline solution, is passed along the canaliculus. If irrigation into the nose is successful, the system is open. If there is shunting of the saline solution through the upper canaliculus and out the punctum, the nasolacrimal duct is probably blocked. If there is any question of a common canalicular block,

the investigation should also be carried out in the upper eyelid. If the canaliculus itself is totally blocked, attempted irrigation will produce a backflow of saline solution around the cannula. When one punctum is occluded and irrigation is attempted through the other, the sac will dilate if the nasolacrimal duct is blocked. In situations in which irrigation is partially successful but difficult to perform, a dacryocystogram will help in uncovering a functional block and demonstrate the possible need for therapy.

Stenosis of the Punctum

In congenital atresia of the puncta a transparent membrane bridges the punctal opening. The rest of the lacrimal system is usually intact and open. The child will have epiphora, but often not a great deal of mucus discharge. Breaking through the membrane with a sharp punctum dilator cures the condition.

Older people have stenosis of the puncta associated with involutional changes. Strong miotics also produce closure of the punctum. Repeated dilatation may be all that is necessary to keep the patient asymptomatic. If this is not successful, a punctalplasty is indicated.

Two-Snip Punctalplasty

Technique (Fig. 16–39)

A. The punctum is dilated as much as possible. One blade of a pair of sharp iris scissors is placed in the distal part of the punctum and the other blade on the tarsal–conjunctival surface. The tissue is cut.

B. A similar incision is made through the proximal part of the punctum, laying bare the punctum on the tarsal–conjunctival surface.

C. The incision is left open. A piece of silicone may be threaded into the canaliculus and sutured to the lid margin for several weeks in order to prevent closure of the new opening.

If both the upper and lower puncta are severely stenosed, indwelling silicone intubation (Quickert-Dryden) for several months is indicated (see next section).

Canalicular Disorders

Canaliculitis

Inflammation of the canaliculus is commonly caused by *Actinomyces israelii.* In acute cases

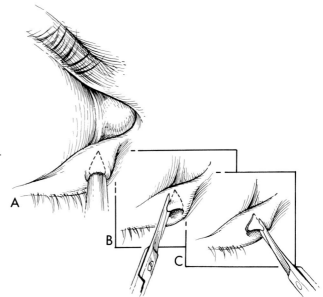

FIGURE 16–39. Two-snip punctalplasty.

the patient complains of a painful, erythematous swelling over the canaliculus. Hot compresses and antibiotics are indicated. *Actinomyces* is usually sensitive to tetracyclines, sulfas, and penicillins.

In the chronic case concretions develop and may cause lacrimal blockage. The concretions can often be milked out by massage. Gentle probing and irrigation may be needed to flush them out. If canaliculitis persists despite the use of antibiotics and manual expression, a canaliculotomy with direct removal of the concretions should be done.

Technique (Fig. 16–40)

A. A probe is placed in the affected canaliculus and an incision is made on the tarsal–conjunctival surface, sparing the punctum.

B. A curette removes the concretions from the dilated canaliculus (inset). The incision can be left open or repaired over a silicone tube.

Canalicular Stenosis

Common Canalicular Stenosis. If the common canaliculus is stenosed, but the nasolacrimal duct is open, the patient may complain of intermittent tearing. In this situation a lacrimal

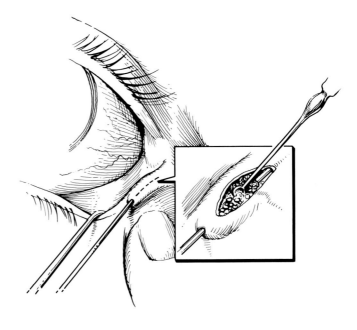

FIGURE 16–40. Canaliculotomy.

cannula passes easily through the canaliculus until just before it enters the sac. Irrigation at this point produces reflux out the opposite punctum; a slight amount of fluid may also enter the nose. If the cannula is able to be forced past the stenosis into the sac, irrigation is easily accomplished. The use of indwelling silicone tubes can serve to dilate the stenotic area.

INDWELLING SILICONE INTUBATION (QUICKERT-DRYDEN)[43]

Technique (Fig. 16–41)

A. Cottonoids (cotton strips 1 × 7.5 cm) soaked in 0.25% or 0.5% phenylephrine are placed in the inferior meatus. A fiberoptic headlight is used to illuminate the nasal cavity. The puncta are dilated maximally to allow easy passage of a wire probe with a silicone tube swaged on one end (Concept #9035, Storz #E5651,

Jed-Med #28-0185). A1. If the punctum is stenotic, a "one snip" is made on the tarsal–conjunctival surface.

B. The probe is then passed into the sac and brought into a vertical position to permit entry into the nasolacrimal duct. The cottonoids are removed from the inferior meatus before the probe is passed into the nose. A nasal speculum opens the nares, and the inferior turbinate is visualized. If the probe cannot be seen in the meatus, a periosteal elevator is placed along the medial side of the turbinate; this, with a small amount of pressure, fractures the turbinate medially toward the nasal septum to open up the meatus. A groove director is slid along the floor of the nose into the meatus and engages the end of the probe. With pressure from above, the probe will slide out the nose within the groove director, which is slowly withdrawn. Once the probe is grasped, it is slowly ad-

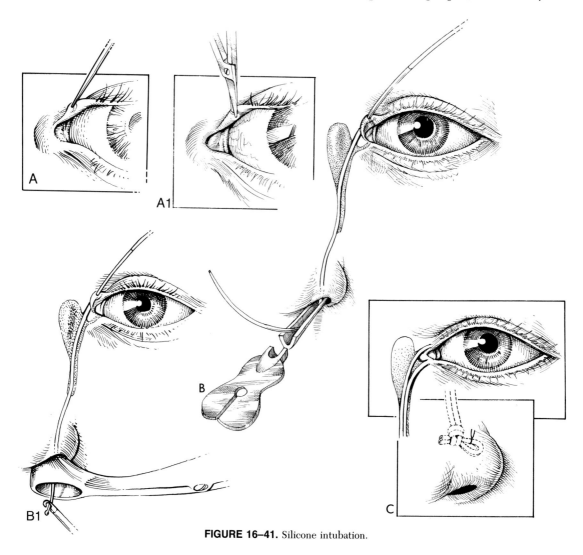

FIGURE 16–41. Silicone intubation.

vanced, making certain the medial eyelid is kept taut to allow the end of the probe with the tube swaged on to pass without being forced off. This is particularly important in the lower eyelid. Because the lower eyelid is more difficult to intubate, owing to its more acute angle to the nasolacrimal duct, it is advisable to do it first. B1. The Crawford intubation set (Jed-Med #28-0185) has probes that are approximately #000 to #0000 in size with a bulbous tip at the end. A hook with a special indentation is placed into the inferior meatus and engages the bulbous tip, and the probe is removed from the nose. This is useful in infants, who have a small space in which to work.

C. After both canaliculi have been intubated the two free ends of the tube are pulled out the nose for about 1 cm, so that the continuous loop becomes snug in the medial fornix. The two free ends of the tube in the nose are tied to each other, forming a small loop. A 5-0 Prolene suture is passed through the loop several times and then passed through the posterior aspect of the inner nares and tied. If the tube is under tension between the upper and lower puncta, the suture should be loosened within the nose. Ideally, there should be no tension on the puncta, and one should usually be able to pull the tubes out several millimeters.

The patient is instructed to avoid picking his nose, to prevent dislodging the suture. If the tube begins to come out of the puncta, it should be repositioned immediately, to prevent its complete extrusion or the distal looped ends from becoming lodged in the nasolacrimal duct or sac.

This technique of silicone intubation can be used in the following situations:

1. Congenital nasolacrimal duct obstruction when probing has failed
2. Trauma to the canaliculi or lacrimal sac
3. Punctal stenosis
4. Canalicular stenosis
5. Partial obstruction of the nasolacrimal duct
6. In combination with dacryocystorhinostomy with or without common canalicular stensosis

Patients are generally less symptomatic with the tubes in place because the tubes act as a wick around which tears can flow. The tubes are generally left in place for approximately 1 year, and can be left in as long as several years as long as the puncta are not being split. The dilatory effect on the stenosed lacrimal system has usually reached its maximum by 1 year.

To remove the tube, the loop in the medial fornix is cut, the suture is removed in the nares, and the tube is pulled out the nose. If the suture has become loose in the nose, the patient is asked to forcefully blow his nose, to bring the tube to the area of the nares where it can be grasped and removed. This technique can also be done in children, but it is occasionally necessary to remove the tube under general anesthesia if it is not well visualized in the nose.

Distal Canalicular Stenosis. After trauma to the canalicular system and despite attempted repair, a stricture can occur in the lower lid, causing epiphora. If the stenosis is in an accessible area of the eyelid, resecting the stenotic area and repairing it over a silicone tube stent is indicated.

RESECTION OF CANALICULAR STRICTURE

Technique (See Indwelling Silicone Intubation, Fig. 16–41)

A. Under the operating microscope the scar is excised to expose uninvolved canaliculus on either side.

B. The indwelling silicone tubes are passed first through the punctum and across the excised area into the proximal canaliculus and then through the rest of the lacrimal system. The other end is passed through the opposite eyelid. The canalicular ends are joined with interrupted sutures of 7-0 chromic catgut or Vicryl. The tubes are left in place for at least 6 months.

Complete Canalicular Stenosis. When both the upper and lower canaliculi are blocked, a bypass procedure is necessary. The most successful procedure has been the Lester Jones conjunctivodacryocystorhinostomy with use of a Pyrex glass tube,[42] described in the section on dacryocystorhinostomy.

Obstruction of the Nasolacrimal Duct

Congenital Nasolacrimal Duct Obstruction

Congenital nasolacrimal duct obstruction is usually due to a membranous obstruction at the valve of Hasner at the distal end of the nasolacrimal duct. It occurs in 5 to 7 per cent of newborns; one-third are bilateral. Some open spontaneously 4 to 6 weeks after birth.[44] Rarely, a blue dilated sac is present at birth; this may be an amniotocele, which is an accumulation of amniotic fluid and inspissated material within the sac and nasolacrimal duct. It may decompress on its own, but may require gentle probing to allow evacuation of the material before it becomes infected.

Conservative management with topical antibiotics, nasal decongestants, and massage is recommended as the first line of treatment. If there is no adequate improvement after 2 to 4 weeks, probing may be considered. General anesthesia is preferred after 6 months of age; before 6 months the procedure can be done merely by restraining the infant, although damage can occur to the lacrimal system by excessive movement. There is much difference of opinion as to the optimum age for probing. Because the great majority of cases clear spontaneously, many ophthalmologists routinely wait until the child is 6 months of age. Those ophthalmologists with an office setup that permits probings in small infants may prefer to do them at an earlier age, but these are still done only after a full trial of medical management. Our experience has been that probing done before 8 months of age will assure a 95 per cent cure rate. After 18 months of age, probing alone provides little chance of cure.

Probing of the Nasolacrimal Duct. The upper canaliculus is preferred, since it is easier to stretch the eyelid upward in passing the probe down the nasolacrimal duct. Also, if the canaliculus should be injured, it would be preferable to leave the lower one untouched. The punctum is dilated, and #00 or #000 Bowman probes are passed along each canaliculus to determine their patency. The lacrimal cannula is passed through the upper canaliculus, and irrigation is attempted. If the sac dilates or reflux is produced out the lower punctum, the nasolacrimal duct is blocked. A #00 probe is passed along the upper canaliculus into the sac. With the probe vertically positioned, gentle forward motion will find the mouth of the nasolacrimal duct. The probe is passed until it meets obstruction or until the floor of the nose is reached. In infants, passage of the probe beyond 2 cm usually indicates that the inferior meatus has been entered. The usual site of obstruction is at the valve of Hasner, which is in the membranous portion of the nasolacrimal duct within the inferior meatus. This block will produce a restriction in the passage of the probe, but a small amount of force will break through this membrane and, occasionally, a "pop" is felt. Irrigation through the upper canaliculus into the nose should now be successful. If there is any question of the patency because of reflux of some of the fluids out the inferior punctum, place a punctum dilator in the lower punctum and then irrigate through the upper canaliculus.

The fluid should now go directly into the nose. Using saline solution colored with fluorescein and recovering it on a cotton pledget in the inferior meatus is definite proof that the system is open. To increase the success rate of probings, we routinely in-fracture the inferior turbinate (see section on Silicone Intubation) at the beginning of the procedure. This increases the vault of the inferior meatus where the valve of Hasner empties.

The child is placed on antibiotic drops and the parents are requested to bring the child to the office 2 weeks later.

If the probe fails to penetrate the nasal mucosa within the inferior meatus, attempt to locate the probe along the lateral wall of the meatus with a periosteal elevator, and cut through the mucosa to the probe. This could turn a failure into a successfully functioning fistula. If a previous probing had been successful but a block recurred, another probing is in order. At the time of the repeat probing the inferior turbinate should be fractured toward the nasal septum to increase the size of the meatal vestibule.

If repeated probings have been technically successful but have otherwise failed, an indwelling silicone intubation (Quickert-Dryden) is indicated (see Fig. 17–32). It these tubes can be passed and left indwelling for 12 months, the membranous portion of the nasolacrimal duct may be permanently dilated and a dacryocystorhinostomy avoided.

Dacryocystorhinostomy is indicated (a) when the nasolacrimal duct is completely blocked and probing is impossible, or (b) after repeated probings and silicone intubation.

Acquired Nasolacrimal Duct Obstruction

After bouts of dacryocystitis a narrowing of the nasolacrimal duct resulting from the chronic infection can occur, leading to complete obstruction. Because of the nasolacrimal duct's proximity to the maxillary sinus and inferior meatus, chronic infection in the area can possibly predispose it to associated or secondary involvement, causing eventual obstruction. Despite the lacrimal sac's insulation by the lacrimal crest, severe trauma to the naso-orbital complex can easily injure the sac because of the bony crush between the nasal and ethmoidal areas. The nasolacrimal duct can also become plugged with the products of medications, such as the melanin casts that follow long-term treatment with epinephrine.

Acute Dacryocystitis. For mild infections topical antibiotics and hot compresses usually suffice; this is particularly true if regurgitation occurs, indicating an external opening to the sac. If frank cellulitis sets in, edema can occur around the common canaliculus, preventing regurgitation and sequestering the infection within the sac. At this point the infection can easily progress, producing a great deal of pain because of the stretching of the periosteum surrounding the sac. Associated signs are erythema and distention of the sac below the medial canthal tendon. Affected patients can become febrile and mildly toxic because of the severity of the infection.

Systemic antibiotics and hot compresses are indicated. Because most infections are caused by staphylococci, an antibiotic effective against the penicillinase-producing variety would be appropriate. Probing of the canaliculi is contraindicated; not only would it be extremely painful, but the probing could spread the infection. In cases of pointing and localization of the infection into an abscess, aspirating with a #18 needle or incising and draining brings instant relief. Placing a drain for 48 hours usually prevents an immediate recurrence or continuation of the process. Such an abscess is perilacrimal, in that the infection breaks through the sac and becomes subcutaneous; therefore, incising and draining usually neither injures the sac nor jeopardizes the success of a future dacryocystorhinostomy.

Nasolacrimal Duct Obstruction. If the primary dye test is negative but the secondary dye test shows fluorescein, a partial obstruction of the nasolacrimal duct is present. This can also be demonstrated by delayed emptying on a dacryocystogram. This is an ideal situation for an indwelling silicone tube; a dacryocystorhinostomy can often be avoided by inserting the tube for up to 12 months in an effort to dilate the membranous portion of the nasolacrimal duct.

DACRYOCYSTORHINOSTOMY. If there is a complete block of the nasolacrimal duct, or if silicone intubation has been unsuccessful in a partial obstruction, dacryocystorhinostomy is indicated. It is necessary to rule out nasal diseases that could compromise the end result. If there is any question of nasal polyps or deviated septum, an otorhinolaryngology examination should be recommended. The patient is also advised to refrain from taking aspirin for at least 2 weeks before and after surgery, to prevent interference with platelet aggregation and subsequent bleeding. A partial thromboplastin time test and prothrombin time are routinely ordered and, if indicated, a bleeding and clotting time, to alert the surgeon to a potential problem. Topical and systemic antibiotics are begun on the day of admission, since infection may be present within the sac. The patient is placed on tetracycline 500 mg every 12 hours, and is given gentamicin or the neomycin combination topically. If cellulitis is present, the surgery is postponed.

Technique (Fig. 16–42)

A. The patient is placed in a reverse Trendelenburg position to reduce venous pressure in the head area. The middle meatus adjacent to the lacrimal fossa is packed with 1×7.5-cm cottonoids soaked in 5% cocaine. An incision is made along the side of the nose 1 cm from the canthus, beginning at the level of the medial canthal tendon and angled toward the nasal alar fold for a distance of 2.5 cm.

B. After the skin incision is made the nasal skin is pulled toward the bridge of the nose to expose the underlying muscle at the different level, in an effort to "step" the incision, avoiding a direct cutaneous-osseous scar. The orbicularis is separated with scissors, with avoidance of the angular vein, which, when identified, can be reflected to one side. Bleeding points are coagulated with the electrocautery.

C. The periostum is incised and a cutting periosteal elevator is used to bare the bone and reflect the periosteum to the lacrimal crest. The blunt-tipped edge of a periosteal elevator is then used to separate the sac from the fossa. Occasionally the medial canthal tendon must be cut to give better exposure of the sac.

D. A Bowman probe is inserted through the superior punctum into the sac to identify its location. A vertical incision is made in the sac, exposing the probe; this prevents missing a full-thickness cut. The incision is placed on the anterior side to leave the posterior flap larger, which facilitates later placement of the sutures.

E. Two 4-0 chromic catgut sutures are placed with a G-2 needle through the anterior flap. Radial incisions are made superior and inferior to the suture placement, to create a flap. A posterior flap is similarly created. Two serrafine clamps of different sizes are placed on the suture ends of the anterior and posterior flaps to aid in their identification.

F. With the sac retracted laterally, an air drill with a 5-mm burr is used to remove the anterior crest. Before reaching the mucosa, the nasal packing is removed.

G. Once the mucosa is exposed, a Kerrison punch is used to enlarge the opening to ap-

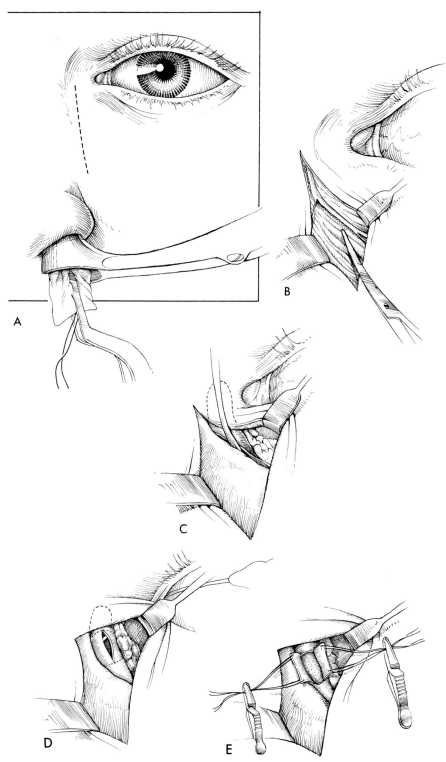

FIGURE 16–42. Dacryocystorhinostomy.

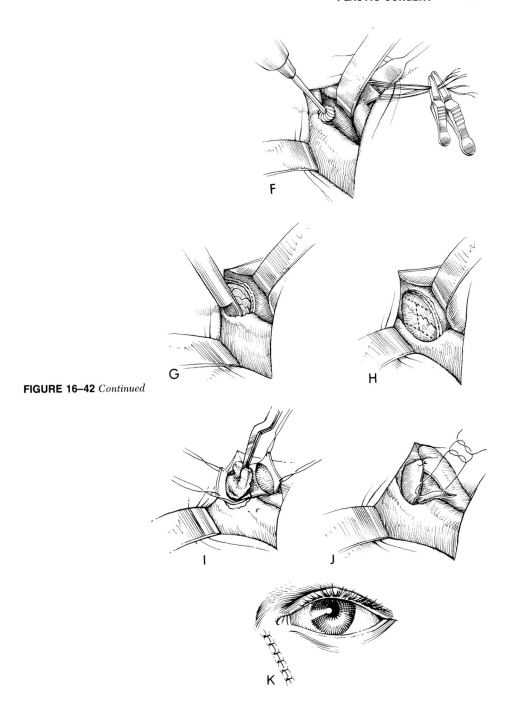

FIGURE 16–42 *Continued*

proximately 12 mm in diameter; the entire area of the lacrimal fossa should be included.

H. With an open, curved hemostat in the nose supporting the nasal mucosa, vertical and horizontal incisions are made to create anterior and posterior nasal flaps. If the mucosa is inadvertently torn or shredded, the bony opening is enlarged to gain greater mucosal length.

I. The posterior flaps of the sac and nasal mucosa are joined with the preplaced 4-0 chromic catgut sutures. Additional sutures can be added, if necessary, to improve the mucosal apposition. At this point two options are available for maintaining hemostasis: (1) Adaptic gauze packing into the rhinostomy site and nose, and (2) Gelfoam packing in the rhinostomy site. If bleeding has not been sufficiently controlled with cautery or intermittent packing with cottonoids, the entire area can be packed with ½-inch Adaptic gauze packing impregnated with Polysporin ointment. This is brought up through the nose to the rhinostomy site, where about 4 inches are brought out. This portion of the gauze is carefully folded within the rhinostomy site. The nasal portion is then folded over and over to pack the nasal cavity all the way.

Ordinarily the Gelfoam packing is sufficient and much simpler.[45] One or two pieces of Gelfoam, $0.7 \times 2.0 \times 6.0$ cm, is soaked in a 5000-unit thrombin solution. The thrombin-soaked Gelfoam pack is then placed in the rhinostomy site. Because thrombin is a protein material, it eventually dissolves and does not need to be removed.

J. The anterior flaps are joined with the preplaced 4-0 chromic catgut suture.

K. The orbicularis is closed with three or four 6-0 plain catgut sutures, which can be used for skin closure as well. A subcuticular 6-0 Prolene suture supplemented by interrupted 6-0 Prolene sutures can also be used to bring the skin edges together. If Adaptic gauze packing is used, it is sutured to the external nares with three or four 4-0 prolene sutures to prevent the nasal pack from falling out.

A folded eye pad is placed over the incision site only. The systemic and topical antibiotics are continued. The patient is usually discharged on the second postoperative day and returns in 7 days for suture removal.

COMPLICATIONS

Bleeding. In the postoperative period the principal problem is bleeding from the rhinostomy site. Packing the site during surgery will prevent this problem; however, removal of gauze packing can bruise newly formed vessels or dislodge clots, which can cause bleeding. It is advisable to leave the pack in for 48 hours, since by then there is less risk of bleeding when it is removed. Moreover, since the packing must make a right-angled turn when being pulled out, it should not be tightly placed within the sac, as this would result in undue trauma to the fresh anastomosis. If infection occurs and worsens despite the use of antibiotics, removal of the pack is indicated. The pack should be removed gently. A little oozing is not uncommon. If active bleeding occurs, the clots within the nose should be removed and cocaine-soaked cottonoids placed against the rhinostomy site. If bleeding persists, the middle meatus can be repacked with Adaptic gauze. If the bleeding cannot be stopped, an otorhinolaryngologist

should be consulted. Postoperative bleeding is a rare problem when the Gelfoam pack is used.

Common Canalicular Stenosis. Recognizing a canalicular stricture preoperatively is important for preventing an unsuccessful functional result from occurring despite a successful anatomical result. The presence of a stricture can be determined by careful probing of the canaliculus to the bony fossa. If the block is in the region of the common canaliculus and is incomplete, the indwelling silicone tubes should be passed through each canaliculus into the nose and tied together near the external nares. If the problem is recognized in the immediate postoperative period, silicone intubation is indicated to salvage a good result.

Closure of the Rhinostomy Site. It is important to recognize nasal problems that may militate against a successful result. These include a deviated septum and polyps, or any other abnormality of the middle turbinate or within the middle meatus. If, after removal of gauze packing, there appears to be some reduction of tear flow, or if irrigation is difficult, the nose should be examined to determine whether there is any retained packing material. If a failure appears evident in the early postoperative period, it is probably due to a fibrovascular occlusive membrane over the rhinostomy. Sometimes salvage of the dacryocystorhinostomy is possible with an intranasal excision of this secondary membrane, as follows.

Technique for Reopening Rhinostomy Site (Fig. 16–43)

A. A probe is introduced through the canaliculus and advanced until it has reached the nasal obstruction. With the probe tenting the membrane, a sharp periosteal elevator is cut into the membrane.

B. The remainder of the membrane is cut away with angled, punch scissors followed by insertion of indwelling silicone tubes.

If failure occurs or has been present for several months, a repeat dacryocystorhinostomy should be done.

Hypertrophic Scar. An unsightly scar results from excessive buried catgut sutures, from failing to "step" the incision to avoid a direct cutaneous-osseous adhesion, or because the patient has a tendency to form keloid. If the incision is too close to the canthus, or is curved along the lacrimal crest, there can be vertical contractures, producing an epicanthal fold or a pulling downward of the medial aspect of the lower lid. Most dacryocystorhinostomy scars are

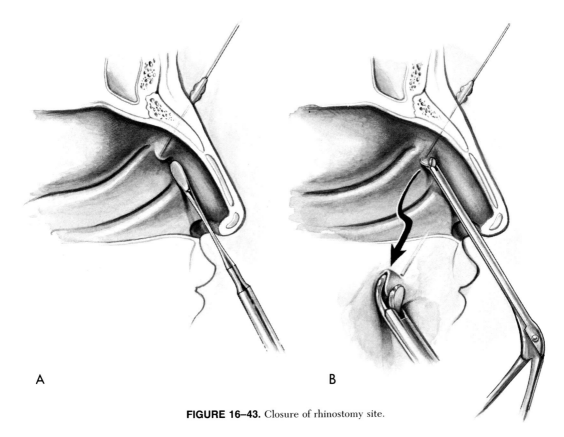

FIGURE 16–43. Closure of rhinostomy site.

somewhat bumpy, but improve in contour within 6 months.

Total Canalicular Block

When both the upper and lower canaliculi are blocked, or when there is a total common canalicular block, a canalicular bypass or conjunctivodacryocystorhinostomy is indicated.[43] This is most effectively accomplished with a Jones Pyrex glass tube, since this material has good capillary traction for tears. The tube is well tolerated by the tissues, and any mucus accumulated can be easily removed. The tube acts as a conduit for tears between the medial fornix and the middle meatus of the nose. The patient, however, must be made aware of the attention that must be paid to the care of the tube and of the need for a lifetime commitment to the tube, since its removal can cause the fistula tract to collapse.

Conjunctivodacryocystorhinostomy (Jones Tube Procedure)

TECHNIQUE (Fig. 16–44)

A. A dacryoscystorhinostomy (see Fig. 16–42) is done through step I. A lid speculum is placed in the cul-de-sac, and the caruncle is excised.

B. At the excision site a knife or sharp scissors is used to make a tract through the medial canthal tissues and lacrimal sac to the area of the common canaliculus.

C. A #1 Bowman probe is used as a guide for the insertion, through the tract, of the polyethylene tube (#240). A collar for the tube is fashioned by flaming one end of the tube, using an ordinary match; the usual length of the tube is 15 to 18 mm. The tube should fit snugly in the medial fornix; the other end should pass over the posterior ledge of the rhinostomy site by several millimeters and rest freely in the middle meatus without abutting the turbinate or nasal septum. The collar is sutured to the medial canthal tissues with several 4-0 silk sutures. The anterior flaps are closed over the tube, and the remainder of the incision is closed as previously described. A Gelfoam-thrombin pack is placed within the rhinostomy site.

D. (Optional) A mucous membrane–lined tract can be created that obviates closure of the tract if the tube should be lost, and may allow permanent removal of the tube sometime in the future.[46]

D1. A full-thickness mucous membrane graft measuring 1.0 × 1.5 cm is removed from the

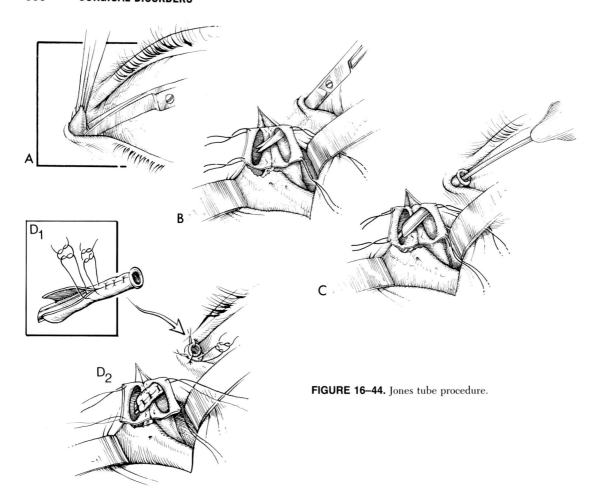

FIGURE 16–44. Jones tube procedure.

lower lip (see Fig. 16–20). The graft is placed around the polyethylene tube, mucosal surface against the tube, and sutured together with 6-0 Vicryl.

D2. The mucous membrane–covered tube is placed in the tract and the mucosa adjacent to the collar joined to the conjunctiva.

Instead of using the polyethylene tube as the initial stent, a Pyrex tube can be placed at the time of surgery. This must be secured to the medial canthus with the suture wrapped around the collar and then through the tissues, or with sutures through small holes in the collar. The collar is usually 4 mm and the tube between 16 and 18 mm in length. This, of course, eliminates the change of tubes necessary in the postoperative period when polyethylene is used.

If a polyethylene tube is used, the exchange is made about 6 weeks postoperatively, with topical anesthesia. If mucous membrane was used, the exchange is made after 8 weeks. The polyethylene tube is removed around a wire guide, which is left in the tract. The Pyrex tube

with a 4-mm collar is run along the wire guide and, with a little pressure, worked into place. If the same size tube is used, it should be seen in the middle meatus of the nose.

CARE OF THE TUBE. It is necessary to caution the patient about holding his finger over the tube or squeezing his lids shut when sneezing; sudden pressure within the nose can force the tube out. If mucus accumulates within the tube, it can be cleaned out with a plastic guide or with a squeeze bottle of saline solution held over the tube.

COMPLICATIONS OF JONES TUBES. If for any reason the tube becomes dislodged or comes out, immediate examination and replacement should be carried out; otherwise, it will be necessary to dilate the tract or even surgically reopen it.

Migration of the tube is an indication that the tract has changed or that bony regrowth has taken place internally. It can also occur from not having had the tube resting freely in the rhinostomy site, away from the bony edges.

The tube may migrate anteriorly in the medial canthus or posteriorly against the globe. When migration occurs, it is necessary to make a new tract, or at least to reposition the distal aspect of the tract to allow the tube to rest without tension in the desired location.

Granulation tissue around the tube can form in the early stages of healing, and possibly block it. Such tissues should be excised and the base cauterized.

Lacrimal Fistula

If the rod of cells—the anlage of the lacrimal duct—that extends from the sac to the skin beneath the medial to the lower punctum does not involute, a lacrimal sac fistula will be present. Jones and Wobig[42] refer to this as the "lacrimal anlage duct." A small dimple can usually be seen below the medial canthal tendon. Although the lacrimal system may be open, many of these patients have tears running out the fistula and down their cheek, producing symptoms that may necessitate repair.

Excision of Lacrimal Fistula

Technique (Fig. 16–45)

A. A probe is placed within the tract as a guide; excision of the tract is carried out to just before it joins with the lacrimal system.

B. An absorbable suture ligature is placed around its distal portion and the tract excised.

C. The incision is closed with fine suture material.

Lacrimal Sac Tumors

Neoplasms of the lacrimal sac are rare but should be suspected when the following triad is found: (1) mass above the medial canthal tendon, (2) chronic dacryocystitis that irrigates freely, and (3) bloody reflux on irrigation. In addition, there can be ulceration of the skin over the sac and regional adenopathy.[47] The most common malignant tumor is transitional cell epidermoid carcinoma.

A computerized tomography scan through the lacrimal sac fossa may show bone erosion, and a dacryocystogram can reveal a dilated sac with partial patency as well as an uneven, mottled density of the contrast media.

The most effective treatment is dacryocystectomy. If there is adjacent spread or bony involvement, a medial canthal exenteration may be necessary. Radiation may also be used, depending on the sensitivity of the tumor. Despite these forms of treatment, the 5-year survival rate is only 50 per cent.

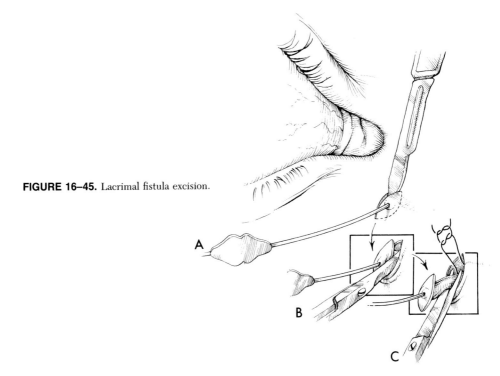

FIGURE 16–45. Lacrimal fistula excision.

Trauma to the Lacrimal System

Laceration of the Canaliculus

All lacerations in the medial canthal area should be carefully inspected for a possible injury to the canaliculus. Many are occult, since edema may join the lacerated edges together, preventing their discovery. A deep laceration between the punctum and canthal angle creates a lateral displacement of the eyelid because the lower arm of the medial canthal tendon has been cut and would invariably involve the canaliculus.

If a canalicular laceration is suspected, gently probe through the punctum to determine if an obstruction is met or if the probe is seen within the laceration. Irrigation produces an extravasation of fluid around the laceration site. It is usually impossible to carry out this examination in conscious children; thus it is necessary to examine any suspected canalicular lacerations under general anesthesia, even when there appears to be good tissue apposition. Although both canaliculi are important, the lower one,

because of its position, may be more effective in draining tears; regardless, every effort should be made to repair any severed canaliculus. The upper canaliculus system may be important to an older person who has punctal stenosis or eversion of the lower lids, which mitigates against a functioning lower canaliculus.

Repair of Canalicular Laceration

TECHNIQUE (Fig. 16–46)

A. The operating microscope or other magnification is almost mandatory for finding the cut ends of the canaliculus, especially with a medially located laceration because of its deeper position. Irrigation with saline solution helps to identify the cut epithelium of the canaliculus by whitening it against the red color of the muscle. The punctum is dilated. A 0.94- or 1.19-mm outside diameter silicone tube is threaded over a #000 or #0000 Bowman probe and passed into the laceration site. The medial end of the canaliculus is located, and the silicone tube with the probe is passed through it into the sac. To make certain it is in the sac,

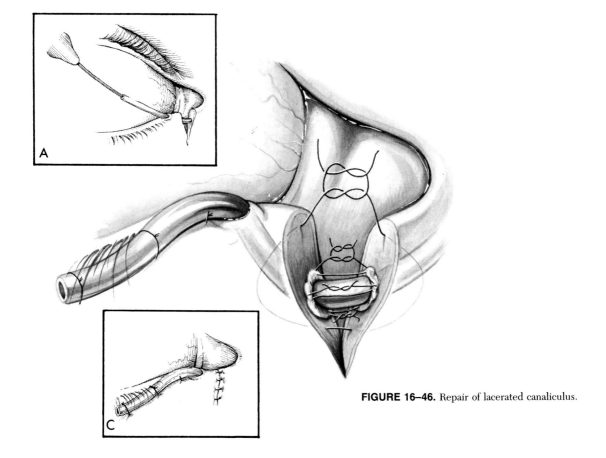

FIGURE 16–46. Repair of lacerated canaliculus.

irrigation is carried out through the tube with a lacrimal cannula.

B. A suture of 6-0 silk is passed through the tube and lid margin, to prevent inadvertent removal of the tube. Three sutures of 7-0 chromic catgut are placed through the lumens of the cut canaliculi. If necessary, a 4-0 chromic catgut suture is placed to reapproximate the lid to the medial canthal tendon. Additional sutures of 6-0 chromic catgut are used to approximate the orbicularis and tendon around the canaliculus, to support it while it is healing.

C. Two additional sutures of 6-0 silk are placed through and around the tube, anchoring it to the lid margin 5 to 7 mm from the punctum. The tube is left in for at least 4 to 5 weeks. During that time patients are instructed to wear a shield at night to prevent them from rubbing the area and loosening the sutures.

For lower canalicular lacerations, particularly in children, the indwelling silicone tubes (see Fig. 16–32) would be preferred. The end-to-end anastomosis is carried out as described above to promote optimal healing. This ensures retention of the stent until its removal is indicated, usually in 3 months; the success rate is more than 90 per cent.

If both canaliculi are cut and the medial ends are located, the indwelling silicone tubes (see Fig. 16–32) are used. The repair of the cut ends of the canaliculi is carried out as previously described. The tubes are left in for at least 1 year.

If it is impossible to find either medial end, a silicone tube 2.5 mm in diameter with a cuffed end (made by Gunter Weiss) can be used as a bypass. The caruncle is removed, and small sharp scissors are used to make a tract in the direction of the lacrimal sac. A probe is placed through the tract, and the silicone tube is passed. An incision is then made in the lacrimal sac, and the tube is threaded into the sac and down the nasolacrimal duct. Polyethylene is too stiff to bend around these corners and will distort the medial canthal angle. Several 6-0 silk sutures will hold the end of the tube in the angle. If lacrimal drainage is not sufficient with the silicone tube, it can be exchanged for a Jones Pyrex tube.

Trauma to the Lacrimal Sac

Trauma to the lacrimal sac is often an associated result of trauma to the naso-orbital area with collapse of the lacrimal fossa. Direct injury to the nasolacrimal duct or sac occurs less frequently. It has been reported as a complication of rhinoplasty.

As a rule, early repair of a damaged lacrimal sac in closed injuries is not feasible. Such damage may not become apparent until the edema disappears and adequate evaluation is possible. With open injuries investigation can be carried out at the time of repair. Elevation of fractures along the lacrimal system, repair of lacerations of the sac, and insertion of the indwelling continuous loop silicone tube (Quickert-Dryden[43]) should be performed in an effort to maintain patency of the system. Dacryocystorhinostomy is necessary for eventual failures or permanent obstruction.

EYELID TUMORS: MANAGEMENT AND REPAIR

The most common eyelid malignancy is basal cell carcinoma.[48, 49] It occurs on the lower lid in 90 per cent of cases, followed in order of frequency by the medial canthus, lateral canthus, and upper eyelid. Squamous cell carcinoma is an infrequent lesion, and meibomian gland carcinoma is also rare. However, because these latter two lesions can metastasize, vigilance must be maintained and prompt biopsy carried out in cases of questionable lesions, chronic ulcerative blepharitis, or longstanding nodules undergoing change.

A biopsy can be done in the office with local anesthesia. If the mass is nodular and involves the eyelid without distorting the margin, it can be shaved flush with the margin and the raw base sealed with a hyfrecator. If the histologic report is benign, the surgery will have successfully rid the patient of his lesion. If it is a basal cell carcinoma, surgery is recommended. Because basal cell carcinoma is usually a slow-growing tumor and does not metastasize, there is no emergency to removing it. If it is a squamous cell or meibomian gland carcinoma, however, prompt eyelid resection should be carried out.

If a mass is obviously malignant, such as one distorting the eyelid margin or one with a large central ulceration, a biopsy can be done in the operating room and the definitive surgery carried out as soon as a report has been received. This spares the patient a separate biopsy procedure in the office. However, there is one advantage to the office biopsy, in that the patient and the surgeon have additional time to contemplate the next step. This is of particular significance in cases that may require extensive resection and complicated repair.

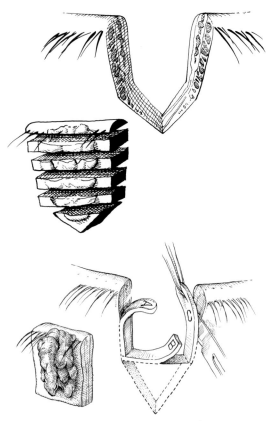

FIGURE 16–47. Frozen section technique.

Frozen Section–Controlled Resection

The operating room microscope or high-power loupes will help in delineating the extent of the tumor by identifying normal meibomian gland orifices that should indicate normal eyelid.[49] The marking pencil is used to draw a line around the tumor, including at least a 0.5-mm space of normal tissue. There are two common means for the pathologist to read the sections.

(Above) In one method India ink is placed at one edge for orientation purposes. Horizontal sections are cut through the specimen, beginning at the lid margin, and are taken well below the extent of the tumor.

(Below) Because it is sometimes difficult for the pathologist to read the margins, owing to crushing of the tissue during processing, the other method involves removal of another 0.5 mm from each side and inferiorly, if necessary (Fig. 16–47). These small strips are labeled according to their location and sent to the pathologist. (Orientation of the strips, except for their location on the lid, is unnecessary, since the presence or absence of tumor is the only information that is needed.) If the pathol-

ogist finds tumor cells, an additional 0.5-mm strip is removed and sent to the laboratory; this process is continued until negative reports are obtained. If a meibomian gland carcinoma is suspected, a fat stain should be requested on fresh tissue. Because there is a tendency for pagetoid spread, suspicious areas in either eyelid or on the bulbar conjunctiva should be sampled.

Small to Moderate Resections of the Eyelid

Primary Closure. For small resections that include approximately one quarter of the upper or lower eyelid, a pentagon-shaped excision can be done with primary closure.

TECHNIQUE (Fig. 16–48). Vertical lines are drawn on either side of the tumor in the pretarsal area and then joined in the cul-de-sac. The vertical length of the resections should be between 1.5 and 2.0 times the horizontal length along the margin, to allow approximation without bunching of the tissues inferiorly. The closure is the same as the basic eyelid closure (Fig. 16–3).

Primary Repair with Canthotomy and Cantholysis. If the edges are difficult to approximate or are under tension, a canthotomy and cantholysis should be done.[30] This can release either eyelid 3 to 5 mm and allow adequate closure.

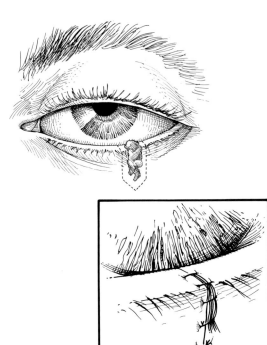

FIGURE 16–48. Primary closure for lid tumor resection.

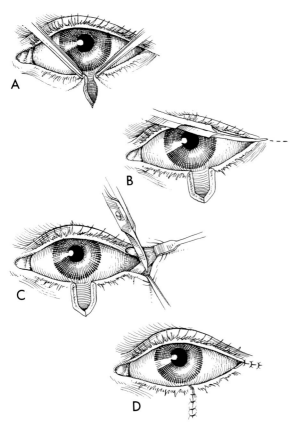

FIGURE 16–49. Primary closure with canthotomy and cantholysis.

TECHNIQUE (Fig. 16–49)

A. After eyelid excision the edges cannot be approximated.

B. A horizontal incision is made through the lateral canthus to the rim.

C. The skin anteriorly and the conjunctiva posteriorly are separated on either side of the lower arm of the canthal tendon before it is cut. An immediate release of the eyelid can be felt. The separation must include all the attachments between the lid and the rim, to allow for maximum relaxation.

D. The closure is carried out as described for the basic eyelid closure (Fig. 16–3). The canthotomy is closed with interrupted 6-0 plain catgut, and the canthal angle is re-formed. The area that has been advanced from the canthus is left unsutured.

Moderate to Large Resections of the Lower Eyelid

Resections that involve from one-third to one-half of the lower eyelid can be repaired by use of a variety of tarsal–conjunctival grafts and periorbital skin flaps or free grafts.

Transpositional Tarsal Grafts with Upper Eyelid Skin-Muscle Flaps. In this procedure the tarsal-conjunctival flap is a single horizontal transpositional flap based in the lateral fornix. The skin-muscle flap is taken from the supratarsal area and is based in the lateral canthus.[50]

TECHNIQUE (Fig. 16–50)

A. The tumor is removed with a free edge of 1 mm followed by the frozen section control as described previously. The skin-muscle flap is outlined in the upper lid by drawing a line in the upper eyelid crease to the lateral canthal area. Estimation of the amount of upper lid skin safely removed is made, and the superior line is drawn parallel to the crease line. This line is taken a little farther laterally for easier rotation of the graft into the lower lid.

B. The upper lid is everted, and the tarsal-conjunctival graft is prepared by making two parallel incisions 2 to 3 mm from the lid margin; the graft is 4 mm wide and is hinged in the lateral fornix. Its length corresponds to the size of the defect.

C. The tarsal-conjunctival graft is rotated into the defect; if there is too much laxity in the graft, a tuck can be taken between the conjunctival pedicle and lateral canthal tendon to firm its lateral base. The shaded area is the donor site, which is left unsutured. The upper eyelid skin flap is removed from the supratarsal area, to avoid, as much as possible, skin removal directly over the donor tarsal graft. The width and length of the flap are governed by the size of the defect, with several millimeters added to allow for shrinkage.

D. The graft is sutured to the inferior conjunctiva with 6-0 chromic catgut. It is lined up with the medial lid segment and sutured to the tarsus with 6-0 chromic catgut. It is important to maintain a firm apposition of the graft to the globe. If the graft is too long, it can be trimmed immediately, or it can be attached to the lateral canthal area with 6-0 chromic catgut suture.

E. The skin-muscle flap is sutured in place with interrupted 6-0 silk with the ends left long, and the two grafts are joined at the new eyelid margin. It is sutured to the tarsus superiorly, with care taken to ensure that the skin edge is away from the globe. A double-armed 6-0 silk suture is brought full thickness through the remaining eyelid medial to the suture line, to be used as a bracing suture for the cotton stent.

F. A cotton roll soaked in antibiotic solution and surrounded by Adaptic gauze is tied over the graft and is extended 1 cm beyond the

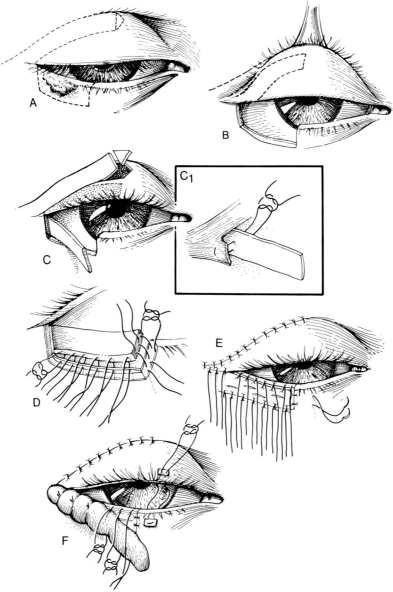

FIGURE 16–50. Transpositional tarsal-conjunctival graft with skin muscle transpositional graft for lower eyelid tumor.

lateral canthus and suture line medially. Sutures through the uninvolved lid medially, and beyond the lateral canthus laterally, are used to tie over the stent. The stent serves to keep the skin graft on stretch while it is healing, and the sutures beyond the graft help to brace the graft and the suture line by anchoring the stent in the uninvolved eyelid. The stent and sutures are removed in 1 week. The patient is asked to wear a shield at night, to avoid the risk of inadvertent trauma to the area. If vision is good in the other eye, an intermarginal suture (see Fig. 16–51) placed medially between the lids

helps to splint the wound while it is healing. The suture is removed after 1 to 2 weeks.

This procedure is suited for lateral lower lid defects that are too large to be closed primarily with a canthotomy and cantholysis. The transpositional tarsal-conjunctival graft and skin-muscle flap from the upper eyelid act as a sling, preventing a lateral lower eyelid sag. This complication can follow temporal rotational flaps or lower eyelid skin advancement flaps. Another important maneuver in preventing vertical shortening of the graft is to separate conjunctiva from the lower eyelid retractors, to prevent downward traction on the tarsal-conjunctival graft.

Because support for a reconstructed eyelid is important, a tarsal-conjunctival graft is the ideal material, since it restores a similar mucous membrane–supported structure. Moreover, it is a pedicle flap with a blood supply, which aids in ensuring its viability. The skin-muscle flap from the upper eyelid purposely includes orbicularis, to ensure a blood supply that will aid in nourishing the underlying tarsal-conjunctival graft, augmenting the circulation originating from the base of the tarsal-conjunctival flap.

The skin-muscle flap should be taken from above the superior tarsal border, so that it does not overlie the donor tarsal-conjunctival flap area. This staggered placement of the two flaps in the upper eyelid is important, as it will prevent a contiguous defect with only a thin layer of orbicularis remaining, which could cause distortion or vertical shortening during healing.

Temporal Skin Flap with or without Tarsal-Conjunctival Transpositional Flap. If the defect is too large for a canthotomy-cantholysis, a temporal flap, similar to a "Mustardé" flap,[51] can be mobilized. For small flaps, conjunctiva from the lateral fornix can cover the flap; larger flaps may require a transpositional tarsal-conjunctival flap for support.

Technique (Fig. 16–51)

A. The horizontal extent of the mass is measured, and vertical incisions twice that length are made on either side of the tumor and joined in the lower cul-de-sac. The medial one is almost vertical. At the lateral canthus an incision is then begun following the upward curve of the lower eyelid. It passes just under the brow and over the zygomatic arch toward the ear. The skin and subcutaneous tissue are undermined inferiorly to a level at least as far as the inferior edge of the resection. It should not go into the deep muscle area, as fibers of the

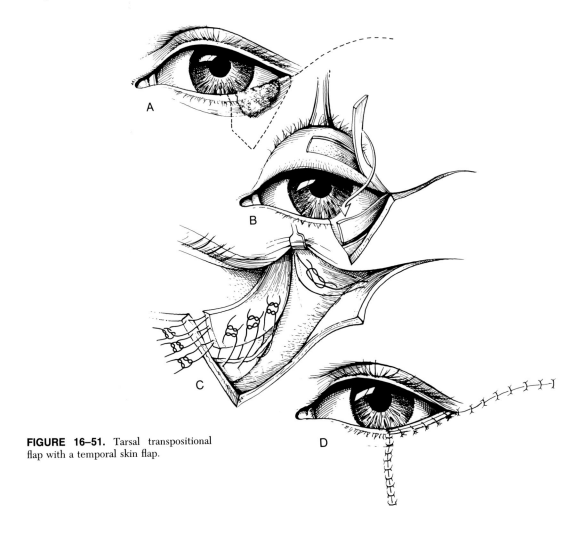

FIGURE 16–51. Tarsal transpositional flap with a temporal skin flap.

seventh cranial nerve could be injured. If the skin is supple, as in older people, only a small flap is necessary, while, conversely, in younger people a larger flap is necessary because of the tautness of the skin. It is wise to make the flaps smaller than needed at first and then to enlarge them as necessary to obtain easy rotation into the defect.

B. The temporal skin flap is pulled into the defect and approximated with the medial lid segment. If there are two free lid margin areas, the basic lid closure is used to join them. If the resection included all the eyelid to the lateral canthus, the free edge of the flap is connected to the remaining lid segment, with 6-0 Vicryl between the tarsus on one side and the subcutaneous tissue on the other; 6-0 silk is used between the skin surfaces. The temporal skin flap is anchored to the lateral rim with a deep suture of 4-0 Vicryl to the periosteum (see Fig. 16–51*B*). At this point the upward curve of the lower lid is overcorrected to account for some postoperative sagging. Conjunctiva is loosened from the lateral fornix to line the flap and is sutured to the temporal skin with 6-0 silk.

C. If more than one-third of the reconstructed lower lid is unsupported, a transpositional tarsal-conjunctival graft from the upper lid to the lower lid can be used (see Fig. 16–50). The outer covering will be provided by the temporal flap as described above. The conjunctiva is separated from the lower lid retractors in the inferior fornix. The graft is sutured to the medial lid segment with 6-0 Vicryl, bringing the graft to the level of the lid margin. It is joined to the conjunctiva in the inferior fornix with 6-0 chromic catgut.

D. The graft is sutured to the skin flap at the new lid margin with 6-0 silk. The canthal angle is re-formed with a deeply placed suture of 5-0 Vicryl, which is externalized. The rest of the incision is closed with deep 5-0 chromic catgut and 5-0 Prolene to the skin.

If tarsus is unavailable for support, nasal septal cartilage and mucosa or upper lateral nasal cartilage and mucosa can be substituted.

Free Tarsal-Conjunctival Graft with Nasally Based Skin-Muscle Flap. This procedure is particularly suited for reconstruction of the medial eyelid because there is little stretch of the medial canthal tissues.[52]

Technique (Fig. 16–52)

A. The tumor is outlined and removed with a clear margin of at least 1 mm.

B. The upper eyelid is everted and a free tarsal-conjunctival graft 4 mm wide and similar in length to the defect in the lower eyelid is removed, leaving at least 3 mm of tarsus at the lid margin. This defect is left unsutured.

C. The graft is sutured in place with interrupted sutures of 6-0 chromic catgut. If the graft is not fairly tight against the globe, it should be trimmed.

D. The skin and orbicularis below the defect form a pedicle flap that is slightly larger than the defect and is based in the medial canthal area.

E. The skin and tarsal-conjunctival grafts are joined with interrupted sutures of 6-0 silk to form the new eyelid margin. Some undermining may be necessary to obliterate traction lines.

F. An ellipse of full-thickness postauricular skin is removed, and the donor site is closed with a continuous 4-0 Prolene suture.

G. In the defect created by the transfer of the skin pedicle flap, the full-thickness postauricular graft is placed and sutured with interrupted 6-0 silk. At the superior edge, where it is sutured to the pedicle graft, bites are taken in the subcutaneous tissue to secure both to the deeper layers. Stab incisions are made in the graft for drainage.

H. This is the immediate postoperative appearance. A cotton stent can be placed over both grafts and tied, with the sutures having been left long at the lid margin and at the inferior edge of the pedicle flap.

If the distal aspect of the canaliculus is intact, an attempt is made to externalize it with sutures, and a silicone tube is left within the orifice for 4 to 6 weeks. When the canaliculus is resected, the tarsal-conjunctival graft is sutured to the lower arm of the canthal tendon with a double-armed suture of 4-0 Vicryl.

The advantage of this procedure is that the lateral canthus is undisturbed and the visual axis is left open, with the repair confined to the medial canthal and nasal area. However, a canthotomy and cantholysis can be done at the lateral canthus to gain further relaxation of the lateral lid segment. If vision is satisfactory in the opposite eye, an intermarginal suture (see Fig. 16–64) lateral to the reconstructed area will splint the wound while it is healing. This suture is removed 1 to 2 weeks postoperatively.

Large Resection of the Lower Eyelid

Modified Hughes Lower Eyelid Reconstruction. For defects involving almost the total lower eyelid, the modified Hughes method is the procedure of choice.[30] This is an advancement tarsal-conjunctival flap from the upper

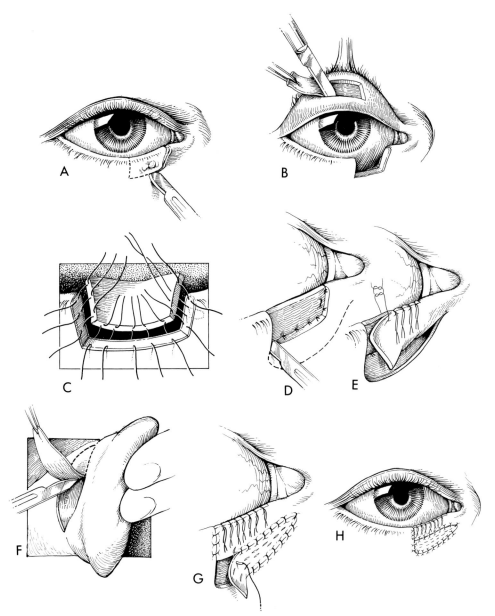

FIGURE 16–52. Medial eyelid reconstruction with free tarsal graft.

eyelid combined with a free skin graft, providing the internal and external lamellae needed to support the new lower eyelid. A disadvantage is the necessity to occlude the fissure for several weeks until the conjunctival flap is released.

TECHNIQUE (Fig. 16–53)

A. The tumor is removed with frozen section control along all edges, with as much conjunctiva left as possible. The upper eyelid is everted, and a horizontal incision is made 3 to 5 mm from the lid margin, depending on

how much tarsal-conjunctival tissue is left in the lower lid. The horizontal length is approximately the same as the amount removed.

B. (Cross section) The tarsus is lifted from the orbicularis to its superior border. Here, Müller's muscle is disinserted, and the dissection is carried into the superior cul-de-sac between Müller's muscle and conjunctiva.

C. In the lower eyelid, conjunctiva is separated from the lower lid retractors to preclude any vertical traction on the grafts.

D. The tarsal-conjunctival graft is brought

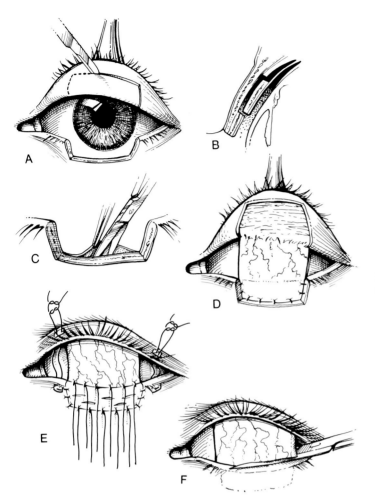

FIGURE 16–53. Modified Hughes procedure.

into the defect and sutured with 6-0 Vicryl to the remaining conjunctiva in the cul-de-sac and the tarsus of the medial and lateral lid edges. Enough tarsus is brought down so that the superior border of the tarsal graft will form the new lid margin. If there is a shortage of conjunctiva, it can be further separated from the retractors to the cul-de-sac and brought up to meet the graft.

E. A full-thickness postauricular graft is placed over the tarsal-conjunctival advancement graft, with the superior border of the skin graft corresponding with the superior border of the tarsal graft. It is sutured with 6-0 silk with the ends left long. Before it is completely sutured in place, a #11 Bard-Parker blade is used to make small stab incisions for drainage. A cotton stent soaked in antibiotic solution is tied over the grafts. If there is lower lid left on either side of the reconstruction, intermarginal sutures of 5-0 Prolene are placed over silicone pegs to splint the lid; they are left in for several weeks.

At the end of 1 week the stent and all sutures are removed.

F. After 4 weeks the conjunctival flap is separated from the tarsal margin and allowed to retract. Some trimming of the new lid margin may be necessary to achieve the desired contour.

The tarsal flap should begin at least 3 mm from the lid margin, to prevent distortion of the margin. Moreover, Müller's muscle should not be advanced with the tarsus; it should be separated from its attachment to the superior tarsal border, as well as from the advancing conjunctiva. This, also, will prevent distortion and entropion of the upper lid.

Moderate to Large Resection of the Upper Eyelid

Temporal Rotational Flap with Conjunctival Lining. When one-third to one-half of the upper eyelid is removed, a primary closure with canthotomy and cantholysis will usually not be adequate. A temporal flap following the downward curve of the upper eyelid will allow rotation of enough tissue to fill the defect. Conjunctiva from the lateral fornix provides the internal covering.

TECHNIQUE (Fig. 16–54)

A. Tumor is resected with parallel incisions through the full height of the tarsus; this is followed by angling of the incision through the orbicularis and skin. The curve of the temporal flap follows the downward curve of the lateral aspect of the upper eyelid. A Z-plasty can be done to gain further advancement, or (box insert

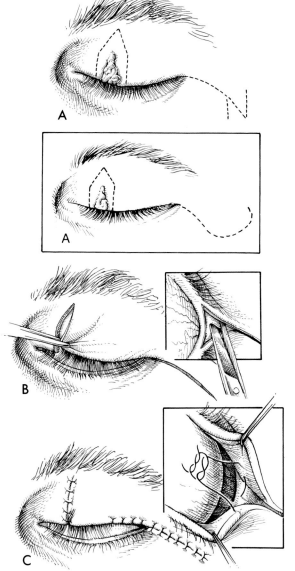

FIGURE 16–54. Upper lid reconstruction with conjunctival lining.

with Fig. 16–54A) the flap can be curved upward, which would give it a longer length.

B. The upper arm of the canthal tendon is cut (box insert with Fig. 16–54B), and the temporal flap is undermined and rotated into the defect.

C. The lid margin is closed in the usual way (basic lid closure, Fig. 16–3). Conjunctiva from the lateral fornix is mobilized to line the flap and is sutured to the new lid margin with 6-0 silk. The flap must be securely fastened to the lateral rim with 5-0 Prolene because the upward pull of the levator muscle may widen the fissure laterally (box insert with Fig. 16–54C). If excessive tension is present, the Z-plasty can be done along the edge of the flap to give it more length.

There is a limitation to the amount of temporal flap that can be rotated into the upper eyelid. The base of this flap is in the area of the eyebrow, which can be turned inward toward the eye when the flap is carried too far inferiorly.

Large Resection of the Upper Eyelid

Cutler-Beard Procedure. Very large upper eyelid defects can be reconstructed with the Cutler-Beard technique, provided the lower lid is normal.[53] This method consists of advancing full-thickness lower eyelid under a bridge of lower eyelid margin into the upper eyelid defect. Depending on the tightness of the tissues, the flap is released in 2 or 3 months; the eye, unfortunately, is occluded during this time.

TECHNIQUE (Fig. 16–55)

A. The tumor is outlined in the upper eyelid. In the lower lid a line similar in length is placed 3 mm from the margin. The line can be smaller, since there should be some medial and lateral stretch in the upper eyelid. Vertical lines are placed from each end to the inferior orbital rim and angled outward to gain greater length of the flap. The tumor is removed, with care taken to salvage as much tarsus as possible, using frozen section control.

B. The lower lid flap is begun by releasing the lower lid completely at a point 3 mm from the margin; this is done by making separate incisions on both the skin and tarsal surfaces and then connecting them, to avoid a miscut and compromise of the marginal artery. Full-thickness vertical incisions are made on either side into the cul-de-sac. If more advancement is necessary, the outward angulated incisions are made to further release the flap.

C. The tarsus of the advancement flap is

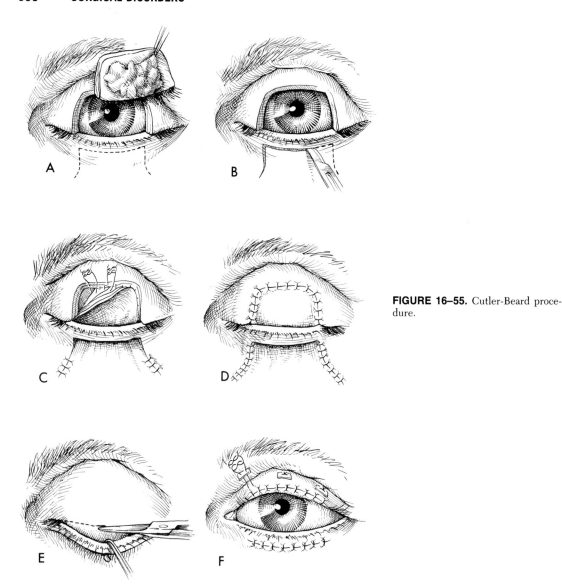

FIGURE 16–55. Cutler-Beard procedure.

sutured to the remaining tarsus or conjunctiva with 6-0 chromic catgut. The levator aponeurosis is approximated to the orbicularis muscle of the flap.

D. The skin edges are joined with 6-0 silk. The raw inferior lower lid surface is left open. The patient is instructed to wear a shield at night, to prevent tension or pulling on the bridge flap. After 2 months the flap may be released if the skin is supple and there is not a great deal of vertical tension present. If there is, waiting another month or so is indicated to allow for further stretching of the flap. During this time the raw surface of the lower eyelid margin epithelializes.

E. The flap is divided in the palpebral fissure, with a little more conjunctiva left inferiorly to bring over the raw upper eyelid margin.

F. At the new lid margin the skin is sutured to the conjunctival edge with 6-0 silk. Three double-armed sutures of 6-0 silk are brought through the upper eyelid 5 mm from the margin and tied over silicone pegs in order to keep the skin edge in a recessed position; this prevents the skin from being pulled over the margin while it is healing. The sutures are removed after 2 weeks. The inferior aspect of the bridge flap, which is epithelialized, is lightly incised, creating an anterior and a posterior edge. The lower lid is reunited to its margin; the deeper tissues are sutured with 6-0 plain catgut and the skin with 6-0 silk.

It is important to leave the flap in place long enough to allow for adequate stretching, to avoid a postoperative lower lid shortening after the lid is reunited to its margin. It is also important to make every attempt to keep the skin edges in the upper eyelid from rolling posteriorly and causing irritation by rubbing against the globe. Through-and-through sutures of 6-0 silk help in preventing this postoperative problem.

Tarsal-Conjunctival Advancement Flaps with Full-Thickness Skin Graft.[54] As opposed to the Cutler-Beard procedure, only the tarsal-conjunctival layer from the lower lid is advanced. The tarsus provides support for the new upper eyelid margin; the remaining tarsus and conjunctiva from the upper eyelid are brought forward to join the lower lid flap. On this conjoined tarsal-conjunctival flap a full-thickness skin graft is placed. This technique is similar to the modified Hughes procedure for lower eyelid reconstruction, in which the superior tarsal edge, which is brought into the lower eyelid defect, remains as the new lower lid margin.

TECHNIQUE (Fig. 16–56)

A. The tumor is outlined in the upper lid and excised with a free edge, as determined by frozen section control. If the entire tumor is not full thickness, as much of the tarsus is salvaged as possible.

B. Vertical incisions are made in the tarsus at the medial and lateral edges of the excision to the superior tarsal border.

C. Müller's muscle is separated from the superior border of the tarsus and conjunctiva (inset with Fig. 16–56C). This is followed by continuation of the vertical incisions in the conjunctiva into the superior cul-de-sac.

D. The lower lid is everted, and an incision is made in the tarsus 1.5 mm inferior to the posterior lid margin corresponding in length to the upper eyelid defect (inset with Fig. 16–56D). The tarsus and conjunctiva are separated from the lower eyelid retractors, and vertical incisions are made to allow for an advancement flap.

E. The lower eyelid tarsal-conjunctival advancement flap is brought into the upper eyelid defect and sutured to the medial and lateral lid margins with 6-0 Vicryl, so that the inferior tarsal edge will form the new upper eyelid margin. The tarsus from the upper eyelid is brought downward to join the lower eyelid flap and sutured with interrupted 6-0 Vicryl and a continuous pull-out suture of 6-0 Prolene.

F. A full-thickness postauricular graft is usually used to fill the defect and sutured in place with 6-0 silk with the ends left long. Several small incisions are placed in the graft for drainage.

G. A cotton stent soaked in antibiotic drops is placed over the graft and the long ends of the 6-0 silk are tied over it. Intermarginal double-arm sutures of 5-0 Prolene tied over #40 silicone bands are placed on either side of the reconstructed area to splint the eyelid in the healing phase.

H. The skin graft sutures are removed in 1 week, and the intermarginal sutures a week later. After 3 to 4 weeks the lower lid advancement flap is severed at the level of the new upper eyelid margin, allowing the flap to retract into the inferior cul-de-sac.

I. If any contour disparities exist in the upper eyelid, the flap can be trimmed at a later date. To avoid lagophthalmos, the upper eyelid must not be shortened vertically.

In this procedure the full-thickness skin graft adheres firmly to the tarsus, preventing the skin from overhanging against the globe. Another advantage of this technique is that the full-thickness portion of the lower lid is not used. Moreover, more of the lower eyelid tarsus can be included in the tarsal-conjunctival advancement flap, leaving only 1.5 mm to maintain support to the lower eyelid margin. Only several millimeters are needed to provide a firmer and more stable upper eyelid margin to keep the skin from rolling inward. There is a potential for secondary lower eyelid shortening after separation of the flap and its retraction into the inferior cul-de-sac. Putting the lower lid on traction with a Frost suture for several days has reduced the likelihood of this occurring.

Resection in the Medial Canthus

Because there is not a great deal of stretch in the medial canthal tissues, it is usually not prudent to attempt primary closure. This could produce traction lines or epicanthal folds within the canthus. Two methods that lend themselves to adequate closure are a free full-thickness skin graft and a glabellar flap.

Tumors in this area carry a poorer prognosis than elsewhere in the orbital area. This is because they usually go undetected for a longer time because they are hidden in the hollow of the medial canthus or are covered by glasses. They are also technically more difficult to remove, owing to the irregular anatomy. Moreover, there is a tendency to be conservative because of the desire to preserve the lacrimal system. It is of vital importance to excise these tumors with meticulous frozen system and me-

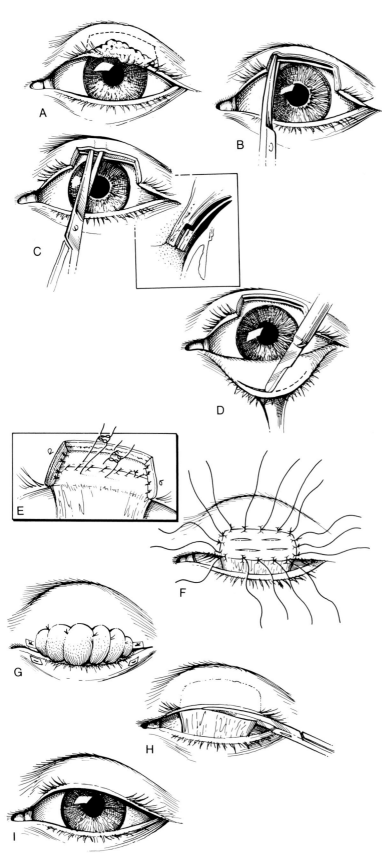

FIGURE 16–56. Tarsal-conjunctival advancement flaps with full-thickness skin graft.

dial wall if necessary. The deep tissues must be free of tumor because recurrent tumors may spread along the medial wall of the orbit before they are recognized externally.

Glabellar Flap, Inverted V to Y. For defects approximately 1 cm in diameter this type of repair is suitable and has the advantage of carrying an abundant blood supply.[40]

TECHNIQUE (Fig. 16–57)

A. From the area of resection an oblique incision is carried through the medial canthus to a point on the forehead 2 to 3 cm above the eyebrow in the midline. Another line is carried from that point into the opposite medial canthus just below the brow. The higher the apex of this inverted V on the forehead, the larger the flap that can be rotated.

B. The flap is lifted from the subcutaneous tissues down to the root of the nose.

C. It is then rotated downward into the defect and sutured with 6-0 silk. The flap is loosely fit into the medial canthal area, to prevent the formation of traction lines. The forehead skin on either side of the bare area is undermined to facilitate closure. Buried 5-0 Vicryl aids in bringing the edges together, and the skin is closed with 5-0 Prolene. Thus the inverted V is converted to an inverted Y.

This procedure confines the surgery to the involved area, and the flap has an abundant blood supply. The disadvantages are the occasional thickened appearance of the flap and the persistent lines of incision in a rather obvious place. In a younger person a full-thickness skin graft is preferred.

Full-Thickness Skin Graft Repair. A full-thickness postauricular skin graft can be used to repair large or small defects in the medial canthal area. This has the advantage of avoiding the vertical scar lines that run into the forehead when a glabellar flap is used.

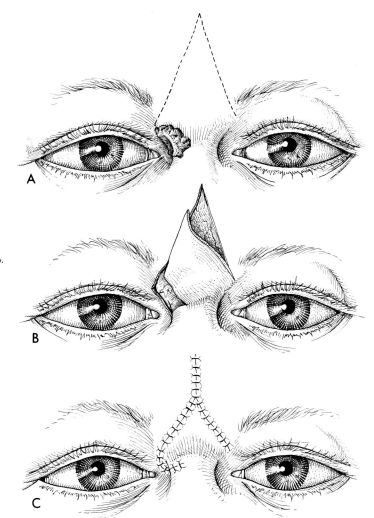

FIGURE 16–57. Glabellar flap.

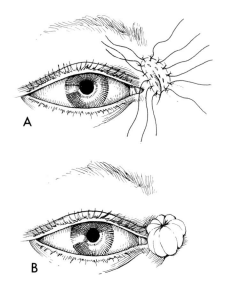

FIGURE 16–58. Full-thickness skin graft in medial canthus.

TECHNIQUE (Fig. 16–58)

A. After the tumor is resected with frozen section control a postauricular graft is taken (see cicatricial ectropion repair, Fig. 16–30) to fill the defect. Multiple stab incisions with a #11 Bard-Parker blade are made for drainage. Many of these stab incisions will create a meshwork, and the graft will have greater stretch and will be able to fill a larger defect. The graft is sutured in place with 6-0 silk with the ends left long.

B. A cotton roll covered with Adaptic gauze and soaked in antibiotic solution is tied over the graft. In the postoperative period the patient is instructed to place antibiotic drops between the cotton roll and the skin several times during the day. The stent and all the sutures are removed in 7 days.

For tumors that invade the deeper medial canthal tissues or involve the periosteum, wide excision of the area, including the lacrimal system and bone if necessary, should be carried out. The defect can be packed with Adaptic gauze and impregnated with antibiotic ointment, and the area allowed to granulate in. This open technique of healing, although lengthy, can produce satisfactory cosmetic results, and recurrences of the tumor are more easily detected. Radiotherapy is usually given postoperatively to eradicate any residual tumor.

Resection in the Lateral Canthus

A tumor at the lateral canthus involving one eyelid can usually be handled by including it in the excision and subsequent reconstruction. If it does not inolve the eyelid, placing a full-thickness skin graft over the defect is preferable, since it avoids the additional incision lines characteristic of flap repairs. Moreover, flaps can place tension on the brow or eyelids and further distort the anatomy.

Periosteal Flaps with Skin Transpositional Flap. When the excision necessitates removing the lateral aspect of both the upper and lower eyelids, lid-sharing procedures are precluded. An alternative to merely joining the eyelids together, and thus automatically shortening the fissure, is to use periosteal flaps as a tarsal substitute covered with a transpositional skin flap.[55]

TECHNIQUE (Fig. 16–59)

A. The area to be removed from the outer aspects of both the upper and lower eyelids is marked. A vertical flap is outlined from the lateral edge of the defect; this is carried upward just lateral to and above the brow.

B. The periosteum of the lateral rim is exposed as well as a temporalis fascia. Two parallel cuts are made 1.5 cm apart, beginning in the temporalis fascia and taken through the periosteum to the inner edge of the lateral rim.

C. The periosteal flap is hinged at the inner edge of the lateral rim, raised, and split horizontally.

D. The flaps are crossed to form an angle that will correspond to the lateral canthal angle. The periosteal edges are sutured to the tarsal-conjunctival layers with 6-0 Vicryl. There must be a moderate amount of tension in the lids; if there is too much laxity, the flaps should be shortened. The skin transpositional flap is mobilized to cover the periosteal flaps.

E. The skin flap, 1.5 cm wide, is raised, including only the subcutaneous tissue. Undermining is done on either side of the donor area to allow for easy approximation of the edges. The flap is transposed into the defect and a split is made in the distal end to separately cover the upper and lower periosteal flaps.

F. The donor edges that have been undermined are sewn with 5-0 Prolene. The periosteal and skin flaps that constitute the new lid margin are approximated with 6-0 silk.

G. To splint the area, an intermarginal suture of 5-0 Prolene over #40 silicone pegs is placed between the lids. A piece of 0.005-inch silicone sheeting is folded over the reconstructed part of the lower lid and secured with a through-and-through double-arm 6-0 silk suture. This keeps the raw edges of the upper and lower lids from adhering to each other. The intermar-

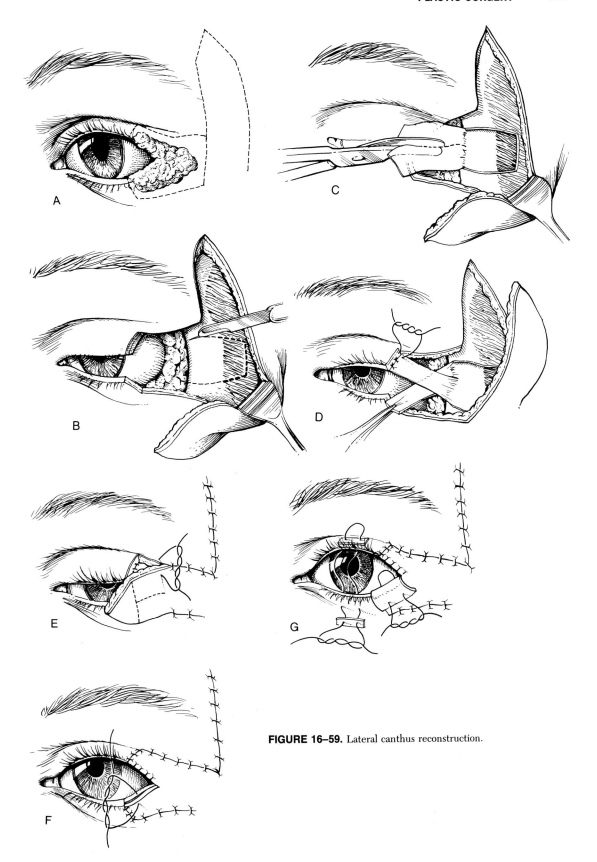

FIGURE 16–59. Lateral canthus reconstruction.

ginal suture and silicone sleeve are removed in 2 weeks.

Rhomboid Flap. When a defect is too large to permit a simple direct closure, a local flap can be used.[56] The technique is useful in an area in which mobility of the skin will not compromise the position of the eyelids. The base of the rhomboid flap should be along the line of greatest skin redundancy; if it is positioned perpendicular to a free lid margin, vertical shortening of the eyelid could occur. The appropriate locations for this flap are the lateral aspect of the brow, cheek, and lateral canthus.

TECHNIQUE (Fig. 16–60)

A. Around the tumor or defect a square with 90-degrees angles or a parallelogram with angles of 60 and 120 degrees is drawn. From one of the angles a line is drawn the same length as one of the sides, followed by another line parallel to the figures.

B. The flap is raised and the surrounding skin, including the defect, is undermined, allowing the flap to move inward 60 to 90 degrees to fill the defect.

C. The flaps are sutured with 5-0 or 6-0 Prolene. If there is tension on the flap, subcutaneous sutures are placed initially.

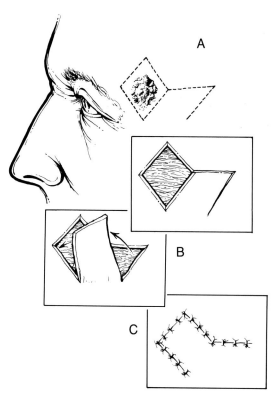

FIGURE 16–60. Rhomboid flap.

If there is too much tension for a satisfactory closure, a rhomboid flap can be brought in from the opposite side with the parallel arm in the opposite direction. The rotated flaps would be joined in the center of the defect, thus reducing the arc of rotation.

Congenital Coloboma

Congenital coloboma is most often found in the medial portion of the upper eyelid.[18] The syndrome with which it is most often associated is Goldenhar's. The defect can range from a scalloping in the lid margin to the absence of the entire medial one-third of the eyelid. The globe can be grossly exposed when the infant is sleeping, but surprisingly, few develop significant keratopathy. There is also the danger of accidental trauma to the constantly exposed eye.

Cases that do show staining should be treated with lubricants until the child is in a safe anesthetic risk category. The technique of repair consists of removing the mucocutaneous lining around the coloboma to create raw edges. It is necessary to have vertical tarsal edges on either side to prevent notch formation.

Technique (Fig. 16–61)

A. Because the lid margin at the edges of the coloboma is generally rounded, it may be necessary to angle the excision of the coloboma outward through the tarsal portion. The tissue above the coloboma should be excised to allow for adequate closure without puckering.

B. When the tarsal edges are brought together (basic closure, Fig. 16–3), the lid margin is forced downward to lessen the chance of notching; if tension is present, a canthotomy and cantholysis may be necessary (Fig. 16–49). Because of possible tethering of the upper eyelid after repair, a ptosis may be produced that may require correction at a later date.

RECONSTRUCTION OF THE CANTHUS

Abnormalities of the canthi may be congenital, acquired, or caused by trauma.

Congenital Epicanthal Folds

The most common congenital epicanthal fold is epicanthus inversus, which arises in the lower

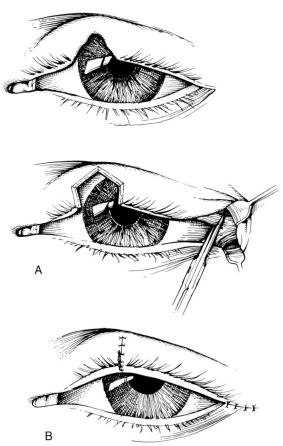

FIGURE 16–61. Coloboma repair.

eyelid and extends upward, partially covering the inner canthus. There are other varieties and positions of epicanthal folds, such as epicanthus tarsalis, which is common in Orientals.

Many patients with epicanthus inversus also have accompanying telecanthus (widening in the intercanthal distance), blepharoptosis, and blepharophimosis. In these cases treatment is initially directed at repairing the epicanthus before the blepharoptosis. The widened intercanthal distance may be reduced at the same time by tucking the medial canthal tendons or by transnasal wiring.

For the mild epicanthal folds seen in infancy it is wise to wait several years to determine if the folds are indeed permanent, since skeletal and soft tissues changes occur as the child grows.

Y-V Operation

The Y-V operation consists of making a Y incision over the fold and then closing it as a V; this serves to flatten out the medial canthus.[57]

Technique (Fig. 16–62)

A. A Y is drawn horizontally on the canthus, with each arm approximately 10 mm long. The point of intersection is 5 mm from the canthal angle, with the arms running parallel with the lid margins and the other part of the Y running along the bridge of the nose.

B. The skin is undermined above and below the horizontal incision, to allow movement of the canthal angle toward the nose.

C. The medial canthal tendon can be exposed and a double-armed suture of 5-0 Prolene used to tuck the tendon. One end is placed through the bony insertion of the tendon and the other near the canthal angle. This will further advance the canthus toward the midline.

D. Buried sutures of 5-0 Vicryl may be necessary to reduce tension on the tissues. The skin is approximated with 6-0 plain catgut or Prolene.

If the intercanthal distance is not widened, the medial canthal tendon does not require tucking. In some cases of telecanthus, transnasal wiring may be indicated to restore a normal position to the medial canthus, as described in the next section.

Mustardé Method of Epicanthal Fold Repair

The Mustardé method is an effective way to eradicate epicanthal folds by breaking up the tight vertical line in the fold.[51] The relatively excessive skin on either side of the fold is utilized to make up for the shortness in the vertical line. The resulting scar thus passes through the inner canthus in a vertical manner, and is prevented from lying in the more obvious nasal skin.

If telecanthus is present, tucking of the medial canthal tendon can be done, or if a greater degree is present, transnasal wiring is done.

Technique (Fig. 16–63)

A. The site of the desired canthus (point x) is marked, with care taken not to pull on the skin of the nose. The general rule is to make the intercanthal distance one-half the interpupillary distance.

B. The second point (point y) is placed at the canthus, and the two points are joined. The line between x and y is measured, giving the basis for the other lines, which are all drawn 1 to 2 mm smaller. The first of these lines begins at the midpoint of the x-y line and is angled 60 degrees toward the eye. At the end of these

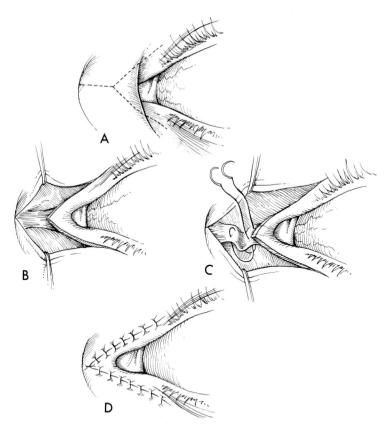

FIGURE 16–62. Y-V epicanthal repair.

two lines additional lines are drawn at a 45-degree angle back toward the nose.

C. From point y, lines are drawn 2 mm from the upper and lower eyelid margin. The flaps are incised and separated from one another.

D. (Optional) Transnasal wiring: The medial canthal tendon is exposed, and a vertical incision is made in the periosteum just anterior to it (upper insert). The periosteum and lacrimal sac are reflected laterally, exposing the anterior lacrimal crest and fossa. The air drill is used to remove the lacrimal crest down to the nasal mucosa (lower insert). The opening is enlarged to at least 5 mm with the Kerrison punch.

E. (Optional) Transnasal wiring: A Keith needle on a #32 wire is passed through the medial canthal tendon tissues. Both needles are passed through the rhinostomy site and nasal septum, coming out through the rhinostomy site on the opposite side. A groove director is used to facilitate removal of the needles. The same thing can be done from the other side with another Keith needle, thus securing the medial approximation from both sides.

F. (Optional) Transnasal wiring: The wire is tied once, pulling both canthi toward the nose and posteriorly. The wire is then twisted until both canthal angles are brought closer together,

attempting to overcorrect by several millimeters using the 2:1 interpupillary-intercanthal ratio as a guide. Postoperatively, some slippage can be expected.

G. After the flaps are incised, the medial canthal tendon is easily exposed and can be imbricated with a buried 5-0 Prolene suture, bringing the canthus closer to the nose (see Fig. 16–62). This step may be omitted when only simple folds exist. The flaps are transposed and may require trimming to adequately fit into place without bunching.

H. The flaps are sutured with 6-0 plain catgut or 6-0 Prolene.

Postoperatively, there is usually obvious scarring for several months; this eventually fades within a year. If blepharoptosis is present, it can be repaired after the scars soften, which is usually 6 months.

Acquired Blepharocanthal Malpositions

Widening of the fissure owing to seventh nerve paralysis is caused by a sag in the lower eyelid and levator overaction resulting from orbicularis paralysis. There is a lack of blinking,

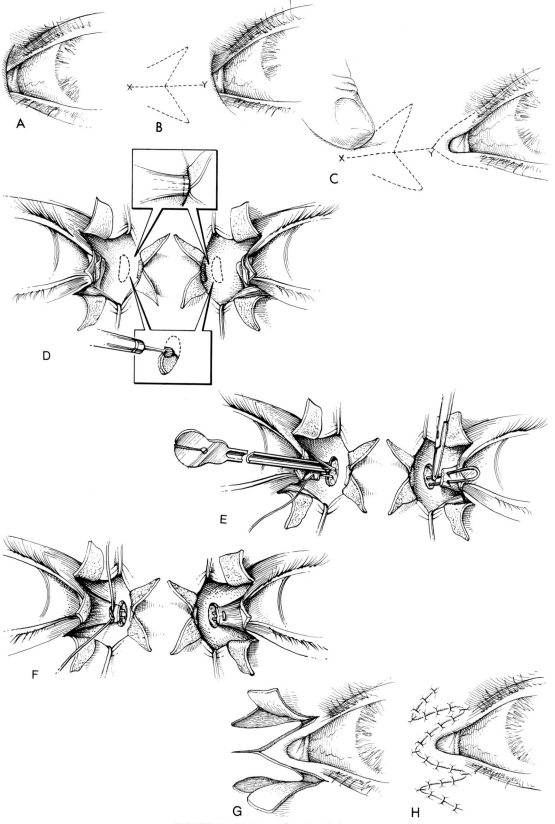

FIGURE 16–63. Mustardé epicanthal repair.

as well as malocclusion of the eyelids, resulting in various degrees of exposure keratopathy, depending on the severity and longevity of the paralysis. If the condition has shown no improvement in 6 months, reducing the size of the enlarged eyelid fissure may be contemplated.

Proptosis secondary to Graves' disease will also increase the dimensions of the fissure. Although orbicularis action is normal, there can still be exposure problems because of upper and lower eyelid retraction in addition to the proptosis, which subjects the eyes to a great deal of drying.

Intermarginal Sutures or Tarsorrhaphy

When protection of the eye is required for only a few weeks, intermarginal sutures tied over silicone pegs can be used. However, in cases of exposure keratopathy that are due to temporary conditions such as Bell's palsy, but in which conservative management is unsuccessful, temporary tarsorrhaphy is indicated.

Technique (Fig. 16–64)

A. (Intermarginal suture) A double-armed 4-0 silk or 4-0 Prolene suture is passed first through a #40 silicone band peg and then through the skin 5 mm below the lash line, catching some epitarsal tissue and coming out the gray line. It is similarly brought through the opposite lid and tied over a silicone peg. It

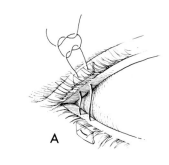

A

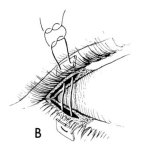

B

FIGURE 16–64. Tarsorrhaphy and intermarginal suture technique.

is usually placed in a position from the lateral canthus to adequately protect the eye. This can be determined by pinching the lids together to ascertain the amount of coverage needed.

B. (Tarsorrhaphy) If a more permanent adhesion is desired, the lid margin is stripped of mucosa to create raw edges, and vertical incisions are made 5 mm into the lid along the gray line. The amount to include in the tarsorrhaphy is determined as described in step A. The sutures are placed as described above, coming through the split in each lid. After 2 weeks they are removed. Splinting the lid with an intermarginal suture medial to this will allow the raw edges to heal without any tension, and can be removed a week after the original suture is taken out.

Lateral Canthorrhaphy

Lateral canthorrhaphy is irreversible and will permanently reduce the fissure. It is appropriate for cases that are stable and require a reduction in the horizontal fissure.

Technique (Fig. 16–65)

A. With the patient in an upright position the lids at the external fissure are pinched together and marked, to determine how far medially the lateral canthus should be removed. The lid margin is split to the canthal angle, and the anterior lid margin, including the lash follicles, is excised.

B. The mucosa from the posterior lid margin is stripped to create a raw edge, and the posterior lamellae (tarsal-conjunctival) are joined with interrupted 6-0 chromic catgut.

C. The anterior lamellae of skin and orbicularis are approximated with 6-0 silk, and an intermarginal suture of 4-0 silk is placed medial to this area, to allow healing without tension on the wound edges. The silk sutures are removed in 10 days, and the intermarginal suture is allowed to remain for at least 2 weeks.

Medial Canthorrhaphy

When there is an increase in the size of the medial eyelid fissure because of a sag in the nasal aspect of the lower eyelid, a medial canthorrhaphy can be done.[58] This condition occurs from longstanding seventh nerve paralysis or any type of vertical shortening of the lid. In most of these cases the caruncle is also more exposed and may appear as an obvious bump in the corner of the eye. This procedure joins the eyelids between the canthal angle and puncta, covering the caruncle and reducing the medial eyelid fissure.

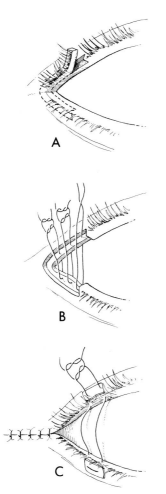

FIGURE 16–65. Lateral canthorrhaphy.

Technique (Fig. 16–66)

A. An incision is made in the mucocutaneous junction, beginning just medial to the punctum, and is carried around the canthal angle to the opposite punctum. A probe is placed in the canaliculus in order to identify the position of the lumen. Magnification is necessary, since the canaliculus is very close to the surface. The conjunctiva and skin are separated into two layers.

B. The conjunctiva and skin are freshened to remove the smooth mucocutaneous tissue. The conjunctival layer, including the fine fibrous tissue overlying the canaliculus, is joined with interrupted sutures of 6-0 chromic catgut, and the skin with interrupted 6-0 silk.

C. To remove tension from the suture line during healing, an intermarginal suture of 5-0 Prolene over silicone pegs is placed lateral to the punctum to splint the eyelids for 2 weeks.

This procedure is often combined with a lateral canthal sling (Fig. 16–67), which produces a hammock effect by supporting and elevating the lid medially and laterally.

Lateral Canthal Sling

The lower eyelid may sag after seventh nerve paralysis or as a result of the weight or atonicity of the prosthesis in an anophthalmic socket. As described by Tenzel, a sling is made from the lower arm of the canthal tendon and its extension into the lateral tarsus, and is reattached at a higher level on the lateral orbital rim.[59]

In seventh nerve paralysis the lid sags because of lack of tone of the orbicularis muscle. The lid may not necessarily be in an ectopic position, but merely lower on the globe, so that more of it is exposed.

After blepharoplasty, trauma, or fracture repair, the orbital septum may contract, causing the lower lid to be pulled downward. In this condition there is not a shortening of skin or conjunctiva, but a vertical shortening of the orbital septum and, possibly, the lower lid retractors.

In the anophthalmic patient the lid commonly sags because of the weight of the prosthesis or loss of the inferior cul-de-sac.

Technique (Fig. 16–67)

A. A 2.5-cm lateral canthotomy is done. The lateral orbital rim is exposed superior and inferior to the insertion of the lateral canthal tendon.

B. The skin and conjunctiva are separated on either side of the lower arm of the canthal

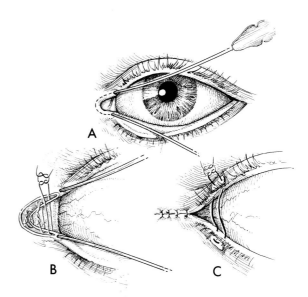

FIGURE 16–66. Medial canthorrhaphy.

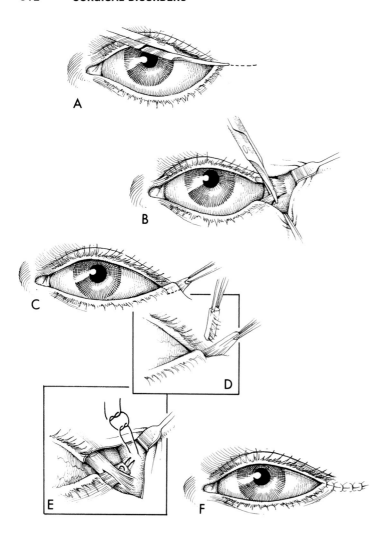

A

B

C

D

E

F

FIGURE 16–67. Lateral canthal sling.

tendon, and the tendon is severed from the lateral rim.

C. The tendon is pulled laterally and upward to raise and tighten the lid, and the area that crosses the upper lid is marked.

D. The lid margin is stripped of the mucocutaneous layer, and the lash area is removed. This area is now the extension of the lower arm of the lateral canthal tendon.

E. The upper arm of the canthal tendon is split with scissors. After the position and tightness of the lid have been determined, the tendon-sling with a 5-0 Prolene mattress suture is brought through the split and sutured through the periosteum. Additional sutures are placed for security.

F. The skin is sutured with interrupted sutures of 6-0 silk.

In severe cases of seventh nerve paralysis a medial canthorrhaphy can be done as well; this brings both ends of the lid to a higher suppor-

tive position and should be done before the lateral canthal sling.

When a contracted orbital septum and lower lid retractors are pulling the lid downward, scissors are passed between the skin and conjunctiva to sever the responsible structure, which can be felt emanating from the inferior orbital rim. In this situation the lid must be kept in an overcorrected elevated position for several weeks by means of a 4-0 silk Frost suture or an intermarginal suture between the eyelids.

Traumatic Telecanthus

Telecanthus is a condition in which the intercanthal distance is widened, resulting in a hooding or hiding of the medial part of the globe.[52] This is usually associated with a reduction in the size of the horizontal fissure. Normally the intercanthal distance is approximately half the pupillary distance. Hypertelorism, on the other hand, is a widening of the interorbital distance without alteration of the canthal-pupillary distance ratio. As a congenital condition, telecanthus is usually associated with blepharoptosis, blepharophimosis, and epicanthal folds. After trauma to the naso-orbital area there can be a splaying outward of the bones, resulting in a flattening of the medial canthal area and lateral displacement of the canthus. In most cases the lacrimal system is disrupted, resulting in a chronic dacryocystitis. Repair consists of moving the canthus medially, combined with a dacryocystorhinostomy.

Technique (Fig. 16–68)

A. Both sides of the nose are packed with 5% cocaine. A vertical incision is made 1 cm from the canthus, extending above and below it, and exposing the lacrimal sac, which is usually dilated.

B. Scar tissue is cut away, and bony irregularities are removed with a burr attached to the air drill until the medial wall is reached. Here, bone is removed as in a dacryocystorhinostomy (see Fig. 16–42) until the mucosa is reached.

C. A larger osteotomy than usual is made, measuring at least 15 mm in diameter, to allow enough room for return of the soft tissues against the side of the nose.

D. Because of the increased distance between the posterior lacrimal sac and the nasal mucosa flaps, the flaps are purposely made long and are joined with 4-0 chromic catgut.

E. The tissue in the area of the medial canthal tendon is grasped with heavy forceps and pulled into the rhinostomy site. Any area of restriction is severed, to allow for a free movement toward the nose.

F. A 1-cm incision is made in the opposite canthus over the bony reflection of the medial canthal tendon. A hand drill with a fine bit and needle eye is used to drill a hole on either side of the tendon through the nasal septum, coming out in the opposite rhinostomy site. The drill bit must be angled slightly posteriorly. A #25 wire threaded on a cutting needle is passed through the remnant of the canthal tendon several times. Each end of the wire is threaded through the eye of the bit and brought back to the opposite side through each hole. Two unattached #28 wires are passed from one side to the other and held out of the way.

G. Sutures of 4-0 chromic catgut are placed between the anterior flaps of the lacrimal sac and the nasal mucosa and tagged with serrafine clamps. The medial canthus is grasped and firmly positioned medially while the fixation wires are tightened on the opposite side. They are carefully twisted until tight and then are cut and bent into one of the drill holes.

H. The lacrimal sutures are then tied. The deep tissue is approximated with 4-0 chromic catgut and the skin with interrupted 6-0 Prolene. Methylmethacrylate canthoplasty buttons (Storz) are placed over each incision, and the two unattached #28 wires are passed through the holes and tightened to maintain the contour of the reconstructed canthal area. The external wires and the sutures are removed in 2 weeks.

Because there is usually some postoperative lateral movement or slippage, it is necessary to overcorrect the position of the canthus. By measuring from the midpoint on the bridge of the nose, the position of the canthus as compared with the normal side can be judged while the wires are being tightened. When both sides are involved, the 2:1 interpupillary-intercanthal ratio is used as a guide. It is also necessary to have the wires come through the nasal septum at a position slightly posterior to the level of the drill holes, to bring the displaced canthus in a normally deep-set position against the nose.

THYROID OPHTHALMOPATHY (GRAVES' DISEASE)*

The most common finding in Graves' disease is retraction of the upper eyelid.[60] This is initially due to hyperactivity of Müller's muscle, which is a sympathetically innervated muscle. In later stages there is also inflammatory infiltration of both Müller's muscle and the levator. Similarly, there can be stimulation of the inferior tarsal muscle, which pulls the lower eyelid downward. Retraction of the eyelids—which principally occurs in the upper eyelid—will expose more of the globe and can give the illusion of exophthalmos. Because Graves' disease is often accompanied by exophthalmos as well, the lid retraction exaggerates the amount of exposure to which the globe is subjected.

Because of inflammatory infiltration and enlargement of the extraocular muscles, proptosis occurs in Graves' disease. Computed tomography clearly demonstrates this finding and aids in ruling out other causes of exophthalmos. This

---

*See Chapter 15 for a fuller discussion of exophthalmos and its surgical management.

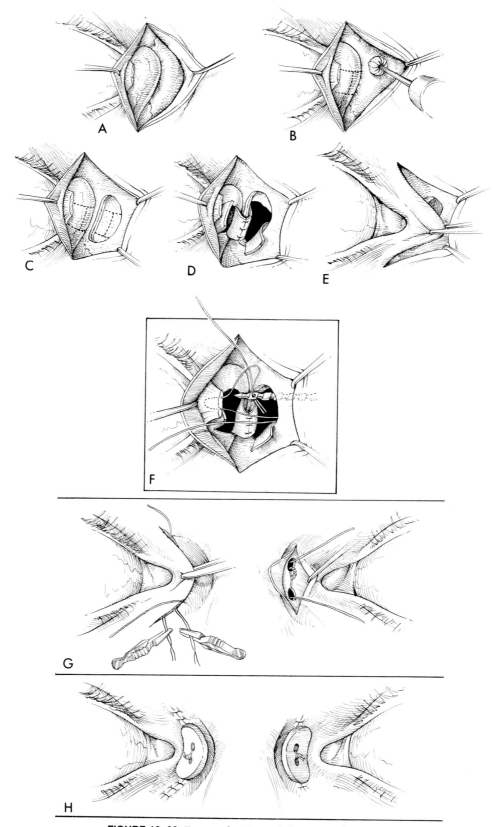

FIGURE 16–68. Transnasal wiring with dacryocystorhinostomy.

happens most commonly in hyperthyroid states, but it can also occur when the patient is euthyroid or even hypothyroid. This aspect of Graves' disease can occur acutely, in which case it is accompanied by a great deal of inflammatory reaction, causing severe proptosis, chemosis, exposure, and compression of the optic nerve. On the other hand, the progression may be slow, without inflammatory signs, but significant enough to cause optic neuropathy owing to increased intraorbital pressure. In either case, vision can be irreparably lost.

Patients with exophthalmos and shallow orbits, as seen in black people, can be subjected to subluxation of the globe between the lids. Just the right amount of pressure on the lids can cause them to slide behind the globe, and with squeezing they can become incarcerated. Grasping the upper lid near the lashes and pulling the lid back over the globe with the patient relaxing will oftentimes reverse the situation. If this is unsuccessful, a Van Lint nerve block may be necessary, or even general anesthesia in extreme cases. Protection of the globe must be maintained during these distressing situations.

Recession or Excision of the Upper Eyelid Retractors

Upper eyelid retraction is the most common surgical problem associated with Graves' disease. Müller's muscle is overacting, and the levator, in severe cases, may be infiltrated with inflammatory cells, causing fibrosis and shortening. There can be exposure symptoms and, if exophthalmos is present, frank exposure keratopathy. Because the eyelid elevator muscles are so tight, it is difficult for the patient to blink adequately, and the eyes may be chronically dry and exposed during sleep. It may also be a cosmetic problem for the patient, especially if it is unilateral, creating an asymmetric appearance. To release the retracted upper lid, a Müller's muscle excision or levator–Müller's muscle recession can be done.

Excision of Müller's Muscle

Excision of Müller's muscle, as described by Putterman and Urist,[61] is done under local anesthesia, the amount of excision being titrated to reach a satisfactory level.

Technique (Fig. 16–69)

A. A frontal nerve block can be done (see Ptosis section, Fig. 16–32); however, if it is unsuccessful, it will be impossible to take advantage of the sensory block with motor function intact. Therefore, the alternative anesthesia is local infiltration with a lidocaine–bupivacaine combination in a 60 per cent–40 per cent mixture with epinephrine and hyaluronidase subconjunctivally in the superior cul-de-sac and a small amount on the anterior skin surface. This is more predictable and should not affect levator function. The upper eyelid is everted over a Desmarres retractor, and a scratch incision is made in the conjunctiva at the superior tarsal border.

B. The conjunctiva is separated with blunt dissection from Müller's muscle to the superior cul-de-sac. This is done with a combination scissors and cotton-tipped applicator. Müller's muscle is cut at its attachment to the superior tarsal border and is lifted away from the levator aponeurosis. Comparison is then made between the two eyelid fissures if the other one is normal. If both eyelids are affected, the lid level achieved should be similar. If the lid level is still elevated, Müller's muscle is separated from the levator aponeurosis to its origin.

C. The lids are again compared, and if they are similar, Müller's muscle is excised. An attempt is made to bring the eyelid to about 1 mm above the desired level, since it will fall when orbicularis function returns.

D. If retraction is still present, the levator aponeurosis fibers are teased apart, depending on where the most retraction remains. Repeated observation is made until the level is satisfactory. The conjunctiva is approximated with a continuous pull-out 6-0 Prolene suture, with both ends tied on the external upper eyelid surface.

E. A 6-0 double-armed silk retraction suture is placed from the upper lid to the cheek, to keep the cut edge of Müller's muscle from reattaching, and is removed in 24 to 48 hours. The Prolene suture is removed in 5 days.

There is usually an overcorrection postoperatively, caused by the surgical trauma and edema. Within 6 weeks the eyelid level will return to a stable position. If it is overcorrected, a Fasanella-Servat ptosis procedure can be done (see Fig. 16–33). If it is undercorrected, another attempt can be made, or a levator recession with sclera can be done.

Levator Recession with Preserved Sclera

Recession of the levator aponeurosis and Müller's muscle can be done from an external approach, similar to the technique for external levator recession. This gives the surgeon the

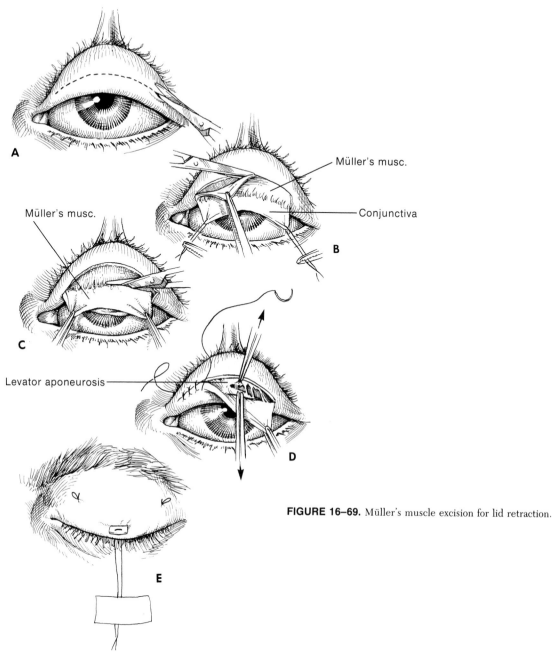

A

B

Müller's musc.

Conjunctiva

Müller's musc.

C

Levator aponeurosis

D

E

FIGURE 16–69. Müller's muscle excision for lid retraction.

advantage of planning the procedure preoperatively, by determining how large a graft will be used, depending on the amount of lid lowering desired. The use of 1.0- to 1.5-mm graft per 1 mm of lowering desired has been the general rule. However, lids that are tightly retracted may need more recession, whereas lids that are loosely retracted may need less. This test is carried out by asking the patient to look down and then grasping the lashes and pulling downward; little give in the eyelid would indicate a tight lid, and vice versa.

Technique (Fig. 16–70)

The procedure is the same as that for external levator resection through the step of separating the levator aponeurosis and Müller's muscle from the conjunctiva (see Fig. 16–31). The aponeurosis is separated medially and laterally far enough to allow peeling of the conjunctiva from Müller's muscle to the point of its origin from the underneath surface of the levator. The preserved scleral graft is cut long enough to match the anterior edge of the aponeurosis, and

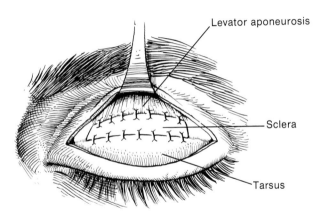

FIGURE 16–70. Levator recession with sclera.

Levator aponeurosis

Sclera

Tarsus

the width of the graft is determined by the preoperative measurements and is cut accordingly. It is sewn in place with 5-0 Vicryl to the superior tarsal border on one side and the aponeurosis on the other. Grasping the epitarsal tissues, the surgeon then places lid crease sutures of 6-0 silk between the skin edges.

The sclera, which is preserved in 90% alcohol, is removed and placed in saline 15 minutes before surgery. At the start of the procedure it is transferred to another container of saline solution for several minutes and then soaked in gentamicin drops until needed.

Recession of the Lower Eyelid Retractors

Recession of the lower eyelid retractors is indicated when the lower lid is pulled downward and backward, leaving the sclera exposed below the limbus.[62] This is caused by overstimulation of the lower eyelid retractors, specifically of the inferior tarsal muscle, which is the counterpart of Müller's muscle in the upper eyelid. This condition can aggravate or cause exposure keratopathy as well as prevent complete closure of the eyelids, particularly if there is upper eyelid retraction as well. Releasing the lower eyelid retractors and placing sclera in the intervening space between them and the lower border of the tarsus will allow the lid to return to a normal level. The general rule is 2 to 3 mm of sclera for every 1 mm of retraction.

Because thin ear cartilage is firmer and shrinks less than sclera, some surgeons prefer it.[63]

Technique (Fig. 16–71)

A. The lower lid is everted over a Desmarres retractor, and a scratch incision is made in the conjunctiva at the lower tarsal border.

B. The conjunctiva is removed with sharp and blunt dissection from the surface of the inferior tarsal muscle to the inferior cul-de-sac.

C. (Cross section) The lower lid retractors are buttonholed laterally below the tarsus, and scissors are passed between the retractors and the orbicularis. The blades of the scissors pass on each side of the retractors, and the retractors are cut loose from the inferior tarsal border.

D. Vertical incisions are made medially and laterally to release the retractors' peripheral attachments.

E. A piece of sclera approximately 2.5 cm long, and corresponding in width to three times the amount of recession desired, is sutured with 6-0 chromic catgut to the tarsus on one side and the recessed lower lid retractors on the other. (Optional) An alternative method is to excise the retractors completely, without using any replacement tissue or graft. The lower lid is kept on upward stretch for at least 2 weeks with a reverse Frost suture.

F. The conjunctiva is replaced with a pull-out suture of 6-0 Prolene, with both ends tied on the skin surface. The lid is placed on stretch for 7 to 10 days, with either a Frost suture taped to the forehead or intermarginal sutures to the upper eyelid.

It is necessary to keep the lower lid on upward stretch, since gravity works counter to this eyelid-lengthening procedure. There could be excessive shrinkage of the graft and the lower lid retractors could reinsert at an undesirable position near the tarsus. There should be an overcorrected position postoperatively that gradually improves to the desired level. If the globe is proptotic, this procedure may need to be combined with a permanent tarsorrhaphy (Fig. 16–65) to achieve a satisfactory result. Repairing lower lid retraction when the globe is proptotic is difficult, since the forward position of the globe forces the lower eyelid downward, militating against a successful result. In

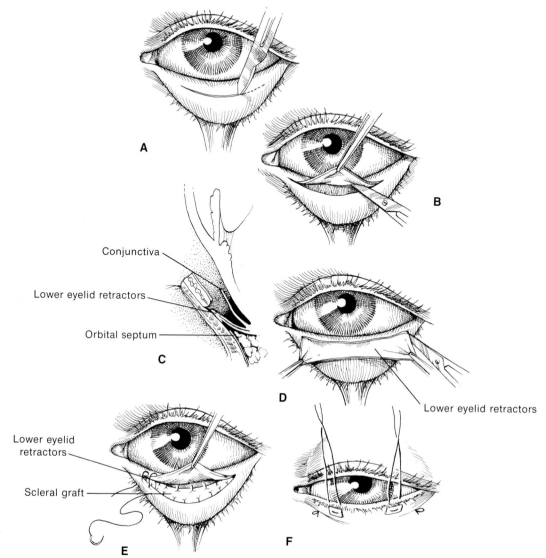

Conjunctiva

Lower eyelid retractors

Orbital septum

Lower eyelid retractors

Lower eyelid
retractors

Scleral graft

FIGURE 16–71. Recession of lower lid retractors with sclera.

these cases it may be appropriate to consider decompression first.

Orbital Decompression

Decompression of the orbit in cases of thyroid ophthalmopathy is done for the following:[64]

1. Compressive optic neuropathy when the patient is refractive to or unable to take steroids

2. Exposure keratopathy owing to exophthalmos with or without eyelid retraction

3. For cosmetic reasons; the patient must be stable for at least 12 months or longer

Dysthyroid optic neuropathy can occur in patients, even in the absence of external inflammatory signs, particularly if the patient is taking steroids. The extraocular muscles may enlarge in the posterior one-third of the orbit, compressing the apical portion of the optic nerve. In these cases it is necessary to decompress the orbit in order to relieve the pressure on the optic nerve.[65, 66] Dysthyroid optic neuropathy has the following clinical profile: 40- to 80-year-old without sex predilection, moderate to severe orbital congestion, visual acuity loss that may occur rapidly, visual field defects, and depression of the visual evoked potential.

The various methods of decompression are removal of the lateral, inferior (floor), or medial wall of the orbit. One, two, or all three of the walls can be removed, depending on how much decompression is desired. Because familiarity with the inferior approach has usually been gained with orbital floor fracture repair, this method is indicated if 3 to 5 mm of decompression is desired. Including the medial wall adds several millimeters and aids in decompressing the posterior orbit; this is important with optic nerve compression. If a larger decompression is desired, such as up to 8 mm, the lateral wall can be removed. Because the temporalis muscle rests within the temporalis fossa, creation of the large space for orbital tissue prolapse is limited. Nevertheless, the aggregate of the various combinations of orbital wall removal is usually sufficient for an adequate decompression, whether it be for dysthyroid optic neuropathy or cosmesis.

Lower Lid Approach

Floor and Medial Wall Decompression

TECHNIQUE (Fig. 16–72)

A. After the patient has been placed under general anesthesia, the lower lid and anterior orbit are infiltrated with lidocaine with 1:100,000 epinephrine for hemostasis. An intermarginal double-armed suture of 6-0 silk over a #40 silicone band is placed through the midportion of the upper and lower eyelids and is used for upward traction. An incision is made 2 mm below the lashes, from the punctum to the lateral canthus, where it is angled downward for 1.0 to 1.5 cm.

B. The plane of dissection is carried between the orbicularis and orbital septum down to the inferior orbital rim. A periosteal cut is made from the lacrimal crest to the lateral canthal tendon. The periorbita is lifted upward, exposing the entire orbital floor. The infraorbital nerve canal is recognized as a raised linear ridge running from the infraorbital fissure to the infraorbital nerve foramen anteriorly.

C. The clear area within the dotted line represents the surgical floor of the orbit, or roof of the antrum, which can be removed in its entirety. The area within the hash marks is the inferior aspect of the medial wall of the orbit, which is adjacent to the ethmoidal sinuses. This area can be removed if further decompression is desired. The thin wall posterior to the lacrimal sac fossa and overlying the ethmoidal sinuses can be removed. Staying below the ethmoidal vessels will prevent inadvertent penetration into the cranial cavity.

D. A chisel or sharp periosteal elevator is used to carefully unroof the infraorbital nerve canal. On either side of the canal the bony floor is fractured.

E. A biting forceps is used to remove the bone and underlying mucosa, as well as the underneath portion of the infraorbital canal. The infraorbital nerve and vessels are protected during these maneuvers.

F. On either side of the belly of the inferior rectus muscle, periosteal slits are made with scissors across the area of decompression and carefully spread apart.

G. The orbital fat prolapses into the antrum while the central strip of periorbita supports the globe.

H. The skin is approximated with 6-0 silk. The deeper tissues are left unsutured. The intermarginal suture is tied to protect the globe and keep the lower lid on stretch, and is removed in 24 hours. In order to reduce postoperative edema, 4 mg of dexamethasone is given intravenously at the end of the procedure and continued every 6 hours intramuscularly for 24 hours, followed by oral administration for 7 to 10 days.

Inferior Cul-de-Sac Approach

This is my preferred approach to the orbital floor. Not only is the exposure as good as the lower lid cutaneous approach, but there is neither skin incision nor risk of vertical shortening. One must, however, adequately re-form the lateral canthal angle; a deformity here is a potential complication. If a three-wall decompression is planned, the lateral wall is removed first, followed by a continuation of the canthotomy incision into the inferior cul-de-sac.

TECHNIQUE (Fig. 16–73)

A. A lateral canthotomy is done to the lateral orbital rim.

B. The lower arm of the lateral canthal tendon is exposed and cut, to release the lower eyelid.

C. Ribbon retractors are placed between the globe and eyelid, exposing the outline of the orbital rim through the inferior cul-de-sac. An incision is made through the conjunctiva to the periosteum across the entire lower cul-de-sac. The retractors must be kept in place to maintain exposure and keep orbital fat out of the operative field. The rest of the procedure is carried out as described in the previous section.

D. The deeper tissues are left unsutured, and the conjunctiva is approximated with a continuous suture of 6-0 plain catgut. The canthotomy is closed with deep bites of several 5-0 Vicryl sutures re-forming the canthal angle.

Lateral Orbitotomy Approach

This is a similar approach one would use to remove a retrobulbar tumor. If the floor is going

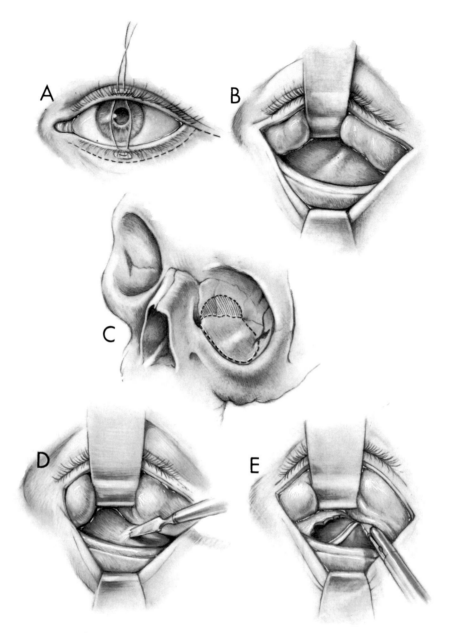

FIGURE 16–72. Orbital decompression through lower eyelid.

to be removed as well, the canthotomy can be extended into the inferior cul-de-sac without additional skin incision.

Removal of the Lateral Wall (Lateral Wall Decompression)

TECHNIQUE (Fig. 16–74)

A. An incision is made through the lateral canthus extending over the lateral rim into the temporal fossa for 4 to 6 cm. The superficial fascia is incised with the cutting Bovie down to and including the temporalis fascia. The lateral rim is exposed and an incision made in the periosteum, beginning at the level of the zygomatic arch to above the zygomatic-frontal suture line; the periorbita is reflected from the lateral wall.

B. With a ribbon retractor against the periorbita, the reciprocating saw makes cuts in the lateral rim at the level of the zygomatic arch and above the level of the zygomatic-frontal suture.

C. The rongeur grasps the lateral rim between the cuts and breaks the rim backward, and the bone is discarded.

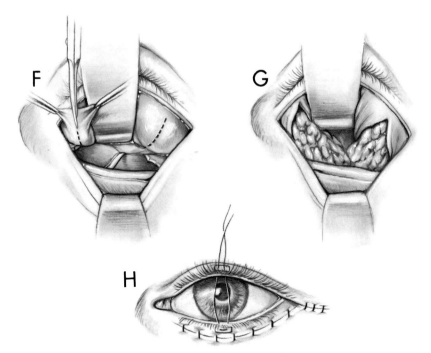

FIGURE 16–72 *Continued*

D. The rest of the lateral wall is removed with the rongeur until the thicker bone of the sphenoid is encountered, which limits any further expansion of the defect.

E. An incision is made in the periorbita.

F. The fat is gently spread to allow its prolapse into the temporal fossa.

G. The lateral aspects of the upper and lower eyelids are reattached with several sutures of 5-0 Vicryl, thus re-forming the lateral canthal angle.

H. To keep a space for the orbital tissue prolapse, only the subcutaneous tissue is closed with 5-0 Vicryl and the skin with 5-0 Prolene.

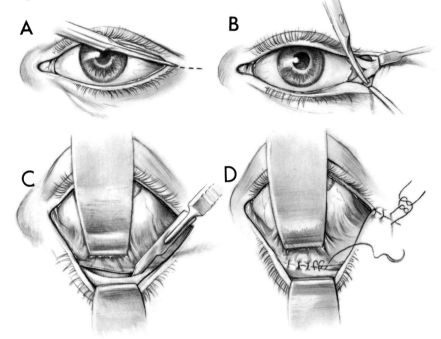

FIGURE 16–73. Cul-de-sac orbital decompression.

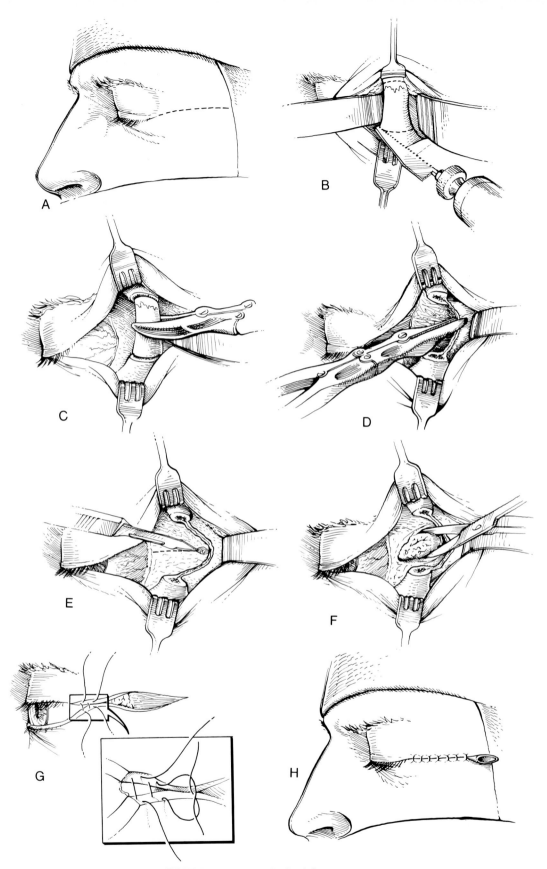

FIGURE 16–74. Lateral orbital decompression.

A Penrose drain is placed in the lateral orbit, coming out through the temporal incision. The drain is removed on the 2nd postoperative day.

Complications from orbital decompression include infraorbital nerve anesthesia and extraocular disturbance and diplopia. Both of these problems usually improve with time; if diplopia is persistent after 6 months, strabismus surgery may be necessary. This occurs more frequently in patients (up to 30 per cent) who already have muscle restriction preoperatively.[67] If inflammation persists postoperatively or soft tissue signs and myopathy worsen, radiotherapy should be considered in an effort to arrest the process. The usual dose is 2000 cGy, 1000 cGy from each lateral port over a 10-day period.[68]

To lend support to the globe and prevent extraocular muscle imbalance, a central hammock of periorbita is left under the inferior rectus and oblique muscles. Periosteal slits are made on either side of the central hammock, allowing the fat to freely prolapse into the maxillary antrum. Occasionally the fat is gelatinous and does not easily prolapse. This may be due to the increase in the mucopolysaccharide content, which causes the fat to be firmer and more adhesive, and which, along with the increased extraocular muscle mass, probably accounts for the less-than-expected recession of the globe.

Despite removal of the orbital floor, the globe does not fall into the antrum because of two anatomical factors: (1) the ligament of Lockwood, which is a thickening of Tenon's capsule, blends with the capsulopalpebral fascia and forms a fascial sling below the globe, and (2) the central strip of periorbita forms the additional support for the globe. Therefore, with the fat prolapsing into the antrum, the globe should move posteriorly along this combined support. Because the periosteal slits are placed on either side of this support, the inferior rectus and oblique muscles are protected from inadvertent incarceration.

ENUCLEATION

Removal of an eye is, for an ophthalmologist, rather like the performance of euthanasia for an internist. Both acts are tacit expressions of failure. The significance of enucleation to the patient must also be recalled; the event, even when not overtly accompanied by the threat of total blindness, can be devastating.

Indications for enucleation include the presence of intraocular malignant tumors (see Chapter 19), severe disruption of the globe with no reasonable chance for visual recovery, persisting marked intraocular inflammation after penetrating injury or surgery, intolerable pain, and unsightly appearance.

It is common practice to attempt to repair badly damaged eyes despite what appears to be a hopeless situation. Many of these eyes become a source of discomfort because of persistent inflammation. Patients are usually grateful for any attempt made to save their eyes; if the attempt proves unsuccessful, they are then more able to accept the prospect of enucleation. Sightless eyes that have gone through various stages of vascular occlusion, glaucoma, and inflammation can become miserably painful, and instant relief is brought about with their removal. As an alternative, retrobulbar injection with several milliliters of absolute alcohol in the region of the ciliary ganglion can produce temporary relief. Unsightly eyes with no hope of visual rehabilitation can be camouflaged with cosmetic scleral shells. If this is unsatisfactory because of buphthalmos or foreign body irritation, removal of the eye is preferred.

In eyes with suspected malignancies the emphasis should be on atraumatic surgery because studies by Fraunfelder and colleagues have shown that melanoma cells can be pushed into the venous circulation by pressure on the eye.[69] Eyes that have retinoblastoma require as long an optic nerve segment as possible, since the tumor extension commonly occurs in that direction.

Many ingenious methods have been proposed and used to impart a lifelike movement to the prosthesis. However, because of ease of bacterial entry into the orbit, the incidence of extrusion is high with any implant that is externalized and connected to the prosthesis. No technique has stood the test of time as well as simple enucleation with placement of a plastic or silicone sphere within Tenon's capsule.

Technique (Fig. 16–75)

A. A peritomy is made at the limbus, separating the conjunctiva and Tenon's capsule from the globe for the full 360 degrees.

B. The rectus muscles are tagged with 4-0 chromic catgut and cut from their insertions.

C. The superior oblique tendon is grasped with a muscle hook and cut.

D. The inferior oblique muscle is clamped with two hemostats side by side for hemostasis, and the muscle between them is cut. The hemostats are released after several minutes.

E. All attachments between Tenon's capsule

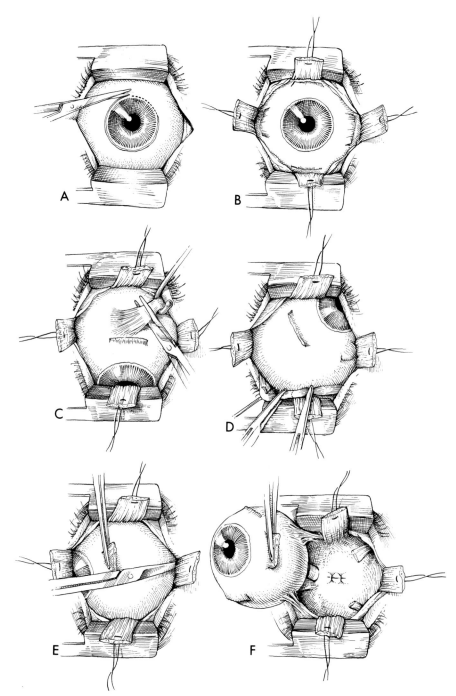

FIGURE 16–75. Enucleation.

and the globe are separated by blunt dissection, allowing the globe to move freely. With a secure hold kept on the medial rectus insertion to steady the eye, the enucleation scissors are passed posteriorly along the globe. A back-and-forth movement should be used to assure location of the optic nerve; the scissors could be referred to as "gently strumming the optic nerve." The scissors are pulled back slightly, opened, and then advanced to engage the nerve. To obtain a long piece of nerve, the scissors are pushed posteriorly into the orbit before the optic nerve is cut.

F. The globe is delivered and the few re-

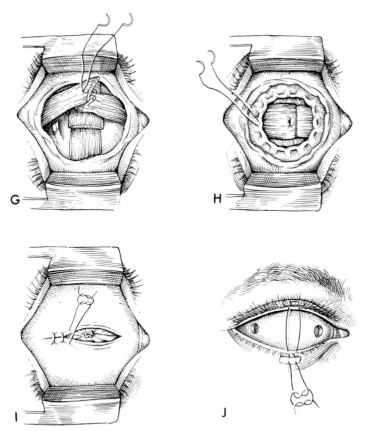

FIGURE 16–75 *Continued*

maining tissue attachments are cut. If bleeding persists, electrocauterization may be necessary. If Tenon's capsule has been lacerated, it should be repaired with interrupted 4-0 chromic catgut.

G. An 18- to 22-mm sphere is placed in Tenon's capsule, and the horizontal and vertical muscles are joined over the implant with mattress sutures of 4-0 chromic catgut.

H. Tenon's capsule is closed with either purse-string or interrupted sutures of 4-0 chromic catgut.

I. The conjunctiva is approximated with interrupted 6-0 plain catgut.

J. A conformer is placed in the cul-de-sac. An intermarginal suture of 6-0 silk may be used to join the lids, which will produce a mild pressure effect on the socket. This suture is removed at the first dressing.

It is imperative to preserve all conjunctiva in order to prevent compromise of the cul-de-sac. Control of bleeding is of paramount importance, and pressure alone may be inadequate to seal the arterial bleeding in the orbit. In that event, careful and coordinated use of sponges and

suction should allow grasping of the bleeding points with forceps, followed by electrocauterization. An implant that is too large, producing tension on Tenon's capsule, is likely to extrude. On the other hand, an implant that does not properly fill Tenon's capsule may result in a socket that appears sunken. In summary, control of bleeding, prevention of infection, and choice of an implant that is not too large are probably the most important factors in preventing extrusion.

Antibiotic ointment is instilled in the socket for several weeks postoperatively. The conformer is not removed during the healing period. A clear methylmethacrylate conformer will allow a view of the suture line, which is not possible with the opaque silicone conformers. At 8 to 12 weeks the edema is generally gone and the suture line well healed, which allows fitting of an artificial eye by the prosthetic technician (ocularist).[70] When the artificial eye has been inserted, the patient should be reexamined in order to evaluate the fitting of the prosthesis and the condition of the socket. The patient is instructed not to remove the prosthesis, since this would allow contaminants to be introduced. If discharge should occur, irrigation around the prosthesis with a squeeze bottle of saline solution is suggested. With persistent discharge, examination by the physician is recommended.

EVISCERATION

Evisceration of the globe refers to removal of the entire contents of the eye within the scleral shell.

Evisceration is indicated in a hopelessly traumatized eye in a young person with no history of previous eye disease. An eye with opaque media may be suitable for evisceration if careful ultrasonography can clearly rule out the presence of an intraocular mass. In all other situations the advisability of performing an evisceration is questionable because of the threat, however, remote, of sympathetic ophthalmia.[71] The danger of spreading an unsuspected intraocular malignancy is always a possibility as well.

The cosmetic result after evisceration is generally superior to that after enucleation; the upper lid sulcus is usually normal and motility of the prosthesis is better. With the modified Burch technique the cornea is retained, leaving the socket relatively undisturbed. Even when the cornea is removed, the extraocular muscles are still attached to the scleral shell, which results in a movable implant, and thus a more natural-appearing prosthesis.[70]

Standard Technique (Fig. 16–76)

A. A peritomy 5 mm from the limbus is made from 3 to 9 o'clock superiorly. An incision the same length is made in the exposed sclera 3 mm from the limbus, through to the uvea.

B. The entire uvea is separated from the sclera by an evisceration spoon and is completely removed.

C. A gauze sponge on a hemostat is rotated within the sclera shell to remove the remaining uvea.

D. The scleral edges are tagged with 4-0 chromic catgut and used to hold open the shell while an 18- to 22-mm implant is inserted by use of a sphere introducer. If tension is present on the wound when the corneal cap is closed, a smaller implant should be inserted.

E. Before closure the posterior surface of the cornea should be scarified with a curette, to reduce its sensitivity. The sclera is closed with interrupted 5-0 Vicryl. The conjunctiva is approximated with interrupted 6-0 plain catgut, and a conformer is placed in the cul-de-sac. A light dressing is applied.

Alternate Method: Keratectomy with Scleral Flaps (Fig. 16–77)

A. The cornea is removed and radial incisions are made in the four quadrants for 1 cm.

B and **C.** A smaller implant 14 to 16 mm in diameter, is placed in the scleral shell, and the flaps are overlapped and sutured with 4-0 Dacron.

D. The conjunctiva is approximated over the sclera with 6-0 plain catgut.

Postoperatively, the patient is placed on topical antibiotics. There is generally less pain postoperatively than with enucleation, since the orbit itself is undisturbed. When the cornea is retained, there are occasional problems with foreign body sensation, as well as chronic pain caused by pressure within the scleral shell. This is remedied by removing the cornea and inserting a smaller implant within the scleral flaps.

SOCKET RECONSTRUCTION

Secondary Implants

Inadequate filling of the socket is a disturbingly frequent complication of enucleation. An unattractive, sunken upper lid is the usual result; furthermore, it may become difficult or even impossible to fit a cosmetically satisfactory prosthesis. A common cause is absence of an implant; one may not have been inserted at the time of enucleation because of an infection or loss or damage to the tissues. Untreated fractures increase the volume of the orbit because of fat displacement, with shrinkage occurring later, despite the presence of an implant. If the implant inserted was too small, it may inadequately fill out the upper eyelid. The orbital tissues may also gradually atrophy.

Whatever the cause of the enophthalmic appearance, the treatment is volume replacement with silicone,[72] methylmethacrylate, or dermal fat grafts.[73]

If an implant was not used at the time of enucleation or evisceration, a secondary sphere implant can be inserted. A solid piece of silicone

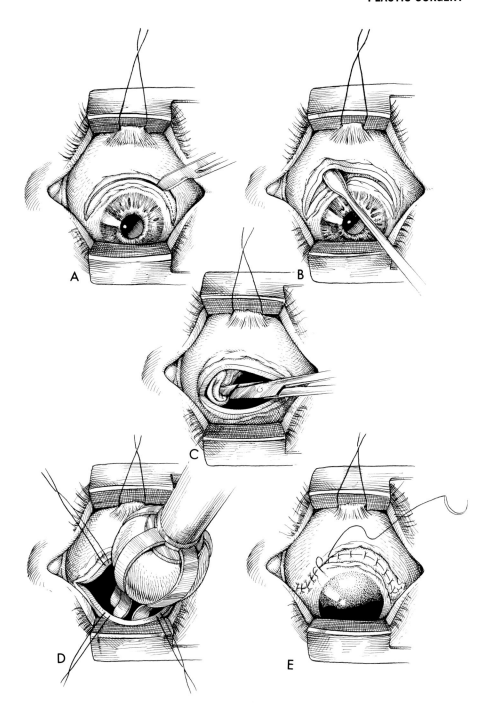

FIGURE 16–76. Eviseration.

that is carved with a ridge at the posterior aspect is placed in the floor of the orbit and can push the remaining orbital tissue superiorly and forward. This would also apply in cases in which an implant was already present; a silicone block would push the implant superiorly to fill out the supratarsal space. An expandable silicone implant can also be used in the same manner; saline solution is injected into a silicone bag after the implant is placed in the orbit.

Sphere Implant

If sclera is used, the implant is placed within the scleral sphere. Several radial incisions are

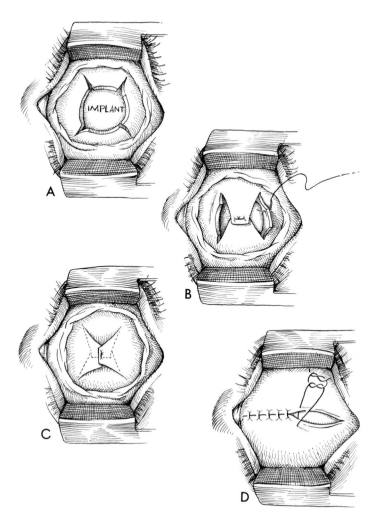

FIGURE 16–77. Evisceration, alternate method.

made, and the flaps are closed over the implant with 5-0 Vicryl sutures.

The implant can be further secured by placement of two 5-0 Prolene sutures through opposite sides of the implant or sclera and then through the horizontal muscle bellies.

Scleral Wrapped Implant

If an implant was not inserted at the time of enucleation, or if one has extruded and there is a sunken appearance to the orbit, a secondary implant can be inserted. This can be either a silicone or plastic sphere. To ensure its position within the orbit, wrapping the implant with preserved sclera provides a fibrous coat and added stability. Because Tenon's capsule is collapsed, the implant is placed in the retrobulbar space.

Technique (Fig. 16–78)

A. A lid speculum is placed in the cul-de-sac, and a horizontal incision is made in the conjunctiva across the fundus of the socket.

B. Tenon's capsule, which is collapsed and thickened unless it is a fresh extrusion, is incised into the posterior orbit. Orbital fat will be seen through the incision, and finger palpation of the apex is possible. If it is a fresh extrusion, the anterior and posterior layers are discernible and are separately tagged with 4-0 chromic catgut.

C. A 16- to 18-mm silicone sphere is inserted into the space.

D. Tenon's capsule is closed in two layers over the implant with interrupted 4-0 chromic catgut sutures.

E. The conjunctiva is closed with interrupted 6-0 chromic catgut sutures.

F. Cross section showing the position of the implant behind a collapsed Tenon's capsule.

In these cases Tenon's capsule is thickened and forms an excellent barrier for the implant. We have not found it practical to search for the extraocular muscles because they are usually contracted and difficult to isolate and do not add a significant advantage to the overall result.

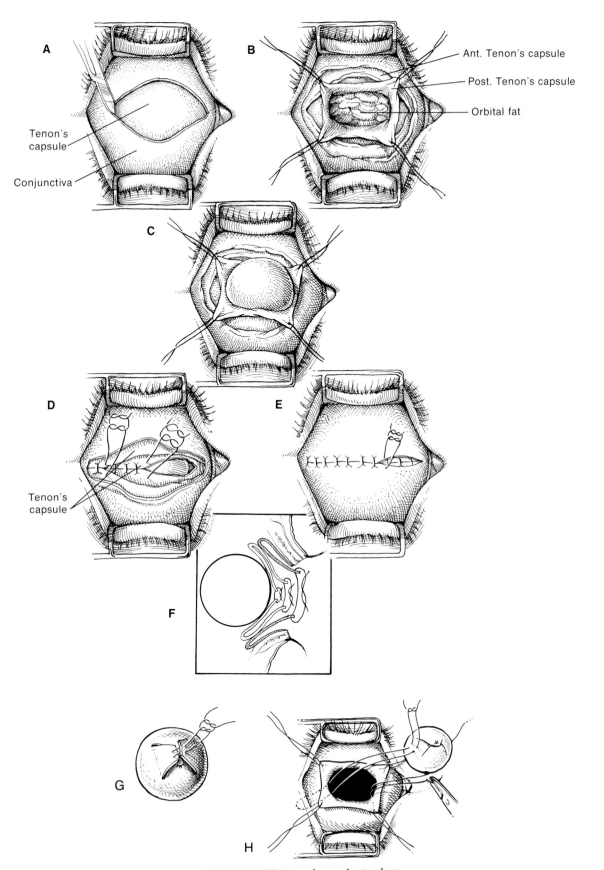

FIGURE 16–78. Secondary socket implant.

G. If sclera is used, the implant is placed within the scleral sphere. Several radial incisions are made, and the flaps are closed over the implant with 5-0 Vicryl sutures.

H. The implant can be further secured by placement of two 5-0 Prolene sutures through opposite sides of the implant or sclera and then through the horizontal muscle bellies.

Silicone Block Implant

In cases of enophthalmos with a deep upper lid recess, and when an implant is present, adding a thick silicone block along the floor of the orbit will push the implant upward and forward. This reduces the upper lid recess. When loss of the eye is associated with orbital fractures, fat is displaced into the maxillary or ethmoidal sinuses. The silicone implant helps to reduce the volume of the orbit and bring the sphere and upper lid forward. The approach is through the inferior cul-de-sac.

Technique (Fig. 16–79)

The initial steps are similar to those shown in Figure 16–73. A block of silicone in the range of 3.0 × 2.5 × 0.5 to 1.0 cm is placed along the floor of the orbit. It is either above or below the periosteum, and is positioned as far posteriorly as possible, to avoid problems of compromise of the inferior fornix. The closure is the same as described in Figure 16–73.

Scleral Patch Graft

When an implant is partially exposed as a result of thinning of Tenon's capsule, a scleral patch graft can, by reinforcing the area, prevent further extrusion.[74] Attempts to suture the

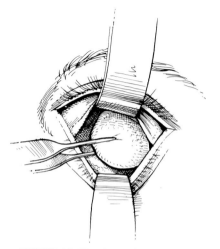

FIGURE 16–79. Silicone block implant.

edges together are usually futile because the tissue is under tension and the sutures usually pull out. This procedure is not indicated when there is almost total exposure of the implant with extrusion a virtual certainty.

Technique

A. The conjunctiva is separated from Tenon's capsule for a distance of at least 1.5 cm around the area of exposed implant, and the edges are freshened to remove ingrown epithelium.

B. A piece of preserved sclera at least twice the size of the defect is sutured over the defect to Tenon's capsule with 6-0 chromic catgut sutures.

C. The conjunctiva is closed with interrupted 6-0 chromic catgut sutures.

Dermal-Fat Graft to Socket

A dermal-fat graft is an ideal implant, since it is autogenous and, therefore, has virtually no reason to be rejected. It must, however, have enough available blood supply to survive. The fat portion has even a greater need for nourishment; otherwise, it will atrophy. Because graft atrophy has been reported to be between 5 and 10 per cent and, rarely, up to 40 per cent,[75] it is necessary to overcorrect by a moderate amount.

The indications for a dermal-fat graft are an extruding implant that is beyond repair with a scleral patch, a socket whose implant is already extruded, a socket that has had multiple extrusions of alloplastic implants, and in a primary enucleation. The first indication is the most appropriate situation. There is usually infection in the area that would decrease the success rate with an alloplastic implant. Moreover, the conjunctiva, which is usually shrinking around the extruding implant, does not need to be approximated with a dermal-fat graft. The dermal-fat graft is left uncovered, since epithelialization occurs from the surrounding conjunctiva.

Technique (Fig. 16–80)

A. The extruding implant is removed from the socket and the cavity is irrigated with saline solution and an antibiotic solution.

B. A dermal-fat graft is removed and prepared as shown in Figure 16–7. The graft should measure 20 to 25 mm in diameter, depending on the patient's age and the redundancy of the tissue. In a child it is difficult to close an abdominal wall excision greater than 1 cm in width. In that case the graft can be cut and

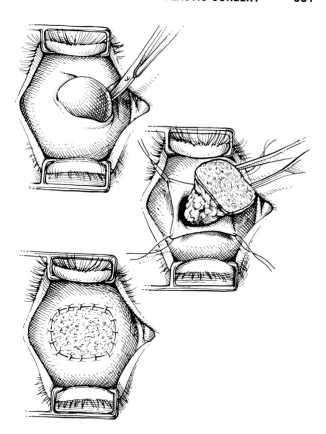

FIGURE 16–80. Dermal-fat graft to socket.

doubled in width. The fat portion should measure at least 2.5 cm. Grafts much larger than this may not acquire the proper vascularization and nourishment and thus may atrophy. A pocket is created through Tenon's capsule so that the graft can be comfortably placed.

C. Tenon's capsule and conjunctiva as well as any muscle stumps are sutured to the dermal edge with 6-0 Vicryl. A conformer steep enough to vault the graft is placed in the socket. The dermal portion usually assumes a lighter color in the first few weeks followed by gradual epithelialization and a redder, more normal color. An artificial eye can be fitted after several months.

Cul-de-Sac Reconstruction

Contracture of the anophthalmic socket may make insertion or retention of a prosthesis difficult. Reducing the size of the prosthesis may solve the problem temporarily. Contracture may be due to poor technique at the time of enucleation, resulting in conjunctival loss, or secondary to loss of tissue associated with

trauma. Chemical injuries, particularly lye burns, result in severe contracture, owing to loss of integrity of the conjunctiva and destruction of the tear glands and goblet cells. Contraction and loss of the inferior fornix commonly develop after any chronic external inflammation. When contracture is so severe that a prosthesis cannot be properly fitted, a mucous membrane graft is necessary to enlarge the socket and re-form the cul-de-sac.[24] In the case of marked contracture of the socket after several failed attempts at reconstruction, or with the elderly or infirm, total obliteration can be considered. The remaining conjunctiva, tarsal-conjunctiva, and lid margin are removed. The skin and muscle flaps from the eyelids are joined with or without a dermal-fat graft to fill out the sunken appearance.[76] This gives a smooth appearance to the orbit and frees the patient from having to care for the area and from any discomfort.

In other cases the appearance of a contracted socket can result from a prolapse of orbital contents into the inferior cul-de-sac, often accompanied by a laxity of the lower lid. If enough conjunctiva is present, and if shrinkage is not a factor, tightening the lower lid may deepen the fornix. The attachment of the lower fornix to the capsulopalpebral fascia may be lost, allowing orbital fat to fill the space. Sometimes this can be corrected with through-and-through double-armed sutures of 4-0 chromic catgut placed from the conjunctiva through the periosteum of the lower rim and out the skin surface. As the catgut sutures dissolve, there may be enough tissue reaction and scarring to keep the cul-de-sac deep enough to retain a prosthesis.

Technique (Fig. 16–81)

A. A lid speculum is placed in the cul-de-sac and an incision is made in the conjunctiva across the fundus of the socket.

B. The conjunctiva is dissected free and, depending on where the contracture is, allowed to fill the needed space. If both upper and lower cul-de-sacs are involved, the conjunctiva is freed to its tarsal attachments.

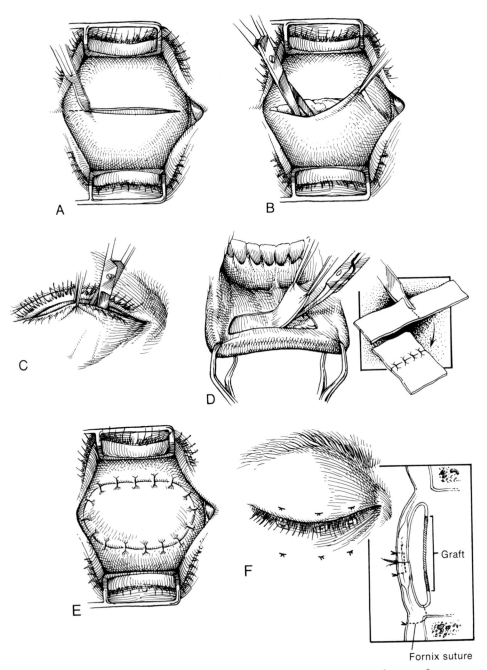

FIGURE 16–81. Socket reconstruction with full-thickness mucous membrane graft.

C. Sharp and blunt dissection through the inferior socket and posterior aspect of the lower lid to the inferior orbital rim creates a lower cul-de-sac. Extreme care must be exercised in the upper cul-de-sac, since the levator aponeurosis could be injured. A flat methylmethacrylate conformer approximately 2.5 to 3 × 2.0 to 2.5 cm is placed in the socket to test the newly created space. The lids should close over the conformer without tension.

D. A full-thickness mucous membrane graft is taken from the lower lip. If more tissue is needed, the upper lip and cheek areas can be used (see section on Cicatricial Entropion). Frequently the graft is too long but not wide enough; if so, the graft is divided across its longer dimension and joined side by side with interrupted sutures of 6-0 chromic catgut to permit its covering the socket defect.

E. The graft is sutured in place between the two edges of conjunctiva with 6-0 chromic catgut. One or two sutures connect the graft to the canthal areas.

F. The conformer is placed in the socket, and the eyelids are approximated with intermarginal sutures of 4-0 silk tied over silicone pegs. To preserve the formation of the lower cul-de-sac, the conformer must be large enough to create a snug fit within the socket. A step that will augment the lower cul-de-sac re-formation is to bring through-and-through 4-0 chromic catgut from the lower cul-de-sac through the periosteum of the inferior rim and out the lower eyelid, where it is tied.

The patient is placed on oral antibiotics for 1 week, and topical antibiotics are continued for as long as the intermarginal sutures are in place. It is necessary to keep the eyelids approximated, in order to exaggerate the cul-de-sac. It is preferable to leave the intermarginal sutures in for at least 3 to 4 weeks. The cul-de-sac sutures are allowed to dissolve on their own to create a scar tissue adherence. In cases of severe cicatricial changes associated with a lack of tear secretion, the prognosis is guarded. Should the result be unsatisfactory in these cases, split-thickness skin can be used.

Symblepharon

Symblepharon is an adhesion between the conjunctival surfaces. It can occur after eyelid or conjunctival surgery, trauma, and chemical injuries, particularly lye burns. Inflammatory conditions, including Stevens-Johnson disease, ocular pemphigoid, and chronic cicatricial conjunctivitis, are also commonly responsible. The adhesions may consist of small bands in the fornices, or they may involve the entire palpebral and bulbar conjunctival surfaces, resulting in loss of the cul-de-sac. With the exception of symblepharon after surgery and trauma, there may also be decreased tear production caused by conjunctival shrinkage involving the ducts of the main and accessory lacrimal glands. Moreover, the cicatricial changes may continue relentlessly despite medication and surgery. With the destruction of the conjunctival goblet cells and obliteration of lacrimal secretory function, the eye becomes dry, the conjunctiva shrinks and becomes keratinized, and total xerophthalmia may develop. Unfortunately mucous membrane grafting is not likely to succeed, for such grafting fails unless there is some moisture present. In severely compromised eyes parotid duct transplantation may offer a chance of survival.[77]

When the condition has been stable for 6 months, surgical repair can be undertaken.[78] In mild cases either a Z-plasty or transposition of the symblepharon band is appropriate. If the entire cul-de-sac is involved, however, split-thickness mucous membrane grafting will be necessary.

Z-plasty

Technique (Fig. 16–82)

A. An incision through conjunctiva and Tenon's capsule is made along the line of tension. This is usually in line with the symblepharon band. At either end, incisions are made in opposing directions at a 60-degree angle from the original line.

B. The conjunctiva is undermined, and the flaps are transposed and sutured with 7-0 chromic catgut.

Transposition of the Symblepharon

Technique (Fig. 16–83)

A. The symblepharon is cut away from the globe, and radial incisions are made on either side to free it completely.

B. A suture of 6-0 double-armed silk is placed through the leading edge of the symblepharon, which is reflected into the cul-de-sac.

C. The suture is brought through the skin and tied over silicone pegs; it is removed after 1 week.

D. The bulbar conjunctiva on either side is undermined and approximated with 7-0 chromic catgut to the inferior cul-de-sac.

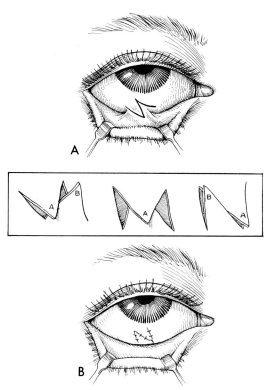

FIGURE 16–82. Symblepharon repair with Z-plasty.

Split-Thickness Mucous Membrane Grafting

Technique (Fig. 16–84)

A. Traction sutures of 6-0 chromic catgut are placed through the sclera at the limbus, and the eye is rotated away from the symblepharon to put the area on traction. The symblepharon is removed from the globe or cornea with a #69 Beaver blade, or separated across the lines of tension with scissors. When all the adhesions are finally severed it becomes possible to rotate the globe further, which exaggerates the defect. The symblepharon is reposited in the cul-de-sac as lining for the eyelid.

B. The lower lip is infiltrated with an anesthetic such as lidocaine with epinephrine; then saline solution is injected to make the inside of the lip firm enough to facilitate removal of the graft. Towel clips can be used to evert and steady the lip during removal of the graft. The Castroviejo mucotome with the 0.4 to 0.5 mm shim is a useful instrument for taking the split-thickness graft. The mucotome is placed parallel to the lip and advanced across at a rate slow enough to allow the graft to be seen coming through the head. Forceps grasp the leading edge of the graft to hold it away from the blade as it comes through. Tissue from the upper lip and cheek can be used if additional mucous membrane is needed. The graft is immediately placed on a wet sponge or a wet gauze sponge with the epithelium up. The donor area is covered with a wet saline sponge.

An additional source of graft material is conjunctiva from the superior-lateral bulbar conjunctiva. A size limit of 1 cm in diameter is a prudent guide. Only conjunctiva is removed, leaving the substantia propria and Tenon's capsule as the framework for epithelialization of the donor area.

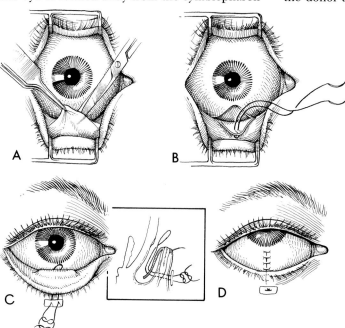

FIGURE 16–83. Transposition technique of symblepharon repair.

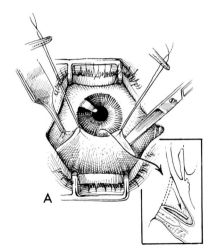

FIGURE 16–84. Symblepharon repair with split-thickness mucous membrane.

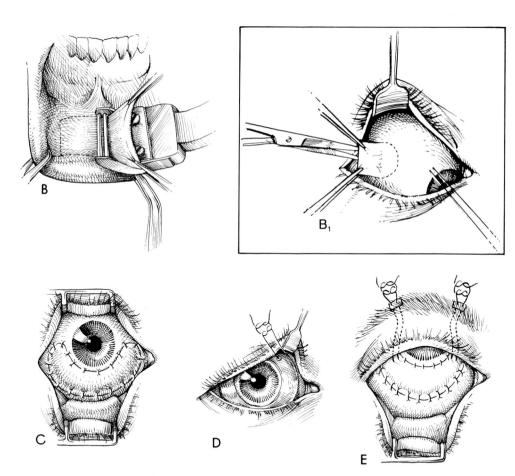

C. With the free conjunctival edge or symblepharon reflected into the fornix, the defect on the globe is made as large as possible. The graft is placed on the globe and into the fornix, and sutured with 6-0 chromic catgut, catching the scleral tissue. It is important to place as much of the graft as possible on the globe itself, since it will heal better and shrink less in that

position, from which it has an immovable frame on which to grow. In contrast, that portion of the graft that lies in the cul-de-sac and in the palpebral areas has a less rigid base and tends to shrink more; therefore, it should be more loosely placed.

D. A scleral donut conformer is inserted in the cul-de-sac. Suturing the conformer to the globe prevents movement of the edge of the conformer across the cornea. An additional technique that can be used to keep the cul-de-sac on stretch is to place intermarginal sutures between the upper and lower lids; judicious observation, however, is necessary to prevent these sutures from causing pressure damage to the globe or cornea. If the double-armed 4-0 silk suture that is placed through each lid is tied with a bow knot, the lid can effectively be joined, but inspection of the eye is still possible by releasing the bow knot.

E. An alternate method of keeping the graft on stretch without the use of a conformer is to use traction sutures. These are 4-0 Dacron sutures placed first through the sclera on either side of the cornea and then through the opposite fornix, catching the periosteum before the needles emerge from the skin surface. They are tied over silicone pegs.

The patient is placed on antibiotic drops for as long as the conformer is present. It is preferable for it to be in place for at least 2 weeks but can be left in for 4 weeks without any untoward effect. The purpose of the conformer is not only to keep the grafts stretched, so that they conform to the shape of the cul-de-sac, but also to prevent contact between the surfaces of the grafts; this contact would tend to lead to unwanted adhesions. When attempts to retain the conformer in position result in too much irritation or in possible damage to the globe, it must be removed earlier. The patient can be given steroids and antibiotic drops after removal of the conformer to reduce inflammation and graft shrinkage.

Although the traction suture shown in Figure 16–71E does indeed keep the graft on tension by mechanically rotating the eye away from the involved area, it is quite painful because of the constant tension. There can also be erosion of the sutures into the sclera. It is difficult for the patient to tolerate these sutures for longer than a week.

REFERENCES

1. Smith, B., Leone, C. R.: General principles of ophthalmic plastic surgery. Eye, Ear, Nose and Throat Mon., 47:589, 1968.
2. Reeh, M. J., Beyer, C. K., Shannon, G. M.: Practical Ophthalmic Plastic and Reconstructive Surgery. Philadelphia, Lea & Febiger, 1976.
3. Wolff, E., Last, R. J.: Anatomy of the Eye and Orbit, 6th ed. Philadelphia, W. B. Saunders Co., 1968.
4. Jones, L. T., Reeh, M. J., Wirtschafter, J. D.: Ophthalmic Anatomy (manual). Rochester, Minn., American Academy of Ophthalmology, 1970.
5. Iliff, C. E.: Dermatochalasis and blepharochalasis of the upper eyelids. Trans. Am. Acad. Ophthalmol., 85:709, 1978.
6. Wilkins, R. B.: Evaluation of the blepharoplasty patient. Trans. Am. Acad. Ophthalmol., 85:703, 1978.
7. Small, R. G.: Supratarsal fixation in ophthalmic plastic surgery. Ophthalmic Surg., 9:73, 1978.
8. Tenzel, R. R.: Correction of brow ptosis. Trans. Am. Acad. Ophthalmol., 85:716, 1978.
9. Schwarz, F., Randall, P.: Conjunctival incision for herniated orbital fat. Ophthalmic Surg., 11:276, 1980.
10. De Mere, M., Wood, T., Austin, W.: Eye complications with blepharoplasty or other eyelid surgery. Plastic Reconstr. Surg., 53:634, 1974.
11. Waller, R. R.: Is blindness a realistic complication of blepharoplasty? Ophthalmology, 85:730, 1978.
12. Llyod, W. C. III, Leone, C. R. Jr.: Transient bilateral blindness following blepharoplasty. Ophthalmic Plast. Reconstr. Surg., 1:29, 1985.
13. Van Gemert, J. V., Leone, C. R. Jr.: Correction of a deep superior sulcus with dermis-fat implantation. Arch. Ophthalmol., 104:604, 1986.
14. Jankovic, J., Havins, W. E., Wilkins, R. B.: Blinking and blepharo-spasm: Mechanism, diagnosis and management. JAMA, 248:3160, 1982.
15. Hankinson, H. L., Wilson, C. B.: Microsurgical treatment of hemifacial spasm. West. J. Med., 124:191, 1976.
16. Shore, J. W., Leone, C. R. Jr., O'Connor, P. S., et al.: Botulinum toxin for the treatment of essential blepharospasm. Ophthalmic Surg., 17:747, 1986.
17. Gillum, W. N., Anderson, R. L.: Blepharospasm surgery: An anatomic approach. Arch. Ophthalmol., 99:1056, 1981.
18. Frueh, B. R., Callahan, A., Dortzbach, R. K., et al.: The effects of differential section of the VII nerve on patients with intractable blepharospasm. Trans. Am. Acad. Ophthalmol., 81:595, 1976.
19. Callahan, A.: Reconstructive Surgery of the Eyelids and Ocular Adnexa. Birmingham, Aesculapius Publ. Co., 1966.
20. Leone, C. R.: Internal tarsus-orbicularis resection for senile spastic entropion. Ann. Ophthalmol., 7:1004, 1975.
21. Jones, L. T., Reeh, M. J., Wobig, J. L.: Senile entropion: A new concept for correction. Am. J. Ophthalmol., 74:327, 1972.
22. Quickert, M. H., Rathbun, E.: Suture repair of entropion. Arch. Ophthalmol., 85:304, 1971.
23. Wies, F. A.: Spastic entropion. Trans. Am. Acad. Ophthalmol. Otolaryngol., 59:503, 1955.
24. Smith, B. C., Nesi, F. A.: Practical Techniques in Ophthalmic Plastic Surgery. St. Louis, C. V. Mosby Co., 1981.
25. Leone, C. R.: Mucous membrane grafting for cicatricial entropion. Ophthalmic Surg., 5:24, 1974.
26. Hecht, S. D.: Cryotherapy of trichiasis with use of the retinal cryoprobe. Ann. Ophthalmol., 9:1501, 1977.
27. Smith, B.: The lazy "T" correction of ectropion of the lower punctum. Arch. Ophthalmol., 94:1149, 1976.
28. Leone, C. R. Jr.: The treatment of entropion and ectropion. Ophthalmic Forum, 1:16, 1983.
29. Leone, C. R.: Repair of cicatricial ectropion by horizontal shortening and pedicle flap. Ophthalmic Surg., 606:47, 1976.
30. Soll, D. B. (ed.): Management of Complications in Ophthalmic Plastic Surgery. Birmingham, Aesculapius Publ. Co., 1976.
31. Beard, C.: Ptosis, 2nd ed. St. Louis, C. V. Mosby Co., 1976.

32. Cogan, D. G.: Neurology of the Ocular Muscles, 2nd ed. Springfield, Ill., Charles C Thomas, 1956.

33. Havener, W. H.: Ocular Pharmacology, 4th ed. St. Louis, C. V. Mosby Co., 1978.

34. Kearns, T. P.: External ophthalmoplegia, pigmentary degeneration of the retina and cardiomyopathy: A newly recognized syndrome. Trans. Am. Acad. Ophthalmol. Soc., 65:559, 1965.

35. Leone, C. R. Jr., Shore, J. W.: The management of the ptosis patient. Part I. Ophthalmic Surg., 16:666, 1985.

36. Epstein, F. A., Putterman, A. M.: Super-maximum levator resection for severe unilateral congenital blepharoptosis. Ophthalmic Surg., 15:1971, 1984.

37. Jones, L. T., Quickert, M. H., Wobig, J. L.: Cure of ptosis by aponeurotic repair. Arch. Ophthalmol., 93:629, 1975.

38. Fasenella, R. M., Servat, J.: Levator resection for minimal ptosis: Another simplified operation. Arch. Ophthalmol., 65:493, 1961.

39. Leone, C. R. Jr., Shore, J. W., Van Gemert, J. V.: Silicone rod frontalis sling for the correction of blepharoptosis. Ophthalmic Surg., 12:881, 1981.

40. McCord, C. D.: Combined frontalis suspension and eyelid fold procedure. Ophthalmol. Times, March 1979, p. 21.

41. Baylis, H. I.: Correction of residual ptosis following levator surgery. Ophthalmol. Times, 10:29, 1982.

42. Jones, L. T., Wobig, J. L.: Surgery of the Eyelids and Lacrimal System. Birmingham, Aesculapius Publ. Co., 1976.

43. Quickert, M. H., Dryden, R. M.: Probes for intubation in lacrimal drainage. Trans. Am. Acad. Ophthalmol. Otolaryngol., 74:431, 1970.

44. Viers, E. R.: Lacrimal Disorders. St. Louis, C. V. Mosby Co., 1976.

45. Leone, C. R. Jr.: Gelfoam-thrombin dacryocystorhinostomy stent. Am. J. Ophthalmol., 94:412, 1982.

46. Campbell, C. B. III, Shannon, G. M., Flanagan, J. C.: Conjunctiva-dacryocystorhinostomy with mucous membrane graft. Ophthalmic Surg., 14:647, 1983.

47. Stokes, D. P., Flanagan, J. C.: Dacryocystectomy for tumors of the lacrimal sac. Ophthalmic Surg., 8:85, 1977.

48. Yanoff, M., Fine, B. S.: Ocular Pathology. Hagerstown, Md., Harper & Row, 1975.

49. Older, J. J., Quickert, M. H., Beard, C.: Surgical removal of basal cell carcinoma of the eyelids utilizing frozen section control. Trans. Am. Acad. Ophthalmol. Otolaryngol., 79:658, 1975.

50. Leone, C. R., Van Gemert, J. V.: Lower eyelid reconstruction with upper eyelid transpositional graft. Ophthalmic Surg., 11:315, 1980.

51. Leone, C. R., Hand, S. I.: Reconstruction of the medial eyelid. Am. J. Ophthalmol., 87:797, 1979.

52. Mustardé, J. C.: Repair and Reconstruction in the Orbital Region. Baltimore, Williams & Wilkins, 1966.

53. Cutler, N., Beard, C.: A method for partial and total upper eyelid reconstruction. Am. J. Ophthalmol., 39:1, 1955.

54. Leone, C. R. Jr.: Tarsal-conjunctival advancement flaps for upper eyelid reconstruction. Arch. Ophthalmol., 101:945.

55. Leone, C. R. Jr.: Lateral canthus reconstruction. Ophthalmology, 94:238, 1987.

56. Bullock, J. D., Koss, N., Flagg, S. V.: Rhomboid flap in ophthalmic plastic surgery. Arch. Ophthalmol., 90:203, 1973.

57. Hughes, W. L.: Surgical treatment of congenital palpebral phimosis: The Y-V operation. Arch. Ophthalmol., 54:586, 1955.

58. Lee, O. S.: An operation for the correction of everted lacrimal puncta. Am. J. Ophthalmol., 34:375, 1971.

59. Tenzel, R. R.: Treatment of lagophthalmos of the lower lid. Arch. Ophthalmol., 81:366, 1969.

60. Jones, I. S., Jakobiec, F. A.: Diseases of the Orbit. Hagerstown, Md., Harper & Row, 1979.

61. Putterman, A. M., Urist, M.: Surgical treatment of upper eyelid retraction. Arch. Ophthalmol., 7:401, 1972.

62. Dryden, R. M., Soll, D. B.: Use of scleral transplantation in cicatricial entropion and eyelid retraction. Trans. Am. Acad. Ophthalmol. Otolaryngol., 83:669, 1977.

63. Baylis, H. I., Rosen, N., Neuhaus, R. W.: Obtaining auricular cartilage for reconstructive surgery. Am. J. Ophthalmol., 93:709, 1982.

64. Leone, C. R., Bajandas, F. J.: Inferior orbital decompression for thyroid ophthalmopathy. Arch. Ophthalmol., 98:890, 1980.

65. McCord, C. D., Moses, J. L.: Exposure of the inferior orbit with fornix incision and lateral canthotomy. Ophthalmic Surg., 10:53, 1979.

66. Leone, C. R.: Management of ophthalmic Graves' disease. Ophthalmology, 91:770, 1984.

67. Shorr, N., Neuhaus, R. W., Baylis, H. I.: Ocular motility problems after orbital decompression for dysthyroid ophthalmopathy. Ophthalmology, 89:323, 1982.

68. Brennan, M. W., Leone, C. R. Jr., Janaki, L.: Radiation therapy for Graves' disease. Am. J. Ophthalmol., 96:195, 1983.

69. Fraunfelder, F. T., Boozman, F. W., Wilson, R. S., et al.: No-touch technique for intraocular malignant melanoma. Arch. Ophthalmol., 95:1616, 1977.

70. Guibor, P., Goubleman, H. P. (eds.): Problems and Treatment of Enucleation, Evisceration, Exposure. New York, Stratton Medical Book Corp., 1974.

71. Green, W. R., Maumenee, A. E., Sanders, T. E., et al.: Sympathetic uveitis following evisceration. Trans. Am. Acad. Ophthalmol. Otolaryngol., 76:625, 1972.

72. Soll, D. B.: Correction of superior lid sulcus deformity with subperiosteal implants. Arch. Ophthalmol., 85:188, 1971.

73. Smith, B., Petrelli, R.: Dermis-fat graft as a movable implant within the muscle cone. Am. J. Ophthalmol., 85:62, 1978.

74. Helveston, E. M.: A scleral patch for exposed implantation. Trans. Am. Acad. Ophthalmol. Otolaryngol., 74:1307, 1970.

75. Smith, B., Bosniak, S., Nesi, F., et al.: Dermis-fat orbital implantation: One hundred eighteen cases. Ophthalmic Surg., 14:941, 1983.

76. Shore, J. W., Burks, R., Leone, C. R. Jr., McCord, C. D. Jr.: Dermis-fat graft for orbital reconstruction after subtotal exenteration. Am. J. Ophthalmol., 102:228, 1986.

77. Bennett, J. E.: The management of total xerophthalmia. Arch. Ophthalmol., 81:667, 1969.

78. Stewart, W. B., et al.: Ophthalmic Plastic Surgery (manual). San Francisco, American Academy of Ophthalmologists, 1984.

17

EXTRAOCULAR MUSCLES

by Robert D. Reinecke

INTRODUCTION

Strabismus surgery departs from other forms of ocular surgery in two distinct ways. First, it is the only form of ocular surgery in which movement of the tissue is the essential feature of the final goal of the surgery. Second, currently and in the foreseeable future there is almost a 20 per cent chance that further surgery

will be necessary. The surgeon should keep these two features in mind in that the technique should generally be designed to avoid excessive restrictions on the eye, and the muscles should be repositioned and altered in a manner that minimally disturbs their strength and leverage. Finally, the procedure should be executed in such a manner that the tissue planes are preserved, thus allowing surgical reintervention to be easily accomplished. The general anatomical factors that are important for these features are obvious for the most part and will not be described in detail, but the variations and clinical cues to assist the surgeon in the procedure will be pointed out whenever possible. For detailed knowledge of anatomy the reader is urged to turn to one of the many texts that treat the subject in depth.[1-3]

The physician about to engage in surgery of the muscles of the eye should note that although excessive bleeding is seldom responsible for excessive scar tissue, an interruption of the muscle sheaths will allow blood, fat, and connective tissue to fuse the muscle tissue in such a mass that future surgery is difficult and adhesions that prevent the muscle antagonist from functioning typically result. Only when the surgeon wants the muscle to retract to an unusual degree should the muscle sheath be interrupted. For example, if the inferior oblique is to retract fully to reduce its action to the maximum extent in a disinsertion procedure, its muscle sheath should be carefully dissected from the belly of the muscle. In most instances it is not advisable to excessively dissect the check ligaments and tissue surrounding a muscle. Only in those cases in which prior surgery has made excessive tissue grow about the muscles are deep dissections appropriate.

The shape and directions of the muscles often give the surgeon clues to appropriate dissections in those secondary operations in which the identity of the muscle mass is obscure. Even for the more common strabismus procedures the surgeon should take care to position the globe accurately and avoid inappropriate deep thrusts of instruments. If one cannot see what is being cut, the chance of damaging tissue is obviously increased. Remember the adage that if things can go wrong in surgery, they will.

Straight, properly functioning eyes are regarded with such delight by the patient and his family that a good result gives the surgeon a degree of satisfaction akin to that achieved with successful cataract surgery. Fortunately for the patient and for the surgeon a result that is not satisfactory can usually be corrected with further surgery, unless a disastrous step has been taken along the way in prior surgery.

EXAMINATION TECHNIQUES

A brief overview of examination technique with suggestions for interpretation follows.

Visual Acuity

Assessment of visual acuity is essential in the strabismus examination and should be faithfully documented at each examination. Neonates frequently are a challenge in this regard, but remember that a face is the best fixation device. The OKN drum is occasionally of use in attracting the neonate's attention, while interesting toys often will do the trick for infants and toddlers.

Differences in the fixation preference, and hence the visual acuity of the two eyes, are determined by fixation and following patterns. Exact quantification of visual acuity is not possible in infants, but differences between the eyes in the ability to hold fixation and to follow patterns are essential in evaluating vision. Does the child hold fixation and follow well with each eye? Does he hold fixation through a blink? Although children often reject attempted patching, a winter hat with ear guards can often be used to cover one eye without complaints. For the 2½-year-old child Allen cards may be used to give the first easily recorded visual acuities, but remember that these are isolated targets as opposed to full-line letters. Monocular and binocular vision is measured and recorded at each examination. Watch for head turns and latent nystagmus. In latent nystagmus the binocular acuity should be recorded and each eye's acuity measured while the fellow eye is occluded with a +5-diopter lens.

Tumbling Es are often substituted for the Allen cards by the time a child is 3½ years of age. Full horizontal lines of the Es are substituted for individual Es as soon as possible, in order to discover whether there is an amblyopia that may have been masked by the crowding phenomenon. For example, a patient's vision with isolated letters may be 6/9 in each eye yet may measure only 6/15 in OD and 6/9 in OS when full lines are used. One should remember that children are less likely to confuse Es in up and down direction than those facing left and right. In older children letter and number charts are substituted for the tumbling E chart.

Nystagmus patients, both children and adults, should have visual acuity measurements recorded at different gaze positions. The null point as to gaze direction should also be noted with such patients.

Whenever suboptimal visual acuity is noted, an attempt should be made to use pinhole vision as an indication of uncorrected refractive error. If pinhole vision improves the visual acuity, a refraction is indicated.

Stereo Testing

Stereoacuity testing as an initial screening examination has proved to be efficient and effective over the past few years. The Random Dot-E (RDE), when held at 1 m, correlates with the number 4 circle on the Titmus test. Increasing the card distance of the RDE from the patient decreases the stereo arc. If the child passes the RDE from a distance of 2 m, the child has good fusion and good vision, and only an intermittent exotropia will be missed. These stereo cards also allow assessment of stereopsis in different positions of gaze. Other stereopsis tests include the Titmus fly and TNO.

Youngsters who fail the RDE card can often be enticed to play the *two-pencil test* (Fig. 17–1). The child must touch the point of one pencil to the point of a pencil held by the examiner. The more accurate he is, the higher the level of stereopsis. Covering one eye of the patient during the test will quickly confirm that visual input from both eyes is helping the child to perform.

Stereo testing is essential in the strabismus examination and should be performed after visual acuity has been tested. If a negative RDE is attained initially, the test should be repeated later if fusion is suspected in a particular field of gaze. Good stereopsis means that the patient has no significant amblyopia, and that any form of occlusion is contraindicated.

Worth 4 Dot

To test for suppression a Worth 4 dot test, consisting of two green, one red, and one white illuminated dots, may be used. Red and green glasses are placed on the child's eyes (red on the right is traditional). Because the red glass filter blocks out the two green lights, making them invisible, only the red and white dots (two dots) on a hand-held Worth 4 dot flashlight can be seen with the eye behind the red glass. With green over the left eye only the green and white dots (three dots) can be seen with this eye. Seeing all four dots represents no

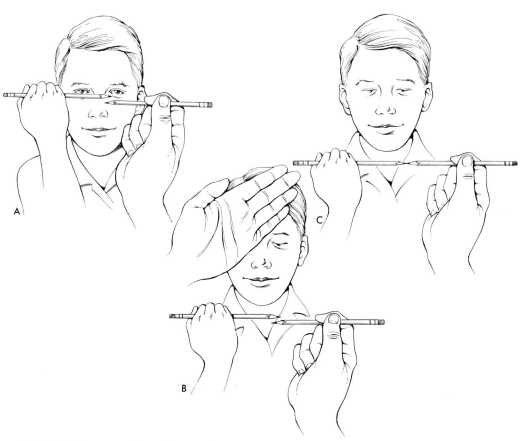

FIGURE 17–1. Two-pencil test showing (*A*) patient with suppression, (*B*) test for accuracy of response by covering one eye, and (*C*) normal response.

suppression; two reds, suppression of the left eye; three greens, suppression of the right eye; and five dots, diplopia. With intermittent exotropes who fuse at near, and therefore see four dots at near, the hand-held Worth 4 dot flashlight is moved away until suppression occurs, at which point the distance is noted. This test gives a crude indication of the status of central binocular fusion. The distance wall-mounted Worth 4 dots are so large that they indicate only peripheral fusion.

Ductions and Versions

The first step in the evaluation of ductions and versions assesses the general appearance of parallelism of the eyes in the primary and extreme positions. If the patient is determined to have strabismus, detailed measurements of heterophorias and heterotropias with prisms in the nine diagnostic fields of gaze should then be done. As careful testing of versions in all directions is performed, underactive and overactive obliques, "A" and "V" patterns, and restrictions should be noted.

A V *pattern* is defined as a heterophoria-tropia of more esotropia 20 degrees below and more exotropia 20 degrees above. An A *pattern* is the reverse, that is, it has more relative esotropia above and more exotropia below. A patient with a V pattern esotropia might have 15 prism diopters esotropia above and 45 prism diopters esotropia below. An overacting inferior oblique causes that eye to elevate and abduct as the fellow eye fixates in extreme lateral gaze just above the horizontal. An overacting superior oblique causes the adducting eye to depress excessively and abduct while the fellow eye is fixating just below the horizontal in extreme lateral gaze.

Typically, overactive inferior obliques give a V pattern, whereas overactive superior obliques give an A pattern. The overacting obliques can be tested most easily at near with a detailed fixation target. To detect these patterns, and therefore make the correct surgical decisions, it is critical to have the patient look in extreme upgaze and downgaze. Alternate cross-cover testing in the nine diagnostic gazes should be performed first *without prisms*, to give a general feeling for the case. Only then should prisms be used to quantitate these findings.

Ductions refer to the movement of each eye alone. Testing of ductions may be misleading in assessing underactions of a muscle that can be correctly evaluated only when seen in conjunction with its contralateral yoke muscle.

Distance and Near Measurements

In a child diagnostic position measurements are easier to evaluate at near, although the 6-m measurement in primary gaze is important, as it can be related to the convergence at near for an estimate of the accommodative convergence–accommodation ratio (AC:A). In exotropes measurements with fixation at 100 m or more are helpful in eliciting the maximal exotropia. A long hallway or window is useful for taking measurements in these patients. While measuring the heterotropia, fixation estimates are essential. If one eye is amblyopic, its quality of fixation should be noted first while occluding the good eye. With this technique the patient is more likely to give a distinctive refixation pattern with the good eye.

4–Prism Diopter (Base-out) Test

Small-angle esotropes with small central suppression scotomas are often difficult to detect. A 4-diopter prism is placed base-out over one eye while fixation is directed to an accommodative target. The prism will cause the patient to see the image toward the apex of the prism. A relatively slow fusional movement nasally will be difficult to see in each eye, as the eyes immediately converge. This takes the fellow eye off target, which will in turn cause a refixation of each eye in the same direction. The opposite eye will move simultaneously an equal amount temporally, according to Hering's law. Each of these movements is equal to only one-half the amplitude of the prism; thus each is small and difficult to detect.

If, on the other hand, suppression is present in an eye, placing the 4-diopter prism base-out moves the image within the scotomatous area, and *no* movement will be seen. When the 4-diopter prism is placed before the nonsuppressing eye, both eyes will move the full 4 diopters, and the movement is easily seen.

Angle of Strabismus

The angle of deviation is initially determined by estimating the light reflex (Hirschberg test) or by centering the light reflex with prisms of increasing size in front of the fixating eye. (One millimeter of deviation approximates 7 degrees, or 15 prism diopters of deviation.) More accurate determinations are evaluated by the cover, cover-uncover, and alternate cover tests.

Cover Test. Heterotropias are determined by covering one eye while looking for *any* movement in the opposite eye. After the occluder has been removed the opposite eye is covered and the examiner again looks for any movement in the uncovered eye.

Cover-Uncover Test. Heterophorias are determined by using a cover-uncover test. The eye is occluded and uncovered while the examiner looks for fusional movement in the eye as it is covered and uncovered. Any movement represents a phoria, that is, a deviation that becomes manifest only when fusion is interrupted and that is evidenced by the fusion movement as the cover is removed from that eye. The other eye does not move as it maintains steady fixation.

Alternate Cover Test. To measure the heterophoria or heterotropia, an appropriate-sized prism is placed over one eye, and the cover is alternated every 2 seconds back and forth between the two eyes. The size of the prism is increased until the movement is neutralized. To assure the best measurement, an opposite movement should be induced first with a larger-sized prism, after which one returns to the next smaller prism.

Cycloplegia

Inducement of full cycloplegia is necessary for determination of refraction in childhood. Although topical atropine used three times a day for 3 days before the next office visit is often recommended, adequate cycloplegia can be obtained at the initial office visit. This can readily be accomplished by using one drop each of proparacaine, 2% cyclopentolate, and 1% tropicamide, in that order. Proparacaine decreases the painful sensations of the cycloplegics and increases their absorption. Retinoscopy should be performed 20 to 25 minutes after instillation. This technique gives cycloplegia within +.25 of a full atropine refraction. The advantage is that the examination can be completed in one office visit, and therapy, whether medical or surgical, can be initiated immediately.

The record should be flagged with the date of the visit on which the cycloplegic refraction was done. The cycloplegic re-refraction should be repeated with the following frequency if a strabismus or amblyopia is being treated and followed:

AGE	FREQUENCY WITH WHICH CYCLOPLEGIA SHOULD BE REPEATED
<1 year	Every 6 months
1–3 years	Every 9 months
>3 years	Once a year

Fixation

A Visuscope or a direct ophthalmoscope with a small star target can be used to assess fixation. The patient fixates the eye being tested on the figure, and the image on the retina is observed to see if it is directly on the fovea or is eccentric to the fovea. Eccentric fixators will invariably have decreased vision in direct proportion to the distance of the image from the fovea. The fellow eye should be occluded during this test. The test is not necessary for an eye that sees 6/6, since that eye must be using the fovea to attain normal vision. The indirect ophthalmoscope is useful for evaluating eccentric fixation in the dilated patient. The examiner positions a pencil in the real image located just anterior to the condensing lens. Because this point in space is coincident with the retina, the patient and the examiner can see the target. The examiner can note the shadow of the pencil tip on the retina, and thus determine the area of the retina the patient is using for fixation.[4]

Diplopia Fields

Paralytic strabismus typically gives diplopia in the field of action of the palsied muscle. A Goldmann perimeter or tangent screen can be used to plot the "diplopia field." In this test a patient is instructed to follow a 3-mm white object with both eyes while keeping his head still, and to report the appearance of the second image. Areas of diplopia and single vision are plotted on one visual field chart. Sequential diplopia fields over time are helpful in following muscle palsies or comparing preoperative and postoperative findings.

Lancaster Red-Green Test

In a haploscope (Lancaster red-green or Hess screen) the visual fields of the two eyes are dissociated so that paralytic conditions can be diagnosed. The Lancaster test uses reversible red-green goggles and two hand-held projectors, one red and one green. The examiner projects one color on the Lancaster screen while the patient superimposes the other colored light directly on the first. This method dissociates the two eyes so that the distance between the lights will exactly correspond to the amount of deviation between the two eyes. Torsion is easily diagnosed by tilting of the patient's light when a strictly vertical or horizontal line has been shown by the examiner. This examination, in a cooperative patient, gives a graphic demonstration of paralytic muscles.

Electro-oculogram

Electro-oculograms (EOGs) may be used to determine saccadic velocities in suspected muscle palsies. In nystagmus patients the frequency, amplitude, and type of eye movement can be quantified and null points of usual nystagmus and periodic alternating nystagmus documented for future comparison. The distinction between manifest latent nystagmus and infantile nystagmus is needed to assess the optimal time for strabismus surgery. Manifest latent nystagmus is relieved by fusion.

Photos and Videotape

Photographs of the eyes in diagnostic fields of gaze may be used for documentation of eye muscle disorders, but videotape recordings of most conditions and particularly of nystagmus and other dynamic eye movements provide more useful documentation.

Both modes of recording are used in the patient with congenital nystagmus. Still photos can clearly document the preferred head position, while videotape and EOGs show the eye movements.

Retinoscopy

To assure fixation, a patch should be placed on the patient's opposite eye when performing retinoscopy. Loose spherical and cylindrical lenses should be placed in a trial frame if possible, to give accurate astigmatic corrections. Visual acuity can be checked with the new net retinoscopic findings. In general, the full spherical and full astigmatic correction should be prescribed to children with esotropia who have a "significant" refractive error.

Retinoscopy can also be used to determine the preferred eye in a patient with a microstrabismus. If a patient is instructed to look directly at the light of a retinoscope from a distance of 2 feet, the eye that is fixating the light will have a darker light reflex because a reflection from the macula area is more darkly pigmented than a reflection from the eccentric fixating nonpreferred eye.

ANATOMY

The surgical anatomy of the tissues under surgical consideration are discussed here in respect to the individual muscles as the techniques are described; thus only those details necessary for the surgeon to note before starting surgery are covered in this section.[5]

Positioning of the Globe

To avoid the surgical error of operating on the wrong muscle, it is essential that the globe be positioned so that the surgeon is correctly oriented with respect to the expected position of the muscle. Several factors that may allow verification of the position of the eye with respect to the orbit are discussed in the following paragraphs.

Preoperative evaluation of the patient's eyes in the primary position should include specific evaluation of torsion of each eye. Ophthalmoscopic appearance of the disc and the position of the fovea in relation to the disc typically will allow detection of significant torsion. If the patient cooperates, plotting of the blind spot will confirm the torsional position of the globe. A further test is the Maddox rod rotated in such a manner as to produce a subjectively horizontal line (see Fig. 17–2).

General anesthesia alters the position of the eye as the depth of the anesthesia is varied. If the patient is lightly anesthetized, the eyes elevate and extort as they are mechanically stimulated. The surgeon should insist that anesthesia be deepened to permit the eyes to be in the primary position before surgery is started. Local anesthetics can affect the muscles independently, depending on the completeness of the retrobulbar block. Because typically the superior oblique may be inadequately anesthetized, care should be exercised to ensure that there is not excessive intortion of the eye under local anesthesia. (See discussion of cardiac irregularities with muscle surgery.)

As the eye is inspected in the primary position, an area can be discerned as a lateral limbal

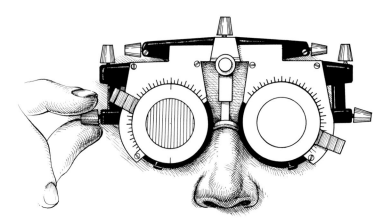

FIGURE 17–2. Patient or examiner rotates the Maddox lens until the patient reports the line from the light of a flashlight to be precisely horizontal. Any nasal deviation of the top of the Maddox rod denotes intorsion; any temporal deviation indicates extorsion.

triangle on most eyes. This landmark can be noted and tagged with a 7-0 silk traction suture. The lateral limbal triangle (Fig. 17–3) is formed by the lessened scleral overlay laterally as compared with superiorly and inferiorly. Usually no similar triangle is seen nasally.

The patterns of muscle insertions with respect to the limbus are fair indicators of the muscle's identity. The distance of the insertions gradually increases from the medial rectus's 5.5 mm to the superior rectus's 7.0 to 7.5 mm, but these distances are not helpful in most instances, since any confusion will be between two adjacent muscles, such as the lateral rectus and the inferior rectus, in which case the differing measurements are small. The direction of the insertions in relation to the limbus serves to distinguish the horizontal recti from the vertical recti. The horizontal recti insert parallel to the limbus. (Any prior surgery negates the usefulness of insertion direction for that particular muscle.) The vertical recti insert at an angle corresponding to their direction from the apex of the orbit to the globe. Thus the temporal margin of the vertical recti's insertion is further from the limbus than the medial edge of the

insertion. A virgin insertion of either the vertical or horizontal rectus will serve to distinguish which is a horizontal rectus muscle (Fig. 17–4).

The oblique muscles are good confirmatory landmarks. The inferior oblique is under the inferior rectus (i.e., close to the floor of the orbit). It then courses laterally and posteriorly beneath the lateral rectus (i.e., closer to the globe than the lateral rectus). When the inferior rectus is operated on, the inferior oblique will be seen coursing perpendicular to the inferior rectus (Fig. 17–5, left diagram). When the lateral rectus is isolated, inspection of the inferior margin of the lateral rectus will reveal the

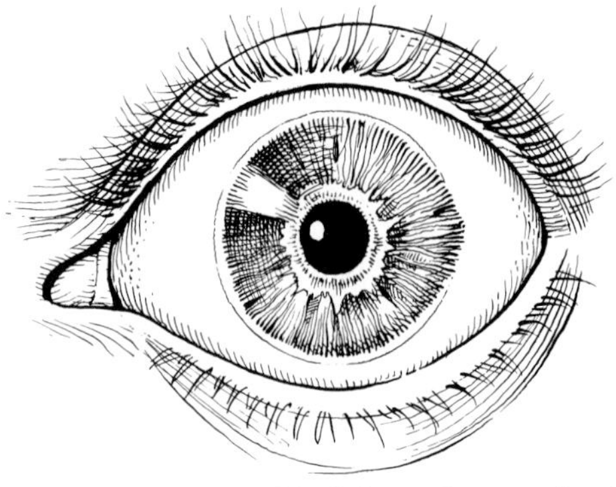

FIGURE 17–3. The lateral limbal triangle. Note the clear space of cornea forming a triangular space laterally.

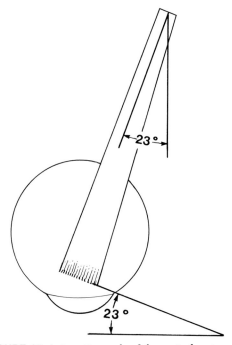

FIGURE 17–4. Insertion angle of the vertical rectus muscles.

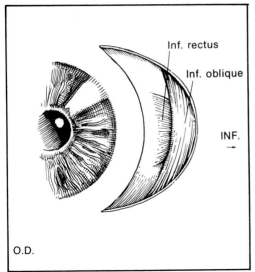
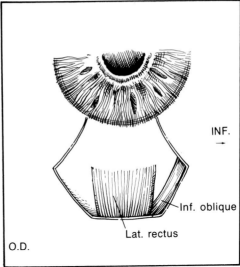

FIGURE 17–5. The inferior oblique muscle as an orienting landmark.

inferior oblique coursing medial to it (Fig. 17–5, right diagram). Because the inferior oblique muscle has no tendon, it can be easily recognized.

The superior oblique tendon and its insertion provide a landmark on the superior half of the globe (Fig. 17–6). The superior oblique tendon is inferior to the superior rectus (as the inferior oblique is inferior to the inferior rectus), but closer to the globe at the equator. The insertion of the superior oblique is at the lateral edge of the superior rectus. A small muscle hook passed laterally and slightly posteriorly under the superior rectus will easily engage the thin tendon.

The superior oblique tendon, medial to the superior rectus, is 12.0 mm posterior to the medial border of the superior rectus insertion, and should not be isolated unless it is to be specifically involved in the surgery. The reason for such avoidance is the susceptibility of that area to form adhesions with any minor trauma.

The direction of the muscle fibers is easily discernible as the muscle is isolated. Any discrepancy in the expected direction of such fibers, and hence in the course of the muscle, should alert the surgeon that the wrong muscle may have been isolated, and the other signs of globe position just mentioned should be used. If any doubt remains, an ophthalmoscope should be used to observe the disc and disc-fovea orientation.

Variations from the expected norm are expected and should be carefully noted on the surgical diagrams, as should the point at which the new insertion is placed. The surgical chart can be conveniently used for this purpose (see

Fig. 17–7A). Figure 17–7B indicates an unusually posterior insertion of a medial rectus and its new insertion.

Conjunctiva

The skill of performing extraocular muscle surgery can be masked or accentuated, depending on the treatment rendered the conjunctiva. If carefully handled, meticulously repaired, and unencumbered by bulky tissue beneath it, the conjunctiva will tolerate repeated manipula-

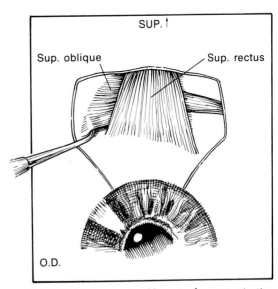

FIGURE 17–6. The superior oblique tendon as an orienting landmark.

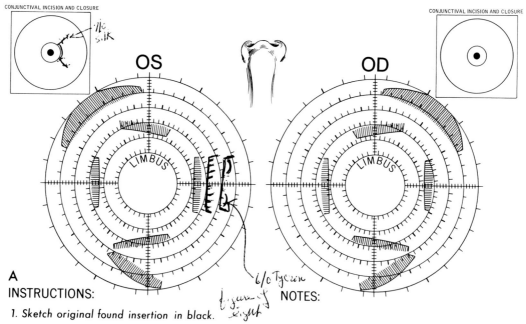

A

INSTRUCTIONS:

1. Sketch original found insertion in black.

2. Sketch new insertion in blue.

3. Sketch original insertion plus red for resection.

4. Sketch sutures in green and label type of material.

NOTES:

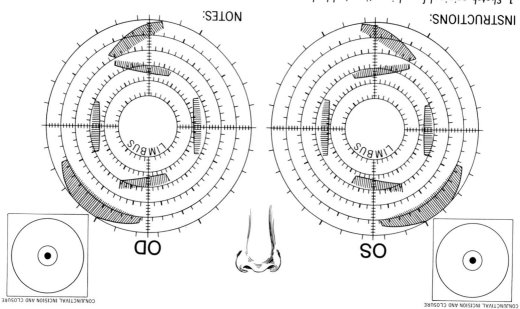

B

FIGURE 17–7. The surgical chart. *A,* Surgical chart indicating a recessed medial rectus. Note that the chart as shown here is inverted to reflect the surgeon's position at the head of the patient. *B,* Subsequent to surgery, the chart can be conveniently mounted in the patient's chart consistent with the face-to-face view of the patient in the examining chair.

tions. Careless closure and trauma to the conjunctiva will cause it to form scars and lose its mucus-producing goblet cells. The scars may well act as check ligaments, simulating paretic muscles. The loss of goblet cells causes the conjunctiva to scar further, appear dull, and react excessively with redness to mildly noxious stimuli. Conjunctiva already compromised by prior trauma or disease can be predicted to scar excessively, and may undo the extraocular muscle surgery.

The conjunctiva normally acts as a covering for the globe and as a lubricating surface for its tarsal portion. Mobility of the conjunctiva in the cul-de-sac is necessary to assure free movements of the globe and lids. The mobility is assured by the lack of global contact, except for that portion approximately anterior to the rectus insertions. Posterior to the muscular insertions, the conjunctiva is reflected over Tenon's capsule and fat. Intrusion into that posterior area in the cul-de-sac almost assures excessive scarring.

Tenon's Capsule

The remarkable free movement of the extraocular muscles and globe is allowed by the glove-like muscle sheaths, with similar loose connective tissue condensations reflected back over the globe and fused between the muscles into the intramuscular septum. Anteriorly, this loose connective tissue condensation, called Tenon's capsule, continues as a condensation to insert on the globe, beneath conjunctiva, 1 or 2 mm behind the limbus (Fig. 17–8). Posteriorly, Tenon's capsule divides to continue as a loose covering of the globe called the fascia bulbi and as muscle sheaths. Trauma to Tenon's capsule causes fibrocytes to migrate to the site and create firm adhesions that limit the mobility of the globe. Blood in the area of Tenon's tissue typically does not result in scarring unless it is accompanied by trauma. The best surgical technique is the one that interferes the least with Tenon's capsule while still producing the desired degree of change in muscle strength or leverage.

Other connective tissue condensations extend from Tenon's capsule and the muscle sheaths both vertically and horizontally. The condensations most easily identified are those that extend medially from the external sheath of the medial recti to the periosteum. Traditionally referred to as "check" ligaments, these condensations typically do not interfere with or limit the mobility of the eye; hence they can safely be ignored. After prior surgery fibrous bands may result from the surgical trauma and mimic check ligaments. These bands must be carefully incised if the surgery is to succeed. If the globe

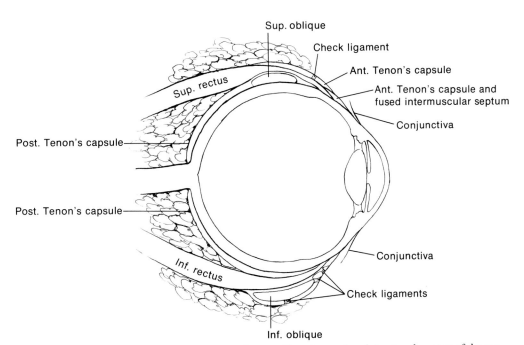

FIGURE 17–8. Vertical section of the eye, emphasizing Tenon's capsule relation to other parts of the eye.

can be passively moved easily, concern for check ligaments is inappropriate and further dissection needless.[3]

Innervation of the Extraocular Muscle

The preceding discussion emphasizes the careful dissections to be made, which should be as restricted in scope as possible while still allowing for adequate muscle strengthening or weakening. Thus the problem of damage to the nerves entering the muscles is minimal, since the nerves enter approximately between the posterior and middle third of the muscle. That point of nerve entry should not be exposed or manipulated during appropriate extraocular muscle surgery. If the surgeon manipulates and cuts only what he can see and identify, there is little chance of damage to the entering nerve.

SURGICAL TECHNIQUES

General Remarks

Anesthesia

General Anesthesia.[6-9] The oculocardiac reflex is especially marked in the young, but is ever present in all age groups. The likelihood of causing a cardiac slowing is somewhat proportional to the abruptness and intensity of the muscle stretch. The reflex can and should be abolished before strabismus surgery in every patient. If general anesthesia is used, atropine should be given and supplemented as necessary to block the reflex. In both children and adults the intramuscular dosage is 0.01 mg/kg. The atropine should be supplemented as needed by intravenous doses of 0.1 mg in children and 0.2 mg in adults. Any slowing of the constantly audible pulse by way of the monitor (or doppler) should alert the ophthalmologist to request the anesthesiologist to administer further atropine. It is clearly inappropriate to give retrobulbar anesthesia as a substitute for atropine, since optic nerves have been damaged, eyes perforated, and even meningeal injections inadvertently introduced. Atropine, given systemically, solves the problem and is safely administered.

Local Anesthesia. If local anesthesia is adequate, atropine is not needed for most patients. However, an occasional young male may have such a sensitive vagal reflex that atropine is indicated and necessary even before the retrobulbar injection.

Surgical Preparation

The ever-present danger of postoperative infection makes it imperative to observe strictest caution in technique and surgical preparation. Any sign of an infection, whether conjunctival or corneal or of the meibomian glands, should be sufficient cause to cancel surgery. Although the effectiveness of preoperative local antibiotics for strabismus surgery has not been verified, the adverse reaction to such use of antibiotics is so minimal that they may be used at the surgeon's discretion. Because the rate of infection for strabismus surgery is only 1 in 2000 cases, with or without antibiotics, patients who are allergic to antibiotics can safely be prepared for surgery without them.

A suitable surgical periocular skin preparation can be effected in a variety of ways. Scrubbing the skin with some detergent followed by scrubbing with an antiseptic, with good irrigation between applications, should suffice. Particular care should be taken to avoid getting soap or alcohol inside the eyelids, since a corneal epithelial defect will produce postoperative discomfort greater than that from the conjunctival and muscle surgery.

Magnification

Although the microscope has been sporadically recommended for extraocular muscle surgery, most surgeons recommend using an operating loupe that provides about $2.2\times$ magnification. Further magnification unduly decreases the operative field and depth perception of the surgeon.

Illumination

Adequate illumination for horizontal muscle surgery is generally provided by ordinary surgical operating lights. Vertical and oblique muscle surgery is greatly enhanced with headlight.

Forced Ductions

Forced ductions should be done on every patient before placement of the surgical incision.[10]

Indications for Strabismus Surgery

When the use of spectacles, patching, and fusion exercises have failed to align the eyes horizontally to within 15 prism diopters and vertically to within 10 prism diopters, a cosmetic deformity will be apparent in most patients. Such a patient will seek and can be offered surgical alignment; a significant number of these patients can expect increased fusion. The younger the patient, the more aggressive the approach should be. Studies have been done that generally delineate the optimal age group for surgical intervention (i.e., alignment of a child's eyes by age two, and certainly by age four if at all possible).[11] As the categories of strabismus are briefly discussed, my personal guidelines are mentioned. (For a summary of specific indications for strabismus surgery, see Table 17–1.)

The question as to the amount of most surgical procedures poses some problems. The adage that a great effect from surgery can be expected in a nonparalytic large-angle strabismus and a lesser effect from surgery in a nonparalytic small-angle strabismus is a good pragmatic rule. The important point is to perform adequate surgery, as there is a great tendency to do a less than effective amount. Once the threshold amount of surgery is determined for a surgeon, further plans can be confidently made. If an overcorrection rate of approximately 7 per cent is not attained, it is an indication that the amount of surgery performed was inadequate for that technique.

If the surgeon uses the techniques recommended in this chapter, the guidelines for amounts of surgery will be generally satisfactory. However, if changes are incorporated, such as the use of various dissections, differing sutures, and many other personal choices, which are perfectly satisfactory, the surgeon will find that the amounts must be changed. The best assurance that appropriate amounts of surgery are being done is for the surgeon to keep a scattergram of his results, with the effect of surgery on the abscissa and the original size of the squint on the ordinate (see Fig. 17–9). A perfect result in all cases would be represented by each case that falls on a diagonal. All cases that fall in the shaded area would represent cases that are cosmetically acceptable. Separate scattergrams should be constructed for esotropes and exotropes, and different markers (e.g., squares versus crosses) used when the technique is altered.

Accommodative Esotropia

Esotropia may be categorized in several ways, but can be discussed most conveniently by age after excluding accommodative esotropia. Those patients who have straight eyes brought to within 8 prism diopters of alignment at distant fixation with plus lenses are defined as having accommodative strabismus, and surgery is sel-

dom indicated. For patients with a significant near heterophoria or heterotropia that is only partially corrected with bifocals, or for patients who cannot tolerate bifocals, specific surgery is mentioned under "esotropia at near"[12] (see Table 17–1).

Esotropia in the Child Under Age Three

Esotropia in the child under age three is treated surgically according to the following schedule, once it is ascertained that hyperopic spectacles will not straighten the eyes:

a. Esotropia of less than 25 prism diopters warrants a recession of a medial rectus of 5 mm and a resection of the same sided lateral rectus of 7 mm. If possible, it is best to operate on the eye that is preferred if the eyes' visual acuities are approximately equal after the amblyopic treatment. If one eye is functionally poor despite adequate amblyopia treatment, the poorer eye is straightened.

b. Esotropia greater than 25 prism diopters in this age group will not be straightened with a single recess-resect. Thus more muscles need to be done at the same time, and 5-mm medial rectus recessions combined with 7-mm lateral rectus resections are recommended on the four horizontal muscles. If the surgeon choses to modify the technique, such as by incorporating large recessions of the conjunctiva, then bimedial recessions of 5 to 6 mm of each medial rectus may suffice.

If these patients have had previous surgery, creation of a surgical pseudotendon for the recession coupled with a resection of 6 mm is recommended.

Esotropia in the Child Age Three Or Older

Esotropia in the child of age three or older is treated with recession-resection of one eye or medial rectus recessions of both eyes. The amount of the surgery is 5-mm recession and 7-mm resection for strabismus of up to 25 prism diopters. For those with esotropia of 25 to 45 prism diopters, the surgery is increased to a 6-mm recession. If the esotropia is greater than 45 prism diopters, three muscles are occasionally done, including a 5-mm recession of both medial recti and one lateral rectus resection of 7 mm. If prior surgery has been done, the same amounts are indicated, with the incorporation of a pseudotendon. Bilateral resections may be of benefit if done no longer than 8 weeks after a bimedial recession has been performed; if done at a later time, isolated resections are often ineffective and are not usually performed

Text continued on page 656

TABLE 17–1. Indications for Strabismus Surgery

CONDITION	AGE (YEARS)	SURGERY—CHOICE IN ORDER OF PREFERENCE	CONSIDERATIONS
Esotropia			
(a) Congenital ET (<25^Δ)	<3	(1) Recess medial rectus 5 mm ⎫ one eye Resect lateral rectus 7 mm ⎭ (2) Recess medial rectus OU 5 mm	*Note:* Measurements are with full cycloplegic refraction. (1) Dominant eye if VA almost equal; nondominant eye if VA poor after extensive patching of dominant eye (2) If undercorrected will need resection of laterals within 6 weeks or, if later, secondary re-recession of medial rectus with lateral resection
(b) Congenital ET (>25^Δ) (*Note:* Most congenital ETs are 40^Δ–60^Δ ET)	<3	(1) Recess medial rectus 5 mm OU and resect lateral rectus 7 mm OU (2) Recess medial rectus 5 mm OU with large conjunctival recessions	(1) Adequate amount of surgery is essential (2) Will typically leave undercorrection requiring second operation

(c) Esotropia
Ortho at distance, 20^Δ ET' at near
High AC/A ratio
Example: 25 ET distance
  45 ET' near
Example: 15 ET distance
  30 ET' near
	<10
	
	>10
		Glasses with bifocals (+3.00 OU)
		
		Bimedial rectus recession 4 mm OU with Faden
		Bimedial rectus recession 5 mm OU with Faden 12 mm from insertion on medials OU
			Note to optician: Bifocals to bisect the pupil—flat top
			Larger deviation at near can be decreased with Faden

(d) Esotropia	>3		*Note:* Surgery on small angle gives small result; surgery on large angle gives large result.
15^Δ–25^Δ		(1) Medial rectus recession 5 mm and lateral rectus resection 7 mm (2) Medial rectus recessions 5 mm OU	(1) Dominant eye if VA about equal; amblyopic eye if VA <20/50 (following intensive occlusion) (2) If undercorrected, will need lateral resections within 6 weeks or re-recession of medial rectus and lateral resection
25^Δ–45^Δ		(1) Medial rectus recession 5 mm and lateral rectus resection 7 mm (one eye) (2) Medial rectus recessions 5 mm OU	(2) More caution needed with older children Larger R & R* on one eye if this eye is severely amblyopic
45^Δ–60^Δ	>3	Medial recession 5 mm OU and lateral resection 7 mm (one eye)	
>60^Δ distance and near	>3	Medial rectus recessions 5 mm OU and lateral rectus resections 7 mm OU	
Nystagmus Blockage			
(a) <35^Δ ET	Any	Medial rectus recessions 4 mm with Faden procedure OU	
(b) >35^Δ ET	Any	Medial rectus recessions 5 mm with Faden OU	

Esotropia Reoperations

(a) S/P bimedial recession 5 mm OU with 15Δ ET'–25Δ ET' (equal distance and near) (or any ET residual ET if patient is under age 2)	<3	(1) Re-recession of medial rectus 5 mm (use pseudotendon for as much of the 5 mm as possible) (2) Re-recessions of both medial recti 2–3 mm OU with pseudotendon	Unless lateral rectus resection is done with 6 weeks of original surgery, lateral resections will not help
(b) S/P & R one eye 15'Δ–30'Δ ET (equal distance and near) (or any ET residual ET if patient is under age 2)	Any	R & R opposite eye 5 mm and 7 mm	
(c) S/P bimedial recession "5 mm" OU 30Δ ET'–50Δ ET' (equal distance and near) (or any residual ET if patient is under age 2)	Any	Forced ductions (look for nystagmus blockage syndrome) Recessions of medial recti an additional 2–3 mm OU with lateral resection 7 mm OU	
(d) Residual ET with near 10Δ > distance (high AC:A)	Any	Bimedial recessions 5 mm with Faden OU (use pseudotendon if necessary)	
(e) S/P R & R OU 15Δ–30Δ ET' (equal distance and near)	Any	—Re-recession of medial recti OU 3 mm OU with pseudotendon (If no Pseudotendon, then add 3-mm recess and 5-mm resectio)	
(f) Esotropia (a) one eye <20/80	4–7	(a) Align cosmetically	—Less chance for fusion *if* eyes have never been aligned —Take into account angle kappa
(g) Esotropia (a) if <20/100 (b) if fusion is breaking	>8	(a) Align cosmetically (b) Align fully	—Adjustable suture on recession

Divergent Paralysis	Usually over 60	Lateral rectus resection 7 mm OU	Typically eso distance, ortho near

A Pattern Esotropia

(a) <25Δ (difference between up- and downgaze)	Any	Treat as usual esotrope	Measure in 20° upgaze and downgaze
(b) 25Δ–35Δ difference in A pattern; estropia in primary position = X	Any	(1) Elevate medial recti one tendon width and recess medial recti OU (2) Recess one medial and elevate one tendon width; resect lateral rectus same eye and lower one tendon width	X = recess medials as in esotropia, depending on deviation in primary position —Expect some additional esotropia in 1° gaze (no change in 1° gaze in children) —Treat X + 40Δ as indicated under "Esotropia"
(c) 35Δ–600Δ difference in A pattern of 40Δ; Eso in 1° position = X	Any	Superior oblique tenotomies OU and appropriate surgery for ET (with expected 40Δ increase in ET)	

Consider the estropia to be treated in 1° position to be X + 40Δ

Table continued on following page

TABLE 17–1. Indications for Strabismus Surgery *Continued*

CONDITION	AGE (YEARS)	SURGERY—CHOICE IN ORDER OF PREFERENCE	CONSIDERATIONS
Exotropia			
(a) <35$^\Delta$ at distance (XT = same at distance and near after ½ hr patching) Treat pseudodivergence excess (XT same distance and near after ½ hr patching) same as comitant XT	Any	(1) Dominant eye, if VA equal or other eye >20/50 —lateral recession 7 mm —medial resection 5 mm (2) Lateral recessions 7 mm OU	(1) Treat nondominant eye if VA <20/50 (2) *Disadvantage of lateral recessions:* If eye goes XT again one must either (a) resect medials within 6 weeks, or (b) re-recess laterals OU or R & R one eye
(b) >35$^\Delta$–55$^\Delta$ at distance	Any	(1) Lateral recession 8 mm; medial resection 6 mm (2) 8 mm recession OU	(1) *Disadvantage of # 1*—may get some lid fissure narrowing; *Advantage of #1*—one eye untouched
(c) >60$^\Delta$ (amblyopic eye)	Any	(1) Medial resection 8 mm $\longrightarrow$ same Lateral recession 8 mm $\longrightarrow$ (2) Adjustable suture on one medial	

(d) >60$^\Delta$ (no amblyopia)	Any	Two eyes
		(1) Recess laterals 7–8 mm OU
		    Reset medials 5 mm OU
		(2) Recess one lateral 8 mm
		    Reset medials OU 5 mm
		    Adjustable suture other lateral rectus	

Convergence Insufficiency			
(a) If associated with intermittent XT	Any	—Convergence exercises —Correct intermittent XT deviation determined by distance numbers —Larger resection, less recession	
(b) If ortho at distance and intermittent X(T)′ at near	Any	(1) Convergence exercises (2) If all exercises and glasses fail, perform bimedial resection 5 mm	
Esotropia with Hypertropia			
(a) Eso with hyper <5$^\Delta$	Any	Eso surgery alone	The larger the esotropia, the more the hypertropia should be ignored in surgical planning. (This presumes surgery is on hypertropic eye.)
(b) Eso with hyper 5–10$^\Delta$	Any	Eso surgery (R & R one eye); lower both horizontal reci one-half tendon width or lower medials one-half tendon width	
(c) Eso with hyper 10$^\Delta$–12$^\Delta$	Any	Eso surgery and lower muscle one full tendon width	

Alternating Sursumduction (Dissociated vertical divergence)	Any	—Superior rectus recession OU 6–8 mm OU —Side with larger sursumduction gets larger recession (Faden OU is a helpful addition if there is a larger alternating sursumduction)
Double Elevator Palsy (Palsy of inferior oblique and superior rectus)	Any	—If forced duction is positive, recess inferior rectus —If no resistance, perform vertical superior transposition of horizontal muscles
Brown's Syndrome (Superior oblique tendon sheath syndrome)	Any	Tenotomy of superior oblique and weakening of inferior oblique
Hypertropia (Alone)		
(a) 15ᐞ hyper	Any	—Superior rectus recession 3 mm inferior rectus resection 3 mm
(b) 20ᐞ hyper	Any	—Superior rectus recession 4 mm Inferior rectus resection 4 mm
(c) 25ᐞ hyper	Any	—Superior rectus recession 5 mm Inferior rectus resection 5 mm
Incomitant Strabismus		
(a) Third Cranial Nerve Palsy	Any	See text (p. 695)
(b) Fourth Cranial Nerve Palsy	Any	(1) *One-muscle-at-a-time procedure* (a) Disinsert inferior oblique on eye of palsy (b) If hypertropia remains, recess inferior rectus on opposite eye (c) If hypertropia and extorsion remain, tuck superior oblique in eye with palsy (d) If torsion is single problem, advance anterior half of superior oblique (2) *Second alteratives* (a) Disinsert inferior oblique on side of palsy alone if deviation <15ᐞ hyper Add tuck (same side) or inferior rectus recession opposite eye during initial operation of >15ᐞ hyperdeviation. If torsion >8° on palsied eye, recommend tuck of palsied superior oblique rather than recession. If <8° torsion on palsied eye, recommend recession of inferior rectus opposite with inferior oblique disinsertion of palsied eye.	Watch for inferior oblique overaction of opposite eye following inferior oblique disinsertion on palsied eye. This represents bialteral superior oblique palsy. *Treatment:* Disinsert overactive inferior oblique on opposite eye.

Table continued on following page

TABLE 17–1. Indications for Strabismus Surgery *Continued*

CONDITION	AGE (YEARS)	SURGERY—CHOICE IN ORDER OF PREFERENCE	CONSIDERATIONS
		(b) Second operation: (1) If still hyper, measure torsion; (2) if torsion, do tuck of superior oblique on eye with palsy; (3) if no torsion, perform inferior rectus recession on opposite eye.	

(c) Sixth Cranial Nerve Palsy	Any	—If incomplete palsy:
		  6 mm medial rectus recession
		  8 mm lateral rectus resection
		—If complete palsy:
		  Operation #1:
		    12 mm medial rectus recession
		    10 mm lateral rectus resection (or combined with Jensen procedure)
		  If eye still has decreased abduction, then:
		  Operation #2: lateral transposition of vertical muscles (6 weeks later)	

(d) Duane's syndrome	Any	—If head turn: Recess medial rectus with small resection (5 mm at most) of lateral recti, if necessary —If eye elevates or depresses in adduction, simulating overactive obliques, a Faden suture on the *lateral* rectus will help stabilize the lateral rectus and decrease incomitancy in adduction	

Adhesive Syndrome

			Ortho' (Null 30° to Right)	20 ET' (Null 30° to Right)
(a) Thyroid	Any	—Recession of appropriate muscle —Often recession of inferior rectus, with adjustable suture —Elevation of lower lid		
(b) Blow-out fracture	Any	—No initial surgery except for trimalleolar fracture —Do *not* advocate Supramid plates initially —Wait 6 months —(a) Treat individually if forced duction is negative; (b) if eye will not elevate and forced duction is positive, perform inferior rectus recession (consider adjustable); (c) if eye cannot depress, do Faden procedure on opposite inferior rectus		
(c) Adherent muscle—S/P multiple surgeries (caused by muscle, blood, and fat being enmeshed together)	Any	Supramid sleeve around muscle after careful dissection of and freeing of muscle from fat. Supramid cap on sclera may help.		
Nystagmus				
(a) Head turn with null point of nystagmus opposite to head turn	Any	Find null point. (*Example:* Null to right, head turned left) —Recess right lateral rectus —Resect right medial rectus —Recess left medial rectus —Reset left lateral rectus	8 mm 6 mm 6 mm 7 mm (Faden all horizontal muscles)	5 mm 5 mm 6 mm 8 mm
(b) If ET >40Δ with head turn (may be cross fixator)	<3	—Correct ET with bimedial recessions coupled with Faden procedure —Correct head turn when child is older		

*R & R, Medial rectus recession with lateral rectus resection.

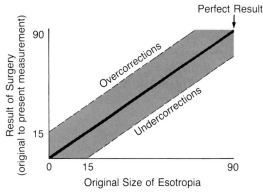

FIGURE 17–9. This type of scattergram chart should be kept by most strabismus surgeons. An × is marked for each final result.

without associated recessions, except in cases of divergence paralysis.

Divergence Paralysis

Divergence paralysis usually occurs in the 60-and-over age group. The esotropia typically measures 15 to 18 prism diopters at distance and ortho at near. Bilateral 5- to 6-mm resections of the lateral recti are indicated.[13] The near phoria will usually not be changed by the surgery.[13]

"A" Pattern Esotropia

"A" pattern esotropias are treated as usual esotropes unless the A pattern is greater than 20 prism diopters. If the A pattern is 20 to 30 prism diopters, the medial recti are elevated one tendon width and recessed 5 mm if the esotropia in the straight-ahead position measures greater than 15 prism diopters. If the A pattern is 35 to 45 prism diopters and overactions of the superior obliques are demonstrated, bilateral superior obliques tenotomies are combined with the surgery indicated for the esotropia as measured in the primary position.[14]

"V" Pattern Esotropia

"V" pattern esotropias greater than 20 prism diopters are best treated with inferior oblique weakening procedures combined with appropriate horizontal recti adjustments indicated by the esotropia measured in the primary position. If, however, any overaction of the superior oblique can be demonstrated, the weakening of the inferior oblique is contraindicated, as such a patient will typically be converted to an A pattern. Large V patterns that are ortho in the up position and eso in the down position can

be corrected with bilateral superior oblique tucks that also correct the overacting inferior oblique.

Convergence Excess

Patients classified as having convergence excess are those esotropes who have a high AC:A ratio. Bimedial weakening procedures are indicated, with an average of 5-mm recession for each medial rectus recession. If the patient has a basic esotropia at distance, that amount of esotropia should be corrected and the excessive action of the medial recti reduced by bilateral posterior fixation sutures (Faden procedure) of the medial recti.

Nystagmus Blockage Syndrome

Nystagmus blockage syndrome is characterized by a congenital nystagmus that is blocked with overconvergence; this is manifested by a variable esotropia and, if vision is equal, a cross-fixational pattern. Treatment consists of a 4-mm recession combined with a posterior fixation suture of each medial rectus.[15]

Exotropias

Exotropias may be corrected by either bilateral lateral rectus recessions or by recession of the lateral recti combined with resection of the medial recti. If bilateral recessions are done and the strabismus is under 35 prism diopters, 8-mm recessions are usually adequate. If the recess-resect is to be done and the exotropia is less than 35 prism diopters, the recession should be 7 mm and the resection of the medial should be 5 mm. If the exotropia is greater than 35 prism diopters, the lateral recti should be recessed 8 mm each, and if recess-resect is to be done, an 8-mm lateral rectus recession and a 6-mm medial rectus resection are advised.[16–18]

Horizontally Incomitant Squints

Sixth Cranial Nerve Palsies. Sixth cranial nerve palsies—if *incomplete*—are successfully treated with 6-mm recession of the medial rectus combined with an 8-mm resection of the lateral rectus muscle. If the sixth nerve palsy is *complete*, the medial rectus should be recessed 10 to 12 mm and either the Jensen procedure done at this time or lateral transpositions of both vertical recti performed at a later date. If the transpositions are to be done, the recession of the medial rectus is accompanied by a 10-mm resection of the lateral rectus, followed in 6 weeks by the lateral transposition of both vertical recti. The 6-week interval is recommended to reduce the likelihood of anterior segment necrosis.[19–23]

Duane's Syndrome. Also known as the retraction syndrome, Duane's syndrome should seldom be treated surgically unless a severe cosmetic problem exists, in which case recession of the medial rectus is done. Only modest, if any, resections of the lateral rectus muscle should be done, as the retraction can be severely worsened with resection of the lateral rectus. The frequent upshoot and downshoot in adduction of such an eye mimics severe overaction of both the inferior and superior oblique muscles. This overshoot in adduction can be minimized with a posterior fixation suture in the lateral rectus 16 mm posterior to its insertion.[24–26] The paralysis of the lateral rectus in Duane's syndrome can be treated by lateral transpositions of the vertical recti.

Third Cranial Nerve Palsies. These are treated by 14- to 16-mm recession of the lateral rectus and either transposition of the superior oblique muscle (after removal of the tendon from the trochlea) to the medial rectus or transposition of the superior oblique tendon to the medial border of the superior rectus. After the desired horizontal eye position has been achieved, a frontalis suspension procedure for the ptosis is done.[27]

Fourth Cranial Nerve Palsies. These may be approached by (a) weakening the antagonist of the superior oblique muscle—the inferior oblique; (b) strengthening the weak superior oblique with a tuck of the tendon of the involved superior oblique; or (c) weakening the yoke muscle of the superior oblique—the inferior rectus muscle of the other eye. Authors have proposed various criteria as to which procedure should be done first, and Table 17–1 details some of these alternatives. I prefer the simple approach of first weakening the inferior oblique; second, tucking the superior oblique; and, finally, weakening the yoke muscle. Each procedure should usually be done separately.[28]

Double Elevator Palsies

Double elevator palsy is treated with vertical transposition of the horizontal rectus muscles, unless there is marked resistance to elevation in the forced duction test. If resistance is prominent, a 6-mm recession of the inferior rectus is advised.[29]

Dissociated Vertical Divergence (Alternating Sursumduction)

Dissociated vertical divergence (or alternating sursumduction) responds best to an 8-mm recession of the superior rectus of the eye with the larger deviation, and a 5-mm recession of the superior rectus of the other eye even though the sursumduction may be predominantly uniocular.[30]

Superior Oblique Tendon Sheath Syndrome

This condition should not be treated surgically unless the cosmetic problem is severe, in which case tenotomy of the superior oblique is done, with a warning to the patient that overcorrection may necessitate a later weakening procedure of the inferior oblique.[31, 32]

Surgical Techniques for the Medial Rectus Muscle

Recession of the Medial Rectus[33]

Primary Surgery. Primary surgery is frequently bilateral or is combined with a resection of the lateral rectus muscle. Medial rectus recession is the most common extraocular muscle procedure.

The globe must be abducted to provide good exposure for isolation of the medial rectus. Until a muscle hook fully engages the muscle, the globe must be held in the abducted position with a traction suture or forceps. A 7–0 silk lateral traction suture can be easily passed to half the depth of clear cornea at the lateral limbus. The admonitions above regarding position of the globe should be considered in the application of the traction suture. The corneal traction suture is passed through a rubber band and tied, and a small clamp is applied. The weight of the clamp is sufficient to keep the eye in the abducted position. A piece of moist Gelfoam about the size of a dime is laid on the cornea. The Gelfoam will keep the cornea hydrated and protect it from abrasions.

CONJUNCTIVAL INCISION. The limbal incision (Fig. 17–10) is most often used.[34–36] Inspection of the area will typically reveal the outline of the medial rectus through the conjunctiva. The older the patient, the thinner the conjunctiva and the easier the muscle is to be seen. The conjunctiva can be moved about with smooth forceps, and the anterior ciliary vessels of the muscle can often be noted as not moving with the conjunctiva. Two radial incisions are made through the conjunctiva and Tenon's capsule, well away from the muscle. The incisions should form an angle of about 90 degrees if imaginary lines were extended to the cornea's center. Bare sclera should be revealed. The two incisions

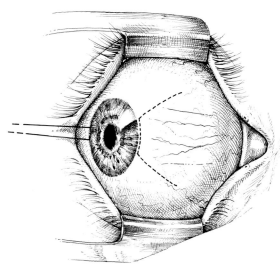

FIGURE 17–10. The conjunctival incision for a medial rectus recession should extend along the dotted line.

can be joined by a peritomy as close to the cornea as possible. One tip of the scissors will easily slide beneath the conjunctiva as the incision is made. No undermining of tissue is necessary, and indeed such undermining should be avoided. Blind undermining of tissue commonly causes serious bleeding and may even result in perforations of the eye.

Blunt-tipped cross-action scissors should be used for the conjunctival incision and for the further exposure of sclera. Smooth forceps are used to grasp conjunctiva and Tenon's capsule

at the apex of the incision, furthest from the cornea as the sclera is exposed (Fig. 17–11).

Isolation of the Medial Rectus. Scissors are used to spread Tenon's capsule away from the sclera under direct inspection. If the scissors are held perpendicular to the globe, the opening of the scissors elevates Tenon's capsule away from the globe, as shown in Figure 17–12A, allowing a clear view of the field; lateral spreading (Fig. 17–12B), on the other hand, obscures the field.

Any significant resistance indicates that the scissors are entering the muscle or sclera. Stop. Go to the other incisional apex, which should be located well away from the muscle. If the two radial incisions are made 90 degrees apart, both of them should be well away from the medial rectus muscle. If, by torsion or misjudgment in making the incision, the insertion is encountered, the 90-degree separation of the two radial incisions should ensure that the other incision is well away from the muscle. Inadvertent dissection into the insertion is the most common cause of bleeding in this procedure. If the correct plane is entered, bare sclera should be seen continuously from the limbus to a point about 14 mm posterior to the limbus. Because the medial rectus muscle inserts approximately 5.5 mm posterior to the limbus, a von Graefe muscle hook (Fig. 17–13) can be placed under the muscle while the hook is directly observed. The hook is brought forward until the insertion is engaged. One should not attempt to include the entire muscle on the first pass, as the muscle

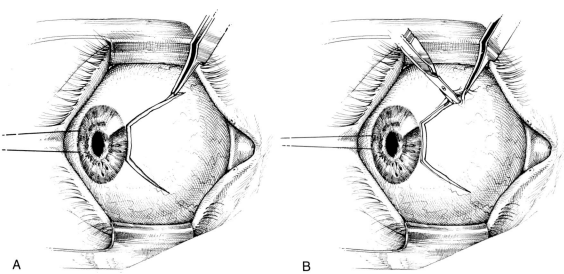

A   B

FIGURE 17–11. *A,* The conjunctiva and Tenon's capsule are elevated slightly at the apex of the incision. *B,* While the tissues are elevated, the sclera is bared, well away from the muscle.

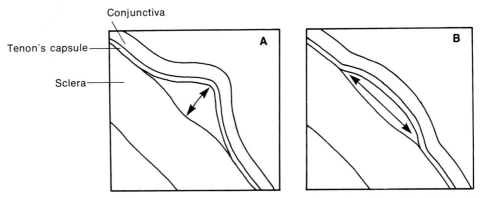

FIGURE 17–12. Vertical spreading (*A*) is appropriate as indicated, whereas lateral spreading (*B*) hides the tissues from the surgeon's view. Lateral spreading, if repeated, may damage the globe.

sheath will usually be pushed forward with such a broad sweep. Rather, a second hook should now be passed from the same side just posteriorly to the small first hook, which has engaged the insertion. The second hook will usually pass

under the muscle and can be identified on the other side of the insertion. The second hook will probably be covered with a filmy white tissue. This is muscle sheath and should not be buttonholed. Another hook is now passed under

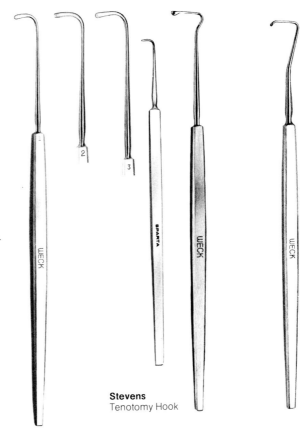

FIGURE 17–13. The principal muscle hooks currently used.

Graefe
Muscle Hook

Stevens
Tenotomy Hook

Jameson
Muscle Hook

Green
Muscle Hook

the muscle and toward the edge of the muscle that was first approached. The two hooks are passed back and forth until one comes out cleanly without tissue on its tip. A Jameson muscle hook is finally passed. The Jameson hook has a small enlargement on its tip that keeps the muscle in place on the hook during the remaining dissection (see Fig. 17–13).

The next step involves dissection of conjunctiva from the muscle sheath. While the surgeon holds the muscle hook in place, the assistant picks up the edges of the conjunctiva from the peritomy incision. The clamp on the traction suture is released, since the globe is securely fixated with the muscle hook. Sharp dissection with blunt-tipped cross-action scissors is used to free the conjunctiva and Tenon's capsule from the muscle sheath. The proper plane is devoid of blood vessels. As the dissection is carried medially, the fibers of the medial rectus can be seen through the filmy muscle sheath. The dissection should continue close to the muscle sheath, with constant care taken to avoid buttonholing either the conjunctiva or the muscle sheath. Blood vessels are visible and should be avoided. If a blood vessel must be severed, it should be cauterized before being cut. If a blood vessel is inadvertently severed and bleeding ensues, that bleeding point should be identified and cauterized before proceeding. When the conjunctiva has been freed about 5 mm past the insertion, the traction of the smooth forceps on the conjunctival edge is no longer adequate for exposure, and two von Graefe muscle hooks are used as retractors for the remaining dissection. One muscle hook is passed on bare sclera above the superior edge of the muscle, and the second is passed over the middle of the muscle. Slight medial traction with the muscle hooks allows the intermuscular septum to be seen and severed. The same maneuver is done below the inferior edge of the muscle. Sharp dissection is

now carried medially and posteriorly. Frequent repositioning of the muscle hooks is necessary. The end point is reached when a white condensation of Tenon's capsule appears. Check ligaments have been severed by the time this point is reached. If the white condensation is entered, orbital fat will be encountered. Disturbed orbital fat tends to allow dense adhesions to form; hence it is generally not advisable to continue the dissection. If further dissection is necessary, proceed by incising the muscle sheath where it is joined by Tenon's capsule. The muscle sheath will keep the orbital fat out of the surgical field, and a better result will occur than if the fat pocket is entered. Point A in Figure 17–14 represents the white condensation referred to above.

If the surgeon inadvertently causes fat to prolapse into the surgical field, a judgment must be made as to whether to excise this fat or to hope that it will not cause excessive scarring. In general, excision of the prolapsed fat should be done. Care must be taken to clamp the fat, cut on the distal side of the clamp, and cauterize the cut end before releasing the clamp. The danger is considerable that a massive retrobulbar hemorrhage may result from a severed blood vessel embedded in the fat. Appropriate care in hemostasis usually can avoid this sight-threatening possibility.

Adhesions or accessory muscle slips may be present between the globe and the muscle posterior to the insertion. To explore this possibility, a second Jameson muscle hook is placed behind the one being used for traction. The second hook is gently pushed posteriorly approximately 12 to 14 mm. If any resistance is encountered, the area should be explored after the muscle is disinserted.

DISINSERTION OF THE MEDIAL RECTUS. After isolation the medial rectus muscle is ready to be disinserted as soon as it is securely fixated.

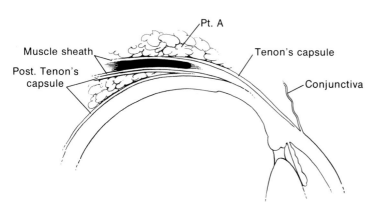

FIGURE 17–14. Tenon's capsule and the muscle sheath relations.

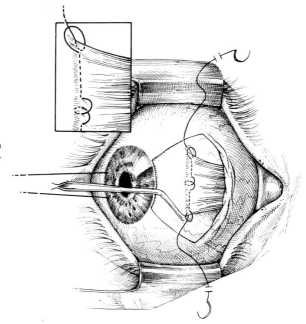

FIGURE 17–15. A double-armed suture is locked in the tendon of the medial rectus muscle before disinsertion.

Either sutures, which are locked in the tendinous portion of the muscle close to the insertion (Fig. 17–15), or a Berens clamp (Fig. 17–16) can be used. If locked sutures are used, a double-armed 6–0 synthetic absorbable suture is recommended. The suture should be stitch-locked in the middle and at each border of the muscle. After the sutures are locked the muscle can be disinserted with blunt-tipped cross-action scissors.

During disinsertion the hook should stay in place with some forward tension to raise the

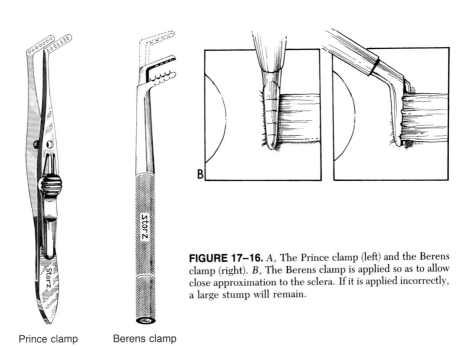

Prince clamp   Berens clamp

A

FIGURE 17–16. *A*, The Prince clamp (left) and the Berens clamp (right). *B*, The Berens clamp is applied so as to allow close approximation to the sclera. If it is applied incorrectly, a large stump will remain.

tendon from the globe. Care must be taken not to cut the sutures. If considerable manipulation has been required to prepare the muscle for disinsertion, the globe may be excessively soft; thus the sclera may tent up easily, and the sclera could be easily buttonholed.

The ever-present potential complication of a lost muscle should be considered at every stage of muscle surgery. Because the disinsertion of the tendon sets the stage for a lost muscle, appropriate instruments should be at hand to manage each contingency. If the sutures should be cut or the muscle start to slip from a clamp, the muscle should be immediately grasped with any convenient forceps and a clamp applied. The Prince muscle clamp is particularly handy for such a problem. The Prince clamp (Fig. 17–16A) can be snapped on the muscle and the sutures reapplied without any undue difficulty. What to do in the case of loss of a muscle is discussed later as other complications are considered.

REINSERTION OF THE MEDIAL RECTUS. Appropriate placement of the sutures in the tendon at the borders and middle often prevents further bleeding from the tendon after disinsertion. If further bleeding occurs from vessels about the sutures, cautery can be applied to the vessel well behind the suture. The cautery can easily sever the suture if an attempt is made to apply the heat to the bleeding point. Smooth forceps can be used to grasp various areas of the muscle or tendon behind the suture to find the appropriate site for cautery.

About 5 mm posterior to the insertion two small blood vessels will be found on the sclera. These should be lightly cauterized, as they frequently start bleeding later, when the muscle has been reattached, and are thus hard to cauterize.

These two vessels normally supply the muscle and are severed as the muscle is disinserted (Fig. 17–17). They are not present at reoperation, since they were severed at the initial surgery. No other ocular muscle has similar vessels.

The stump of the insertion usually bleeds, and appropriate light cautery can be used. If the stump is large or if extra tissue remains around the stump, the area should be trimmed down to bare sclera. Excessive tissue will cause a red area in the conjunctiva that may last for years.

The amount of recession should have been determined before the surgery. That amount set on the calipers allows an indentation mark to be made on the sclera. Firm pressure gives a mark that persists for several minutes. The two vessels mentioned above provide a 5-mm landmark to verify the accuracy of the calipers' scleral mark (Fig. 17–18).

A variety of needle placements can be used to reinsert the muscle to the globe. The spatula needle should be placed to a depth of about 0.1 mm. The outline of the needle should be seen as it is in the sclera. It is not necessary to bring the suture through the insertion stump. The simplest technique that results in the least amount of suture material buried consists of placing the scleral bite parallel to the limbus. If the muscle is noted to sag excessively, a bite can be taken through the center of the muscle (Fig. 17–19).

The Berens clamp figure-of-eight technique

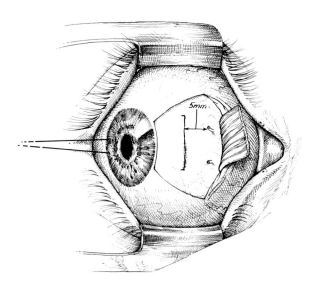

FIGURE 17–17. Two small blood vessels are usually present under the medial rectus muscle, which are severed as the muscle is disinserted.

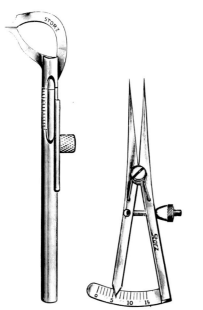

FIGURE 17–18. Two commonly used calipers. Markings indicate millimeters.

(Figs. 17–20 and 17–39) uses a single-armed, nonabsorbable suture. The advantage of the figure-of-eight is that it is a technique specifically designed for nonabsorbable suture material. The knot is tied in such a way that it can be tucked under the muscle.

The advantage of the nonabsorbable suture is the avoidance of tissue resection and unpredictable absorption. Catgut sutures should be avoided, as they produce a high incidence of tissue reactions, which may continue for as long as 18 months after surgery. The synthetic absorbable sutures also have disadvantages, as they drag tissue excessively, have allowed muscles to slip days to weeks after surgery, and produce some tissue reaction.[37]

The Berens clamp is applied to the muscle and tightened securely, and the muscle is disinserted.

After the muscle is disinserted the cut end of the muscle in the jaws of the clamp, the stump of the muscle, and the two scleral arteries 5 mm posterior to the stump of the medial rectus insertion are cauterized.

A nonabsorbable 6-0 braided Dacron suture, silicone-coated (Tycron), with a spatula needle, is used. The measurement from insertion stump to new insertion is done with calipers, and the first scleral bite is taken away from the middle of the planned insertion (see Fig. 17–20). (See also Fig. 17–30 for detailed views of the figure-of-eight suture.) The needle is passed through the aperture in the clamp, thus imbricating muscle. Care should be taken to pass the needle along the floor of the clamp to assure an adequate bite of muscle. The needle is then passed back through the adjacent opening of the clamp toward the cut end of the muscle. As this bite is taken, the needle again should be aimed along the floor of the clamp, to ensure that an adequate bite of muscle tissue is taken. The next scleral bite is taken—once again parallel to the limbus and from the middle of the desired insertion toward the site where the border of the muscle is to be. Before the Berens clamp is loosened the needle should be passed under the suture, as shown in Figure 17–20. This passage will allow the knot to be tucked under the muscle. Failure to tuck the knot and ends of suture under the muscle will result in a suture that is forever visible through the conjunctiva. Furthermore, the ends of the suture may protrude, producing discomfort and a possible route for infection. Because a suture such as braided Dacron is truly permanent, great care must be taken to be sure the knot and suture ends are precisely where you want them to be.

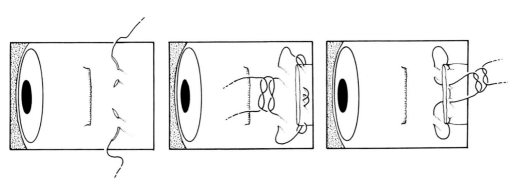

FIGURE 17–19. Suture placement for recession. If the muscle sags, the middle of the muscle should be incorporated, as shown in the sketch at the right.

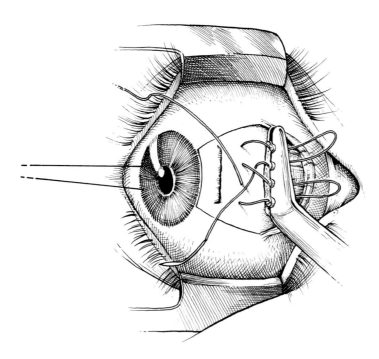

FIGURE 17–20. Suture placement in the figure-of-eight technique.

The Berens clamp can now be removed. The suture is tightened by a two-stage maneuver after an overhand loop has been tied. The suture's ends are pulled toward you, and then the knot is tightened. This procedure should be gentle, but may be repeated until the muscle is secure. During the tightening of the suture care should be taken to avoid tissue drag. If tissue is seen to drag, the assistant should use a hand-over-hand technique with two pairs of smooth-tipped forceps to free the adherent tissue. When the suture is satisfactorily tightened, the assistant grasps the overhand throw with smooth forceps and the knot is tied. If you want to avoid having the sutures held by the assistant, a surgeon's knot with the extra initial overhand throw will usually prevent slippage. After the knot has been tied two more overhand throws are placed to ensure a knot that will not untie.

A word of caution should be mentioned against excessive tightening of the sutures. Not only is there a danger of breaking the suture, but annoying astigmatism will be created that will take up to 6 weeks to abate. When correctly placed the muscle will lie flat on the globe and there will be no buckling of sclera.[38]

After the knot is tied the suture ends are cut about 2 to 3 mm from the knot. The long ends will lay flat as the knot is tucked under the muscle. Short suture ends will tend to stick straight up and erode through the conjunctiva.

At this point you may want to spread the muscle end so that it is flat and evenly distributed over the new insertion.

CLOSURE OF CONJUNCTIVA. Closure of the conjunctiva should be meticulous. Smooth forceps are used to position the conjunctiva in its desired place. If there is doubt as to whether the tissue is conjunctiva or Tenon's capsule, the area should be briefly irrigated with saline solution, which will turn Tenon's capsule white but has no effect on conjunctiva.

Conjunctiva should be closed with 7-0 black interrupted silk. If catgut or other suture material is used, frequent dellen and uncomfortable eyes will result. Do not use 8-0 silk for this procedure, for the sutures will not fall out. Tie the 7-0 silk tightly with only a single square knot and cut the ends close to the knot. The suture will fall out in 5 to 7 days.

Four to six interrupted sutures placed as drawn in Figure 17–21 are usually needed to assure a good closure of a limbal conjunctival incision.

RECESSION OF THE CONJUNCTIVA. If the conjunctiva is tight, or if a large esotropia is present or the lateral rectus is weak, the effect of a medial rectus recession can be enhanced with a recession of the conjunctiva. All that is needed is to secure the conjunctiva to sclera or episclera with the interrupted silk sutures. To maintain the recessed conjunctiva in the correct position, the central free edge of conjunctiva should

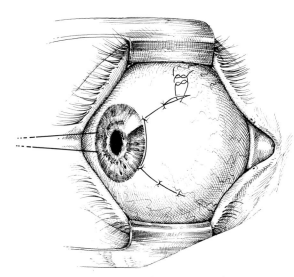

FIGURE 17–21. Conjunctival suture placement.

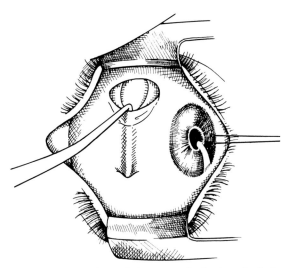

FIGURE 17–23. The medial rectus tendon has been hooked from below.

be secured to the sclera as shown in Figure 17–22.

Recession of the conjunctiva leaves an area of bare sclera. Fortunately this bare sclera is comfortable, heals well, and results in a white eye. The surgeon must be careful to leave a perfectly bare sclera. If loose tissue is left to heal, a red eye will result.

Excessive recessions of conjunctiva should be avoided, as the conjunctiva will fold on itself and produce a poor cosmetic result. Typically a recession of about 4 mm will not cause such a complication, yet will be adequate to enhance the muscle recession. The conjunctival reces-

sion, although elective in primary muscle surgery, becomes almost mandatory in reoperations, which will be discussed later.[39]

THE CONJUNCTIVAL FORNIX INCISION. The desire to have the incision hidden under the lids led Parks to devise this incision (Figs. 17–23 through Fig. 17–30).[40] Because the conjunctival fornix incision will be hidden in the inferior cul-de-sac, the incision must be pulled up to the muscle insertion. The assistant rotates the eye superiorly to allow the surgeon to make the incision. The incision is made between the insertion of the medial and inferior rectus muscles through conjunctiva and Tenon's capsule down to bare sclera. The incision should be

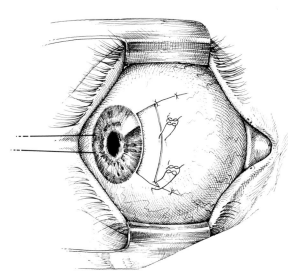

FIGURE 17–22. Recession of conjunctiva.

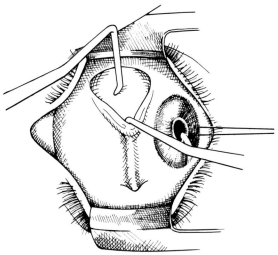

FIGURE 17–24. The second muscle hook is positioned for placement to ensure that the complete tendon has been hooked.

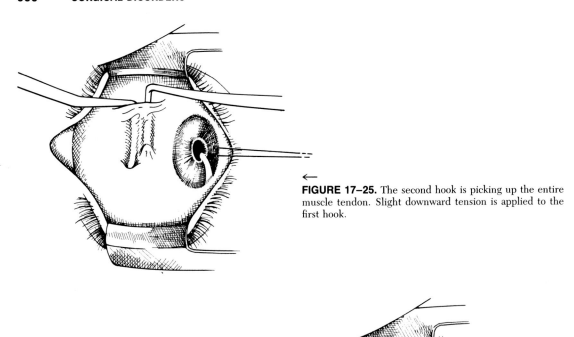

←

FIGURE 17–25. The second hook is picking up the entire muscle tendon. Slight downward tension is applied to the first hook.

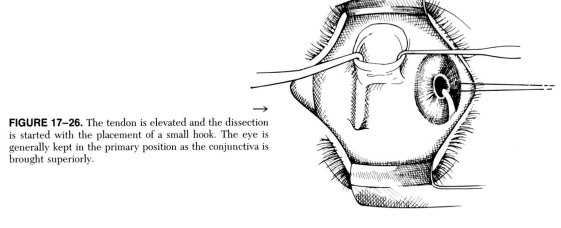

FIGURE 17–26. The tendon is elevated and the dissection is started with the placement of a small hook. The eye is generally kept in the primary position as the conjunctiva is brought superiorly.

→

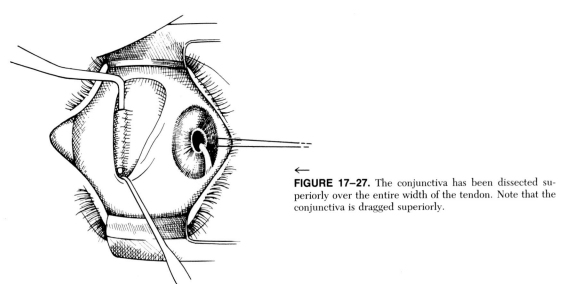

←

FIGURE 17–27. The conjunctiva has been dissected superiorly over the entire width of the tendon. Note that the conjunctiva is dragged superiorly.

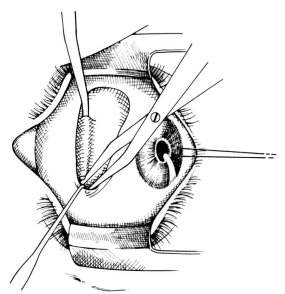

FIGURE 17–28. Scissors are used to undermine Tenon's and conjunctiva in the superior nasal quadrant, staying well away from the tendon and insertion.

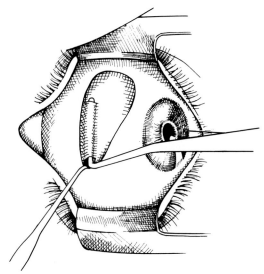

FIGURE 17–30. The tendon is now isolated, the muscle can be isolated and the appropriate procedure performed on the muscle.

approximately parallel to the lower border of the medial rectus muscle and should be no more than 10 mm behind the limbus to avoid entering the fat pockets. (If the fat pockets are entered and the fat disturbed, bleeding and severe scarring often result. This scarring may be so severe that uncorrectable restrictions may occur.)

To isolate the muscle, the eye is maintained

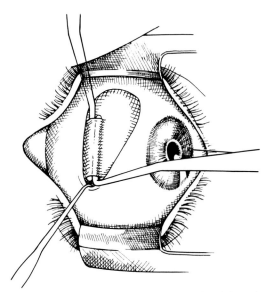

FIGURE 17–29. Another muscle hook is placed from the superior edge of the tendon. The hook should pass easily and not pick up any tissue as it comes out inferiorly.

in the primary position as muscle hooks are passed under the muscle until the entire muscle is engaged. First, a small muscle or tendon hook is used to lift the conjunctiva and Tenon's capsule to allow direct identification of the lower edge of the insertion. The Green muscle hook is used to pass along the sclera under the insertion of the medial rectus. With that in place a second muscle hook is passed to ensure that the complete tendon has been engaged. With the medial rectus muscle tendon firmly engaged the eye is pulled down as the conjunctiva is pulled up while gentle and careful dissection exposes the entire insertion. Care must be taken to ensure that the entire tendon is isolated and not split. After the insertion is dissected free the muscle can be further isolated in the conventional manner and the recession or resection carried out in the favorite manner of the surgeon.

Secondary Surgery. Secondary recessions of the medial rectus are similar in most details to the primary operation described above. The complexity of this procedure is inversely related to the care with which the primary procedure was executed.

The conjunctival incision should be limbal in most circumstances. This approach allows the easiest dissection. If the conjunctiva is firmly adherent to the globe, it may be necessary to use a scleral knife to carefully dissect the conjunctiva from the conjunctiva. As you proceed posteriorly with the sharp dissection, have the assistant retract the conjunctiva with smooth forceps, holding the conjunctiva perpendicular to the sclera. At about 5 to 6 mm the original muscle insertion may be seen. Keep your dissection just subconjunctival. You often will see what appears to be muscle or tendon growing from the old insertion posteriorly. Do not dissect this tissue now, but proceed with the conjunctival dissection.

As the dissection proceeds the plane will dive posteriorly. Follow the curvature of the globe to a reasonable extent. The muscle fibers will soon be visible, as well as the sclera. This is a slow and tedious procedure, and constant attention to hemostasis is necessary. After 4 to 5 mm of conjunctiva is dissected free from the sclera, the dissection into the quadrants well away from where the medial rectus is anticipated to be can usually be done with relative ease. One should be sure that bare sclera is identified in the quadrants.

At this point a muscle hook can frequently engage the recessed muscle. If successful, passage of hooks back and forth may allow a clean tip to emerge. If the muscle hook cannot be easily passed, temporarily abandon that effort and return to dissection of superior and inferior edges of the muscle. Muscle hooks or Ragnel retractors may be necessary to give an adequate view. Do not enter the medial fat pocket, but continue along the surface of the muscle.

Because you have already bared the sclera superiorly and inferiorly you can now pass a muscle hook under direct visualization about 12 to 14 mm posterior to the limbus.

If the prior surgery has left the muscle sheath intact, the passage of the muscle hook is quite easy. If the muscle sheath was interrupted, it

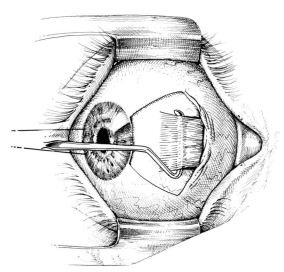

FIGURE 17–32. Muscle hook at last surgical insertion. Pseudotendon extends forward to original insertion.

is necessary to be behind the equator for placement of the hook (Fig. 17–31).

This point posterior to the equator, where a muscle hook can be passed, is about 12 mm posterior to the original insertion or about 17 mm posterior to the limbus. After the muscle hook is in place it will dissect its way forward to a point close to the last surgical insertion (Fig. 17–32).

Because the muscle has now been isolated, you are now ready to either place the Berens clamp (or imbricating sutures) to recess the muscle further or, more commonly, to dissect the pseudotendon from the sclera, beginning at the original insertion.

A scleral knife is the best tool to isolate the pseudotendon from the original insertion to the insertion created by the last surgery (Fig. 17–33).

Place the Berens clamp or imbricating sutures in the pseudotendon before completing the dissections from the globe (Fig. 17–34). Proceed to disinsert the muscle from the globe. Free all adhesions to the extent that a muscle hook will easily pass posteriorly without meeting resistance and without causing the globe or medial rectus muscle to move. Next check the retractability of the medial rectus muscle. It should easily retract as its tension is relieved.

Reinsert the muscle on the sclera the desired amount, using either the figure-of-eight nonabsorbable technique or the imbricating sutures.

Close the conjunctiva with at least a 4-mm recession of the conjunctiva. Be sure to dissect

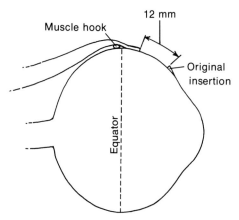

FIGURE 17–31. The expected point of adherence if muscle sheath has been stripped in prior surgery.

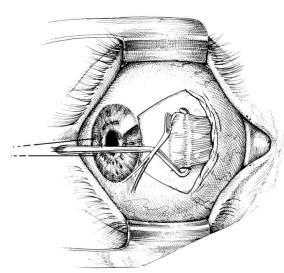

FIGURE 17–33. Dissection of pseudotendon.

all loose tissue from the scleral area to be left bare and control all bleeding before closure. Tack the conjunctiva to sclera with interrupted 7-0 silk. Because the sutures are further from the limbus here than with a primary case, you can safely use absorbable sutures, but they will not be as comfortable as the 7-0 silk.

Do not use interrupted 8-0 silk sutures to close the conjunctiva because they do not fall out spontaneously as do the 7-0 silk.

DIFFICULT DISSECTIONS. The dissections just discussed hold for about 8 out of 10 re-recessions of the medial recti. The other 20 per

cent are the most difficult. The key to such difficult dissections is careful hemostasis with constant attention to finding the muscular-appearing tissue. Keep the curvature of the globe in mind. The muscle is only 1.5 to 2 mm thick and will be on the sclera. If you proceed more medially, you will enter the fat pocket and cause further problems. When in doubt in respect to the dissection move well away from the muscle, first superiorly and then inferiorly, until bare sclera is seen with gradual delineation of the muscle. There are no other landmarks such as the oblique muscles to assist you in the localization of the medial rectus. The earlier admonitions regarding careful positioning of the globe are most important with regard to allowing proper orientation throughout these difficult procedures. Narrow malleable retractors of 6 to 16 mm are valuable to push the loose tissue out of the way and allow definite visualization of the muscle. Above all else, do not rush the procedure.

ADJUSTABLE SUTURES FOR RECESSIONS. The cooperative older child or adult can tolerate the postoperative adjustment of the muscles' position quite easily if the following steps are taken. A variety of techniques allow the muscle to be adjusted under topical anesthesia either at the time of surgery, a few hours or 1 day after the surgery has taken place. With the advent of same-day surgery it is typically most convenient to adjust the sutures 2 to 3 hours after the surgery, when the local anesthesia or general anesthesia has worn off. The following list of materials and medications are useful.

A. Medications
   1. Topical anesthesia, such as tetracaine or proparacaine (a sterile fresh bottle)
   2. Atropine 0.4 mg for IV use
   3. Topical antibiotic drops of your choice
B. Materials
   1. Sterile cotton-tip applicators
   2. Sterile towel
   3. Sterile 7-0 silk suture with needle
C. Surgical instruments
   1. Self-retaining lid speculum
   2. Tying forceps
   3. Forceps with teeth
   4. Cross-action scissors
   5. Needle holder
   6. Headlight with loupes for illumination and magnification at the bedside

At the time of surgery the resections are typically carried out in the usual manner, although an adjustable suture can be used to

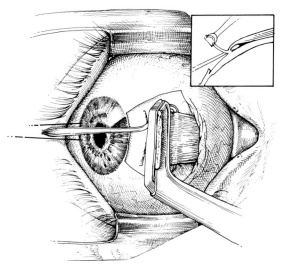

FIGURE 17–34. Berens clamp on pseudotendon; muscle hook at last surgical insertion.

place the resection at the desired point, yet adjust them with a recession if needed. The same general technique as that described here for recessions is used to place the adjustable suture for resections.

A limbal approach is used with the fornix-based flap turned in the manner described above for medial rectus recession. The medial rectus is imbricated on the arms of a 6-0 braided Dacron suture coated with silicone or a 6-0 Dexon noncoated suture, locking it in the middle, upper, and lower borders of the muscle. The muscle is disinserted and the sutures are passed through the insertion. A bow knot is tied with the appropriate recessed amount (see Fig. 17–35A). It is advisable to recess the muscle slightly more than the usual surgical amount because advancing the muscle at the time of adjustment is somewhat easier than further recessing it. The suture is tied in the

bow knot manner, and the ends of the suture, which are cut to about 3 inches, are coiled in the conjunctival cul-de-sac. A 6-0 braided Dacron suture is placed in the bare sclera and tied in a loose loop so that it can be grasped for fixation in the event the muscle will not easily slip; the patient has to look strongly in the direction of the medial rectus while the eye is held laterally to cause the muscle to slip back further. The traction suture is also useful in patients who have difficulty fixating at the desired point. The upper portion of the conjunctiva is closed with interrupted 7-0 silk sutures, and a single eye pad is applied (see Fig. 17–35B).

After the patient awakens or the local anesthesia wears off, topical anesthesia is instilled in the conjunctival cul-de-sac for about 10 applications at about 15- to 20-second intervals. This will give complete anesthesia of the area,

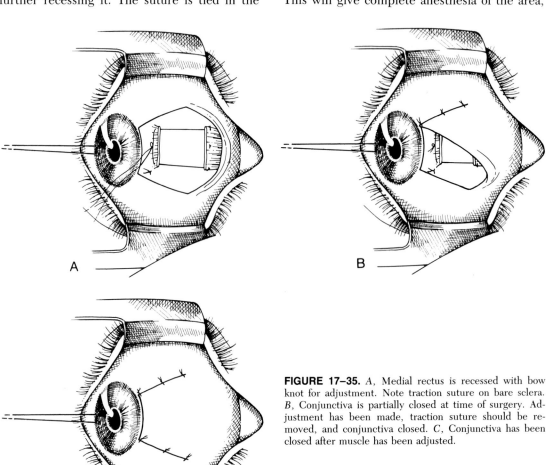

FIGURE 17–35. *A,* Medial rectus is recessed with bow knot for adjustment. Note traction suture on bare sclera. *B,* Conjunctiva is partially closed at time of surgery. Adjustment has been made, traction suture should be removed, and conjunctiva closed. *C,* Conjunctiva has been closed after muscle has been adjusted.

and the patient can have the adjustment done without discomfort. The patient is screened for near and distance for the desired position of the eye. If the patient is exo, the medial rectus should be advanced. If the patient is eso, the medial rectus should be recessed. The bow knot is untied, and either the suture is pulled up, or the knot is loosened and the muscle allowed to recede. When the desired position is attained the suture arm, coming from the single bow knot, is cut close to the knot and the suture simply pulled through and tightened so that no slippage of the knot will occur. One or two extra single throws are placed in the knot to ensure a nonslipping knot. The arms of the suture should be cut so that they are approximately 1.5 to 2.0 mm long and tucked under the suture so that they lie flat against the globe. Otherwise, the suture ends have a tendency to errode through the conjunctiva and produce discomfort. The braided Dacron offers the advantage of being a nonabsorbable suture so that late slippage will not occur. Several patients have had the muscles slip from their intended position days to weeks after the surgery at a time coincident with absorption of the sutures. This slippage is particularly prone to occur if any steroids are administered to the patient postoperatively. The traction suture is removed and the conjunctival closure completed with interrupted 7-0 silk sutures (see Fig. 17–35C). Antibiotic drops are placed. The lid speculum is removed, and the patient discharged.[41]

Before the adjustment administer an appropriate dose of atropine intravenously to avoid the vasovagal response during the adjustment. The patient should be warned that this will make his mouth slightly dry, but will make him more comfortable during the adjustment. The adjustment is most conveniently carried out with the patient in bed to avoid the instability of the patient and occasional syncope of the patient sitting in an examining chair.

With the use of short-acting narcotics (such as fentanyl citrate) and sedatives (such as medazolon hydrochloride), topical anesthesia can be used for recessions and the muscles adjusted at the time of surgery.

Resection of the Medial Rectus

Primary Surgery. Primary resection of the medial rectus is usually done only (a) after the lateral rectus has been recessed, or (b) if the patient has convergence insufficiency and shows orthophoria during distance fixation. As a rule, do not try to correct an exotropia with isolated resection of a medial rectus muscle.

The technique is similar to that described for recession of the medial rectus, with the obvious exception that the muscle clamp is placed at the desired position to allow a portion of the tendon and muscle to be removed. The limbal conjunctival approach is usually recommended. The muscle is isolated in the manner described for recession. A Berens clamp is applied to the muscle, just ahead of the measured resection (Fig. 17–36).

If a Prince clamp is applied before placement of catgut sutures, the same points for measurement are used as with the Beren's clamp. After the clamp has been securely applied the muscle is disinserted reasonably flush with the sclera. If the two-suture technique is used, a slightly larger stump should be left. If the figure-of-

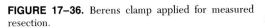

FIGURE 17–36. Berens clamp applied for measured resection.

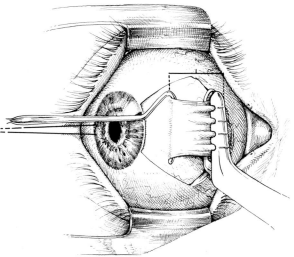

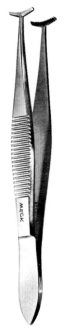

FIGURE 17–37. Green forceps—fixation forceps that are also convenient for grasping the free muscle to be resected.

eight technique is used, the stump should be as small as possible. The piece of muscle to be removed is grasped with the Green forceps and excised (Fig. 17–37).

The two-suture technique is preferred by many surgeons if absorbable sutures are to be used. Two double-armed sutures of 5-0 or 6-0 absorbable sutures with spatula needles are passed through the muscle, immediately behind the clamp. One should leave the clamp on the muscle until both double-armed sutures are ready for tying. The needles are passed through the stump of the muscle, emerging from the sclera about 5 mm behind the limbus. The clamp is removed and the sutures tied as shown in Figure 17–38.

If nonabsorbable sutures are to be used, the figure-of-eight suture with the Berens clamp is recommended. The figure-of-eight suturing technique for resections is identical to that used for recessions. Only the placement of the scleral sutures varies. In the resection the needle is

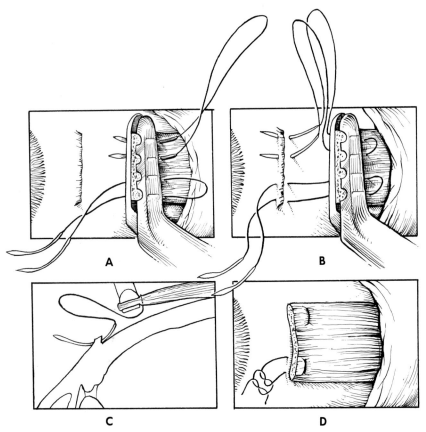

FIGURE 17–38. The two-suture technique for resection. *A,* Two double-armed sutures are passed just posteriorly to clamp. *B,* Scleral bites are taken under the insertion stump. *C,* Side view of scleral bites. *D,* Second suture is tied.

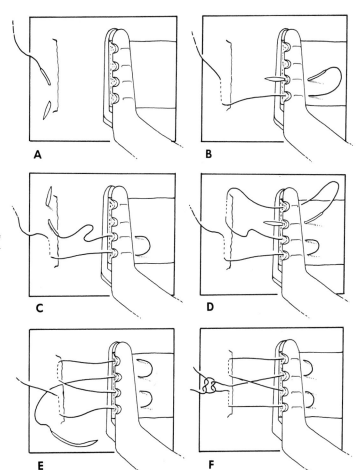

FIGURE 17–39. The figure-of-eight suture technique used for either resection or recession. (Resection is shown here.)

passed just anterior to the stump, parallel with the limbus, as shown in Figure 17–39.

The scleral bite should be sufficiently anterior to be in the sclera—not in the cut end of the tendon. A suture placed perpendicular to the fibers of the tendon has a tendency to split the fibers of the tendon and pull out. Remember to start the figure-of-eight suture with a bite away from the middle of the proposed insertion, just as recommended for the recession. The single knot and the loose ends must be carefully tucked under the end of the muscle, for the insertion is sufficiently anterior that a suture, if visible through conjunctiva, will result in a poor cosmetic appearance.

The conjunctiva is closed in the usual manner. Recessions of the conjunctiva are seldom done with primary resections. If additional effect from the resection is sought, the conjunctiva can be resected. No data are available as to the absolute effects of such a resection. If it is done, care should be exercised to be sure

that no restriction of eye motion is created by excessive resection of the conjunctiva, unless such restriction is desired. The resection is accomplished by simply excising that amount of conjunctiva deemed excessive and closing the conjunctiva in the usual manner, as indicated in Figure 17–40.

Secondary Surgery. The details of identification and localization of a medial rectus in a secondary resection procedure differ little from those discussed in the section on secondary surgery for recession of the medial rectus. Usually a prior resection results in less scar tissue, and therefore the muscle can be isolated more easily than the muscle involved in a prior recession.

The same careful hemostasis and dissection should be done in all reoperations. In addition, the insertion will be found to be relatively large if the prior resection procedure has been done within 2 years. Often absorbable sutures will still be present after a 1½- to 2-year interval.

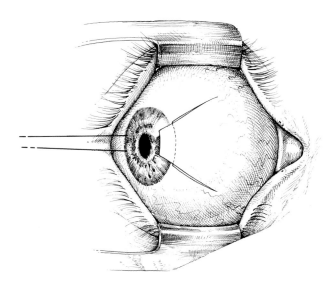

FIGURE 17–40. Resection of conjunctiva.

The exuberant tissue should be excised and the new insertion applied to a bare sclera. If the prior suture material was nonabsorbable, all remnants of it should be removed as well.

If the medial rectus has been recessed, the identification difficulties are those already described. The medial rectus in such an instance should not be further resected, but advanced an amount equal to the desired resection. In general, a muscle should not be advanced closer than 5.5 mm from the limbus. The chances of developing a red eye or even a slight conjunctival bump so close to the limbus are significant. Because there is no mechanical advantage to an excessive advancement, the recommendations about the usual anterior limit should be followed. If the muscle is found 8 mm from the limbus, only a 2.5-mm advancement should be done; a 6-mm resection would be accomplished with the 2.5-mm advancement combined with a 3.5-mm resection. The surgeon should further realize that each disinsertion and reinsertion will usually necessitate a 2.5-mm resection. If excessive scarring is present, the amount of unavoidable resection may be somewhat larger. Although the above affect the calculation, resections generally have much less effect than recessions in changing the alignment of the eyes. Any such considerations have much more importance in recessions.

After reattachment of the muscle be sure to test the mobility of the eye before closing the conjunctiva. If the eye will not rotate the desired amount at the time of anesthesia, definitive restrictions will certainly exist postoperatively. If the resection or advancement has created restrictions, the muscle should be dis-

inserted and an appropriate recession performed. After the motility has been assured without any conjunctival closure, the conjunctiva should be closed and the globe tested again for its motility. You may want some restrictions for unusual cases, but any restriction so created tends to remain after surgery.

Vertical Transposition of the Medial Rectus

In surgery designed to correct V pattern esotropias the medial rectus muscles may be displaced inferiorly; another method is to displace the medial rectus muscle inferiorly and the lateral rectus superiorly during a recess-resect procedure. In order to have a significant effect the medial rectus should be displaced vertically an amount at least equal to the width of the muscle (Fig. 17–41). Because the width of the muscle is about 10 mm, the minimal transposition should be 10 mm. Another way of stating the same thing is to place the superior border of the muscle where the inferior border would be in the usual state.

The effect from vertical displacement of both medial recti will be about 25 prism diopters' correction of the V pattern. Similarly if a recess-resect procedure is done with the medial rectus muscle being moved down and the lateral rectus muscle being moved up, about the same 25 prism diopters of V pattern correction can be expected.[42, 43]

If an A pattern is to be treated, the medial rectus or recti should be moved superiorly. The same principle is followed: the muscle should be moved at least 10 mm vertically if an effect is to be achieved.

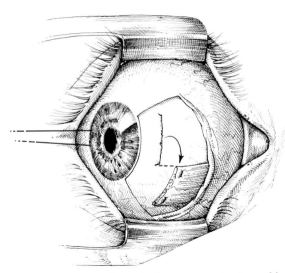

FIGURE 17–41. Inferior displacement one tendon width of the medial rectus muscle, combined with recession.

A corollary of the above is that if small errors are made in the vertical position of the muscle as it is reattached, one will not expect significant motility problems to be created.

Remember the rule that to correct A pattern and V pattern esotropias, the horizontal rectus muscles should be moved in the direction in which weakening is needed. For example, in a V pattern the medial rectus should be moved inferiorly, whereas in an A pattern the medial rectus should be moved superiorly.

If the purpose of the surgery is to change the action of the medial rectus muscle from an adductor to an elevator, a more drastic transposition is required. Typically the lateral rectus is moved in the same direction to create better elevation or depression. For example, in a double elevator palsy both the medial and lateral rectus muscles may be moved superiorly to create an elevating force. The new position of the medial rectus muscle should be adjacent to the superior rectus muscle (Fig. 17–42).[44]

In such a transposition the surgeon must place the medial rectus adjacent to the superior rectus insertion or even slightly beneath it. Failure to transpose the medial rectus fully will not create the desired elevating force. The surgeon performing this type of surgery for the first time may be concerned that a limitation of adduction or a horizontal strabismus will be created. Interestingly, neither of these complications occurs if, concomitantly, the same surgery is done on the lateral rectus muscle.

The measurements regarding the new insertion are made from the limbus, as noted in Figure 17–42. The new insertion will be parallel to the limbus.

Inferior transposition to change the force of the medial rectus partially to a depressor is accomplished much in the same manner as the supraplacement, only inferiorly. The medial rectus is reinserted adjacent to the medial border of the inferior rectus, so that the new insertion is parallel to the limbus. Only rarely is the inferior rectus muscle palsied, but in such a case both the medial and lateral rectus muscles would be transposed inferiorly, as the medial rectus is diagrammed in Figure 17–43.

Marginal Myotomy of the Medial Rectus

Occasionally the surgeon will want to weaken the medial rectus without altering its insertion. In such a case the muscle can be incised in a variety of ways to weaken it. To achieve any significant weakening, all the muscle fibers should be cut, with sufficient strands left between the muscle cuts to prevent pulling apart of the muscle.

A clamp is usually applied to crush the muscle before the incision. Cautery can also be applied to the crushed muscle before the incision, to prevent bleeding as the incision is made.

The decision as to which pattern of myotomy cuts to use is made at the time of surgery, as it is based on the width of the muscle and the

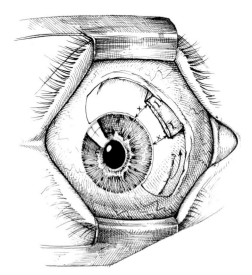

FIGURE 17–42. Superior transposition of medial rectus muscle.

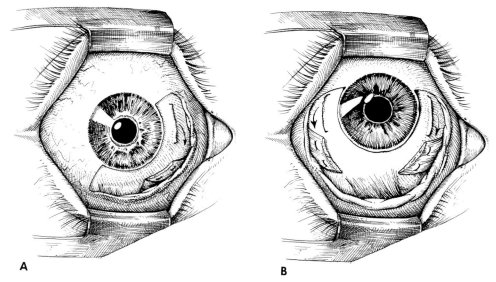

FIGURE 17–43. *A,* Medial rectus is transposed inferiorly to enhance depression. *B,* Medial rectus and lateral rectus are transposed inferiorly to enhance depression.

scarring pattern. In a fresh case the pattern shown in Figure 17–44*B* gives somewhat better results.

Posterior Fixation Suture of the Medial Rectus (Faden Procedure) [45]

When the medial rectus is to be selectively weakened in adduction without changing its strength in the straight-ahead or abducted position, the posterior fixation suture, using nonabsorbable suture material, is indicated. Typical conditions that require this procedure are the nystagmus blockage syndrome and a weakness of the yoke muscle (i.e., a weak lateral rectus of the other eye).

The posterior fixation suture is often combined with a recession of the medial rectus. While the muscle is disinserted, two double-armed sutures are used to secure the muscle to a point 12 mm posterior to the original insertion (i.e., 17 mm behind the limbus).

Figure 17–45*A* and *B* demonstrate a recession combined with a posterior fixation suture. Note that the distance from the clamp to where the muscle is sutured must be calculated in consideration of the recession. Similarly, if a resection were to be combined with such a procedure, the amount of the resection should be disregarded and the sutures placed 12 mm posterior to the muscle clamp after the muscle tissue has been resected. Figure 17–45*C* shows

a Faden procedure after reinsertion, without recession of the medial rectus.

In most instances, if no recession or resection is to be combined with the posterior fixation suture, the muscle need not be disinserted. Because, at best, the exposure is difficult when the sutures are placed quite posteriorly, occasionally the medial rectus muscle is disinserted and reinserted at its original insertion. For those patients who do not require disinsertion of the medial rectus, a single-armed suture is usually used and the muscle fixated at the edges of the muscle with only a single bite at each site, as noted in Figure 17–46.

The sutures should be loosely tied and the ends trimmed close to the knots. In the event that removal of the suture is indicated this can be easily done and the function will return as if the suture had not been applied. Failure to place the suture at least 12 mm posterior to the limbus will result in no effect.

After placement of the posterior fixation suture and before conjunctival closure passive forced ductions should be done. The operation depends on the direction of pull of the posterior portion of the medial rectus and should not impose any passive restriction to motility. If such restrictions are found, the procedure has been technically flawed and the sutures should be removed and replaced. The most common error is the entrapment of tissue other than that intended as the suture is tightened and tied.

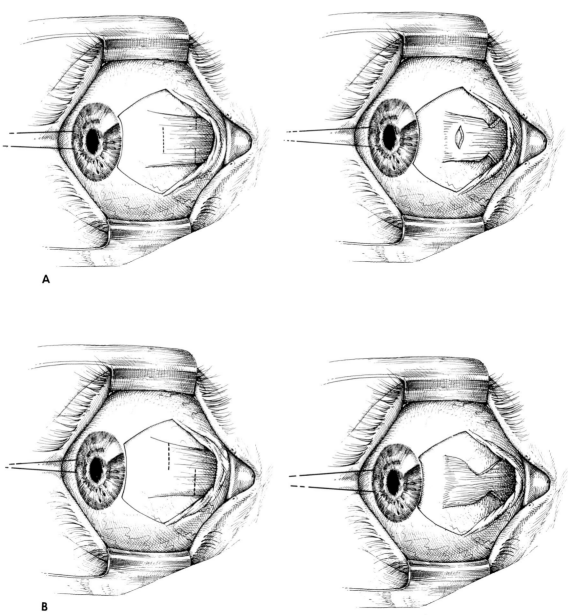

A

B

FIGURE 17–44. *A*, Three-cut marginal myotomy. *B*, Two-cut marginal myotomy.

Surgical Techniques for the Lateral Rectus

Recession of the Lateral Rectus

Recessions of the lateral recti are often done to correct exotropia. Both lateral recti may be recessed or only one if the one is combined with a resection of the medial rectus. The technique of recession of the muscle is basically the same as for that for recession of the medial rectus. For details of the recession procedure refer back to the section on medial rectus recession. The following discussion focuses on specific features of the lateral rectus recession procedure, which may differ from the procedure for recessions of the medial rectus.

Primary Surgery. The prior admonitions regarding correct positioning of the eye to allow accurate orientation of the surgeon are especially important, as serious errors in operating on the wrong muscle are more common with lateral rectus surgery than with medial rectus

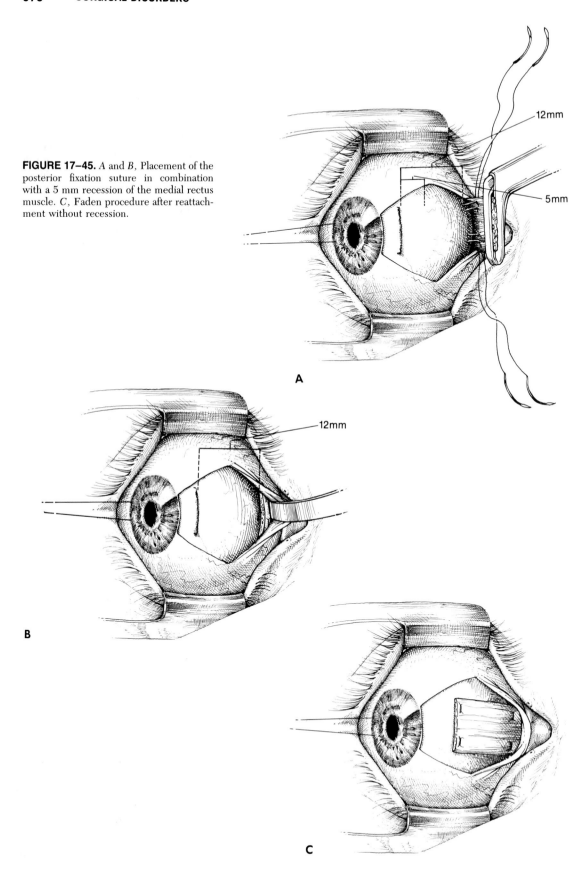

FIGURE 17–45. *A* and *B*, Placement of the posterior fixation suture in combination with a 5 mm recession of the medial rectus muscle. *C*, Faden procedure after reattachment without recession.

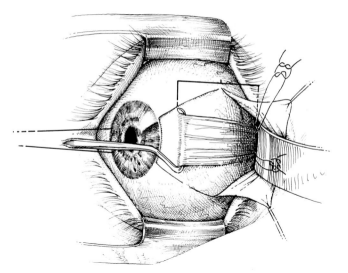

FIGURE 17–46. The posterior fixation suture application to the medial rectus muscle.

surgery. This is true even though more positioning signs are present laterally than medially, such as the lateral limbal triangle and insertions of the inferior and superior oblique.

The conjunctival incision may be of the surgeon's choice, but for most cases the limbal incision offers better exposure and is technically the easiest. Recall the rule to open the conjunctiva well away from the muscle, that is, in the quadrants, so that the muscle will not be inadvertently split and the muscle sheath interrupted. The fixation suture that has been placed laterally in clear cornea is used to adduct the eye fully. The conjunctival incision should be continued with sharp dissection, with the surgeon taking care to stay in the avascular tissue plane and to keep the muscle sheath intact.

The muscle is isolated from below by passage of the muscle hook under direct visualization. Muscle hooks are passed alternately from above and below the muscle until one emerges clear of tissue on its tip. No buttonholing is necessary. Care should be taken to pass the hooks no more than about 10 to 14 mm behind the limbus. Deep passage will pick up portions of the inferior oblique that may be inadvertently incorporated in the clamp, which can cause inferior oblique adhesive traction patterns with limitation of motility.

The Jameson muscle hook is passed to ensure good fixation of the globe during further dissection. The intermuscular septum is severed 5 to 10 mm posterior to the insertion; about 10 mm of muscle should be free of check ligaments. A second hook is passed under the muscle and slid posteriorly to ensure freedom of the lateral rectus from the underlying inferior oblique muscle. A slight resistance can readily be overcome, and the hook should easily pass along the globe to a depth of 25 mm from the limbus.

The Berens clamp is applied, the muscle is disinserted, and a 6-0 figure-of-eight nonabsorbable suture is placed the required amount behind the original insertion. Reattachment of the muscle may also be done by the alternate techniques mentioned for recession of the medial rectus. Recessions of the lateral recti less than 4 mm are seldom indicated. Large recessions greater than 10 mm are used only when limitation of function of the lateral rectus is desired. Such an indication would be a paralysis of the medial rectus in a palsy of the third cranial nerve.

At some point in the recession of the lateral rectus it is a good practice to retract the tissue and identify the inferior oblique muscle coursing parallel to the limbus in the inferior temporal quadrant (Fig. 17–47). This is further insurance that the lateral rectus muscle is the one being recessed as diagrammed. Further details on identification and isolation of the inferior oblique are given in the discussions under surgery of the inferior oblique.

After recession of the muscle forced ductions are done as recommended after each muscle reattachment before the conjunctival closure. If any restriction is noted, look for incarceration of the tissues adherent to the inferior oblique.

Be careful to have any nonabsorbable suture or suture ends well buried, as they become readily visible after healing. Because the lateral aspect of the globe is more visible than the

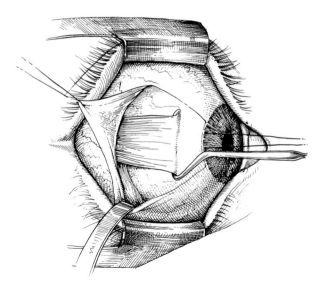

FIGURE 17–47. Note the direction of the inferior oblique muscle fibers as compared with that of the lateral rectus fibers.

medial, special care must be taken in the excision of redundant tissue before conjunctival closure and the burying of nonabsorbable suture material.

Closure of the conjunctiva is done with interrupted 7-0 silk, for the reasons mentioned under Closure of Conjunctiva (p. 664). If the conjunctiva is tight and closing under stress when the eye is adducted, it should be recessed, leaving the sclera bare. However, it is best not to recess the conjunctiva unless it is definitely required because the excessively loose conjunctiva that results from unneeded recession will fold on itself, leaving a pseudocaruncle that will remain red and unsightly for many years.

Secondary Surgery. Secondary recessions of the lateral recti are often time-consuming. Not only must the lateral rectus muscle be isolated with care and with good hemostasis, but further isolation may be required where the inferior oblique has become adherent to the medial side of the lateral rectus. This portion of the dissection has to be done after the muscle is in the clamp and has been disinserted.

The dissection of a pseudotendon from the original insertion to the muscle is usually possible and provides tissue for an effective further recession. In the dissection of the pseudotendon the thinness of the sclera behind the original insertion of the lateral rectus must be regarded with caution. Similarly, the passage of muscle hooks in reoperations must never be forceful and must always be under direct observation. Note: *Failure to follow this rule may result in a perforated globe.*

Placement of the needle in the reattachment

of the muscle is similarly somewhat hazardous, owing to the thinness of the sclera in the lateral portion of the globe. Thin spatula needles have made this maneuver quite safe, but the danger for perforation is always present. If perforation is suspected, the needle is replaced, the procedure temporarily halted, and the pupil dilated. Indirect ophthalmoscopy is used to inspect the site of the possible perforation while the suspected area is depressed with a cotton-tipped applicator. Most of the time the retina will not have been perforated, and the needle will have passed only into the suprachoroidal space. No treatment is indicated. If retinal holes are found, cryocautery is applied about the holes. No scleral flap is turned or an implant done unless a retinal tear is seen accompanied by vitreous traction. The need for such treatment (i.e., scleral buckle) in such cases is rare.

Resection of the Lateral Rectus

Primary Surgery. Resection of the lateral rectus should seldom be done as an isolated procedure, but it commonly is done in combination with recession of the medial rectus for an esotropia. After the muscle is isolated, identified, and freed from adhesions the Berens clamp is applied at the point desired, and the muscle between the clamp and insertion is excised. The amount of muscle resected varies from 7 to 12 mm. The muscle is reattached in the manner described for the medial rectus.

If excess conjunctiva is present, some may be excised before closure, or if a slight restriction of adduction is sought, the conjunctiva may be resected.

Secondary Surgery. Secondary resections of

the lateral rectus technically are similar to those described for the medial rectus. If the lateral rectus insertion is found posterior to the usual 6.5-mm distance from the limbus, it can be advanced to its original insertion site and the clamp applied to make up the difference in the resection. For example, if the insertion can be advanced 4 mm to its original insertion, only a 4-mm resection need be done to obtain the effect of an 8-mm resection. If the muscle is found 8 mm back, or about 14 mm from the limbus, an advancement to the original insertion site should suffice.

In advancements care must be taken to avoid pulling up nonmuscular tissue that will tether the eye. Thus, in any advancement procedure, forced ductions after attachment of the muscle (and before conjunctival closure) are essential.

Vertical Transposition of the Lateral Rectus

Vertical transpositions of lateral recti are done following the same rules mentioned in regard to the medial rectus. The muscle should be isolated and freed to a greater extent than that required for a recession, as the muscle should lie free of restrictions in its new site. The minimal amount of vertical transposition required to achieve an effect is 10 mm or the tendon width. The muscle should be moved in the direction in which weaker action is sought. For example, in an A pattern the lateral rectus should be moved inferiorly, whereas in a V pattern the lateral rectus should be moved superiorly.

The amount of vertical movement is greater than the amount of recession or resection required for the basic straight-ahead deviation. For example, in an A pattern exotropia the lateral recti may be recessed and moved inferiorly as well.

Standard Procedure. If the lateral rectus is moved vertically to change its force from that of an abductor to that of an elevator or depressor, the entire muscle should be moved to join the lateral margin of the superior or inferior rectus muscle, respectively, just as described for the medial rectus muscle transposition. With such major transpositions the muscle is strengthened as it is effectively advanced. The amount of such an effect can be estimated to be about 5 mm. If further strengthening is required, some additional muscle is resected before reattaching the muscle adjacent to either the superior or the inferior rectus muscle.[46]

Jensen Procedure. The Jensen procedure is a compromise of the transposition of the full

insertion. In the past the vertical rectus muscles were split and the lateral half of each muscle was disinserted and reinserted down and laterally near the insertion of the lateral rectus. This technique, known as the Hummelscheim operation, fell into well-deserved disrepute, for it seldom was successful. The failure was caused by the scarring to the globe of the entire transposed muscle. The Jensen procedure, although it also involves the splitting of muscles, seems often to work successfully. To treat a palsied lateral rectus, the medial rectus is recessed 8 to 10 mm and the inferior, lateral, and superior recti are isolated. Each of the three rectus muscles is split longitudinally 20 mm from its insertion into equal halves. The medial halves of the superior and inferior recti are not manipulated further. The lateral halves of the vertical recti are joined to the adjacent half of the lateral recti with a loop of 4–0 nonabsorbable suture at the equator of the globe (see Fig. 17–48).

The 4-0 sutures should be anchored to the sclera. Because the lateral rectus is paralyzed, it will passively stretch. Unless the suture is anchored the lateral rectus will migrate to the superior and inferior recti as they slowly return to their original positions. The same effect can be attained without involving the lateral rectus simply by placing the vertical recti in the Jensen position and anchoring them to the sclera. Operations on the lateral and vertical muscles subsequent to a Jensen procedure are difficult, owing to the split edges of the muscles becoming fibrosed to the sclera. Because greater abduction can be attained with lateral transposition of the intact vertical recti, fewer surgeons are using the Jensen procedure.

The conjunctiva is closed with interrupted black 7-0 silk sutures. The advantage of the procedure is that it can be accomplished in one operation, whereas the full-width transposition must be staged 6 weeks after a recess-resect operation because of the potential for anterior segment necrosis. Anterior segment necrosis may occur after the Jensen procedure as well, but this is uncommon.

Marginal Myotomy of the Lateral Rectus

Marginal myotomy of the lateral rectus muscle is most commonly indicated when surgery is necessary on either the inferior or superior rectus of that eye and when the lateral rectus is to be weakened as well. As a rule, adjacent rectus muscles are not disinserted during the same surgical procedure because of the risk of

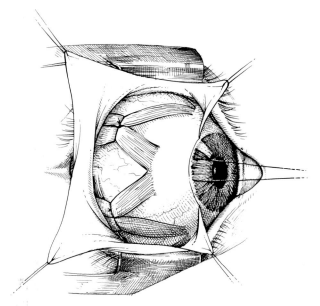

FIGURE 17–48. The Jensen procedure. The looping sutures must be nonabsorbable.

anterior segment necrosis. The marginal myotomy can be used to weaken the muscle while leaving the blood supply relatively intact.[47]

The procedure for the marginal myotomy entails isolation of only that portion of the muscle that will be myotomized and making the incisions such as those described for marginal myotomy of the medial rectus muscle. One should recall that to achieve any significant weakening, all the fibers of the muscle should be cut, while leaving sufficient strands between the muscle cuts to prevent pulling apart of the muscle (see Fig. 17–44).

Posterior Fixation Suture of the Lateral Rectus

The posterior fixation suture technique with respect to the lateral rectus muscle is accomplished in the same manner as that described for the medial rectus, with the one important exception of placing the suture at least 16 mm posterior to the usual insertion of the lateral rectus. In doing this the anterior border of the inferior oblique insertion will often be seen and can be used to advantage. A single bite into the insertion of the inferior oblique will frequently suffice for the fixation suture as shown in Figure 17–49.

Surgical Techniques for the Superior Rectus

The traction suture recommended for horizontal muscle surgery is not adequate for vertical muscle surgery. An additional suture placed in the medial portion of clear cornea will augment the usual laterally placed traction suture in a satisfactory manner for most vertical rectus procedures. Each 7-0 silk suture should have a rubber band tied to it, to give a gentle traction and prevent the fixating suture from tearing the tissue. Both sutures can be used together to elevate or depress the globe, as shown in Figure 17–50. The elevation and depression obtainable with these sutures will

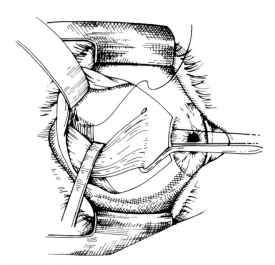

FIGURE 17–49. Posterior fixation suture being placed in the insertion of the inferior oblique and lateral rectus muscles. The double-armed nonabsorbable suture is brought through the lateral rectus muscle and loosely tied. Measurements on the muscle should be such that after tying the fixation suture the muscle is under slight tension against the globe. Appropriate placement of the fixation suture in recession or resection of the lateral rectus should be calculated as described with the posterior fixation suture of the medial rectus.

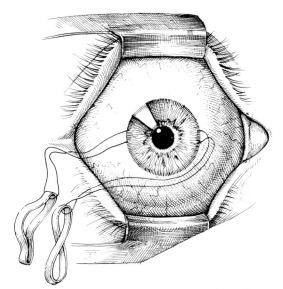

FIGURE 17–50. Traction sutures for vertical muscle surgery.

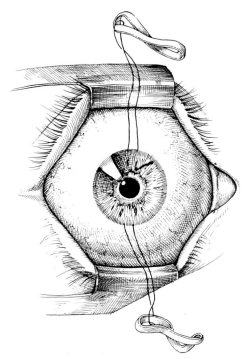

FIGURE 17–51. Traction sutures for vertical rectus surgery when extensive visualization is required.

typically allow muscle hooks to easily be passed under the superior or inferior rectus muscle. Further elevation or depression can be easily done after placement of the muscle hooks. In the patient who requires reoperation on the vertical rectus muscles, generous exposure is necessary before the muscle hooks can be used. In the latter cases a corneal suture is placed to achieve better traction and allow better visualization. This is placed at 12 o'clock for exposure of the superior rectus and at 6 o'clock for exposure of the inferior rectus muscle. The recommended suture is 7-0 silk placed in clear cornea close to the limbus but here in the vertical meridian (see Fig. 17–51).

Recession of the Superior Rectus

Primary Surgery. The conjunctival incision may be limbal or just anterior to the muscle insertion (Fig. 17–52). The limbal incision gives better exposure and is recommended for most cases. The two arms of the incision are made approximately 90 degrees to each other, and a peritomy joins the two. The arms of the incision should extend about 7 mm for primary recession of the superior or inferior rectus.

If no conjunctival recession is planned, an incision just anterior to the insertion can be used (Fig. 17–53). Because the superior rectus inserts about 7 mm from the limbus, the conjunctival incision should be about 5 mm behind the limbus. If a larger conjunctival incision is needed, the incision can be extended toward the quadrant.

If the more posterior conjunctival incision is used, care should be taken to expose bare sclera at the ends of the incision rather than in the middle. In this way the insertion will not be split. The superior rectus inserts with the nasal

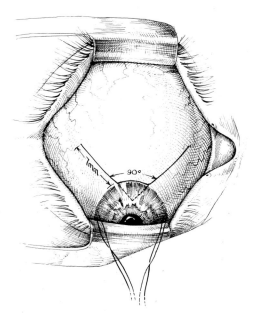

FIGURE 17–52. Conjunctival incision for superior rectus exposure if conjunctival recession is planned.

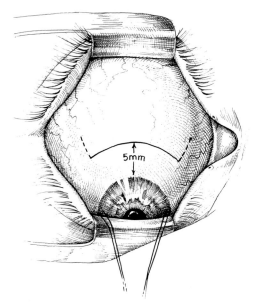

FIGURE 17–53. Conjunctival incision for superior rectus if no conjunctival recession is to be done.

edge closer to the limbus than to the lateral border. Hence it is good practice to pass the hook from the temporal aspect. The temporal approach also allows the hook to be passed in the same direction as the fibers of the superior oblique, sliding over the insertion of the superior oblique rather than hooking the insertion, as one might if approaching it from the medial side.

The superior rectus is isolated in the same manner as described for the medial rectus, with care taken to pass the muscle hooks under direct visualization. Because the superior oblique passes under the superior rectus, any posterior blind hooking maneuvers may catch a portion of the superior oblique and produce a restrictive pattern if not corrected at the time of surgery.

After the muscle is isolated by the to-and-fro passage of hooks until one comes out free of tissue over an area of bare sclera, the conjunctiva is dissected away from the insertion. Unless a large recession is planned the dissection should be carried at least 10 mm posterior to the insertion. The intermuscular septum is similarly cut about the same amount.

The usual recession of the superior rectus is combined with resection of the inferior rectus. The effect from the vertical recess-resect procedure is about 7 prism diopters per millimeter of recession. The resection should be approximately the same amount. If only a recession is done, the effect will be about two-thirds that achieved when combining it with a resection.

A large recession is occasionally needed. For example, in alternating sursumduction (often called dissociated vertical divergence, or DVD) the superior rectus should be recessed 6 to 9 mm, and both superior recti should be so recessed.

Before the muscle is disinserted or placed in the Berens clamp the superior oblique should be identified, to ensure that a portion of the superior oblique tendon is not drawn down to the insertion. The insertion of the superior oblique can be easily identified by pulling the eye down and nasally while passing a hook first medially and then posteriorly and laterally to engage the anterior portion of the superior oblique tendon (see Fig. 17–54).

After the superior rectus has been isolated either a locking suture or the Berens clamp is applied at the insertion, and the muscle is disinserted. The scleral reinsertion should parallel the original insertion angle, with the temporal reinsertion being more posterior than the nasal, as indicated in Figure 17–55. The conjunctiva may be closed with 7-0 black silk interrupted sutures, or it may be recessed if indicated when the opening has been limbal.

Secondary Surgery. Secondary recessions of the superior recti deserve the same general considerations discussed in respect to secondary procedures on the horizontal recti. If the muscle was previously resected, the procedure will usually differ little from a primary procedure.

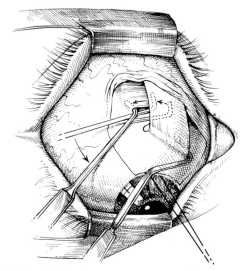

FIGURE 17–54. The anterior insertion of the superior oblique is identified and pulled laterally to ensure its freedom from the hook under the superior rectus tendon.

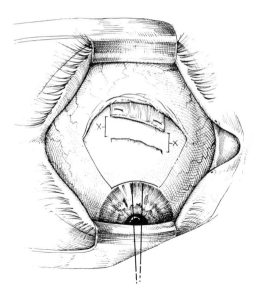

FIGURE 17–55. Recession of superior rectus X amount, with emphasis on angular reinsertion parallel to original insertion.

Resection of the Superior Rectus

This resection is preceded by isolation of the muscle in the manner just described for recession. No extra dissection is required between the superior rectus and levator muscles. A ptosis will not be created unless the resection is extremely large and excessive nonmuscular tissue is brought forward. Because resections of the superior rectus larger than 6 mm are seldom, if ever, indicated, extra dissection is similarly not needed. The muscle should be reattached at the original insertion, with appropriate regard for the natural slant of the insertion as mentioned in regard to recession. The conjunctiva is closed with the techniques described under primary surgery for recession of the superior rectus.

Horizontal Transposition of the Superior Rectus

Horizontal transposition of the superior rectus may occasionally be indicated in A patterns in which the secondary adduction force of the superior rectus is to be weakened. The superior rectus should be moved laterally for A patterns and medially for V patterns. No effect can be expected unless the insertion is changed the full width of the original insertion (i.e., about 10 mm). The rule mentioned with regard to the horizontal recti also applies here: If a major adduction or abduction force is needed, the muscle insertion should be transferred respectively to abut the insertion of the medial or

lateral rectus at its superior border. In such cases the inferior rectus insertion is transposed to the lower border of the medial or lateral rectus tendon.

Marginal Myotomy of the Superior Rectus

Marginal myotomy of the superior rectus is mentioned here only to condemn the procedure. This procedure is *not* advised because of its effect on the underlying superior oblique. Whenever a muscle is myotomized the cut edges of the muscle adhere to whatever tissue is closest. Where the medial and lateral recti are concerned, this tissue is typically the sclera, and no great harm will be done. However, if the superior rectus is myotomized, the muscle will adhere to the sclera and superior oblique in such a manner that any future superior oblique surgery will be difficult, if not impossible.

Posterior Fixation Suture of the Superior Rectus

The posterior fixation suture of the superior rectus is used with some regularity. If the following suggestions are heeded, the procedure is not overly difficult, and no serious problems will be generated. The superior rectus is isolated in the usual manner, but the conjunctival incision is made over the insertion of the muscle and carried into the quadrants, to give an adequate opening that will not tear as the traction necessary for exposure is applied (see Fig. 17–56). If the conjunctiva is to be recessed, the conjunctival incision should be limbal with generous quadrantic relaxing incisions.

After the muscle has been isolated, with care taken not to invade the muscle's sheath, it is clamped in the Berens clamp and disinserted from the globe. The muscle is held in place (with the eye depressed by the corneal traction sutures), and the superior oblique is picked up with the Hardesty superior oblique tendon hook. This is a small tendon hook with a marking indentation 12 mm posterior from the hook. The hook is passed medial to the superior rectus until the indentation marker is at the insertion of the superior rectus. Mild elevation of the tissue over the hook will usually allow visualization of the superior oblique tendon as it is picked up. The tendon is brought forward, with care taken to ensure that the splayed-out portion of the superior oblique tendon is not caught in the clamp applied to the superior rectus. The downward traction on the superior oblique

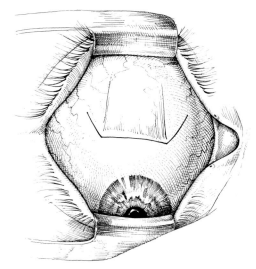

FIGURE 17–56. Conjunctival incision for placement of posterior fixation suture in the superior rectus muscle.

gives further depression of the globe. A 6- or 16-mm malleable retractor between the superior rectus and the superior oblique gives excellent exposure. The posterior fixation suture is placed 14 to 16 mm posterior to the original insertion of the superior rectus (see Fig. 17–57). The traction on the superior oblique pre-

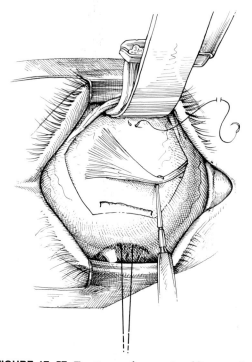

FIGURE 17–57. Traction on the superior oblique tendon allows adequate visualization and appropriate placement of the posterior fixation suture to the superior rectus muscle.

vents its imbrication in the superior oblique tendon, an iatrogenic cause of a superior oblique tendon sheath syndrome.

A double-armed nonabsorbable suture is used, and one or two bites of sclera are taken with appropriate placement of the needle through the superior rectus, with due regard to any planned recession of the superior rectus. If the superior rectus is to be recessed, that amount should be subtracted from the point at which the needle is passed through the muscle. A single suture has been found adequate if passed through the center of the muscle.

If the posterior fixation suture is to be removed because of having had too great an effect, the exposure technique is the same as that discussed above. The suture is cut as it emerges from the sclera, a muscle hook is passed to assure freedom of the muscle from the globe, and the wound is closed. No exploration to look for pieces of the cut suture is advised, as the pieces will cause no difficulties, but excessive exploration may.

Surgical Techniques for the Inferior Rectus

The traction sutures generally used are identical to those described for the superior rectus: 7-0 silk sutures through clear limbal cornea at 9 and 3 o'clock for most cases. If the patient has had prior surgery on the inferior rectus that makes it necessary for much of the dissection to be done before a muscle hook can be placed under the inferior rectus, then an additional individual 7-0 silk suture through the clear limbal cornea at 6 o'clock may be necessary. Incorporating a rubber band in the 7-0 silk suture prevents sudden excessive traction.

Recession of the Inferior Rectus

Primary Surgery. Primary recessions are usually technically no more difficult than those of the other rectus muscles, with the exception of those done for restrictions owing to dysthyroid myopathies. Special notes regarding the latter are made under Recessions for Restricted Upward Gaze, below.

The conjunctival incision should be limbal if recession of the conjunctiva is anticipated or if the surgeon is not a frequent operator on this muscle. The limbal incision is 3 hours of the clock (i.e., from 4:30 to 7:30), thus making the quadrantic incisions 90 degrees to one another (see Fig. 17–58). As emphasized at the beginning of this chapter, the surgeon should care-

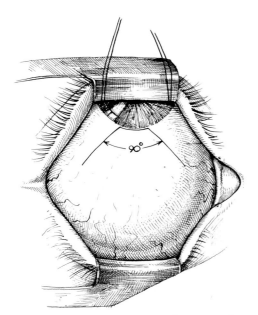

FIGURE 17–58. Limbal conjunctival incisions for approaching the inferior rectus muscle.

fully orient himself with regard to the position of the globe before placing the corneal fixation sutures. The conjunctiva and Tenon's capsule are undermined and the muscle is isolated by repeat passages of muscle hooks to prevent perforation of the muscle's sheath. Remember that the temporal side of the insertion is further from the limbus than the nasal edge of the insertion. The order of muscle hook passage that is cleanest is to place a tendon hook under the temporal insertion. This brings the insertion into easy viewing and a larger muscle hook can be passed from this side toward the nose. If the initial maneuver is made from the nasal side, the muscle insertion may be inadvertently divided at about the juncture of the middle and temporal third of the insertion.

The dissection is carried out for about 10 mm for the usual recession of up to 4 mm. If a more extensive recession is to be done, the dissection should be extended. The extended dissection will involve the inferior oblique–inferior rectus adhesion. One or two large veins are typically present. Careful dissection will permit identification of these veins, and cautery should seldom be necessary. Inadequate dissection for large recessions will produce lagophthalmos of the inferior lid.

The procedure for reattachment may be either the free double-armed locked sutures or the Berens clamp with the figure-of-eight technique. These techniques are described earlier in this chapter. Be sure to reattach the muscle parallel to its original insertion, with the temporal edge more posterior than the nasal side of the insertion. As the sutures are tightened, inspect the edge of the insertions, as sometimes an excessive amount of Tenon's capsule will be drawn along the suture.

Secondary Surgery. Secondary recessions of the inferior rectus are often difficult, as the prior surgery frequently causes fibrous adhesions to form between the inferior oblique, the inferior rectus, and the globe. The principal admonition is to use careful hemostasis, slow deliberate dissection, and a limbal conjunctival approach. The dissection should be done first in the quadrants well away from the muscle; it can be carried toward the inferior rectus from each side, and the muscle can usually be easily identified. This method results in less bleeding than occurs if you proceed over the anticipated insertion. There is also a lessened chance of entering the fat pockets or of confusing a portion of the inferior oblique with the inferior rectus. For the difficult dissection, 6- and 16-mm malleable retractors are essential.

Recessions for Restricted Upward Gaze. Recessions of the inferior rectus for dysthyroid ophthalmopathy are often difficult. The patient has retraction of the upper lid secondary to the restricted elevation caused by the tight inferior rectus. Forced ductions are positive, and the globe frequently cannot be sufficiently elevated to allow good visualization of the inferior rectus. In such cases the tissues must be retracted inferiorly, since the globe cannot be elevated. It may be necessary to remove the self-retaining lid retractor and to retract the lid, conjunctiva, and tissues with malleable retractors. In the occasional case the exposure is so limited that only the edge of the muscle can be imbricated with a suture, and the muscle must be disinserted with a knife by cutting down on the muscle hook. After disinsertion the globe should be readily elevated. If restrictions remain, a strip of the inferior rectus is still attached—usually a lateral third. Continue to explore until the globe can be elevated.

Lagophthalmos of the lower lid may be created after recessions of the inferior rectus. To avoid such lagophthalmos, (a) the dissection should be adequate, and (b) the closure should approximate the lower lid in the correct position with respect to the globe. With respect to the dissection, the adhesions between the inferior rectus and the lid must be severed; otherwise, a recession of the inferior rectus will predictably result in a lagophthalmos. To verify the ade-

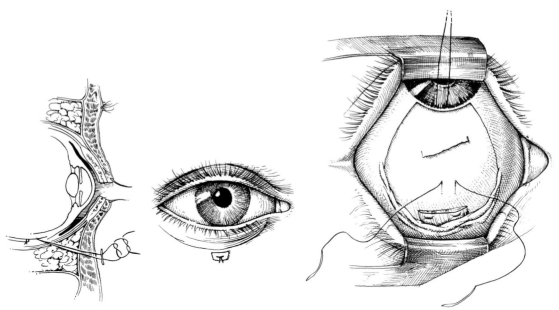

FIGURE 17–59. Globe-to-lid suture to prevent lagophthalmos of lower lid after large recession of the inferior rectus muscle.

quacy of the dissection, check that movement of the inferior rectus after disinsertion does not affect the position of the lower lid. If no further steps are taken at the time of surgery, often no lagophthalmos of the lower lid occurs. In frequent cases, however, it will appear, and most of these could have been prevented had the surgeon reestablished appropriate connections with either the lid and the inferior rectus or the globe and the lid (see Fig. 17–59). If the inferior rectus is recessed more than 8 mm, the tissues of the lid should be approximated directly to the globe, anterior to the recessed muscles. The conjunctiva is closed with interrupted silk sutures.

Resection of the Inferior Rectus

Resection of the inferior rectus differs from resection of other rectus muscles in only a few details. As with the other procedures, the conjunctival incision should be limbal, unless specific reasons exist for an incision immediately anterior to the insertion. There is seldom justification for incisions medial or lateral to the insertion.

Primary Surgery. Primary resections should be initiated in the usual manner, by identifying bare sclera medially and laterally to the inferior rectus, and passing muscle hooks repeatedly until the tip of the hook emerges clean. No buttonholing of any tissue should be necessary. The insertion is not parallel to the limbus, but at about a 23-degree angle to it, hence note the prior admonitions regarding potential splitting of the tendon. After dissection is carried down to the condensation of Tenon's capsule at the surface of the interior oblique and inferior rectus muscles, the Berens clamp is applied at the desired point and the muscle reattached in a figure-of-eight manner with a 6-0 nonabsorbable suture.

If the dissection of the lid tissues from the inferior rectus is inadequate, the lower lid may be too high on the globe. The inferior rectus normally has some connections to the lower lid. As the inferior rectus is resected, it may draw the lower lid superiorly. Check for freedom of movement of the inferior rectus after it has been disinserted from the globe. A reasonable amount of movement of the inferior rectus should not cause the lower lid to move to any extent. Always check the position the lid has with respect to the globe in the primary position. If it is too high or too low, it should be adjusted with a lid-globe suture before closure of the conjunctiva. The conjunctiva is closed with interrupted 7-0 black silk sutures.

Secondary Surgery. Secondary resections of the inferior rectus are easy if the primary procedure was done without interruption of the sheath. If earlier surgery or trauma has interrupted the sheath or the fat pockets, dissection will be tedious. Sharp dissection with careful hemostasis is the key to success. The required dissection may be extensive and may require entering the inferior oblique–inferior rectus interface.

Horizontal Transposition of the Inferior Rectus

Horizontal transposition of the inferior rectus is usually done in conjunction with a similar temporal or nasal transposition of the superior rectus. The inferior rectus is adherent to the inferior oblique, and this adherence should be broken so that the inferior rectus can be directed medially or laterally, in order that it may sufficiently change a major portion of its depressor force to that of an adductor or an abductor.

After the muscle has been freed with appropriate dissection, if abducting force is desired, the insertion is moved so that the lateral edge of the inferior rectus is adjacent to the lower edge of the lateral rectus, and the medial border of the inferior rectus is applied a similar distance from the limbus; the new insertion should appear as shown in Figure 17–60.

A vertical squint can be corrected by recessing or resecting the superior rectus or inferior rectus appropriately in combination with the transposition. If a vertical rectus is to be recessed, it should be moved further posteriorly while its lateral insertion is kept even with the proximal border of the lateral rectus.

The same principles can be applied to medial transpositions of the inferior rectus with respect

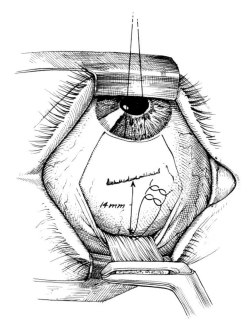

FIGURE 17–61. Placement of a posterior fixation suture to an inferior rectus muscle. Knot is tied between muscle and globe.

to the medial rectus muscle when the function of the inferior rectus is to be changed to include adduction in the primary position.

Marginal Myotomy of the Inferior Rectus

Marginal myotomy of the inferior rectus is seldom done, but if it is required, it should be done in the manner described for the other rectus muscles, with the inferior rectus myotomized anterior to the inferior oblique condensation.

Posterior Fixation Suture of the Inferior Rectus

The posterior fixation suture or Faden procedure is difficult to do with respect to the inferior rectus. The methods of exposure are those cited for the other muscles. Good traction of the globe, disinsertion of the inferior rectus, malleable retractors, and good illumination are important. Unless the suture is placed 14 to 16 mm posterior to the original insertion, no effect is to be expected. Because the inferior oblique blocks access to the sides of the inferior rectus, the inferior rectus should be removed from the globe. Instead of passing the double-armed suture through the inferior rectus and tying it on the outside of the muscle, a bite of the muscle can be taken at the desired point and the suture tied between the muscle and the globe (see Fig. 17–61). The measured place-

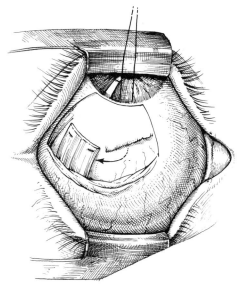

FIGURE 17–60. Lateral transposition of the inferior rectus muscle insertion to the lower edge of the lateral rectus insertion.

ment on the muscle should correspond to the new position of the inferior rectus if it is to be recessed or resected. For example, if the muscle is to be recessed 4 mm, the suture should be placed 10 mm posteriorly in the muscle (14–4) to correctly position the muscle on the globe.

Surgical Techniques for the Inferior Oblique

Surgery on the inferior oblique is usually limited to weakening procedures.[48] Because the inferior oblique is seldom paralyzed or symptomatically weak, strengthening procedures are not needed, and if they were, they would be difficult because the insertion is difficult to visualize and is located over the macular area. Its location over the macular area should give cause for caution as to all surgical procedures on the insertion of the inferior oblique. The three procedures most commonly used for weakening of the inferior oblique are disinsertion, recession, and myotomy or myectomy.

Disinsertion of the Inferior Oblique

Disinsertion of the inferior oblique is difficult only if the surgeon obliterates the landmarks by careless steps early in the procedure. This is the only procedure in muscle surgery in which intentional dissection of the muscular sheath from the muscle is indicated; hence excessive dissection is not necessary to isolate the muscle.

The globe must be turned superiorly and nasally to bring the inferior oblique into view in the inferior temporal quadrant of the orbit. The globe may be grasped with forceps, rotated, and held in a superior-nasal direction by the assistant while the surgeon opens the conjunctiva. The incision should be 8 to 10 mm posterior and parallel to the limbus, with care taken to direct the incision toward the globe. If the dissection is directed inferiorly, the fat pockets of the orbit will be encountered, and excessive postsurgical scarring will result. Bleeding should be controlled with cautery before proceeding. Tenon's capsule is incised, baring the sclera. A Ragnel retractor is introduced to give good exposure of the sclera, and a Jameson muscle hook is placed under the insertion of the lateral rectus muscle. The assistant may now release the fixation forceps. The surgeon should place a 4-0 black silk suture armed with a round needle along the path of the muscle hook, piercing the conjunctiva at the superior border of the lateral rectus, close to its insertion

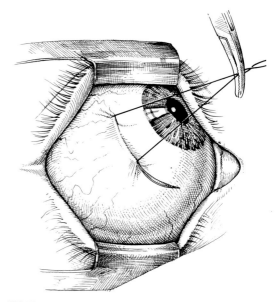

FIGURE 17–62. A 4-0 silk suture has been passed under the lateral rectus tendon and is used as a traction suture for visualization of the inferior oblique muscle.

(Fig. 17–62). The muscle hook may be removed and the suture either held by the assistant or affixed to the drape to hold the eye in a maximally adducted and elevated position.

The 6-mm malleable retractor is used to expose the inferior oblique. The muscle will be seen coursing parallel to the limbus, rather deep in the incision. If it cannot be seen, use two smooth forceps "hand over hand" to gently pull Tenon's capsule forward; the inferior oblique will thereby be exposed. The next objective is to bring the entire muscle forward. A common mistake is the inadvertent anterior hook placement, which brings forward only the anterior one-half to two-thirds of the muscle, leaving the remainder, which nullifies the goal of the procedure. To avoid this mistake, a second retractor (6 mm) is slid along the globe. The complete width of the inferior oblique can now be visualized, and a muscle hook should engage the posterior border of the inferior oblique. As the muscle is brought forward, care should be exercised to avoid pulling fat or other tissues with the muscle. A second muscle hook can be placed close to the first hook. The second hook usually will engage only the muscle and allow any excess tissue to drop back into the orbit. The muscle sheath can now be stripped from the muscle. The tissue will fall away. Any splitting of the muscle can be identified and the remaining strands of muscle engaged with another hook. The dissection of the muscle sheath should extend superiorly to the insertion and inferiorly to the lateral border of the inferior rectus muscle.

To disinsert the muscle, use blunt-tipped scissors to cut the attachment at the globe under direct visualization. Because no blood vessels traverse the insertion of the inferior oblique, bleeding will not be encountered unless the muscle is cut more than about 2 mm from the insertion. If the dissection has been adequate, the muscle will fully retract into its sheath beneath the inferior rectus. If the muscle does not retract, further dissection should be done until the muscle can be tucked well under the inferior rectus. At this point the muscle sheath's lateral opening can be closed with an absorbable synthetic suture if it is necessary to ensure that the inferior oblique will not reattach to the globe.

The conjunctiva is either closed with interrupted black silk sutures or simply repositioned in the inferior fornix without sutures. If sutures are not used, only eye drops and no ointments should be used.

If the procedure above is to be additive to lateral rectus surgery, the initial opening may be limbal in the usual manner and the operation may proceed as if the lateral rectus surgery were to be done until the time for application of the Berens clamp. At this point the 4-0 black silk suture should be passed under the lateral rectus, the eye maximally elevated nasally, and the procedure of isolation and disinsertion of the inferior oblique done as described.

Recession of the Inferior Oblique

Recession of the inferior oblique is carried out after the muscle has been isolated in the manner described above. After the muscle has been disinserted it should retract under the inferior rectus. The end of the muscle is readily identified and a suture passed through the end. The suture may be absorbable synthetic or nonabsorbable. The end of the muscle is sutured to the sclera 3 mm posteriorly and 3 mm laterally to the lateral edge of the inferior rectus insertion. Some surgeons place the suture in the muscle before its disinsertion, but there is no need to do this, as the suture gets in the way while the muscle is being disinserted and may be cut by the cautery if any bleeding is to be controlled. If the muscle should happen to retract to the extent that the end cannot be located for suturing, the procedure will be adequate and no suture is needed. The conjunctiva is closed as mentioned above.

Myotomy, Myectomy, or Biopsy of the Inferior Oblique

Myotomy, myectomy, or biopsy of the inferior oblique is carried out by isolating the inferior oblique as described above to disinsert it. Just before the step of cutting the muscle at its insertion, a small hemostat is used to crush the inferior oblique in the area of muscle exposed over the muscle hooks. If only a myotomy is to be done, one hemostat is used. If a piece of the inferior oblique is to be removed, two hemostats are used. The hemostats are left in place for about 15 seconds and then removed, after which cautery is placed along the crushed tissue and the muscle incised along the cautery line or lines.

If a biopsy is to be done without a weakening procedure, a few posterior strands of the muscle are allowed to remain. No paresis will be created by such a biopsy.

In performing a biopsy, myotomy, or myectomy it is important to inspect the ends of the cut tissue and be certain that there is adequate hemostasis before closure. There may be significant postoperative bleeding if this step is not done. On occasion sutures may be necessary to control the bleeding from the cut ends of muscle.

Myotomy or Myectomy of the Inferior Oblique, Medial to the Inferior Rectus

A myotomy or myectomy of the inferior oblique muscle, medial to the inferior rectus, is not recommended for the usual case. If it is to be done, an incision is made in the skin just superior to the lower medial orbital rim. The origin of the inferior oblique can usually be palpated through the skin. The incision should be along natural skin folds. Careful hemostasis is necessary, as the incision is carried through the skin, orbicularis, and orbital septum to the muscle. The muscle is easy to identify, and traction on the muscle confirms its action. If any question as to its identity is raised, the inferior rectus should be isolated through the usual conjunctival approach and the globe and inferior rectus moved to ensure that the muscle will not be damaged. After the inferior oblique is identified and isolated a crushing clamp (or clamps) is applied and then removed, and the tissue is cauterized along the crush line. The crush lines are incised, further cautery is applied as necessary, and the skin is closed. No closure of the orbital septum is necessary unless the dissection has been extensive.

Surgical Techniques for the Superior Oblique

These include tenotomy or tenectomy, tucking, selective tucking, and transposition of the insertion. Because these procedures may involve alternative approaches to the superior oblique tendon from the temporal, global, or nasal side of the superior rectus muscle, the three isolation procedures are described separately from the superior oblique manipulations.[49]

Nasal (to the superior rectus) isolation of the superior oblique tendon is usually done by way of a conjunctival incision placed just nasally and superiorly to the insertion of the superior rectus. The eye is depressed with either fixation forceps or corneal fixation sutures, as described for isolation of the superior rectus procedures. Conjunctival bleeding is controlled, and the incision is carried through Tenon's capsule down to bare sclera. A small muscle hook is used to locate the medial border of the insertion of the superior rectus. With the small hook the border of the superior rectus is held slightly away from the globe as a Jameson hook is placed under the complete insertion of the superior rectus (Fig. 17–63). The Jameson hook should not be swept posteriorly, as other tissues may be brought forward that will later obscure the identity of the superior oblique. The Jameson

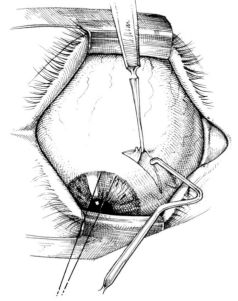

FIGURE 17–63. The medial border of the superior rectus is elevated to allow a muscle hook to be placed under direct visualization.

hook is used to fixate the globe in the depressed position. A Ragnel retractor will conveniently hold the conjunctiva out of the way while a small tendon hook with a mark 12 mm from its tip (H. Hardesty's superior oblique hook) is placed posteriorly until the 12-mm mark is at the nasal border of the insertion of the superior rectus (Fig. 17–64). The muscle hook should be inserted with the tip applied on the surface of the sclera. The tip is rotated up (from the position of the tip pointing nasally) and the tendon of the superior oblique brought forward. The tendon is easily identified by its silvery appearance and by its direction; its identity may be verified by palpating the tendon through the upper lid as it goes to the trochlea. Tugging on the tendon will cause intorsion, depression, and further abduction.

If the procedure above is not successful, do not blindly try to hook the superior oblique tendon, but stop, keep the Jameson hook in place under the superior rectus, and remove the lid speculum (Fig. 17–64). Place a 6-mm malleable retractor in the incision, elevate the tissues from the globe, and inspect for the superior oblique tendon. Typically it can be easily seen and picked up with a tendon hook; the lid speculum can then be reapplied and the procedure continued. If this move is unsuccessful, however, discontinue the attempts through this incision and approach the superior oblique through the temporal approach, returning to this incision after successful isolation of the insertion temporally.

Global (to the superior rectus) isolation of the superior oblique tendon is often done through the incision for isolation of the superior rectus. The conjunctival incision is as described in one of the maneuvers described for isolation of the superior rectus. The superior rectus is isolated and disinserted from the globe. The superior rectus is reflected superiorly, and the anterior edge of the superior oblique tendon will either remain flat on the globe about 10 to 12 mm posterior to the superior rectus insertion or it may be partially reflected with the superior rectus. The distinctive direction of the glistening superior oblique tendon should be apparent to the surgeon. The tendon fans out temporally toward its insertion. The anterior edge of this fan can be followed to its insertion by slipping a smooth spatula under the tendon. The vortex vein will be apparent anterior to the insertion of the superior oblique. If the vortex vein is inadvertently severed, hemostasis is a problem, and a scleral suture may be necessary to control the bleeding.

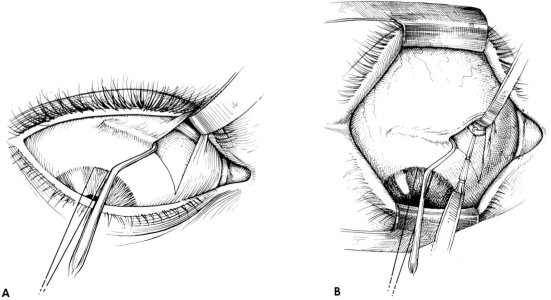

FIGURE 17–64. *A,* The superior oblique can be visualized directly with adequate retraction of tissues. Removal of the lid speculum is helpful. *B,* The Hardesty hook is withdrawing the superior oblique tendon under direct visualization. The indentation mark should not have passed posterior to the insertion of the superior rectus tendon.

Temporal (to the superior rectus) isolation of the superior oblique tendon is approached through a conjunctival incision placed in the quadrant temporal and superior to the insertion of the superior rectus. The eye is depressed with forceps or corneal stay sutures. Conjunctival bleeding is controlled, and the incision is carried through Tenon's capsule to bare sclera. The superior rectus is hooked in the manner described earlier with respect to the nasal approach. The technique should include the use of a small tendon hook to raise the margin of the superior rectus tendon before placement of the Jameson hook under direct visualization without posterior hooking. Retraction of the temporal margin of the superior rectus permits direct visualization of the fan-shaped tendon in the same manner described for such identification of the tendon on the global side of the superior rectus. If the tendon is not readily identified, search for it on the retracted superior rectus (see Fig. 17–65).

Tenotomy or Tenectomy of the Superior Oblique

Tenotomy or tenectomy of the superior oblique should be done without extensive dissection. The superior oblique tendon should be isolated on the nasal side of the superior rectus in the manner already described. As the tendon is brought forward, it is cleaned by gently pushing aside the tissue with smooth-tipped forceps; hooks are reapplied as necessary in order to see that the entire width of the tendon is on the hook. No effort to dissect away the sheath is necessary. The tendon and its sheath are simply severed with scissors. If a portion is

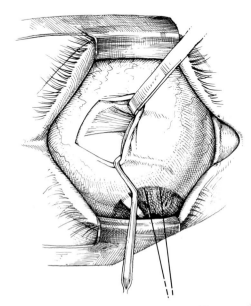

FIGURE 17–65. Isolation of the superior oblique tendon insertion.

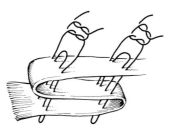

FIGURE 17–66. Suture placement for tucking of the superior oblique tendon.

to be removed (tenectomy), the tendon is grasped with a hemostat before making the first incision, and cuts are then made on both sides of the hemostat. If the correct surgical plane has been established, no bleeding will be seen. The tenectomy or tenotomy should be done only on the nasal side of the superior rectus, where the tendon is compact, because if it is done here, overaction is relieved and no paralysis will occur. If the superior oblique tendon is severed completely as it fans out beneath the superior rectus, a complete paralysis of the superior oblique is likely to be seen postoperatively.

Tucking of the Superior Oblique

Tucking of the superior oblique refers to a folding over of the tendon on itself (Fig. 17–66). The procedure may be done through either a nasal or a temporal approach. Both are prone to produce some restriction of elevation in adduction, but when the tucks are done temporally such restrictions usually disappear. Various instruments have been designed to facilitate the tuck of tendons (see Fig. 17–67). If the tuck is done on the nasal side of the superior rectus, care should be taken to make the tuck close to the superior rectus, so that the bulk of the tuck in the tendon will not abut the trochlea as the superior oblique contracts. An occasional report of such a complication has made most surgeons favor the temporal tuck of the tendon. When the tuck is done temporally, care must be taken to engage the *entire* tendon and not just the anterior portion; otherwise, an exclusive torsion effect will be obtained. (The latter may be desired in some instances, as described under Selective Tucking of the Superior Oblique, below.)

Nonabsorbable sutures should be used in the tucking, or the effect will dramatically lessen as the sutures absorb. One suture is placed when the muscle is folded on itself, tied, and passed through the tendon again to be tied finally on the original side (see Fig. 17–68). The tucking tool is removed, and the free loop of tendon is sutured to the tendon on the arm of the tendon distal to the trochlea (i.e., toward the insertion), as shown in Figure 17–66.

Selective Tucking of the Superior Oblique

Selective tucking of a portion of the superior oblique is done to achieve strengthening of a

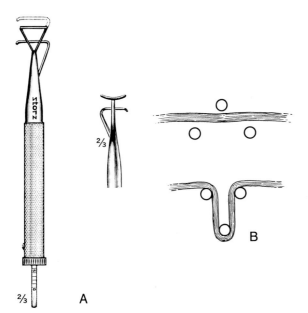

FIGURE 17–67. *A,* Tendon-tucking instrument. *B,* Cross section of placement of tucking instrument (above) and tightening of tuck (below).

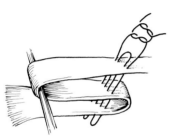

FIGURE 17–68. Placement of first suture for tucking of superior oblique tendon. The free fold should be sutured as shown in Figure 17–66.

specific function of the superior oblique—intorsion. Because the portion of the superior oblique that inserts anteriorly is mainly responsible for torsion, any maneuver that selectively strengthens this anterior portion as it fans out in its insertion will accomplish the desired result. The tendon of the superior oblique is isolated on the temporal side of the superior rectus. A small tendon hook is used to split the tendon into an anterior half and a posterior half. The anterior half can be strengthened by one of four methods.

1. A conventional tuck of only this portion may be done as described above for the whole tendon, but in this instance only the anterior portion is tucked.

2. The anterior half may be brought forward and sutured close to the insertion of the superior rectus. This results in a functional stretching of the tendon and anterior placement to increase the torsional effect (see Fig. 17–69).

3. The insertion of the anterior half may be advanced. This in effect is similar to the procedure shown in Figure 17–69B except that the suture is placed in the anterior portion close to the end of the insertion (see Fig. 17–69C).

4. An adjustable 6-0 synthetic absorbable suture may be used for the torsion effect, by continuing the sutures from the end of the anterior portion of the tendon, through scleral bites and out through the conjunctiva. After the effects of anesthesia have disappeared the torsion of the eye is adjusted according to the patient's subjective response. A 6-0 synthetic absorbable suture is used for this procedure.

Transposition of the Superior Oblique

Transposition of the superior oblique is the treatment of choice for paralysis of the third cranial nerve,[50] a condition that presents a special problem in that no readily available intact

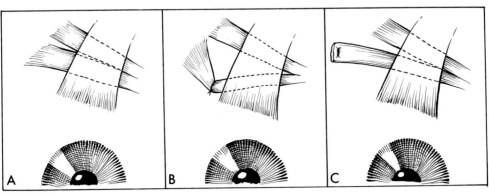

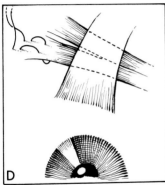

FIGURE 17–69. *A,* Splitting of the superior oblique tendon. *B,* Anterior placement of half of superior oblique tendon to increase torsion. *C,* Advancement of anterior half of superior oblique tendon. *D,* Selective tucking of anterior half of superior oblique tendon.

muscle can be transposed to give a tonic force to keep the eye aligned. Because the lateral rectus in such a case is intact, it will eventually contract to a point at which the eye will turn out again. Such secondary contracture can be prevented by application of a tonic force even though the force may not be coordinated with movement. The only intact muscle to oppose the lateral rectus in third nerve paralysis is the superior oblique. To treat such a patient, the lateral rectus muscle is recessed approximately 16 mm and the superior oblique repositioned to act as an abductor. The superior oblique can be changed from an abductor to an adductor by moving the insertion of the tendon from its original location to the nasal border of the insertion of the superior rectus. A more effective procedure is to dissect the superior oblique from the trochlea and bring it directly to the insertion of the medial rectus.

In the first alternative the superior oblique tendon is isolated on the medial side of the superior rectus. The tendon is severed and brought forward to the medial border of the superior rectus insertion. The tendon is sutured to that point, with sufficient shortening of the tendon achieved to maintain the eye in about 10 degrees adduction (see Fig. 17–70). A non-absorbable suture is used. The disadvantage of this technique is that considerable intorsion will be caused by the placement just described. The

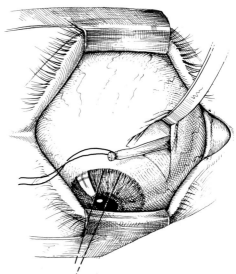

FIGURE 17–71. The cut end of the superior oblique tendon is imbricated with 4-0 silk to provide traction during removal of the tendon from the trochlea.

advantages of the technique are its simplicity as well as the fact that if a satisfactory alignment is not attained, the following technique may be used to attain it at a later date.

In the second alternative, that of transferring the superior oblique tendon out of the trochlea and directing it to the insertion of the medial rectus, the superior oblique tendon is isolated on the medial side of the superior rectus. The tendon is cut as far laterally as is convenient, to give a tendon long enough for manipulation. The tendon is grasped with a small hemostat before being cut laterally. After it has been cut a traction suture of 4-0 silk is imbricated in the end of the tendon and securely tied, leaving long ends for traction (see Fig. 17–71).

The lid speculum is removed, and a 6-mm malleable retractor is inserted to provide exposure along the tendon, toward the trochlea. (A head-mounted light is necessary for good visualization of this portion of the procedure.) It is helpful to alternate the 6- and 16-mm malleable retractors for this difficult exposure problem. When the trochlear area is reached the tendon will be seen to disappear into a fibrous unit I term the "trochlear tunnel." If the patient is past 40 years of age, the tunnel will be calcified and somewhat brittle and may be broken by opening it with force using a small hemostat. Some cutting will be necessary, with care taken to ensure that the tendon not be severed. The trochlear tunnel is firmly attached to the periosteum and may be loosened artifactually along with the periosteum. The tendon

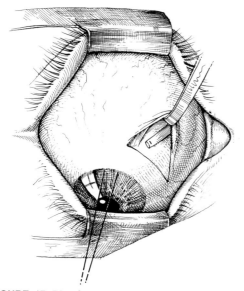

FIGURE 17–70. The transposition of the tendon of the superior oblique to the medial side of the superior rectus muscle insertion. Excess superior oblique tendon has been excised.

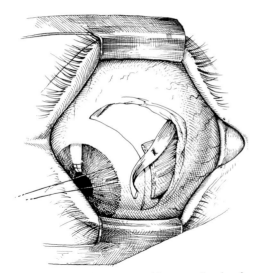

FIGURE 17–72. The superior oblique tendon has been removed from the trochlea, allowing the muscle to be brought anteriorly and inferiorly so that the muscle can be sutured to the medial rectus insertion.

can be pulled down in such a case, but with time it will be drawn back to its position with the periosteum, thereby producing a bad result.

Meticulous cutting will eventually free the tendon from the trochlear tunnel. Once this is done the superior oblique tendon will be free to be brought down to lie along the superior border of the medial rectus (Fig. 17–72). The conjunctival incision should be extended to allow isolation of the medial rectus. The medial rectus is resected 6 mm, and the superior oblique is incorporated in the figure-of-eight reattachment of the medial rectus. The superior oblique should have been sufficiently free to permit the muscle tissue to be attached to the globe and the entire tendon of the superior oblique excised. The conjunctiva is closed with 7-0 black silk interrupted sutures. At the end of surgery the eye should be in 10 degrees adduction.

Intraoperative Problems

Intraoperative problems can largely be avoided if the suggestions given under each procedure are followed. However, irrespective of the skill, care, and knowledge of the surgeon, some of the following problems will become evident if sufficient strabismus surgery is done.

Anatomical Variations. Anatomical variations in the extraocular musculature are reasonably rare. When variations are seen check the land-marks mentioned under Anatomy in this chapter to be absolutely sure that the intended area is being inspected. If possible, take photographs. If a camera is not available, make careful sketches, interrupting the procedure if necessary to confirm or make the sketches. If the muscle is thought to be absent and this absence conforms to the ocular movements, proceed as if the muscle were completely paralyzed, recess its antagonist, and plan appropriate transpositions. When the muscle is found to be extremely large and forming a syncytium, it is usually a vestige of the retractor bulbi and can be fashioned to approximate a muscle, but will act poorly. Most variations are iatrogenic, stemming from the prior surgery. Careful charting of each surgical procedure will prevent most surprises.

Lost Muscles. The losing of muscles during surgery can come about in ways varying from cutting the muscle on the wrong side of the clamp to a broken suture. Whatever the cause the net effect is the same: the muscle is seen to suddenly retract into the tissues. Often as the muscle starts to slip away it can be grasped and no further significant problems occur. Once the muscle has disappeared, however, the rule to be followed is to "do no harm." If the muscle is frantically searched for, not only will it not be found, but also the orbital fat pockets will be invaded and a frozen orbit may result. When the muscle has slipped out of sight one should stop for a moment to be sure adequate retractors are available. Place an additional fixation suture in the insertional stump on the globe. Remove the lid speculum and replace it with lid sutures. If the procedure has been attempted through a small conjunctival opening, enlarge that incision. Rotate the globe maximally away from the muscle being sought. If the medial rectus has been lost, fully abduct the eye with the suture that has been placed in the insertion of the medial rectus. Use 6- or 16-mm malleable retractors to give adequate exposure of the more superficial tissues. Typically the muscle sheath opening can be seen, and by holding this open the cut end of the muscle will be apparent. Do not look back along the globe itself, for that is not the usual direction of the muscle. Recall that once the greater circumference of the globe is passed as the muscle goes posteriorly, the muscle is headed for the orbital apex, which is almost directly posterior for the medial rectus, nasal for the lateral rectus, inferior for the superior rectus, and superior for the inferior rectus.

If the maneuver above is not successful,

extend the dissection in the direction you estimate to be the path of the muscle. When tissue has been identified tentatively as muscle, it may be verified by its appearance, or by having the anesthesiologist give succinylcholine and note the contraction or the use of an electrical stimulus. If no muscle stimulator is present, the Bovie cautery will cause muscle to contract. A nerve stimulator is useless, as the electrical power is too low to cause a muscle contraction.[51–53]

If the muscle cannot be found, a stay suture should be used to fix the globe in the position of full contraction of the lost muscle (e.g., full adduction if a medial rectus is lost). Such a stay suture should be scleral, with bites taken of the insertion of the vertical recti. The sutures are passed through the conjunctiva and lids, to be tied over cotton bolsters. The eye should remain in that position for 2 weeks. If no function is present after that period, the deviation should be treated as any completely palsied muscle—that is, with a crippling recession of its antagonist and transposition of the appropriate two adjacent rectus muscles.

Muscles lost at the time of previous surgery are sought in the manner just described. Hemostasis is difficult but must be complete. Care in dissection is just as important here as in the first instance because a frozen orbit can be created with the reoperation even more easily than at the original surgery. In addition to looking for the lost muscle in the locations that seem logical, look along the globe surface as well. If the original surgeon did not use stay sutures, the muscle may have reattached itself to the globe quite posteriorly and will be seen as a round mass. It may insert so far posteriorly that the use of an indirect ophthalmoscope is necessary to localize the site of insertion to be sure the tissue does not include the optic nerve.

In both the primary and secondary searches for the lost muscle, the blind grasping and suturing of unidentified tissues to the globe is not useful, and only contributes to a frozen orbit.

Bleeding. Excessive bleeding is usually the result of making blind deep incisions without providing consecutive control of blood vessels in each plane of tissue. The only recourse when this occurs is to use suction and sponging to clear the field and cauterize the bleeding points. The wet-field cautery is occasionally particularly helpful in that continuous irrigation will make the bleeding vessel visible for use of that cautery. If bleeding is a frequent problem with a surgeon, careful assessment of technique is in order. A primary case should bleed little if the appropriate surgical planes have been developed. Excessive bleeding may be venous, and if so, the anesthesiologist should be queried as to whether there was any pressure in the airway system during the expiratory phase. It is not uncommon for the anesthesiologist to unwittingly apply some pressure to the bag throughout this phase, and if this is the case, the venous pressure will build up and manifest itself by excessive bleeding. This is the usual reason for bleeding to be a problem when only "certain" anesthetists or anesthesiologists administer the anesthesia.

Scleral Perforation. Scleral perforation has become rare with the use of small flat spatula needles. The size and shape of the needles permit them to perforate the sclera without causing retinal holes. If perforation is suspected, the pupil should be dilated and the site of the suspected perforation inspected. If no retinal holes are present, no treatment is necessary. If a tiny hole is seen, cryotherapy should be applied. Only if a retinal tear is present should scleral buckling be considered. If vitreous loss is encountered, the wound should be closed with a mattress suture. The fundus should be evaluated and the wound treated with an implant and diathermy if retinal holes with vitreous traction are found. If the wound is in the pars plana, simple closure of the wound with careful follow-up will suffice.[54, 55]

Operation of the Wrong Eye. In many cases in which the wrong eye was operated on, the patient will often actually be benefited. For instance, if the surgery was planned to be done on the more frequently deviating eye, the postoperative temporary astigmatism associated with strabismus surgery may encourage further use of the nonpreferred eye with further treatment of any amblyopia. The main problem in such cases, then, is that of properly explaining the situation to the patient's parents, and assuring them that there is no cause for concern. Obviously, if the wrong eye is operated in a paralytic strabismus patient, then the patient may require further surgery, but even here, if the surgery was a horizontal recess-resect, the patient may benefit significantly from such a procedure.

Performance of the Wrong Procedure. If the wrong procedure has been done, such as recessing the lateral rectus and resecting the medial recti, the operation should be redone as soon as the surgeon becomes aware of this mistake. Such an error typically becomes apparent to the surgeon as the second muscle is being resected. If the muscle has not been resected, it should be recessed and the other muscle resected. If the second muscle has already been resected, it should be recessed 2 mm more than the amount that is maximal for good function. With the technique described in this chapter good function can be expected with recession of the lateral recti 10 mm, the medial recti 6 mm, the inferior recti 5 mm, and the superior recti 6 mm. The muscle that was recessed, but should have been resected, is redone and resected 1 mm less than the planned amount.

Operation of the Wrong Muscle. Surgery on the wrong muscle, such as on an inferior rectus instead of medial rectus, creates severe problems and should be corrected as soon as the surgeon realizes his mistake. If that realization occurs during surgery, the correction should be made then—in other words, the sooner, the better.

Postoperative Problems

Postoperative problems with strabismus surgery are typically few and trivial; most can be minimized with good patient communication regarding what the patient should expect as to discomfort, redness, discharge, vision, and position of the eyes.

The four most common types of postoperative problems are discussed in more detail below.

Decreased Muscle Function. Minimal eye muscle function may mimic or indicate a slipped muscle. If the muscle has been stretched a lot during surgery, the function will slowly return over a week or so. Often the patient will "splint" eye movements because of discomfort, and this, too, may mimic a slipped muscle. Remember that ocular vestibular stimulation is a powerful driving force for eye position. Sudden repositioning of the head will drive the muscle to the opposite side, and a decision can then be made as to whether the muscle is functioning. If splinting is severe, wait an hour and retest the patient. Velocity studies are usually not necessary, since *any* function—not reduced function—is the question at hand. If, after consideration of the possibilities above, you are forced to conclude that the muscle has slipped, exploration is indicated, and the muscle should be searched for in the manner described for the same muscle lost during surgery. The muscle slippage typically occurs during the first 24 hours after surgery, but occasionally will happen as long as 4 weeks later. Whenever slippage occurs intervention is necessary.

Allergic Reactions. Allergic reactions seldom occur with the techniques described here, particularly if nonabsorbing sutures are used on the muscle and silk on the conjunctiva. Absorbable sutures made of synthetic material cause infrequent reactions. The redness of the eye with such sutures is more commonly due to the rough wirelike ends of those sutures, which either have been placed in the conjunctiva or have eroded through the conjunctiva. Catgut sutures frequently cause reactions. The severity of the reaction may vary and is not related to the expected duration. If a reaction is due to catgut, repeat use of catgut will predictably cause a similar, if not severer, reaction. The treatment is topical corticosteroids.

Infection. Infections are rare after strabismus surgery. Estimates of 1 case per 2000 operations would seem reasonable. The principal problem is distinguishing the infection from an allergic suture reaction. The latter is self-limiting and causes no long-term problem, whereas the infection, if not treated, can result in loss of sight. Pain is a distinguishing factor, as well as localized tenderness. If an infection is thought to be present, the patient should be surgically explored and the suture (or any other foreign material) removed and cultured. No fear as to muscle slippage is justified. The reaction will easily hold the muscle in place. Removal of the suture accompanied by appropriate systemic antibiotics will result in a prompt cure. If, however, procrastination has led to an endophthalmitis, a poor visual result, which spares enucleation, may be the best that can be hoped for. Because with an endophthalmitis the prognosis for good vision is poor, any suspicion that an infection is developing should cause prompt treatment as outlined above.

Overcorrections or Undercorrections. Large overcorrections or undercorrections may cause considerable consternation in the patient, family members, and surgeon, but must be expected to occur occasionally. Once the possibility of a slipped muscle is ruled out, the usual treatment for undercorrections and overcorrections (e.g., alternate occlusion, spectacles, prisms, and miotics) is begun as appropriate. Do not immediately return the patient to surgery, as in some of these patients there will be a reduction of this untoward result without surgical manipulation.

Postoperative Care

Usual postoperative care in the hospital includes application of an antibiotic solution topically at the conclusion of surgery. Patches are never applied to both eyes, as they are unnecessary and produce severe anxiety in some patients. Most patients complain if any pressure is applied to the patch. Because pressure to prevent swelling is the only justification for a patch, patches are seldom used. Instructions are given for home care. Any nausea and vomiting from general anesthesia are controlled with systemic medication before discharge.

Home care instructions include how to place antibiotic ointment in the operated eye(s) at bedtime and antibiotic solutions in the morning. Foreign-body sensation is emphasized as usual, but any severe pain should prompt at least a telephone call. The patient should be encouraged to engage in normal activities as soon as possible, except for swimming, which should not be done for 10 days after the operation. The patient is given an appointment for 3 to 5 days post operation for examination, and is seen subsequently as necessary for follow-up treatment of eye position, amblyopia, and fusion.

REFERENCES

1. Wolff, E.: Anatomy of the Eye and Orbit. 7th ed. Revised by R. Warwick. Philadelphia, W. B. Saunders Co., 1976, pp. 248–274.
2. Duke-Elder, W. S. (ed.): System of Ophthalmology. Vol. VI: Ocular Motility and Strabismus. St. Louis, C. V. Mosby Co., 1973, pp. 3–28.
3. Parks, M. M.: Ocular Motility and Strabismus. Hagerstown, Md., Harper & Row, 1975, pp. 1–12.
4. Rife, C. J.: Pleoptics by the indirect ophthalmoscope. Arch. Ophthalmol., 73:607, 1965.
5. Helveston, E. M.: Atlas of Strabismus Surgery. 2nd ed. St. Louis, C. V. Mosby Co., 1977.
6. Quigley, H.: Mortality associated with ophthalmic surgery. A 20 year experience at the Wilmer Institute. Am. J. Ophthalmol., 77:517, 1979.
7. Duncalf, D., Gartner, S., Carol, B.: Mortality associated with ophthalmic surgery. Am. J. Ophthalmol., 69:610, 1970.
8. Gartner, S., Billet, E.: A study on mortality rates during general anesthesia for ophthalmic surgery. Am. J. Ophthalmol., 45:847, 1958.
9. Ap, L., Isenberg, S., Gaffney, W. L.: The oculocardiac reflex in strabismus surgery. Am. J. Ophthalmol., 76:533, 1973.
10. Stephens, K. F., Reinecke, R. D.: Quantitative forced ductions. Trans. Am. Acad. Ophthalmol. Otolaryngol., 71:324, 1967.
11. Parks, M. M.: Early operations for strabismus. Transactions of the First Congress of the International Strabismological Association, London, 1971, pp. 29–36.
12. Breinin, G. M.: Accommodative strabismus and the AC/A ratio. Am. J. Ophthalmol., 71:303, 1971.
13. Cunningham, R. D.: Divergence paralysis. Am. J. Ophthalmol., 74:630, 1972.
14. Knapp, P.: Vertically incomitant horizontal strabismus: The so-called "A" and "V" syndrome. Trans. Am. Ophthalmol. Soc., 57:666, 1959.
15. von Noorden, G. K.: Nystagmus compensation syndrome. Am. J. Ophthalmol., 82:283, 1976.
16. Burian, H. M.: Exodeviations: Their classification, diagnosis and treatment. Am. J. Ophthalmol., 62:1161, 1966.
17. Burian, H., Spivey, B.: The surgical management of exodeviations. Am. J. Ophthalmol., 59:603, 1965.
18. Cooper, E. L.: The surgical management of secondary exotropia. Trans. Am. Acad. Ophthalmol. Otolaryngol., 65:595, 1961.
19. Ernest, J. T., Costenbader, F. D.: Lateral rectus muscle palsy. Am. J. Ophthalmol., 65:721, 1968.
20. Jensen, C. D. F.: Rectus muscle union: A new operation for paralysis of the rectus muscles. Trans. Pacific Coast Otolaryngol. Ophthalmol. Soc., 45:359, 1964.
21. Helveston, E. M.: Muscle transposition procedures. Surv. Ophthalmol., 16:92, 1971.
22. Uribe, L. E.: Muscle transplantation in ocular paralysis. Am. J. Ophthalmol., 65:600, 1968.
23. von Noorden, G. K.: Anterior segment ischemia following the Jensen procedure. Arch. Ophthalmol., 94:845, 1976.
24. Duane, A.: Congenital deficiency of abduction associated with impairment of adduction retraction movements, contraction of the palpebral fissure and oblique movements of the eye. Arch. Ophthalmol., 34:133, 1905.
25. Huber, A.: Duane's retraction syndrome: Consideration of pathogenesis and aetiology of the different forms of Duane's retraction syndrome. *In* Hugonnier, R., Hugonnier, S. (eds.): Strabismus, Heterophoria, Ocular Motor Paralysis: Clinical Ocular Muscle Imbalance. St. Louis, C. V. Mosby Co., 1969, p. 36.
26. Scott, A. B., Wong, G. Y.: Duane's syndrome. Arch. Ophthalmol., 87:140, 1972.
27. Reinecke, R. D.: Surgical results of third cranial nerve palsies. N.Y. State J. Med., 72:1255, 1972.
28. Knapp, P.: Paretic squints. *In* Transactions of the New Orleans Academy of Ophthalmology: Symposium on Strabismus. St. Louis, C. V. Mosby Co., 1978, pp. 252–253.
29. Knapp, P.: The surgical treatment of double elevator paralysis. Trans. Am. Ophthalmol. Soc., 67:304, 1969.
30. Braverman, D. E., Scott, W. E.: Surgical correction of dissociated vertical deviations. J. Pediatr. Ophthalmol., 14:337, 1977.
31. Crawford, J. S.: Surgical treatment of true Brown's syndrome. Am. J. Ophthalmol., 81:289, 1976.
32. Scott, A. B., Knapp, P.: Surgical treatment of superior oblique tendon sheath syndrome. Arch. Ophthalmol., 88:282, 1972.
33. Reinecke, R. D.: The figure of eight suture for eye muscle surgery. Ophthalmol. Digest, 34:22, 1972.
34. von Noorden, G. K.: The limbal approach to surgery of the rectus muscles. Arch. Ophthalmol., 80:94, 1968.
35. von Noorden, G. K.: Modification of the limbal approach to surgery of the rectus muscles. Arch. Ophthalmol., 82:349, 1969.
36. Parks, M. M.: Fornix incision for horizontal rectus muscle surgery. Am. J. Ophthalmol., 65:907, 1968.
37. Dunlap, F. A.: Survey of sutures used in strabismus surgery. Am. J. Ophthalmol., 74:625, 1972.
38. Thompson, W. E., Reinecke, R. D.: The changes in refractive state following routine strabismus surgery.

Fifth Annual Ped. Ophthalmol. Symposium, Toronto, Canada, 1979.

39. Cole, J. G., Cole, H. G.: Recession of the conjunctiva in complicated eye muscle operations. Am. J. Ophthalmol., 53:618, 1962.

40. Parks, M. M.: Rectus muscle surgery. *In* Parks, M. M. (ed.): Atlas of Strabismus Surgery. Philadelphia, Harper & Row, 1983.

41. Nelson, L. B., Wagner, R. S., Calhoun, J. H.: The adjustable suture technique in strabismus surgery. Int. Ophthal. Clin., 25:4, 1985.

42. Viller, J. E.: Vertical recti transplantation in the A and V syndromes. Arch. Ophthalmol., 64:175, 1960.

43. Goldstein, J. H.: Monocular vertical displacement of the horizontal rectus muscles in the A and V patterns. Am. J. Ophthalmol., 64:265, 1967.

44. Reinecke, R. D.: Surgical management of third and sixth cranial nerve palsies. Int. Ophthal. Clin., 25:4, 1985.

45. Cuppers, C.: The so-called "Faden operation." *In* Fells, P. (ed.): The Second Congress of the International Strabismological Association. Paris-Marseille, Division Générale de Librairie, 1976.

46. Scott, A. B.: Active force tests in lateral rectus paralysis. Arch. Ophthalmol., 85:397, 1971.

47. Helveston, E. M., Cofield, D. D.: Indications for marginal myotomy and technique. Am. J. Ophthalmol., 70:574, 1970.

48. Parks, M. M.: The weakening surgical procedures for eliminating overreaction of the inferior oblique muscle. Am. J. Ophthalmol., 73:107, 1972.

49. Parks, M. M., Helveston, E. M.: Direct visualization of the superior oblique tendon. Arch. Ophthalmol., 84:491, 1970.

50. Peter, L. C.: The use of the superior oblique as an internal rotator in third nerve paralysis. Am. J. Ophthalmol., 17:297, 1934.

51. Isenberg, S. J., Ap, L.: The oculocardiac reflex as a surgical aid in identifying a slipped or "lost" extraocular muscle. Fifth Annual Ped. Ophthalmol. Symposium, Toronto, Canada, 1979.

52. Rosenbaum, A. L., Metz, H. S.: Diagnosis of lost or slipped muscle by saccadic velocity measurements. Am. J. Ophthalmol., 77:215, 1974.

53. Scott, A. B.: Disinserted extraocular muscles. Am. J. Ophthalmol., 79:289, 1975.

54. McLean, J. M., Galin, M., Baras, I.: Retinal perforation during strabismus surgery. Am. J. Ophthalmol., 50:1167, 1960.

55. Havener, W. H., Kimball, O. P.: Scleral perforation in strabismus surgery. Am. J. Ophthalmol., 50:807, 1960.

18

THERAPEUTIC APPROACHES TO INTRAOCULAR TUMORS*

by Jerry A. Shields

This chapter considers current modalities for the management of intraocular tumors, with emphasis on their application to specific types of tumor.[1]

GENERAL CONSIDERATIONS

Diagnosis

Tumors in the eye present special diagnostic problems. Because the treatment of an intraocular mass may vary considerably with the type of tumor, it is important to establish an accurate diagnosis before proceeding with therapy. The use of indirect ophthalmoscopy has greatly improved the clinician's ability to diagnose tumors accurately, especially when combined with ancillary studies such as trans-

illumination, fluorescein angiography, ultrasonography, the radioactive phosphorus uptake (^{32}P) test, and needle biopsy in selected cases.[1-4]

Management

Important considerations in making a therapeutic decision include the type of tumor, whether it is benign or malignant, the location of the lesion, the age of the patient, the health of the patient, and the condition of the opposite eye. In general, benign tumors are managed more conservatively than malignant lesions. Tumors located near the fovea or the optic disc that have produced visual loss are often managed differently from asymptomatic lesions located in the peripheral fundus. Treatment is often deferred for older or chronically ill patients or for patients who have a tumor in their only useful eye.

Newly developed methods of treatment have improved management of intraocular tumors. In the past the generally accepted management of malignant tumors was enucleation of the

---

*Most of the material in this chapter is modified from Shields, J. A.: Intraocular Tumors, St. Louis, C. V. Mosby Co., 1983.

involved eye. There was no satisfactory treatment for benign tumors; consequently these sometimes caused significant visual loss. Improved therapeutic modalities such as irradiation, photocoagulation, cryotherapy, and better surgical techniques, combined with new knowledge regarding the biological behavior of certain tumors, have resulted in a variety of reasonable therapeutic alternatives. Depending on the overall clinical situation, a particular tumor can now be managed by simple observation, photocoagulation, radiotherapy, cryotherapy, local resection, enucleation, orbital exenteration, chemotherapy, or immunotherapy.[1, 5–7]

OBSERVATION

There are a number of instances in which simple periodic observation of an intraocular tumor is justified. Most benign lesions, for example, have little or no tendency to grow and no potential to metastasize. Examples of benign conditions that do not usually require treatment include uveal nevi, congenital hypertrophy of the retinal pigment epithelium, and retinal astrocytomas. Some benign tumors, however, are more likely to require treatment because of visual symptoms. The capillary hemangioma of the retina and the cavernous hemangioma of the choroid are examples of benign tumors that may require treatment.

In most instances some form of treatment other than simple observation is appropriate for malignant intraocular tumors. In recent years, however, it has been recognized that certain small malignant lesions, particularly small choroidal melanomas, may have little or no potential to cause local tissue damage or to metastasize. Consequently an increasing number of authorities are advocating only periodic observation of suspect nevi and small to medium-sized melanomas for evidence of change before initiating treatment.[7, 8]

If it is elected to observe an intraocular tumor periodically, records of baseline studies should be kept so that change may be detected in the future. Careful drawings, photography, fluorescein angiography, and ultrasonography may be useful. The ^{32}P test, which often involves a surgical procedure,[9] should not be performed if the clinician has decided to manage the lesion by periodic observation alone. It may provide useful information, however, in cases in which the differentiation between a benign and malignant tumor is difficult.

PHOTOCOAGULATION (XENON ARC AND LASER)

For more than 30 years, light has been used to treat certain intraocular lesions. The principle of such therapy is that light is absorbed by pigment and, in the process, light energy is converted to heat energy. When enough heat is generated to raise the temperature of the tissue to the point at which protein is coagulated, a thermal effect, or burn, is produced. This process is called photocoagulation.[10]

For ocular photocoagulation to be effective, it is necessary to have both a source of light, and pigment to absorb the light. The light sources for ophthalmic use include xenon arc tube and various types of laser (*Light Amplification by Stimulated Emission of Radiation*). The retinal pigment epithelium and the uveal pigment within the eye are ideal for the absorption of light. Examples of lesions that may be managed by photocoagulation include selected cases of choroidal melanoma, retinoblastoma, retinal capillary hemangioma, and choroidal hemangioma.

Choroidal Melanoma

Xenon arc photocoagulation and more recently the argon laser have been used to treat selected choroidal melanomas.[11]

Indications. My current indications for considering photocoagulation in the management of a choroidal melanoma are as follows: (1) the diagnosis should be suggested by indirect ophthalmoscopy, fluorescein angiography, and ultrasonography; (2) the lesion should show documentation of growth by serial fundus photographs or strong evidence of growth on the initial examination; and (3) the lesion should not exceed 10 mm in diameter or 3 mm in thickness as measured by A-scan ultrasonography.

There has been controversy as to whether photocoagulation should be used for lesions that are within 1 mm of the optic disc or foveola, or that have produced extensive retinal detachment. Use of photocoagulation is probably justified in selected situations, but the visual prognosis in such cases is guarded.

Technique. The patient's pupil should be widely dilated. Retrobulbar anesthesia is usually necessary when the melanoma is treated with xenon photocoagulation, but topical anesthesia will often be adequate when the argon

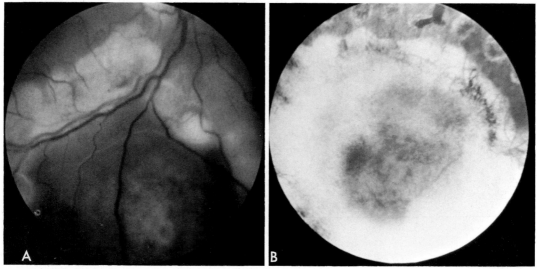

FIGURE 18–1. Photocoagulation of a choroidal melanoma. *A,* Photograph after initial treatment, showing photocoagulation burns around tumor. *B,* Photograph after final treatment, showing flat chorioretinal scar.

or krypton laser is used. With the latter lasers, a Goldmann fundus contact lens or a panfunduscope lens is applied to the patient's cornea. During the first session two rows of treatment are applied around the margins of the tumor in normal retina (Fig. 18–1*A*). With the argon laser one can use a spot size of 500 μm, with duration of 0.5 to 1.0 second, and power of 500 to 1000 mW. The intensity of treatment will necessarily vary with the degree of pigmentation of the fundus.

About 3 weeks later the same area is treated again, using similar settings. A third treatment, using similar settings, is applied to cover the tumor surface about 3 weeks after the second treatment. Subsequent treatments every 3 to 4 weeks should cover the tumor surface again. Between four and ten treatments are usually necessary to produce a circular area of scar tissue through which the yellow sclera is clearly visible, surrounding a dark central lesion (Fig. 18–1*B*). When this central pigmentation is hypofluorescent with fluorescein angiography, no further treatment is necessary. The residual central pigmentation generally regresses over the next 2 years.

Complications. Among the main complications of photocoagulation of choroidal melanomas are hemorrhage, iris damage, cystoid foveal edema, branch vascular obstruction, preretinal fibrosis, choroidovitreal fibroneovascularization, and tractional retinal detachment. Bleeding from photocoagulation can occur on the surface of the tumor, or in the retina or vitreous.

It most often occurs at the time of photocoagulation and usually resorbs within a few weeks.

Damage to the iris can occur at the time of photocoagulation, particularly if the pupil is not widely dilated. This can result in focal or sector iris atrophy and an irregular pupil secondary to damage to the sphincter or dilator muscles.

Cystoid foveal edema can develop after photocoagulation, particularly if the xenon arc is used. It may result from subclinical vitreous traction or from increased permeability of the perifoveal capillaries. Although the cystoid foveopathy may partially resolve, it can lead to permanent visual distortion.

Branch obstruction of a retinal artery or vein can occur after photocoagulation, particularly if a large vessel passes over the tumor being treated. The obstruction of a large retinal vein can lead to retinal or prepapillary neovascularization. Heavy treatment, particularly with xenon photocoagulation, can lead to preretinal fibrosis, which can result in a macular pucker. If Bruch's membrane is disrupted by heavy photocoagulation, choroidovitreal neovascularization can occur. This may lead to vitreoretinal traction and subsequent retinal detachment.

Retinoblastoma

Photocoagulation is the treatment of choice for selected small retinoblastomas.[12, 13] Because of its availability, xenon arc photocoagulation is most commonly used. It may be used either as

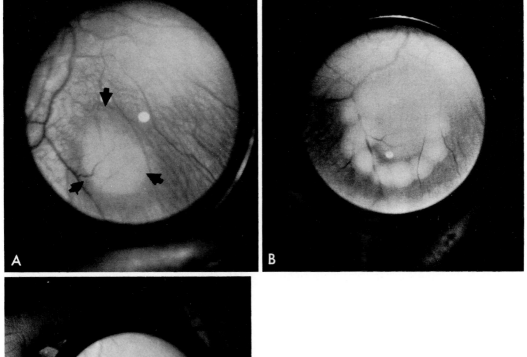

FIGURE 18–2. Photocoagulation of retinoblastoma. *A*, Pretreatment photograph showing small tumor (arrows). *B*, Photocoagulation burns around tumor. *C*, Final appearance, showing depressed scar but no evidence of viable tumor.

the primary treatment or, in cases that were initially treated with irradiation or cryotherapy, as a supplementary treatment. When administered properly, photocoagulation has fewer complications than does irradiation.

Indications. Photocoagulation is indicated for small tumors confined to the retina that do not involve the optic disc or the fovea (Fig. 18–2A). It is contraindicated if there is ophthalmoscopic evidence of vitreous seeding, choroidal invasion, or involvement of the fovea, optic disc, or pars plana. This technique will not eliminate tumor cells in the vitreous. It will not destroy tumor cells in the choroid, but it could possibly promote dissemination of the tumor in such

cases. If it is used on the optic disc or fovea, photocoagulation will result in marked visual loss. In such cases, irradiation is preferable.

Technique. A portable xenon arc photocoagulator, which can be transported to the operating room, is commonly used. One or two rows of confluent xenon burns should be placed around the tumor, using enough power to whiten the surrounding retina and close the retinal vessels that supply the tumor (Fig. 18–2B). The treatment should be heavy enough to obliterate the retinal vessels but not so heavy that it disrupts Bruch's membrane. Within a few weeks the tumor should regress into a depressed scar (Fig. 18–2C). It may be necessary to apply second and third treatments in some cases, waiting 3 to 4 weeks between sessions.

Complications. Significant complications of photocoagulation of retinoblastoma are not common. Vitreoretinal traction may lead to macular pucker or retinal detachment if treatment is too heavy. If Bruch's membrane is ruptured by heavy photocoagulation, choroidovitreal neovascularization may occur. Minor complications such as small retinal or vitreous hemorrhages at the time of treatment usually do not produce serious problems.

Retinal Capillary Hemangioma

Retinal capillary hemangioma (von Hippel's tumor) is a benign lesion that can lead to progressive retinal detachment, macular exudation, and profound visual loss. This tumor may be treated in selected cases with either argon laser or xenon photocoagulation.[14]

Indications. Photocoagulation of a retinal capillary hemangioma may be indicated when the tumor is less than 5 mm in diameter, has produced little or no retinal detachment, and is causing visual loss as a result of macular exudation.

Technique. There is some controversy as to the best technique for treating retinal capillary hemangioma with argon laser or xenon photocoagulation. Small tumors (less than 2 mm in diameter) can be managed by heavy photocoagulation directed to the entire tumor. If the tumor is larger than 3 mm in diameter, photocoagulation should be used to surround the tumor and encroach on the feeder vessels. It is important that the feeding arteriole be closed off first and the draining vein closed off at a later session. On subsequent sessions the tumor margins are encroached on, as are the feeder vessels. When the macular exudate and retinal detachment have resolved, no further treatment is necessary.

Complications. The complications of photocoagulation for retinal capillary hemangioma include hemorrhage, retinal detachment, and vitreoretinal traction. Hemorrhage can occur from direct treatment to the tumor surface or from obliteration of the feeder vein before closure of the artery.

The most common type of retinal detachment that can occur after photocoagulation for retinal capillary hemangioma is an exudative response known as ablatio fugax. This transitory detachment usually resolves spontaneously in a few weeks.

Vitreoretinal traction is uncommon after argon laser treatment but occurs more frequently when xenon arc photocoagulation is used.

Choroidal Hemangioma

Choroidal hemangiomas are benign vascular tumors that may produce visual loss as a result of a serous detachment of the fovea. Photocoagulation may help to resolve this detachment and improve the visual acuity.[15]

Indications. If a choroidal hemangioma is asymptomatic, treatment can usually be deferred. However, if there is a secondary retinal detachment that involves or threatens the fovea, photocoagulation is indicated (Fig. 18–3A).

Technique. The technique for photocoagulating a choroidal hemangioma differs considerably from that used for a choroidal melanoma or retinoblastoma. The procedure is to use argon laser photocoagulation over the entire hemangioma surface (Fig. 18–3B). The objective is to create a chorioretinal adhesion over the surface of the tumor, which prevents further accumulation of subretinal fluid and encourages resorption of the subretinal fluid already present. The treatment should be just intense enough to create a distinct burn on the surface of the tumor at the level of the retinal pigment epithelium (Fig. 18–3C). This usually requires a spot size of about 200 μm, a duration of about 0.2 to 0.5 second, and a power of about 200 to 500 mW, depending on the degree of fundus pigmentation and the amount of subretinal fluid over and around the tumor. It may be necessary to repeat the treatment on two or three occasions, at 3- to 4-week intervals.

Complications. The complications of photocoagulation of a choroidal hemangioma are similar to those resulting from photocoagulation of other tumors. If treatment is too heavy over the tumor surface, leading to rupture of Bruch's membrane, choroidal neovascularization with secondary exudation can occur. Because many choroidal hemangiomas are located near the fovea, contraction of the internal limiting membrane of the retina can lead to visual distortion.

RADIOTHERAPY

Although irradiation sometimes damages normal intraocular structures, certain intraocular tumors can be successfully treated with radiotherapy. These include selected malignant mel-

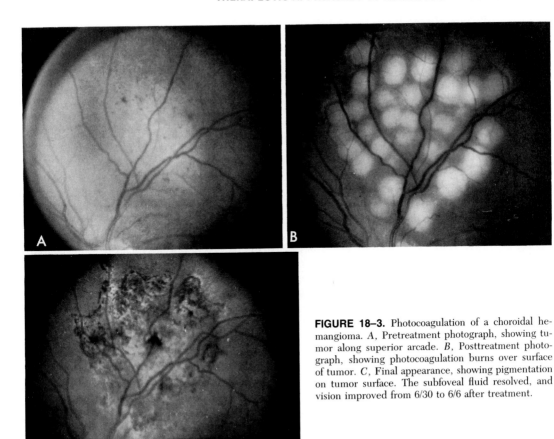

FIGURE 18–3. Photocoagulation of a choroidal hemangioma. *A*, Pretreatment photograph, showing tumor along superior arcade. *B*, Posttreatment photograph, showing photocoagulation burns over surface of tumor. *C*, Final appearance, showing pigmentation on tumor surface. The subfoveal fluid resolved, and vision improved from 6/30 to 6/6 after treatment.

anomas of the uveal tract, retinoblastomas, metastatic tumors to the uvea, and lymphoid tumors. The two methods of radiotherapy that are generally used for intraocular tumors are external beam irradiation and the local application of a scleral plaque.[16]

There are several methods for treating intraocular tumors with external beam irradiation, such as orthovoltage and supravoltage techniques. Orthovoltage has the ability to deliver radiation to the entire eye and may be more applicable for the diffuse neoplastic processes. Supravoltage, with use of a betatron or linear accelerator, has the advantage of a sharp beam and more precise focus, and is more applicable for isolated or solitary tumors.

More recently other methods such as helium ion irradiation and proton beam irradiation using a Bragg peak have been used.

Radioactive plaques are particularly suitable for retinoblastomas and malignant melanomas of the posterior uvea. My colleagues and I have recently used a variety of plaques, including cobalt-60, ruthenium-106, iridium-192, and io-

dine-125. These are manufactured in several shapes and sizes, depending on the type and size of the tumor.

Melanoma

Scleral Plaque Irradiation

Today most clinicians recommend a scleral plaque rather than external beam irradiation for treating posterior uveal melanomas.[16]

Indications. The indications for treating a choroidal melanoma with plaque radiotherapy are somewhat controversial. Until recently we routinely employed cobalt-60 for tumors greater than 7 mm in thickness, ruthenium-106 for tumors 5 to 7 mm in thickness, iridium-192 for tumors 3 to 5 mm in thickness, and iodine-125 for tumors 2 to 3 mm in thickness. More recently we have used more low energy plaques, particularly the iodine-125 plaques, for the majority of tumors. The patient should have either useful or salvageable vision in the involved eye. Tumors that are even larger can be treated with a plaque if the tumor is located in the patient's only useful eye.

Technique. As part of the preoperative evaluation, careful A-scan ultrasonography is performed to obtain the maximum height of the tumor. Because each plaque delivers a specific number of rad per hour, calculations can be made to determine the time necessary to deliver about 40,000 cGy to the base of the melanoma. Depending on the strength of the plaque and the thickness of the tumor, this may take from 3 to 10 days.

Insertion of the plaque may be done under local or general anesthesia (Fig. 18–4). A peritomy is performed and the quadrant of the tumor is exposed. The tumor is localized by either transillumination or indirect ophthalmoscopy, and superficial diathermy marks are placed on the sclera corresponding to its margins. A dummy plaque is then placed on the sclera precisely over the base of the tumor, and 4-0 nonabsorbable sutures on a spatula needle are aligned with the holes in the dummy plaque. Once the scleral sutures are aligned, the dummy plaque is removed and the radioactive plaque is positioned. The sutures are tied and cut, and the positioning of the plaque is rechecked. The conjunctiva is closed with interrupted 6-0 plain catgut sutures.

Postoperatively, the patient is kept in a private room. When approximately 40,000 cGy have been delivered to the base of the tumor, the patient is returned to the operating room and, usually under local anesthesia, the peritomy is opened. The sutures holding the plaque are exposed and cut, and the plaque is removed.

The conjunctiva is closed with 6-0 absorbable sutures. The patient is discharged on the same day and advised to use antibiotic drops three times daily.

Decrease in the size of the tumor is slow, but when the melanoma is sensitive to irradiation it should become markedly smaller 6 to 12 months after treatment (Fig. 18–5).

Complications. The most serious complications from a scleral plaque are radiation retinopathy and cataract. Radiation retinopathy is characterized by obliteration of retinal capillaries, telangiectasia, exudates, and superficial retinal hemorrhages. When the radiation retinopathy involves the optic disc or fovea, profound irreversible visual loss can result. Radiation retinopathy may become clinically apparent between 6 and 24 months after treatment. Although cataracts occur after irradiation of ciliary body melanomas, they appear to be relatively uncommon after therapy for choroidal melanomas.

Retinoblastoma

Retinoblastoma is more radiosensitive than the posterior uveal melanoma. This tumor can be treated with either external beam irradiation or scleral plaque irradiation.[1, 13, 17]

External Beam Irradiation

External beam irradiation is required when it is necessary to treat the entire globe with radiotherapy in order to sterilize the preexisting

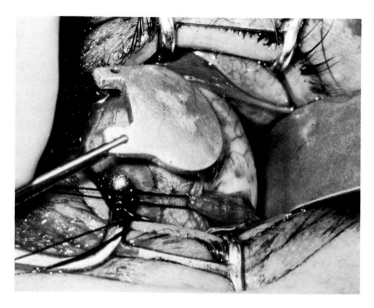

FIGURE 18–4. Insertion of radioactive plaque for treatment of a choroidal melanoma. The technique for treating retinoblastoma with a plaque is similar.

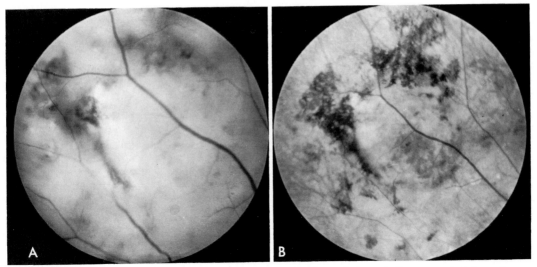

FIGURE 18–5. Response of choroidal melanoma to radioactive plaque therapy. *A*, Pretreatment photograph, showing tumor that measures 7 × 7 × 4 mm. *B*, Photograph of same lesion 6 months later. It is now flat, and the surrounding retinal detachment has resolved.

retinoblastoma and to prevent the occurrence of new tumors. With the advent and refinement of episcleral plaque radiotherapy,[17] my colleagues and I employ external beam irradiation less frequently today.

Indications. External beam irradiation is most frequently indicated for treatment of the second eye after the eye with the more advanced tumor has been enucleated. It is often used if the second eye has a large tumor filling more than one-third of the globe, if it has multiple tumors (Fig. 18–6*A*), or if extensive vitreous seeding of tumor cells is present. If there are moderately advanced tumors in both eyes with sparing of half of the retina, bilateral external beam irradiation may be justified.

External beam irradiation is also indicated if, after enucleation, the tumor is found histologically to extend into the optic nerve to the line of surgical transection. This method of treatment can also be used when there is orbital recurrence of the tumor.

Irradiation is probably contraindicated in cases in which the tumor fills the entire globe and is producing secondary glaucoma. Such eyes should generally be enucleated.

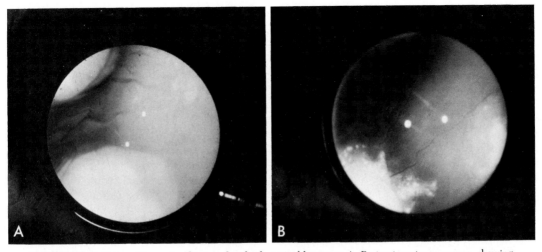

FIGURE 18–6. External beam irradiation of multiple retinoblastomas. *A*, Pretreatment appearance, showing large viable tumors. *B*, Same lesions 3 months after irradiation, showing shrunken, calcified masses.

Technique. For retinoblastoma the method of external beam irradiation most commonly used is a combined anterior and temporal portal approach with a linear accelerator, using gamma rays. Although 7000 to 8000 cGy were previously used, it is now believed that 3500 to 4000 cGy delivered in divided doses over a 3-week period is the treatment of choice. The anterior portal technique involves a greater risk of producing a radiation-induced cataract but does provide irradiation to the ora serrata region. The temporal portal approach is less likely to produce a cataract, but it may miss the anterior aspects of the retina, especially on the nasal side.

A successfully treated retinoblastoma usually appears as a shrunken white retinal mass (Fig. 18–6B). There may be pigmentary alterations and scar tissue around the regressed tumor. Three patterns of regression after irradiation of retinoblastoma are recognized.[13] Type I is characterized by a white calcified mass that resembles cottage cheese. Type II has a pink translucent appearance that resembles fish flesh. It may be extremely difficult ophthalmoscopically to differentiate type II regression from residual viable tumor. Type III represents a combination of types I and II.

Complications. The main complications of external beam irradiation for retinoblastoma are radiation retinopathy and cataract. Radiation retinopathy is characterized by telangiectasia, retinal edema, exudate, and disappearance of the small retinal vessels, which may lead to preretinal neovascularization and vitreous hemorrhage from 6 months to several years after treatment. In some cases the retinal vessels appear to be highly sensitive to irradiation, and extensive vascular shutdown can occur. Other complications include a dry eye, a sunken orbit with atrophy of the temporal fossa, and optic atrophy.

Perhaps the most important long-term complication of external irradiation is the development of a radiation-induced tumor. Radiation-induced orbital sarcomas, usually in the field of irradiation, are the most common, but other malignancies such as lymphomas and leukemias have also been recognized. The incidence of such tumors has greatly decreased since the radiation dose was reduced from 8000 to 3500 cGy. More recently the development of new tumors distant from the site or irradiation has been noted,[17] and neoplasms have also been recognized in patients who had no irradiation.[18] It is known that patients with bilateral retinoblastoma have a greater chance of developing a number of other malignancies later in life.

Scleral Plaque Irradiation

An alternative method of irradiation for retinoblastoma is the application of a radioactive scleral plaque. Any of the plaques described for melanomas can also be used for selected retinoblastomas.

Indications. Radioactive plaques were initially used for retinoblastomas between 6 and 15 mm in diameter and located at least 3 mm from the optic disc or the fovea (Fig. 18–7A). This treatment was used for such tumors in unilateral cases or for treatment of the second eye in bilateral cases. Recurrent or residual tumors that have been uncontrolled with external beam irradiation, photocoagulation, or cryotherapy can also be treated by this method.

More recently, we have employed the technique of sequential paired opposing plaques (rotating plaques) when the retinoblastoma has severe vitreous seeds, for multiple tumors, and for some solitary tumors in the macular area. Radiation oncologists believe that this technique may entail fewer complications in selected cases.

Technique. The tumor to be treated is carefully localized with indirect ophthalmoscopy. By means of scleral depression with a diathermy tip, the sclera is lightly marked 1 mm outside the margins of the tumor. A dummy plaque is then sutured over the base of the tumor, using the technique previously described for a malignant melanoma. In the case of retinoblastoma only about 3000 to 4000 cGy are delivered to the apex of the tumor.

With the more recently used paired opposing plaque technique, two shielded iodine-125 plaques are applied in the equatorial region of the eye and subsequently moved to the two remaining quadrants. This technique permits irradiation to the intraocular structures but minimizes irradiation to the surrounding orbital tissues.

Most tumors show a dramatic response to irradiation. Shrinkage occurs within the first 3 weeks after removal of the plaque (Fig. 18–7B). The regression patterns that are noted are similar to those seen with external beam irradiation.

Complications. The complications of radioactive plaque therapy, such as cataract and radiation retinopathy, are the same as those that occur with external beam irradiation. Although it is a rare complication, scleral necrosis may occur at the site of the plaque after many months. It is uncertain, however, whether radiation-induced sarcomas occur after radioactive plaque therapy. As more follow-up becomes available, it is possible that such complications will appear.

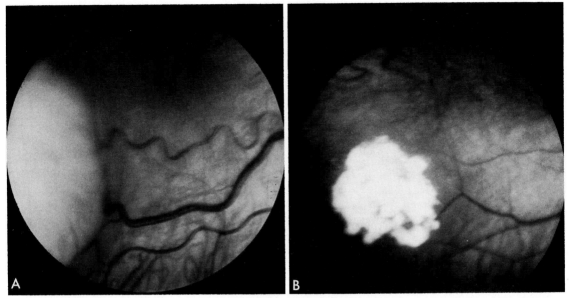

FIGURE 18–7. Radioactive plaque therapy of retinoblastoma. *A*, Pretreatment appearance of lesion temporal to macular area. *B*, Photograph of same lesion 4 months after radioactive plaque application, showing marked resolution of tumor.

Metastatic Tumors of the Uvea

Chemotherapy/External Beam Irradiation

Chemotherapy is the fundamental treatment for metastatic tumors to the uvea. In certain instances this may be combined with irradiation.[20]

Indications. About one half of metastatic tumors are either asymptomatic or are controlled systemically with chemotherapy alone. In such cases irradiation is usually withheld until visual symptoms occur. I believe that a metastatic tumor to the uvea should be treated with irradiation if it has caused visual loss either because of its location beneath the fovea or because of a retinal detachment that involves the fovea.

Technique. The technique for irradiating metastatic tumors to the uvea is external beam irradiation to the whole eye, usually through a lateral portal approach. About 3000 to 4000 cGy are delivered in divided doses over a 3-week period. The visual improvement after such treatment is often dramatic.

Complications. The complications of irradiating metastatic tumors are the same as those for other tumors that are radiated. In our experience there have been fewer complications with metastatic tumors than with treatment of choroidal melanoma or retinoblastoma. Many patients do not survive long enough to develop the late complications of radiation therapy.

CRYOTHERAPY

Cryotherapy is of value in the management of selected intraocular tumors. It has been used in the treatment of retinal capillary hemangiomas and retinoblastomas. It is occasionally used for small peripheral choroidal melanomas.

Retinal Capillary Hemangioma

Indications. In selected cases of retinal capillary hemangioma, cryotherapy is the treatment of choice. A capillary hemangioma of the retina can be treated with cryotherapy if it is less than 6 mm in diameter and is producing a retinal detachment or exudation (Fig. 18–8). Lesions in the peripheral fundus can be treated without surgery, whereas those located more posteriorly may require a conjunctival incision to reach the tumor.

Technique. The cryotherapy technique for a retinal capillary hemangioma is to use the cryoprobe as a scleral depressor and to freeze the tumor while observing it with indirect ophthalmoscopy. If the tumor is less than 3 mm in diameter, it may be possible to freeze it completely with one application. However, when the tumor is greater than 3 mm in diameter sometimes it is impossible to accomplish this. The technique in these latter instances is to position the cryoprobe so that it covers the

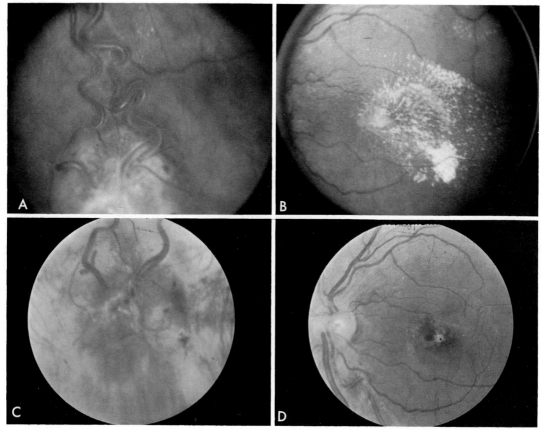

FIGURE 18–8. Capillary hemangioma of peripheral retina in a 13-year-old girl treated with several sessions of cryotherapy. *A,* Clinical photograph of tumor near the inferior equator of the left eye. *B,* Macular exudate, producing a vision of 6/60. *C,* Appearance of the lesion after treatment. *D,* Macular area, showing resolution of exudate after treatment. Vision returned to 6/9.

margin of the normal retina adjacent to the tumor. In either case, freezing should be applied until an ophthalmoscopically visible iceball envelops the tumor. It should be allowed to thaw for a few seconds and then should be refrozen. This cycle should be repeated three times. The patient is reexamined after 3 weeks, at which time the treatment may be repeated. The goal of treatment should be to obtain the best possible visual acuity and not necessarily to destroy the tumor totally. Thus, even if the tumor is not eradicated, one may withhold further treatment if the macular exudation is resolving.

Complications. The main complications of cryotherapy for retinal capillary hemangioma are hemorrhage and retinal detachment. Hemorrhage can occur at the time of cryotherapy as a sudden event; the retinal detachment (ablatio fugax) can occur several hours after treatment. In most cases both resolve spontaneously in a matter of weeks.

Retinoblastoma

Cryotherapy can be an effective method for eradicating small retinoblastomas.[13, 21] It is occasionally used as the primary treatment, but is more frequently used to supplement other treatment modalities. Cryotherapy has the advantage of preserving Bruch's membrane as well as the internal limiting membrane of the retina, which may be natural barriers to the spread of tumor cells into the choroid and vitreous, respectively. Cryotherapy should generally not be used if there are tumor cells in the choroid or in the vitreous cavity. In such instances plaque radiotherapy is usually more effective.

Indications. Cryotherapy is the primary treatment for small peripheral retinoblastomas located near the ora serrata. Sometimes it is used to treat residual or recurrent tumors in the peripheral fundus after incomplete eradication with external beam irradiation, provided there is no clinical evidence of vitreous seeding.

Technique. Cryotherapy for retinoblastoma should be administered by the triple freeze-thaw technique, which is similar to the technique used for treating retinal capillary hemangioma. With the cryoprobe used as a scleral depressor, the tumor is elevated on the tip, and freezing is applied until the surrounding retina turns white and ice crystals appear in the overlying vitreous. After freezing for 10 to 15 seconds the tumor is allowed to thaw. It is then immediately refrozen and the sequence is repeated. Three successive freeze-thaw applications are usually adequate. It may be necessary to repeat the treatment in 3 to 4 weeks if there is still ophthalmoscopic evidence of viable tumor.

Complications. The complications of cryotherapy for retinoblastoma are the same as those for treating retinal capillary hemangioma. Local vitreous hemorrhage can occur at the time of treatment, but this usually resolves within a few days to a few weeks.

DIATHERMY

Before the development of photocoagulation and cryotherapy, diathermy was used to treat selected cases of choroidal melanoma, retinal angioma, and certain other tumors. Because it involves considerable damage to the sclera, it is seldom used today. The only possible exception is retinal capillary hemangioma associated with a large retinal detachment. In such cases a scleral buckling procedure with penetrating diathermy to the angioma can be an effective method.[14]

IRIDECTOMY

Iridectomy removes a portion of the iris. A sector iridectomy, most commonly used to excise iris tumors, involves removal of a portion of the iris extending from the pupillary margin to the iris root. It is mainly used for selected cases of melanoma of the iris and is not commonly indicated for other iris tumors.

Indication. Most melanomas of the iris are relatively benign, slow growing or nongrowing tumors that pose no major threat to the patient's eye or life. If a suspicious iris tumor demonstrates unequivocal evidence of growth, however, an iridectomy may be justified. It may also be indicated for diffuse iris tumors with secondary glaucoma. In such cases the clinician may want to know whether the diffuse lesion is a nevus or a melanoma before making a therapeutic decision.

In rare instances it may be necessary to perform an iridectomy for a suspected metastatic tumor to the iris when no tissue diagnosis of metastatic disease has been established systemically.

Preoperative Care. There is little specific preoperative care before an iridectomy for an iris tumor. In cases with glaucoma, use of acetazolamide or osmotic agents to lower the intraocular pressure may be advisable.

Anesthesia. Local or general anesthesia may be used for iridectomy. If local anesthesia is used, one should give a facial and retrobulbar nerve block; mepivacaine 2% is an appropriate agent, followed by retrobulbar anesthesia. This may dilate the pupil somewhat, but it does not interfere with the surgical procedure. General anesthesia is preferable when the patient is unusually apprehensive or if there is a possible bleeding abnormality.

Technique. Use of the operating microscope is preferable for iridectomy and the other resection techniques to be discussed shortly. A peritomy is performed. A 180-degree corneoscleral limbal incision is made in the area of the tumor. This incision may be larger or smaller, depending on the anticipated size of the iridectomy; however, it is far better to err on the larger side than on the smaller. Preplaced sutures may be used. The cornea is retracted by means of a single suture through the corneal margin. Radial incisions are made in the iris on either side of the tumor (Fig. 18–9A). The lens must be meticulously avoided. The iris root is gently torn free or cut with the iridectomy scissors, and the specimen is gently removed (Fig. 18–9B). The preplaced corneoscleral sutures are then tied and additional corneoscleral sutures added in order to secure the wound. Any fine suture is appropriate, such as 9-0 virgin silk or 10-0 nylon. Removal of the tumor by this method leaves the patient with a keyhole-shaped pupil (Fig. 18–10).

The specimen is kept flat and allowed to dry on a thin piece of cardboard for a few minutes. It is then gently placed into 10% formalin solution. This prevents rolling or folding of the specimen and facilitates proper orientation for pathologic study.

Postoperative Care. The patient should be given a topical cycloplegic such as homatropine,

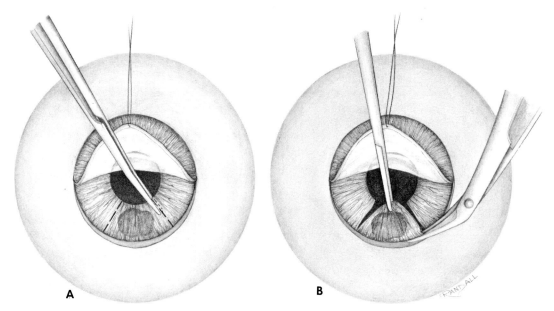

FIGURE 18–9. Technique of sector iridectomy for iris tumor. *A,* A limbal incision has been made for 180 degrees, and two radial cuts are made from the pupillary margin to the iris root (dotted lines). *B,* After the radial incisions are made, the iris is cut at its base to free it from the anterior portion of the ciliary body.

and a corticosteroid-antibiotic combination. The patient should be examined daily and is usually discharged on the second or third day. Intraocular pressure should be checked daily, especially if it has been elevated preoperatively. Timolol and the carbonic anhydrase inhibitors should be used when pressure control is required. The first postoperative visit is usually after 1 week. The patient is then seen monthly for 3 months. The topical medications can usually be discontinued in 1 to 2 weeks. Reevaluations should be made every 6 months to 1 year, and should include applanation tonometry, indirect ophthalmoscopy, slit-lamp biomicroscopy, and gonioscopy to look for recurrence of the tumor in the anterior chamber or in the angle.

Complications. The complications of iridec-

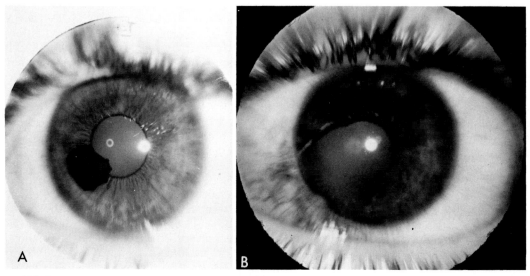

FIGURE 18–10. *A,* Iris tumor, which was documented to be changing in size. *B,* Postoperative appearance after sector iridectomy, showing keyhole-shaped pupil.

tomy include hemorrhage into the anterior chamber, iridodialysis, and, rarely, vitreous loss. The postoperative hyphema usually resolves in a few days. An iridodialysis is permanent but seldom causes problems unless it is extensive.

IRIDOCYCLECTOMY

Iridocyclectomy is the surgical removal of a portion of the iris and ciliary body.

Indications. The major indication for iridocyclectomy is a melanoma that involves the iris and ciliary body. The tumor should involve no more than 4 clock hours of the limbus. The treatment of tumors larger than 4 clock hours by iridocyclectomy usually leads to such poor visual results that enucleation or scleral plaque radiotherapy may be preferable. Occasionally tumors other than melanoma may also be appropriately treated with iridocyclectomy.

Preoperative Care. The preoperative care for iridocyclectomy is essentially the same as that for iridectomy. Because of the greater chance of vitreous loss, however, preoperative osmotic agents are usually used. Pressure on the eye to reduce the vitreous volume is *not* indicated because of the possibility of forcing tumor cells out of the eye.

Anesthesia. Either local (facial and retrobulbar block) or general anesthesia can be used for iridocyclectomy. I prefer general anesthesia because of the extended duration of the surgery.

Technique. Although there are several techniques for iridocyclectomy, the approach that is usually preferred on the Oncology Service at the Wills Eye Hospital is to make a fornix-based conjunctival flap and to locate the tumor by transillumination. A square or rectangular scleral flap involving four-fifths of the sclera is cut, allowing a 2-mm margin, if possible, around the tumor (Fig. 18–11A). This flap is dissected forward to the limbus. A second small flap is designed in the remaining sclera, and diathermy is placed on the remaining inner scleral fibers around the tumor. The anterior chamber is entered surgically at the limbus, and an iridectomy is performed by the method already described. Instead of cutting the iris at its root, however, the radial incisions are continued posteriorly into the inner flap of the sclera, including the inner wall of the sclera and the underlying ciliary body around the wall of the tumor (Fig. 18–11B). The iris and ciliary body containing the tumor are then removed *in one piece*.

The sclera is sutured with interrupted or running 5-0 Mersilene sutures (Fig. 18–11C). Fine sutures such as 9-0 or 10-0 nylon may be used. The handling of the specimen is the same as described for the iridectomy specimen.

Postoperative Care. The postoperative care for iridocyclectomy patients is the same as that for those who have undergone iridectomy. The patient should be followed more closely for a wound leak and hypotony because the scleral sutures can be relatively insecure.

Complications. The complications of iridocyclectomy include those that can occur with iridectomy—hemorrhage into the anterior chamber, iridodialysis, and vitreous loss. In addition, because of the more posterior incision, an iridocyclectomy is more likely to result in subluxation of the lens and vitreous hemorrhage. If the tumor extends to the ora serrata, an iridocyclectomy can result in retinal dialysis and detachment.

PENETRATING SCLEROUVEORETINOVITRECTOMY

Penetrating sclerouveoretinovitrectomy, also referred to as sclerochorioretinal resection (SCRR), or full-thickness eye wall resection, is a technique that has been used to remove melanomas of the peripheral choroid.[22, 23]

Indications. Some authorities believe that SCRR is never indicated, and that peripheral choroidal melanomas that show signs of growth should be managed by irradiation or enucleation. I have found it useful, however, in selected cases. The melanoma should be located in the peripheral choroid and should show evidence of growth. Findings of fluorescein angiography, ultrasonography, and the ^{32}P test should all be compatible with the diagnosis of malignant melanoma. In general, the tumor should not exceed 8 mm in diameter and 6 mm in thickness. There should be minimal retinal detachment, and the vitreous must be clear, to enable preoperative photocoagulation.

Preoperative Care. Preoperative care for SCRR includes dilation of the pupil with the mydriatic of choice and administration of topical corticosteroids.

Technique. SCRR requires preparatory photocoagulation or cryotherapy surrounding the lesion to provide a chorioretinal adhesion for 2 to 3 mm around the tumor. It may take from two to four treatment sessions to achieve a satisfactory result. Later, at the time of defini-

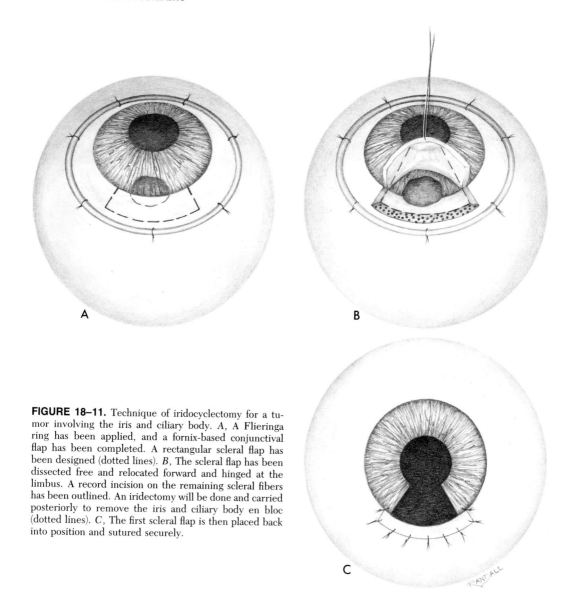

FIGURE 18–11. Technique of iridocyclectomy for a tumor involving the iris and ciliary body. *A,* A Flieringa ring has been applied, and a fornix-based conjunctival flap has been completed. A rectangular scleral flap has been designed (dotted lines). *B,* The scleral flap has been dissected free and relocated forward and hinged at the limbus. A record incision on the remaining scleral fibers has been outlined. An iridectomy will be done and carried posteriorly to remove the iris and ciliary body en bloc (dotted lines). *C,* The first scleral flap is then placed back into position and sutured securely.

tive surgery, a specially designed eye basket is used to stabilize the globe, with the ring of the basket sutured to the sclera outside the margins of the tumor (Fig. 18–12*A*).

Alternating cutting and diathermy are used to penetrate the sclera almost to the bare choroid around the tumor (Fig. 18–12*B*). A piece of sclera from a donor eye is cut to fit the defect where the eye wall is to be removed. The choroid is then cut gently and the full-thickness eye wall is removed, including the sclera, the choroidal tumor, and the retina. A vitrectomy is performed through the defect, using any of the standard vitrectomy instruments, and the

scleral graft is sutured into the defect with permanent 4-0 or 5-0 sutures (such as Mersilene) (Fig. 18–12*C*). Postoperative ophthalmoscopy reveals a clear view of the scleral graft and the surrounding photocoagulation (Fig. 18–12*D*).

Postoperative Care. The patient should be given sub-Tenon's antibiotics (gentamicin, 20 mg) and corticosteroids (Celestone, 3 mg or similar), which should be supplemented by topical antibiotics and corticosteroids. Carbonic anhydrase inhibitors may be given daily. A daily slit-lamp examination should be performed and the intraocular pressure measured. About 3

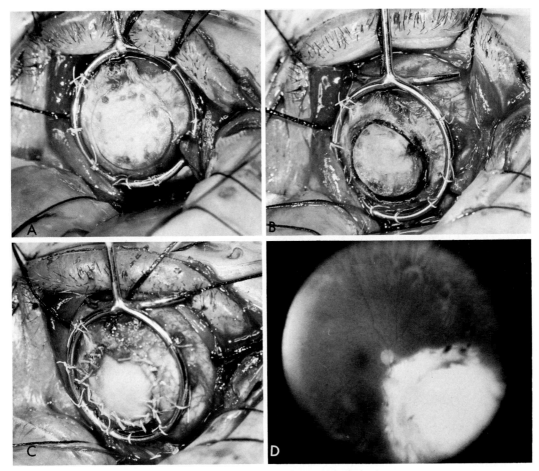

FIGURE 18–12. Technique and results of eye wall resection for choroidal melanoma. The choroidal tumor had been previously surrounded by photocoagulation. *A*, Eye basket sutured in place; diathermy marks the margins of the tumor, and a round scleral incision is made 1.5 mm outside the tumor. *B*, The scleral incision has been extended to the choroid. *C*, The eye wall containing the tumor has been removed, and a scleral graft has been applied to fill the defect. *D*, Postoperative appearance taken with wide-angle lens. Note that the scleral graft occupies most of the inferonasal quadrant, and the disc and macula are not altered.

days after surgery the patient is discharged with orders of restricted activities.

Complications. There are many potential complications of SCRR for choroidal melanomas. Because preoperative photocoagulation is necessary, all of the complications of photocoagulation can also occur. If xenon photocoagulation is used, there is a high incidence of cystoid foveal edema.

Operative complications include vitreous hemorrhage and retinal detachment. They are most likely to occur when one is cutting through the area of previous photocoagulation. Postoperative complications include vitreoretinal fibrosis, tractional retinal detachment, cataract, and anterior segment ischemia.

LAMELLAR SCLEROUVECTOMY

My colleagues and I have recently modified our technique of resecting posterior uveal melanomas. Instead of performing a full-thickness eye wall resection (SCRR), we have used a modification of the technique popularized by Stallard and Foulds, which I call a partial lamellar sclerouvectomy.[24] The indications, complications, and postoperative care are similar to those of SCRR described above, and the details of the technique have been enumerated in a recent article.[24] Therefore, only a summary of the technique is discussed and shown here.

Technique

A lid speculum is inserted and a conjunctival peritomy is made at the limbus for 360 degrees. The rectus muscles are gently hooked and isolated with 4-0 black silk traction sutures. All episcleral blood vessels are cauterized until bare sclera is exposed over a wide area in the quadrant of the tumor.

Transillumination is performed by placing a bright focal light against the sclera on the side of the eye exactly opposite the tumor. The margins of the tumor are outlined on the sclera with a sterile marking pencil. At this point note should be taken of the location of the insertion of the adjacent rectus muscles. If a rectus muscle insertion is less than 3 to 4 mm from the tumor margin, the muscle should be temporarily detached and tagged with a long 5-0 absorbable suture and reflected out of the operating field until the end of the procedure.

A circular or octagonal incision is then outlined on the sclera around the previously marked tumor shadow, leaving the most posterior portion unmarked, as this will be the base of the posteriorly hinged scleral flap (Fig. 18–13A). The octagon should ideally be at least 5 mm from the tumor margin, but sometimes limited space will permit only a 3- to 4-mm margin. In cases in which the tumor extends anteriorly through the ciliary body to the iris root, the flap can be hinged anteriorly instead of posteriorly in the peripheral portion of the cornea to permit entrance into the anterior chamber in order to perform an iridectomy and gain access to the angle structures to facilitate complete tumor excision.

At this time a supporting device such as a Flieringa ring may be sutured to the sclera around the octagon. If space will not permit its application, however, the procedure can usually be performed without the ring.

A #57 Beaver blade is then used to make a superficial groove in the sclera along the circular line. This groove is gently deepened until the blue color of the underlying uvea is evident throughout its extent. In general, the depth of the groove should be about 80 per cent thickness of the sclera.

Beginning anteriorly, a scleral flap is then developed with the Beaver blade and carried posteriorly 4 to 5 mm beyond the posterior

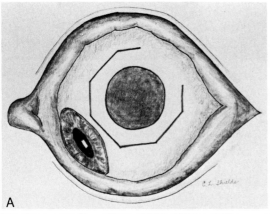

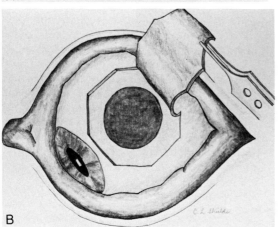

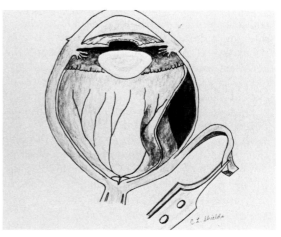

FIGURE 18–13. *A,* The shadow of the round tumor has been marked and an octagonal incision has been outlined about 4 mm outside the mass. *B,* Development of the scleral flap. Left, direct view; right, side view.

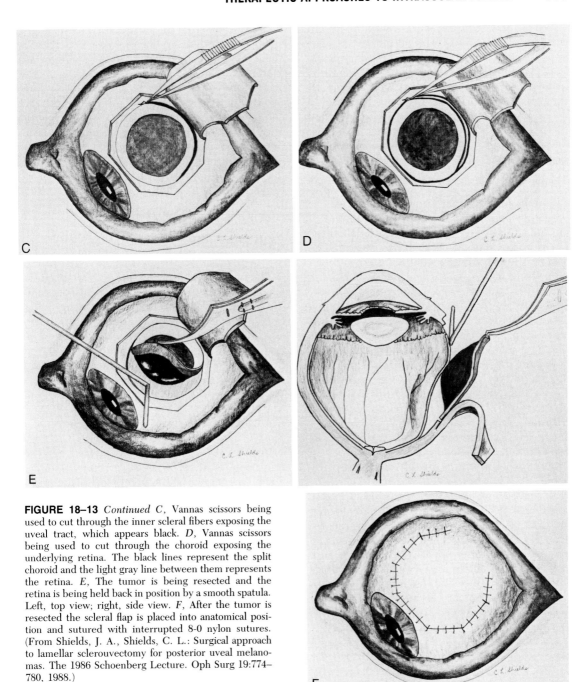

FIGURE 18–13 *Continued C*, Vannas scissors being used to cut through the inner scleral fibers exposing the uveal tract, which appears black. *D*, Vannas scissors being used to cut through the choroid exposing the underlying retina. The black lines represent the split choroid and the light gray line between them represents the retina. *E*, The tumor is being resected and the retina is being held back in position by a smooth spatula. Left, top view; right, side view. *F*, After the tumor is resected the scleral flap is placed into anatomical position and sutured with interrupted 8-0 nylon sutures. (From Shields, J. A., Shields, C. L.: Surgical approach to lamellar sclerouvectomy for posterior uveal melanomas. The 1986 Schoenberg Lecture. Oph Surg 19:774–780, 1988.)

extent of the tumor, which corresponds to the hinge of the flap (Fig. 18–13*B*). During the course of scleral dissection the vortex veins or other small emissary vessels may be encountered, and bleeding from these can usually be adequately controlled with bipolar cautery.

When the flap is fully developed, transillumination should be repeated and the margins of the tumor outlined on the remaining thin inner scleral tissue with a marking pencil or low-power diathermy. A scratch-down circumferential incision using a small razor blade knife is then outlined on the inner scleral fibers 3 mm outside the margin of tumor. Once a small area of the underlying choroid is exposed, the remaining inner scleral fibers can be gently cut along the previously marked circumferential outline without entering the choroid by using a knife needle or small microsurgical scissors, such as the Vannas scissors (Fig. 18–13*C*).

When the last of the inner scleral fibers are cut and the choroid is exposed for 360 degrees around the tumor, the choroid will typically bulge slightly outward. Prominent choroidal blood vessels may be evident at this time. If they are in the area to be resected, they should be cauterized until they are entirely blanched by gentle application of the eraser tip of the unipolar cautery. If the cautery is too hot, holes may develop in the choroid, exposing the underlying retina and vitreous.

The next step is to cut through the choroid and separate it from the overlying retina. To accomplish this, the choroid is gently lifted in one piece with fine forceps, and a small slit is made in the choroid with a knife needle. The Vannas scissors are then gently placed with one blade into the slit beneath the choroid and the choroid is lifted away from the retina and cut, hopefully leaving the overlying sensory retina intact (Fig. 18–13D). If a retinal detachment surrounding the tumor is present, this step is greatly facilitated, since the subretinal fluid decreases the chance of inadvertently perforating the retina. When the thin gray retina is exposed for 360 degrees around the tumor, the inner scleral fibers over the tumor are grasped with forceps and lifted away from the retina. A small spatula or other smooth instrument is used to hold the retina in its correct anatomical position when the tumor is lifted out (Fig. 18–13E).

If removal is successful, the sensory retina remains intact and the vitreous cavity is not entered. When the anterior border of the resected area is in the ciliary body region, the anterior edge of the retina will be unsupported within the resected area, since the nonpigmented ciliary epithelium generally adheres to the resected specimen. As long as the hyaloid face remains intact, this unsupported retina will remain in the correct anatomical position postoperatively. If vitreous is lost anteriorly, then a superficial localized open-sky vitrectomy is carefully performed through the ciliary body region, taking care not to touch the unsupported ora serrata. If a hole should develop in the retina during tumor resection, it can generally be disregarded at that time, since the perforated retina will usually adhere to the scleral flap after completion of the surgery.

The scleral flap is then gently placed over the retina and sutured back into its original position with multiple interrupted 8-0 silk sutures until the wound is secure (Fig. 18–13F). Indirect ophthalmoscopy should be performed at the termination of the scleral closure to examine the status of the retina. If a postoperative retinal detachment is detected, then a standard scleral buckling procedure with cryotherapy should be considered.

Any previously detached rectus muscles are resutured to their original insertion and the conjunctiva is reapproximated to the limbus with 6-0 absorbable sutures. Subconjunctival injections of an antibiotic and corticosteroid are given, and the patient is placed on systemic or local antibiotics and corticosteroids as well as cycloplegics.

ENUCLEATION

The subject of enucleation is discussed in Chapter 16. Because this chapter deals specifically with intraocular tumors, however, additional aspects of the procedure specifically related to such lesions will be reviewed here. The two introcular tumors most commonly managed by enucleation are retinoblastoma and malignant melanoma of the uvea.

Retinoblastoma

Enucleation of the involved eye has been the traditional method for treating retinoblastoma. Early enucleation after the clinical diagnosis is probably the main reason for the marked improvement in survival rates during the past 50 years. In recent years more eyes with retinoblastoma have been salvaged by more conservative treatment modalities. Today only about two thirds of affected eyes are enucleated.[25]

Indications. Enucleation is probably indicated for all unilateral cases in which the tumor fills most of the globe, and in which there is little hope of salvaging any viable retina or useful vision. If half of the retina is free of tumor, then other methods of treatment may be considered, so long as the parents have been fully informed as to the possibilities of metastasis and the complications of treatment.

In bilateral cases the eye with the most advanced tumor is usually enucleated, and the less involved eye is managed with irradiation or other methods. If the eye with the most advanced disease has sparing of more than one-half of the retina, an attempt may be made to salvage both eyes with treatment other than enucleation.

If both eyes have far-advanced tumors and there is no hope of any vision, bilateral enucleation may be advisable. Bilateral irradiation with close follow-up in children may be justified if the parents are fully informed and choose such a course of treatment in preference to bilateral enucleation.

Technique. The technique of enucleation for retinoblastoma is slightly different from the standard enucleation performed by most ophthalmic surgeons. Because retinoblastoma is a loosely cohesive malignant tumor, precautions should be taken to be extremely gentle during the procedure. An attempt should be made to obtain as long a section of optic nerve as possible. This may be accomplished by placing 4-0 silk traction sutures on the stumps of the four rectus muscles and severing the oblique muscles and other attached tissue from the globe. This will permit the globe to be gently pulled forward, putting the optic nerve on stretch at the time that it is cut deep in the orbit.

Complications. There are few significant complications of enucleation. Hemorrhage at the time of surgery may be controlled with orbital compression. Postoperative ecchymosis of the eyelids usually subsides with a pressure patch. Patients who are receiving chemotherapy may develop recurrent infections of the socket, which are easily managed with appropriate antibiotic therapy. Long-term complications such as a sunken orbit may be managed by adjustments of the prosthesis by an ocularist or by reconstructive surgery by the ophthalmologist.

Melanoma of the Uvea

Although enucleation has long been considered the treatment of choice for most melanomas of the posterior uvea, this method of treatment has recently been challenged by some authorities.[26] I believe, however, that there are specific indications for enucleation of an eye that harbors a uveal melanoma. The technique of standard enucleation has also been challenged, and more recently some authorities have advocated the use of a freezing no-touch technique.[27] The value of this technique is not proven, and in recent years most physicians who treat uveal melanomas have modified or even abandoned the technique. I believe that a standard enucleation performed in a gentle manner is most appropriate. Nevertheless, the no-touch technique is briefly described here.

Indications. Indications for enucleation in cases of uveal melanoma include (a) a diffuse iris melanoma that is producing severe secondary glaucoma and is too large to resect surgically, (b) a ciliary body or choroidal melanoma that has produced significant visual loss and is too large to treat with irradiation or resection, and (c) any posterior uveal melanoma that has produced a total retinal detachment, dense cataract, and secondary glaucoma.

Technique. The conjunctiva is opened at the limbus for 360 degrees, and the subconjunctival connective tissues are gently dissected in the four quadrants. The rectus muscles are identified, gently hooked, and carefully cut at their insertion. A retractor is then placed between the sclera and Tenon's capsule in the quadrant of the tumor. A special cryo-ring is inserted between the retractor and the adnexa. Its tip is lightly apposed to the sclera overlying the tumor. The cryoprobe is then activated in order to freeze the tumor and attach the globe firmly to the probe. When a satisfactory iceball has formed, the enucleation scissors are inserted, the optic nerve is cut, and the eye is gently removed by pulling upward with the cryoprobe. The oblique muscles and other tissues are cut, and the eye is delivered. After achieving hemostasis a 16- or 18-mm silicone sphere is inserted into the socket. Some surgeons prefer not to use such an implant. Tenon's capsule is closed with 4-0 chromic catgut sutures, and the conjunctiva is closed with running 6-0 plain catgut sutures. A conformer is placed on the closed conjunctiva and a pressure patch applied.

The usual technique of enucleation may be somewhat modified under special circumstances. If invasion of the optic disc is suspected clinically, it is necessary to obtain as long a section of optic nerve as possible. Cutting all the rectus and oblique muscles and placing traction sutures on the rectus muscle stumps before cutting the optic nerve may facilitate obtaining a long section. If there is gross evidence of extraocular extension of a melanoma or retinoblastoma, it may be necessary to remove Tenon's capsule or other adjacent tissues with the globe.

ORBITAL EXENTERATION

Although orbital exenteration is commonly used for certain primary malignant tumors of the orbit, its role in the management of intraocular tumors remains controversial. Some authors, however, strongly advocate orbital exenteration as the treatment of choice in eyes with malignant melanomas that have any degree of extrascleral extension.[28, 29] I prefer a lid-sparing enucleation for cases involving considerable extraocular extension.[1, 30] The technique of orbital exenteration is discussed in Chapter 16.

CHEMOTHERAPY AND IMMUNOTHERAPY

Chemotherapy and immunotherapy have not proved to be beneficial in preventing or controlling metastasis from malignant intraocular tumors. Such therapy seems reasonable, however, in patients who are considered to be at a high risk to develop metastasis. Chemotherapy is often used in cases of retinoblastoma, in patients with tumors metastatic to the eye, and in patients with leukemic or lymphomatous intraocular involvement. Sometimes immunotherapy is used with patients who have uveal melanomas, but its effectiveness is not yet established. Chemotherapy and immunotherapy should be managed by a physician experienced in their use.

REFERENCES

1. Shields, J. A.: Diagnosis and Management of Intraocular Tumors. St. Louis, C. V. Mosby Co., 1983.
2. Shields, J. A., McDonald, P. R.: Improvements in the diagnosis of posterior uveal melanomas. Arch. Ophthalmol., 91:259, 1974.
3. Shields, J. A., McDonald, P. R., Leonard, B. C., et al.: The diagnosis of uveal melanomas in eyes with opaque media. Am. J. Ophthalmol., 82:95, 1977.
4. Shields, J. A.: Accuracy and limitation of the ^{32}P test in the diagnosis of ocular tumors. An analysis of 500 cases. Ophthalmology, 85:950, 1978.
5. Joffe, L., Shields, J. A.: A practical approach to the diagnosis and therapy of common malignant tumors of the ocular fundus. Perspect. Ophthalmol., 2:307, 1978.
6. Shields, J. A., Young, S. E.: Malignant tumors of the uveal tract. Curr. Prob. Cancer, 5:1, 1980.
7. Shields, J. A.: Current approaches to the diagnosis and management of choroidal melanomas. Surv. Ophthalmol., 21:443, 1977.
8. Zimmerman, L. E., McLean, I. W., Foster, W. D.: Does enucleation of the eye containing a malignant melanoma prevent or accelerate the dissemination of tumor cells? Br. J. Ophthalmol., 62:420, 1978.
9. Shields, J. A., Sarin, L. K., Federman, J. L., et al.: Surgical approach to the ^{32}P test for posterior uveal melanomas. Ophthalmic Surg., 5:13, 1974.
10. Zweng, H. C., Little, H. L., Peabody, R. R.: Laser Photocoagulation and Retinal Angiography. St. Louis, C. V. Mosby Co., 1969, p. 15.
11. Shields JA, Meiler W, Shields CL: Photocoagulation treatment of choroidal melanomas (submitted).
12. Shields, J. A., Shields, C. L., Parsons, H., and Giblin, M. E.: The role of photocoagulation in the management of retinoblastoma (in press).
13. Shields, J. A., Augsburger, J. J.: Current approaches to the diagnosis and management of retinoblastoma. Surv. Ophthalmol., 25:347, 1981.
14. Annesley, W. H., Leonard, B. C., Shields, J. A., et al.: Fifteen year review of treated cases of retinal angiomatosis. Trans. Am. Acad. Ophthalmol. Otolaryngol., 83:446, 1977.
15. Anand, R., Augsburger, J. J., Shields, J. A.: Circumscribed choroidal hemangiomas. Arch Ophthalmol 107:1388–1342, 1989.
16. Shields, J. A., Augsburger, J. J., Brady, L. W., et al.: Cobalt plaque therapy of posterior uveal melanomas. Ophthalmology 89:1201–1207, 1982.
17. Shields, J. A., Giblin M. E., Shields, C. L., Markoe, A. M., Karlsson, U., Brady, L. W.: Episcleral plaque radiotherapy for retinoblastoma. Ophthalmology 96:530–537, 1989.
18. Abramson, D. H., Ellsworth, R. M., Zimmerman, L. E.: Non-ocular cancer in retinoblastoma survivors. Trans. Am. Acad. Ophthalmol. Otolaryngol., 81:454, 1976.
19. Abramson, D. H., Ronner, H. J., Ellsworth, R. M.: Second tumors in nonirradiated bilateral retinoblastoma. Am. J. Ophthalmol., 87:624, 1979.
20. Stephens, R., Shields, J. A.: Diagnosis and management of cancer metastatic to the uvea. A study of 70 cases. Ophthalmology, 86:1336, 1979.
21. Shields, J. A., Shields, C. L., Parsons, H., Giblin, M. E.: The role of cryotherapy in the management of retinoblastoma. Am J Ophthalmol. (in press).
22. Peyman, G. A., Erickson, E. S., Axelrod, A. J., et al: Full-thickness eye wall resection in primates. An experimental approach to the treatment of choroidal melanoma. Arch. Ophthalmol., 89:410, 1973.
23. Shields, J. A., Augsburger, J. J., Stefanyszyn, M. A., Connor, R. W.: Sclerochorioretinal resection of choroidal melanoma. A clinicopathologic correlation of a postmortem eye. Ophthalmology, 91:1726, 1984.
24. Shields, J. A., Shields, C. L.: Surgical approach to lamellar sclerouvectomy for posterior uveal melanomas. The 1986 Schoenberg Lecture. Oph Surg 19:774–780, 1988.
25. Shields, J. A., Shields, C. L., Sivalingam, V.: Decreasing frequency of enucleation in patients with retinoblastoma. Am J Ophthalmol 108:260–264, 1989.
26. Zimmerman, L. E., McLean, I. W., Foster, W. D.: Does enucleation of the eye containing a malignant melanoma prevent or accelerate the dissemination of tumor cells? Br. J. Ophthalmol., 62:420, 1978.
27. Wilson, R. S., Fraunfelder, F. T.: "No touch" cryosurgical enucleation: A minimal trauma technique for eyes harboring intraocular malignancy. Ophthalmology, 85:1170, 1978.
28. Shammas, H. F., Blodi, F. C.: Orbital extension of choroidal and ciliary body melanomas. Arch. Ophthalmol., 95:2002, 1977.
29. Shields, J. A., Augsburger, J. J., Corwin S., et al.: The management of uveal melanomas with extrascleral extension. Orbit, 5:31, 1986.
30. Shields, J. A., Shields, C. L.: Massive orbital extension of posterior uveal melanomas. Submitted.

19

OPHTHALMIC CONDITIONS REQUIRING PROMPT CARE

by George L. Spaeth

Usually the first appropriate act when a patient presents with an ophthalmic symptom or sign is to determine urgency of care. Since emergency and urgency mean different things to different people, before proceeding further I will define what I mean here by these terms. *Emergencies* are conditions that require care within an hour or less of the time of the onset of the problem. *Urgent* cases are those in which therapy can be delayed several hours without undue concern. Because different conditions with differing degrees of urgency may have similar signs and symptoms, the need for *evaluation* may be an emergency, even if the need for therapy is not.

Some of the ophthalmic conditions requiring prompt care are listed in Table 19–1. There are surprisingly few true therapeutic emergencies in ophthalmology.

There are relatively few situations that demand that care be administered within an hour or less of the onset of the ocular problem. On the other hand, some people become markedly anxious when they believe that their eyes or sight are threatened. Thus, some conditions that do not actually require immediate treatment may seem urgent from the patient's point of view. Other conditions that *are* true emergencies may not be regarded as such by the patient. The physician, receptionist, or paramedical person first contacted should remember that the patient usually does not know how

TABLE 19–1. Urgency with Which Ocular Symptoms or Conditions Require Care

BY SYMPTOM

A. *Needing immediate care:*
  Sudden loss of vision (see Table 19–2)
  Sudden onset of pain
  Sudden anisocoria
B. *Needing evaluation within several hours:*
  Sudden blurring of vision
  Ocular trauma
  Foreign body sensation
C. *Needing evaluation within 24 hours:*
  Acute red eye

BY CONDITION

A. *Needing instantaneous care:*
  Retinal vascular occlusion
  Chemical burns
B. *Needing care within several hours:*
  Acute glaucoma
  Cavernous sinus thrombosis
  Lacerated or ruptured globe
C. *Needing care within the day, although the sooner the better:*
  Corneal ulcer
  Orbital cellulitis
  Intraocular foreign body
  Adnexal injuries (lid lacerations, and so on)
  Corneal erosions
  Anisocoria
D. *Needing evaluation as soon as feasible* (therapy may be urgent or delayed, depending on findings):
  Retinal detachment
  Hyphema

Modified from Spaeth, G. L., and Purcell, J.: Examination of the eye and its adnexa. *In* Schwartz, G. R., et al. (eds.): Principles and Practice of Emergency Medicine, 2nd ed. Philadelphia, W. B. Saunders Co., 1987.

rapidly care needs to be given. Informed, re-assuring guidance is important in such a situation.

By and large, the more sudden the onset, the more urgent the evaluation. Thus, the second question in taking a history is usually, "When did the trouble first start?" The first question, of course, is directed toward the nature of the trouble, the "chief complaint." This complaint must always be taken at its face value. However, the probable correctness of the patient's comments must be evaluated, for there may well be discrepancies between the perceived and the actual time of onset. For example, it is not uncommon for a patient with no ocular problem other than a unilateral cataract to state that he noted a sudden loss of vision. In actuality the visual loss was gradual. But the patient's *awareness* of the visual loss was not gradual; it was sudden. Hence the patient perceived that something had suddenly gone awry. Thus, only after thoughtful listening and sometimes only after examination can the physician come to a valid conclusion regarding the proper urgency of therapy.

SUDDEN LOSS OF VISION

Central Retinal Artery Occlusion

Cessation or marked diminution of flow in the central retinal artery requires virtually instantaneous attention. Visual acuity is typically limited to light perception, and the pupil is sluggish or even nonreactive. This sudden, unilateral extreme visual loss is usually painless. However, central retinal artery occlusion may occur secondary to some other cause, such as marked elevation of intraocular pressure or temporal arteritis, in which case it may be associated with discomfort. Differential diagnosis of sudden visual loss includes the entities listed in Table 19–2.

The major causes for occlusion of the central retinal artery include arteriolar sclerosis, embolus (platelet, arteriosclerotic plaque, septic, and the like), temporal arteritis, trauma, sickle-cell disease, and carotid artery insufficiency.

The retina in the posterior pole of the involved eye is edematous and whitish in appearance, except for the macula, which has a "cherry red" spot. The retinal arteries are narrowed.

Central retinal artery occlusion may be treated successfully when appropriate therapy

TABLE 19–2. Differential Diagnosis of Sudden Visual Loss

Central retinal artery occlusion
Temporal arteritis
Acute anterior optic neuropathy
Central retinal vein occlusion
Migraine
Intracranial disease
Retinal detachment
Vitreous hemorrhage
Optic neuritis
Solar retinitis
Acute glaucoma
Corneal decompensation
Traumatic or spontaneous hyphema
Ruptured or lacerated globe
Malingering or hysteria

is instituted within a few minutes of the onset of the sudden visual loss. The goal, obviously, is restoration of blood flow prior to death of the retina. Four ways in which restoration of blood flow can be helped are: (1) dilatation of the retinal artery, (2) decrease of the external pressure on the arteriole wall (that is, diminution of intraocular pressure), (3) increase in the blood pressure within the artery, and (4) increase in activity or administration of factors causing clot dissolution.

Dilatation of the retinal arterioles may be accomplished by raising the blood level of carbon dioxide through the rebreathing of expired air or administration of carbon dioxide. An appropriate mixture is 5 per cent carbon dioxide with 95 per cent oxygen. Pure oxygen alone should not be given, as it tends to cause vasoconstriction, which is clearly counterproductive.

Intraocular pressure may be decreased by immediate administration of acetazolamide (500 mg per 70 kg body weight) or 20 cc of mannitol 50 per cent (per 70 kg adult). However, these measures are more useful in maintaining rather than initiating the rapid decrease of intraocular pressure that is required. Anterior chamber paracentesis will obtain the quickest and largest decrease of intraocular pressure; as such, it is both indicated and appropriate treatment in patients having recent onset of central retinal artery occlusion. Even after 30 minutes or more, it may still be helpful if occlusion has not been complete. The technique of paracentesis is discussed in Chapter 4.

There are presently no feasible ways to increase the blood pressure in the retinal artery. Since hypotension can produce further ischemia, and since it is amenable to treatment, blood pressure should be monitored and appropriate therapy given as needed.

The value of anticlotting agents is not established. Heparin, dicoumarol, or aspirin may possibly prevent extension of an existing thrombus but will not lyse a thrombus already present. Fibrinolytic agents have troublesome side effects and have not been shown to help. Low molecular weight dextran 10 per cent has been recommended by some. This is thought to reduce blood viscosity, but such treatment has not been proved beneficial. Heparin and dicoumarol are also associated with considerable hazard to the patient, especially since most individuals developing a central retinal artery occlusion have an underlying vascular problem.

An additional procedure that may be helpful in some instances is to compress the eye vigorously for a second or two, and then release the pressure suddenly. The purpose of this maneuver is to cause a sudden increase and decrease in the intraocular pressure, in the hope that this will dislodge an embolus from its position and permit it to pass further out the arterial tree.

In patients with central retinal artery occlusion, the possibility of carotid insufficiency should be considered, and appropriate diagnostic steps taken, including palpation of the carotids, auscultation over the carotid arteries, the obtaining of a pertinent history, and non-invasive blood flow studies.

The intraocular pressure should always be determined rapidly in patients with central artery occlusion. It is usually adequate to estimate the pressure with the fingers. Acute glaucoma with elevation of intraocular pressure to a level that will produce a central retinal artery occlusion is frequently painful. However, elevation of pressure to the range of 60 mm Hg or more may occur without discomfort and without the usual signs of acute congestive glaucoma: corneal edema, a dilated pupil, and a red eye.

The possibility that the sudden visual loss is the result of temporal arteritis should be considered. Usually this is associated with severe headache or ocular pain. Blood should be drawn promptly so that an erythrocyte sedimentation rate may be obtained. This may be normal in the early stages of the disease, especially if the patient is receiving large doses of pain-relieving drugs such as Butazolidin or aspirin. If the ESR is higher than expected for the patient's age, treatment with systemic corticosteroids should usually be instituted immediately and further diagnostic and therapeutic measures taken as appropriate (Table 19–3).[1]

TABLE 19–3. Values for Erythrocyte Sedimentation Rate

	NORMAL (Westergren Technique)	
	Male	*Female*
Newborn	0–2	0–2
Child (1–14 years)	0–13	3–13
Adult	0–15	0–20
65–80	0–35	0–50

ABNORMAL

Sedimentation rate 20–100 mm per hour
  Acute and chronic infectious diseases
  Acute localized infections
  Reactivation of a chronic infection
  Rheumatic fever
  Rheumatoid arthritis
  Acute glomerulonephritis
  Myocardial infarction
  Malignant tumors with necrosis
  Hyperthyroidism
  Lead and arsenic intoxication
  Nephrosis
  Internal hemorrhage
  Acute hepatitis (viral)
  Unruptured ectopic pregnancy after third month
  Ruptured ectopic pregnancy, late
  Menstruation
  Normal pregnancy after third month
  Ingestion of oral contraceptives
  Anaphylactoid purpura
  Hb C disease

Sedimentation rate 100 mm or more per hour
  Multiple myeloma and Waldenström's
    macroglobulinemia
  Malignancy
  Severe anemia
  Acute severe bacterial infection
  Collagen diseases
  Portal or biliary cirrhosis
  Ulcerative colitis
  Severe renal disease

Modified from Miale, J. B.: Laboratory Medicine: Hematology, 5th ed. St. Louis, C. V. Mosby Co., 1977, p. 419.

Retinal Vein Occlusion

Complete occlusion of the central retinal vein of the eye may cause severe but painless visual loss.[2] The rapidity and severity of the loss are less prominent than with central retinal artery occlusion. The appearance of the fundus of the eye in the individual with a central retinal vein occlusion is striking: Retinal hemorrhages abound, the optic disc may be swollen, there may be hemorrhage into the vitreous, and the retinal veins are dilated and tortuous. The condition is usually unilateral, the most common cause being hypertensive-arteriosclerotic disease, though other conditions may also be responsible, such as leukemia, diabetes mellitus, carotid disease, or diseases associated with hyperviscosity of the blood. Most patients who have severe visual loss in association with a central retinal vein occlusion also have an element of arterial insufficiency. Paracentesis may be indicated in some cases.

A detailed discussion of retinal vein occlusion is found on pages 388 to 391 and in Reference 2.

Migraine

The sudden onset of visual symptoms caused by migraine can be very disturbing to the affected patient. The symptoms are so highly characteristic that proper diagnosis is usually possible merely on the basis of the history itself. The patient complains of scintillating scotomas and zigzag lines, usually off to one side. There may be severe reduction of visual acuity, though this is unusual. The attack passes spontaneously after a few minutes but leaves the patient apprehensive and wondering when the next attack may occur. Headaches and other symptoms of migraine may be present, but often are not (see Table 19–4).

Although usually benign, migraine can be incapacitating. The immediate treatment is reassurance. However, referral may be indicated. A variety of treatment programs are available, including propranolol, 20 to 40 mg 3 times daily. Many attacks are triggered by food allergy.

Intracranial Disease

In cases in which sudden visual loss is a reflection of intracranial disease, associated neurologic deficits are often found. The usual eti-

TABLE 19–4. Symptoms of Migraine

I. Prodromal features
  A. Aura
    1. Flashing lights, dots, or stars (usually in peripheral temporal field)
    2. Spreading scotoma (may extend to involve central vision)
    3. Glowing "light bulb" (usually paracentral)
    4. Zig zag lines
    5. Brilliantly colored visual hallucinations
  B. Homonymous hemianopia
  C. Metamorphopsia
  D. Photophobia
  E. Ocular motor nerve palsy (usually third nerve)
II. After effects
  A. Headache (absent with ocular migraine)
  B. Nausea
  C. Permanent field defects

TABLE 19–5 Neurological Signs Associated with Visual Loss Due to Intracranial Disease

Speech disturbances
Seizures
Skeletal muscle abnormalities
Extraocular muscle movement disturbances
Nystagmus
Diplopia
Visual hallucinations
Visual field loss
Visual-verbal dissociation syndromes
Visual disorientation
Visual agnosia

ology is vascular insufficiency. The nature of the associated neurologic symptoms or signs depends upon the region of the brain affected. Should the lesion be in the occipital lobe, the only finding may be a loss of sight (Table 19–5).

Papilledema may also cause a reduction of visual acuity, which is usually mild and may be intermittent. Examination of the optic disc usually makes the correct diagnosis immediately apparent (Table 19–6).

Optic Neuritis

Inflammation of the optic nerve may cause rapid diminution of central visual acuity. Pain is frequent in young patients but uncommon in the elderly. A central scotoma is almost always present.

When the anterior optic nerve is involved, edema of the optic disc, hemorrhages at the rim of the optic disc, and cellular reaction in the posterior vitreous are typical findings. In retrobulbar neuritis there may be no visible changes in the fundus at the time of the acute episode, although optic atrophy develops later.

TABLE 19–6. Differential Diagnosis of Papilledema

Papilledema
  Space-occupying lesion
  Interference with venous return from brain
  Obstruction to flow of cerebrospinal fluid
  Primary diffuse cerebral edema (pseudotumor)
  Secondary diffuse cerebral edema:
    Hypertension, lead intoxication, etc.
  Orbital lesions
  Hypotony of the globe
Pseudopapilledema (usually hypermetropia)
Opaque optic nerve fibers
Drusen
Juxtapapillary chorioretinitis
Optic neuritis

TABLE 19–7. Differential Diagnosis of Unilateral and Bilateral Optic Neuritis

UNILATERAL OPTIC NEURITIS
Idiopathic
Multiple sclerosis
Orbital infection
Sarcoid
Systemic lupus erythematosus
Infectious mononucleosis
Herpes zoster
Secondary syphilis

BILATERAL OPTIC NEURITIS
Demyelinating conditions
Leber's hereditary optic atrophy
Toxic disorders
    Methyl or ethyl alcohol
    Tobacco
    Quinine
Deficiency of vitamin B_{12}
Diabetes mellitus
Bilateral optic neuritis of childhood

UNILATERAL OR BILATERAL OPTIC NEURITIS
Ischemic optic neuropathy
Optic nerve compression
    Meningioma
    Aneurysm
    Chiasmal mass
Tumor of the optic nerve

When optic neuritis is unilateral, the presence of the Marcus Gunn pupillary response is evidence of optic nerve damage.

Evaluation by a neurologist is often appropriate. Treatment is medical and related to the presumed etiology. Corticosteroids may be helpful in certain cases (Table 19–7).

Glaucoma

The diagnosis and management of glaucoma are discussed in detail in Chapter 11. However, the rapidity with which visual loss can occur in glaucoma must be stressed. When intraocular pressure rises above the systolic pressure in the retinal arteries, the stage is set for rapid visual deterioration. Intraocular pressure should be lowered as rapidly as is feasible. A paracentesis is usually not indicated. Medical means are usually adequate, and the shallowness of the anterior chamber and the edema of the cornea may make the paracentesis excessively hazardous.

Chemical Burns

Almost without exception, the treatment of chemical burns of the eye consists of prompt, copious, and continuing irrigation. The sooner the irrigation starts and the more completely the toxic chemical is washed away, the more complete will be the recovery. The treatment of chemical burns is discussed in more detail in reference 7.

Malingering and Hysteria

Nonorganic conditions may cause sudden visual loss. The malingerer knows that his visual loss is not real but attempts to fool the examiner. In contrast, visual loss in a hysterical patient is real, although emotionally caused. The malingering patient may act as if he is completely blind. He may be aggressive and uncooperative, especially when repeated testing is requested. In contrast, the hysterically blind individual tends to show a lack of concern: "la belle indifférence."

Since in malingering and hysteria the ocular examination shows no apparent abnormalities, the differential diagnosis is fairly well limited to retrobulbar neuritis and occipital lobe cerebrovascular insufficiency (Table 19–8). Associated signs will often be present when there is bilateral visual loss. In the patient with unilateral visual loss, a careful search for an afferent pupillary defect, defective red color vision, or an upper quadrant temporal visual field defect should help eliminate an organic cause.

Thoughtful visual field examination usually allows differentiation of these conditions. The patient with retrobulbar neuritis will usually have a fairly full visual field in which there is a dense central or paracentral scotoma. Occipital lobe lesions usually cause dense, congruous hemianopic field loss, often limited to the central visual field. When a visual field using a tangent screen or perimeter is measured in hysterical or malingering patients, the patient often responds only to test objects in the central 5 to 25 degrees of the visual field. Yet such a patient will not show the incapacitation that is typical for patients with such marked loss of peripheral vision.

TABLE 19–8. Differential Diagnosis of Sudden Visual Loss Without Apparent Other Abnormalities

Hysteria
Malingering
Optic neuritis
Visual agnosia
Solar retinitis
Optic nerve compressive lesion

There are a variety of ways of testing the patient in order to determine if the visual field loss is real or faked. Measurement of the field at 1 and 2 meters is one of the most helpful procedures. Two isopters are determined using two different test objects at 1 meter. The patient is then retested with the same test objects at 2 meters. Normally, when a patient is moved from 1 to 2 meters the position of the isopter on the tangent screen is almost the same in terms of degrees of visual angle, which means that the isopter at 2 meters should be almost twice as far from the point of fixation as the isopter determined at 1 meter (Fig. 19–1). Therefore, if there is little or no change in the area of visibility, a nonorganic cause for visual loss must be considered. Thus a "tubular visual field," especially one with sharp, steep margins, is characteristic of the hysterical or malingering patient. A spiral or star-shaped visual field is

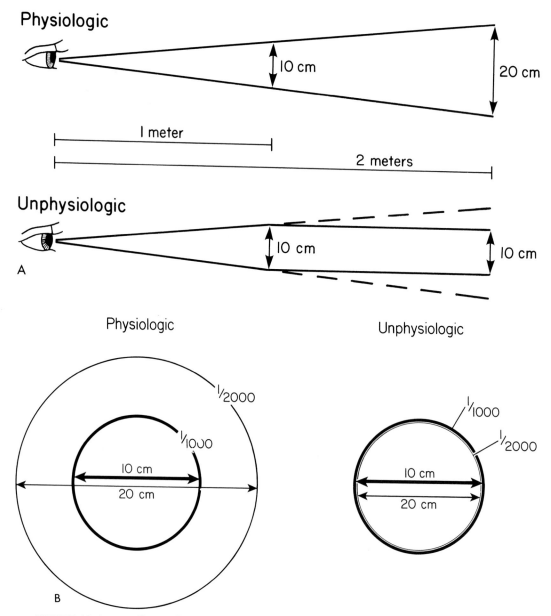

FIGURE 19–1. *A,* Difference between the normal visual field (top) and the tubular visual field of the hysterical or malingering patient (bottom). *B,* In contrast to the cone-shaped field of the normal subject (left), the steep-margined tubular field of the hysterical patient measures the same at 1 and 2 meters. Such a tubular field is not possible organically.

TABLE 19–9. Common Causes for Anisocoria

Congenital variant	Topical drugs
Disease of third cranial nerve (oculomotor nerve)	Horner's syndrome
Disease of second cranial nerve (optic nerve)	Syphilis
Unilateral blindness	Active iridocyclitis
Adie's tonic pupil	Old iridocyclitis
Trauma to pupillary sphincter	Dislocated lens
Glaucoma	

Modified from Spaeth, G. L., Purcell, J.: Examination of the eye and its adnexa. *In* Schwartz, G. R., et al. (eds.): Principles and Practice of Emergency Medicine, 2nd ed. Philadelphia, W. B. Saunders Co., 1987.

also typical of the hysterical patient, although it may also be a sign of fatigue. If there are questions regarding the correctness of visual acuity, the acuity can be checked while the patient is looking through a Phoroptor. The patient should be refracted so that the proper lenses can be inserted to assure the best refractive correction. The addition of plus lenses should then blur the acuity. The examiner can also rapidly and asymmetrically occlude one or the other eye. In the case of unilateral visual complaint a ten degree prism may be placed base-out in front of the defective eye and the patient asked to read. If in fact the eye has good vision it will deviate medially; removal of the prism will allow the eye to return to its normal position. Such a deviation would not be expected to occur unless binocular vision were actually present.

Other tests that may be employed include the visual-evoked response and the determination of optokinetic nystagmus.

TABLE 19–10. Prophylactic Treatment of Tetanus

		State of Tetanus Immunization		
		Complete		
TYPE OF WOUND	**Incomplete**	*Years Since Last Booster*		
		1*–5	5–10	More than 10
Clean; minor	Begin or complete immunization per schedule: Tetanus toxoid, 0.5 cc	None	Tetanus toxoid, 0.5 cc	Tetanus toxoid, 0.5 cc
Clean; major or tetanus-prone	BOTH Human tetanus immune globulin, 250 mg, in one arm† AND Tetanus toxoid, 0.5 cc, in other arm† PLUS Complete immunization per schedule	Tetanus toxoid, 0.5 cc	Tetanus toxoid, 0.5 cc	BOTH Tetanus toxoid, 0.5 cc, in one arm† AND Human tetanus immune globulin, 250 mg, in other arm†
Tetanus-prone; delayed or incomplete debridement	BOTH Human tetanus immune globulin, 500 mg, in one arm† AND Tetanus toxoid, 0.5 cc, in other arm† PLUS Complete immunization per schedule PLUS Antibiotic therapy	Tetanus toxoid, 0.5 cc	Tetanus toxoid, 0.5 cc PLUS Antibiotic therapy	BOTH Tetanus toxoid, 0.5 cc, in other arm† AND Human tetanus immune globulin, 250 mg, in other arm† PLUS Antibiotic therapy

Modified from Spaeth, G. L., Purcell, J.: Examination of the eye and its adnexa. *In* Schwartz, G. R., et al. (eds.): Principles and Practice of Emergency Medicine, 2nd ed. Philadelphia, W. B. Saunders Co., 1987.
*No prophylactic immunization is required if patient has had a booster within the previous year.
†Use different syringes, needles, and sites.
NOTE: With different preparations of toxoid, the volume of a single booster dose should be modified as stated on the package label.

TRAUMA

The management of trauma to the globe and the adnexa is fully discussed in Chapters 15 and 16. Two points will be discussed here: the significance of anisocoria and the prophylactic treatment for tetanus.

Anisocoria. Careful examination of the pupils is important in all cases with ocular or head trauma. A unilaterally dilated pupil may result from trauma directly to the globe or may be the sign of orbital or intracranial pathology. These matters are further discussed in Chapter 15. The anisocoria may be unrelated to the trauma and other causes should be considered (Table 19–9).

Prophylaxis for Tetanus. The incidence of tetanus has decreased markedly in the United States. However, cases still occur and carry with them an extremely high mortality. Appro-

TABLE 19–11. Differential Diagnosis of the "Red Eye"*

CONDITION	PAIN	PHOTOPHOBIA	VISION	OCULAR INJECTION
1. Conjunctivitis (see Table 19–12)	Minimal	None to mild	Slightly blurred by discharge	Lid and eye
2. Episcleritis	Moderate	None	Normal	Deep vessels of sclera, often focal
3a. Bacterial or fungal corneal ulcer	None to severe	Variable	Usually decreased, often markedly	Diffuse
3b. Viral corneal ulcer	Foreign body sensation	Moderate	Mildly reduced	Mild to Moderate
4. Corneal erosion or foreign body	Mild to moderate foreign body sensation	Moderate to marked	Normal or slightly reduced	Mild
5. Nonalkali corneal burn (ultraviolet or other)	Moderate	Severe	Reduced	Moderate
6. Uveitis	Mild to moderate	Mild to severe	Normal or moderately reduced	Next to limbus
7. Glaucoma (acute)	Severe or mild	Moderate	Decreased by corneal edema	Diffuse
8. Orbital cellulitis	None to severe	None	Normal or reduced	Diffuse with chemosis
9. Endophthalmitis	Severe	Moderate to marked	Drastically reduced	Severe

	OCULAR DISCHARGE	LID SWELLING	PUPIL	ANTERIOR CHAMBER	MANAGEMENT PLAN
1. Conjunctivitis	Marked (except allergic type)	Varies	Normal	Normal	See Table 19–12
2. Episcleritis	Minimal	None	Normal	Normal	Usually topical steroids
3a. Ulcer-B	Present	None to moderate	Normal	Inflammatory reaction, often hypopyon	Specific diagnosis and vigorous specific antimicrobial therapy topically and periocularly
3b. Ulcer-V	Tearing	None	Normal	Mild flare and cells	Topical antiviral drop or ointment
4. Foreign body	Tearing	None	Normal or miotic	Normal or mild flare and cells	Instillation of cycloplegic, antibiotic and then patch
5. Burn	Tearing	Varies	Normal or miotic	Normal or mild flare and cells	Instillation of cycloplegic, antibiotic and then patch
6. Uveitis	None	None	Miotic	Flare and cells	Usually steroids and cycloplegics
7. Glaucoma	None	None	Dilated	Flare and cells	Prompt medical reduction of intraocular pressure, then surgery (see text)
8. Orbital cell	None	Diffuse (confined to orbit)	Normal	Normal	X-rays, culture and vigorous systemic antibiotic therapy (see text)
9. Endophthalmitis	Varies	Moderate to marked		Hypopyon	See Chapter 6

Modified from Spaeth, G. L., Purcell, J.: Nontraumatic ophthalmic emergencies. *In* Schwartz, G. R., et al. (eds.): Principles and Practice of Emergency Medicine, 2nd ed. Philadelphia, W. B. Saunders Co., 1986.

*The intensity of the sign varies depending upon many factors, including stage of development. For example, vision is not reduced in the earliest stage of endophthalmitis.

TABLE 19–12. Features of Commonly Occurring Conjunctivitis

	DISCHARGE	TEARING	ITCHING	INJECTION	PAPILLAE	FOLLICLES	TREATMENT*
Allergic	+	+ + +	+ + +	+	+ +	0	None or anti-inflammatory agents†
Bacterial	+ + +	+	+	+ +	+	+ −	Appropriate antibiotic
Viral	+ (watery)	+	+	+ +	0	+ +	Usually none

Modified from Spaeth, G. L., Purcell, J.: Nontraumatic ophthalmic emergencies. *In* Schwartz, G. R., et al. (eds.): Principles and Practice of Emergency Medicine, 2nd ed. Philadelphia, W. B. Saunders Co., 1986.

*Hot compresses are helpful in most instances of bacterial or viral conjunctivitis.

†Decongestant, corticosteroid, or Chromylin.

priate prophylactic treatment is almost invariably successful.

Even with minor wounds about the eye, the possibility of tetanus must be considered. Inquiry regarding the state of immunization should be made and treatment given as shown in Table 19–10.

THE ACUTE RED EYE

Correct diagnosis is essential for proper management of the patient with an inflamed eye of recent onset. Basic points of the differential diagnosis are given in Tables 19–11 and 19–12.

More extensive discussion of corneal disease is found in Chapter 8, of glaucoma in Chapter 11, or orbital cellulitis in Chapter 15, and of endophthalmitis in Chapter 6.

REFERENCES

1. Jahr, D. A.: Rheumatic diseases. *In* Ryan, S. (ed.): Retina. St. Louis, C. V. Mosby Co., 1989, pp. 471–473.
2. Clarkson, J. E.: Central retinal vein occlusion. *In* Ryan, S. (ed.): Retina. St. Louis, C. V. Mosby Co., 1989, pp. 421–426.
3. Rose, F. C.: Medical Ophthalmology. St. Louis, C. V. Mosby Co., 1976. (See entire section on Neuro Ophthalmology, by various authors, pp. 69–224.)
4. Scherr, S. A., Blum, M. D., Laigon, E. E.: Tetanus of the head and neck. Trans. Penna. Acad. Ophthalmol. Otolaryngol., 33:55, 1980.
5. Spaeth, G. L., Purcell, J.: Examination of the eye and its adnexa. *In* Schwartz, G. R., et al. (eds.): Principles and Practice of Emergency Medicine, 2nd ed. Philadelpia, W. B. Saunders Co., 1987.
6. Spaeth, G. L., Purcell, J.: Nontraumatic ophthalmic emergencies. *In* Schwartz, G. R., et al. (eds.): Principles and Practice of Emergency Medicine, 2nd ed. Philadelphia, W. B. Saunders Co., 1986.
7. Purcell, J., and Spaeth, G. L.: Ocular trauma. *In* Schwartz, G. R., et al. (eds.): Principles and Practice of Emergency Medicine, 2nd ed. Philadelphia, W. B. Saunders Co., 1986.

INDEX

Note: Page numbers in *italics* refer to illustrations; page numbers followed by t refer to tables.